THE UNOFFICIAL GUIDE TO
PAEDIATRICS

FIRST EDITION

Zeshan Qureshi BM BSc (Hons) MSc MRCPCH
Academic Clinical Fellow, Great Ormond Street Hospital,
UK and Institute of Global Health, UCL, UK
Paediatric Registrar, London Deanery, UK

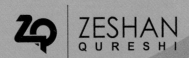
ZESHAN QURESHI

ISBN 978-0957149953

Edited by Zeshan Qureshi.

Original design Anne Bonson-Johnson and Zeshan Qureshi. Page make-up by Amnet-systems.

Illustrated by Anchorprint Group Limited.

Clinical Photography
Steven Kenny, Medical Photographer, Lewisham and Greenwich NHS Trust – 3.2 and 3.4. Modelling by Amy Moran, Angad Singh Kooner, Paarus Kaur Johal, Ishminder K Johal, Sorcha Mullen, Sion Santos, Annabelle Santos, Rachel Luke, Micah Ayos Mahinga, Marie Jasim, Ilyaas Jasim and Terouz Pasha.

Medical illustrations
Caitlin Monney, and Emily McDougall. 1.2: Fig 2-4, 1.3: Fig 1-6, 1.6: Fig 2, 4, 5, 7, 11, 12, 14, 15-7, *Table 11*, 1.7: Fig 1-2, 4-6, 1.8: Fig 13, 1.9: Fig 1-4, 1.10: Fig 1-2, 1:12: Fig 2, 1:14: Fig 4, 1.16: Fig 3-10, 14-26, *Table 7*, 1.17: *Table 5*, Fig 1-2, 1.18: Fig 5, 7. 1.21: Fig 1-4, 6-7. 1.22: Fig 2-6, 8. 1.23: Fig 1, 8. 1.23: Fig 2, 5, 1.25: Fig 1-3, 1.26: Fig 3, 5-9, 11, 3.2: Fig 5, 7-24, 26, 33, 40, 66, 73-4, 78, 86, 109, 110, 123, 126, 136-7, 153, 155, 157. 3.4: Fig 2, 34, 40, 74.
Peter Gardiner. 1.3: Fig 7-11, 1.4: Fig 1-4. 1.5: Fig 1-5, 1.11: Fig 2, 4-6, 1.15: Fig 2-5, 22-25, 29, 31, 46, 1.18: Fig 1-3, 1.19: *Table 1*, 1.22: Fig 1. 3.2: Fig 6, 154

Clinical photographs
Alex Rothman. 1.5: Fig 6, 1.6: Fig 10, 1.8: Fig 14, 1.9: Fig 5, 1.15: Fig 8, 1.16: Fig 26.
Centers for Disease Control and Prevention Image Library. 1.8: Fig 1 – 2631, Fig 15 – 15408/15403, 1:15: Fig 20 – 2632, 32 – 15115.
D@nderm. 1.11: Fig 1, 3, 1.15: Fig 8, 1.19: Fig 12. 1.21: Fig 5. 1.23: Fig 2-7, 9-14, 1.26: Fig 15.
Auckland district health board – adhb.govt.nz. 1.15: Fig 6-15, 17-19, 21.
NHS Fife. 3.2: Fig 72.
John Offenbach. David Osrin review photo.

X Rays
Mark Rodrigues. 1.7: Fig 3, 1.18: Fig 9, 1.19: Fig 2-11, 13. 1.22: Fig 7, 10.
Radiopedia. 1.15: Fig 37, 1.16: Fig 11-13, 3.4: Fig 56.
A catalogue record for this book is available from the British Library.

Zeshan Qureshi's Acknowledgements
I would like to thank my colleagues, mentors, friends, and most of all, my parents for their unwavering support through the years, without which none of this would have been possible. I have been inspired and trained by Paediatricians throughout the years, all of which cannot be named but particularly Ewen Johnston, Julie-Clare Becher, Jason Gane, Shahid Karim, Ella Aidoo, Susanna Sakonidou, Grant Marais, Tobias Hunt, Chris Harris, Simon Broughton, Kamal Ali, Terrence Stephenson, and Ildilko Schuller.

Printed and bound by Nutech Print Services - India

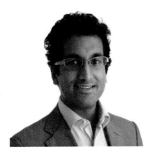

Introduction

It has been a privilege to work with so many Paediatricians, and to serve as part of the big teams that deliver the excellent care that every child deserves. Whilst my career to date has involved challenging situations, I have invariably been able to unite with colleagues and parents around the fact that above anything else, the wellbeing of a child should not be compromised.

It has been a privilege to work with so many Paediatricians, and to serve as part of the big teams that deliver the excellent care that every child deserves. Whilst my career to date has involved challenging situations, I have invariably been able to unite with colleagues and parents around the fact that above anything else, the wellbeing of a child should not be compromised.

Editing this book, and working closely with my professional colleagues has really made me reflect on what the true definition of a Paediatrician might be. I'm on a Paediatric training programme, but I don't think this is necessary to be a Paediatrician. I am privileged to say that I have passed the MRCPCH membership examinations, but again don't think that is necessary to be a Paediatrician. I am now delighted to say that I've edited a Paediatrics textbook. But this doesn't qualify me as a Paediatrician.

So what is the core essence of this profession? Who can be a Paediatrician, in the true spirit of the word? And who should decide? In my humble opinion, it comes down to one simple litmus test. Can you do what is necessary, within the limitations of your knowledge, to be an advocate for a potentially sick child? Are you willing to try your utmost to communicate with a child and family to identify what their possible concerns are, and tease out any relevant pathology? If something goes wrong, or you are unhappy with something that is done regarding a child's care, regardless of any contextual factors, will you speak up on behalf of the child?

There is no substitute for clinical experience. Reading this book will inform you about Paediatrics. But to me, the most important thing in Paediatrics comes down to caring for the child, and when it comes down to this there should be no hierarchy: be tactful, use the appropriate channels, but never hesitate to speak up whenever you are worried that patient care is being compromised, regardless of who it might offend.

Anyone can be a Paediatrician. A medical student on a Paediatric rotation; the student will often take the opportunity to spend more time listening to the patient then any healthcare professional that day: and I'm always grateful when a student comes up to me relaying valuable patient concerns and diagnostic information: they are a Paediatrician. The primary care physician that follows a child from womb to adulthood: they are a Paediatrician. Their knowledge of the family and the

'...the most important thing in Paediatrics comes down to caring for the child, and when it comes down to this there should be no hierarchy'

child throughout their life course is indispensable in identifying when things might go wrong in advance. The academics that improve the evidence on which care can be delivered: they are Paediatricians. The managers and policy makers that turn ideas into a reality: they are Paediatricians. And the Emergency Medicine doctor that sees a frightened parent and sick child for the first time, the ENT surgeon, the orthopaedic surgeon, the paediatric surgeon, the geneticist, the immunologist, the physiotherapist, the art therapist, the play specialist, the nurse, the dietician, the pharmacist, the social worker, the teacher, the police, every specialist, every person, every advocate that helps identify and address concerns and potential concerns to a child's wellbeing: they are all Paediatricians.

I am indebted to all their guidance and help in helping me provide care to children that I cannot fully provide on my own. It's up to you to decide what a Paediatrician is. But in my humble opinion, you can all be a Paediatrician today.

Zeshan Qureshi
Chief Editor
Unofficial Guide to Paediatrics

The Unofficial Guide
to Medicine Project

Additionally, we want you to get involved. This textbook has mainly been written by junior doctors and students just like you because we believe:

...that fresh graduates have a unique perspective on what works *for students*. We have tried to capture the insight of students and recent graduates to make the language we use to discuss this complex material more digestible for students.
...that texts are in *constant* need of being updated. *Every student* has the potential to contribute to the education of others by innovative ways of thinking and learning. This book is an open collaboration with you.

You have the power to *contribute* something valuable to medicine; we welcome your suggestions and would love for you to get in touch.

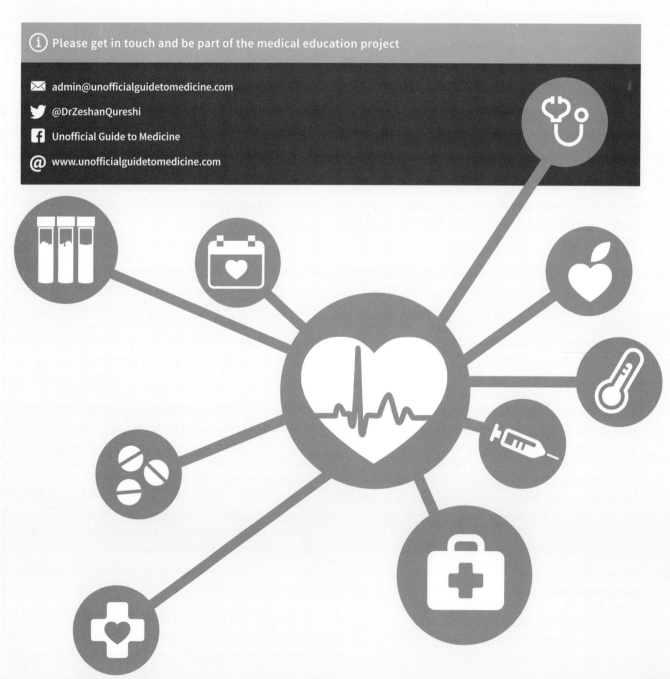

ⓘ **Please get in touch and be part of the medical education project**

✉ admin@unofficialguidetomedicine.com

🐦 @DrZeshanQureshi

f Unofficial Guide to Medicine

@ www.unofficialguidetomedicine.com

Foreword

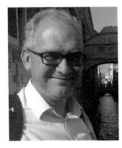

Dr Simon Broughton PhD FRCPCH
- Consultant Paediatrician,
  King's College Hospital NHS
  Foundation Trust
- Senior Lecturer, King's College
  London – Course Director, MSc
  in Advanced Paediatrics
- Training Programme Director

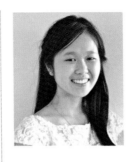

Beryl Lin
- President, University of New
  South Wales Medical Society
- Co-chair, University of New
  South Wales Paediatrics Special
  Interest Group

Congratulations to Zeshan and his colleagues on producing 'The Unofficial Guide to Paediatrics'. It is a huge piece of work by trainees and experts for anybody who has an interest in paediatrics, from medical students to established consultants and anybody interested in caring for children.

This book covers paediatrics in a traditional system based approach, but also has sections on the expanding speciality of adolescent healthcare, child health and the law, and public health. In addition, with sections on undergraduate and postgraduate assessments, starting out as a junior doctor and career sections, it provides useful advice to medical students and junior doctors wherever they are in their own career.

So, why do we need another textbook on paediatrics? There are already plenty of excellent texts on this subject, however none have created a book like this. The inspiration behind this book is the working together of junior doctors, medical students, and experts to pull together a textbook that is accessible to all types of learners. We now live in a world where knowledge is so widely and freely available, that simply reprinting knowledge is becoming unnecessary. If knowledge is to be pulled together in a textbook, then every effort should be made to make that knowledge as relevant and accessible to the reader as possible, and that is what the Unofficial Guide to Paediatrics achieves.

Every effort has been made to make this textbook as up to date as possible. However, inevitably, new research and guidance will be published. The genius behind this book however, is in empowering readers or users of this book to write to Zeshan with updates and suggestions for future editions.

Being a Paediatrician is an absolute privilege, caring for children and young people and their families at very difficult times in their lives is an unbelievably rewarding challenge. One of the challenges that busy paediatricians struggle with, is keeping themselves up to date in all areas of paediatrics. The Unofficial Guide to Paediatrics will help with that, providing guidance to paediatricians of the future and assist in providing excellent care to children, young people and their families.

Paediatrics is a 'big' topic about 'little' people. It is intellectually challenging and an exciting field for research and learning, but it can also be daunting when medical school is often set up to focus on adult medicine. Caring for children is different – both in a purely scientific sense, but also the way a sick child and their family should be approached, the dynamic of the hospital and multidisciplinary team, the ethical and sociocultural considerations involved, and even the career pathways that present are unique – all of which are covered in this book.

The Unofficial Guide to Paediatrics features an easy-to-read overview of paediatrics, broken down by systems. Each chapter describes core conditions by beginning with aetiology and clinical features, and progresses through investigations, differential diagnoses, management, complications, and finally prognosis. Furthermore, this book covers history taking, examination, communication, and practical skills – all supplemented with clinical cases, labelled diagrams, and information about common examinations and assessment criteria. The authors have also provided illustrations of common procedures and medical devices in clinical practice. As a book produced and written by trainees for other trainees, it captures key information in a digestible manner. With extensive collaboration from renowned academics and specialists, the content is reliable and based on up-to-date evidence.

This textbook is part of an international medical education project, which embodies a passion for peer teaching, and the empowerment of young people who are making a positive impact. Congratulations to Zeshan's team for this award-winning series of textbooks that will help others in their medical journey.

In the wonderful world of paediatrics, this is a wonderful resource for students, junior doctors, and paediatric trainees alike - or anyone looking for a simple and reliable complement to learning from the literature and clinical encounter. The development and success of this has been no child's play - one might even say, it's a milestone of an achievement!

Abbreviations

4C compound	4-carbon compound
5C compound	5-carbon compound
17OHP	17-Hydroxyprogesterone
A	Airway
ABG	Arterial blood gas
ABPA	Allergic bronchopulmonary aspergillosis
ACE	Angiotensin-converting enzyme
ACE	Antegrade colonic enema
Acetyl CoA	Acetyl coenzyme A
Ach	Acetylcholine
ACTH	Adrenocorticotropic hormone
ADA	Adenosine deaminase
ADEM	Acute disseminated encephalomyelitis
ADH	Antidiuretic hormone
ADHD	Attention Deficit Hyperactivity Disorder
AED	Anti-epileptic drugs
AFP	Alpha fetoprotein
AI	Adrenal insufficiency
AIDS	Acquired immunodeficiency syndrome
AKI	Acute kidney inury
ALL	Acute lymphoblastic leukaemia
ALP	Alkaline phosphatase
AMH	Anti-Mullerian hormone
AML	Acute myeloid leukaemia
ANA	Antinuclear antibody
ANCA	Antineutrophil cytoplasmic antibody
AP	Anteroposterior
APLS	Advanced Paediatric Life Support
APS1	Autoimmune polyendocrine syndrome 1
APTT	Activated partial thromboplastin time
ART	Antiretroviral therapy
AS	Aortic stenosis
ASD	Atrial septal defect
ASD	Autism spectrum disorder
ASOT	Antistreptolysin O antibody titres
ATG	Anti-thymocyte globulin
ATP	Adenosine triphosphate
AV	Arteriovenous
AVP	Arginine vasopressin
AVPU	Alert, voice, pain, unresponsive
AVSD	Atrioventricular septal defect
B	Breathing
BC	Blood culture
BCG	Bacillus Calmette-Guérin
BiPAP	Bi-level Positive Airway Pressure
BMA	Bone marrow aspirate
BMD	Becker's muscular dystrophy
BMI	Body mass index
BNF	British National Formulary
BNFc	British National Formulary for Children
BP	Blood pressure
BPM	Beats per minute
BTS	British Thoracic Society
BVM	Bag-valve mask
BXO	Balanitis xerotica obliterans
C	Circulation
CAFCASS	Children and Family Court Advisory and Support Service
CAH	Congenital adrenal hyperplasia
CAKUT	Congeital anomalies of the kidney and urinary tract
CAMHS	Child and Adolescent Mental Health Service
CA-MRSA	Community-associated methicillin resistant Staphylococcus aureus
CBA	Collagen binding activity
CBD	Case-based discussion
CBS	Cystathionine beta synthase
CBT	Cognitive behavioural therapy
CCAM	Congenital cystic adenomatoid malformation
CD	Crohn's disease
CDC	Centers for Disease Control and Prevention
CDH	Congenital dislocation of the hip
CDGP	Constitutional delay of growth and puberty
CEX	Clinical evaluation exercise
CF	Cystic fibrosis
CFAM	Cerebral function analysing monitor
CFTR	Cystic fibrosis transmembrane conductance regulator
CFRD	Cystic fibrosis related diabetes
CGD	Chronic granulomatous disease
CGH	Comparative genomic hybridization
CHARGE syndrome	Coloboma of the eye, heart defect, atresia of the choanae, retarded growth and/or development, genital and/or urinary abnormality, ear abnormality and deafness
CHD	Congenital heart defect
CHL	Conductive hearing loss
CK	Creatine kinase
CKD	Chronic kidney disease
CLL	Chronic lymphoblastic leukaemia
CMP	Cow's milk protein
CMV	Cytomegalovirus
CMV	Controlled mandatory ventilation
CNS	Central nervous system
CO$_2$	Carbon dioxide
CP	Cerebral palsy
CPAP	Continuous positive airway pressure
CPR	Cardiopulmonary resuscitation
CRH	Corticotropin releasing hormone
CRP	C-reactive protein
CSF	Cerebrospinal fluid
CT	Computed tomography
CTG	Cardiotocography
CVID	Common variable immunodeficiency
CVL	Central venous line
CVS	Chorionic villous sampling
CXR	Chest X-ray
CYP450	Cytochrome P450 enzyme
D	Disability
DAT	Direct antigen test
DDAVP	Desmopressin
DDH	Developmental dysplasia of the hip
DEJ	Dermo-epidermal junction
DEXA	Dual energy X-ray absorptiometry
DI	Diabetes insipidus
DIC	Disseminated intravascular coagulation
DIDMOAD	Diabetes insipidus, diabetes mellitus, optic atrophy and deafness
DIOS	Distal intestinal obstruction syndrome
DHEAS	Dehydroepiandrosterone sulphate
DHT	Dihydrotesterone
DKA	Diabetic ketoacidosis
DM	Diabetes mellitus
DMARD	Disease-modifying antirheumatic drug
DMD	Duchenne muscular dystrophy
DMSA	Dimercaptosuccinic acid
DNA	Deoxyribonucleic acid
DOPA	Dihydroxyphenylalanine
DOPS	Direct observation of procedural skills
DRESS	Drug Reaction (or Rash) with Eosinophilia and Systemic Symptoms
DSD	Disorder of sexual development
dsDNA	Double stranded DNA
DVT	Deep Vein Thrombosis
E	Exposure
EBV	Epstein-Barr virus
ECG	Electrocardiogram
ECMO	Extracorporeal membrane oxygenation
ED	Emergency department
EDH	Extradural haemorrhage
EEG	Electroencephalogram
EHEC	Enterohaemorrhagic Escherichia coli
EIEC	Enteroinvasive Escherichia coli
EMA	Endomysial antibody
EMG	Electromyography
ENaC	Epithelial sodium channel
ENT	Ear, nose and throat
EO	Eosinophilic oesophagitis
EPEC	Enteropathogenic Escherichia coli
EPLS	European Paediatric Life Support
ERT	Enzyme replacement therapy
ESR	Erythrocyte sedimentation rate
ESWL	Extracorporeal shock wave lithotripsy
ET	Endotracheal
ETC	Electron transport chain
ETEC	Enterotoxigenic Escherichia coli
EVD	Extraventricular drain
FAH	Fumarylacetoacetase
FBC	Full blood count
FEV$_1$	Forced expiratory volume in one second
FFP	Fresh frozen plasma
FGFR	Fibroblast growth factor receptor
FiO$_2$	Fraction of inspired oxygen
FISH	Fluorescence in situ hybridisation
fMRI	Functional magnetic resonance imaging
FODMAP	Fermentable Oligo-Di-Mono-saccharides and Polyols
FPG	Fasting plasma glucose
FSH	Follicle stimulating hormone
FUO	Fever of unknown origin
FVC	Forced vital capacity
G6PD	Glucose-6-phosphate dehydrogenase
GA1	Glutaric aciduria type 1
GABA	Gamma-aminobutyric acid
GAD	Glutamic acid decarboxylase
GAGs	Glycosaminoglycans
GALT	Gut-associated lymphoid tissue
GALT	Galactose-1-phosphate uridyl transferase
GARS-2	Gilliam Autism Rating Scale

GAVI	Global Alliance for Vaccines and Immunisation	ITP	Idiopathic thrombocytopenic purpura	OGTT	Oral glucose tolerance test
GBM	Glomerular basement membrane	IUD	Intrauterine device	OME	Otitis media with effusion
GBS	Group B streptococcus	IUGR	Intrauterine growth restriction	OP	Oropharyngeal
GBS	Guillain-Barré syndrome	IUS	Intrauterine system	ORS	Oral rehydration solution
GCS	Glasgow coma scale	IV	Intravenous	OSCE	Objective structured clinical examination
GFR	Glomerular filtration rate	IVA	Isovaleric acidaemia	OT	Occupational therapy
GH	Growth hormone	IVH	Intraventricular haemorrhage	PA	Propionic acidaemia
GHD	Growth hormone deficiency	IVIG	Intravenous immunoglobulin	PALS	Patient advice and liaison service
GLUT-1	Glucose transporter 1	JIA	Juvenile idiopathic arthritis	PANDAS	Paediatric autoimmune neuropsychiatric disorders associated with streptococcal infections
GOR	Gastro-oesophageal reflux	JVP	Jugular venous pressure		
GORD	Gastro-oesophageal reflux disease	KDOQI	Kidney Disease Outcomes Quality Initiative		
GP	General practitioner	KUB	Kidney-ureter-bladder	PAPP-A	Pregnancy-associated plasma protein-A
GnRH	Gonadotropin-releasing hormone	LARC	Long acting reversible contraception	PCD	Primary ciliary dyskinesia
GSDs	Glycogen storage disorders	LCH	Langerhans cell histiocytosis	PCDAI	Paediatric Crohn's Disease Activity Index
GvHD	Graft-versus-host disease	LDH	Lactate dehydrogenase		
HAART	Highly active antiretroviral therapy	LFT	Liver function test	PCP	Pneumocystis carinii (jirovecii) pneumonia
		LH	Luteinising hormone		
Hb	Haemoglobin	LP	Lumbar puncture	PCR	Polymerase chain reaction
HbA1c	Glycated haemoglobin	LTOT	Long term oxygen therapy	PCV	Packed cell volume
HbS	Sickle cell haemoglobin	MAG3	Mercaptoacetyltriglycine	PDA	Patent ductus arteriosus
HcG	Human chorionic gonadotropin	MAP	Mean arterial pressure	PE	Pulmonary Embolism
		MAP	Mean airway pressure	PEEP	Positive end expiratory pressure
HD	Hodgkin's disease	MCAD	Medium-chain acyl-CoA dehydrogenase	PEF	Peak expiratory flow
HDU	High dependency unit			PEG	Percutaneous endoscopic gastrostomy
HFNC	High flow nasal cannulae	MCADD	Medium-chain acyl-CoA dehydrogenase deficiency		
HFOV	High-frequency oscillatory ventilation	MC&S	Microscopy, culture and sensitivity	PEG-J	Percutaneous endoscopic gastro-jejunostomy
HH	Hypogonadotropic hypogonadism	MCUG	Micturating cystourethrogram	PET	Positron emission tomography
		MCV	Mean cell volume	PG	Plasma glucose
HiB	Haemophilus influenza type B	MCV	Molluscum contagiosum virus	PHEX	Phosphate regulating endopeptidase homolog
		MDGs	Millennium Development Goals		
HIE	Hypoxic-ischaemic encephalopathy	MDI	Metered-dose inhaler	PICC	Peripherally inserted central catheter
		MDR	Multi-drug resistant		
HIV	Human Immunodeficiency Virus	MDT	Multidisciplinary team	PICU	Paediatric intensive care unit
		MEN	Multiple endocrine neoplasia	PIP	Peak inspiratory pressure
HLA	Human leucocyte antigen	MenC	Meningococcus C	PKU	Phenylketonuria
HLH	Haemophagocytic lymphohistiocytosis	MG	Myasthenia gravis	PMTCT	Prevention of mother-to-child transmission
		MIBG	Metaiodobenzylguanidine		
HPA	Hypothalamic-pituitary-adrenal	MIS	Müllerian-inhibiting substance	PNET	Primitive neuroectodermal tumour
HPV	Human papilloma virus	MMA	Methylmalonic acidaemia		
HPG	Hypothalamic-pituitary-gonadal	MMR	Measles, mumps and rubella	PORCN	Porcupine homolog
		MODY	Maturity onset diabetes of the young	PP	Precocious puberty
HR	Heart rate			PPHN	Persistent pulmonary hypertension of the newborn
HRCT	High resolution computed tomography	MPS	Mucopolysaccharidoses		
		MRCPCH	Membership of the Royal College of Paediatrics and Child Health	PPV	Patent processus vaginalis
HS	Hereditary spherocytosis			PR	Per rectum
HSCT	Haemopoietic stem cell transplantation			PRO	Parental Responsibility Order
		MRI	Magnetic resonance imaging	PROM	Premature rupture of the membranes
HSP	Henoch Schönlein Purpura	MRSA	Methicillin resistant Staphylococcus aureus		
HSV	Herpes simplex virus			PRN	Pro re nata i.e. as required
HUS	Haemolytic uraemic syndrome	MSUD	Maple syrup urine disease	PS	Pulmonary stenosis
		NAD	Nicotinamide adenine dinucleotide	PT	Prothrombin time
HVA	Homovanillic acid			PTV	Patient triggered ventilation
IBD	Inflammatory bowel disease	NAI	Non-accidental injury	PTH	Parathyroid hormone
IBS	Irritable bowel syndrome	NBM	Nil by mouth	PT	Physiotherapy
IC	Indeterminate colitis	NEC	Necrotising enterocolitis	PTSD	Post-traumatic stress disorder
ICD	Implantable cardioverter defibrillator	NF	Neurofibromatosis	PUCAI	Paediatric Ulcerative Colitis Activity Index
		NF1/2	Neurofibromatosis type 1 or 2		
ICP	Intracranial pressure	NG	Nasogastric	PUJ	Pelvi-ureteric junction
ICU	Intensive care unit	NHL	Non-Hodgkin lymphoma	PUV	Posterior urethral valve
Ig	Immunoglobulin	NICE	National Institute for Health and Care Excellence	PVL	Periventricular leukomalacia
IgA	Immunoglobulin A			PWS	Prader-Willi syndrome
IGF1	Insulin-like growth factor 1	NICU	Neonatal intensive care unit	RBC	Red blood cell
IGF2	Insulin-like growth factor 2	NIPE	Newborn and infant physical examination	REM	Rapid eye movement
IL-2	Interleukin-2			ReSoMal	Rehydration solution for malnutrition
IL-4	Interleukin-4	NIPPV	Non-Invasive Positive Pressure Ventilation		
IL-5	Interleukin-5			RF	Rheumatoid factor
IL-13	Interleukin-13	NKF	National Kidney Foundation	RiCOF	Ristocetin cofactor
ILAE	International League Against Epilepsy	NLS	Newborn life support	RIF	Right iliac fossa
		NMDA	N-methyl-D-aspartate	RNA	Ribonucleic acid
IIH	Idiopathic Intracranial hypertension	NPA	Nasopharyngeal aspirate	RR	Respiratory rate
		NSAIDS	Non-steroidal anti-inflammatory drugs	RSV	Respiratory syncytial virus
IM	Intramuscular			RUTF	Ready-to-use therapeutic food
INR	International normalised ratio	NSPCC	National Society for the Prevention of Cruelty to Children	SAH	Subarachnoid haemorrhage
IO	Intraosseous			SALT	Speech and language therapy
IPS	Infantile pyloric stenosis			SBAR	Situation, background, assessment and recommendation
IQ	Intelligence quotient	NTD	Neural tube defect		
IRT	Immunoreactive trypsinogen	O_2	Oxygen		
ISS	Idiopathic short stature	OA	Osteoarthritis	SBR	Serum bilirubin
ITP	Immune thrombocytopenia	OAE	Oto-acoustic emissions	SC	Sickle cell anaemia

SCAD	Short-chain acyl-CoA dehydrogenase	SUFE	Slipped upper femoral epiphysis	UAC	Umbilical artery catheter
SCBU	Special care baby unit	SVCO	Superior vena cava obstruction	UC	Ulcerative colitis
SCID	Severe combined immunodeficiency	SVD	Spontaneous vaginal delivery	UDT	Undescended testes
SD	Standard deviation	SVT	Supraventricular tachycardia	U&E	Urea and electrolytes
SDGs	Sustainable Development Goals	SWAN	Syndrome without a name	UO	Ureteric orifice
SDH	Subdural haemorrhage	SWS	Sturge-Weber syndrome	UN	United Nations
SEDU	Specialist eating disorders unit	T1DM	Type 1 diabetes mellitus	URTI	Upper respiratory tract infection
SENCO	Special Educational Needs Coordinator	T2DM	Type 2 diabetes mellitus	USS	Ultrasound scan
SGA	Small for gestational age	Te	Expiratory Time	UTI	Urinary tract infection
SHOX	Short Stature Homeobox gene	Ti	Inspiratory Time	UV	Ultraviolet
SIADH	Syndrome of inappropriate antidiuretic hormone secretion	TAC	Team around the child	UVC	Umbilical vein catheter
SIDS	Sudden infant death syndrome	TAPVD	Total anomalous pulmonary venous drainage	VACTERL association	Vertebral defects, anal atresia, cardiac defects, tracheo-oesophageal fistula, renal anomalies and limb abnormalities
SIGN	Scottish Intercollegiate Guidelines Network	TB	Tuberculosis		
SIMV	Synchronised intermittent mandatory ventilation	TCA	Tricarboxylic acid	VHL	Von Hippel-Lindau disease
SLE	Systemic lupus erythematosus	TDS	Ter die sumendum ie. Three times a day	VLCAD	Very-long-chain acyl-CoA dehydrogenase
SMA	Spinal muscular atrophy	TFT	Thyroid function test	VMA	Vanillylmandelic acid
SNHL	Sensorineural hearing loss	Tg	Thyroglobulin	VMAT	Vesicular monoamine transporter
SPECT	Single-photon emission computed tomography	tTGA	Tissue transglutaminase antibody	VP	Ventriculoperitoneal
SpO2	Oxygen saturation	Th2	Type 2 Helper T-Cell	VSD	Ventricular septal defect
SROM	Spontaneous rupture of membranes	Thal	Thalassaemia	VT	Ventricular tachycardia
SRS	Social Responsiveness Scale	TIA	Transient ischaemic attack	VTEC	Verotoxin producing Escherichia coli
SSPE	Subacute sclerosing panencephalitis	TIBC	Total iron binding capacity	VUJ	Vesicoureteric junction
SSRI	Selective serotonin reuptake inhibitor	TLS	Tumour lysis syndrome	VUR	Vesico-ureteric reflux
STEC	Shiga Toxin-Producing E. coli	TNF	Tumour necrosis factor	VZV	Varicella zoster virus
SUDEP	Sudden unexpected death in epilepsy	TORCH	Toxoplasmosis, Other, Rubella, CMV, Herpes	WAS	Wiskott-Aldrich syndrome
SUDI	Sudden unexpected death in infancy	TPO	Thyroperoxidase	vWD	von Willebrand disease
		TPMT	Thiopurine methyltransferase	vWF	von Willebrand factor
		TPN	Total parenteral nutrition	WCC	White cell count
		TRH	Thyrotropin-releasing hormone	WHO	World Health Organisation
		TSH	Thyroid-stimulating hormone		
		TST	Tuberculin skin test		
		tTG	Tissue transglutaminase		
		TTN	Transient tachypnoea of the newborn		

Contributors

Chief Editor

Zeshan Qureshi BM MSc BSc (Hons) MRCPCH
Academic Clinical Fellow, Great Ormond
Street Hospital, and Institute of Global
Health, UCL, UK

Associate Editor

Tina Sajjanhar MBBS DRCOG DCH FRCPCH
FCEM
Consultant in Paediatric Emergency
Medicine, Divisional Director for Children
and Young People Services, Lewisham and
Greenwich NHS Trust, UK

Authors

John Jungpa Park MB ChB MTh
BMedSci (Hons)
Junior Doctor, North Central Thames
Foundation School, UK

Chi Hau Tan MBBS (Hons) GDipSurgAnat
Neurosurgery Registrar, Monash Health,
Melbourne, Australia

Anand Goomany MbChB BSc
Core Surgical Trainee, Bradford Teaching
Hospitals Foundation Trust, West
Yorkshire, UK

Amy Mitchell MBChB BSc (Hons) MSc
DipClinEd MRCPCH
Consultant Paediatric Oncologist,
Southampton University Hospital Trust,
Southampton, UK

David K K Ho MBChB DTM&H MRCPCH
Clinical Research Fellow, Institute of Child
Health, University College London, UK

Christopher Harris MBChB MRCPCH
Paediatric Neonatal Registrar, King's College
Hospital, London, UK

Marylyn-Jane Emedo MBBS BSc MRCPCH
Paediatric Registrar, London Deanery,
London, UK

Maxine Wilkie
Medical Student, Keele University, UK

Anna Capsomidis BSc MBChB (Hons)
MRCPCH PGDip (Med Ed) PGC (Healthcare
Ethics and Law)
Clinical Research Fellow, UCL, Great Ormond
Street Institute of Child Health, UK

May Bisharat MBBS (Hons) MSc FRCS
(Paed Surg)
Registrar in Paediatric Surgery, Evelina
Children's Hospital, London, UK

Rachael Mitchell MRCPCH MA (Cantab)
Paediatric Registrar, London Deanery,
London, UK

Alexander Young MBChB MSc MRCS PGCME
Trauma and Orthopaedic Surgery Registrar,
Severn Deanery, UK

Marie Monaghan MBBS BSc (Hons) MRCPCH
Paediatric Registrar, London Deanery, UK

Antonia Hargadon-Lowe BMBS BMedSci
MRCPCH MSc
Paediatric Registrar, London Deanery,
London, UK

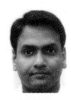
Sadhanandham Punniyakodi
MBBS MRCPCH MSc
Senior Training Fellow in Paediatric
Endocrinology, The Great North Children's
Hospital, Royal Victoria Infirmary, Newcastle
upon Tyne

Stephen D Marks MD MSc MRCP
DCH FRCPCH
Consultant Paediatric Nephrologist, Great
Ormond Street Hospital for Children NHS
Foundation Trust, London, UK.

Hannah Linford BMBS MRCPCH
Paediatric Registrar, KSS Deanery, UK

Anita Demetriou MBBS BSc MRCPCH DTMH
Paediatric Registrar, London Deanery, UK

Christopher Grime MBChB MRCPCH
Paediatric Registrar, London Deanery, UK.

Debasree Das MBBS BSc MRCPCH
Paediatric Registrar, London Deanery, UK

Philippa King BSc MBChB MRCPCH MSc
Academic Clinical Fellow, Medical
Microbiology, East of England Deanery, UK

Isabel Mawson MBBS BSc MRCPCH
Paediatric Registrar, London Deanery, UK

Claire Bryant BMedSc BMBS
Junior Doctor, South Thames Foundation
School, London, UK

Anna Chadwick MBBS BSc MRCPCH
Paediatric Registrar, London Deanery, UK

Andrew Hall MBChB MRCS DOHNS
ENT Specialist Registrar, Great Ormond Street
Hospital, UK

Amy Moran MBBS MRCPCH
Paediatric Registrar, London Deanery, UK

Michael Malley MA (Hons) Cantab
MBBS MRCPCH
Paediatric Registrar, London Deanery, UK

Alice Armitage MBBS BSc MRCPCH
Academic Clinical Fellow, Paediatrics, London
Deanery, UK

Vaitsa Tziaferi MD MRCPCH MSc
Consultant in Paediatric Endocrinology &
Diabetes, Leicester Royal Infirmary, UK

Kunal Babla BSc(Hons) MBBS MSc
MRCPCH MAcadMEd
Neonatal Registrar, London Deanery, UK

Maanasa Polubothu BSc MBChB MSc
MRCPCH PGDip (Genomic Medicine)
Academic Clinicial Fellow, London
Deanery, UK

Sam Thenabadu MBBS MRCP DRCOG DCH
MA Clin Ed FCEM MSc (Paed) FHEA
Consultant Adult & Paediatric Emergency
Medicine. Honorary Senior Lecturer, King's
College London

Stephanie Connaire
Final Year Medical Student, Cardiff University,
Cardiff, UK

 Zainab Kazmi BSc (Hons) MBChB
Academic Foundation Doctor and Honorary
Clinical Fellow, University of Glasgow

 Pooja Parekh MBBS
Paediatric Trainee, London Deanery, UK

Expert Reviewers

Dr Vandy Bharadwaj
Consultant Paediatric Haematologist, Southampton
Children's Hospital, Southampton, UK

Prof. Robert Tulloh MA DM FRCP FRCPCH
Consultant Paediatric Cardiologist, Bristol Royal Hospital
for Children, UK. Honorary Professor of Congenital Cardiology
and Pulmonary Hypertension, University of Bristol

Prof. David Walker
Professor of Paediatric Oncology, Children's Brain Tumour
Research Centre, Nottingham, UK

Mr RA Wheeler MS FRCS LLB (Hons) LLM
Consultant Neonatal & Paediatric Surgeon. Director,
Department of Clinical Law. University Hospital of
Southampton, UK.

Mr Theo Joseph FRCS
ENT Consultant, Royal National Throat Nose and Ear
Hospital, London, UK

Dr Victoria Jones MRCPCH
Consultant Paediatrician, North Middlesex University
Hospital, UK

Dr Anne-Marie Ebdon MBBS MRCPCH FRACP
Consultant Paediatrician, Queen Mary's Hospital for Children,
Epson & St.Hellier University Hospitals NHS Trust, UK

Dr Sarah K Clegg MBChB BSc MRCPUK MRCPCH
Consultant Paediatrician, Department of Community Child
Health, Edinburgh, UK

Dr Solomon Kamal-Uddin MBBS BMedSci
Paediatric Registrar, London Deanery, UK

Dr Delan Devakumar MBChB MSc MRCPCH DTM&H
MFPH PhD
Public Health Registrar, London Deanery, UK

Dr Khadija H Aljefri MBChB MRCP (UK) MRCP (Derm)
Dermatology Registrar, Royal Victoria Infirmary, Newcastle
upon Tyne, UK

Mr Neil Tickner MRPharmS PGDip. Clin. Pharm
Lead Pharmacist Paediatrics, St Mary's Hospital, London, UK

Stephanie Connaire
Final Year Medical Student, Cardiff University, Cardiff, UK

Dr Pooja Parekh MBBS
Paediatric Trainee, London Deanery, UK

Bianca Davis
School Teacher, Head of Personal Social and Health
Education, London, UK

Dr Sreena Das MB ChB MRCPCH
Consultant Paediatrician, King's College Hospital, London, UK

Dr Simon Chapman BA BM FRCPCH
Consultant Paediatrician, King's College Hospital, London, UK

Dr Isabel Farmer MBBS MRCPCH
Haematology Registrar, Queen Elizabeth Hospital, London, UK

Tabatha English BSc (Hons) RM
Midwife, Lewisham Hospital, London, UK

Kelly Frogbrook PgDip RN
Paediatric Nurse, Queen Elizabeth Hospital, London, UK

Dan Purnell
Lead Resuscitation Officer, Lewisham and Greenwich
Healthcare NHS Trust

Dr Daniel Langer BSc (Hons) MRCPCH DPID
Consultant in Acute & Ambulatory Paediatrics.
Special interest in paediatric infectious diseases
(SPIN ID) and global child health
Epsom & St Helier NHS Trust, UK

Lydia Shackshaft
Medical Student, King's College London, UK

Sammie Mak
Medical Student, Leeds University, UK

Ben Evans
Medical Student, University of Newcastle, UK

Contents

SECTION 2: CLINICAL CASES

SECTION 3: CLINICAL SKILLS

SECTION 4: BECOMING A PAEDIATRICIAN

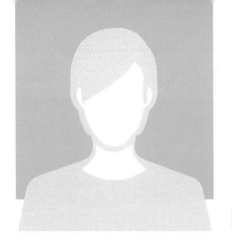

1.01

ADOLESCENT MEDICINE

ALICE ARMITAGE

CONTENTS

APPROACH TO THE ADOLESCENT CONSULTATION

Adolescence is the transitional phase of growth and development between childhood and adulthood. An adolescent is defined by the World Health Organisation as a person between 10 and 19 years of age. There is increasing recognition of the specific problems of this age group, including trauma, mental health issues, pregnancy and sexually transmitted diseases. The rise in healthcare usage in adolescence is multifactorial; increasing survival from chronic childhood conditions, use of drugs and alcohol, and risk-taking behaviour all play a role, and advances in perinatal care and immunisation have shifted the burden of disease away from the under-fives. Understanding the unique needs of this age group is a core skill for any physician. The law relating to children and adolescents is covered in Chapter 1.13.

Adolescent History Taking

It is important to adapt the approach to the needs of the adolescent age-group. At the start of a consultation, consider the following:

- Always speak to the patient, not to their parent or carer, unless there is no alternative.
- Ask the patient if they would like to speak to alone or ask them if they would like someone to be present, such as a parent or friend.
- For any examination, offer a chaperone.
- Talk in an age-appropriate fashion. It is easy to alienate an adolescent patient by appearing patronising or by using medical jargon.
- Try to anticipate issues around consent and confidentiality.

The psychosocial history is vital to the adolescent history. Many presentations will stem from an issue like drug use, a fight with a partner or worries about sexuality. A useful aide-memoire is the HEADSS tool, shown in *Table 1*. In general, start with more open questions and then focus questions to the information given. A common reason for missing important issues is making assumptions; for example, thinking that all young people live at home with their parents or that all young people are heterosexual.

TABLE 1: Key aspects of adolescent history taking (HEADSS tool)

Domain	Example Questions	Importance
Home and environment.	• How are things at home? • Has anything changed recently? • Who are you living with at the moment? • What is your relationship like with your foster parents? • Who would you talk to if you're worried about something?	Young people may be living with family, in foster care or living independently. Relationships with people they live with are likely to have a major impact on their health and well-being. Someone to confide in is vital to emotional well-being.
Education and employment.	• Are you at school or college at the moment? • Do you have a job? How is that going? • What are your plans for when you finish school?	A young person may be struggling in education because of problems with their mental or physical health or problems such as bullying or domestic violence at home. Young people may need support to re-engage with education or to start applying for jobs.
Activities.	• What kind of thing do you enjoy doing? • Do you play any sports or have hobbies? • Are you in a group or a gang? • How much time do you spend playing computer games or on social media?	Young people may be obese or have nutritional problems linked to their activities. There may be mental health problems, bullying or involvement in gangs.
Drugs and alcohol.	• Do you drink alcohol? How often do you drink? • Do you or any friends take drugs? What kind? • Have you ever regretted something you have done after taking drugs or alcohol?	There are links with risk-taking behaviour, isolation and damage to relationships. Addiction may indicate a need for psychological input.
Sexual health.	• Do you have a boyfriend or girlfriend? • How old were you when you first had sex? • Have you ever had or thought about having a partner of the same sex? • Have you ever been for a sexual health screen?	Giving contraceptive and sexual health screening advice is important. There may be concerns about sexual exploitation or another abusive relationship. Mental health problems can arise from worrying about gender identity or sexuality.
Suicide and depression.	• Most of the time do you feel down or depressed? • Have you ever done anything to hurt yourself like cutting your arms or taking pills? • Do you ever think about hurting yourself?	Young people may have mental health problems and need psychological interventions. It is important to assess suicide risk.

Asking Difficult Questions

Some of these questions can feel difficult to ask directly, and are even more difficult to answer directly. One useful tip is to use scenarios as a way into difficult questions. For example:

> "It's quite common for young people to experiment with drugs; is that something you've had experience with?"
> "Some of the work I do with young people is about choosing types of contraception and talking about sexual health; has anyone ever talked to you about this?"

This is also a good way to address more specific concerns that may have arisen during the consultation. For example:

> "Some young people I work with have told me that their parents fight a lot and sometimes it gets violent; is that something that happens in your home?"
> "One thing that can happen in a relationship is feeling pressured into acting or behaving in a certain way; sometimes people feel they don't have any choice about it. Have you ever felt like that?"

Questions need to ensure the young person will feel supported but not accused. For example, with the drug question, a young person may not admit to usage if they believe the police will immediately be called. The more comfortable the child, the more likely they are to give an honest response. When questioning, the doctor must remain aware of nonverbal language, e.g. changes in body language when talking about home (breaking eye contact, fidgeting and shorter responses).

Puberty, Growth and Development

Any consultation with an adolescent patient should include assessment of height, weight and pubertal status. This assessment is often forgotten, particularly in older teenagers transitioning to adult care. Young people with chronic health needs may have delayed growth and puberty compared with their peers. This is also a good opportunity to highlight problems such as obesity, eating disorders or neglect.

Autonomy, Consent and Confidentiality

One of the challenges of working with adolescents is managing their emerging autonomy as they move into adulthood. The ability to develop and maintain trust and rapport with patients relies on sensitive handling of these complex issues.

Remember:

> Each adolescent should be assessed on an individual basis without prejudice.
> There is no lower age limit to Gillick competence, and even younger children may be able to consent for their own medical care.

> There is no lower age limit on confidentiality but there are limits to this confidentiality, such as if there is a concern that the patient is in danger. If there is a duty to break confidentiality, tell the patient beforehand, except in rare, exceptional circumstances where this may result in significantly more harm than good.

RELATIONSHIPS, SEXUAL HEALTH AND CONTRACEPTION

Before bringing up sex and relationships, give patients an opportunity to talk alone and reassure them about confidentiality. If a young person is having sex or considering having sex, it is important to talk to them about healthy relationships, sexual health and contraception. As with drugs and alcohol, some of this may have been covered at school. Do not make assumptions based on age, culture, disability or diagnosis. If a patient is not sexually active, they may well wish to be and have questions about this. Chronic health conditions and disabilities impact on sex and relationships; therefore, doctors are potentially in a position to address these issues.

Sexual Health

Globally, young people have disproportionately high rates of sexually transmitted infections (STIs), with chlamydia, gonorrhoea, viral warts and syphilis being particularly common. The best protection is through use of condoms; these are often freely given out in health care settings and should be discussed with all young people even if on another form of contraception. Some STIs can by asymptomatic, particularly in women, so regular sexual health screening should be recommended for anyone who is sexually active. Walk-in services allow for easy, anonymous access to sexual health advice and testing. Similarly, the sending of results of STI testing by text messaging is convenient and helps preserve anonymity.

Contraception

In addition to condoms, forms of long-acting reversible contraception (LARC) are a good option for adolescent patients, and providing leaflets and counselling will allow them to choose the method that they feel is most appropriate for them. Some examples of LARCs include:

> Intrauterine device (IUD). This is also called a coil; this can stay in place for five to ten years but can be removed at any time.
> Intra-uterine system (IUS). This coil releases a small amount of progestogen locally. It can stay in place for five years.
> Contraceptive injection. This lasts for eight or twelve weeks; it delivers systemic progestogen.
> Contraceptive implant. This sits under the skin and releases a small amount of systemic progestogen. It can stay in place for up to three years.

All these forms are over 99% effective, and normal fertility returns as soon as they are removed. However, unless sex is with a regular partner and both have had recent sexual health screening, it is important to recommend additional barrier methods of contraception, like condoms. Doctors in the UK and elsewhere are legally allowed to provide contraception to females under 16 without parental consent, providing certain conditions are met (p174).

Teenage Pregnancy

Globally, over 10% of births are to girls 15 to 19-years-old. Although the majority of these are in low and middle-income countries, both the UK and the USA continue to have high rates of teenage pregnancy. This remains a significant cause of morbidity and mortality in this age-group, particularly in younger adolescents (13 to 15-years-old) who experience higher rates of pregnancy complications and pre-term births.

Risk factors for teenage pregnancy include:
> Low socioeconomic status.
> Low level of educational attainment.
> Having been a baby of a teenage parent.

Any young person who becomes pregnant should be offered counselling covering abortion and adoption to allow them to make an informed choice. Remember that for some young people, particularly in certain ethnic groups, having a baby as a teenager can be a positive choice.

An important part of antenatal care for younger patients is a focus on health promotion, including reducing drug and alcohol intake and optimising nutritional status. It is important to involve social care and consider the needs of both the mother and the unborn child.

MENTAL HEALTH

Half of all mental illnesses begin before 14-years-old, and 75% begin before 24-years-old. Young people suspected or known to have mental health problems should be formally assessed by a child and adolescent mental health service (CAMHS). CAMHS teams involve a range of professionals including psychiatrists, psychologists, family therapists, social workers, counsellors and nurses. Some common mental health problems are discussed below.

Depression

The three core symptoms of depression are low mood, low energy levels and loss of interest in activities that were previously pleasurable (anhedonia). Other symptoms are shown in *Table 2*.

Approximately five percent of teenagers suffer from depression at some point. Most young people will go through periods of feeling "down" or anxious. However, depression is longer lasting and interferes with the patient's ability to function.

3

TABLE 2: Symptoms of depression		
Core Symptoms	Biological Symptoms	Cognitive Symptoms
Low mood. Low energy levels. Loss of interest.	Sleep disturbance. Reduced appetite. Weight loss or weight gain. Constipation. Loss of libido.	Worthlessness/low self-esteem. Poor memory. Poor concentration. Guilt. Tearfulness. Agitation.

In addition to the symptoms listed above, depression in adolescents may present with symptoms such as:

- Extreme sensitivity to criticism.
- Irritability and anger.
- Worsening performance at school.
- Unexplained aches and pains.

In young people, the signs of depression may be: taking drugs, going missing or getting involved in fights. A presentation of depression can be secondary to another problem; examples in adolescence are bullying, undisclosed sexual assault or maltreatment.

Management of depression in adolescent therapy involves initially identifying possible precipitants (e.g. bullying) and addressing them where possible. Cognitive behavioural psychotherapies are used more commonly than with adults. However, in moderate to severe depression, doctors may choose to prescribe medication, e.g. a selective serotonin reuptake inhibitor (SSRI). Fluoxetine is the preferred choice in adolescents, although it may be associated with an increased risk of suicide. Both approaches can be used simultaneously.

Self-harm

Common forms of self-harm in adolescence include:

- Cutting the arms or legs with a sharp object.
- Taking an overdose of medications (commonly paracetamol).
- Alcohol or illicit drug intoxication.

Self-harm is linked with attempted suicide, but this is not always the case. Depression is a common comorbidity.

In assessing and managing these children, perform a risk assessment and explore the intent of suicide. Then explore the circumstances leading to the self-harm episode. Bear in mind that even those who self-harm frequently may have different reasons for each episode. Young people who present to hospital with acute self-harm will need to be formally assessed by the mental health team and will have a clear follow-up plan in place on discharge.

Suicide Risk

Any patient with depression or presenting following self-harm should have their suicide risk assessed. Never be afraid to ask directly about suicide. Questions to ask include:

- Have you ever tried to hurt yourself?
- Have you had thoughts about wanting to kill yourself?
- Have you ever tried to kill yourself?
- Have you ever made plans to kill yourself (for example, collecting tablets or writing a note)?

Any concerns about patient safety need to be escalated following child protection procedures, ideally with an assessment by someone trained in child and adolescent mental health.

Psychosis

The definition of psychosis is when a person "loses touch with reality" and may be characterised by:

- Hallucinations. When a person sees, hears or otherwise perceives things that are not present; for example, hearing voices.
- Delusions. When a person holds a belief that is untrue despite logical evidence to the contrary; for example, believing that their parent is trying to kill them.

Psychosis is a symptom of several conditions, including schizophrenia, bipolar disorder, autoimmune disease and meningoencephalitis. Schizophrenia has a prevalence of 1% in middle to late adolescence. Many more people will have at least one psychotic episode in their lives and the first episode of psychosis commonly occurs in adolescence or in the early 20s.

Psychosis is an extremely distressing experience for patients and their families. Despite antipsychotic medications, psychotic illness such as schizophrenia continues to have a poor prognosis, with multiple relapses and high rates of suicide.

Drug and Alcohol Abuse

Many young people experiment with drugs and alcohol and, for some, this can become an addiction.

Warning signs include:

- Change in behaviour.
- Hanging out with a new group of friends.
- Deterioration in academic performance.
- Getting involved in fights or shoplifting.

Beyond the direct health effects of drugs and alcohol, these substances can isolate young people from their friends and family and increase risk-taking behaviour. These problems can be easily missed, as young people will often try to hide drug and alcohol use.

Medically Unexplained Symptoms

Adolescent patients may present with symptoms such as pain, tiredness or dizziness, for which, despite investigations, no medical cause is evident. This is also called "somatisation disorder". These symptoms are more common in women, patients with depression, those who have recently had a significant medical problem or those who have experienced a bereavement. This is a difficult diagnosis to make as it is a diagnosis of exclusion, making these patients very challenging to manage. Rarely, the patient or their carer may be knowingly fabricating symptoms (this is known as factitious or fabricated illness). If the motivation is a reward for feigning or exaggerating illness, such as financial benefit or attention, this is specifically known as malingering. However, the majority are not "faking it", and if they feel judged or disbelieved, their condition is likely to worsen rather than improve.

The best approach is for a single consultant to coordinate the patient's care, working closely with the primary care physician and offering psychological support.

Management of Mental Health Problems in Adolescence

As with adults with mental health problems, adolescent patients can be managed in an inpatient or outpatient setting depending on their diagnosis and needs. In younger patients, the focus is more on treating the family unit (e.g. through family therapy), and medication is used less frequently. The two broad categories are talking therapies and medication.

Talking Therapies

> Counselling. This gives young people with mental health problems an opportunity to talk about their problems one-to-one with an empathetic listener. This is useful for young people with most types of mental health or behavioural problems.
> Family therapy. This may be helpful for behavioural problems or addiction, where difficulties or conflicts may exist within the family as a whole. It may help family members to see each other's perspectives and be honest with each other.
> Cognitive behavioural therapy (CBT). This may be helpful for many mental health problems including depression, anxiety and psychosis. CBT teaches techniques for overcoming or controlling thoughts or behaviours.
> Psychotherapy. This seeks to address the root causes of thoughts and behaviours by talking about the past; for example, childhood experiences.

Medication

> Antidepressants. These can be used with other therapies to treat depression and anxiety symptoms. Various types are available but commonly used drugs include selective serotonin reuptake inhibitors (SSRIs) such as fluoxetine and sertraline. Side effects are common and include dry mouth, tiredness and headache.
> Antipsychotics. These are used to treat psychosis and can have benefit as mood stabilisers as well. Examples include haloperidol, risperidone and clozapine. Side effects include autonomic effects, movement disorders and weight gain.

> Stimulants. These are helpful for controlling symptoms of Attention Deficit Hyperactivity Disorder (ADHD) and can reduce inattention and impulsiveness. The most common example is methylphenidate (Ritalin).

SAFEGUARDING IN ADOLESCENCE

The adolescent age group presents its own safeguarding challenges. Overlap may exist between victims and perpetrators; for example, a teenage parent who is on a child protection plan and is neglecting her own child.

Bullying

A National Society for the Prevention of Cruelty to Children (NSPCC) study found that almost half of all children have been bullied at some point in their lives. As such, bullying represents a major cause of maltreatment in the adolescent group. It may involve physical assault but can also include verbal, non-verbal, exclusion, racial and sexual bullying. It may also take place online or via text messaging. All adolescent patients should be asked about cyberbullying, social networking sites and sexual bullying, which is an increasing problem.

Children who are bullied may show a range of symptoms and, at worst, may present to health services following physical assault or self-harm. It should be part of the differential diagnosis in any adolescent presentation, particularly with mental health problems and self-harm.

Sexual Exploitation and Assault

Sexual exploitation remains a largely hidden problem worldwide. It can manifest as physical, sexual, emotional and financial abuse or as coercive control. It may occur within young people's relationships and may be influenced by hierarchies within and external to any relationships. Typically, those in a position of power coerce a young person into sexual activities. Both boys and girls are at risk and many young people are unaware that abuse is taking place. One in four girls and one in ten boys are likely to experience sexual abuse in the UK. Notably, the figures for boys may be underestimated as some evidence indicates that many do not seek help, feeling too ashamed to admit victimhood.

Signs that a young person may be being exploited include:
> Relationships with older men.
> Behavioural changes (including sexual promiscuity).
> Going missing.
> Self-harm.

In the UK, over one-third of all presentations of rape and sexual assault are in the adolescent age bracket. Globally, up to one-third of girls report their first sexual experience as being forced. Fear of being judged or not believed may prevent young people from seeking help. Sexual assault by partners or relatives is significantly less likely to be reported.

5

Any young person who presents after sexual assault should be referred to a sexual assault referral centre. These are one-stop specialist medical and forensic services where a patient can receive acute medical and emotional support, have forensic samples taken if necessary, and be referred on for counselling or tests. After assault, patients have high rates of psychological morbidity, particularly post-traumatic stress disorder (PTSD).

TRANSITION FROM PAEDIATRIC TO ADULT SERVICES

Transitional care relates to children and young people with or without chronic disorders being transferred to adult services at a certain age. This process is a challenge in the healthcare of young people. Variable policies and health systems structures often leave patients "in limbo" between services and unsure of where to turn for help. Further challenges are presented by the increasing numbers of patients surviving into adulthood with what were previously considered paediatric conditions, such as congenital heart disease and metabolic conditions.

Good practice in transitional care includes:

› Introducing the concept of transition early (for example, at 13 or 14-years-old).
› An individualised age of transition (depending on the needs of the patient, their disease control and level of maturity).
› A transitions coordinator or keyworker (who remains in contact with the patient throughout transition).
› A written transition plan individualised to each patient.
› "Transition clinics" with the paediatric and adult team together, so that a more formal handover of the patient occurs.
› Access to staff with training in the needs of adolescents and young adults.

REFERENCES AND FURTHER READING

1 Cohen E et al. HEADSS, a psychosocial risk assessment instrument: Implications for designing effective intervention programs for runaway youth. J Adolesc Health, 1999; 12: 539-44.
2 Dick B, Ferguson JB. Health for the world's adolescents: A second chance in the second decade. J Adolesc Health. 2015; 56:3-6.
3 Ford T, Goodman R, Meltzer H. The British child and adolescent mental health survey 1999: the prevalence of DSM-IV disorders. J Amer Acad Child Adolesc Psychiatry. 2003; 42:1203-11.
4 Cawson P et al. Child maltreatment in the United Kingdom: a study of the prevalence of abuse and neglect. London: NSPCC. 2000.
5 Berelowitz S et al. I thought I was the only one. The only one in the world. The Office of the Children's Commissioner's Inquiry into Child Sexual Exploitation in Gangs and Groups: Interim report. 2012.
6 Viner R. Transition from paediatric to adult care. Bridging the gaps or passing the buck? Arch Dis Child. 1999; 81:271-5.
7 Crowley R et al. Improving the transition between paediatric and adult healthcare: a systematic review. Arch Dis Child 2011: archdischild202473.
8 NICE CG16. Self-harm: The short-term physical and psychological management and secondary prevention of self-harm in primary and secondary care. 1994. https://www.nice.org.uk/guidance/cg16.
9 Courvoisie H, Labellarte MJ, Riddle MA. Psychosis in children: diagnosis and treatment. Dialogues Clin Neurosci. 2001; 3:79-92.

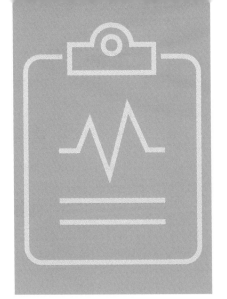

1.02

ASSESSMENT AND MANAGEMENT OF THE ACUTELY UNWELL CHILD

CHRISTOPHER HARRIS

CONTENTS

INTRODUCTION

Clinicians are fearful of treating children and infants in the Emergency Department (ED), and, more generally, of making medical decisions concerning children. Junior doctors manage children in many settings (*Box 1*).

Box 1: Settings in which unwell children may be encountered

- Primary Care.
- Emergency Department.
- Paediatric Emergency Department.
- Paediatric wards.
- Adult specialties with paediatric cover (surgery, orthopaedics, ENT and dermatology).

This chapter provides a framework for assessing any child that presents for medical attention to ensure they receive timely and effective care, with a particular focus on dealing with the very sick child.

When approaching a potentially sick child, bear in mind that children are not just small adults. Different challenges and techniques must be addressed to get to the bottom of the problem quickly.

Consider the following:

➤ The parents or carer may not have the whole story if the child has been in the care of someone else, and so a collateral history may be necessary.

➤ The parents' "sixth sense" regarding their child should always be taken seriously, but equally, parents may underestimate the seriousness of their child's condition.

➤ Younger children may not be able to give any history, or the history given may be misleading.

➤ All children, but particularly younger infants, may have underlying congenital abnormalities that have remained undetected until presentation in extremis.

> Examination interpretation depends on the cooperation of the child, and this can lead to signs being missed or misinterpreted.

> Children can compensate physiologically for severe illness, meaning that signs of deterioration may not be evident until late in the illness.

> Children are dependent on adult carers for many things, particularly in early life. This can lead to opportunities for abuse, which can be easily missed if not assessed for specifically.

> Decisions made during childhood with regards to health can impact all areas of development.

RAPID ASSESSMENT

The initial approach should begin with a comprehensive review of the child's ABC: Airway, Breathing and Circulation. This should be done on all children and can be done during the introduction to the patient and their family. If a baby is crying with no stridor or a child is able to say their name, it can be assumed that their airway is patent. Clues on respiratory status are evident from an assessment of how comfortable the child is, whether they can speak in sentences, and their colour. A child who is running around the waiting room and interested in playing with all the toys and equipment will probably have little in the way of circulatory issues. This initial screen can be useful in deciding whether the child needs immediate resuscitation or whether there is time to get a more detailed history before deciding on a management plan. If there are any signs of compromise to A, B or C, these should be addressed immediately, and help should be sought.

"Red flag" signs that might be identified are summarised in *Table 1*.

History

A focused history is an important part of the assessment of a sick child. However, when a child is very sick, the emotional distress of the parents can make this difficult. If a child requires immediate medical intervention, this should be addressed while another member of the medical team establishes the history from the family member.

Key questions are summarised in *Table 2*.

Examination

An assessment of airway, breathing and circulation should be performed in any encounter. Following this assessment, if the child is stable, a full examination of the child should be done.

Often, the system responsible for illness is not clear because of an uncertain history or the global effect of serious illness. Attention to red flag signs is important, as well as a screening of all systems. Do not cut short an examination due to fears of making a child cry. This is particularly true of babies and young children, who must be examined fully, looking at the entire body, whilst still making efforts to protect the child's modesty.

Parents or a chaperone should be present during examinations. It is common for physical signs, such as non-blanching rashes, to appear on the background of a fairly benign history, and these signs may develop quickly; for example, a non-blanching rash appearing in the groin since the parents last changed the baby.

General

Observing the general condition of a child is vital. A child running around in the waiting area is unlikely to require emergency intervention, but a child who is lethargic and not interested in their surroundings may be seriously unwell. The interaction of the child, the hygiene status and the appropriateness of the clothing can yield important information. Any medical devices or equipment may give clues to underlying conditions and therapy compliance. For example, an inhaler may suggest asthma, but if it is being carried without a spacer device, it may highlight concerns regarding inhaler technique.

Respiratory

Inspect the chest wall and nares for signs of respiratory distress and cyanosis. Listen for stridor or a barking cough. Palpate the trachea to ensure it is central and not displaced like in pneumothorax. Percuss the chest wall, particularly at the lung bases, to identify consolidation or effusion in the older child (>5-years-old). Auscultate for wheeze or added sounds, indicating obstruction or consolidation.

Cardiovascular

Inspect for signs of congenital cardiac disease, such as clubbing of the fingers, shortness of breath or cyanosis. In the older child, it may be possible to see a raised jugular venous pressure (JVP). Palpate the apex beat and the femoral pulses. Auscultate the heart: some heart murmurs may be undetectable at birth and may only be heard at 2 to 4-weeks-old when the left ventricular pressure becomes greater, allowing flow across some heart lesions. Palpate the abdomen for an enlarged liver and auscultate the lung fields. Measure the blood pressure and compare it to age-related normal values.

Abdominal

Inspect the size of the abdomen and any visible peristalsis. Palpate the whole abdomen for tenderness and masses. Palpate and percuss for abdominal organomegaly and ascites. Listen for bowel sounds. Also note "tinkling" sounds in obstruction or absent sounds in perforation. The acute abdomen presents with a child reluctant to move or with a distended abdomen tender to palpation, with possible rebound tenderness. Remember to look at the face of the child when palpating the abdomen to see if it is tender. Distracting questions may help to discern between voluntary and involuntary guarding.

TABLE 1: Red flag signs needing urgent intervention

Red Flag	Possible Cause	Assessment	Management
Non-blanching rash.	• Meningococcal sepsis. • Leukaemia. • Henoch-Schönlein purpura. • Thrombocytopaenia.	• Assess the rash, and areas affected. • Full blood count (FBC), blood film, coagulation, blood cultures, CRP, meningococcal PCR.	• Urgent antibiotics if possible meningococcal sepsis. • Fluid resuscitation.
Traumatic injury.	• Internal bleeding. • Head injury.	• Full trauma assessment regardless of how well the child looks.	• Contact trauma team and immobilise the cervical spine.
Soot around the mouth or nose.	• Smoke inhalation.	• Chest X-ray (CXR). • Oxygen saturations. • Carbon monoxide levels.	• Consider securing the airway early.
Major burns.	• House fire. • Accident. • Chemical exposure.	• Airway assessment. • Calculate percentage of surface area affected. • Intravascular fluid volume. • Circumferential burns.	• Consider securing the airway. • Release circumferential burns (to remove constriction effect) if respiration compromised. • Fluid resuscitation. • IV antibiotics. • Discussion with local burns centre and the paediatric intensive care unit (PICU).
Faltering growth.	• Underlying medical abnormality. • Child protection issues.	• Careful examination and social history.	• Close observation due to risk of deterioration.
Unexplained bruising or bleeding.	• Leukaemia. • Child protection issues. • Thrombocytopaenia.	• Careful examination and social history. • FBC, coagulation and blood film.	• Stop massive bleeding. • Ideally take blood samples pre transfusion of products.
Sudden onset coughing, wheezing or stridor.	• Foreign body inhalation (even if not directly observed).	• Unilateral polyphonic wheeze. • CXR may be normal, consider inspiratory/expiratory films.	• Keep child calm. • Oxygen as required. • Examination by ENT specialist. • Consider PICU transfer if needed.
Delayed central capillary refill time (>2secs).	• Septic shock. • Hypovolaemic shock. • Cardiogenic shock. • Anaphylactic shock.	• Identify underlying cause, e.g. swollen lips/urticaria. • Temperature. • Inflammatory markers.	• 20ml/kg 0.9% saline bolus (10ml/kg boluses in trauma, diabetic ketoacidosis (DKA), neonates, raised intracranial pressure, cardiac conditions).
Tachycardia.	• Sepsis. • Shock. • Supraventricular tachycardia (SVT).	• Identify underlying cause. • ECG.	• Vagal manoeuvres. • Adenosine. • Electrocardioversion or chemical cardioversion may be required if SVT causing deterioration.
Bradycardia.	• Pre-terminal event. • Heart block.	• Ensure pulse present. • Identify underlying cause. • ECG.	• CPR if no pulse. • Discuss with cardiologist urgently if heart block.

TABLE 2: Key questions in a focused history

Question	Explanation
What happened?	Mechanism of injury. Cause of deterioration.
How long has your child been unwell?	Acute or rapid worsening versus more gradual decline.
Any illnesses in the past or PICU/NICU admissions?	Underlying conditions, such as asthma, diabetes, allergy, cardiac conditions or metabolic conditions.
Any medications?	Potential overdose, missed medication (e.g. diabetes and insulin), allergies (e.g. new antibiotics).
Anyone unwell in the family?	Potential infectious cause of illness, potential medication available for accidental ingestion.

(Continued)

TABLE 2: (*Continued*)

Question	Explanation
Any family history of illness?	Sudden deaths in the family (long QT syndrome), atopy (asthma), systemic lupus erythematosus (SLE) (heart block in infants born of mothers with anti-Rho antibodies).
Any foreign travel in the last year?	Helps to widen or narrow the differential diagnosis and subsequent investigations, e.g. malaria, Ebola.
Any discussions regarding resuscitation or end of life care?	It is common for children with life-limiting conditions to be rushed into hospital in the final stages as parents get worried or find they are unable to cope with events unfolding. They may want support at end-of-life rather than immediate life-prolonging measures. Examples include terminal cancer, severe genetic conditions such as spinomuscular atrophy, and heart disease not amenable to surgical correction.
If time permits: • Immunisations up to date? • Who was caring for the child when they became unwell? • Any other witnesses to the event? • Other services involved, e.g. police, social services? • Any other casualties and are they being cared for? • Are there any other children in the house and are they being cared for? • Can I call someone to support you?	These questions build a picture of the overall health of the family and provide more information to piece together what has happened. It is important to recognise how difficult it can be for the parents or other members of the public to see and manage an unwell child until help arrives. This is an opportunity to safeguard others involved in an accident or those forgotten at home in the rush to get to hospital.

Neurological and Developmental

In an emergency, the AVPU scale can be helpful in quickly assessing neurological status. A paediatric GCS will give more information if time allows. Examine the power, tone and reflexes. Cranial nerves should also be examined. New focal neurological signs are an important indicator that further imaging is warranted. Assess if the child responds appropriately and has reached their gross motor, fine motor, social and language developmental milestones.

INITIAL MANAGEMENT

The initial management of a child identified as peri-arrest or very unwell shares a common pathway, regardless of aetiology. Perform life-saving management prior to initiating treatment of the underlying condition. Although meningococcal sepsis requires antibiotic therapy, if the child is not breathing and has no circulation, antibiotics will have little effect.

Resuscitating a Patient Using the DR ABCDE Approach

Once you have identified that a child might be seriously unwell, ensure it is safe to approach them for assessment. In other words, assess for danger (D). The next thing to do is to assess if they are responsive (R). This can be done by asking them a question, followed by gentle shaking if there is no response. A sternal rub can be used if there is still a doubt. The next step is to assess the airway (A), breathing (B), circulation (C), disability (D) and then exposure (E). The assessment and management at each stage is summarised in *Tables 3-7*. Throughout, the cervical spine should be immobilised if there is a concern about potential injury due to trauma. Address any abnormalities in airway, breathing or circulation, in this order. Do not be distracted by other injuries until 'A, B and C' are stable. Don't ever forget to measure glucose, as hypoglycaemia is an important cause of reversible decline.

Advanced Paediatric Life Support

The Advanced Paediatric Life Support (APLS) algorithm is a useful tool for managing the unresponsive patient, and is summarised in *Figure 1*. Important differences, when compared to the advanced life support algorithm for adults, are:

> In a child under 2-years-old, the airway is opened by putting the child's head in a neutral position and a chin lift is used. For older children, head tilt and chin lift is used, also known as the "sniffing the morning air position".

> In neonates/smaller children, oropharyngeal airways (if used) are directly placed in the mouth in the position they are intended to sit. This contrasts to older children/adults, where oropharyngeal airways are put in upside down, and then twisted round to the correct position after being advanced. They are sized identically, i.e. from the angle of the mandible to the incisors. Nasopharyngeal airways are used identically as in adults.

> Cardiopulmonary resuscitation (CPR) begins with five ventilation breaths, then compressions to ventilation breaths at a rate of 15:2. This is because children are more likely to have a respiratory rather than cardiac problem.

> Technique for chest compression is different to adults (*Figure 2 and 3*). Compressions are also given at a faster rate, of 100-120 per minute.

> Ventilation breaths are given at a rate of 10-12 per minute, once the airway is secured.

TABLE 3: Airway

Assessment	Cause of compromise	Management
• Talk to the child. • Listen for stridor. • Consider obstruction in the airway, e.g. vomit, foreign body, swelling. • Check air entry in the chest.	• Croup. • Epiglottitis. • Foreign body. • Tumour. • Reduced consciousness.	• Keep the child calm, if the child is conscious and maintaining own airway – do not lay the child down if conscious. • If unconscious, place those <2-years-old in the neutral position, and those >2-years-old in the "sniffing the morning air" position (head tilt and chin lift). • Airway adjuncts such as oropharyngeal or nasopharyngeal airways. • Intubation by skilled person only.

TABLE 4: Breathing

Assessment	Cause of compromise	Management
• Respiratory rate, oxygen saturation. • Look at chest movement, and work of breathing, e.g. accessory muscles, intercostal recession, grunting. • Palpate the trachea. • Percuss the chest wall. • Auscultate the chest.	• Pneumothorax. • Haemothorax. • Consolidation. • Flail chest. • Respiratory splinting due to pain. • Anaphylaxis.	• Oxygen. • Relieve any pneumothorax or haemothorax. • Pain relief, if appropriate. • Ventilation. • Treat anaphylaxis/sepsis.

TABLE 5: Circulation

Assessment	Cause of compromise	Management
• Pulse (rate, rhythm, and volume). • Central capillary refill time. • Blood pressure. • Heart sounds. • Cardiac monitor.	• Sepsis. • Arrhythmia. • Shock. • Congenital cardiac disease. • Hypoxia. • Electrolyte abnormality. • Cardiac tamponade. • Anaphylaxis.	• Chest compressions, if no pulse. • Fluid bolus 20mL/kg (10 mL/kg boluses in trauma, diabetic ketoacidosis (DKA), neonates, raised intracranial pressure, cardiac conditions). • Inotropes. • Treat sepsis. • Electrocardioversion or chemical cardioversion. • Correct electrolytes. • Drain pericardial effusion.

TABLE 6: Disability

Assessment	Cause of compromise	Management
• AVPU score/GCS. • Pupillary responses. • Focal neurological signs. • Blood glucose.	• Seizure. • Space occupying lesion. • Intracranial bleed. • Raised intracranial pressure. • Drug overdose. • Sepsis.	• Intubate if AVPU score is P (GCS <8). • Correct hypoglycaemia. • Treat seizures. • Intubation and ventilation. • Arrange imaging once safe to do so if required.

TABLE 7: Exposure

Assessment	Cause of compromise	Management
• Body temperature. • Full head-to-toe examination.	• Hypothermia. • Covered injuries (e.g. internal bleed/fracture).	• Rewarm slowly if hypothermic. • Prevent hypothermia during resuscitation.

> Drug doses (e.g. adrenaline) are calculated based on weight, as is defibrillation current (up until 8-years-old, where adult defibrillation doses can be used).

For non-shockable rhythms, adrenaline is given as soon as intravenous access is established, and then every 3-5 minutes, at a dose of 10 micrograms/kg or 0.1 mL/kg of a strength of 1:10,000.

Shockable rhythms are rare in children (ventricular fibrillation/pulseless ventricular tachycardia). They require adrenaline and amiodarone (5 mg/kg) to be given after the third shock, not at the start. If the patient remains in a shockable rhythm, adrenaline can then be repeated every 3-5 minutes, and amiodarone can be repeated one further time after the fifth shock.

11

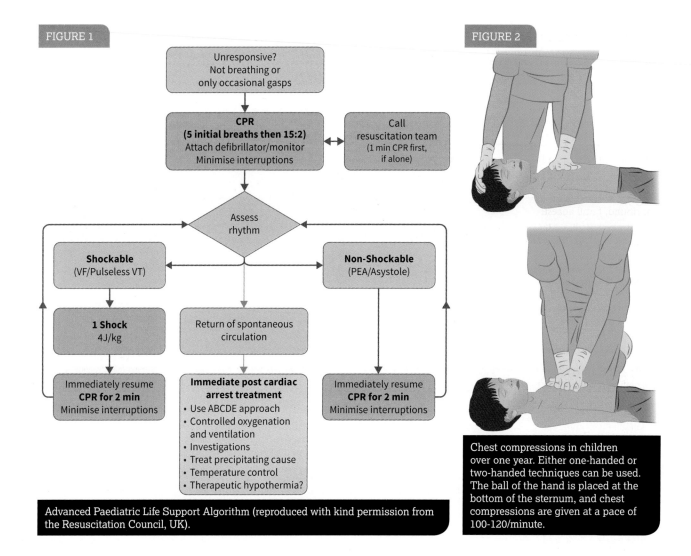

FIGURE 1

Unresponsive?
Not breathing or
only occasional gasps

CPR
(5 initial breaths then 15:2)
Attach defibrillator/monitor
Minimise interruptions

Call
resuscitation team
(1 min CPR first,
if alone)

Assess
rhythm

Shockable
(VF/Pulseless VT)

Non-Shockable
(PEA/Asystole)

1 Shock
4J/kg

Return of spontaneous
circulation

Immediately resume
CPR for 2 min
Minimise interruptions

Immediate post cardiac
arrest treatment
• Use ABCDE approach
• Controlled oxygenation
  and ventilation
• Investigations
• Treat precipitating cause
• Temperature control
• Therapeutic hypothermia?

Immediately resume
CPR for 2 min
Minimise interruptions

Advanced Paediatric Life Support Algorithm (reproduced with kind permission from the Resuscitation Council, UK).

FIGURE 2

Chest compressions in children over one year. Either one-handed or two-handed techniques can be used. The ball of the hand is placed at the bottom of the sternum, and chest compressions are given at a pace of 100-120/minute.

FIGURE 3

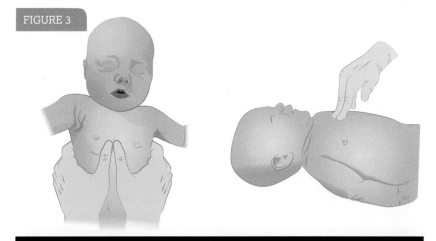

Chest compressions in children under 1-year-old. Either both hands are used, encircling the baby, with both thumbs on the sternum (left), or two fingers are used (right). The latter approach is more helpful if there is no assistant, and ventilation breaths need to be delivered.

As with adults, reversible causes should be considered throughout: hypoxia, hypovolaemia, hyper/hypokalaemia (and other electrolyte disturbances), hypothermia, tension pneumothorax, tamponade, thromboembolism and toxins.

In the event of return of spontaneous circulation, post-cardiac arrest treatment should be initiated. This involves close monitoring and supportive care. The underlying cause of the cardiac arrest needs to be investigated and managed. Evidence is growing for a role for therapeutic hypothermia after cardiac arrest to reduce adverse neurological outcomes.

Other Important Considerations during Resuscitation

Establishing Intravenous Access

Unwell children can be very difficult to cannulate, particularly those between 6 and 18-months-old. Intraosseous (IO) needle insertion is a quick and easy way to get central access for drug delivery and placement only takes seconds (*Figure 4*). Reluctance to insert an IO needle can lead to delays in treatment. As such, IO access should be considered if venous access is difficult, even if the patient is not completely moribund. Local anaesthetic can be used if the patient is conscious, and all medications, fluids and blood can be given via this route, except for infusions. The needle is commonly inserted into the medial aspect of the tibia but can also be inserted into the humerus, femur and pelvis, if needed.

Communication with Nursing Staff and Medical Colleagues

A designated team leader should coordinate the resuscitation team. The team leader should take advice from any necessary specialists, delegate tasks to appropriate team members, and keep an overview of the resuscitation process. It is vital that communication is clear and understanding is checked at each stage. Recap events regularly to ensure nothing has been missed.

Communication with the Child and the Parents

Children who are conscious but very unwell will be understandably frightened. Communication with both the child and the parent is incredibly important. If possible, a member of staff should be dedicated to this. In the event of an unconscious child, a careful decision must be made by the resuscitation team whether the parents should be present during all aspects of the resuscitation.

Factors that may influence this are:

> Research suggests that parents benefit from observing the resuscitation process, especially if the child ultimately dies.
> Team members may be less able to do their jobs when faced with the emotional responses of the parent.
> Parents may unintentionally impede resuscitation.
> There may be insufficient space available in the resuscitation area.

If the parents cannot be present or do not wish to be present during the whole resuscitation, it is important to keep them updated regularly.

Documentation of Events

A team member should be dedicated to documenting the timing of important events during resuscitation. This is vital to ensure an accurate record. All parties should take real-time notes, labelled with the patient information, immediately following resuscitation. If the child dies, an examination of the whole child should be performed immediately and a body map used to document any injuries, cannula sites and iatrogenic marks.

KEY INVESTIGATIONS

Closely monitor respiratory rate, heart rate, blood pressure and temperature throughout resuscitation and recovery. Blood tests can be crucial for further information, but getting these samples can be very difficult from a shocked child. If taking investigations is not possible, it is vital not to delay essential treatment, such as antibiotics. Below are some investigations that form a "first line" of investigations, but this list depends on facilities available at the treating hospital and the specific presenting symptoms.

Blood Glucose

Hypoglycaemia is a clinical emergency and should be corrected immediately. High blood glucose can be a normal response to severe illness or physiological stress. However, in combination with urinary/blood ketones and an acidotic blood gas, it may represent diabetic ketoacidosis.

Blood Gas

Useful information can be gained from arterial, venous or capillary blood gas analysis. They can indicate the severity of the overall condition, as well as direct management of airway and breathing. A child with high blood carbon dioxide will likely need ventilation support. Carbon dioxide levels will be most accurate on an arterial sample and highest on a venous sample, especially if perfusion is poor. Oxygen levels are only reliable when measured from arterial blood. Most blood gas analysers can also give figures for some electrolytes, blood glucose and lactate; these figures can guide initial treatment, pending formal laboratory values.

FIGURE 4

Patella
Tibial tuberosity
Femur
Tibia
90°
Epiphyseal plate

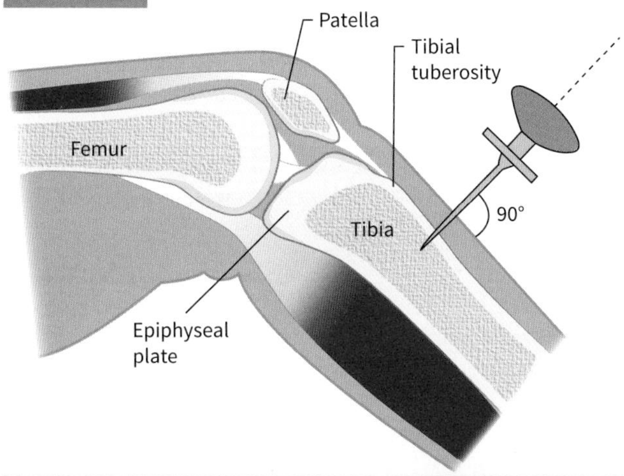

Insertion of an intraosseous needle into the tibial plateau.

Venous Blood Samples

> Blood culture and CRP. This can aid the diagnosis of an infection, and may guide the length of treatment if specific bacteria are isolated. Ideally, it should be taken before antibiotics are started, as bacterial growth in culture will be suppressed once antibiotics are started.

> Full blood count (FBC). Of particular help in the acute setting are white cells (sepsis, leukaemia), haemoglobin (trauma) and platelets (leukaemia, infection, or autoimmune). It should be noted that initial haemoglobin measurements may be normal in a trauma setting despite significant blood loss.

> U&Es. As well as hinting at an underlying condition, correcting some biochemical abnormalities may be essential to early treatment. High serum potassium can be a cause of cardiac arrhythmia. Abnormal sodium, calcium or magnesium can all cause seizures. Marrow from I/O needle insertion can be sent for simple biochemistry only and should be marked as a marrow sample for the lab to analyse appropriately.

> Coagulation. These tests take approximately 20 minutes to obtain results. Although it does not guide immediate resuscitation, abnormal coagulation can guide the use of blood products in prolonged resuscitation and is essential in those with liver failure or known clotting disorders, and in those who have received multiple fluid boluses or massive blood loss.

> Blood cross match. O-negative blood is often available in the emergency situation, with group matched blood available approximately 20 minutes after a sample is received by the laboratory. A full crossmatch with extended antibody screen takes one hour or more. Taking a cross match sample before giving O-negative blood helps the cross matching process and ensures the most appropriate blood product is given.

Additional investigations in special circumstances are shown in *Table 8*.

Radiological Imaging

A chest X-ray is useful in children with an oxygen requirement or in those with abdominal pain but normal abdominal examination. In very small children, diagnosing pneumonia and even pneumothorax can be difficult by examination alone. In trauma, a full trauma series of X-rays should be done to include the pelvis, cervical spine and long bones.

Having definitive imaging of the brain is important if new onset focal neurological signs are present. This is particularly true in trauma where, in cases of intracranial bleeding, the time to neurosurgical correction is the key to outcome. CT scans are commonly used for emergency brain imaging, as CT is far more readily available and quicker than MRI. It is essential to ensure the patient has been resuscitated and the airway secured before attempting any scan outside the resuscitation area.

TABLE 8: Specific investigations in special circumstances

Condition	Investigation
Paracetamol overdose.	• Paracetamol level - Be aware of polypharmacy overdose. Compare against nomogram to guide treatment with N-acetyl cysteine. • Coagulation studies.
Heavy metal poisoning (iron, mercury and lead).	• Blood film. • Heavy metal blood levels. • Abdominal imaging to look for obstruction in acute abdomen presentation. • Brain imaging.
Other poisons.	• ECG. • Urine toxicology. • Blood pressure. • Cardiac monitoring. • Biochemistry. • Coagulation. • Expert advice.

TRAUMA

Trauma is a common cause of death amongst the paediatric population. Prompt assessment and treatment by the trauma team (*Box 2*) remain the primary goals of care. An ABC approach is vital, taking care to stabilise the cervical spine, arrest any major blood loss and look for any immediately life-threatening conditions. Always be aware of the potential for non-accidental injury in any child presenting with an injury.

Trauma assessment should consist of the following components:
> Primary survey (ABCDE) - including C-spine immobilisation.
> Resuscitation.
> Secondary survey.
> › "AMPLE" history - allergy, medications, past medical history, last meal, events/environment.
> › Examination of whole body.
> Definitive care for any identified injury, e.g. fractured femur.

Life-threatening injuries, such as major bleeds, must be prioritised over non-urgent injuries, such as stable fractures and wounds. Blood products should be given early in resuscitation if significant blood loss is suspected.

Box 2: Members of a trauma team

• ED doctor and nurses.
• General surgeon.
• Orthopaedic surgeon.
• Anaesthetist.
• Paediatrician.
• Neurosurgeon/cardiothoracic surgeon if required.

ONGOING CARE

The decision whether a patient can be discharged, requires admission to hospital, or even needs the services of paediatric intensive care is one that requires experience to make safely. A good handover is important to ensure good ongoing care. A clear summary of the case should be given when handing over to another team that will take on responsibility for the patient. The summary should include:

- The diagnosis.
- How the patient presented.
- Results of investigations.
- Investigations with results outstanding.
- What treatment has been given.
- Specialists involved.
- Current plan for ongoing care.
- Discussions had with the patient or their carers.

The Child Requiring Admission

Reasons for admission include:

- Need for specialist medical care.
  - IV medication.
  - Fluids.
  - Operative care.
- Potential for deterioration.
  - High risk patients.
- The diagnosis is uncertain.
  - A fever where there is no focus.
  - Continued observation.
- The safety of the child.
  - Awaiting further social services or police input.
- To facilitate urgent investigations or await results.
  - Blood tests.
  - Urgent imaging.
  - Specialist review.

Paediatric Intensive Care (PICU)

The need for intensive support should be considered as soon as possible, as the nearest PICU may be some distance away from the referring hospital.

PICU provides:

- Airway support. e.g. severe croup, anaphylaxis, unconscious patient.
- Ventilation. e.g. sepsis, neurological conditions.
- Haemofiltration. e.g. cardiac or renal failure.
- Intensive observation. Where rapid deterioration is possible.
- Facilitate transfer to specialist centres. e.g. burns/surgical patients.
- Coordination of the care. For the critically ill child who requires care between multiple specialties.

Sending a Patient Home

After a full assessment and initial treatment, a child may improve enough to be discharged. This should occur if there is a likely diagnosis (even if this is "no illness"), stable observations, and assessment by someone experienced in assessing children. Treatment of conditions unlikely to rapidly deteriorate can be done at home. In all cases, the team sending the child home should ensure that the parents or carers understand the diagnosis and the treatment plan prescribed. Explain that children can sometimes get worse, and if this was to occur they should re-attend, even if this is soon after going home. This advice is referred to as "safety-netting" and is a vital part of the care of children being discharged.

Care in the Community

Increasingly, children with even the most complex illnesses are being managed at home with the close support of community care teams. This involves both chronic illness and acute illness (e.g. the administration of intravenous antibiotics by a community nurse for infection). Good communication between the hospital team, primary care physician and community team is essential, with a clear plan for escalation in place.

Specialist Follow Up

Many conditions require specialist follow up, particularly those of a complex or chronic nature. An example would be a child with wheeze which completely settles with salbutamol. This child can be discharged, but would require ongoing support from an asthma clinic in the primary or secondary care setting. Hospitals also may have setups whereby patients can attend a rapid access clinic for early review (e.g. faltering growth), or rebook into the ED for a follow up the next day (e.g. a jaundiced baby with a bilirubin level close to the phototherapy threshold).

THE DEATH OF AN INFANT OR CHILD

If a child dies, the consultant should be informed, whatever the time of day. The discussion with the parents should be led by the most senior doctor on duty. Death is rightly an emotive subject, but care should be taken not to form any judgments and to remain impartial, even in the face of apparent evidence of wrong doing. It is the job of the clinician to provide excellent medical care, not to assign blame or responsibility. Support from senior nursing staff is vital for this conversation. Remember that parents are individuals and their reactions and expectations will vary accordingly. Key to these discussions is giving time and empathy to the parents. They will likely ask questions with unclear answers, either clinical or procedural. In these cases, never guess or speculate.

All child deaths in the UK must be reported to the child death overview panel, and similar setups exist elsewhere. It is important to notify all medical professionals who are involved in the care of the child. Of note, the patient's primary care physician must be told as soon as possible. This, amongst other things, helps the primary care physician offer support to the parents. Every department has a proforma and post child death procedures to be followed.

Most child deaths will be unexpected and will therefore be referred to the coroner. All lines and tubes placed during resuscitation should be left in situ, unless directed otherwise by the coroner or a consultant. Once death has been declared, further investigation should be discussed with a coroner. Initial investigations vary according to local policy, but may include:

> Routine bloods. FBC, U&Es, bone profile, LFTs, CRP and coagulation are helpful to send as, although difficult to interpret, they may identify an underlying pathology.
> Toxicology. Urine and blood samples should be considered to look for evidence of drug intoxication.
> Microbiology. Stool, urine, CSF and blood cultures may identify a source of infection. Any lesions should be swabbed. A nasopharyngeal aspirate (NPA) should be sent for virology.
> Metabolic screen. Urine and blood samples may help identify a possible inherited metabolic disease. A screen may include blood gas, lactate, ammonia, urine/plasma amino and organic acids, free fatty acids, and glucose.
> Chromosomes. These should be evaluated if the child had any dysmorphic features.

In some cases, all additional investigations are done at post-mortem by the coroner, rather than the attending doctor in ED. It is often advisable to broach the subject of a post mortem examination with the parents as soon as possible, to ensure these examinations are done in a timely fashion, with sensitivity to religious beliefs and legal requirements.

The infant or child should be examined from head to toe, with a body map used to document any marks or bruises. If the death is suspicious or a suspected suicide, further investigations should not be done without the consent of the police or coroner. Post mortem investigations may include further blood samples, urine samples and cerebrospinal fluid samples, as well as biopsies of skin, muscle and liver.

Sudden Unexpected Death in Infancy

Sudden unexpected death in infancy (SUDI) (previously referred to as Sudden Infant Death Syndrome) refers to the sudden death of an infant which remains unexplained after a thorough investigation of the clinical history, a review of the circumstances of death and a complete autopsy.

SUDI can affect children up to their first birthday, but the majority of cases occur between 0 and 6 months. The exact pathophysiology is unknown. The incidence in the UK has dramatically reduced following the "Back-to-Sleep" campaign, started in 1994, now known as "Safe to Sleep". A number of cases of SUDI were analysed and a series of risk factors were identified. As a result, guidance is now given to every new parent regarding how best to promote safe sleep at home in these first few months (*Table 9*). The most recent UK statistics show the rate of SUDI to be 0.35 per 1000 live births.

Debriefing

Lastly, it is important, if possible, to have a post resuscitation debrief for all those involved in the episode. These can be incredibly difficult times for everybody. Recognise that it is a normal response to feel sad at these times and not a sign of weakness. Help and support should be readily available in every hospital for those who feel affected by these traumatic experiences.

TABLE 9: Advice to reduce the incidence of SUDI	
Interventions Shown to Reduce the Risk of SUDI	**Comment**
Always put babies to sleep on their backs, with their feet at the bottom of the bed/cot.	This is for all periods of sleep. Ideally, the baby should be in the same room as the parents.
Use a hard or safety approved surface.	Not a car seat, sofa, pillow or on top of a duvet. Child safety approved mattresses are preferred.
Do not co-sleep with your baby in the same bed or on a chair.	The risk of SUDI is increased if the adult has consumed alcohol/drugs or smokes whilst co-sleeping.
Keep soft objects out of the baby's crib or bed.	Only one blanket should be in the cot with the baby. This should be tucked in and must not cover the face.
Do not smoke.	Parental smoking and smoking around babies has been shown to increase the risk of SUDI.
Do not allow the room to get too hot or cold.	A comfortable temperature for an adult is ideal.
Do not use a pacifier with a string or cord attached.	Pacifiers may reduce the risk of SUDI, but cords attached to some pacifiers may become entangled with the baby and cause serious harm.
Apnoea mattresses and other products are unnecessary and have no safety data to support their use.	Relying on untested equipment has no benefit and may potentially cause harm.
Seek medical attention if the baby becomes unwell.	Parents must feel able to access medical care if their baby is unwell.

REFERENCES AND FURTHER READING

Paediatric Emergencies

1 Wyatt JP, Illingworth RN, Graham CA, Hogg K, Clancy MJ, Robertson CE. Paediatric Emergencies. Oxford, UK: Oxford University Press; 2006.

2 Group ALS. Advanced Paediatric Life Support the Practical Approach. Hoboken: John Wiley & Sons; 2011. Available from: http://kcl.eblib.com/patron/FullRecord.aspx?p=712138.

3 Cameron FJ, Wherrett DK. Care of diabetes in children and adolescents: controversies, changes, and consensus. Lancet. 2015; 385:2096-106.

4 Lacroix J, Demaret P, Tucci M. Red blood cell transfusion: decision making in pediatric intensive care units. Semin Perinatol. 2012; 36:225-31.

5 National Poisons Information Service (NPIS). 2015. Toxbase. Available from: https://www.toxbase.org.

PICU and Child Death

1 Bronner MB, et al. Course and predictors of posttraumatic stress disorder in parents after pediatric intensive care treatment of their child. J Pediatr Psychol. 2010; 35:966-74.

2 Cvetkovic M, et al. Timing of death in children referred for intensive care with severe sepsis: implications for interventional studies. Pediatr Crit Care Med. 2015; 16:410-7.

3 Bateman ST, Dixon R, Trozzi M. The wrap-up: a unique forum to support pediatric residents when faced with the death of a child. J Palliat Med. 2012; 15:1329-34.

4 Robert R, Zhukovsky DS, Mauricio R, Gilmore K, Morrison S, Palos GR. Bereaved parents' perspectives on pediatric palliative care. J Soc Work End Life Palliat Care. 2012; 8:316-38.

5 O'Meara M, Trethewie S. Managing paediatric death in the emergency department. J Paediatr Child Health. 2016; 52:164-7.

SUDI

1 Task Force on Sudden Infant Death S, Moon RY. SIDS and other sleep-related infant deaths: expansion of recommendations for a safe infant sleeping environment. Pediatrics. 2011; 128:1030-9.

2 Saiki T, Hannam S, Rafferty GF, Milner AD, Greenough A. Ventilatory response to added dead space and position in preterm infants at high risk age for SIDS. Pediatr Pulmonol. 2011; 46:239-45.

ASSESSMENT AND MANAGEMENT OF THE ACUTELY UNWELL CHILD

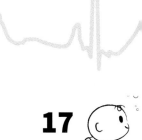

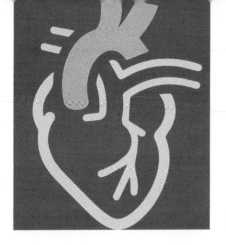

1.03
CARDIOLOGY
HANNAH LINFORD

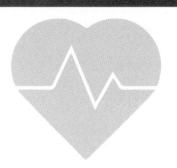

CONTENTS

CARDIAC RHYTHMS

Normal Cardiorespiratory Parameters

In children, the normal range for heart rate, blood pressure and respiratory rate vary significantly with age. *Table 1* summarises these features.

The Paediatric ECG

Interpreting an electrocardiogram (ECG) in children is not the same as with an adult because the heart is physiologically different. Points to note are:

› Normal heart rate is much higher. A heart rate of over 150 bpm is normal in a newborn. Conversely, for a newborn, a heart rate less than 100 needs further assessment.

› Normal marked sinus arrhythmia. This is because the heart rate varies dramatically with breathing.

› Cardiac axis is deviated to the right in the newborn. This is because there is marked right ventricular hypertrophy, as the right ventricle pumps blood against a high-resistance collapsed lung in utero. Often, the right ventricle is captured by placing an additional lead (V4R) in the fifth intercostal space, at the mid clavicular line on the right. V1 (looking directly at the right ventricle) and V2-V3 often have a dominant R wave.

› Possible partial right bundle branch block. This manifests as a normal QRS complex, plus an RSR pattern (M shape) in V1.

› T wave inversion. This is normal in leads V1-3 and potentially V4 as well.

› Q waves. These are normal in the inferior (AVF, II, II) and left precordial leads (V5-6).

The normal ranges for ECG interpretation change with age. *Table 2* and *Table 3* show the QRS complex and corrected QT interval. *Figure 1* shows a normal ECG and *Figure 2* shows the calculation of the QT interval.

TABLE 1: Normal values for heart rate, blood pressure and respiratory rate in children. Source: Advanced Paediatric Life Support, the practical approach. Fifth edition – Advanced Life support group.				
Normal ranges of routine observations in children.				
	<1 year.	2-5 years.	5-12 years.	12-18 years.
Heart rate.	110-160bpm.	95-140bpm.	80-120bpm.	60-100bpm.
Systolic blood pressure (50th centile).	80-90mmHg.	85-100mmHg.	90-110mmHg.	90-120mmHg.
Respiratory rate.	30-40 breaths/min.	25-30 breaths/min.	20-25 breaths/min.	15-20 breaths/min.

TABLE 2: QRS ranges in children	
Age	Cardiac Axis
1 week – 1 month.	+ 110° (range +30° to +180°).
1 month – 3 months.	+ 70° (range +10° to +125°).
3 months – 3 years.	+ 60° (range +10° to +110°).
Over 3 years.	+ 60° (range +20° to +120°).
Adult.	+ 50° (range -30° to 105°).

TABLE 3: Corrected QT interval	
Age	QT Interval
< 6 months.	<0.49 seconds.
>6 months.	<0.44 seconds.

FIGURE 1

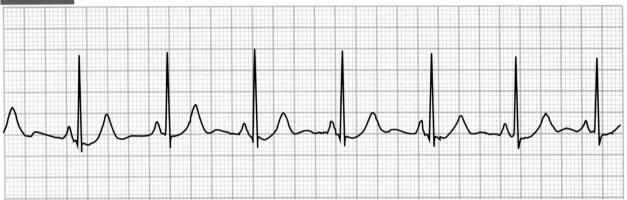

Normal sinus rhythm.

FIGURE 2

R-R interval

QT interval

Location of the QT interval, from beginning of Q to end of T in the same cycle. Note that this needs to be compared to the preceding RR interval to get the corrected QT interval (QT/ √RR).

Tachycardia

Tachycardia may result from physiological processes that alter the sympathetic/ parasympathetic tone, resulting in a sinus tachycardia. Such causes include:

› Excessive activity.
› Crying/being upset.
› Stress.

It may also be caused by a secondary problem outside the heart, like fever, infection, hyperthyroidism, anaemia or any other problem causing a high metabolic rate. It is rarely due to a primary cardiac cause. A primary cause is more likely if tachycardia is particularly high or an isolated finding.

Bradycardia

Bradycardia is commonly encountered in paediatrics and is usually physiological, occurring particularly in athletes and during sleep. Other causes include:

› Drugs. e.g. beta blockers.
› Cushing reflex. The combination of bradycardia, hypertension, reduced consciousness and irregular respiration is a sign of raised intracranial pressure.
› Shock/sepsis.
› Heart block.

Supraventricular Tachycardia

Supraventricular tachycardia (SVT) is a narrow complex tachycardia originating at or above the atrioventricular node. It is the most common tachyarrhythmia encountered by paediatricians and can be difficult to differentiate from a simple sinus tachycardia.

Aetiology

A re-entry mechanism is the most common cause of an SVT, and this can occur anywhere along the atrioventricular junction. This mechanism results in rapid acceleration of the heart rate, as it does not rely on a new impulse to be generated by the sino-atrial node. Children who develop re-entry tachycardia will generally have an anatomical abnormality or variant, such as an accessory conduction pathway or abnormal division of an existing conduction pathway. An example of this is the Bundle of Kent in Wolff-Parkinson-White syndrome.

Clinical Features

Presentation of an SVT varies with the age of the child and the severity of the condition. It usually presents with palpitations, although some patients may present in heart failure, as moribund or in cardiorespiratory arrest. This is summarised in *Table 4*.

Investigations

If the child is stable, elicit a history from them or their caregiver. The history will often indicate a certain diagnosis and can guide and focus further investigations.

› ECG. This is the primary diagnostic test. The ECG will show narrow complex tachycardia. The rate will generally be above 220 bpm for an infant and above 180 bpm for an older child. There will be no discernible P-waves and there will be no rate variability (*Figure 3*).
› Chest X-ray. This investigation can serve as a useful indicator of heart failure as it may show plethoric lungs. It can also help to exclude pulmonary causes of shortness of breath (e.g. consolidation, pneumothorax, pleural effusion).
› Blood gas. This is a good investigation to do for an unwell child, as it can indicate how systemically compromised they are with lactate levels, carbon dioxide and base excess. Electrolyte levels, including potassium and calcium, are often available from the blood gas machine.
› Blood glucose. It is very important to check this value in any unwell child, as hyper- or hypoglycaemia can cause or worsen many presentations.

TABLE 4: Presentation of SVTs		
	Infant	**Child**
Palpitations.	• HR >220 bpm. • Irritable. • Inconsolable crying/ quiet. • Pallor.	• HR >180 bpm. • Irritable. • Complaining of chest pain/fluttering heart. • Dizziness. • Nausea.
Heart failure.	• Shortness of breath (especially when feeding). • Initially poor weight gain. • Oedema/weight gain. • Enlarged liver.	• Shortness of breath. • Initially poor weight gain. • Oedema/weight gain. • Enlarged liver. • Diffuse crepitations across the chest.

FIGURE 3

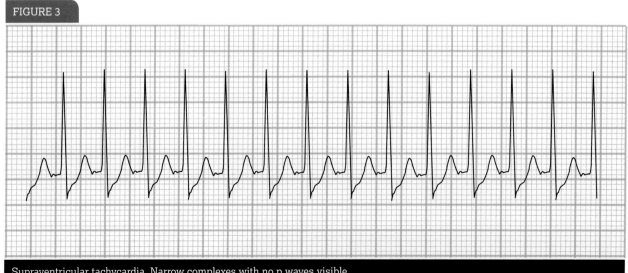

Supraventricular tachycardia. Narrow complexes with no p waves visible.

▸ Haematology and biochemistry tests. These are useful in determining the underlying health of the patient and the effect their condition is having on the rest of their body. Anaemia, infection or dehydration may exacerbate a tachycardia. Imbalances of electrolytes (e.g. potassium, magnesium, calcium) or thyroid dysfunction may also trigger an arrhythmia. Magnesium levels have to be specifically requested as they are not part of a normal electrolyte work up.

▸ Echocardiogram. This is used to identify any underlying structural cardiac abnormalities.

Differential Diagnoses

Sinus tachycardia is the main differential diagnosis. The key features that distinguish SVT from sinus tachycardia are:

▸ Sudden onset.

▸ No rate variation.

▸ Very fast rate (>220 bpm in an infant and >180 bpm in a child).

▸ Not responsive to a fluid bolus.

▸ No P waves visualised on the ECG reading.

Management

Stable Child

If the patient is relatively well, vagal manoeuvres can initially be attempted. These vary depending on the age of the patient. The child must be attached to a heart monitor/ECG so that cardioversion can be captured and sent to the local tertiary unit. In infants, ice immersion can be attempted. This involves wrapping the infant and immersing its face into a basin of ice for approximately 10 seconds. This stimulates the diving reflex and can trigger the heart rate to return to normal. A variation of this is placing a bag containing crushed ice onto an infant's face for 15–30 seconds.

In children, a Valsalva manoeuvre can be attempted. One way of getting children to successfully comply with this is by asking them to blow into an empty 10 mL syringe.

Unstable Child

In patients that are more acutely compromised or in those in whom initial vagal manoeuvres don't work, adenosine may be given or DC cardioversion may be needed.

Complications

In the acute setting, SVT can lead to cardiovascular compromise, insufficient cardiac output, shock and ultimately death. Treatment also has complications. Vagal manoeuvres and adenosine can lead to asystole and should be done under careful monitoring, with full resuscitation facilities available.

Following resolution of SVT, further ECG abnormalities may be detected. An example of this would be Wolff-Parkinson-White syndrome (*Figure 4*). This is characterised by a slurred R wave, known as a delta wave, across all leads. The delta wave is caused by an accessory conduction system which bypasses the AV node, thereby shortening the PR interval and making the patient prone to episodes of re-entry tachycardia.

Prognosis

In general, patients that have a single episode of SVT have a good prognosis, particularly with an uncomplicated presentation.

SVT episodes may be recurrent. In the long-term, particularly if a patient has frequent episodes, prophylactic measures should be considered under the advice of a paediatric cardiologist. This would initially involve advice with regard to vagal manoeuvres and when to summon help. The patient may also be commenced on anti-arrhythmic medication. Those on longer term medications may suffer side effects, although SVTs can generally be well controlled, and medications are stopped after having an ablation. Patients may undergo radiofrequency ablation of their accessory pathway when they are teenagers, which renders that pathway nonfunctional.

FIGURE 4

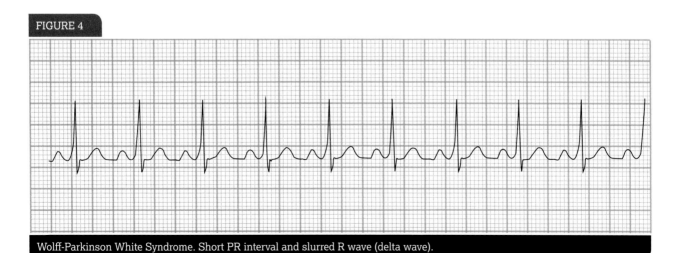

Wolff-Parkinson White Syndrome. Short PR interval and slurred R wave (delta wave).

Ventricular Tachycardia

Aetiology

Ventricular tachycardia (VT) is a broad complex tachycardia. The complexes are wide because the electrical activity originates within the ventricles themselves, resulting in a slower conduction than via the specialist conducting fibres within the heart (bundle of His and Purkinje fibres).

Clinical Features

Although it may be possible to have short runs of VT and be asymptomatic, VT usually presents in a very compromised, tachycardic, hypotensive patient who may go on to have a cardiac arrest.

Investigations

It is important to review these patients frequently and to look for reversible causes of arrhythmia in their histories, examinations and biochemical evaluations. Investigations are similar to that for SVT. *Figure 5* shows the ECG appearance of ventricular tachycardia.

Management

Any patient without a pulse requires cardiopulmonary resuscitation (CPR), cardiac defibrillation and possibly adrenaline/amiodarone administration. Patients with a pulse are divided into those in shock and those who are not.

> For patients not in shock, treatment with amiodarone is recommended.

> For those in shock, synchronized DC cardioversion is preferred.

The senior clinician must always make the treatment decisions and, if possible, following discussion with a tertiary cardiac specialist.

Complications

VT is associated with sudden death, and any suggestion of VT on ECG needs prompt evaluation by a senior clinician as the risks of cardiac arrest and further deterioration to ventricular fibrillation are high.

Prognosis

This is highly dependent on the aetiology and clinical situation. Short runs of asymptomatic VT could go unnoticed over an entire lifetime, whereas VT could also be first noted at a cardiac arrest.

Heart Block

As with adults, children can get first degree (slowed conduction of atrial impulses to ventricles, causing prolonged PR interval), second degree (some atrial impulses are conducted to the ventricles, causing "dropped beats") or third degree heart block (complete dissociation between atrial and ventricular activity (*Figure 6*)).

FIGURE 5

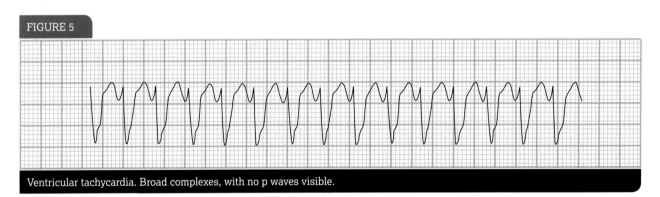

Ventricular tachycardia. Broad complexes, with no p waves visible.

FIGURE 6

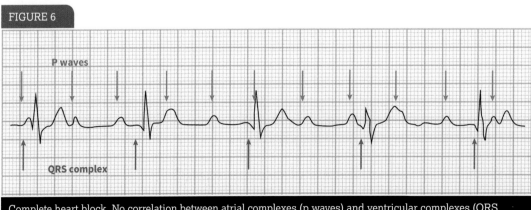

Complete heart block. No correlation between atrial complexes (p waves) and ventricular complexes (QRS complexes)

Treatment involves identifying and correcting any possible causes (e.g. Lyme disease), and focusing on maintaining a heart rate tolerated by the patient. Acutely, the most compromised patients might require isoprenaline (a β agonist that increases heart rate) or temporary pacing wires. The most severe cases may require a permanent pacemaker, but most patients require no active intervention.

Congenital Heart Block

Congenital heart block is most often encountered in a baby whose mother suffers from connective tissue disorders with anti-Ro or anti-La antibodies (e.g. systemic lupus erythematosus; SLE). These antibodies are thought to attack the conduction system within the developing heart and cause atrophy of the AV node. This faulty node causes heart block, or sometimes intrauterine death or a hydropic foetus. Whenever a maternal history of connective tissue disorder is encountered or when anti-Ro or anti-La antibodies are found, an ECG must be performed on the baby after birth.

Long QT Syndrome

Long QT syndrome is a syndrome in which the QT interval measured on ECG is prolonged. The corrected QT interval or QTc (from the beginning of the Q wave to the end of the T wave) should last less than 440 ms (or 490 ms if <6 months old). A long QT can also precipitate more dangerous rhythms. One such rhythm is Torsades de Pointes (literally "twisted points"). This rhythm causes a degree of cardiovascular compromise and can quickly progress to ventricular tachycardia.

Aetiology

Causes of Long QT syndrome include:
- Congenital. Mutation in the LQTS 1 gene.
- Acquired. Secondary to electrolyte imbalance.
- Iatrogenic. Due to medication, including anti-psychotic agents.

In congenital long QT syndrome, a malfunctioning ion channel within myocardial cells is thought to give rise to the prolongation. During periods of exercise or stress (increased sympathetic tone), this fault within the cell can trigger arrhythmias and sudden death.

Clinical Features

Often, these children are asymptomatic but are investigated because of the diagnosis of a close family member with long QT syndrome. If symptomatic, these children can present following a faint or collapse, which is often misdiagnosed as simple vasovagal syncope or a seizure. Long QT syndrome should be excluded when assessing a child who presents with a collapse, especially if the collapse happened during an episode of exertion.

Management
Initial Management
This involves:
- Correcting underlying electrolyte abnormalities.
- Addressing any acute rhythm disturbance.

Long-term Management
Long-term management depends on the underlying risk of sudden cardiac death. This is determined by factors such as family history of sudden cardiac death, the length of the QT interval, and prior cardiac events. Treatment options include medication to reduce the QT interval (e.g. β Blockers), and, in very high risk patients, implantable cardioverter defibrillator (ICD) placement.

Prognosis

Risk of fatal arrhythmia is low once appropriate therapy is instigated. Even when Torsades de Pointes happens, it is usually self-limiting. Patients that have serious cardiac events despite optimal medical therapy usually have an ICD, which markedly improves prognosis.

CONGENITAL HEART DISEASE

Congenital heart disease is increasingly diagnosed antenatally, particularly with the advent of obstetric ultrasound and foetal MRI. In some centres, oxygen saturations are routinely checked in newborn babies, increasing the early identification of cyanotic congenital heart disease even further.

Causes of congenital heart disease include:
- Chromosomal heart disease. e.g. Down syndrome (AVSD, ASD, VSD), Turner syndrome (coarctation of the aorta, aortic stenosis), Williams syndrome (aortic stenosis, peripheral pulmonary stenosis), Noonan syndrome (pulmonary stenosis).
- Intrauterine infection. e.g. rubella.
- Maternal disease. e.g. diabetes (all congenital heart defects [CHDs]), SLE (congenital heart block).
- Drugs in pregnancy. e.g. alcohol, anticonvulsants.

Presentation is usually as cyanosis, shock, or heart failure. Investigations involve ECG, chest X-ray, echocardiogram and cardiac catheterisation. Complications of heart disease vary depending on the underlying aetiology. Very broadly, patients can develop heart failure (left, right or congestive) and cardiac arrhythmias. Management is led by tertiary cardiac specialists.

Heart disease may also present later in life due to an underlying multisystem disorder. For example, both Marfan syndrome and Ehlers-Danlos syndrome increase the risk of aortic dissection.

Tetralogy of Fallot (TOF)
This is the most common cyanotic congenital heart disease.

TABLE 5: The features of Tetralogy of Fallot (TOF)	
Infundibular Pulmonary Stenosis.	This causes a "right outflow tract obstruction" making it difficult for the right ventricle to pump enough blood to the lungs for oxygenation. This, in turn, leads to right ventricular hypertrophy.
Right Ventricular Hypertrophy.	This is secondary to the right ventricle being exerted to pump adequate amounts of blood into the pulmonary circulation.
Ventricular Septal Defect.	This defect allows deoxygenated blood to flow from the right ventricle (which is operating at a higher than normal pressure due to the outflow tract obstruction) into the left.
Overriding Aorta.	This abnormality of the insertion of the aorta simply means that its opening lies directly over the ventricular septal defect, so both the left and right ventricles pump blood into it.

FIGURE 7

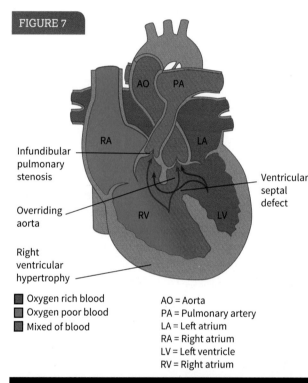

Infundibular pulmonary stenosis

Overriding aorta

Right ventricular hypertrophy

Ventricular septal defect

■ Oxygen rich blood
■ Oxygen poor blood
■ Mixed of blood

AO = Aorta
PA = Pulmonary artery
LA = Left atrium
RA = Right atrium
LV = Left ventricle
RV = Right atrium

Tetralogy of Fallot (TOF).

Aetiology

Four abnormalities make up the condition of TOF (tetra= four). *Table 5* and *Figure 7* summarise the features.

Investigations

Electrocardiogram (ECG) shows right axis deviation and right ventricular hypertrophy (dominant R wave in V1-4R). Chest X-ray (CXR) shows a boot-shaped heart from right ventricular hypertrophy and oligemic lung fields due to pulmonary stenosis. Definitive diagnosis is made based on echocardiogram.

Clinical Features

Antenatal Detection

TOF is often picked up during routine antenatal scanning. This allows better preparation at birth and, if possible, delivery at a specialist cardiac unit.

Postnatal Detection

For patients that present postnatally, particularly those without antenatal care, presentation is dependent upon the degree of outflow tract obstruction (i.e. the severity of pulmonary stenosis).

› If the pulmonary stenosis is critical, the baby will present soon after birth with cardiovascular compromise and cyanosis.

› If outflow tract obstruction is moderate, TOF will likely be detected during secondary evaluation of a heart murmur picked up on the routine baby check. The murmur heard in TOF is due to the pulmonary stenosis rather than the VSD (systolic murmur heard best over the left upper sternal edge).

› In cases with moderate pulmonary stenosis, the child may also present with hypercyanotic spells. These spells are moments of acute right ventricular outflow tract obstruction brought on by agitation or exertion, during which the child will appear cyanotic and compromised.

› In cases with only mild obstruction, presentation may coincide with heart failure.

Management

Emergency Management

Acutely Unwell Neonate

An acutely unwell neonate may be commenced on a prostaglandin infusion. This keeps the ductus arteriosus patent, allowing blood to shunt from the aorta to the pulmonary artery, bypassing the pulmonary stenosis. This should be followed by referral to a tertiary cardiology unit for urgent cardiac surgery.

Hypercyanotic Spells

In an older child with a hypercyanotic spell, treatment initially starts by positioning the child in the "knees–to-chest" position. This increases systemic vascular resistance, thereby reducing blood flow from right to left through the VSD, and therefore increasing blood flow through the pulmonary artery. High flow oxygen and morphine should also be administered to act as a pulmonary vasodilator and systemic vasoconstrictor. If these conservative measures fail, consider IV treatment with morphine or beta blockers.

Surgical Repair

All children with TOF require surgical repair to close the VSD and widen the right ventricular outflow tract. Previously, babies with TOF would have a palliative surgical procedure before definitive surgical repair that involved placing a shunt (Blalock-Taussig shunt) between the subclavian artery and the pulmonary artery. This works in a similar fashion to a patent ductus arteriosus (PDA), allowing blood to shunt from the systemic circulation to the pulmonary artery. Complications include thrombosis and infection. Although complete surgical repair in the first year of life is now standard practice, babies that are too small or compromised may have a temporary shunt placed first.

Future surgery may be required if the patient develops pulmonary regurgitation: this is a complication of widening the ventricular outflow tract.

Prognosis

Children with simple forms of the disease who undergo early surgery have excellent long-term outcomes, although a small risk of life threatening ventricular arrhythmias remains.

Without surgery, mortality steadily increases with age. Tetralogy of Fallot associated with pulmonary atresia has the worst prognosis.

Other Cyanotic Congenital Heart Disease

Table 6 summarises the key features of other important cyanotic heart diseases.

Acyanotic Congenital Heart Disease

Table 7 (left-to-right shunts) and *Table 8* (outflow obstructions) summarise the key features of acyanotic diseases. VSDs are the commonest type of congenital heart disease, and PDAs are the second most common.

Einsenmenger Syndrome

Einsenmenger syndrome is an important complication of a left–to-right shunt. It occurs due to a large left-to-right shunt (e.g. from a large ventricular septal defect), either in isolation or as part of a wider complex cardiac disease. This leads to right ventricular hypertrophy, and therefore increased pressure in the pulmonary vessels, causing pulmonary hypertension.

TABLE 6: Key cyanotic heart diseases			
Disease	**Definition**	**Presentation**	**Management**
Transposition of the great arteries (TGA) (*Figure 8*).	The aorta attaches to the right ventricle and the pulmonary artery connects to the left ventricle. This results in two separate, unconnected circuits where oxygenated blood is pumped between the left atrium, ventricle and lungs, and deoxygenated blood is pumped through the right atrium, right ventricle and around the body.	• This is the most common cyanotic heart disease to present in the neonatal period. • It is incompatible with life unless further defects permit shunting of blood across the heart to allow oxygenated blood into the systemic circulation. • It presents neonatally with cyanosis and circulatory compromise. • The ECG is normal. • Chest X-ray shows cardiac outline of "egg on side" and increased pulmonary vascular markings.	• A prostaglandin infusion is started initially to maintain duct patency. • Urgent transfer to a specialist cardiac unit is needed. • Initially a balloon atrial septostomy is life-saving (creating an ASD to allow mixing). • Corrective surgery involves switching the aorta and the main pulmonary artery (the arterial switch procedure).
Truncus Arteriosus.	Only one great vessel arises from both ventricles. The aorta and the pulmonary artery both originate from this structure. It is always accompanied by a VSD.	• Initial mild to moderate cyanosis may be the only finding. • Later signs of pulmonary congestion and heart failure occur over the next few days/weeks.	• Urgent transfer to a specialist cardiac unit is needed. • Surgical repair comprises closure of the VSD, separation of the pulmonary artery from the single truncal vessel and the formation of a conduit between the pulmonary artery and the right ventricle.
Total Anomalous Pulmonary Venous Drainage (TAPVD).	The four pulmonary veins drain into the right atrium (or into the brachiocephalic veins or superior vena cava) instead of the left atrium. This means that oxygenated blood is pumped back into the lungs rather than into the systemic circulation and that the child has two separate non-communicating circulation systems. The only chance of survival for these children is mixing of the blood via a VSD, ASD or PDA.	• This presents antenatally with cyanosis and circulatory compromise. • The ECG is normal in the neonate. • Chest X-ray shows a cardiac outline of "snowman in a snowstorm" or "cottage loaf" from congested atria and pulmonary veins, giving rise to pulmonary oedema.	• A prostaglandin infusion is initially started to maintain duct patency. • Urgent transfer to a specialist cardiac unit is needed. • Surgical correction involves reconnecting the four pulmonary veins to the left atrium and closing any associated defects.

(Continued)

TABLE 6: *Continued*

Disease	Definition	Presentation	Management
Hypoplastic left heart syndrome.	A group of defects affecting the left side of the heart (valves and chambers) in which the structures are too small to support systemic output.	• This is usually antenatally diagnosed – with an aim for delivery at a cardiac centre. • It presents as a breathless, severely cyanotic and compromised neonate soon after birth. • ECG shows absent ventricular forces.	• A prostaglandin infusion is initially started to maintain duct patency. • Urgent transfer to a specialist cardiac unit is needed. • There is a three stage surgical treatment (e.g. Norwood, Glenn, then Fontan). The ultimate aim is for the right ventricle to remain the systemic ventricle, with blood passively flowing to the lungs. Heart transplant is another option.
Tricuspid atresia.	The tricuspid valve (between the right atrium and right ventricle) is blocked or absent. Therefore, deoxygenated blood cannot flow into the pulmonary circulation from the right ventricle. This defect is incompatible with life unless it is accompanied by both a VSD and an ASD or a PDA.	• Cyanosis is present soon after birth. • A systolic murmur is heard at the left lower sternal edge if a VSD is present or a continuous murmur below the left clavicle if a PDA is present.	• Surgical correction occurs by a course of several staged procedures. Initial palliation may involve inserting a systemic-pulmonary shunt (e.g. Blalock-Taussig shunt). • Systemic venous return is connected to the pulmonary artery, bypassing the right ventricle (Fontan circulation).
Complete atrioventricular septal defect (AVSD).	A large ASD which is continuous with a large VSD; all four chambers of the heart are communicating with one another. This causes increased blood flow to the lungs as well as less effective drainage, thereby promoting pulmonary hypertension and heart failure. Note that smaller AVSDs may be acyanotic.	• Heart failure and cyanosis. • This is the abnormality most often associated with Down syndrome. • Ejection systolic murmur at left upper sternal edge (pulmonary flow murmur). • Pansystolic murmur at the apex (mitral regurgitation). • Fixed splitting S2 (ASD). • Loud S2 (pulmonary hypertension).	• The heart failure is medically managed. • The VSD and ASD are surgically closed and the atrioventricular valve is surgically repaired (to fashion separate mitral and tricuspid valves).

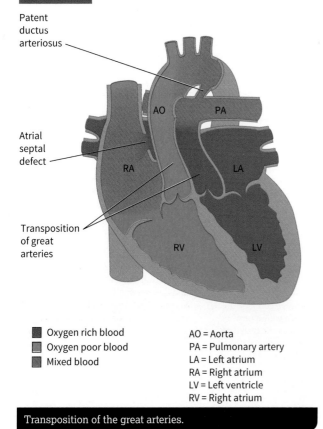

Patent ductus arteriosus

Atrial septal defect

Transposition of great arteries

AO
PA
RA
LA
RV
LV

■ Oxygen rich blood
■ Oxygen poor blood
■ Mixed blood

AO = Aorta
PA = Pulmonary artery
LA = Left atrium
RA = Right atrium
LV = Left ventricle
RV = Right atrium

Transposition of the great arteries.

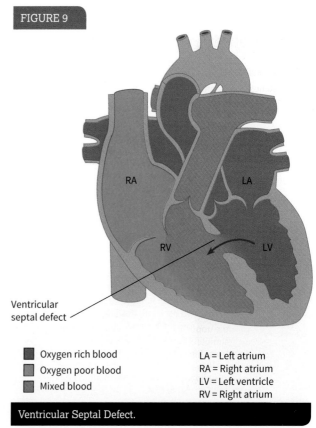

RA
LA
RV
LV

Ventricular septal defect

■ Oxygen rich blood
■ Oxygen poor blood
■ Mixed blood

LA = Left atrium
RA = Right atrium
LV = Left ventricle
RV = Right atrium

Ventricular Septal Defect.

TABLE 7: Left to right shunting heart defects

Defect	Definition	Presentation	Examination	Management	Associations
Ventricular septal defect (VSD) (*Figure 9*).	A communication between the ventricles causing a left to right shunt of blood across the defect.	• Small – Well child with incidental finding of murmur. • Large – Heart failure.	• A systolic murmur is heard at the lower left sternal edge. It is louder with a smaller defect, as there is greater turbulent blood flow. • Pulmonary plethora on CXR indicates significant shunting.	• Small VSDs will close spontaneously. • Medical management consists of diuretics, captopril and extra calories. • Surgical correction of large VSDs should be performed by 12 months of age to prevent the development of pulmonary hypertension. The defect is closed with a synthetic patch.	• Mostly idiopathic. • Foetal alcohol syndrome. • Trisomy 21.
Atrial septal defect (ASD) (*Figure 10*).	A communication between the atria causing left to right shunting of blood across the defect. It may be ostium primum (inferior portion of atrial septum) or secundum (usually arises from an enlarged foramen ovale).	• Small – Well child. • Large – Heart failure. • Ostium primum may be associated with mitral regurgitation.	• A soft systolic murmur in the upper left sternal edge is heard, with fixed splitting of S2. • Pansystolic murmur may be heard if there is associated mitral regurgitation.	• If significant, correction is usually performed at 3-5 years of age. • Closure may be surgical or non-surgical by placing a device during cardiac catheterisation, although this is not possible if there is associated mitral regurgitation.	• Trisomy 21. • Foetal alcohol syndrome.
Patent ductus arteriosus (PDA) (*Figure 11*).	A failure of the ductus arteriosus to close following birth.	• Usually a well child, but may also present with left heart failure or recurrent infection.	• A continuous machinery murmur is heard midway below the left clavicle, and/or an early systolic murmur in the left sternal upper edge. Bounding pulses may also be felt.	• Diuretics and fluid restriction in neonates. • Surgical ligation or percutaneous coil closure.	• Prematurity.

TABLE 8: Outflow obstructions

Defect	Description	Presentation	Examination	Management	Associations
Aortic stenosis (AS).	Commonly a malformation of the aortic valve itself, with two leaflets (bicuspid) forming rather than three. It may also be secondary to rheumatic fever.	• If mild-moderate, it is asymptomatic. • 10% will develop heart failure within the first year. • Older children may report chest pain or syncope. • Patients with congenital valvular AS are at risk of sudden death and endocarditis.	• A harsh ejection systolic murmur over the right upper sternal edge may be heard. • Slow rising pulse. • Narrowed pulse pressure. • Soft S2 heart sound.	• Balloon valvuloplasty/valvotomy or open surgical replacement. • If presenting with neonatal cyanosis, prostaglandin therapy may be commenced.	• Turner syndrome. • Williams syndrome.
Coarctation of the aorta.	A narrowing of the descending aorta. It is characterised by weak femoral pulses and relative hypertension in the upper limbs compared to the lower limbs. It is associated with Turner syndrome.	• Neonates may initially be asymptomatic if the coarctation is accompanied by a PDA. • Severe coarctations present with early cardiovascular collapse. • Duct-dependent lesions present after a few days of life when the duct begins to close.	• There is usually no murmur – but it is often accompanied by a PDA (continuous machinery murmur left upper sternal edge).	• Balloon angioplasty or open surgical repair. • If presenting with neonatal cyanosis, prostaglandin therapy may be commenced.	• Turner syndrome.

(Continued)

TABLE 8: *Continued*

Defect	Description	Presentation	Examination	Management	Associations
Pulmonary stenosis (PS).	Narrowing of pulmonary valve outflow tract.	• Severe PS presents soon after delivery, sometimes with cyanosis secondary to a large right-to-left shunt via a patent foramen ovale. • Mild or moderate PS is asymptomatic but often detected during a routine neonatal exam.	• An ejection systolic murmur is heard at the left upper sternal edge, radiating into the back. An ejection click may also be heard.	• Treatment includes balloon valvuloplasty/ valvotomy or open surgical replacement. • If presenting with neonatal cyanosis, prostaglandin therapy may be commenced.	• Noonan syndrome. • Williams syndrome. • Alagille syndrome.

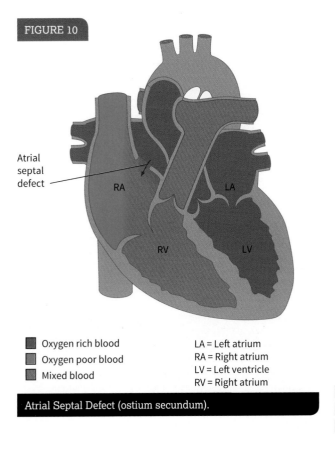

FIGURE 10

- Oxygen rich blood
- Oxygen poor blood
- Mixed blood

LA = Left atrium
RA = Right atrium
LV = Left ventricle
RV = Right atrium

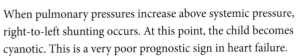

Atrial Septal Defect (ostium secundum).

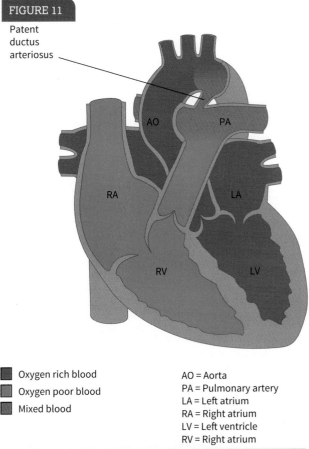

FIGURE 11

Patent ductus arteriosus

- Oxygen rich blood
- Oxygen poor blood
- Mixed blood

AO = Aorta
PA = Pulmonary artery
LA = Left atrium
RA = Right atrium
LV = Left ventricle
RV = Right atrium

Patent Ductus Arteriosus.

When pulmonary pressures increase above systemic pressure, right-to-left shunting occurs. At this point, the child becomes cyanotic. This is a very poor prognostic sign in heart failure.

HEART MURMURS

Innocent Murmurs

The first question to ask when a patient presents with a murmur is whether it is an innocent murmur or one which requires further evaluation. *Table 9* summarises the key characteristics of an innocent murmur.

Examples of innocent murmurs include the following. They all originate from hyperdynamic states.

- ▸ **Venous hum.** Continuous murmur below the right clavicle. Decreases when the patient is in a supine position.

- ▸ **Still's murmur.** Early soft systolic murmur heard over the lower left sternal edge. Louder when the patient is in a supine position.
- ▸ **Pulmonary flow murmur.** Ejection systolic murmur, heard at the upper left sternal edge in toddlers and adolescents. Does not radiate to the back.

Pathological Murmurs

Pathological murmurs are worrying and they should always be investigated. Factors increasing clinical suspicion include:

TABLE 9: Characteristics of innocent murmurs	
The Seven S's of an innocent murmur	
Systolic.	Diastolic murmurs are always pathological.
Soft.	It is never above grade II intensity.
Small.	It does not radiate to a large area.
Short.	The murmur is short in duration.
Single.	Never accompanied by additional noises (S3, clicks, etc.).
Sweet.	Never harsh sounding.
Sensitive.	The sound varies with respiration and movement.

> A child with symptoms.
> Cyanosis.
> Grade III or higher on Levine scale.
> Associated thrill.
> Diastolic murmur.
> Abnormal heart sounds.
> Abnormally strong or weak pulse.

Table 10 gives some examples of pathological murmurs and the associated potential diagnoses.

Grading Murmurs

Murmurs can be graded on a Levine scale as shown in *Table 11*. If the murmur is grade IV-VI, it is more likely to be a pathological murmur.

HEART FAILURE

Heart failure, in simple terms, is the inability of the heart to supply oxygenated blood to vital organs.

Aetiology

Many different conditions can lead to heart failure, as summarised in *Table 12*.

Clinical Features

Presentation of heart failure can be non-specific and is age-dependent.

Infants

Infants may present with poor feeding and poor growth. Parents may report that the infant takes a longer time to complete feeds but seems hungry. This is due to both respiratory difficulties being exacerbated by activity and the increased calorie requirement of the body secondary to the heart failure itself. Parents may also report increased sweatiness of the baby when feeding or that the baby looks "puffy". As heart failure progresses, the baby will experience increasing respiratory difficulties and sudden/

TABLE 10: Pathological murmurs		
Timing	Location	Pathology
Ejection Systolic.	Right side/aortic region, accentuated if the patient exhales/sits up.	Aortic stenosis (radiates to carotids).
	Left side/pulmonary area.	Pulmonary stenosis (S2 soft).
	Between the scapulas.	Coarctation of the aorta (also assess for radio-femoral delay).
Pansystolic.	Left lower sternal edge.	VSD.
	Radiating to the axilla, accentuated if patient rolls onto the left side.	Mitral regurgitation.
Early Diastolic.	Lower left sternal edge/ upper right sternal edge, accentuated if the patient exhales/sits up.	Aortic regurgitation.
Mid Diastolic.	Apex, accentuated if patient rolls onto the left side.	Mitral stenosis.
Continuous.	Below left clavicle.	PDA "Bounding pulse".
	Across chest.	Over shunt.

TABLE 11: Grading of murmurs		
Grade	Thrill	Auscultation
I.	No.	Only faintly audible with a stethoscope.
II.	No.	Faint, but easily audible on auscultation.
III.	No.	Moderately loud and easily heard on auscultation.
IV.	Yes.	Loud, but not audible without a stethoscope.
V.	Yes.	Very loud, but not audible without a stethoscope.
VI.	Yes.	Extremely loud and audible without a stethoscope.

significant weight gain (fluid retention), oedema and hepatomegaly.

Older Children

Older children may also have difficulty with weight gain. They will often report tiredness and can show more shortness of breath than their peers during usual activities. They may also describe chest pain or palpitations and can be prone to recurrent chest infections. *Table 13* summarises the clinical features. The severity of symptoms in heart failure can be thought of in terms of the modified Ross criteria, listed in *Table 14*.

TABLE 12: Causes of heart failure

	Left Ventricular Pump Failure	Volume Overload	Pressure Overload
Structurally normal heart.	• Cardiomyopathies. Diseases of the heart muscle itself are the most common cause of left ventricular pump failure in structurally normal hearts. • Myocarditis. Infection (usually viral) of the myocardium can resolve and bring normal heart function, or it can lead to secondary dilated cardiomyopathy. • Myocardial infarction. This is rare in the paediatric population and is due to malformed coronary arteries, rather than atherosclerosis and degenerative change. • Arrhythmias. These can cause inadequate cardiac output due to disjointed and uncoordinated ventricular contraction.	• Renal failure. This can cause fluid overload, overwhelming the cardiac pump.	• Systemic Hypertension. This increases afterload on the heart due to increased vascular resistance.
Structurally abnormal heart.	• Congenital cardiac defects. These are usually surgically corrected at a young age, although these repairs have a limited life expectancy. Surgical failure can result in ventricular pump failure.	• VSD, PDA, ASD, AVSD. • There is a reasonably sized communication (shunt) between the pulmonary and systemic circulations, which reduces the efficacy of the cardiac contractions. • Valvular insufficiency. This reduces the efficacy of cardiac contractions.	• Aortic stenosis, pulmonary stenosis, coarctation of the aorta. There is a ventricular outflow obstruction.

TABLE 13: Features of heart failure

Feature	Comments
Faltering growth.	Faltering growth occurs secondary to poor feeding and additional calorific demands.
Sweating.	Excess sweating occurs around the forehead and face of the infant—often when feeding.
Tachycardia.	Increased heart rate compensates for the defect and allows adequate amounts of oxygenated blood to be circulated.
Respiratory distress.	This is due to fluid overload and poor oxygenation.
Poor peripheral perfusion.	Cool hands or feet occur when the body has selected to prioritise its perfusion to more important organs (i.e. the brain).
Hepatomegaly.	Backflow of blood causes congestion in the inferior vena cava and engorgement of the liver.

TABLE 14: Modified Ross criteria

Ross staging criteria for infants and children with heart failure	
Stage I.	No symptoms of heart failure are present.
Stage II.	Infants: Mild tachypnoea or sweating occurs when feeding. Older children: Dyspnoea occurs on exertion.
Stage III.	Infants: Significant tachypnoea and sweating occur when feeding. Growth is poor and feeding times are prolonged. Older children: Significant dyspnoea occurs on exertion.
Stage IV.	Tachypnoea, respiratory distress, grunting and sweating occur when at rest.

Investigations

Clinical diagnosis is generally adequate, but confirmation can be gained through an echocardiogram. This investigation shows the volume of blood successfully pumped out of the ventricles (ejection fraction), as well as the pressures within the heart. It can also help to identify any abnormal cardiac anatomy which could be causing the heart failure.

Chest X-ray may reveal cardiomegaly and plethoric lung fields, and ECG may show ventricular hypertrophy.

Management

Following an ABC approach and when the patient is stable, initial treatment would be administration of a diuretic to offload the heart. ACE inhibitors are useful in patients with ventricular dysfunction. The cause for the heart failure would need investigation and correction if possible, and the child would require referral to a paediatric cardiologist. When caring for children with heart failure, their increased calorific requirements need consideration. For this reason, advise parents on dietary supplements or high energy milk formulas to ensure healthy growth velocity.

Prognosis

Prognosis is very dependent on cause. A correctable structural problem identified at an early stage has an excellent outlook.

INFECTION AND INFLAMMATION IN THE HEART

Infective Endocarditis

Aetiology

Infective endocarditis is uncommon in children, but it is more likely in those who already have valvular pathology or in those with an indwelling central venous catheter. The turbulent blood flow caused by these abnormalities can lead to local inflammation of the vascular endothelium and a localised non-infective thrombus. Following transient bacteraemia (which can commonly occur in all children), this thrombus can become infected and rapidly proliferate, throwing off micro emboli and causing both systemic upset and local damage.

Clinical Features

Diagnosis is made based on Duke Criteria (*Table 15*). The clinical diagnosis of infective endocarditis requires either:

➤ Two major criteria OR

➤ One major and three minor criteria OR

➤ Five minor criteria.

Management

At least two sets of blood cultures are taken, ideally before commencing antibiotics. If diagnosed, patients require a four to eight week course of antibiotics.

Prognosis

Prognosis is good if appropriate antibiotics are started early. However, many infections are diagnosed late and are caused by resistant organisms: the mortality rate is extremely high in these cases.

Kawasaki Disease

Aetiology

This is the most common systemic vasculitis of childhood. It is an acute febrile vasculitis, involving small and medium sized arteries. Kawasaki disease tends to affect children between six-months-old and six-years-old and is more prevalent in people of Japanese and Afro-Caribbean origin.

Clinical Features

Children will present with a high fever, which is difficult to control, and irritability. Biochemically, they will have elevated inflammatory markers but no clear focus of infection. Children may also report abdominal pain, diarrhoea and vomiting and may have a characteristic thrombocytosis on full blood count, although this does not usually occur until at least a week later. Younger infants are more likely to be affected by significant complications and can present with "incomplete" or atypical symptomology.

TABLE 15: Modified Duke criteria for diagnosis of infective endocarditis

Major criteria

1 Typical microorganism consistent with infective endocarditis from two separate blood cultures.
   - *Viridans streptococci, Streptococcus bovis* or HACEK group (*Haemophilus, Actinobacillus, Cardiobacterium hominis, Eikenella corrodens* and *Kingella*).
   - *Staphylococcus aureus* or *enterococci* without primary focus.

2 Evidence of endocardial involvement (as seen on echocardiogram).
   - New dehiscence of prosthetic valve.
   - 'Oscillating intracardiac mass' on valve.
   - Abscess.

Minor criteria

1 Predisposition.
   - Predisposing heart condition, prosthetic valve or intravenous drug use.

2 Fever.
   - Temperature of >38°C.

3 Vascular phenomena.
   - Septic pulmonary infarcts.
   - Intracranial haemorrhage.
   - Conjunctival haemorrhages.
   - Major arterial emboli.
   - Janeway lesions (small non-tender erythematous/macular lesions found on the soles of the feet or palms of the hands only).

4 Immunologic phenomena.
   - Osler nodes (small, painful and tender swellings found on the palms of the hands and soles of the feet only).
   - Roth Spots (retinal haemorrhage).
   - Glomerular nephritis.

5 Microbiological evidence.
   - Positive blood culture not typical of endocarditis.

6 Echocardiographic findings.
   - Consistent with diagnosis but do not meet major criteria.

Diagnostic Criteria

Kawasaki disease is defined by a fever lasting more than five days without any clear focus of infection, plus any four of the following:

➤ Bilateral non-purulent conjunctivitis.

➤ Mucositis. Dry red lips / strawberry tongue.

➤ Cervical lymphadenopathy.

➤ Extremity changes. Red or indurated hands or feet, eventually leading to desquamation (peeling).

➤ Polymorphous rash.

Coronary Artery Disease

The vasculitis can affect the coronary arteries, leading to coronary artery aneurysms. These may rupture; however, they more often resolve but leave behind scar tissue. This scar tissue causes narrowing of the arteries and can lead to ischaemic damage to the myocardium.

31

Management

Treatment consists of high dose aspirin (acting as an anti-platelet and anti-inflammatory) and intravenous immunoglobulin (IVIG). Aspirin therapy is continued for several weeks—and longer if any abnormal findings are observed on echocardiograms. Children must be followed up with regular ECGs and an echocardiogram to look for the presence of coronary artery aneurysms.

Prognosis

With prompt treatment, prognosis is good, especially in older children. 20% of cases are IVIG resistant and higher risk patients may need IV high dose steroids or infliximab (anti TNF).

Rheumatic Fever

Aetiology

This is an autoimmune inflammatory process occurring approximately 20 days following acute infection with a group A beta haemolytic streptococcal organism (most commonly, group A strep pharyngitis). The prevalence of rheumatic fever in Europe has vastly decreased since the widespread use of effective antibiotics during streptococcal infections.

Clinical Features

The Jones diagnostic criteria for acute rheumatic fever require recent infection with a *group A streptococcus,* plus two major or one major and two minor criteria (*Table 16*).

Management

Acute rheumatic fever can be treated with anti-inflammatory medications and antibiotics if a *group A streptococcus* growth has been identified.

Prognosis

Following prompt and adequate treatment, patients will have no long-term ill effects. If, however, recurrent or prolonged inflammation occurs, this can cause fibrotic changes and long-term complications, especially within the heart.

Myocarditis

Aetiology

This is an inflammation of the heart muscle itself, which may be caused by an autoimmune process, a toxin or an infective process. The most common aetiology is viral infection (often adenovirus or enterovirus, commonly Coxsackie virus).

Clinical Features

Children with myocarditis can present with a wide spectrum of symptoms, and these are all largely non-specific.
Signs and symptoms can include:
- Gallop rhythm.
- Abnormal ECG (non-specific ST changes and decreased QRS voltage).
- New cardiomegaly.
- Difficulty in breathing.
- Arrhythmias.

Young children can present with cardiovascular collapse, arrhythmia and sudden death. In a shocked child, be wary if they worsen following a fluid bolus, as they may have been pushed into heart failure.

Management

Diagnosis is largely clinical, although some centres use cardiac MRI for detailed imaging.

Simple measures, such as diuretic therapy and ACE inhibitors to reduce afterload, can be instigated initially. These patients will often require management in an intensive care setting. Treatments have included intravenous immunoglobulin therapy, as well as corticosteroid therapy, to alter inflammatory processes and damage occurring within the myocardium.

Prognosis

With the correct treatment, the majority will have complete recovery. Neonates have the poorest prognosis.

Pericarditis

Aetiology

This is an inflammation of the fibroelastic tissue covering of the heart, often with accompanying pericardial effusion. It is usually secondary to a viral infection. However, recurrent pericarditis or prolonged inflammation can lead to more significant issues, such as constrictive pericarditis.

Clinical Features

It presents with pleuritic central chest pain that improves on leaning forward. Examination may reveal a pericardial rub, which is the squeaky sound made when the two layers of inflamed pericardium move against each other. This will also be louder as the patient sits forward.

Management

In general, anti-inflammatory medicines and supportive care are all that are needed. An echocardiogram should be performed to look for possible effusions. ECG may show

TABLE 16: Modified Jones criteria	
Major Criteria	**Minor criteria**
• Carditis. • Arthritis (generally involving the large joints). • Erythema marginatum. • Sydenham chorea. • Subcutaneous nodules.	• Arthralgia. • Increased PR interval. • Fever. • Increased ESR/CRP.

saddle-shaped ST elevation, although the most specific finding for pericarditis is PR depression.

Prognosis

Viral pericarditis is usually self-limiting, with no long-term sequelae. Bacterial pericarditis can be life threatening, particularly if diagnosis is delayed.

CARDIOMYOPATHIES

A cardiomyopathy is a disease of the heart muscle itself. This differs from myocarditis in that the muscle is altered by the condition and it is not necessarily an acute inflammation.

Aetiology

The cause is often genetic, but cardiomyopathy can also be associated with certain drugs and toxins, connective tissue disorders, post viral complications, sarcoidosis and amyloidosis. There are three main categories of cardiomyopathy:

- **Dilated cardiomyopathy.** The ventricles become dilated and less able to pump blood around the body.
- **Hypertrophic cardiomyopathy.** The ventricles become thickened and lack the capacity to pump blood adequately around the body.
- **Restrictive cardiomyopathy.** The muscle itself does not change in size or shape, but its compliance decreases as the ventricles become stiff.

Clinical Features

Each pathology can initially present with non-specific symptoms of shortness of breath and increased fatigability. They can then progress on to heart failure.

Management

Symptoms can largely be treated with medical therapies, like diuretics and inotropes. Sometimes pacemakers are needed to help control arrhythmias caused by the faulty cardiac muscle. Heart transplant is reserved for cases in which symptoms remain resistant to medical management.

Prognosis

Predicting the long-term outlook is difficult, but hypertrophic cardiomyopathy tends to have better outcomes than dilated or restrictive cardiomyopathies.

REFERENCES AND FURTHER READING

Cardiac Rhythms

1   Advanced Life Support Group. Advanced Paediatric Life Support. Fifth edition. Hoboken NJ: Wiley-Blackwell Publishing; 2005.
2   Tasker R, McClure R, Acerini C. Oxford Handbook of Paediatrics. Second edition. Oxford UK: Oxford Medical Publications; 2013.

The Paediatric ECG

1   Chan T et al. ECG in Emergency Medicine and Acute Care. St. Louis MO: Elsevier Mosby; 2005.
2   Hampton J. The ECG Made Easy. Seventh edition. London UK: Churchill Livingstone; 2008.
3   Park M. Pediatric Cardiology for Practitioners. Fifth edition. St Louis MO: Mosby 2007.
4   Surawicz B, Knilans T. Chou's Electrocardiography in Clinical Practice. Sixth edition. Philadelphia PA: Saunders Elsevier; 2008.

Arrhythmias

1   Doniger S, Sharieff G. Pediatric dysrhythmias. Pediatr Clin North Am. 2006; 53:85.
2   Josephson M, Wellens H. Differential diagnosis of supraventricular tachycardia. Cardiol Clin. 1990; 8:411.
3   Fleming S, Thompson M, Stevens R, et al. Normal ranges of heart rate and respiratory rate in children from birth to 18 years of age: a systematic review of observational studies. Lancet. 2011; 377:1011.
4   Samuels M, Wieteska S. Advanced Paediatric Life Support the practical approach. Fifth edition. Hoboken NJ:Wiley-Blackwell Publishing; 2005.
5   Wren C. Catheter ablation in paediatric arrhythmias. Arch Dis Child. 1999;81:102-4

Congenital Heart Disease

1   Marino B, Bird G, Wernovsky G. Diagnosis and management of the newborn with suspected congenital heart disease. Clin Perinatol. 2001; 28:91.
2   Sasidharan P. An approach to diagnosis and management of cyanosis and tachypnea in term infants. Pediatr Clin North Am. 2004; 51:999.
3   Blaz W et al. Estimation of usefulness of non-invasive cardiovascular diagnostic screening methods in early detection of critical congenital heart defects in newborns. Arch Dis Child. 2014; 99:a120.
4   Perloff J. Ventricular septal defect. In: The Clinical Recognition of Congenital Heart Disease, Fifth edition. Philadelphia PA:W.B. Saunders Company; 2003. 311.
5   Van Der Linde D et al. Birth Prevalence of congenital heart disease worldwide: a systematic review and meta-analysis. J Am Coll Cardiol. 2011; 58:2241.

Heart Murmurs

1   Frank J, Jacobe K. Evaluation and management of heart murmurs in children. Am Fam Physician. 2011;84:7.

Heart Failure

1   Rosenthal D et al. International Society for Heart and Lung Transplantation: Practice guidelines for management of heart failure in children. J Heart Lung Transplant. 2004; 23:1313.
2   Madriago E, Silberbach M. Heart failure in infants and children—Pediatrics in review. Am Acad Pediatr. 2010; 31:1.

3 Kantor P, Mertent L. Heart failure in children. Part I: Clinical evaluation, diagnostic testing, and initial medical management. Clinical practice. Eur J Pediatr. 2010; 169:269-79.

Infection and Inflammation of the Heart

1 Eleftheriou D, Levin M, Shingadia D. Management of Kawasaki disease. Arch Dis Child. 2013; 0:1-10.
2 NICE. Prophylaxis against infective endocarditis: Antimicrobial prophylaxis against infective endocarditis in adults and children undergoing interventional procedures. 2008. https://www.nice.org.uk/guidance/cg64

3 Hoyer A, Silberbach M. Infective endocarditis—Pediatrics in review. Am Acad Pediatr. 2005; 26:11.

Cardiomyopathies

1 Steven D, Colan M. Hypertrophic cardiomyopathy in childhood. National Institutes of Health. Heart Fail Clin. 2010; 6: 433-44.
2 Burch M et al. Dilated cardiomyopathy in children: determinants of outcome. Br Heart J. 1994; 72:246-50.

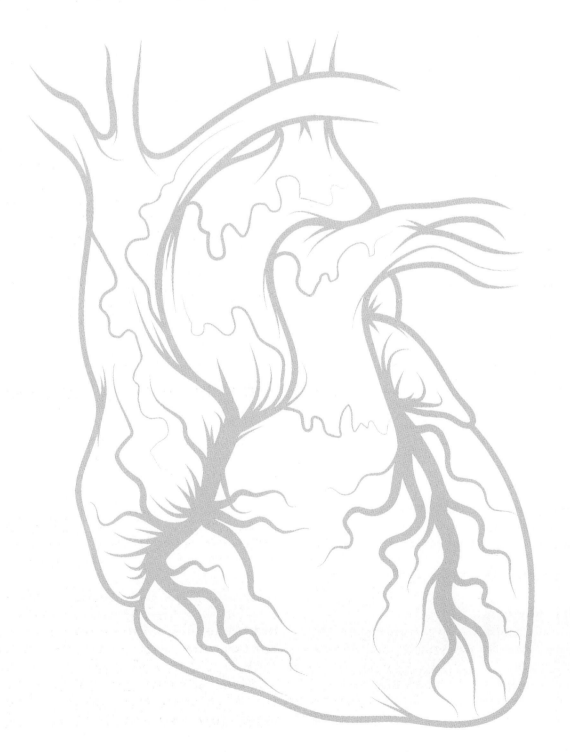

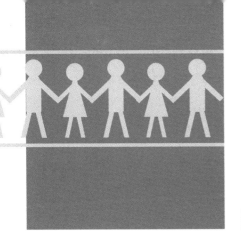

1.04

COMMUNITY PAEDIATRICS

ANTONIA HARGADON-LOWE

CONTENTS

DEVELOPMENT

Normal Development and the Developmental Assessment

Developmental history is often missed when seeing children in acute settings or in primary care. This may be due to time constraints in a busy Emergency Department (ED) or outpatient clinic. However, some information can be gathered quickly with adequate knowledge and practice. Picking up developmental problems early can have a significant impact on that child's outcome. The time taken and depth of questioning on development depends on the clinical scenario (*Table 1*).

TABLE 1: Developmental assessment in different settings	
Scenario	**Suggested Approach**
3-year-old child presenting to ED with a fever and ear pain, and no known developmental concern.	Brief questioning about milestones and parental concerns, e.g. • Do you feel your child is able to do the same things other 3-year-olds can? • At what age did she smile, say her first word and walk?
Outpatient clinic review of 2-year-old boy who has had three seizures in the last few months.	More in-depth questioning is required as relevant to the presenting complaint. The number of questions will depend on the answers and whether concerns emerge. Ascertain whether he is similar to other children of his age. Developmental regression should also be enquired about, i.e. has he lost any skills previously developed. To start, ask a couple of questions in each developmental domain to assess whether he is meeting expected targets for his age: • Gross motor. Is he able to jump? Is he able to climb stairs, and if so, how does he do it? • Fine motor. Can he draw a straight line? How big a tower block can he build with building blocks? • Language/hearing. Can he speak in short sentences? Can he obey simple commands? • Social/Self-Care. Can he eat with a fork/spoon? Does he socially interact (good eye contact and smiles) with adults and other children? • General. Has he lost any skills that he could previously do?
Community paediatric outpatient appointment following a referral from nursery school with concerns of development.	In this situation, the reason for the referral is "developmental concerns", so a full assessment taking approximately one hour is necessary using one of the available tools.

Developmental Milestones

Development is usually categorised into distinct areas; commonly the following domains are used: "Gross Motor", "Fine Motor/Vision", "Language" and "Social/Self-Care" (*Table 2*). This is done because developmental milestones can often be grouped together, and if one sector is affected but not the others, it may indicate a particular group of pathologies. For example, language delay may be secondary to hearing loss, whereas hearing loss is unlikely to cause isolated gross motor delay.

TABLE 2: Average developmental milestones

	Gross Motor	Fine Motor / Vision	Language/Hearing	Social / Self-Care
6 weeks.	• Holds head briefly in ventral suspension. • Some head lag. • Primitive reflexes. • Symmetrical limb movement.	• Holds fists closed. • Turns to light. • Fixes and follows through 90 degrees – especially faces.	• Cries. • Responds to mother's voice. • Startles to noise.	• Smiles.
3-4 months.	• No head lag. • Raises chest (resting on elbows) when prone. • More vigorous limb movements.	• Holds object placed in hand. • Reaches for objects. • Fixes and follows through 180 degrees.	• Cooing. • Quietens to mother's voice.	• Laughs.
5-6 months.	• Sits supported / unsupported with curved back. • Lifts chest on extended arms when prone. • Rolls front to back and later back to front.	• Brings objects to midline. • Transfers between hands. • Consciously releases objects. • Starts mouthing objects.	• Early babbling (with consonants).	• Screams (happy). • No stranger anxiety.
8-9 months.	• Sits unsupported with a straight back. • May crawl / bum shuffle.	• Early pincer grip (uses thumb with all fingers). • Looks for fallen objects.	• Developed babbling – repetitive consonants. • Says "Mama" and "Dada" non-specifically.	• Stranger anxiety develops. • Plays peekaboo.
10 months.	• Pulls to stand. • Cruising.	• Developed pincer grip – picks 'grains of rice' off the floor.	• Understands "No".	• Understands concept of "bye-bye".
12 months.	• Early walking – unsteady / broad based gait.	• Bangs objects together. • Casts objects. • Object permanence – looks for hidden toys. • Points at things.	• Few individual words. • Imitates sounds and speaks jargon with conversational intonation. • Understands names and simple objects.	• Finger feeds. • Can hold spoon and attempt use. • Waves bye-bye / claps. • Points to convey desire, shortly followed by pointing for excitement.
15 months.	• More confident walking.	• Builds tower of two or three bricks. • Turns thick cardboard pages.	• Obeys simple commands. • Can identify common objects.	• Uses cup and spoon.
18 months.	• Squats to pick up object. • Running.	• Builds tower of four blocks. • To and fro scribble. • Points to pictures in books. • Turns pages in book a few at a time.	• 10-20 words including common objects. • Common two word phrases e.g. "all-gone". • Points to body parts.	• Removes socks / shoes. • Imitative play / domestic mimicry (copies parents' actions at home).
2 years.	• Jumping. • Kicks ball. • Climbs stairs two feet per step / holding on.	• Circular scribble. • Draws straight line (at 2.5 years). • Builds tower of six blocks.	• Has 50+ words. • Links words together to make two or three word sentences. • Understands functions of objects (which one do you eat with? [said whilst pointing to a fork and a pencil]), and verbs (who is running?). • Obeys two-part commands.	• Feeds with fork + spoon. • Starts toilet training. • Temper tantrums. • Plays alongside other children (parallel play). • Symbolic play.
3 years.	• Rides a tricycle. • Goes upstairs with one foot per step, and downstairs with two feet per step.	• Copies a circle. • Builds a tower of nine bricks. • Copies a bridge and stairs with six bricks.	• Knows several nursery rhymes. • Complex four to five word sentences. • States first and last name. • "What" and "Who" questions. • Understands prepositions e.g. under / behind. • Understands sizes e.g. big/little, tall/small.	• Washes hands. • Plays with other children. • Understands concept of sharing. • Pretend play.

(Continued)

TABLE 2: *Continued*

	Gross Motor	Fine Motor / Vision	Language/Hearing	Social / Self-Care
4 years.	• Hops. • Walks up and down steps like adult.	• Copies a cross. • Copies stairs with 10 bricks.	• Can tell descriptive account of events. • Uses "why", "when" and "how". • Understands negatives (e.g. which one is not a boy?) / three-part commands.	• Undresses but cannot dress independently. • Understands turn-taking.
5 years.	• Skips. • Catches ball.	• Copies a triangle / square.	• Tells a complex story using all tenses – future and past.	• Dresses, including buttons and zips. • Can eat with knife and fork. • Chooses and names best friends. • Imaginative play including role playing and made up stories.

Figure 1 shows the progression of grip and *Figure 2* shows the progression of gross motor control.

Milestones are important but sometimes difficult to learn, mostly because the "normal" ages vary. It is also important to distinguish between "average" and "when to be worried". As a child gets older, the "normal" range for a milestone spans a greater period. Note also that corrected gestational age needs to be calculated in premature babies less than 2-years-old. Corrected gestational age is calculated as:

$$\text{Corrected gestational age} = \text{Chronological age} - (\text{number of weeks premature})$$

Therefore, a 10-month-old child born two months early has a corrected gestational age of 8-months-old. Developmentally, the child should only be expected to perform in line with an 8-month-old child, not a 10-month-old child.

Certain thresholds for referral are important to recognise, as summarised in *Table 3*.

Routine Childhood Surveillance

Children and their families are assessed at various key points during their early years. *Table 4* summarises the current assessments carried out in the UK based on the 2009 Department of Health "Healthy Child Programme". The aim is to pick up

FIGURE 2

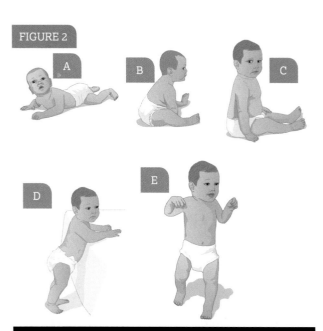

Gross motor progression in first year. (A) Raises chest when prone (three to four months). (B) Sits unsupported with curved back (five to six months). (C) Sits unsupported with straight back (eight to nine months). (D) Cruising (10 months). (E) Early walking (12 months).

any developmental concerns early and implement a package of support tailored to that child to address the underlying issues.

Growth and Development

Until 5-years-old, the child's feeding, growth and development should be monitored. The "Red Book" or parent held health record is given in the first few weeks of life in the UK. This contains a record of vaccinations, early midwife and health visitor assessments, growth charts and general advice on the care of a young child. At each of the screening points, the weight can be plotted on their growth chart. Through the first year, this may be done frequently to ensure they are growing adequately, and then less frequently thereafter. All practitioners

FIGURE 1

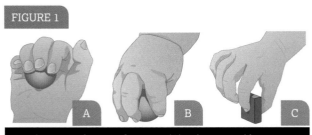

Development of grip in first year. (A) Palmar grip (three to four months). (B) Early pincer grip (eight to nine months). (C) Fine pincer grip (10 months).

should ensure vaccinations are up-to-date at any encounter with a child from birth to 5-years-old.

Vision

Routine visual screening is done initially at the newborn and six-to-eight week check with a red reflex. It is then performed at pre-school or during school entry at 4 to 5-years-old. Concerns outside of these checks will lead to a referral to either an optometrist, ophthalmologist (medically qualified) or an orthoptist.

TABLE 3: Some important situations where referral for further specialist paediatric assessment is indicated	
Age	**Feature**
6-8 weeks.	• Asymmetrical Moro reflex. • Unable to fix and follow. • Not smiling. • Excessive head lag. • No startle to sound.
12 weeks.	• Persistent squint.
8 months.	• Persistent primitive reflexes. • Not vocalising.
1 year.	• Hand preference. • Not responding to their own name.
18 months.	• Not walking.
2 years.	• No or few words spoken by child.
3 years.	• Not speaking in sentences. • Not interacting with other children. • Not following simple commands. • Unable to use the toilet. • Unable to use a spoon.

Squints

"Neonatal misalignments" are common in the first two months (where the eyes do not focus on the same spot) but this usually reduces in the second month. If it is persistent at 10-12 weeks, specialist referral is warranted, as it may represent a squint. The earlier the detection and referral, the more likely specialists are able to correct the squint, allow binocular vision and depth perception to develop as normal, and prevent amblyopia (a lazy eye where the brain chooses to ignore its image), thereby minimising visual dysfunction.

Red Reflex

The "red reflex" can be assessed at any age but is routinely done at the newborn and six-to-eight week check. This term refers to the red reflection of light from the retina when looking through an ophthalmoscope. This test is routinely done at birth to screen for problems such as cataracts and retinoblastomas (where the red reflex is absent and instead there is a "white reflex" or leukocoria). The absence of the red reflex should prompt urgent referral to an ophthalmologist or paediatrician.

Fixing and Following

Fixing and following across the midline up to 180 degrees occurs by three-months-old. The visual pathway then continues to develop during infancy, with rapidly improving acuity in the first six months, reaching near adult levels at approximately 12 months. Colour vision is well developed by six months. Visual acuity tests, summarised in *Table 5*, are age dependent.

The "Ishihara tests" for colour vision are usually used for those more than 10-years-old but have been adapted for use on children from 3-years-old using shapes instead of numbers.

TABLE 4: Routine surveillance of children		
Time Frame	**Assessor**	**Monitoring**
Newborn examination.	Paediatric doctor or midwife.	The baby is examined from head to toe, looking for any obvious abnormalities. The eyes are assessed for a red reflex. Feeding is checked, as is whether the baby is passing urine and has opened their bowels. Weight and head circumference are checked. Hips are assessed and the heart is auscultated for the presence of a heart murmur. A newborn hearing screen is usually carried out and it is ensured that the parents have a basic understanding of how to look after a baby, and when to seek help.
Early newborn baby review 7–14 days.	Health visitor or midwife.	The baby is reassessed to ensure adequate feeding and to identify any parental anxieties or mental health concerns (e.g. postnatal depression) that may have emerged. Such reviews are usually frequent, and in the UK, this is also when the Guthrie test is performed (p210).
6–8 week review.	Primary care doctor.	An assessment similar to the newborn assessment is repeated, particularly focusing on identifying problems with the eyes, hips, heart and testicles. General matters of concern are also addressed.
8–12 months.	Primary care doctor.	Full developmental check is carried out. Growth and feeding are looked at. Any problems identified are addressed as they arise.
2–2.5 years.	Health visitors.	Full developmental check is carried out. Social developmental concerns that may affect a child's ability to access the educational curriculum are usually more obvious at this age. Any children with concerns will be referred on for a specialist assessment.

The shapes are made up of multiple dots of one colour on a background of dots of various other colours.

Hearing

The critical age for intervention in sensorineural hearing loss (SNHL) is before six-months-old; therefore, it is important to assess hearing early. In the UK, the Newborn Hearing Screen has been in place since 2006, replacing the distraction test at 8-months-old. If the child fails the test, or has certain risk factors, they should be referred to an audiologist. *Table 6* summarises hearing testing.

Developmental Delay

Developmental delay is a broad term and covers delay in any of the four main areas, whilst the term global developmental delay indicates that two or more areas are delayed.

Aetiology

Causes include:

> Neurological
>> Congenital. e.g. embryological disorders of brain development, antenatal vascular event.
>> Acquired (static). e.g. hypoxic ischaemic encephalopathy (from birth asphyxia), intraventricular bleeds, prolonged hypoxia (arrest, seizure) or hypoglycaemia, traumatic brain injury, ischaemic stroke.
>> Acquired (progressive). e.g. brain tumour, subsclerosing panencephalitis.
> Infection
>> Congenital. e.g. TORCH (Toxoplasmosis, Other, Rubella, CMV, Herpes) infections, HIV.
>> Acquired. e.g. meningitis, herpes encephalitis.

TABLE 5: Summary of visual acuity tests in children		
Test	**Age Range**	**Description**
Cardiff Acuity Test.	1 to 3-years-old/Those with developmental delay.	Works on the principle of preferential looking; i.e. a child will prefer looking at an image of an object, when compared to a plain image.
Stycar Letter Matching Test.	3 to 5-years-old.	There are versions with shapes and balls for younger children. The child is given a key card of letters and is presented with single letters of reducing size at three metres and asked to point to the matching letter on their key card. It uses only five letters at first (VTOHX) and then increases to seven then nine letters. The "Sheridan Gardiner test" is very similar.
Snellen Chart.	5-years-old and older.	Many letters on one chart (of varying font size) are presented to the child at a distance of 6 metres. The child is asked to either point to a matching letter or say the letter.

TABLE 6: Summary of hearing tests in children		
Test	**Age Range**	**Description**
Oto-acoustic emissions (OAE).	From birth.	Used for neonatal screening (first line) and work on the basis that the inner ear produces a sound in response to noise, which is recorded. It will therefore miss sensorineural hearing loss (SNHL) if the cochlear function is normal.
Auditory brainstem responses.	From birth.	Used if OAE fails. For this, clicks are presented to each ear and electrodes on the scalp pick up responses. Auditory brainstem responses do not distinguish between conductive hearing loss (CHL) and SNHL, and is not possible to carry out if the infant is moving.
Distraction testing.	6 to 9-months-old (although can be used up to 24-months-old).	Involves a parent and two examiners – one gains the child's attention whist the other makes a noise behind the child. In a positive test, the child should move their head towards the noise.
Performance testing.	2-years-old.	Requires the child to respond to different instructions/tasks at various frequencies and volumes. It does rely on appropriate receptive language development so needs careful interpretation.
Discrimination testing, e.g. "McCormack Toy Discrimination test".	2-years-old.	Asks the child to identify objects or pictures using words that sound similar.
Pure tone audiometry.	4-years-old.	Headphones are placed on the child and sounds of different volumes and frequencies are created. The child must indicate when they hear a noise and on which side. It can differentiate between CHL and SNHL.
Tympanometry.	All ages.	Tests for middle ear pathology – a sound is passed into the ear, the amount reflected back is measured and then the compliance is determined by repeating this procedure at varying pressures. The results are then graphed.

> Neuromuscular disorder. e.g. Duchenne Muscular Dystrophy.
> Endocrine abnormalities. e.g. hypothyroidism.
> Genetic. e.g. Down syndrome, phenylketonuria.
> Pervasive developmental disorders. e.g. autism.
> Nutritional. e.g. vitamin deficiencies and malnutrition.
> Others. e.g. isolated speech and language delay, prematurity, metabolic disorders, idiopathic.

Investigations

Tables 7 and 8 summarise investigations that might be considered in global developmental delay.

Management

If concerns are raised about possible developmental delay, the child should be referred to a community paediatrician. The majority of referrals come from health visitors, nurseries, schools, or speech and language therapists, with some coming from primary care physicians or hospital doctors – either with concerns picked up by them or from the parents. The community paediatrician will see the patient for a much longer period (usually at least an hour) and will perform a detailed developmental assessment and wider assessment of the well-being of the child and the family.

TABLE 7: Routine investigations in Global Developmental Delay

Investigations	Justification
Full blood count (FBC) + Haematinics.	Iron deficiency, folate / B12 deficiency — can cause developmental delay and learning difficulties.
Urea and electrolytes (U&Es).	Renal failure and hyponatraemia both may cause poor growth. Renal osteodystrophy can lead to gross motor delay. A baseline is also useful for any future tests.
Creatinine kinase.	Early detection of Duchenne Muscular Dystrophy.
Thyroid function tests.	Hypothyroidism is a well-documented cause of developmental and intellectual delay. If treatment is delayed, its effects are irreversible.
Liver function tests (LFTs).	Abnormalities may suggest further investigations such as those to look for an underlying metabolic disorder.
Bone profile (+ Vitamin D).	Vitamin D deficiency can cause motor delay. Hypocalcaemia can represent this or another underlying disorder with delayed development (e.g. 22q11 deletion).
Hearing test.	Speech and language delay may be as a result of a hearing defect, but genetic disorders with global delay may also involve conductive or sensorineural hearing loss.

TABLE 8: Second-line investigations in Global Developmental Delay

Investigations	Justification
Karyotype.	Karyotyping may identify trisomy disorders or Turner syndrome.
DNA testing.	The FMR1 DNA test can determine if Fragile X Syndrome is present. Fragile X can cause developmental delay, without necessarily showing obvious dysmorphism early on.
Array comparative genomic hybridization (CGH).	Array CGH can identify chromosomal microdeletions or microduplications and may explain previously unknown causes of developmental delay. If a defect already recognised is detected, it may help with prognosis, but if not, then it may contribute to research and help future children. Testing of other family members is offered to clarify if the genetic abnormality is a new finding in the child or inherited from a parent.
Metabolic screen.	Inborn errors of metabolism, e.g. mucopolysaccharide disorders, peroxisomal disorders (both usually dysmorphic), organic and aminoacidaemias, and mitochondrial disorders. These are found in a very small proportion of developmental delay (approximately 1%).
Lead.	Lead toxicity could be found in children with developmental delay and no other symptoms, and is treatable.
Biotinidase.	Biotinidase deficiency can present as developmental delay as its only sign and is treatable.
Brain magnetic resonance imaging (MRI).	This may identify a structural abnormality or damage resulting from a static event (e.g. infection, trauma, etc.) or a progressive neurological disorder. This may require a general anaesthetic in younger children.
Electroencephalogram (EEG).	For children with developmental regression, or associated seizures, an EEG may show typical features of an epilepsy syndrome, e.g. West syndrome, Landau-Kleffner syndrome.

Various assessment tools are available for measuring the developmental level:

- The Griffiths assessment is one of the most comprehensive developmental assessment tools and is often used in the UK, though it requires additional training so is not expected knowledge of a non-specialist.
- Specialised testing kits are also available to facilitate developmental testing of children with a sensory impairment, e.g. the Reynell Zinkin assessment kit for children with a visual impairment.

There are only a few causes of reversible developmental delay. This means most children with developmental delay suffer chronic morbidity. In all cases, the underlying cause needs to be treated, if possible. However, many cases are of unknown aetiology, with management centred on supportive therapy and the aim of maximising the underlying potential in that individual child. *Table 9* summarises specialists that may be involved.

IMPORTANT CONDITIONS

Autistic Spectrum Disorder

Autistic Spectrum Disorder is a developmental disorder characterised by symptoms in three domains:

- Social interaction. Lack of ability to have normal social interactions.
- Social communication. Significant speech delay, with some never acquiring speech, and lack of non-verbal communication (e.g. eye contact, social smiling, facial expressions, gestures).

TABLE 9: Specialists that may be involved in the care of a child with developmental delay	
Specialist	**Role**
SALT (speech and language therapist).	Provide assessment and intervention for children with swallowing and communication disorders.
Occupational therapist.	Identify and manage fine motor problems, coordination, sensory processing difficulties and executive functioning. They can advise on and coordinate adaptation of the house and equipment to the child's needs.
Physiotherapist.	Identify and manage gross motor disorders. They can advise on and coordinate provision of any necessary equipment to the child to aid these skills.
Health visitor.	General health surveillance, screening and advice to parents and their children under 5-years-old.
Geneticist.	Provide advice on possible genetic disorders, testing and implications for future family planning.
Neurologist / Neurodisability specialist.	Provide a specialist neurological opinion on possible aetiology, arranges and interprets specialist investigations, and provides specific therapies (for example, in cerebral palsy, prescribe baclofen injections for reducing spasticity).
Audiologist.	Through a variety of tests, they can provide information on the child's hearing and any associated defect. They coordinate treatment, if indicated.
Social worker.	Disability social workers specialize in working with children with disabling conditions. Social workers are also involved with a family if there are child protection concerns.
Educational psychologist.	Carry out specific assessments on a child's ability to learn and perform in various learning functions. They will provide a summary of the child's relative IQ in all these areas.
Hospice / Respite care.	This may be necessary if the child's condition is terminal.
Ophthalmologist.	Assess and offer treatment for visual difficulties.
CAMHS (Child and Adolescent Mental Health Services).	CAMHS offer psychiatric support and therapy to children with possible mental health disorders including severe behavioural difficulties.
Hospital paediatrician.	May be required for basic management of things such as enuresis, constipation, reflux, pain or specific organ involvement.
Community paediatrician.	Assess the development of a child in detail, including emotional and behavioural aspects. Generally, community paediatricians co-ordinate all the care of the child and ensure no issue is left unaddressed. Advocacy for vulnerable families is a significant part of the role of the community paediatrician.
School teachers/staff.	There may be a Special Educational Needs Coordinator (SENCO) for the school, who ensures every child's learning needs are met including those with developmental delay and/or learning difficulties. This is often provided by the school with extra support. However, if additional support and funding are required, a "Statement of Special Educational Needs" should be applied for. This is granted by the local council and states that a full assessment has been carried out and the child is entitled to extra monetary support to enable them to access the curriculum. The school also may host Team around the Child (TAC) meetings: this is where all personnel involved in a child's care meet and discuss best courses of action.

> Rigidity of thought and behaviour (social imagination). Dislike of routine change, need for stereotyped and repetitive activities, and lack of ability to imagine.

Aetiology

Autism is apparently increasing in the UK population. This could reflect increased awareness, earlier recognition and improved diagnosis. Autism is currently estimated to affect approximately 30–60 per 10,000 people. The exact aetiology is unknown but genetic associations are being increasingly recognised. There are theories regarding environmental factors but no strong evidence. Extreme emotional deprivation can produce autistic features in children and safeguarding concerns should be carefully looked for in the history. Attachment Disorder and Autism Spectrum Disorder can present in a very similar fashion, but "sensory sensitivities" are more common in autism. This refers to difficulty in processing information from sensory channels, e.g. smell, taste and touch, and is a feature of autism.

In 1998, a link was suggested between autism and the measles-mumps-rubella (MMR) vaccine, but this has subsequently been discredited. Nevertheless, the initial publication led to a reduction in MMR vaccinations and a subsequent increase in cases of measles. Parents should be opportunistically advised that no link exists between the MMR vaccine and autism and they should be encouraged to still vaccinate.

Ten to fifteen percent of cases of autism have a diagnosable underlying cause, including:
> Tuberous sclerosis.
> Fragile X syndrome.
> Phenylketonuria.
> Associations with chromosomal microdeletion syndromes.

Primary autism can also be associated with depression, ADHD and other behavioural disorders, as well as Tourette syndrome. People with autism frequently have lower IQs than average, but this is not always the case.

Clinical Features

Children may present:
> At birth, with minimal social skills (limited social smiling, limited eye contact and minimal enjoyment in games).
> Following regression or arrest of social skills, having initially been a sociable baby with normal development.
> Much later, following a social challenge such as progression to senior school (more common in girls). The spectrum of severity ranges from those who are able to function with just a little extra support in mainstream schools and will go on to have normal relationships and jobs, to those who never develop any speech, never become toilet trained and always have severe learning difficulties.

Common features include:
> Delayed or lack of pointing. Children with autism may use the carer's hand to point to things instead.
> Delayed speech. Children may have limited language development to varying degrees.
> Lack of response to name. This is noticeable from an early age.
> Poor eye contact. Often children with autism are described as being "in their own world".
> Delayed and disordered play development. Children may be observed not playing with or interacting with other children (in a conventional way). They may have rituals or certain play that is repetitive in nature, including lining things up or being obsessed with a certain toy or topic. These children lack imagination and often do not demonstrate make-believe play or role-playing games.
> Strong dislike for routine change. This may include things like the route to school or an order in which things happen, and change will lead to a tantrum.

> Motor mannerisms. Examples include hand flapping or jumping.
> Sensory symptoms. There may be a dislike of loud noises and certain textures – most commonly of food and clothing. Children may display sensory seeking behaviour such as excessive play with water/sand or touching/stroking people's skin or hair.
> Regression. Some parents will report apparently normal language progression until around 15-months-old, followed by loss or regression of language skills. It is very important to ask about possible regression in the history, as this can be a feature; i.e. normal initial development does not rule out autism. However, developmental regression needs further investigation to rule out other causes, e.g. Rett Syndrome.

Children with higher functioning autism may have an exceedingly high level of knowledge about a peculiar topic, or an aptitude to remember details or numbers above that of children their age or even adults.

Investigations

Investigations vary depending on the clinical findings, but are broadly similar to that for developmental delay. There are no known biomarkers for autism, but screening tools include:
> Gilliam Autism Rating Scale (GARS-2) for pre-school children.
> Social Responsiveness Scale (SRS) for older children.
> Modified Checklist for Autism in Toddlers.

Clinical assessment and diagnosis is based on an in-depth history and prolonged clinical observation through a variety of tasks and assessments. Multi-disciplinary assessment by both a community paediatrician and a speech and language therapist are recommended for autism assessment and diagnosis. The "Autism Diagnostic Interview" and "Autism Diagnostic Observation Schedule" are considered gold standards for this.

Management

The management is multi-agency and complex. With certain strategies, children with autism can potentially achieve a higher functional level and quality of life. Since many professionals are involved, a "keyworker" usually coordinates and plans individually tailored care for each child (including outreach, one-on-one and group interventions).

Some possible therapies for the child include:

› **Speech and Language Therapy (SALT).** These professionals form the mainstay of management and provide ongoing support and therapy, often teaching the child and family Makaton (a language programme using signs and symbols) in order to communicate.
› **Psychosocial intervention.** Techniques can be employed to try and increase the child's attention, interaction, engagement and reciprocal communication. This may include play-based therapies. Cognitive behavioural therapy may be appropriate in older children if they have the verbal and cognitive ability to engage with it.
› **Behavioural intervention.** This includes assessing factors which might contribute to challenging behaviour, e.g. the physical environment, and making adaptive changes (for example making the environment less noisy). Co-existing medical disorders may also contribute to challenging behaviour and therefore need to be addressed. Psychological and psychiatric illness, e.g. depression or anxiety, can co-exist and need to be identified and therapy instituted where required.
› **Sleep problems.** This is common in autism, and triggers should be identified, e.g. background noise, irregular bedtimes or potentially co-morbidities such as hyperactivity. Medication, such as melatonin, can be considered.
› **Adaptation skills.** It is helpful also to think about general support for development, and access to community services; for example, public transport and leisure facilities. Education needs to be supported, and it may be the case that such children require a statement of special educational needs.
› **Pharmacological intervention.** If psychosocial interventions are unhelpful, and if behaviour remains very challenging, then antipsychotic medication can be considered and started by a specialist. This is very rarely done.

The needs of carers and families should also be identified. They may require personal, social and emotional support, as well as practical support in providing care.

Attention Deficit Hyperactivity Disorder

Attention deficit hyperactivity disorder (ADHD) is a condition characterised by three themes:

1 **Hyperactivity.** Fidgety, constantly on the move, reduced sleep requirement.
2 **Inattention.** Easily distracted, poor concentration.
3 **Impulsiveness.** Acts without reflection, impatient.

Aetiology

Genetic and environmental factors have been implicated in the aetiology. There are common co-existing and not mutually exclusive diagnoses including:

› Mood disorders.
› Conduct disorders.
› Learning difficulties.
› Communication disorders (including autism).
› Anxiety disorders.
› Movement disorders (including Tourette syndrome and tics).

As a result, care must be made in diagnosis. There is also an increased frequency in underlying conditions including:

› Neurofibromatosis.
› Angelman syndrome.
› Fragile X syndrome.
› Foetal alcohol or drug exposure.
› Very low birth weight/extremely premature infants.

Investigations

ADHD is diagnosed clinically, by a child psychiatrist or community paediatrician, without any biochemical tests unless alternate diagnoses are being considered. Children suffering from ADHD tend to be either the predominantly hyperactive and inattentive type or the impulsive type.

For diagnosis, the condition must:

› Have an early onset.
› Have moderate impairment to emotional, educational and social functioning.
› Demonstrate chronicity.

Features should occur in two or more settings (e.g. at home and at school) to demonstrate that the behaviour is not specific to one environment. Diagnosis is supported with scoring charts, assessing for traits in the three themes described above. The most common method uses a Conner's questionnaire. From this, a score will be generated which strongly supports but does not make the diagnosis.

Management

Management involves an MDT approach, with education, behavioural intervention, medication and ensuring a healthy, nutritionally balanced diet. If a link is found with specific food groups, including artificial colourings/additives, then exclusions/adaptations to the diet may be indicated; however, this should be done in conjunction with dietetic advice. The first line medication is usually methylphenidate (a dopamine/noradrenaline reuptake inhibitor).

School Refusal

Stressful life events can often trigger school refusal. This may manifest in a number of chronic symptoms with no organic basis, such as headaches, stomach aches, nausea or diarrhoea, but can also present with tantrums, difficult behaviour or separation anxiety. This may represent a normal part of development and may be short lived, or it may represent more underlying problems, including an emerging underlying anxiety disorder or safeguarding concerns. Each case should be individually assessed, with consideration given to referral to child and adolescent mental health services if needed.

Toddler Tantrums

Temper tantrums can start at around 18-months-old and are very common in toddlers. One reason they might occur is that children experience frustration because they have desires they want to express but do not have the language to express them. Management involves trying to understand the reason for the tantrum (for example, being hungry or feeling frustrated at something) and finding distractions for the child. The temptation to shout back at the child should generally be resisted, as this may worsen the situation. Temper tantrums are self-limiting and become less frequent as the child grows older.

Sleep Disorders

Nightmares

Nightmares occur during Rapid Eye Movement (REM) sleep and so usually occur in the second half of the night. They are common at 5 to 10-years-old, and children often remember the content of the nightmare. If they occur less than once a week, parents should be reassured, but if they are high frequency, contain repetitive themes, or disrupt sleep, this would warrant further attention, especially to look for psychosocial triggers.

Night Terrors

Night terrors involve partial arousal from non-REM sleep, usually early in the night, and peak at 4 to 7-years-old. The child will wake abruptly, screaming and appearing terrified. Then they appear to go back to sleep. Their eyes are usually open but they are not fully awake. Children can usually remember the content of the dreams, but there is no recollection of episodes of night terrors. Night terrors are usually benign and self-limiting, so no specific management is generally required.

Sleepwalking

Sleepwalking occurs in older children, usually at 8 to 12-years-old, and, like night terrors, is not remembered. At the time, they will look wide awake and can often travel significant distances. Safety is an issue and stair gates or locks may be needed. It can also be associated with micturition. No specific management is usually required, although ensuring adequate sleep, reducing stress and avoiding excess stimulation before sleep may be helpful.

Learning Difficulties

Learning difficulty describes the restriction that a child has within an area of their learning development. Learning difficulties can be general or be specific to certain areas, including literacy, numerical reasoning, non-verbal and verbal reasoning, and memory. They can be subcategorised as mild, moderate or severe. The terms "learning disability" and "learning difficulty" are used interchangeably.

Aetiology

Learning difficulties may be idiopathic, particularly if mild, and may also be a result of neglect or lack of mental stimulation. Other potential causes are broadly similar to those which cause developmental delay, and include:

> **Genetic.** e.g. Down syndrome, Fragile X syndrome.
> **Neonatal complications.** e.g. congenital infection, hypoxic ischaemic encephalopathy, prematurity.
> **Acquired illness/injury.** e.g. neurovascular insult, road traffic accident, child abuse.

Investigations

Learning difficulties are usually identified by school teachers due to failure to meet academic standards. It is most accurately assessed by educational psychologists but the child often also sees a community paediatrician to rule out an undiagnosed developmental disorder. They may also exist in those with pre-existing conditions where learning difficulties were predicted.

Investigations may be helpful in identifying an organic cause for the learning difficulty, which may be reversible. They are broadly similar to that for developmental delay.

Management

No medical treatments are available for learning difficulties, unless they are the result of an underlying medical disorder. The emphasis is on providing greater support. The child may have an "Individual Educational Plan" formulated, where specific targets are identified realistic to their capabilities. Certain measures are then put in place to help achieve this, such as small group work, extra support in certain areas, or some one-to-one work. The child may also benefit from going to a school that specialises in providing support for those with additional learning needs.

At a young age, children are often mislabelled as having behavioural problems despite their symptoms being related to the discrepancy between their functioning age and their chronological age. Without extra support for the child, consequences include poorer academic performance, anxiety, depression, behavioural problems, and unemployment and financial instability when older. This may also trigger truancy and bullying.

SAFEGUARDING

Categories of Abuse

Child protection is relevant in every aspect of paediatrics, and more generally for anyone dealing with children. According to the National Society for the Prevention of Cruelty to Children (NSPCC), in the UK approximately two children die per week from homicide, neglect or "undetermined intent".

Abuse can be divided into four categories:

> Physical abuse.
> Neglect.
> Sexual abuse.
> Emotional abuse.

These are not mutually exclusive and often co-exist.

Physical Abuse

Physical abuse encompasses any physical harm caused to a child. *Figure 3* shows the typical sites of accidental and non-accidental injury (NAI). *Figure 4* shows specific non-accidental injuries. This may involve hitting, biting, burning or scalding, shaking, throwing, poisoning, suffocation, drowning, or any cause of physical harm to a child. It includes fabricated or induced illness. Note:

> These injuries can present as bruises, burns, lacerations, bite marks, petechiae, fractures or neurological signs suggesting intracranial injuries.
> Specific patterns of bruising are more suspicious than others:
>> Marks that are well demarcated, have the appearance of a specific implement (such as a belt), or look like finger marks from hitting or gripping.
>> Bruises that are not on bony prominences (inner/ posterior thighs, buttocks, trunk, chest, behind or on ears, neck or shoulders, intra-oral), or bilateral.
> Bruises cannot be aged accurately.
> In burns, look for splash marks and irregular edges to support a story of accidental burns.
> There should be a strong suspicion of NAI in spiral, oblique or metaphyseal fractures, but a consistent and good story could explain these, particularly in older children.
> NAI should be strongly suspected and actively excluded in any non-mobile child or child under 1-year-old with a fracture unless there is a very plausible mechanism of injury.

Neglect

This is the persistent failure to meet a child's basic physiological and psychological needs and has a negative impact on their health and development. It can include:

> Poor diet.
> Meeting health needs.
> Educational achievement.
> Hygiene.
> Protection from danger and prevention of harm.

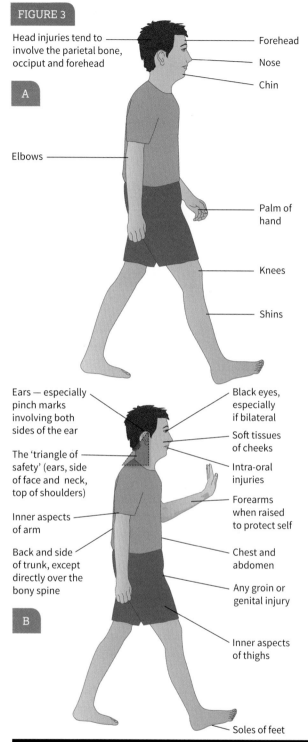

FIGURE 3

Head injuries tend to involve the parietal bone, occiput and forehead

A

Forehead
Nose
Chin

Elbows

Palm of hand

Knees

Shins

Ears — especially pinch marks involving both sides of the ear

The 'triangle of safety' (ears, side of face and neck, top of shoulders)

Inner aspects of arm

Back and side of trunk, except directly over the bony spine

B

Black eyes, especially if bilateral

Soft tissues of cheeks

Intra-oral injuries

Forearms when raised to protect self

Chest and abdomen

Any groin or genital injury

Inner aspects of thighs

Soles of feet

Typical sites of A) accidental injury and B) non-accidental injury.

> Protection from witnessing violence.
> Provision of emotional warmth.

Sometimes, neglect is the only concern preceding a child death from abuse, and therefore the significance of neglect should not be underestimated. Every paediatrician assessing children should be alert to signs of neglect of a child's welfare. One of the best ways to chart wellbeing is through growth parameters,

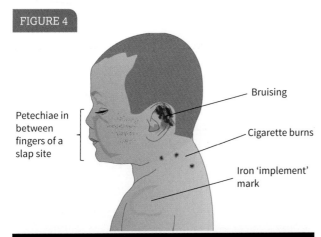

FIGURE 4

Petechiae in between fingers of a slap site

Bruising

Cigarette burns

Iron 'implement' mark

Classic NAI injuries: 1. Slapped cheek with space between fingers seen demarcated by petechiae. 2. Pinna bruising. 3. Cigarette burns. 4. Clear demarcation in a shape suggesting use of implement (iron).

so it is vitally important that heights and weights are recorded accurately and, where available, compared along a timeline to ensure that children are growing adequately. Failure to gain weight and to grow may well be due to failure of basic feeding and nutrition.

Sexual Abuse

This involves forcing or enticing a child or young person to take part in any sexual activity regardless of whether they are aware of what is happening. This includes any physical contact, both penetrative and non-penetrative, oral sex and prostitution. It may also involve non-contact activities such as looking at or being involved in the production of pornography, being forced to watch sexual activity, or being encouraged to behave in a sexually inappropriate way.

In an ever-expanding world of social media, cyber bullying and gang related crime, it is important to explore these issues in depth even if on the surface it seems consensual. There may be grooming, blackmailing or other unlawful behaviours that lead to the sexual activity.

In the UK, sexual intercourse is illegal with those under 16-years-old, but with consent, and partners of similar age, power balance, and where both have capacity to consent (no learning difficulties), legal proceedings rarely occur. Any sexual intercourse with a child under 13-years-old is considered statutory rape, even if there is apparent consent.

Sexual abuse may present with:
- A disclosure.
- Genitourinary symptoms.
- Unexpected pregnancy.
- Inappropriately sexualised behaviour in a young child.

However, sexual abuse commonly goes unnoticed by anyone and becomes apparent later on in life, often with mental health problems and is then disclosed by the adult.

Emotional Abuse

This is the persistent emotional maltreatment of a child to cause severe and persistent adverse effects to their well-being and emotional development. This may involve:
- A lack of emotional warmth and love.
- Constant criticism and being made to feel unworthy, unloved or inadequate.
- Placing developmentally inappropriate expectations upon them.
- Bullying, leading to constant fear.
- Witnessing or hearing of other maltreatment.
- Exploitation/ corruption of a child.

There is some level of emotional abuse in all other categories.

Presentation of Child Abuse

Concerns may be picked up through school, nurseries or presenting to a healthcare provider. The most obvious presentation of abuse is a concerning injury without a fitting explanation. The explanation may be implausible, inadequate or inconsistent and must be taken in the context of the child's developmental age and any background medical conditions. Quite commonly, determining whether it is NAI can be unclear and very challenging. A burn mark in the shape of an iron on the buttocks is obvious. However, a child on a protection plan for neglect with a bruise on their cheek that has a reasonable but not completely obvious explanation is a much harder decision to make and pursue.

Other more subtle presentations include:
- Inappropriate attachment to their caregiver, including attachment disorders.
- Inappropriate affection towards strangers.
- Poor school attendance.
- Poor presentation at school (ill-fitting or dirty clothing, unwashed, smelling of urine/faeces).
- Persistent infestations with lice.
- Persistent severe nappy rash with broken skin.
- Enuresis and/or encopresis.
- Wide ranging behavioural problems.
- Poor educational achievement.
- Early developmental delay.
- Consistently failing to present for medical appointments.
- Children can often disclose physical abuse (and occasionally sexual abuse) at nursery or school.

The following situations are known to place children at increased risk of abuse:
- Domestic violence – an important and often underestimated risk.
- Mental health problems in either parent or caregiver.
- Parental drug and/or alcohol abuse.
- Previous maltreatment of other children within the family, or parents themselves.
- Disability in the child.

- Known maltreatment of animals by parents or carers.
- Parents who have suffered sexual abuse themselves.
- Vulnerable and/or unsupported parents, including but not limited to particularly young parents, those with learning difficulties, asylum seekers, and those with significant financial concerns.

This highlights the importance of considering safeguarding issues in every child. These more subtle presentations can suggest any category of abuse. It is important to also remember that maltreatment can occur in any setting, without any known risk factors.

Management of Abuse

Initial Assessment

If a child presents to the ED and there is strong suspicion of physical abuse by their primary caregiver, the child should remain in hospital as a place of safety, until it is deemed safe to return home or alternative arrangements are made. Social services should be involved early. Management of child abuse is multidisciplinary and follows a clear pathway (*Figure 5*).

It is important to speak alone to any verbal child (usually three to four-years-old) and document verbatim their account, if they have one. Find out whether they feel happy and safe at home, remembering to avoid using leading questions. One increasingly common way is to ask "If you had three wishes, what would they be?"

This process must maintain an open and honest two-way dialogue throughout with the parents/caregivers. Although medical conditions are ruled out simultaneously, this is not the main reason for admission so should not be conveyed as such. The parents must know that NAI is being considered and that social services and the police may be involved. The clinician can explain that it is their legal duty of care to explore this avenue further in any situation where the injury cannot conclusively be explained accidentally. Safeguarding is one of the few circumstances where confidentiality with the child or the parent may have to be broken. The child's right to be protected from abuse overpowers the right to confidentiality.

Always remember siblings and consider their welfare.

Child Protection Medical

Often injuries are noted or disclosed at school or nursery. In this scenario, social services are notified prior to the medical team. They then arrange a "child protection medical" to be carried out.

A "child protection medical", carried out by a senior paediatric doctor, involves:

- Documenting full and explicit details of the story.
- Comments on the child's behaviour, appearance and interaction.
- A body map drawn with every mark measured and documented (this necessitates fully undressing the child).
- Details of all carers and school/nursery noted, including full names and addresses.

Investigations

During any hospital admission when NAI is suspected, a child may also have the following investigations:

- A skeletal survey where all the bones of the body are X-rayed to look for current or old fractures.
- A CT head to rule out any intracranial bleed or specific patterns of injury associated with NAI –more often in infants.
- An ophthalmology review to look for ophthalmological signs of "shaken baby" (retinal haemorrhages).
- Blood testing to check that coagulation is normal and to exclude any metabolic bone disease in a child with fractures.

Social Services

Social services will gather information from all sources (for example, primary care physician, school nurse, school teachers, midwife and health visitor) and make a decision as to what is in the best interests of the child.

In the UK, this can range from:

- Social services removing the child (or children) from their environment.

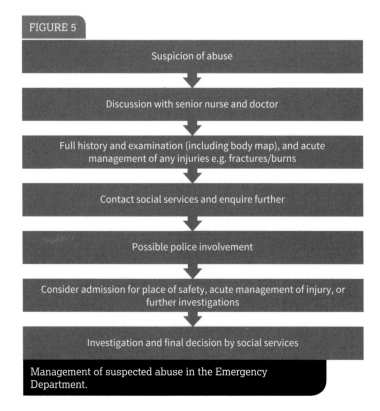

Suspicion of abuse

Discussion with senior nurse and doctor

Full history and examination (including body map), and acute management of any injuries e.g. fractures/burns

Contact social services and enquire further

Possible police involvement

Consider admission for place of safety, acute management of injury, or further investigations

Investigation and final decision by social services

Management of suspected abuse in the Emergency Department.

> The child being made subject to a "child protection plan" (a detailed plan identifying how the child is going to be kept safe).

> The child being made subject to a "child in need plan" (usually for vulnerable children where increased support may be needed but no immediate risk is identified).

> No further involvement.

Sexual Abuse

If sexual abuse is suspected, there are specific pathways to follow. The child should not be examined by an untrained professional. This usually means that if a child presents to the ED and concerns are raised, details of anything disclosed and a general examination of the rest of the body should be documented, including assessment of any risk to immediate health (for example, bleeding after penetrative rape). The story should not be explored in detail.

Sexual Abuse Unit

Once any immediate management has been provided, the child should be referred to the local sexual abuse assessment unit if it is within the last 72 hours (post-pubertal) or the last week (pre-pubertal). If the abuse is longstanding or outside this time frame, the examination is carried out by a trained community paediatrician, but does not need to be time-sensitive. At all times, it must be considered who the possible perpetrator is and whether or not home is a place of safety.

The local sexual abuse assessment unit will be able to offer emergency contraception, sexually transmitted infection (STI) screening and treatment, HIV prophylaxis, hepatitis B vaccinations, forensic evidence collection, counselling and follow up appointments.

Barriers to Appropriate Safeguarding Management

There are many barriers to appropriate recognition of and acting on safeguarding concerns.

> Fear of missing a treatable condition and then being criticised.

> Discomfort of medical professionals in believing parents would lie or cause harm to their child, or fear of wrongly accusing them.

> Cultural beliefs with respect to discipline.

> A desire to maintain positive professional relationships.

> Fear of complaints.

> Stress.

> Personal safety.

> Feeling that there was a justifiable reason for the action which led to maltreatment, with no actual intent to cause harm.

Appropriate Placement of a Child

Decisions about how and where a child should be cared for can be extremely difficult and must take into account positive as well as negative factors at home. There may be many factors that have led to parents maltreating their children, e.g. been in care themselves, poor parenting role models, mental health problems, and learning difficulties, but professionals must advocate for the child. In many cases, increasing support to the parents and providing education can help them provide better for their child's needs. However, if the harm is deemed severe enough, the child/ children may need to be removed and put into foster care. These children are known as "Looked After Children" in the UK.

REFERENCES AND FURTHER READING

Development

1   Bellman M, Lingam S, Aukett A. Schedule of Growing Skills II: User's Guide. Second Edition. London: NFER Nelson Publishing Company Ltd.; 2008.

2   Gardiner M, Eisen S, Murphy C. Training in Paediatrics. Oxford Speciality Training. Oxford UK: Oxford University Press; 2009.

3   Stephenson T, Wallace H, Thompson A. Clinical Paediatrics for Postgraduate Exams. Third Edition. London: Churchill Livingstone; 2003.

4   Shribman S, Billingham K. Healthy Child Programme: Pregnancy and the first 5 years of life. Department of Health. 2009.

5   Weinstock V, Weinstock D, Kraft S. Screening for Childhood Strabismus by primary care physicians. Can Fam Physician. 1998; 44:337-43.

6   Scott O. Vision Testing and Screening in Young Children. 2012. http://patient.info/doctor/Vision-Testing-and-Screening-in-Young-Children.htm.

7   Ansons A, Davis H. Diagnosis and Management of Ocular Motility Disorders. Fourth Edition. Oxford: Wiley Blackwell; 2014.

8   Waggoner T. New Pediatric Color Vision Test For Three to Six Year Old Pre-School Children. http://colorvisiontesting.com/color5.htm.

9   Cardiff Acuity Test. http://www.cardiff.ac.uk/optometry-vision-sciences/research/research-themes/visual-rehabilitation/cardiff-acuity-test.

Developmental Delay

1   Shevell M, et al. Practice Parameter: Evaluation of the child with global developmental delay: Report of the quality standards subcommittee of the American Academy of Neurology and the Practice Committee of the Child Neurology Society. Neurology. 2003; 60:367-80.

2   McDonald L, Rennie A, Tolmie J. Investigation of global developmental delay. Arch Dis Child. 2006; 91:701-5.

3   Cleary M, Green A. Developmental delay: When to suspect and how to investigate for an inborn error of metabolism. Arch Dis Child. 2005; 90:1128-32.

Autistic Spectrum Disorder

1 Kim S. Recent update of autism spectrum disorders. Korean J Pediatr. 2015;58; 8-14.

2 Rutter M. Incidence of autistic spectrum disorders: changes over time, and their meaning. Acta Paediatr. 2005; 94:2-15.

3 NICE Guidelines. CG128. Autism diagnosis in children and young people: Recognition, referral and diagnosis of children and young people on the autism spectrum. 2011. https://www.nice.org.uk/guidance/cg128.

4 NHS Immunisation Information. MMR The Facts. Department of Health Publications. 2004.

5 Dyer C. Lancet retracts Wakefield's MMR paper. BMJ. 2010; 340:c696.

Behavioural Problems

1 NICE Guidelines. CG72. Attention Deficit Hyperactivity Disorder: Diagnosis and management of ADHD in children, young people and adults. 2008. https://www.nice.org.uk/guidance/cg72.

2 McCann D, Barrett A, Cooper A, et al. Food additives and hyperactive behaviour in 3 year olds and 8/9 year olds in the community: a randomised double blinded placebo-controlled trial. Lancet. 2007; 370:1560-7.

Safeguarding

1 NICE Guidelines. CG89. When to Suspect Child Maltreatment. 2009. https://www.nice.org.uk/guidance/cg89.

2 Department for Education. Statutory Guidance: Working together to Safeguard Children. DfE;Ref:DFE-00130-2015; 2015.

3 Maguire S, Mann M. Systematic reviews of bruising in relation to child abuse – what have we learnt: an overview of review updates. Evid. Based Child Health. 2013; 8:255-63.

4 Maguire S, Moynihan S, Mann, M et al. A systematic review of the features that indicate intentional scalds in children. Burns. 2008; 34:1072-81.

5 Maguire S, Cowley L, Mann M, Kemp A. What does the recent literature add to the identification and investigation of fractures in child abuse: an overview of review updates 2005-2013. Evid. Based Child Health. 2013; 8:2044-57.

6 Naughton A, et al. Emotional, behavioural and developmental features indicative of neglect or emotional abuse in preschool children: a systematic review. JAMA Pediatr. 2013; 167:769-75.

7 Core Info – Cardiff Child Protection Systematic Reviews: www.core-info.cardiff.ac.uk.

8 NSPCC. Child Protection Fact Sheet – The definitions and signs of child abuse. NSPCC Inform. 2009.

9 Jutte S, Bentley H, Miller P, Jetha N. How safe are our children? London: NSPCC. 2014.

49

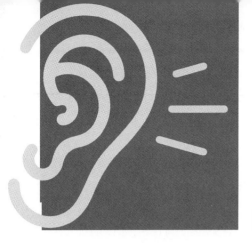

1.05
ENT

ANDREW HALL

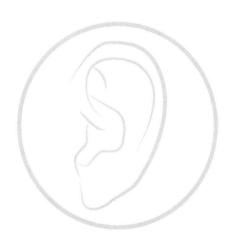
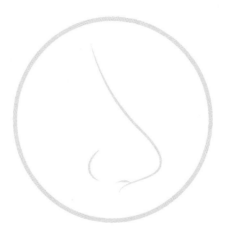
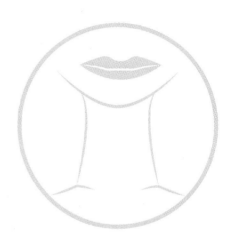

CONTENTS

EAR PATHOLOGY

Hearing Loss

Early detection and intervention of hearing loss allows maximisation of future language and intellectual development. About one to two children in 1000 have at least moderate permanent hearing loss.

Aetiology

Hearing loss is broadly broken down into conductive, sensorineural or mixed:

> Conductive hearing loss (CHL). Sound waves are unable to pass from the opening of the external auditory canal to the inner ear structures. The underlying pathology can involve the external ear canal, tympanic membrane, middle ear or ossicles.

> Sensorineural hearing loss (SNHL). This affects the vestibulocochlear nerve, inner ear structures (cochlea) or the brain itself. There is either a failure in the conversion of acoustic energy received by the cochlea or a failure of neural transmission to the central nervous system.

> Mixed hearing loss. This involves concurrent conductive and sensorineural pathology.

Causes of hearing loss are summarised in *Table 1*. Most children with severe congenital hearing loss have a mutation in the Connexin 26 protein on the GJB2 gene. In addition, some form of hearing loss is found in 75% of all children with Down syndrome. This could be due to developmental abnormality of the inner ear or recurrent otitis media with effusion (OME).

Investigations

Hearing loss is identified through screening tests, as detailed on p39. It may also be specifically screened when hearing loss is suspected, such as in developmental delay or an accidental ingestion of a toxic dose of gentamicin.

Management

Management depends on both the underlying cause and the severity of hearing loss. Formal paediatric audiological input may lead to consideration of cochlear implantation in individuals with profound sensorineural hearing loss who do not benefit from a three month trial of hearing aids.

Otitis Media

Acute middle ear infections are common in the paediatric population, particularly in those 6-months-old to 2–years-old.

Aetiology

The paediatric Eustachian tube is shorter, wider and more horizontal than in adults, making it easier for infection to spread up the tube. Viral infections are more common, but they are difficult to accurately distinguish from bacterial infections on symptoms alone. Bacterial causes include *Streptococcus pneumoniae*, *Haemophilus influenzae* and *Moraxella catarrhalis*, whilst viral causes include respiratory syncytial virus, rhinovirus, adenovirus and parainfluenza virus.

Clinical Features

Symptoms include:

> Otalgia. Children who are unable to vocalise pain may be seen tugging on their affected ear.

> Pyrexia.
> Systemic illness.

A buildup of pus behind the tympanic membrane may lead to spontaneous rupture (perforation) that may discharge blood and fluid. This rupture may be associated with a relief of pain.

On examination with an otoscope, a red, bulging tympanic membrane or perforation of the tympanic membrane may be evident.

Management

Management is based on symptomatic relief. Pain levels should be assessed, and if required, simple analgesia should be prescribed. This is usually all that is required, as most infections are viral and self-limiting. Antibiotic prescribing patterns vary between clinicians. Antibiotic therapy is generally warranted in patients with bilateral otitis media, patients that are systemically unwell, neonates/the very young, and those with persistent non-resolving infection. Penicillins, e.g. amoxicillin, are commonly used.

Complications

> Tympanic membrane perforation. This may occur secondary to the buildup of pus behind the eardrum, resulting in rupture. This may be associated with a conductive hearing loss and risk of future infections.
> Chronic otitis media with effusion.
> Labrynthitis. Infection of the inner ear resulting in vertigo.
> Mastoiditis. See below.

Rarely, intracranial complications are seen from spread of infection, such as abscess formation or meningitis.

Prognosis

Full recovery is usually expected, with no long-term sequelae.

Mastoiditis

Mastoiditis is a result of infection of the mastoid process and is treated aggressively due to potential intracranial spread of infection.

TABLE 1: Causes of hearing loss		
	Conductive (CHL)	Sensorineural (SNHL)
Congenital.	• Down syndrome. • Craniofacial abnormalities e.g. Treacher Collins syndrome.	• Genetic, e.g. Alport syndrome (also associated with nephritis) or Connexin 26 mutation. • Prenatal infection, e.g. toxoplasmosis, rubella, CMV, syphilis.
Acquired.	• Otitis media with effusion. • Wax deposition.	• Perinatal, e.g. birth trauma, hypoxia. • Meningitis. • Ototoxicity, e.g. Gentamycin/Cisplatin.

Clinical Features

Mastoiditis is most commonly seen as a complication of otitis media. It presents with:

> Significant systemic malaise.

> Fever.

> A red, hot, tender swelling over the mastoid.

The pinna itself may protrude anteriorly due to these processes.

Management

This condition warrants urgent Ear, Nose and Throat (ENT) review for assessment. Initial treatment is with broad spectrum intravenous antibiotics, but incision and drainage of the mastoid may be required if an abscess has formed. A CT scan may be organised if there is a concern about a possible intracranial abscess or if the child fails to improve with initial intravenous broad-spectrum antibiotics.

Chronic Otitis Media with Effusion (OME)

This is a painless, chronic inflammation of the middle ear mucosa leading to the buildup of mucus behind the tympanic membrane. It is therefore also called "glue ear". It has a bimodal age incidence, peaking at two and five-years-old.

Aetiology

OME may be caused by infection (acute otitis media is an important risk factor), or fluid may accumulate in the middle ear secondary to Eustachian tube obstruction or dysfunction. It is the most common cause of hearing loss in children.

Clinical Features

Symptoms may include school or parental recognition of hearing loss that may be associated with speech and behavioural problems. Intermittent otalgia can be a feature.

Investigations

Evaluation of hearing (audiometry), eardrum compliance (tympanometry) and an assessment of the ear (otoscopy) allow the diagnosis to be made. On otoscopy, there may be a dull appearance to the eardrum, with a fluid level sometimes visible behind the tympanic membrane.

Management

Intervention is recommended in the presence of:

> Significant symptoms.

> If there is a persistent hearing loss of 25 dB or more in the affected ear for three months.

Insertion of ventilation tubes (i.e. grommets) improves hearing in children with OME for up to 12 months after surgery. A grommet is a hollow tube that punctures the tympanic membrane, and remains in place to prevent the buildup of fluid behind the ear. Another treatment option is hearing aids. This is preferred in children with Down syndrome, where narrow ear canals can make grommets more difficult to insert and subsequently monitor.

Complications

Cholesteatoma is a potential complication of untreated OME. This abnormal collection of skin cells grows and expands within the middle ear and mastoid process, potentially damaging the ossicles. If identified, it is treated with surgery.

Prognosis

OME resolves spontaneously in 90% of children within one year.

NASAL PATHOLOGY

Rhinosinusitis

Rhinitis (inflammation of the nasal lining), rhinosinusitis (inflammation of the nose and paranasal sinuses) and sinusitis (inflammation of the sinuses) represent a spectrum of disease that can be acute or chronic. A majority of paediatric nasal complaints are related to symptoms of nasal obstruction, rhinorrhoea (runny nose), sneezing and snoring. An important potential complication of acute rhinosinusitis is periorbital cellulitis. Most infective cases of rhinosinusitis are viral and self-limiting, whilst allergic causes usually respond to simple antihistamines.

Nasal Polyps

Nasal polyps are rarely found on clinical examination in children, and if present, cystic fibrosis and primary ciliary dyskinesia should be investigated. Most commonly, a diagnosis of nasal polyposis is made in error due to failure to recognise the normal anatomy of the inferior turbinate which can be particularly bulky in children.

Epistaxis

Nosebleeds are commonly encountered in childhood affecting between one-third and two-thirds of all children at some time. It is important to recognise that, in patients less than two-years-old, non-accidental injury is a possible cause.

Management

Paediatric epistaxis is generally idiopathic and can be managed largely in the outpatient setting. There is generally no underlying systemic vascular or haematological abnormality. Despite this, it is important to take a thorough bleeding history of these patients to assess whether the haematology team needs to be involved in their investigation and management.

Topical antiseptic cream in the form of bactroban or naseptin is used as first line therapy. If unsuccessful, nasal cautery of blood vessels can be performed.

UPPER AIRWAY OBSTRUCTION

Stertor and Stridor

Paediatric airway obstruction can range from noisy breathing in an otherwise well child to a respiratory arrest. Identification of the approximate level of obstruction from the nose to the bronchi may be achieved by recognising the distinction between stertor and stridor.

Upper airway obstruction is a medical emergency that can evolve quickly and is best managed by a multidisciplinary team involving paediatricians, ENT surgeons and anaesthetists.

Stertor

This is partial obstruction of the airway with low-pitched snoring produced by vibrations above the level of larynx. *Table 2* shows the differential diagnosis.

Chronic stertor is often caused by adenoid and tonsillar hypertrophy and may indicate the presence of obstructive sleep apnoea. This requires referral to ENT surgeons for consideration of adenotonsillectomy. It is also important to inquire regarding nasal symptoms as to the possibility of a nasal foreign body.

Stridor

This is an audible change in airflow at the level of larynx, trachea or bronchi. Inspiratory stridor indicates turbulent airflow above the vocal cords. Expiratory stridor indicates turbulent airflow in the trachea or bronchi (comparable with wheeze). Biphasic stridor has an inspiratory and expiratory component and is related to pathology located at the level of the vocal cords or subglottis (just beneath the vocal cords).

The differential diagnosis for acute stridor includes croup, epiglottitis, bacterial tracheitis, anaphylaxis and foreign bodies. These will be explored in detail in this chapter. *Table 3* summarises the common causes of chronic stridor. Differentiating between acute and chronic causes of paediatric stridor on history and examination alone can be difficult.

Where there is diagnostic uncertainty or clinical concern, a referral to the ENT team is appropriate for consideration of microlaryngobronchoscopy to evaluate the airway.

Airway Foreign Body

Airway foreign bodies are commonly encountered in children.

Nasal Foreign Body

When identified in the nose, the potential for migration further into the airway necessitates early removal, under anaesthetic if required. A foreign body can usually be removed using simple forceps or by making a seal over the lips, occluding the unaffected nostril, and blowing in the mouth (often done by the mother). This is known as the "kissing technique" or "parent's kiss" (*Figure 1*). Unilateral, offensive nasal discharge may be a presenting symptom of a chronic nasal foreign body.

Distal Foreign Body

A child with a history of coughing or choking on feeding should be carefully evaluated for an airway foreign body. Symptoms are dependent on location and can range from audible stridor and respiratory distress to an asymptomatic child. The bronchus is a worrying site for lodging of an inhaled foreign body, and in older children, this more commonly occurs in the right main bronchus.

A chest X-ray (both inspiratory and expiratory films) allows assessment of the foreign body itself and of any associated airway collapse or air trapping-associated obstruction. In chronic obstruction, there may be a secondary infection.

Bronchoscopic airway evaluation and removal may be required.

Choking

This is usually witnessed in preschool children with a sudden attack of stridor and respiratory distress, secondary to food or foreign body obstruction.

Effective Cough

A conscious child with an effective cough (audible cry/speech, loud cough) should be regularly observed and encouraged to cough.

Ineffective Cough

If the cough is ineffective (inaudible cry/speech, unable to breathe, cyanotic), assistance is required. Five back blows

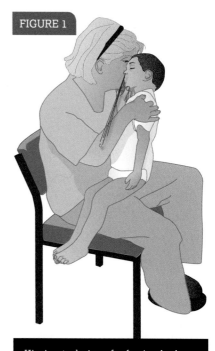

FIGURE 1

Kissing technique for foreign body removal from nostril. A good seal is made around the mouth, the other nostril is occluded and the parent blows forcefully into the patient's mouth.

TABLE 2: Differential diagnosis for stertor		
STERTOR	**Acute**	**Chronic**
Obstruction at level of nose/pharynx.	Tonsillitis.	Enlarged adenoids/tonsils.
	Peritonsillar abscess.	Nasal foreign body.
	Infectious mononucleosis.	
	Nasal foreign body.	

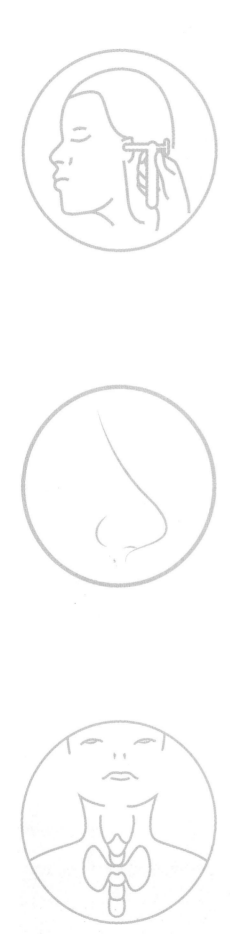

TABLE 3: Causes of chronic stridor

	Laryngomalacia	Subglottic Stenosis	Subglottic haemangioma	Tracheomalacia	Vocal Cord Palsy	Chronic obstruction with foreign body
Age group affected.	• From birth, usually resolved by 2-years-old.	• Any age.	• Typically 2-4 months of age.	• First year of life.	• Any.	• More likely in younger children.
Presentation.	• Stridor worse on feeding/crying.	• Recurrent episodes of stridor. • Poor exercise tolerance.	• Progressively worsening stridor. • Barking cough.	• Cyanotic episodes.	• Altered cry. • Rarely sole cause of stridor.	• Recurrent chest infection (although significant obstruction presents acutely, with breathlessness and stridor).
Risk factors.	• Prematurity. • Neuromuscular disorders.	• Previous intubation. • Down syndrome.	• Cutaneous haemangiomas.	• Prematurity — congenital deformity of tracheal rings. • Extrinsic pressure — neighbouring blood vessels. • Previous repair of oesophageal atresia.	• Intra-thoracic surgery/pathology.	• Learning difficulties. • Parental neglect.
Findings.	• Aryepiglottic folds "indraw" on inspiration.	• Narrow subglottis.	• Haemangioma in subglottis.	• Tracheal compression, e.g. from thymoma.	• Vocal cord in intermediate position.	• Stridor. • Wheeze. • Difficulty breathing.
Treatment.	• Not required in 90% of cases. • Anti-reflux. • If faltering growth-surgical evaluation.	• Varies from observation to ballooning of the stenosis or laryngotracheal reconstruction.	• Propranolol. • May have adjuvant laser debulking to reduce the size.	• May be managed conservatively but if severe surgery can be performed (aortopexy) to relieve pressure on trachea.	• Conservative.	• Removal of foreign body- in ED or under general anaesthetic.

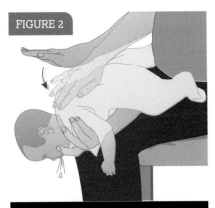

FIGURE 2

Back blow. The infant is placed over the leg to allow gravity to assist. The centre of the infant's back is struck firmly with the palm of the hand five times. In an older child, this is done keeping them upright, but bending them forward at the waist.

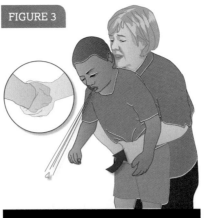

FIGURE 3

Abdominal thrust. Previously called the Heimlich manoeuvre. The person performing the manoeuvre makes a fist with one hand, and grabs it with the other. They then rapidly pull back and upwards through the abdomen to deliver each thrust.

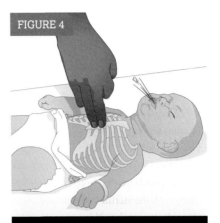

FIGURE 4

Chest thrusts. This has a similar technique to chest compressions. Two fingers are placed at the base of the sternum. Five thrusts are then delivered, compressing downward about 1.5 inches.

(*Figure 2*) should be delivered, followed by five abdominal thrusts in children more than one–year-old (*Figure 3*), or five chest thrusts in children less than 1–year-old (*Figure 4*). The patient should be reassessed after each intervention, and the process should be repeated as necessary.

Unconscious Child

In a very severe obstruction, the child may become unconscious. In this case, attempt to remove anything seen in the mouth with one finger sweep, and then follow the paediatric basic life support, giving rescue breaths.

INFECTION

Periorbital and Orbital Cellulitis

Periorbital Cellulitis

Periorbital cellulitis is infection and inflammation of the skin and eyelid anterior to the orbital septum (unlike orbital cellulitis). This condition can be secondary to a sinus infection, but can also be due to a minor scratch or insect bite. In its most minor form, there is mild eyelid swelling without any systemic symptoms.

Orbital Cellulitis

Progress of periorbital cellulitis can lead to intra-orbital spread of infection causing orbital cellulitis, with red flag signs of proptosis (bulging of the eye), limitation of eye movement and chemosis (conjunctival swelling). Colour vision and visual acuity are important to document, as these are sensitive features of optic nerve inflammation. A paramount concern is the potential for optic nerve injury and permanent loss of sight. Intracranial spread of the infection can occur on rare occasions.

Management

This condition is best managed with a multi-disciplinary approach involving paediatric, ENT, maxillofacial and ophthalmology teams.

Minor cases of periorbital cellulitis usually settle with oral antibiotics. Moderate cases need intravenous therapy. If concerns exist of intra-orbital infection, a computed tomography (CT) scan of the brain/orbit needs to be arranged urgently. Surgical intervention may require either an external or endoscopic approach to drain the pus, depending on the extent and position of the pathology.

Tonsillitis

Aetiology

Tonsillitis involves inflammation of the tonsils. It may be viral or bacterial in origin. Bacterial causes are more likely in the absence of cough, tender cervical lymphadenopathy, high fever and tonsillar exudates. Classically, bacterial infection is with group A streptococcus.

Clinical Features

Clinical features include:
› Sore throat.
› Pain on swallowing (odynophagia).
› Fever.
› Headache.
› Reduced oral intake.

On examination, the tonsils are red and enlarged with possible tonsillar exudate (*Figure 5*). Cervical lymph nodes may also be enlarged and tender. Simple analgesia, antipyretics and adequate

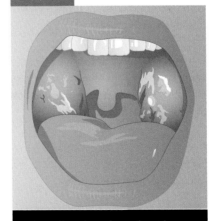

FIGURE 5

Bilaterally enlarged tonsils with exudate.

hydration are required. Antibiotics are not routinely indicated, as the majority of cases are viral.

Management

If group A streptococcus is suspected or found on a throat swab, a ten day course of penicillin V should be prescribed.

Rarely, severe swelling may precipitate stertor and dysphagia. In such cases, IV antibiotics (e.g. benzylpenicillin) are warranted, and IV fluids may be required for maintenance of hydration. Corticosteroids may be initiated to reduce mucosal oedema and reduce both the stertor and pain associated with swallowing.

Tonsillectomy should be considered if the episodes are recurrent (i.e. five or more cases a year), and the episodes are disruptive to everyday functioning.

Peritonsillar Abscess (Quinsy)

Clinical Features

The patient classically appears toxic with a high temperature and may suffer from trismus (inability to open the mouth), making assessment very difficult. On speaking, patients characteristically have "hot potato voice", where their vowels are distorted. Due to difficulty swallowing, drooling may also be present. Other features include lethargy, pain on swallowing, and malaise. If there is airway obstruction, cyanosis/breathing abnormalities may also occur.

The affected tonsil, soft palate and uvula are pushed towards the centre of the mouth.

Management

Quinsy is the most common ENT emergency. Treatment typically includes aspiration/drainage of the abscess by the ENT team and intravenous antibiotics.

Infectious Mononucleosis (Glandular Fever)

Infectious mononucleosis (glandular fever) can affect children of any age, but is more common in teenagers.

Aetiology

It is caused by the Epstein-Barr virus (EBV). It is sometimes called "kissing disease" as the virus can spread by droplet infection and direct contact.

Clinical Features

Patients present with generalised malaise, enlarged exudative tonsils, cervical lymphadenopathy, fever and hepatosplenomegaly.

Investigations

To confirm infectious mononucleosis, a Monospot test or EBV serology can be performed.

Management

Treatment is largely supportive, with fluids and analgesia, but antibiotics may be recommended to treat any superadded bacterial infection. Amoxicillin and ampicillin should not be prescribed as they can cause a generalised, itchy, salmon pink rash. Steroids may be considered in the event of dysphagia to reduce inflammation.

Croup

Croup (acute laryngotracheobronchitis) occurs as a result of a viral infection, most commonly parainfluenza and influenza virus in children under the age of two.

Clinical Features

Classically, croup presents with a barking cough, which can particularly distress parents. Symptoms are more severe at night, but the onset is insidious over several days with an initial viral coryzal prodrome. Mucosal inflammation results in airway narrowing and increased secretions within the larynx, trachea and bronchi.

Management

Treatment of croup is based on severity (*Table 4*). Most croup is mild and managed in primary care or the ED. Moderate cases require corticosteroid treatment to reduce airway inflammation. In more severe cases, with significant airway narrowing, adrenaline and supplemental oxygen may be given. In the worst cases, intubation and ventilation or an emergency surgical airway may be required.

Acute Epiglottitis

Aetiology

This condition describes acute severe swelling of the epiglottis and aryepiglottic folds secondary to a *Haemophilus influenzae* type b (Hib) bacterial infection. This is now very rare due to widespread vaccination. It mainly affects children three to five-years-old and can progress rapidly over several hours.

Clinical Features

Epiglottitis is usually rapid in onset, with severe symptoms, including high fever, drooling/dysphagia, and significant distress. There may be stridor, laboured breathing and a muffled/quiet voice.

Management

Never do anything to upset a child with epiglottitis as this may precipitate full airway obstruction. This includes examining their throat or ears, taking blood or inserting a cannula (without an anaesthetist being present).

Treatment of acute epiglottitis involves protecting the airway as the first priority. This may require intubation or even a surgical airway if there is significant swelling. Broad spectrum antibiotics (e.g. a third generation cephalosporin) should be promptly started, and steroids or adrenaline nebulisers may be needed.

Table 5 summarises key differences between croup and acute epiglottitis.

TABLE 4: Croup assessment (Modified Westley Clinical Scoring System)		
Symptom/Sign	**Degree**	**Points awarded**
Inspiratory stridor.	Not present.	0
	When agitated/active.	1
	At rest.	2
Intercostal recession.	Mild.	1
	Moderate.	2
	Severe.	3
Air entry.	Normal.	0
	Mildly decreased.	1
	Severely decreased.	2
Cyanosis.	None.	0
	With agitation/activity.	4
	At rest.	5
Level of consciousness.	Normal.	0
	Altered.	5

Total score <4=mild croup, 4-6=moderate croup, >6=severe croup

TABLE 5: Comparison of croup and acute epiglottitis		
	Croup (acute laryngotracheobronchitis)	**Epiglottitis**
Voice.	Hoarse.	Muffled/quiet.
Coryzal.	Yes.	No.
Fever.	<38.5°C.	>38.5°C.
Cough.	Barking, prominent feature.	Slight, not prominent feature.
Appearance.	Well.	Toxic.
Drooling.	Unlikely.	Yes, very painful to swallow.
Treatment.	Dependent on severity: Mild: no specific treatment. Moderate: oral steroids. Severe: may require adrenaline, oxygen, intubation, surgical airway.	Steroids, adrenaline nebulisers and IV antibiotics – usually ceftriaxone. Urgent involvement of senior anaesthetist and ENT surgeons with early intubation under general anaesthetic. Occasionally urgent tracheostomy is the only way to secure the airway.

Bacterial Tracheitis (Pseudomembranous Croup)

This is caused by *Staphylococcus aureus* infection and presents with similar clinical features to acute epiglottitis. Bacterial invasion of the trachea results in pseudomembrane formation with purulent secretions unresponsive to conventional management. These patients require broad spectrum antibiotics and may require prolonged intubation, with endoscopic removal of the secretions.

PAEDIATRIC NECK MASSES

Most cervical lymphadenopathy in paediatrics is non-malignant. Utilising a structured method of clinical assessment ensures that the correct diagnosis is made whilst rationalising the number of investigations required.

Red flags for urgent senior help/ENT referral include:
- Sepsis.
- Unwell child.
- Stridor/airway compromise.
- Difficulty swallowing.
- Change in voice quality.
- Rapid progression.

There are a wide variety of causes for palpable neck masses in paediatrics. Key differential diagnoses to consider and subsequent investigations are summarised in *Table 6*. Neck lumps can be very large as with the example of a cystic hygroma in *Figure 6*.

FIGURE 6

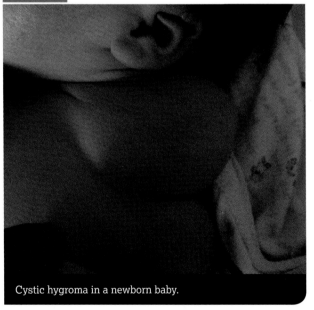

Cystic hygroma in a newborn baby.

TABLE 6: Causes of paediatric neck lumps				
Diagnosis	Description	Clinical Features	Key Investigations	Management
Lymphadenitis (Reactive lymph node swelling)	Infective.	• Generalised cervical lymphadenopathy. • Upper respiratory tract infection.	• Elevated white blood cell count secondary to acute infection.	• Consideration of antibiotics, and surgical drainage of any abscess.
Infectious Mononucleosis (Glandular fever)	Infective.	• Teenagers. • Large, tender, bilateral lymphadenopathy. • Sore throat and malaise. • May be associated hepatosplenomegaly and axillary lymphadenopathy.	• Elevated neutrophils secondary to acute infection. • Positive Monospot. • Liver/splenic USS may show hepatitis/splenomegaly.	• Rehydration and supportive treatment.
Mycobacterium tuberculosis	Infective.	• Painless neck lump. • Can develop discharge/abscess. • Sinus formation. • Associated fever/history of TB risk factors.	• Mantoux test. • CXR: apical consolidation/ cavitation/nodules.	• TB treatment. • Avoid surgical excision as it can result in chronic infection.
Atypical Mycobacterium	Infective.	• Classically occurs at 2 to 5-years-old, likely ingested from soil. • Bright red, enlarged lymph node.	• Mantoux test. • Avoid biopsy as can lead to chronic sinus — remove whole node.	• Spontaneous resolution in most cases but scarring prominent. • Surgical excision of whole node.
Branchial cyst	Congenital.	• Teenagers and young adults. • Located at anterior border of the sternocleidomastoid at the junction of the upper and middle thirds.	• USS will identify a cystic mass.	• Antibiotics to treat any acute infection. • Excision under general anaesthetic.
Thyroglossal cyst	Congenital.	• 90% of midline neck swellings in children. • Embryologically derived from the thyroid gland which descends from the tongue in utero. • Failed atrophy of tract- lump moves on tongue protrusion.	• USS visualises tract and establishes presence of underlying thyroid gland.	• Antibiotics to treat any acute infection. • Excision if recurrent infections.
Lymphatic malformation (cystic hygroma)	Vascular.	• Rare, sponge-like lesions in neonatal period or early infancy. • They can fluctuate in size due to infection and some cause facial disfigurement and airway obstruction.	• USS demonstrates underlying anatomy.	• May need tracheostomy if airway compromised although rare. • Sclerotherapy and possible surgical excision.
Malignancy	Neoplastic.	• Systemic symptoms — fever, weight loss, night sweats. • Often isolated, firm, enlarging, painless lymph node swelling. • Axillary/inguinal lymphadenopathy. • Hepatosplenomegaly.	• Anaemia/Immature blast cells on blood film. Normal blood film does not exclude diagnosis. • Excision biopsy to formally exclude if suspected.	• Dependent on diagnosis. • May include surgery, chemotherapy or radiotherapy.

REFERENCES AND FURTHER READING

Hearing Loss

1   Wilson C, Roberts A, Stephens D. Aetiological investigation of sensorineural hearing loss in children. Arch Dis Child. 2005;90:307-9.

Otitis Media

1   Coker TR et al. Diagnosis, microbial epidemiology, and antibiotic treatment of acute otitis media in children: a systematic review. *JAMA*. 2010; 304:2161-9.

2   Wald ER. To treat or not to treat. Pediatrics. 2005; 115:1087-89.

Otitis Media with Effusion

1   Browning GG et al. Grommets (ventilation tubes) for hearing loss associated with otitis media with effusion in children. Cochrane Database Syst Rev. 2010 6; CD001801.

2   NICE guideline CG60. Otitis media with effusion in under 12s. http://www.nice.org.uk/guidance/cg60 /resources.

Mastoiditis

1 Cohen-Kerem R et al. Acute mastoiditis in children: is surgical treatment necessary? J Laryngol Otol. 1999; 113:1081.

Rhinosinusitis

1 Jones NS. Current concepts in the management of paediatric rhinosinusitis. J Laryngol Otol. 1999 Jan; 113:1-9.

Nasal Polyps

1 Gysin C, Alothman GA, Papsin BC Sinonasal disease in cystic fibrosis: clinical characteristics, diagnosis, and management. Paediatr Pulmonol. 2000; 30:481ysti.

Epistaxis

1 McGarry G. Nosebleeds in children. Clin Evid. 2006;15:496-9.

Periorbital Cellulitis

1 Baring DE, Hilmi OJ. An evidence based review of periorbital cellulitis. Clin Otolaryngol. 2011; 36:57-64.

Stertor and Stridor

1 Kuo M, Rothera M. Emergency Management of the Paediatric Airway. In: Graham JM, Scadding GK, Bull PD. Paediatric ENT First Edition. Berlin: Springer-Verlag; 2007. 183-7.

Airway Foreign Body

1 Rodray Fo, H., Passali, GC, Gregori D., et al, Management of foreign bodies in the airway and oesophagus. Int. J. Pediatr. Otorhinolaryngol. 2012;76:84.

2 Benjamin E. Harcourt J. The modified 'Parent's Kiss' for the removal of paediatric nasal foreign bodies. Clin Otolaryngol. 2007; 32:120-1.

Choking

1 ALSG Paediatric Choking Algorithm. 2015. https://www.resus.org.uk/EasySiteWeb/GatewayLink.aspx?alId=6458

Tonsillitis

1 Burton MJ, Glasziou PP. Tonsillectomy or adeno-tonsillectomy versus non-surgical treatment for chronic/recurrent acute tonsillitis. Evid Based Child Health. 2009; 4:1291.

2 Wilson JA et al. Tonsillectomy: a cost-effective option for childhood sore throat? Further analysis of a randomized controlled trial. Otolaryngol Head Neck Surg. 2011; 146:122-8.

Peritonsillar Abscess

1 Hsiao HJ, Huang YC, Hsia SH, Wu CT, Lin J.J. Clinical features of peritonsillar abscess in children. Pediatr Neonatol. 2012; 53:366-70.

Glandular Fever

1 Luzuriaga K, Sullivan JL. Infectious mononucleosis N Engl J Med. 2010; 362:1993-2000.

Croup

1 Bjornson C, Russell K, Foisy M, Johnson DW. The Cochrane Library and the treatment of croup in children: an overview of reviews Evid Based Child Health. 2010; 5: 1555d.l

Acute Epiglottitis

1 Acevedo JL, Lander L, Choi S, Shah RK. Airway management in pediatric epiglottitis: a national perspective. Otolaryngol Head Neck Surg. 2009 140(4):548-51.

Bacterial Tracheitis

1 Al-Mutairi B, Kirk V. Bacterial tracheitis in children: Approach to diagnosis and treatment. Paediatr Child Health. 2004; 9: 25.

Neck Masses

1 Hartley B. Head and Neck Masses. In: Graham JM, Scadding GK, Bull PD. Paediatric ENT First Edition. Berlin: Springer-Verlag; 2007. 111-22.

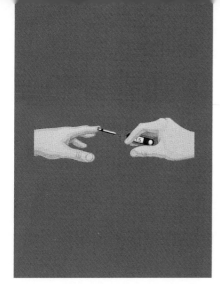

1.06
ENDOCRINOLOGY

ZESHAN QURESHI, VAITSA TZIAFERI, SADHANANDHAM PUNNIYAKODI, MARYLYN-JANE EMEDO AND CLAIRE BRYANT

CONTENTS

GLUCOSE REGULATION

Type 1 Diabetes Mellitus

Diabetes mellitus (DM) is a condition of elevated plasma glucose. There are two main types:
- Type 1 diabetes (T1DM). An absolute deficiency of the pancreatic hormone insulin.
- Type 2 diabetes (T2DM). Failure to appropriately make use of insulin to metabolise glucose.

The vast majority of cases in childhood are T1DM, although with the increasing obesity rates, T2DM is becoming more common. The World Health Organisation (WHO) has formulated a set of diagnostic criteria based on blood glucose measurements, dependent on the presence or absence of typical symptoms of the disorder (*Figure 1*).

Aetiology

T1DM is characterised by autoimmune T-cell mediated damage to the β islet cells of the pancreas. The β cells are responsible for insulin production and their destruction leads to insulin deficiency. Normally, insulin acts to reduce blood glucose through stimulating glucose uptake from the blood,

Diagnosis of diabetes (WHO criteria)

Symptomatic
- FPG> 7.0mmol/L <u>OR</u>
- random PG> 11.1mmol/L

Asymptomatic
- 2 FPGs > 7.0mmol/L OR
- 2 random PG > 11.1mmol/L OR
- 1 of each of the above OR
- OGTT-PG>11.1mmol/L 2 hours post ingestion of 75g glucose
- HbA1C > 48 mmol/mol (6.5%)

FIGURE 1

WHO criteria for diagnosis of Type 1 diabetes (FPG=Fasting Plasma Glucose, PG= Plasma Glucose, OGTT=Oral Glucose Tolerance Test). Adapted from "Definition and diagnosis of diabetes mellitus and intermediate hyperglycaemia": Report of a WHO/IDF consultation.

stimulating glycolysis, reducing liver gluconeogenesis and glycogenolysis. *Table 1* summarises the role of insulin in glucose regulation. Note that insulin also stimulates triglyceride production from blood lipids and reduces lipolysis.

Glucagon is the main counter regulatory hormone to insulin. Its predominant role is to raise blood glucose by stimulating glycogen breakdown in the liver. The interaction of the two hormones is summarised in *Figure 2*.

The insulin deficiency of T1DM leads to elevated glucose concentration in the blood (hyperglycaemia). The cause of the lack of insulin is not entirely clear. It is multifactorial, resulting from an interaction between genetic predisposition and environmental triggering factors:

➤ **Genetic susceptibility.** Genetic factors are suggested by the familial nature of DM. Concordance between identical twins has been found to be 30-50%. Those with a first degree relative with diabetes have an approximately six percent risk of developing the disorder compared to the less than one percent background risk. The HLA-DR3 and HLA-DR4 regions of the genome are associated with an increased risk of developing T1DM. HLA-DR2 and HLA-DR5 appear to be protective.

➤ **Environmental factors.** Studies have indicated that exposure to certain viruses (e.g. enteroviruses, cytomegalovirus [CMV] and mumps), early cow's milk consumption and other dietary factors (e.g. early gluten exposure) may act as triggers in

children with an underlying genetic predisposition.

Clinical Features
Often children are diagnosed with DM following a short history (weeks) of the classic symptoms and signs. A formal oral glucose tolerance test (OGTT) is rarely required for T1DM. Some children may have a first presentation of DM with diabetic ketoacidosis (DKA) and may present extremely unwell.

The 4Ts Mnemonic may help remember the classical signs of diabetes: Toilet, Thirsty, Thinner, Tired.

Classic Signs
➤ Toilet. Polyuria (+/- secondary enuresis).
➤ Thirsty. Polydipsia.
➤ Thinner. Weight Loss.
➤ Tired. Fatigue.

Additional Signs
➤ Polyphagia. Excess hunger/eating.
➤ Recurrent infections.
➤ Abdominal pain. As a presentation of DKA.

Investigations
Although blood glucose level is sufficient to diagnosis DM, further tests can help establish possible aetiology, possible associations and baseline biochemical parameters before starting any treatment.
➤ Full blood count (FBC). There may be anaemia (with chronic disease, poor nutrition or associated pernicious anaemia), or an elevated white cell count (as part of the DM disease process, or an infection).
➤ Urea and electrolytes (U&Es). It is important to gauge baseline renal function, as this may become compromised.
➤ Liver function tests/Bone profile. This is useful as a baseline parameter. There may be later liver damage.
➤ Glycated haemoglobin (HbA1c). This can be used to identify average blood glucose levels over a three month interval. It is a good baseline

TABLE 1: Actions of insulin on glucose regulation	
Inhibition of processes that raise plasma glucose	Stimulation of processes that lower plasma glucose
• Reduced gluconeogenesis (production of glucose from non-glucose substrates) primarily in the liver.	• Increased glucose uptake into fat/muscle cells.
• Reduced glycogenolysis (breakdown of glycogen to glucose).	• Increased conversion of glucose to glycogen in the liver and muscles.

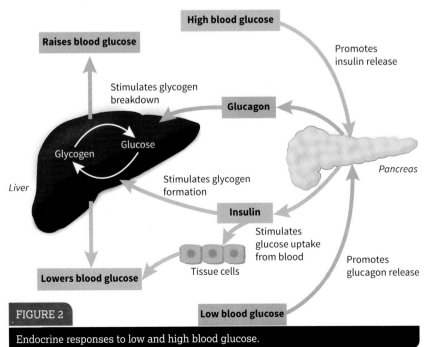

FIGURE 2
Endocrine responses to low and high blood glucose.

to assess glucose control over the coming months.

> Thyroid-stimulating hormone (TSH), thyroid auto-antibodies and coeliac autoantibodies. Hypothyroidism and coeliac disease are both associated with T1DM.
> Anti-islet cell antibodies and anti-glutamic acid decarboxylase (GAD) antibodies. These are associated with T1DM, and are particularly useful if the diagnosis is not clear.

Differential Diagnosis

The diagnosis is usually clear from the history, but polyuria and polydipsia may be associated with compulsive water drinking or diabetes insipidus.

Management

Children with T1DM require exogenous insulin, delivered either by subcutaneous injection several times a day or by continuous infusion via an insulin pump. The types of insulin are summarised in *Table 2*.

Choosing the insulin regimen is dependent on the individual (*Table 3*).

> Multiple daily injections (MDI). The multiple daily injection regime is usually first choice for young people who can take ownership of monitoring their blood glucose. It involves adjusting insulin dosage based on glucose readings, meal contents, and lifestyle choices (e.g. exercise). A twice daily injection regime may be considered in those not able to cope with the demands of MDI despite appropriate education and psychosocial support.
> Insulin pump therapy. Insulin pump therapy is recommended where multiple daily injection regimes have failed, and there is high commitment from the family to use it properly. It may also be considered if there is a strong patient preference, and it matches lifestyle needs.
> Pancreatic transplantation. In the future, pancreatic transplantation is a potential definitive treatment for T1DM, but has major risks, and requires lifelong immunosuppressive therapy.

Wider Management

Children with DM will usually be managed in secondary or tertiary care, by a multidisciplinary team experienced in working with young people and families (*Figure 3*). Long-term control is monitored by measuring HbA1c levels, which reflect average glycaemic control over the lifespan of an erythrocyte (two to three months). The level recommended for children is usually <7.5% (58mmol), which is desirable if this level of control does not induce severe recurrent hypoglycaemia. An HbA1c of persistently >7.5% is associated with a greater risk of long-term complications.

DM is a chronic condition, requiring active management by the child's caregivers. Thus one of the most important steps is educating children and their families:

TABLE 2: Insulin types

Insulin type	Common brand names	Onset of action	Peak	Duration
Rapid acting.	• NovoRapid, Humalog, Apidra.	• 10-15mins.	• 1 hour.	• 2-5 hours.
Short acting.	• Actrapid, Humulin S.	• 30-60 mins.	• 2-4 hours.	• 8 hours.
Intermediate acting.	• Insulatard, Humulin I.	• 1-2 hours.	• 4-12 hours.	• 12-18 hours.
Long acting.	• Lantus, Levemir.	• 2-4 hours.	• Plateaus.	• 12-24 hours.

TABLE 3: Insulin regimens

Regimen	Insulin	Advantages	Disadvantages/ Challenges	Indication
Multiple daily injections (MDI) aka "basal bolus" regimen.	• A long acting insulin plus a short/rapid acting insulin are given to cover meals.	• It is flexible and can be adjusted according to meals. • It is more physiological.	• This requires more injections throughout the day.	• Good for those with variable diets/exercise patterns. • Good for those comfortable with multiple injections and with adjusting insulin doses.
Insulin pump.	• A continuous subcutaneous infusion of short acting insulin with boluses for meals.	• This improves quality of life. • There is a reduction in severe hypoglycaemic episodes. • It is the most physiological.	• This requires a high level of family commitment.	• When the MDI regimen has failed.
2 injections per day.	• A short/rapid acting insulin mixed with intermediate acting insulin.	• Fewer injections are required per day.	• This is less flexible. • It is more difficult to control blood glucose.	• This is rarely used nowadays. • Good for those unable to give multiple injections throughout the day.

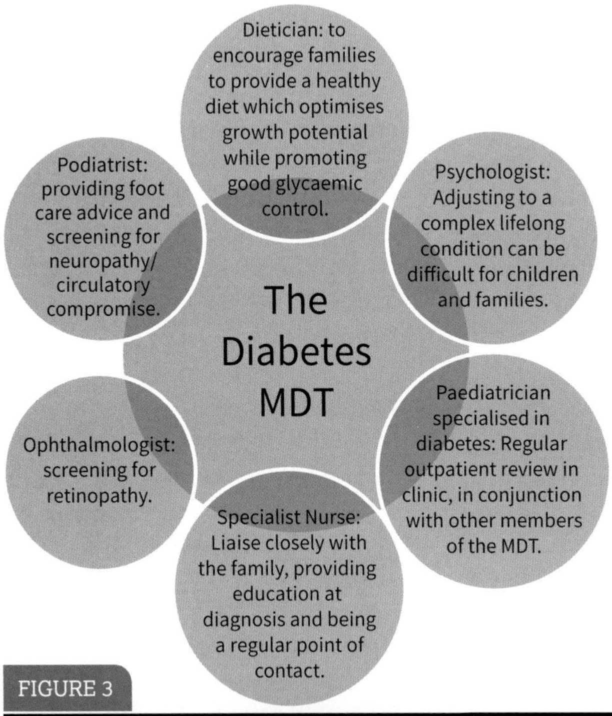

FIGURE 3

Multidisciplinary approach to managing diabetes. (MDT: multidisciplinary team).

> Insulin regimes and dietary advice. Some families learn to "carbohydrate count", titrating insulin dosage to carbohydrate intake.
> Subcutaneous injection. Instruct on the correct technique, and importance of rotating sites.
> Blood glucose monitoring. Families should know when to check glucose, and how to respond to high and low glucose. Children should aim for a blood glucose between 4-8 mmol/L, and <10 mmol/L after meals.
> Short-term glucose control. Give advice regarding avoidance, recognition and management of hypo and hyperglycaemia in the short term.
> Sick day rules. Give advice regarding DM during acute illness. The physiological stress of infection can cause temporary insulin resistance, with reduced oral intake making glucose excursions unpredictable. Blood glucose should be monitored more closely, with correction doses of insulin given if hyperglycaemic.

Complications

Diabetic Ketoacidosis (DKA)

DKA is the triad of ketonaemia, hyperglycaemia and acidosis. It is dealt with on p64.

Hypoglycaemia (blood glucose <4mmol/L)

Low blood glucose can be caused by a number of factors, including:
> Relative excess of insulin.
> Increased utilisation of glucose such as during physical activity.
> Inadequate consumption of glucose containing foods.

TABLE 4: Symptoms of hypoglycaemia

Stimulation of sympathetic nervous system (sympathomimetic).	Anxiety.
	Tachycardia.
	Headache.
	Abdominal pain.
CNS effects (neuroglycopaenic).	Ataxia.
	Weakness.
	Confusion.
	Personality change.
	Seizures.
	Coma.

This can often be prevented by having high carbohydrate meals before strenuous exercise and by carefully monitoring blood glucose levels. *Table 4* summarises the symptoms of hypoglycaemia. Note that neuroglycopaenic symptoms come after sympathomimetic symptoms.

Management of hypoglycaemia depends on level of consciousness.

If the patient is conscious:
> Give 10–20g of rapidly absorbed glucose orally, e.g. three to four glucose tablets, a glass of fruit juice or three teaspoons of sugar/jam. Giving glucose preparation (e.g. Glucogel) into the buccal mucosa may also be considered.
> Re-check glucose within 15 minutes and repeat if necessary.
> Consider following on with complex carbohydrate, e.g. digestive biscuit, toast.

If the patient has a depressed level of consciousness, treatment may involve:
> Intramuscular or subcutaneous glucagon (if out of hospital/ difficult IV access).
> 2mL/kg of 10% glucose, followed by a glucose infusion.

Long-term Complications

Long-term complications with DM are classified as microvascular and macrovascular disease. They are much more common in type 2 DM, partly because there is usually a greater lag time between onset of disease and formal diagnosis.

Microvascular Disease

> Retinopathy. This is screened for annually from 12-years-old. Diabetic retinopathy is the most common cause of blindness in young adults in the UK. Cataracts are also more common in patients with DM.
> Nephropathy. One in three people with DM develop a degree of renal impairment. Annual renal screening looks for protein leakage into the urine (urine albumin/ creatinine ratio).

> Neuropathy. Sensory, autonomic and motor neuropathy result from high blood glucose damaging the blood vessels supplying nerves. Particularly examine the foot.

Macrovascular Disease
Compared to people without DM, diabetic patients have twice the risk of developing cardiovascular disease such as stroke, coronary artery disease, and peripheral vascular disease in later life. They are also at higher risk of hypertension and hyperlipidaemia.

Foot problems, e.g. ulcers, arise due to a combination of vascular disease and neuropathy. Infections are also more prevalent: hyperglycaemia creates an attractive environment for bacteria and fungi to proliferate. These complications occur in later life.

Prognosis
Outcomes in T1DM have dramatically improved with earlier diagnosis, better control of blood glucose levels, and early identification of complications. Life expectancy is still reduced compared to the general population, and outcomes are worse in those with poor glycaemic control.

Diabetic Ketoacidosis
Diabetic ketoacidosis (DKA) is a potentially fatal condition that occurs due to poorly controlled T1DM.

There is a triad of:
> Hyperglycaemia. Glucose >11mmol/L.
> Acidosis. pH<7.3 and bicarbonate <15mmol/L.
> Ketones in the blood. Finger prick ketones>3mmol/L, although urine ketones may be measured if blood ketone monitoring is not available.

Aetiology
It results from an absolute or relative insulin deficiency, most commonly due to infection, poor concordance with diabetes management or a first presentation of T1DM

Although there are high blood glucose levels, glucose cannot be taken up by tissue cells due to the insulin deficiency. This leads to an energy deficit and consequently, fats are broken down as an alternative energy substrate. This produces ketones which are acidotic in nature, creating metabolic acidosis. The high blood glucose (which is not taken up by tissues) results in an osmotic diuresis, leading to severe fluid and electrolyte imbalances.

Clinical Features
Clinical signs may include:
> Dehydration.
> Nausea and vomiting. No associated diarrhoea.
> Deep sighing respiration. This is also known as Kussmaul breathing, and arises due to compensatory respiratory alkalosis. May also get acetone ("pear drop") breath odour.
> Abdominal pain.
> Reduced level of consciousness.
> Tiredness.

Investigations
> Blood glucose. This should be checked using near-patient testing, but also a formal biochemistry laboratory sample.
> Blood/urine ketones. This can be checked using finger prick ketone sticks.
> Blood gas. This will define the degree of metabolic acidosis (low bicarbonate), and will usually show partial respiratory compensation by a low carbon dioxide level. Chloride levels are also helpful, and these may become elevated with fluid therapy, giving a hyperchloraemic acidosis.
> U&Es. This is helpful to assess baseline kidney function, which may be impaired in diabetes. Any degree of renal impairment will mean that potassium replacement would have to be more cautiously done.
> FBC. There may be an increased white cell count purely from DKA, or from an infectious precipitant.

Differential Diagnosis
DKA is often a first presentation of T1DM and can be due to relative lack of insulin in a child with known T1DM. Note that fever is not expected as part of the pathophysiology of DKA, and if present, an infective precipitant should be suspected. Other features of infection include hypotension, lactic acidosis, and any refractory acidosis. If DKA is a first presentation of diabetes, initial investigations as per T1DM should also be performed.

Management
In patients who are not significantly acidotic and are only minimally dehydrated, management consists of subcutaneous insulin and oral rehydration.

Resuscitation
Many cases need more aggressive treatment, which should start with an ABCD assessment:
> Airway. Ensure the airway is patent, and if there is a reduced GCS, insert an airway adjuvant. A nasogastric tube should be inserted and placed on open drainage if there is vomiting/reduced consciousness.
> Breathing. Give 100% oxygen via face mask.
> Circulation. The presence of tachycardia may be an indicator of shock. The child should be placed on a cardiac monitor: there may be hyperkalaemia, which can be detected early on an ECG.
> Disability. Assess any reduction in GCS: cerebral oedema is an important complication to identify early in DKA.

Managing Hyperglycaemia, Dehydration and Acidosis
> Assessment of fluid status. A 5% fluid deficit can be assumed if the pH is above 7.1 (mild/moderate DKA), and a 10% fluid deficit can be assumed if the pH is below 7.1.
    > Fluid boluses should not be given in mild/moderate cases. In severe DKA, up to three 10mL/kg 0.9% sodium chloride boluses may be given, each over 30 minutes, but only if absolutely necessary. This

is half the typical fluid boluses for children (20mL/kg) due to risk of cerebral oedema.

› Maintenance fluids should be commenced (with adjustments for level of dehydration, and fluid boluses already given). These fluids are also given cautiously, and any dehydration is corrected slowly over 48 hours. Fluid of choice would initially be 0.9% sodium chloride (NaCl) with 20mmol potassium in 500mL. Maintenance fluids are lower volume than usual:

  › 2mL/kg/hr (if under 10kg)
  › 1mL/kg/hr (if 10-40kg)
  › 40mL/hr (if over 40kg)

▸ **Insulin therapy.** This should be started at least one hour after initiating fluid therapy, at an initial rate of 0.05-0.1units/kg/hour. Delayed therapy is felt to reduce the risk of cerebral oedema (as starting insulin earlier alongside fluids may result in rapid fluid and electrolyte shifts). The role of the insulin is to suppress plasma glucose levels, but also to suppress ketone production. Long acting subcutaneous insulin may also be commenced/continued at this stage to avoid rebound hyperglycaemia after discontinuation of glucose therapy.

▸ **Sodium bicarbonate therapy.** This should not be given as fluid and insulin should correct the acidosis.

Note that if the child is alert, not clinically dehydrated and not nauseated/vomiting, DKA can be managed with oral fluids and subcutaneous insulin.

Monitoring During Treatment

Monitoring involves:

▸ **Hourly assessments.** Check blood glucose, level of consciousness, heart rate, blood pressure, temperature and respiratory rate. In those under 2-years-old, or with severe DKA, observations should be every 30 minutes due to the high risk of cerebral oedema.

▸ **Continuous ECG monitoring.** This is to detect signs of hypokalaemia (ST depression, U waves).

▸ **Blood tests.** 2 hours post treatment, and then at least four hourly check:

  › **Laboratory blood glucose and blood ketones.** This will inform fluid and insulin therapy.

  › **Renal function.** Urea and creatinine should be checked as part of ensuring adequate fluid input.

  › **Potassium.** Hypokalaemia may occur from insulin driving potassium intracellularly.

  › **Sodium (corrected).** Corrected Na mmol/L = Na mmol/L + 0.4 ([Glucose mmol/L] - 5.5). The corrected sodium should rise as glucose falls: if this is too fast or too slow, there is a risk of cerebral oedema secondary to rapid osmolarity changes. If the corrected sodium is increasing by too much, there is too much fluid loss, and therefore the fluid rate may need to be increased. Conversely, if the corrected sodium is falling by too much, there is too much fluid gain, and therefore the fluid rate may need to be decreased. If suboptimal changes in sodium are associated with cerebral oedema, a hypertonic saline bolus may be required.

  › **Chloride.** If the chloride is high, fluid may need to be changed to 0.45% NaCl, or slowed down in rate.

▸ **Fluid balance.** Fluid balance needs to be carefully documented, including strict urine volumes and monitoring the weight of the child. Consider a urinary catheter if needed for accurate fluid balance.

Adjusting Fluids and Insulin

▸ When the glucose falls to <14mmol/L, the fluids can be changed to 0.9% sodium chloride with 5% dextrose and 20mmol KCL/500mls. If the ketones are less than 3mmol/L, and the pH is above 7.3, reduce or maintain the insulin rate to 0.05 units/kg/hour. These measures help reduce the risk of hypoglycaemia.

▸ If the blood glucose falls <6mmol/L, increase the concentration of glucose in the fluids. 2mL/kg boluses of 10% dextrose may be required if glucose is significantly low (<4mmol/L). However, if there is persistent ketosis, insulin should be maintained at a rate of at least 0.05 units/kg/hour. Insulin has a role in switching off ketogenesis, which is still necessary even with a normal glucose.

Management Post Resolution of Ketosis

▸ Once ketoacidosis is resolving (e.g. ketones < 1mmol/L), and oral fluids are tolerated, subcutaneous insulin can be started.

▸ Subcutaneous insulin should be given at least 30 minutes before stopping the insulin infusion.

Complications

▸ **Cerebral oedema.** The cause is not definitively known but rapid rehydration causing hyponatraemia and influx of fluid into cells is thought to be one factor. The mortality from cerebral oedema is 25%. The risk is reduced by cautious fluid boluses, by correcting dehydration slowly over 48 hours, and by using 0.9% sodium chloride initially (instead of any lower sodium concentrations). Management of cerebral oedema is summarised on p229.

▸ **Hypokalaemia.** Insulin also allows uptake of potassium into cells. In DKA patients have high extracellular potassium but low intracellular concentration. Therefore as soon as the patient is treated with IV insulin, potassium starts to move into cells and hypokalaemia can occur. This is overcome by adding potassium to fluid, and adjusting it based on plasma potassium levels.

▸ **Hyperkalaemia.** This may be present initially with a lack of insulin.

▸ **Aspiration pneumonia.** This is of special concern in children who are drowsy or comatose. A nasogastric tube should pre-emptively be placed to reduce this risk in high risk groups.

65

> Hypoglycaemia. This is a common complication of insulin treatment, more commonly occurring in those more sensitive to insulin such as newly diagnosed young children. It should be avoided in DKA by adding glucose to the fluids when the blood glucose has fallen.

> Venous thromboembolic events. Risk is increased, particularly in those with central venous catheters.

Prognosis

DKA is the most common cause of death in diabetes, and mortality is 100% without insulin therapy. Appropriate management is key, and many complications such as hypoglycaemia, hypokalaemia and fluid overload, are generally avoidable.

Other Types of Diabetes in Childhood

Although the vast majority of DM in children is T1DM, certain risk factors (obesity, Afro-Caribbean/Asian ethnicity, no or very low insulin requirements, systemic illness, young age, or evidence of insulin resistance e.g. acanthosis nigricans) should raise suspicion of other forms of DM.

Type 2 DM

This is due to insulin resistance and is the classic form of DM seen in adults. The single most important risk factor for this is obesity, particularly abdominal obesity. Other risk factors include family history, ethnic group (e.g. higher risk in Asians/African-Americans) and female gender. There is usually enough residual insulin function to not have episodes of DKA and to not require insulin replacement therapy. These children may present incidentally with high blood glucose on a background of obesity and signs of insulin resistance including acanthosis nigricans (velvety, hyperpigmented thickening of the skin often seen on the back of the neck, axilla or the groin) and polycystic ovarian syndrome in girls.

Initial management of T2DM involves the modification of risk factors through encouraging healthy eating and exercise. First-line medication is metformin, an insulin sensitiser. If DM control is not achieved with metformin and lifestyle changes, then insulin therapy is initiated. In symptomatic children or when HbA1C is above 9% at presentation, insulin is usually started at diagnosis.

Maturity Onset Diabetes in the Young (MODY)

This is a rare type of DM, representing 1-2% of people with the disease. MODY usually presents in patients under 25-years-old. It has an autosomal dominant mode of inheritance due to various single gene defects affecting insulin production. MODY is usually managed with dietary modification and oral medication. Due to its rarity, the vast majority of cases are misdiagnosed.

The four most common subtypes are:

> HNF1-alpha. Genetic defect reducing insulin production.

> HNF4-alpha. There is usually a high birthweight, and hypoglycaemia around birth.

> HNF1-beta. This is associated with renal cysts, gout and uterine abnormalities.

> Glucokinase. There is a defect in the gene required for detecting hyperglycaemia. Therefore people with this condition regulate glucose levels at a higher level than normal, typically 5.8-8mmol/L.

Cystic Fibrosis Related Diabetes

This is mainly related to insulin deficiency but has a multifactorial pathogenesis. By 30-years-old, 50% of people with cystic fibrosis will have developed DM. Children are screened annually from 10-years-old.

Genetic Syndromes

A number of genetic syndromes are sometimes associated with diabetes. These include:

> Trisomy 21.
> Turner syndrome.
> Laurence-Moon-Biedl syndrome.
> Prader-Willi syndrome.
> Wolfram syndrome (DIDMOAD: diabetes insipidus, DM, optic atrophy and deafness).

Drug-induced DM

Many drugs can potentially lead to DM, particularly corticosteroids through antagonist effects on insulin. Other implicated drugs include statins, beta-blockers and thiazide diuretics.

Neonatal Diabetes

This rare form of DM appears in the first six months of life. It can be transient or permanent. Implicated genes are KCNJ11 and ABCC8. It may be associated with developmental delay and recurrent seizures.

Hypoglycaemia

Hypoglycaemia is a common clinical problem in neonates but becomes less common as children grow older. The most common cause of hypoglycaemia in children is related to insulin treatment in type 1 DM (p60), but it can be caused by other conditions, particularly during the neonatal period.

The definition of hypoglycaemia is controversial. Suggested thresholds to be aware of are:

> 2.6 mmol/L in neonates.
> 2.8 mmol/L in older children.
> 4 mmol/L in those on insulin therapy.

Aetiology

Sepsis is one of the most important life threatening illnesses associated with hypoglycaemia and should be excluded in the early stages. *Table 5* summarises other conditions.

Newborns at risk of developing hypoglycaemia should be screened:

> Prematurity.
> Low birth weight.
> Infants of diabetic mothers.
> Large for gestational age.

Hypoglycaemia in neonates generally has a different mechanism compared to older children and is usually related to hyperinsulinaemia. Causes of hyperinsulinism include:

> Primary hyperinsulinism.
> Intrauterine growth restriction.

TABLE 5: Conditions associated with or causing hypoglycaemia	
Causes of Hypoglycaemia	
Endocrine.	• Adrenal insufficiency. • Hypopituitarism. • Congenital hyperinsulinism. • Insulin therapy.
Metabolic.	• Medium-Chain Acyl-Coenzyme A Dehydrogenase Deficiency (MCADD). • Glycogen storage disease.
Poisoning/dosing error.	• Salicylates. • Insulin.
Systemic disease.	• Sepsis. • Polycythaemia. • Liver disease.
Other.	• Idiopathic ketotic hypoglycaemia. • Drug related.

TABLE 6: Symptoms of hypoglycaemia in older children	
Autonomic symptoms	**Neurogylcopaenic symptoms**
• Hunger. • Sweating. • Flushing. • Tachycardia/palpitations. • Anxiety. • Tremor.	• Poor concentration. • Confusion. • Behavioural changes. • Weakness. • Drowsiness. • Seizures.

> Maternal gestational diabetes mellitus.
> Hypoxic ischaemic encephalopathy.

Clinical Features

Symptoms of hypoglycaemia present in two stages (*Table 6*); first, those due to activation of the autonomic nervous system, then those due to neuroglycopaenia. As always, symptoms in children vary according to the age of the patient. Neonates may be jittery, lethargic, irritable and may become apnoeic, hypotonic or develop seizures.

Family history may reveal known inborn errors of metabolism that run in the family or history of unexplained infant death. Metabolic conditions are more likely to present in consanguineous families. Clinical examination must include features of sepsis, weight, examination of the liver (hepatomegaly in glycogen storage disease), observation for hyperpigmentation (adrenal insufficiency), and appearance of the genitalia (hypopituitarism).

Investigations
Urine

> **Ketones.** Ketones in the urine or blood imply that fatty acids are being broken down to provide energy. This will not happen in diseases such as MCADD, where fat cannot be mobilised as an energy source. Hyperinsulinism also turns off ketogenesis and therefore ketones won't be seen.
> **Toxicology.** Hypoglycaemia may be associated with an overdose e.g. aspirin and blood salicylate level should be measured.
> **Urine organic acids.** This is to identify organic acidaemia.

Bedside Blood Tests

> **Glucose.** This is useful, although it may be inaccurate at low glucose concentration. A low blood glucose should be confirmed by laboratory testing.
> **Ketones.** Blood ketones (betahydroxybutyrate) can be tested for at the bedside.

> **Blood gas.** Metabolic acidosis may be present if there is reduced end organ perfusion, and in certain metabolic conditions.

Laboratory Tests

> **Glucose.** This is more accurate than bedside tests to diagnose hypoglycaemia.
> **Lactate.** This assesses degree of anaerobic respiration. If it is significantly elevated, it may indicate a metabolic condition e.g. mitochondrial disease.
> **Insulin and C peptide.** Insulin is elevated in states of hyperinsulinism. C peptide is a marker of endogenous insulin, and therefore if C peptide is not also elevated, hyperinsulinism is likely due to exogenous insulin administration.
> **Cortisol and growth hormone.** Adrenal insufficiency and hypopituitarism may be detected.
> **Ammonia.** This is elevated if there is liver failure or increased protein breakdown (e.g. urea cycle defect).
> **LFTs.** There may be associated liver disease, e.g. glycogen storage disease.
> **U&Es.** These may be deranged if there is dehydration, or electrolyte disturbances associated with endocrine disorders.
> **Beta-hydroxybutyrate, Acylcarnitine profile, and free fatty acids.** Beta-hydroxybutyrate and free fatty acids are low in MCADD and in hyperinsulinism. Acylcarnitine profile is abnormal in MCADD.

It is critical for accurate diagnosis to collect these samples at the time of hypoglycaemia (since derangements may recover when the hypoglycaemia resolves), but this is often not possible when the child is very sick. In this case a controlled diagnostic fast when the child has improved can help establish the diagnosis.

Management

Management is divided into management of the acute hypoglycaemia and treatment of the underlying cause. Any hypoglycaemia of unknown cause must be admitted and the underlying cause should be sought prior to discharge.

Acute Symptomatic Hypoglycaemia in a Child

- If the child is able to tolerate oral fluids, give 10-15g of fast acting oral carbohydrate such as juice or energy drinks.
- If the child will not co-operate with oral fluids but is conscious, a glucose gel can be used on the buccal mucosa.
- If the child is unable to tolerate oral fluids or is unconscious, give a 2mL/kg bolus of 10% dextrose followed by a continuous infusion. Intramuscular (IM) glucagon may be given as an alternative if cannulation is not possible.

Acute Hypoglycaemia in a Neonate

- A top-up feed is given, with repeat blood glucose test one hour later.
- If this does not sufficiently raise the blood glucose or the baby is symptomatic, then the baby is likely to need admission to the neonatal unit. If the baby is not vomiting, blood glucose might be maintained on hourly nasogastric feeds. However if the glucose is very low, or the baby is not tolerating oral feeds, consider starting maintenance 10% dextrose fluids, or giving a 2mL/kg bolus of 10% dextrose.

Treating the Underlying Cause

This varies dramatically according to cause. *Table 7* lists some examples.

Complications

The major long-term complication of hypoglycaemia is neurocognitive defects with, for example, developmental delay and reduced intellect. Often children are asymptomatic during the hypoglycaemic episodes, making diagnosing hypoglycaemia retrospectively very difficult.

Prognosis

Hormonal deficiencies and inborn errors of metabolism require life-long medication and careful management. Certain conditions like hyperinsulinism in the newborn period may resolve with age.

GROWTH

During the first year of life, linear growth is very rapid (25 cm/year). It is mostly influenced by nutrition, whilst in the prepubertal child, growth hormone becomes the predominant determining factor. Throughout infancy, childhood and adolescence, a stable psychosocial environment is a prerequisite for normal growth.

Prepubertal children grow between 4 and 8 cm/year. The slowest rate of growth occurs just before puberty starts. Girls experience their growth spurt in puberty about six months to one year before the onset of periods (menarche), whilst boys experience their growth spurt two years later than girls. After menarche, growth gradually declines over a period of two years.

Assessment of Abnormal Stature

The most important component of height assessment is accurate height and weight measurements correctly plotted on the growth charts (*Figure 4*). Specific growth charts exist for specific conditions (such as Down syndrome and achondroplasia), where growth is not expected to follow a normal trajectory.

Measurement

From birth to 2-years-old, children should be measured in the supine position on a length board. After 2-years-old, children's height should be measured on a stadiometer, which consists of a vertical ruler and a sliding horizontal plane which sits on top of the head. Given the difficulties in obtaining length and height measurements in small children, it is important to assess growth over a specific period. Head circumference should also be measured, but only in younger children, as the rate of head growth rapidly declines.

TABLE 7: Possible management strategies for specific causes of hypoglycaemia	
Cause	**Management**
Type 1 DM on insulin.	• Check concordance with therapy, food diary, and exercise patterns. Consider adjusting insulin dosages as necessary.
Sepsis.	• Identify the source of infection and treat it. Hypoglycaemia should resolve as the infection improves.
Hyperinsulinism.	• Requires careful attention to feeding in the short term. • May require treatment with diazoxide.
MCADD.	• Needs a lifelong management plan. General principles include frequent feeding and avoiding periods of fasting.
Congenital hyperinsulinism.	• Diazoxide, which inhibits pancreatic secretion of insulin, stimulates glucose release from the liver and stimulates catecholamine release. Octreotide, which inhibits insulin secretion may also be used. In severe cases, total pancreatectomy might be needed. Partial pancreatectomy in focal lesions is curative.
Focal tumours such as insulinomas.	• Require surgery for definitive treatment. Insulinomas are rare and chemotherapy is given if they metastasise.

FIGURE 4

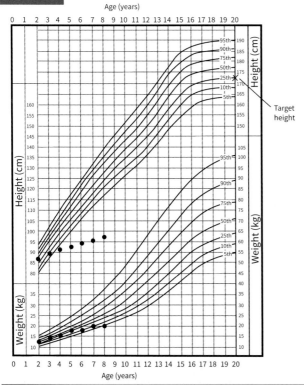

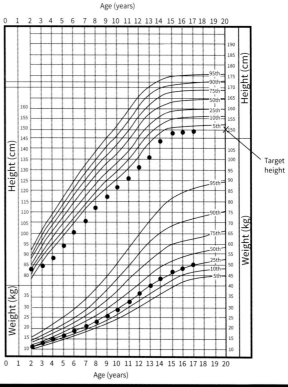

Two examples of short stature. Left shows stature rapidly falling below the centile lines, and fits with growth hormone deficiency, given the timing. On the right, stature is following a consistent centile line. This may be due to familial short stature, or idiopathic short stature, although other causes cannot be ruled out.

Mid-parental Height

Calculation of the mid-parental height is very important as it gives the healthcare provider an indication of the genetic height potential. Several ways exist to do this, one is shown below. This should be corrected for gender (add 13 cm for boys, and subtract 13 cm for girls), as follows:

$$\text{Midparental height (girl)} = \frac{\text{fathers height} - 13 + \text{mothers height}}{2}$$

$$\text{Midparental height (boy)} = \frac{\text{fathers height} + \text{mothers height} + 13}{2}$$

Obesity

Obese children usually grow faster and are taller than their genetic potential, as shown by the mid-parental height. However, if an obese child is short, an endocrine cause should be ruled out.

Short Stature

Short stature is defined as a stature that is less than two standard deviations (SD) below the mean for the age, sex and ethnic-matched population. This essentially represents height below the 2.3rd percentile. The majority of children presenting with short stature do not have an underlying pathology. The most important diagnostic tool is the growth chart and calculation of mid-parental height.

The possibility of an organic cause is greater with:

➤ Lower height centiles.

➤ Larger disparities of the child's height to mid-parental height.
➤ Dysmorphic features.
➤ Signs of chronic illness.
➤ Increased weight:height ratio (the short fat child).
➤ Disproportionate upper:lower segment ratios.
➤ Rapid reduction in height velocity.

Clinical Assessment

A good history is essential. Consanguinity may point to genetic or endocrine causes. Drug history could identify high doses of corticosteroids which may have led to Cushing's syndrome. Consider the heights of the extended family: this might give wider evidence of familial short stature, or of a potentially undiagnosed genetic condition. A social and nutritional history is also important to identify psychosocial factors that may impact on health. Age at the start of puberty should be documented as well.

A full multisystemic examination should be done looking out for signs of dysmorphism, chronic disease, nutritional and pubertal status. Those who are disproportionately heavy for their height should be assessed for an endocrine cause. Dysmorphic features point to a potential genetic abnormality. Splitting height into "upper segment" (pelvis to top of head) and "lower segment" (pelvis to foot) is helpful, as abnormalities in this ratio point to possible skeletal abnormalities (*Figure 5*).

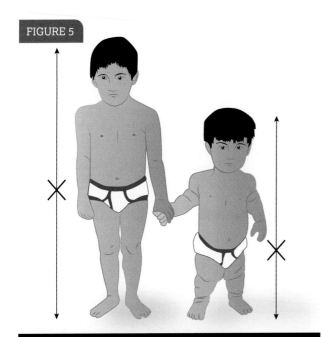

FIGURE 5

Reduced lower segment due to shortened limbs in achondroplasia.

Aetiology
Constitutional Causes of Short Stature
Familial Short Stature

The child is short for the population, but not for the family. Having short parents does not always exclude pathology on its own, as some pathological disorders are inherited (e.g. some skeletal dysplasias and the Short Stature Homeobox (SHOX) gene mutations), so it is worthwhile assessing the parents as well.

Constitutional Delay of Growth and Puberty (CDGP)

Children with CDGP are short, with delayed bone maturation (delayed bone age) and delayed puberty. This is one of the commonest causes of short stature. It is more common in boys, and is often present in the father's history as well. The progression in puberty is late. At the end of their growth, children usually reach their target height, with rapid acceleration in height.

Idiopathic Short Stature

Children with idiopathic short stature (ISS) are short both for the population and the family. These children are often investigated more rigorously and no organic cause is found. In some countries, growth hormone (GH) is prescribed for ISS.

Small for Gestational Age

Children born with a weight less than two standard deviations below that expected for their gestation usually show catch-up growth after birth. Those who fail to catch up by 4-years-old can be offered GH therapy. Children born small for gestational age (SGA) may have other diagnoses as well, such as Turner syndrome or Russell Silver syndrome.

Endocrine Causes of Short Stature
Growth Hormone Deficiency

GH acts mainly via Insulin-like growth factor 1 (IGF1), which is produced by the liver and acts on the growth plate to promote linear growth.

Growth hormone deficiency (GHD) usually presents with poor linear growth after the first year of life. Children with GHD are generally heavier for their height; if the diagnosis is delayed, classical features such as an immature appearance of the face and abdominal adiposity may be noted.

GHD in children is usually congenital; however, a space-occupying lesion needs to be excluded. Therefore, an MRI of the hypothalamo-pituitary area is mandatory in any child with a diagnosis of GHD. Craniopharyngioma is the most common tumour in childhood presenting with hypopituitarism. Another cause of GHD is cranial irradiation for cancer. GHD is most commonly isolated, i.e. without other pituitary hormone deficiencies, but it can be combined with other pituitary hormone deficiencies (hypopituitarism).

Diagnosis of GHD in a short child is made when growth velocity is poor, IGF1 is low and GH fails to rise in two GH stimulation tests. Children with GHD also have delayed skeletal maturation.

Abnormalities of the GH-IGF1 Axis

These are also causes of short stature and are currently very rarely diagnosed. However, with further research, many patients currently labelled as ISS will have a more specific diagnosis and targeted treatment may become possible.

Other Endocrine Causes

These include hypothyroidism, delayed puberty and Cushing's syndrome.

Genetic Causes of Short Stature

Human height is determined by a number of genetic and epigenetic factors. Genome-wide association studies have revealed several hundred single nucleotide polymorphisms influencing human height. SHOX gene mutations are associated with ISS. The most common syndromes associated with short stature are Turner syndrome (p124), Down syndrome (p120), Noonan syndrome, and Russell-Silver and Prader-Willi syndromes.

SHOX Gene

Mutations in the Short Stature Homeobox gene (SHOX), located on the short arm in the pseudo-autosomal region of the X and Y chromosomes, account for a number of children with ISS. SHOX mutations may lead to ISS without obvious skeletal malformations. Individuals with SHOX mutations may have a characteristic deformity of their wrist (Madelung deformity), which is sometimes more obvious in the affected parent rather than the child. Poor growth and skeletal abnormalities in girls with Turner syndrome are largely related to SHOX haploinsufficiency (i.e. one copy of the gene).

SHOX mutation is an indication for GH therapy in many countries.

Noonan Syndrome

Individuals with this syndrome have several phenotypic similarities with Turner syndrome. They may have right-sided cardiac defects (pulmonary stenosis). A trial of GH may be offered.

Russell-Silver Syndrome

Russell-Silver syndrome is a condition characterised by failure to grow pre- and postnatally. Children with this condition may have feeding problems after birth, hypoglycaemia and distinctive facial features that include a triangular head shape, micrognathia, hemihypertrophy (asymmetrical growth of one side of the body) and café-au-lait lesions. In 60% of cases of Russell-Silver Syndrome, a genetic cause is found involving an imprinting defect in genes located on chromosomes 7 or 11.

Children with this condition may be offered GH treatment, as they are born SGA.

Prader-Willi Syndrome

Prader-Willi syndrome (PWS) is a syndrome associated with feeding difficulties early in life and hypotonia, short stature, hypogonadism and developmental delay. Later on in life, it is associated with increased appetite, leading to hyperphagia and excessive weight gain. It is due to an imprinting defect in genes located on chromosome 15.

GH is not only offered to optimise height but for its metabolic effects in fat reduction and increase in muscle mass. Presence of obstructive sleep apnoea is an absolute contraindication for GH treatment, as sudden deaths in children with PWS on GH treatment have been reported.

Skeletal Dysplasias

This is a heterogeneous group of disorders characterised by disproportionate short stature. More than 200 skeletal dysplasias exist. The terminology used is usually descriptive, for example when the proximal part of the limbs is more severely affected the term "rhizomelia" is used, when the middle part is affected "mesomelia", and when the distal part is affected "acromelia". Spinal involvement is indicated by the term "spondylo".

Achondroplasia and hypochondroplasia are the most common skeletal dysplasias. These are autosomal dominant conditions related to mutations in the Fibroblast Growth Factor receptor 3 (FGFR3) gene. Patients with achondroplasia are severely affected with a mean adult height of 100–140cm. They have a prominent forehead, macrocephaly, flat nasal bridge and rhizomelia. They may suffer from frequent ear infections, obstructive sleep apnoea and hydrocephalus.

Chronic Illness

Chronic illness may affect linear growth. Inflammatory bowel disease (IBD) in children can present with poor growth prior to the onset of gastrointestinal manifestations. Diseases controlled by steroids impact adversely on growth. Some diseases such as Crohn's disease and renal failure are associated with GH insensitivity. GH is routinely offered in children with renal failure.

Investigations

A simple diagnostic algorithm is shown in *Figure 6*. Once an initial differential is arrived at, diagnostic tests may be helpful (*Table 8*).

Initial blood tests should include FBC, U&Es, LFT, Vitamin D, thyroid function tests and a coeliac screen. Further tests should be targeted to the history. Remember that any chronic disease may result in faltering growth, and therefore additional investigations should be targeted to this e.g. checking HBA1c in suspected diabetes, or screening for immunodeficiency in a patient with recurrent infections.

Bone age X-ray can help narrow the differential. Bone maturity is delayed with endocrine disorders such as growth hormone deficiency, but also in constitutional delay of growth and puberty.

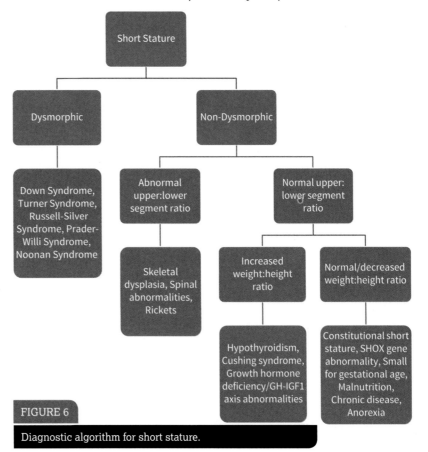

FIGURE 6

Diagnostic algorithm for short stature.

TABLE 8: Investigations in short stature		
Category	Suspected diagnosis	Investigation
Chronic disease.	• Anaemia.	• Full blood count.
	• Chronic liver/kidney disease.	• Liver function test (LFT)/renal function.
	• Vitamin D deficiency.	• Bone profile/Vitamin D levels.
	• Coeliac disease.	• Anti-tissue transglutaminase antibodies/Anti-endomysial antibody.
	• Cystic Fibrosis.	• Sweat test/DNA test.
	• UTI.	• Urine dipstick/Microscopy, culture and sensitivities (MC&S).
	• Renal tubular acidosis (in babies).	• Blood gas.
	• Chronic inflammatory conditions e.g. inflammatory bowel disease.	• C-reactive protein (CRP)/erythrocyte sedimentation rate (ESR).
	• Cardiac disease.	• Echocardiogram.
	• Malnutrition.	• Albumin (may also have anaemia).
Endocrine conditions.	• Hypothyroidism.	• Thyroid function tests.
	• Cushing Syndrome/Disease.	• Cortisol levels/dexamethasone suppression test.
	• Hypopituitarism.	• Pituitary function tests. IGF1 and IGFBP-3 to identify growth hormone deficiency, or a problem in the GH-IGF1 axis. GH stimulation tests and a subsequent pituitary MRI may be required for further evaluation.
Genetic conditions.	• Genetic condition e.g. Turner syndrome.	• Karyotype.
	• SHOX mutation.	• Molecular genetics.
Skeletal conditions.	• Skeletal dysplasia e.g. achondroplasia.	• Skeletal survey.

Management

Management is with a multidisciplinary approach and may include clinical geneticists, paediatric endocrinologists and dieticians. Further evaluation by a psychologist may be required if there is a suspected eating disorder, and social services will need to be informed if neglect is a contributory factor.

Prognosis

Prognosis is cause-specific, but generally short stature has a good outlook. For many conditions, as described above, growth hormone therapy is used successfully.

Tall Stature

Tall stature is more widely accepted by society; thus, tall children are less commonly referred for assessment than those with short stature. Most tall children have familial tall stature, which does not need any treatment. Tall stature may also be related to obesity. However, it is important to establish the possibility of an underlying cause that needs treatment.

The possibility of an organic cause is greater with:

▸ Recent growth acceleration (outside of normal puberty).
▸ Large disparities of the child's height to mid-parental height.
▸ Dysmorphic features.
▸ Signs of chronic illness.
▸ Disproportionate upper:lower segment ratios.

Clinical Assessment

A detailed history and examination will usually exclude the need for further investigations. As with short stature, splitting height into "upper segment" (pelvis to top of head) and "lower segment" (pelvis to foot) is helpful in evaluating dysmorphic children (for example, the ratio may be increased in Klinefelter syndrome). Increased arm span ratio (relative to height) is seen in Marfan syndrome and Homocystinuria (*Figure 7*). Assessing BMI will identify a nutritional contribution, and an assessment of both pubertal and thyroid status are mandatory, as precocious puberty and hyperthyroidism are important causes of tall stature. Head circumference should also be measured, as conditions like Soto syndrome are associated with a large head and tall stature.

Aetiology

Endocrine Causes

Precocious puberty, via the action of sex hormones on growth plates, causes rapid linear growth in childhood. In boys especially, as the first sign of puberty is usually undetected by the families (increase in testicular volume to 4mL), rapid growth might be the presenting

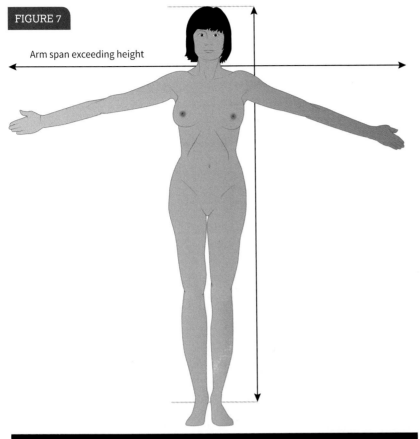

FIGURE 7

Arm span exceeding height

Increased arm span exceeding height in Marfan syndrome.

Homocystinuria

This is an autosomal recessive disorder, characterised by increased homocysteine levels in the blood and urine. These patients have a marfanoid appearance, with associated learning difficulties, psychological disorders and thromboembolic tendencies.

Soto Syndrome

Children with Soto syndrome have very rapid growth during the first few years of life that appears to improve as they grow older. Facial features include: prominent forehead, hypertelorism, down-slanting palpebral fissures and a pointed chin. It is also associated with learning difficulties.

Beckwith-Wiedemann Syndrome

Beckwith-Wiedemann syndrome is an imprinting disorder characterised by large birth weight, long length and rapid growth, especially during infancy and childhood. It is also associated with hypoglycaemia, macroglossia and exomphalos.

Investigations

Figure 8 summarises a diagnostic algorithm. Investigations vary depending on the suspected cause (*Table 9*). Bone age X-ray may also be helpful. Bone maturity may be accelerated in precocious puberty, obesity, hyperthyroidism and familial tall stature. Accelerated bone age means that growth plates are likely to close at an earlier age, thereby hastening growth.

Management

The majority of children require simple reassurance and no active management. Projected final height can be calculated, although it comes with wide confidence intervals. If intervention is required, management is controversial, but one option is:

> ‣ **Epiphysiodesis**. This surgical intervention destroys the growth plate around the knee, preventing further bone growth.

manifestation. It is important not to miss precocious puberty, especially in boys, as it can be due to an underlying brain tumour, whilst in girls, it is usually idiopathic. Deficiency in sex hormones (e.g. Kallmann syndrome), or resistance to sex hormones (e.g. androgen receptor insensitivity) can also cause tall stature, due to delayed closure of growth plates.

Excess of adrenal androgens, such as in premature adrenarche and late onset congenital adrenal hyperplasia, promote linear growth. GH excess is very rare in children, but if it occurs before growth plate fusion, it can result in gigantism. Hyperthyroidism can also cause accelerated bone age and tall stature.

Genetic Causes
Klinefelter Syndrome

This is a chromosomal abnormality (47, XXY) associated with male infertility, tall stature with long legs, gynaecomastia, small testicles and a varying degree of learning difficulties. Tall stature is related to an extra copy of the SHOX gene and delayed bone maturation due to hypogonadism. It is the commonest sex chromosome aneuploidy causing tall stature. Note that other syndromes with extra X chromosomes (e.g. XXX syndrome, or mosaicism with an extra X) will also have an extra SHOX gene and predisposition to tall stature.

Marfan Syndrome

Marfan syndrome is an autosomal dominant connective tissue disorder characterised by a specific body habitus with long limbs, joint laxity, arachnodactyly and chest deformities. It is also associated with dilatation of the aorta, aortic dissection and sudden death in adults. Patients with Marfan syndrome may have mutations in the fibrillin gene.

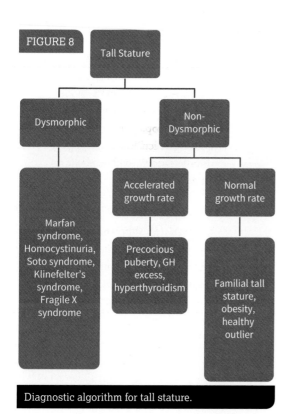

FIGURE 8

Tall Stature

Dysmorphic → Marfan syndrome, Homocystinuria, Soto syndrome, Klinefelter's syndrome, Fragile X syndrome

Non-Dysmorphic → Accelerated growth rate → Precocious puberty, GH excess, hyperthyroidism

Non-Dysmorphic → Normal growth rate → Familial tall stature, obesity, healthy outlier

Diagnostic algorithm for tall stature.

TABLE 9: Investigations in tall stature

Category	Suspected diagnosis	Investigations
Genetic.	• Chromosomal disorder, e.g. Klinefelter (47 XXY) syndrome.	• Karyotype.
	• Beckwith-Wiedemann syndrome.	• Glucose (low in neonatal period).
Endocrine.	• Hyperthyroidism.	• Thyroid function tests.
	• Homocystinuria.	• Serum homocysteine levels.
	• Growth hormone/ growth hormone axis abnormalities.	• IGF-1 and IGFBP-3. • Gold standard is glucose suppression test. • Brain MRI. • Check other pituitary function tests for associated pathology.
	• Precocious puberty.	• Luteinising hormone (LH), follicle stimulating hormone (FSH), testosterone, oestradiol, steroid profile. • Pelvic ultrasound. • Pituitary MRI.

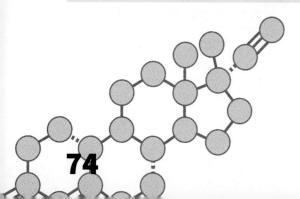

Prognosis

Prognosis is pathology dependent, but tall stature is not generally associated with any long-term increase in morbidity or mortality.

Puberty

Puberty is the progression of a child's body into an adult's body capable of sexual reproduction. Increased frequency and amplitude of gonadotrophin-releasing hormone (GnRH) pulses indicate the onset of puberty. Testosterone is the main sex hormone in males, whereas oestradiol is the main sex hormone in females.

Pubertal Characteristics

This process is associated with development of primary and secondary sexual characteristics. This is separate from growth, which begins at conception and ends in a mature adult. Growth occurs rapidly in the first half of puberty and slows nearing puberty completion. Key features of puberty in boys and girls are summarised in *Table 10*. Tanner staging can be used to identify stages of puberty (*Table 11*). Note that penile length is rarely used for pubertal stages, as it does not change early in puberty. There are also measurement difficulties/awkwardness and ethnic variations.

Abnormal Puberty

Abnormal puberty can either be precocious or delayed. Precocious puberty is defined as the onset of puberty before 8-years-old in girls and 9-years-old in boys. Delayed puberty is defined as absence of any signs of puberty beyond age 13.5-years-old in girls or 14-years-old in boys. *Table 12* lists causes of abnormal puberty.

Clinical Assessment

Assessment should involve:

› History. Focus on previous growth and development throughout childhood, milestones and behavioural changes, height and weight, and family history of abnormal puberty, as well as a full medical and surgical history.

› Pubertal Milestones. Note the age of onset of puberty, but also the order of pubertal milestones: males should begin with testicular enlargement, females with breast enlargement. If androgenic features come first (e.g. pubic hair development), then a source of adrenal androgens should be sought.

› Specific features. It is also important to enquire about sense of smell, as hypogonadotrophic hypogonadism may be associated with anosmia (e.g. Kallmann syndrome).

Clinical examination of the breasts, genitalia and body habitus, and examination of the neurological and endocrine systems are also very important. In cases of precocious puberty, examination of the testes may suggest an underlying

TABLE 10: Progress of puberty in boys and girls

	Male	Female
Age of onset (years).	• 12–13	• 8.5–12
Initial signs.	• Testicular enlargement to > 4mL (due to increased FSH). This can be measured using an orchidometer.	• Breast enlargement (thelarche – mediated by oestrogen), which may just be unilateral.
Growth spurt.	• Age 14 to 16-years-old. • Occurs when testicular volume is 12-15 mL.	• Age 10 to 14-years-old. • Rapid and occurs early, with thelarche.
Progress.	• Enlargement of the penis and scrotum, with pubic hair (due to adrenal androgens). • Growth usually occurs one to two years later.	• Hair growth in the pubic and axillary regions (due to adrenal androgens) occurs after thelarche. • Approximately two years following thelarche, menarche (the first menstrual cycle) occurs.
Common Features.	• Other signs of puberty in both sexes are body odour, mood changes and acne.	

cause: bilaterally small suggests an adrenal pathology, bilaterally enlarged suggests excess gonadotrophins and unilaterally enlarged suggests a gonadal tumour. Café-au-lait lesions are seen in neurofibromatosis or McCune-Albright syndrome. Growth charts should also be reviewed.

Precocious Puberty

Precocious puberty is defined as the onset of puberty before 8-years-old in girls and 9-years-old in boys. Precocious puberty can cause a variety of problems, including emotional distress for both children and their families. Early growth spurts can result in tall stature during

TABLE 11: Tanner stages of puberty. Testicular volume on the orchidometer scale is shown in blue

	Males	Females
Tanner I (Prepubertal).	**Testicles.** < 1.5 mL. **Pubic Hair.** None.	**Breast.** No glandular tissue. **Areola.** Follows chest contour.
Tanner II.	**Testicles.** 1.6-6 mL. **Pubic Hair.** Small amount of downy hair.	**Breast.** Buds develop, with small area of surrounding glandular tissue. **Areola.** Begins to widen.
Tanner III.	**Testicles.** 6-12 mL (with enlarging scrotum). **Pubic Hair.** Coarser, curly hair.	**Breast.** Becomes elevated **Areola.** Continues to widen but still not elevated from surrounding breast.

(Continued)

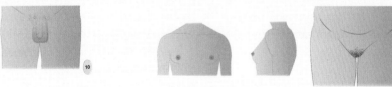

TABLE 11: *(Continued)*

	Males	Females

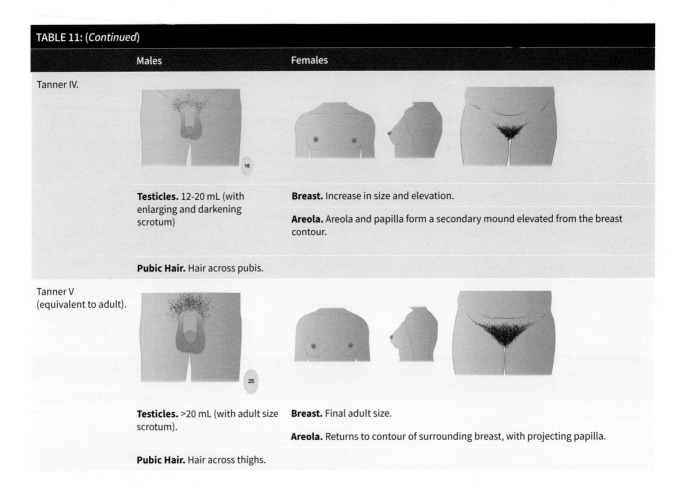

Tanner IV.

Testicles. 12-20 mL (with enlarging and darkening scrotum)

Pubic Hair. Hair across pubis.

Breast. Increase in size and elevation.

Areola. Areola and papilla form a secondary mound elevated from the breast contour.

Tanner V (equivalent to adult).

Testicles. >20 mL (with adult size scrotum).

Pubic Hair. Hair across thighs.

Breast. Final adult size.

Areola. Returns to contour of surrounding breast, with projecting papilla.

TABLE 12: Causes of abnormal puberty

Precocious	Delayed
• Gonadotrophin-dependent precocious puberty, e.g. idiopathic or pituitary tumours. • Gonadotrophin-independent precocious puberty, e.g. adrenal/ovarian/testicular tumours, late onset CAH. • Isolated premature thelarche. • Isolated premature adrenarche. • Isolated premature menarche.	• Constitutional delay. • Hypogonadotrophic hypogonadism, e.g. Kallmann syndrome or pituitary tumour. • Hypergonadotrophic hypogonadism, e.g. Turner syndrome or gonadal trauma.

(CAH: Congenital adrenal hyperplasia)

childhood, but result in short adult stature since growth ceases at the end of puberty. It is more common in girls and in those with an elevated BMI. In boys, precocious puberty is more likely to have an organic cause and is more likely to justify investigation. Categories of precocious puberty are shown in *Table 13*.

Investigations

Precocious puberty is more likely to be benign in girls, but invariably needs to be investigated in both genders. Tests include:

› **Baseline and stimulated FSH/LH hormone concentration, oestrogen/testosterone.** In central precocious puberty baseline and stimulated LH and FSH are elevated (as seen

in pubertal children), whilst in gonadotrophin-independent puberty they are suppressed. Stimulation with gonadotrophin releasing hormone (GnRH) increases the sensitivity of the test. If LH and FSH are suppressed but sex hormones are high, this suggests gonadotrophin-independent precocious puberty. Low, but detectable early morning oestradiol (girls) or testosterone (boys) suggests that puberty is imminent.

› **Adrenal androgens.** These will be elevated in precocious puberty but grossly elevated in adrenal tumours. A urine steroid profile is very helpful in diagnosis of gonadal or adrenal tumours or adrenal biosynthetic defects, such as congenital adrenal hyperplasia (CAH) (p81).

› **TFTs.** Hypothyroidism may be a cause of precocious puberty.

› **Imaging.** Pelvic/testicular ultrasounds are helpful to assess for ovarian/testicular tumours or cysts. An adrenal ultrasound scan (USS) or magnetic resonance imaging (MRI) may identify adrenal pathology. Brain MRI is indicated in all children with evidence of central precocious puberty from GnRH stimulation test, as it may identify a pituitary tumour.

› **Bone age X-Ray.** If bone age is advanced in precocious puberty, the child may benefit from medical inhibition of their puberty.

Management

Treatment for various causes of precocious puberty are shown in *Table 13*.

TABLE 13: Categories of precocious puberty	
Condition	**Features**
Gonadotrophin dependent precocious puberty ("true" or "central" PP).	• This involves the entire hypothalamo-pituitary gonadal (HPG) axis, thus all hormonal and physical changes of puberty occur as normal, and in sequence. • It may be idiopathic, or due to a pituitary tumour. • Central idiopathic precocious puberty is managed with GnRH analogues (which paradoxically suppresses gonadotrophin release). • The decision to treat is based on the age of presentation, whether early puberty has an adverse psychological impact on the child and if adult height is impaired. Surgery may be required for a pituitary tumour.
Gonadotrophin independent precocious puberty ("false" or "pseudo" PP).	• This is due to causes such as congenital adrenal hyperplasia (CAH), tumours of the adrenal gland/ovaries/testicles, Cushing syndrome and hyperthyroidism. • A rarer cause is McCune-Albright syndrome, characterised by autonomous hormone excess in various glands including the gonads, fibrous dysplasia and café-au-lait lesions. Virilisation (e.g. pubic hair growth) may occur early and out of sync with the rest of puberty. • Management is targeted to the underlying diagnosis.
Premature thelarche (isolated premature breast development).	• This is common and benign, occurring in girls usually between 6-months-old and 2-years-old. • There may be transient breast development in a newborn baby owing to maternal oestrogens. • Boys may also develop a transient gynaecomastia in adolescence—this again is usually benign.
Premature pubarche (also known as adrenarche—isolated public hair development).	• This is more common in Asian and black children. It should be investigated as it may suggest increased adrenal androgen production; but is usually not pathological.
Premature menarche.	• Rarely menarche may be the first sign of puberty. Other causes of bleeding must be investigated and excluded, but it is usually benign. • It may be a sign of a pituitary tumour.

Prognosis

Prognosis is generally good, particularly in mild cases that have not required treatment. Those that start treatment with GnRH require close follow up of growth, bone age and pubertal features to ensure that the progression of puberty has arrested.

Delayed Puberty

Constitutional delay of growth and puberty is the commonest cause of delayed puberty. It is covered on p70. Emotional distress may occur, but children reach their target height eventually. If the family and the young person are keen, a short course of hormonal induction (with androgen or oestrogen) may be offered.

Pathological causes of delayed puberty can be divided into low gonadotrophin and high gonadotrophin disease:

Low gonadotrophins (hypogonadotrophic hypogonadism)

This result in the ovaries/testicles being understimulated. This may be due to:
▸ Disorders of the hypothalomo-pituitary-gonadal axis e.g. Kallmann syndrome, pituitary tumour.
▸ Systemic disease e.g. cystic fibrosis, anorexia nervosa, hypothyroidism.

High gonadotrophins (hypergonadotrophic hypogonadism)

This is a normal physiological response to low levels of oestrogen/testosterone in the context of gonadal failure. The primary problem may be:

▸ **Congenital.** Chromosomal abnormalities affecting the gonads, such as Klinefelter (resulting in reduced testosterone production) or Turner syndrome (resulting in reduced oestrogen production). Rarely, there may be a steroid hormone enzyme deficiency.
▸ **Acquired.** Gonadal damage. This could be due to torsion, chemotherapy/radiotherapy, infection e.g. Mumps, or an autoimmune process.

Investigations

These are not necessary in every patient, particularly if there is a strong family history of constitutional delay and the patient is systemically well. Investigations may include:
▸ **Baseline bloods.** FBC, ferritin, TFTs, U&Es, LFTs, coeliac screen, looking for evidence of chronic disease.
▸ **X-Ray of the wrist.** Delayed bone age in settings such as hypothyroidism, and constitutional delay of puberty.
▸ **Baseline and stimulated FSH/LH concentrations, oestrogen/testosterone.** To identify pituitary hormone deficiencies. FSH and LH may be elevated in primary gonadal failure, but very low in hypogonadotrophic failure. LH may be high in polycystic ovarian syndrome, which in severe cases may present with primary amenorrhoea. Other anterior pituitary hormones should also be tested in hypogonadotrophic hypogonadism to look for hypopituitarism. Note that in constitutional delay of growth and puberty, LH levels are low, but classically rise when Luteinising Hormone Releasing Hormone (LHRH) is given, thus differentiating itself from hypogonadotrophic hypogonadism.

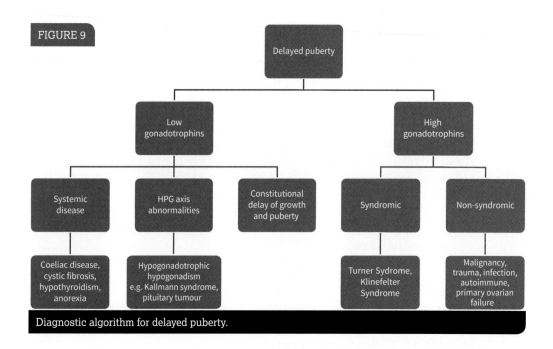

FIGURE 9

Delayed puberty

Low gonadotrophins

High gonadotrophins

Systemic disease

HPG axis abnormalities

Constitutional delay of growth and puberty

Syndromic

Non-syndromic

Coeliac disease, cystic fibrosis, hypothyroidism, anorexia

Hypogonadotrophic hypogonadism e.g. Kallmann syndrome, pituitary tumour

Turner Sydrome, Klinefelter Syndrome

Malignancy, trauma, infection, autoimmune, primary ovarian failure

Diagnostic algorithm for delayed puberty.

> Chromosomes. This is essential in girls, as delayed puberty may be the only presenting feature of Turner syndrome.

> Imaging. Pelvic ultrasound is helpful particularly in girls with suspected gonadal failure. MRI of the pituitary should be considered if there is a concern about a pituitary lesion.

A diagnostic algorithm is shown in *Figure 9*.

Management

In those presenting with delayed puberty, it is important to exclude serious organic disease and chromosomal disorders. Hormonal induction will induce breast development in girls, penile development in boys and secondary sexual characteristics and growth spurt in both sexes. However in hypogonadotrophic hypogonadism, testes will not grow with testosterone replacement. Administration of pulsatile LHRH or injections of hCG and FSH may induce fertility in such cases.

Prognosis

Outlook for reproduction is generally good in hypogonadotrophic hypogonadism, but in cases of gonadal failure chances of reproduction are severely impaired.

DISORDERS OF SEXUAL DEVELOPMENT

Disorders of sexual development (DSD) are a complex group of disorders relating to hormones involved in the development of the gonads. The foetal gonad is initially undifferentiated. A testis-determining gene on the Y chromosome (SRY) results in the gonad differentiating into a testis in the second month of foetal life. In the absence of SRY, the gonads become ovaries, and secondary female sexual characteristics develop. In males, the three key hormones involved in sexual development are:

1 Testosterone. For internal genitalia.

2 Dihydrotestosterone. For external genitalia.

3 Anti-Mullerian hormone. To inhibit uterus and fallopian tube development.

Problems that arise in the above process may result in a disorder of sexual development. These are now classified into three distinct categories (*Table 14*). The most common cause is congenital adrenal hyperplasia, resulting in virilisation of a 46XX female. Maternal drug ingestion in the first trimester may also result in virilisation. There may be a family history of infertility, ambiguous genitalia or sudden death.

Clinical Features

Presentation is usually at birth with ambiguous genitalia, but this not always the case (*Figure 10*). Ambiguous genitalia may be due to:

> Virilisation from excessive androgens in a female. For example, due to congenital adrenal hyperplasia (CAH).

> Undervirilisation from insufficient androgens in a male. For example, due to 5 alpha reductase deficiency, which converts testosterone to dihydrotestosterone.

> Gonadotrophin insufficiency. For example, hypopituitarism.

DSDs may also present with secondary sexual characteristics inconsistent with apparent sex (e.g. gynaecomastia associated with testicles), with primary amenorrhoea, infertility later in life, or unexpected changes in puberty.

Investigations

Disorders of sexual differentiation are rare and are often distressing for parents, who will be eager for their child's

TABLE 14: Classification of disorders of sexual development according to the Chicago consensus on disorders of sex development (DSD)

Classification	Examples
Sex Chromosome DSD.	• **45,X.** Turner syndrome. • **47,XXY.** Klinefelter syndrome. • **46,XX/46,XY.** Chimerism, where both male and female sex chromosome sets are present in different cells.
46,XX DSD.	**Disorders of ovarian development.** • Gonadal dysgenesis, leading to ovarian failure. • The presence of a small Y fragment in the genetic material: 46,XX SRY+ **Androgen excess.** • Congenital adrenal hyperplasia e.g. 21-hydroxylase deficiency.
46,XY DSD.	**Disorders of testicular development.** • Gonadal dysgenesis, leading to testicular failure. **Androgen insufficiency.** • Disorders of androgen synthesis e.g. 17-hydroxysteroid dehydrogenase deficiency, 5 alpha reductase deficiency. • Disorder of androgen receptor e.g. partial or complete androgen insensitivity.

FIGURE 10

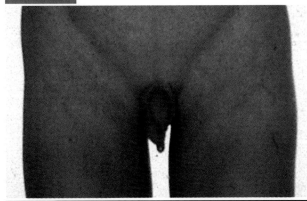

Boy with bilateral absent testicles.

sex to be assigned. Assessment starts from careful clinical examination, including identifying any secondary sexual characteristics.

Important tests to consider include:

▸ **Chromosomal analysis.** To assess the genotype. Results of fluorescence in situ hybridisation (FISH) analysis to look for the SRY gene on a Y chromosome fragment usually come back within 24 hours.

▸ **Glucose, electrolyte, cortisol and 17-hydroxyprogesterone (17OHP) levels.** These are important in identifying congenital adrenal hyperplasia. 17OHP measurement is not reliable before 36 hours of age. Urine steroid profile, adrenocorticotropic hormone (ACTH) levels and renin are also helpful in determining this diagnosis. An ACTH stimulation test will further assess adrenal biosynthesis.

▸ **HcG (human chorionic gonadotropin) stimulation test.** This will assess androgen biosynthesis.

▸ **AMH (anti-Mullerian hormone).** This inhibits uterine and fallopian tube development, and therefore should be suppressed in females, and raised in males.

▸ **Molecular analysis of the androgen receptor gene.** Low levels or androgen receptor insensitivity may result in under-virilisation.

▸ **Dihydrotestosterone.** 5 alpha reductase deficiency results in undervirilised males. The enzyme is required in the production of dihydrotestosterone (DHT) from testosterone. Penile development is dependent on DHT.

▸ **Abdominal and pelvic USS.** This is important for the identification of a uterus and fallopian tubes. The adrenals may be bulky in congenital adrenal hyperplasia.

▸ **Laparoscopy and biopsies of gonadal tissue.** This may reveal mullerian structures (uterus and fallopian tubes), ovarian tissue, testicular tissue, mixed ovarian/testicular tissue, or streak gonads.

Management

Children with DSD should be managed by a multidisciplinary team. This team includes: neonatologist/paediatrician, paediatric endocrinologist, clinical psychologist, clinical geneticists, paediatric urologist, specialist nurse, paediatric radiologist, clinical endocrine biochemist and a gynaecologist.

Medical therapy depends on the underlying cause. Supplementary hormone therapy may be indicated. Psychological input for the parents and the child is very important throughout the process.

The sex assigned in early childhood may not correlate with the child's gender preference in adulthood. The brain plays a large role in determining sex, and this is impossible to assess in the neonatal period. Therefore, while corrective surgery may be required in the infant period, definitive surgery should be done later in life when gender is clearer. Virilised females may have a feminising genitoplasty (including a vaginoplasty and clitoroplasty), whilst undervirilised males often have hypospadias requiring surgical correction (p350).

Terms such as "hermaphrodite" and "intersex" are generally abandoned, as they are often considered stigmatising.

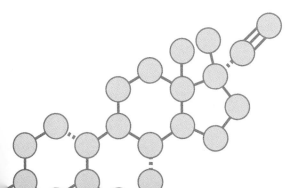

ADRENAL DISORDERS

The adrenal glands are located on top of the kidneys and each adrenal gland has a cortex and medulla. The adrenal cortex consists of three distinct layers: the zona glomerulosa, zona fasciculata and zona reticularis (*Figure 11*):

> **Zona glomerulosa (outer layer).** This produces mineralocorticoids (aldosterone) under the control of the renin-angiotensin system for maintaining salt and water balance.

> **Zona fasciculata (middle layer).** This produces glucocorticoids (cortisol) under the control of the Hypothalamic-Pituitary-Adrenal (HPA) axis through corticotropin releasing hormone (CRH) and Adrenocorticotropic hormone (ACTH). Cortisol production has diurnal variation with a peak value at around 8 a.m. and a trough value around midnight. Importantly, there is a negative feedback loop, whereby elevated cortisol downregulates ACTH and CRH production (thus reducing cortisol), and conversely a positive feedback loop, whereby low cortisol upregulates ACTH and CRH production (thus increasing cortisol). Cortisol is important for glucose regulation, blood pressure control and inflammatory mediation. *Figure 12* summarises cortisol regulation.

> **Zona reticularis (inner layer).** This matures late in childhood and secretes sex steroids (androgens). This includes testosterone, but also dihydrotestosterone (DHT) and androstenedione (a precursor to oestradiol and testosterone).

The adrenal medulla produces catecholamines (predominantly adrenaline/epinephrine, but also noradrenaline/norepinephrine).

Adrenal Insufficiency

Aetiology

Adrenal insufficiency (AI) results in low cortisol. AI can be primary or secondary. Low ACTH is the key difference in diagnosing secondary AI (ACTH is high in primary adrenal insufficiency).

Primary AI

In primary AI, the adrenal cortex is dysfunctional or non-functional. Addison's disease (autoimmune adrenalitis) is an example of this. Other examples include infection (tuberculosis [TB], human immunodeficiency virus [HIV], meningococcemia), and congenital adrenal hyperplasia (p81). Since the pituitary is functioning normally, low cortisol results via the positive feedback loop in higher ACTH secretion. As there is a primary problem in the adrenals, mineralocorticoid (aldosterone) production is also affected.

Low cortisol can result in hypoglycaemia and low blood pressure. High ACTH results in increased skin pigmentation, giving patients with primary AI a sun-tanned appearance.

Lack of aldosterone results in hyponatraemia, hyperkalaemia and hypotension, as aldosterone is required for sodium/water

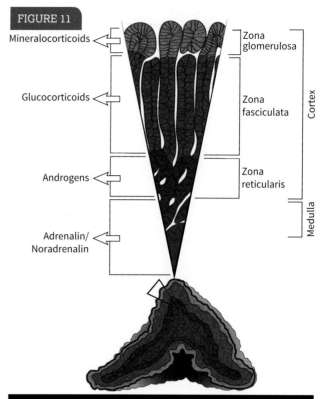

Hormone production in the adrenal glands.

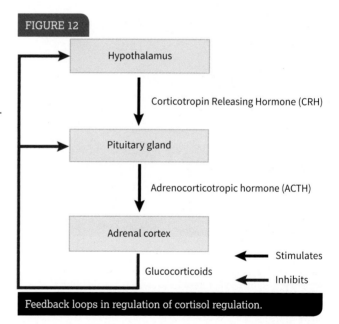

Feedback loops in regulation of cortisol regulation.

reabsorption and potassium excretion in the kidneys. This results in high renin in an effort to compensate. In congenital adrenal hyperplasia, specific markers can be tested for (p82).

Secondary AI

This is due to primary ACTH deficiency, hence both cortisol and ACTH levels are low. This most commonly occurs due to rapid discontinuation of long-term exogenous corticosteroids.

Other causes include congenital panhypopituitarism, cranial irradiation and pituitary tumours. ACTH deficiency is most often part of multiple pituitary hormone deficiencies, whilst isolated ACTH deficiency is rare. Mineralocorticoid function is preserved in secondary adrenal insufficiency, since aldosterone secretion is independent of ACTH.

Clinical Features
Presenting features vary depending on whether this occurs in the neonatal period or in infancy/childhood (*Table 15*).

Investigations
Table 16 summarises the investigation results in primary compared to secondary AI.

Management
Acute Management
Children can present in adrenal crisis profoundly unwell, with hypotension, hypoglycaemia, hyperkalaemia and hyponatraemia. This is classically in the context of an infection or rapid withdrawal of steroid treatment. Such children need prompt resuscitation, along with correction of any hypoglycaemia and hyperkalaemia. Intravenous hydrocortisone should be started initially and once the patient is clinically

stable, physiological doses of oral hydrocortisone are initiated. If mineralocorticoid deficiency is confirmed, this needs to be replaced as well with fludrocortisone. It is often necessary in primary AI but not secondary AI.

Long-term Management
Children on hydrocortisone and fludrocortisone replacement require regular growth and blood pressure monitoring. Hydrocortisone is the preferred choice of corticosteroid in paediatrics as it does not have adverse effects on growth if not over-replaced. Periodic measurements of cortisol, ACTH and renin concentrations are useful in optimising the treatment doses. The usual maintenance dose of hydrocortisone in primary AI is $10-12$ mg/m²/day; in secondary AI, lower doses are usually sufficient. Because of its short half-life, hydrocortisone needs to be given three or four times a day.

An emergency treatment plan for stressful situations should be given to all patients on hydrocortisone replacement therapy. Patients are advised to double their corticosteroid replacement dose during illnesses and are provided with hydrocortisone intramuscular injections for emergencies. Patients with AI should have a Medic-alert bracelet.

It is important also to think about how adrenal crisis can be prevented. Any child started on a long course of steroids (e.g. for asthma or nephrotic syndrome) should have their dose gradually weaned. High dose corticosteroids result in ACTH and CRH suppression, and therefore reduction of endogenous steroid production. Thus, rapid discontinuation of treatment may precipitate an adrenal crisis.

Prognosis
Mortality is usually related to cardiovascular instability and electrolyte derangement. However, with proper treatment and rapid identification of illness, outlook is good.

Congenital Adrenal Hyperplasia
Aetiology
Congenital Adrenal Hyperplasia (CAH) is a deficiency of enzymes involved in the synthesis of cortisol and aldosterone. It occurs in one in 5000 births and encompasses a group of autosomal recessive disorders involving a deficiency of an enzyme involved in the synthesis of cortisol, aldosterone or both. As with most autosomal recessive disorders, it is more prevalent in the offspring of consanguineous couples. The most common cause of CAH is 21-hydroxylase deficiency (95%). 11β-hydroxylase is the second commonest enzyme defect, whilst other forms are rare.

Impaired cortisol production results in an increase in ACTH through a positive feedback mechanism involving the HPA axis. ACTH stimulation triggers the pathways in the adrenals which normally produce cortisol. This results in adrenal hyperplasia. However, CAH is characterised by an enzyme deficiency preventing the production of cortisol

TABLE 15: Clinical features of adrenal insufficiency		
	Neonatal period	**Infancy and childhood**
Presenting features.	• Hypoglycaemia. • Hyponatraemia. • Hyperkalaemia. • Adrenal crisis. • Conjugated hyperbilirubinaemia. • Disorders of sexual development.	• Anorexia. • Fatigue. • Muscle weakness. • Vomiting, diarrhoea. • Weight loss. • Craving for salt. • Hypotension. • Behaviour changes. • Poor concentration. • Increased skin pigmentation (primary AI). • Adrenal crisis.

TABLE 16: Differentiating primary and secondary AI using blood tests. The most sensitive marker is ACTH levels, although preserved aldosterone function may serve as a further clue		
	Primary AI	**Secondary AI**
Cortisol.	• Low.	• Low.
ACTH.	• High.	• Low.
Aldosterone.	• Low.	• Normal.
Renin.	• High.	• Normal.
Sodium.	• Low.	• Normal.
Potassium.	• High.	• Normal.
Glucose.	• Low.	• Low.

and aldosterone; consequently, the precursors to them build up in the adrenals. A raised level of the cortisol/aldosterone precursor 17-hydroxyprogesterone (17OHP) in the blood is used to diagnose CAH. Since these substrates cannot be used for cortisol/aldosterone production, they are diverted to other biosynthesis pathways, resulting in androgen production, particularly dehydroepiandrosterone (DHEA) and androstenedione, which result in virilisation. *Figure 13* summarises these reactions.

Symptoms result from:

1 Low cortisol. Hypotension, hypoglycaemia.
2 Low aldosterone. Hypotension, hyponatraemia, hyperkalaemia.
3 Elevated androgens. Virilisation.

Clinical Features

CAH can be classified into classic CAH and non-classic CAH. In classic CAH, the enzyme defect is more severe. Approximately 75% of patients with classic CAH have severe aldosterone deficiency, presenting in the neonatal period with a salt-losing crisis. Girls with classic CAH usually present with genital ambiguity at birth, whilst boys present with salt-losing crisis. The non-classic form is late onset, presenting in childhood, with precocious puberty in boys and virilisation in girls.

Salt-Losing Crisis

A salt-losing crisis manifests in the neonatal period with vomiting, poor feeding, weight loss, dehydration, hypotension, hyperkalaemia, hyponatraemia and hypoglycaemia.

Genital Ambiguity

High androgens in girls cause virilisation of the external genitalia: clitoral enlargement and scrotalisation and hyperpigmentation of the labia majora skin. In boys, it may result in a large phallus and hyperpigmentation of scrotal skin. *Figure 14* shows the spectrum of genital changes in females.

Investigations

Despite the emergency of a salt-losing crisis, the correct specimens should be taken before initiation of corticosteroid replacement:

› Cortisol. This will be low.
› 17OHP. This will be elevated, as it is a precursor to cortisol/aldosterone.
› ACTH and renin (if possible). ACTH and renin will both be elevated to try and compensate for low aldosterone and cortisol.
› Urine steroid profile. This quantifies metabolites of different steroids, and can therefore point towards any changes in steroid profile.

However, if blood sampling is difficult and CAH is strongly suspected, then treatment should be initiated without delay. Diagnosis can be established later, when the baby is stable, with a synacthen test.

Management

Acute Management

Acute management of a salt-losing crisis involves:

› Fluid resuscitation.
› Intravenous hydrocortisone.
› Slow correction of hyponatraemia.
› Rapid correction of hyperkalaemia and hypoglycaemia.

Long-term Management

The main goals of the treatment are to replace glucocorticoid and mineralocorticoid deficiencies and suppress excess

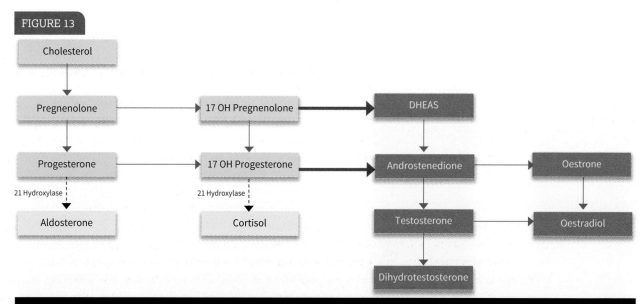

FIGURE 13

Adrenocorticotropic hormone (ACTH) stimulation in Congenital Adrenal Hyperplasia (CAH), resulting in elevated androgens (dehydroepiandrosterone sulphate [DHEAS] and androstenedione), low cortisol and low aldosterone.

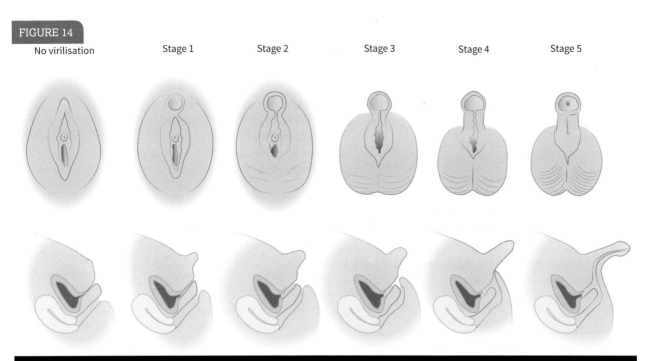

FIGURE 14

| No virilisation | Stage 1 | Stage 2 | Stage 3 | Stage 4 | Stage 5 |

Prader Scale reflecting the degree of virilisation of the external genitalia in girls.

adrenal androgen production. Children with CAH need regular follow up to monitor growth, skeletal maturation, weight gain, blood pressure, electrolytes, 17OHP, adrenal androgens and renin to ensure optimal corticosteroid and mineralocorticoid replacement. An emergency treatment plan for stressful situations should be given to all patients on hydrocortisone replacement therapy, similarly to other conditions of AI. Children with genital ambiguity require surgical evaluation.

Prognosis

Prognosis is good with adequate treatment. It is important to emphasise the importance of stress doses of steroids during times of illness. There are also commonly significant psychological difficulties in those with genital abnormalities.

Cushing Syndrome

Aetiology

Cushing syndrome is a result of excess corticosteroids. The most common cause of Cushing syndrome is excess exogenous/iatrogenic glucocorticoid. Endogenous Cushing syndrome can be classified into ACTH independent and ACTH dependent (Cushing disease). Causes vary with age:

▸ In children less than 7-years-old, adrenal causes are the commonest cause. These include adrenal adenoma, adrenal carcinoma and bilateral adrenal hyperplasia. Adrenal tumours should be suspected if a child presents with features of Cushing syndrome of a short duration.

▸ In children over 7-years-old, Cushing disease accounts for approximately 75% of Cushing syndrome. Cushing disease is caused by an ACTH-secreting pituitary adenoma.

▸ Ectopic ACTH production from tumours is very rare in childhood.

Clinical Features

Onset of Cushing syndrome is usually insidious, with weight gain and slowing of growth. Common features of Cushing syndrome are a moon-like face, acne, easy bruising, central obesity, abdominal striae, hirsutism and hypertension (*Figure 15*). Long-term Cushing syndrome may cause osteopenia and vertebral fractures, which can present as back pain.

Investigations

In Cushing syndrome, there is loss of diurnal variation (as measured by early morning and midnight cortisol and ACTH) and 24-hour urinary free cortisol is high. In Cushing disease, ACTH is also elevated, whereas in non-pituitary disease, the ACTH would be suppressed. Symptomatically, the elevated ACTH may manifest as increased skin pigmentation.

Dexamethasone Suppression Test

Dexamethasone suppression tests are used to establish the diagnosis. Dexamethasone results in inhibition of ACTH, and therefore suppression of cortisol. Patients that are disease free usually suppress their cortisol production with a low-dose test, whereas with Cushing syndrome they will not.

High-dose tests are then used to subcategorise Cushing syndrome. In the high-dose test, the dose of dexamethasone is large enough to suppress ACTH secretion in Cushing disease (ACTH dependent). However, in ACTH independent Cushing syndrome, since ACTH secretion is already very low, there is

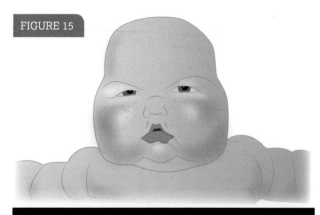

FIGURE 15

Cushingoid baby.

TABLE 17: Identifying Cushing disease and Cushing Syndrome			
	Normal	ACTH Dependent Cushing Syndrome (Cushing Disease)	ACTH Independent Cushing Syndrome
24-hour urinary free cortisol.	• Normal.	• High.	• High.
ACTH levels.	• Normal.	• High.	• Low.
Diurnal variation in ACTH level.	• Present.	• Absent.	• Absent.
Low dose dexamethasone suppression test.	• Cortisol production suppressed.	• Cortisol production NOT suppressed.	• Cortisol production NOT suppressed.
High dose dexamethasone suppression test.	• Cortisol production suppressed.	• Cortisol production suppressed.	• Cortisol production NOT suppressed.

little room for further downregulation. Thus, no suppression of cortisol production occurs.

Table 17 summarises results interpretation.

Imaging
Imaging (CT or MRI scans) of adrenal and pituitary glands is required to rule out adrenal and pituitary tumours.

Management
Management is directed at the specific cause. Surgery is usually indicated if a tumour is identified at either site. Adrenal steroid inhibitors (e.g. metyrapone) may be required. If a bilateral adrenalectomy is required, lifelong hormone replacement is needed.

Prognosis
Excess steroids increase the risk of obesity, and cardiovascular problems such as hypertension and coronary artery disease in older age. Those with benign lesions and curative surgery have the best outcomes. However, those having surgery are also at risk of adrenal insufficiency.

THYROID DISORDERS
Thyroid hormone is essential for normal brain development, linear growth and normal metabolism throughout life. Iodine is essential for thyroid hormone production. Thyrotropin releasing hormone (TRH), secreted by the hypothalamus, stimulates release of thyroid stimulating hormone (TSH) from the anterior pituitary gland. TSH stimulates the synthesis and release of thyroid hormone from the thyroid gland. The thyroid hormones are T4, thyroxine (the metabolically active thyroid hormone), and T3 (the thyroxine precursor). Thyroid hormone has a negative feedback control over TSH/TRH secretion i.e. as thyroid hormone goes up, TSH and TRH go down, as summarised in *Figure 16*.

Thyroid hormone is important for:
> Increasing the basal metabolic rate.
> Increasing the body's sensitivity to catecholamines.
> Regulation of growth as well as protein, fat and carbohydrate metabolism.

Table 18 shows the interpretation of the thyroid function test (TFT).

Hypothyroidism
Aetiology
Congenital Hypothyroidism
Congenital hypothyroidism affects about one in 4000 babies. If untreated, it can lead to severe learning difficulties; therefore, newborn screening programmes are available worldwide. During foetal life, the placenta is permeable to T3 and T4 but not to TSH. Therefore, maternal euthyroid status gives a relative protection of brain development to the hypothyroid infant.

Congenital hypothyroidism may be due to:
> **Thyroid dysgenesis.** This is a developmental abnormality of the thyroid gland, either agenesis (no thyroid gland) or dysgenesis (a small, poorly formed thyroid gland that may be ectopic).
> **Thyroid dyshormonogenesis.** Less commonly, congenital hypothyroidism is due to an enzymatic defect in thyroid hormone production.

Acquired Hypothyroidism
Causes of acquired hypothyroidism include:
> **Autoimmune thyroiditis (Hashimoto disease).** There are often circulating anti-thyroid antibodies, most commonly anti-thyroid peroxidise antibodies (anti-TPO Ab) and anti-thyroglobulin (anti-Tg Ab). Children with Type 1 Diabetes are regularly screened for autoimmune hypothyroidism.
> **Iodine deficiency or iodine excess.**

FIGURE 16

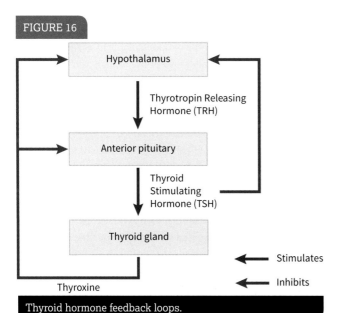

Thyroid hormone feedback loops.

TABLE 18: Thyroid Function Tests			
TSH	Free T4	Free T3	Diagnosis
• High.	• Low.	• Low.	• Primary hypothyroidism. • Low thyroid hormone triggers an increase in TSH but it is not sufficient.
• High.	• Normal.	• Normal.	• Subclinical hypothyroidism. • It is compensated for by elevated TSH.
• Low/Normal.	• Low.	• Low.	• Central hypothyroidism. • Low TSH secretion resulting in low thyroid hormones.
• Low.	• High.	• High.	• Hyperthyroidism. • Autonomous production of thyroid hormones not controlled by TSH.

> Drugs. Carbimazole, propylthiouracil, amiodarone, antiepileptic medications.
> External radiation therapy.
> Thyroidectomy.
> Radioactive iodine treatment.

Central Hypothyroidism

This can be due to TSH deficiency (pituitary or secondary hypothyroidism) or TRH deficiency (hypothalamic or tertiary hypothyroidism). Acquired central hypothyroidism can occur as a late effect of cranial irradiation for CNS tumours. It can also occur due to trauma, tumours, infiltrative conditions like sarcoidosis, and infections like tuberculosis and syphilis. Central hypothyroidism is rare and usually associated with other pituitary hormone deficiencies and midline defects.

Investigations

Newborn screening tests, usually done between the fifth and eighth day of life, measure TSH to identify congenital hypothyroidism. If TSH is elevated, free T4 and TSH need to be formally measured. Low free T4 and high TSH confirm the diagnosis of hypothyroidism. Once diagnosis is confirmed, a nuclear scan of the thyroid is performed to differentiate potential causes of congenital hypothyroidism. Auditory assessment is also required, since hypothyroidism may be associated with sensorineural deafness (Pendred syndrome).

Hypothyroidism may also be picked up later in life, either due to a child becoming symptomatic, or as part of a screening programme (e.g. T1DM). Central hypothyroidism is diagnosed when T4 is low with a low or normal TSH.

Clinical Features

Clinical features of congenital hypothyroidism are summarised in *Table 19*, but it is usually picked up in asymptomatic infants on screening. Screening programmes have dramatically reduced intellectual impairment in congenital hypothyroidism because of early recognition and treatment.

The clinical features of acquired hypothyroidism are often subtle, depending on the severity and duration of hypothyroidism. They may include:

> Poor growth.
> Weight gain.
> Lethargy and excessive sleepiness.
> Impaired school performance.
> Muscle weakness.
> Coarse hair and patchy hair loss.
> Goitre.
> Slow relaxation of deep tendon reflexes.
> Pubertal abnormalities.
> Low mood.

Management

In congenital hypothyroidism, Levothyroxine (L-Thyroxine) replacement therapy is necessary for life. Neurocognitive development is significantly improved if L-Thyroxine replacement is started within 10–14 days of life. Regular monitoring of growth, neurodevelopment and thyroid function should be undertaken in the first two years of life, with less frequent monitoring after this age.

TABLE 19: Clinical features of congenital hypothyroidism	
Symptoms	Signs
• Poor feeding. • Lethargy. • Constipation. • Prolonged jaundice. • Hoarse cry.	• Macroglossia. • Coarse facies. • Hypotonia. • Bradycardia. • Umbilical hernia. • Wide fontanelle. • Goitre.

In acquired hypothyroidism, L-Thyroxine replacement is also required, and in many cases this treatment is also lifelong. The aim is to normalise the TSH and maintain T4 in the upper half of the normal range. When treating central hypothyroidism, cortisol deficiency must be excluded before starting L-Thyroxine because a co-existent ACTH deficiency together with thyroxine replacement can precipitate an adrenal crisis.

Hyperthyroidism
Aetiology
Hyperthyroidism is rare in children. The most common cause is Graves' disease, which is six times more common in girls than boys. It is caused by antibodies (TRAb) directed against TSH receptors. TRAb acts like TSH and stimulates the thyroid gland to produce excessive thyroid hormones. Other causes include:
> Toxic adenoma.
> Toxic multinodular goitre.
> Sub-acute thyroiditis.
> Functioning pituitary adenoma.
> Factitious hyperthyroidism.
> Metastatic thyroid cancer.

Clinical Features
Table 20 summarises the signs and symptoms of hyperthyroidism.

Investigations
Hyperthyroidism is biochemically characterised by high free T3 and T4 and low or undetectable TSH. If hyperthyroidism is confirmed, an ultrasound scan of the thyroid gland should be carried out. This will identify any changes in the morphology of the thyroid gland, including any nodules. Measurement of anti-thyroperoxidase antibodies (Anti-TPO Ab), anti-thyroglobulin antibodies (Anti-Tg Ab) and TRAb is also useful to identify an autoimmune cause.

Management
Antithyroid drugs (carbimazole, methimazole and propylthiouracil) remain the first line treatment for hyperthyroidism and these drugs

TABLE 20: Clinical features of hyperthyroidism

Symptoms	Signs
• Hyperactivity.	• Goitre.
• Restlessness.	• Fine tremor.
• Emotional lability.	• Hyperreflexia.
• Anxiety.	• Moist, warm skin.
• Declining school performance.	• Tachycardia, rarely SVT.
• Palpitations.	• Lid lag.
• Dyspnoea.	• Exophthalmos.
• Excessive sweating.	• Ophthalmoplegia.
• Heat intolerance.	• Proximal muscle wasting.
• Increased appetite.	• Hair loss.
• Weight loss.	• Osteoporosis.
• Diarrhoea.	• Hypercalcaemia.
• Oligo or amenorrhoea.	

suppress the overactive thyroid gland. Propranolol (beta blocker) is helpful in controlling acute symptoms. If antithyroid drug treatment fails or side effects of medication are unacceptable, a definitive therapy needs to be considered with either total thyroidectomy or radioactive iodine treatment.

CALCIUM DISORDERS
The plasma concentration of calcium depends on the net balance of intestinal and renal reabsorption, and the bone mineral deposition and resorption. This process is tightly regulated by a complex system involving parathyroid hormone (PTH), calcitonin, vitamin D and the calcium sensing receptor.

PTH is produced by the chief cells of the parathyroid glands. It raises calcium concentration by enhancing the activity of 1-alpha hydroxylase in the kidneys, the enzyme implicated in the conversion of 25-hydroxyvitamin D to its active form: 1,25-dihydroxyvitamin D (calcitriol). This increases calcium reabsorption in the distal collecting tubule, mobilises calcium from the bones and increases gut absorption. The calcium sensing receptor is the "calcistat". Essentially, it senses changes in ionised calcium concentration: a decrease in its concentration triggers PTH release, while an increase in its concentration suppresses PTH production.

Calcitonin is a hormone produced by the parafollicular cells of the thyroid gland in response to high calcium levels. However, its role is not very significant in calcium regulation, with PTH being the major player.

The majority of calcium (55%) is usually bound to albumin or other cations, with the rest being ionised, in the form of unbound, active calcium. Measurement of total and ionised calcium is important because in some diseased states (e.g. hypoalbuminaemia), total calcium levels can decrease while the ionised calcium level remains normal. Investigation of hypocalcaemia should also include measurements of the magnesium level because low magnesium inhibits PTH bioactivity. *Figure 17* summarises calcium homeostasis.

Hypocalcaemia
Aetiology
The most common cause of hypocalcaemia is vitamin D deficiency (p251). Hypoparathyroidism-related hypocalcaemia can be genetic or acquired. Genetic causes of hypoparathyroidism are mostly related to abnormal development of the parathyroid glands (e.g. Di George syndrome, where there is aplasia or hypoplasia of the parathyroid glands) or to mutations in genes affecting PTH synthesis. Acquired causes include parathyroidectomy, thyroidectomy, autoimmune causes and haemosiderosis.
> **Thyroidectomy.** This can be complicated with usually transient hypocalcaemia. More rarely, if the parathyroid glands are not preserved, it can lead to permanent hypoparathyroidism.
> **Autoimmune hypoparathyroidism.** This is usually part of autoimmune polyendocrine syndrome 1 (APS1, also known as APECED [autoimmune polyendocrinopathy-candidiasis-ectodermal dystrophy]). It manifests with hypoparathyroidism, Addison's disease and chronic mucocutaneous candidiasis.
> **Haemosiderosis.** Iron overload related to frequent transfusions, such as in

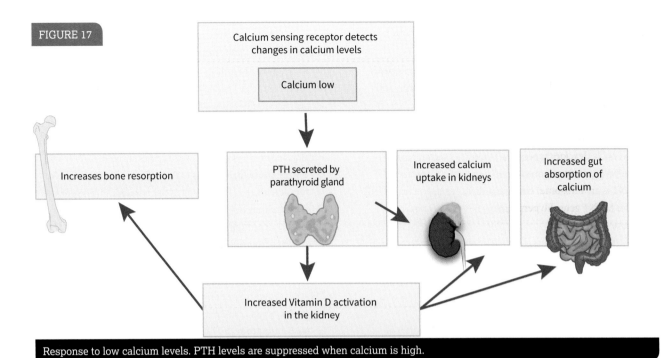

FIGURE 17

Calcium sensing receptor detects changes in calcium levels

Calcium low

Increases bone resorption

PTH secreted by parathyroid gland

Increased calcium uptake in kidneys

Increased gut absorption of calcium

Increased Vitamin D activation in the kidney

Response to low calcium levels. PTH levels are suppressed when calcium is high.

patients with thalassaemia, can cause hypoparathyroidism due to iron deposition (haemosiderosis) on the parathyroid glands.

Pseudohypoparathyroidism consists of a group of disorders characterised by resistance to the action of PTH. PTH concentration is high, but PTH itself is ineffective. Another rare cause is activating mutations of the calcium sensing receptor. This results in the calcium threshold at which PTH production is switched off being set too low, meaning inappropriate PTH suppression and hypocalcaemia.

Clinical Features
Hypocalcaemia may be asymptomatic or present with:
› Tetany (involuntary muscle spasms).
› Seizures.
› Numbness, muscle pains and cramps.
› Stridor.
› Dilated cardiomyopathy.

In evaluating hypocalcaemia, a thorough history and examination coupled with measurement of serum calcium, vitamin D, PTH, albumin, phosphate, magnesium and renal function is indicated. Blood tests are summarised in *Table 21*. Phosphate is usually elevated, as it is generally sacrificed for calcium reabsorption.

In older children the characteristic signs of Chvostek and Trousseau can be elicited.
› Chvostek sign. When the facial nerve is tapped at the angle of the jaw, the ipsilateral facial muscles twitch.
› Trousseau sign. A blood pressure cuff is inflated to a pressure above systolic blood pressure, and this is maintained for three minutes. In the context of hypocalcaemia, this will lead to spasm in the muscles of the hand/forearm.

Management
Hypocalcaemia is managed with calcium supplementation. Intravenous calcium is rarely given. If vitamin D deficiency is present, this should be supplemented as well.

TABLE 21: Blood test results in hypoparathyroidism				
	Hypoparathyroidism.	Pseudohypoparathyroidism.	Vitamin D deficiency.	Activating calcium sensing receptor mutations.
Description.	• The primary problem is deficiency/low levels of PTH.	• The primary problem is PTH resistance.	• Vitamin D deficiency.	• Inappropriate PTH suppression.
PTH.	• Low.	• High.	• High.	• Low.
Calcium.	• Low.	• Low.	• Low (may increase with PTH).	• Low.
Phosphate.	• High.	• High.	• Low.	• High.
Urinary Calcium.	• Low.	• Low.	• Low (may increase with PTH).	• Low.

Hypercalcaemia

Aetiology

Hypercalcemia in children is rare. The most common causes of hypercalcaemia in children are hyperparathyroidism and inactivating calcium sensing receptor mutations.

› Hyperparathyroidism. This can be isolated or part of multiple endocrine neoplasia. Patients with MEN1 almost universally develop hyperparathyroidism and may also develop pituitary adenomas and pancreatic tumours. MEN1 is an autosomal dominant disorder due to mutations in the MEN1 gene. Hyperparathyroidism may also be a feature in MEN2.

› Inactivating mutations of the calcium-sensing receptor. In this condition, the threshold to switch off PTH production is set too high, i.e. PTH is suppressed at a much higher ionised calcium concentration.

Cancer-related hypercalcaemia is found less commonly in children in comparison to adults, where it is due to circulating PTH-related proteins. Children with Williams syndrome, a genetic condition characterised by distinctive "elfin" facies, supravalvular aortic stenosis and learning difficulties, may also present with hypercalcaemia in infancy. Hypercalcaemia may be present in subcutaneous fat necrosis, such as seen in newborns following birth trauma. The mechanism is not clear, but is thought to be related to rapid conversion of 25-hydroxy vitamin D to 1,25-dihydroxyvitamin D, stimulated by the macrophages accumulated in the necrotic area.

Clinical Features

Hypercalcaemia can manifest with:
› Abdominal pain.
› Constipation.
› Irritability.
› Renal stones.
› Bone pains.
› Soft tissue calcification.

Some key features of hypercalcaemia can be recalled by the mnemonic "stones, bones, thrones, abdominal moans, psychiatric overtones".

Management

Hypercalcaemia is managed with intravenous fluid hydration, with or without diuretics. If persistent, bisphosphonates and corticosteroids may be used. Bisphosphonates act by reducing bone resorption. Their action to reduce calcium is slow. Diuretics like furosemide increase renal calcium excretion. In severe cases, calcitonin may also be used. In primary hyperparathyroidism, treatment is parathyroidectomy.

SODIUM DISORDERS

Water and sodium disturbance is one of the commonest derangements occurring in the paediatric inpatient population.

Plasma osmolality is tightly controlled by thirst and antidiuretic hormone (ADH). ADH controls the urine concentration. Both hyper and hyponatraemia can cause non-specific symptoms, like irritability, tiredness, headache, nausea, vomiting and confusion. They can potentially cause seizures and respiratory arrest.

Hyponatraemia

Clinical assessment in patients with hyponatraemia involves:

1 Assessing body fluid status (hypovolaemia, euvolaemia or hypervolaemia). If the patient is dehydrated, this implies fluid loss, either through the kidneys or elsewhere. Sodium may be lost through this. Hypovolaemic patients may be experiencing fluid shifts away from the intravascular compartment, thus losing sodium from the blood.

2 Measuring serum osmolarity, electrolytes and glucose. Dilutional hyponatraemia may occur in the setting of hyperglycaemia or increased plasma osmolality. This is due to fluid shifts from the intracellular space to the blood stream caused by osmosis.

3 Measuring urinary sodium and osmolality. In the setting of normal renal function, sodium should be conserved by the kidneys in a hyponatraemic child. Therefore, suspect a renal pathology if the sodium is unexpectedly high in the urine.

Figure 18 summarises assessment. Further evaluation is then related to the cause. It is important to review medications, as many medications, e.g. diuretics, can cause hyponatraemia.

Symptomatic hyponatraemia is a medical emergency and requires intensive treatment. Hypertonic sodium chloride (2.7%) can be used initially in children with severe symptomatic hyponatraemia. Once asymptomatic, fluid restriction should be reinstituted to achieve further correction in serum sodium level.

No matter the cause of hyponatraemia, correction of serum sodium should be done cautiously, as rapid changes can cause cerebral demyelination and brain damage.

Syndrome of Inappropriate Secretion of Antidiuretic Hormone (SiADH)

Inappropriate secretion of ADH (SiADH) is commonly seen in children with severe pulmonary or CNS infections and immediately after neurosurgical procedures. The most common cause for severe hyponatraemia is SiADH. The mechanism for SiADH is not fully understood. When triggered, ADH acts on the distal convoluted tubule and collecting ducts of the kidney to increase sodium and water reabsorption. SiADH is usually acute and transient in children and responds very well to fluid restriction.

Hypernatraemia

Clinical assessment for body fluid status is the first step and the contributing factors for hypernatraemia should be evaluated. Measuring serum electrolytes, serum osmolality, glucose, urine osmolality and urinary sodium is the next step in finding out the cause for hypernatraemia in children (*Figure 19*). In hypovolaemia, the normal response of the kidneys should be to reabsorb both sodium and fluid. Therefore, urinary sodium should be low and urinary osmolality should be high. If this is not the case, then a pathological cause is likely.

Correcting the serum sodium and circulatory volume is the cornerstone of hypernatraemia management. In cases of severe dehydration, normal daily fluid requirement plus fluid deficit should be corrected over 48–72 hours. This is because over-rapid correction can precipitate cerebral oedema.

FIGURE 18

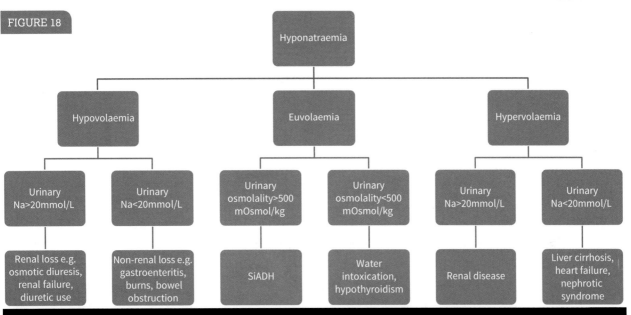

Flow chart for the assessment of hyponatraemia.

FIGURE 19

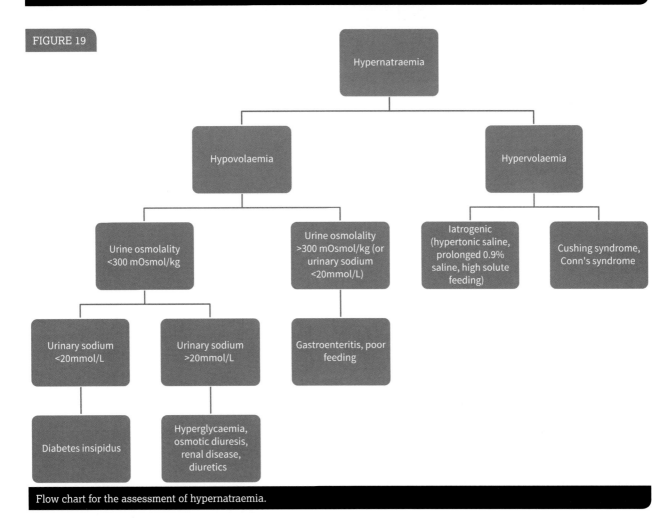

Flow chart for the assessment of hypernatraemia.

Diabetes Insipidus

Central Diabetes Insipidus (DI) occurs when ADH production is reduced by more than 90%, resulting in increased water loss through the kidneys. In nephrogenic DI, ADH production is normal but the kidneys are unresponsive to it. As the body has insufficient ADH activity, renal diuresis is increased, with water and sodium loss. Therefore, the urine osmolality remains low, despite a high serum osmolality. The way to differentiate nephrogenic and central DI is to give ADH: in central DI, the urine will become more concentrated and sodium will start to fall, whilst in nephrogenic DI, the kidneys do not respond to ADH.

Children with DI present with polyuria, polydipsia, enuresis and/or nocturia. It is important to exclude diabetes mellitus.

Central DI can be idiopathic, but possible causes may be congenital or acquired:

▸ Congenital. Septo-optic dysplasia, midline cranial defects.
▸ Acquired. Neoplasms (brain tumour, leukaemia and lymphoma), histiocytosis, CNS infections (especially TB), head trauma, CNS surgery.

Nephrogenic DI may be related to drug therapy, e.g. lithium.

Treatment for central DI is synthetic vasopressin. Nephrogenic DI is more difficult to manage. The combination of a thiazide diuretic and amiloride is most commonly used. Any underlying cause needs to be removed or treated. Adequate calorie and fluid intake is essential in nephrogenic DI to avoid dehydration and ensure good growth. A low salt diet is also advisable.

REFERENCES AND FURTHER READING

Diabetes

1   The World Health Organization and International Diabetes Federation. Definition and Diagnosis of Diabetes Mellitus and Intermediate Hyperglycaemia. Available at: http://whqlibdoc.who.int/publications/2006/9241594934_eng.pdf?ua=1
2   Delli AJ et al. Type 1 Diabetes. In: Holt RIG, Cockram CS, Flyvbjerg A et al. (eds.) Textbook of Diabetes. Fourth edition. Oxford: Wiley-Blackwell; 2010.
3   Zeitler P et al. ISPAD Clinical Practice Consensus Guidelines 2014 Compendium Type 2 diabetes in the child and adolescent. Pediatr Diabetes. 2014; 15 (Suppl. 20): 26–46.
4   Diabetic genes. Maturity-Onset Diabetes of the Young (MODY). Available at http://www.diabetesgenes.org/content/mody
5   NICE guidelines NG 18: Diabetes (type 1 and type 2) in children and young people. Diagnosis and management. 2015. https://www.nice.org.uk/guidance/ng18.
6   Diabetes UK. www.diabetes.org.uk
7   British Society for Paediatric Endocrinology and Diabetes http://www.bsped.org.uk

Hypoglycaemia

1   Canadian Paediatric Society. Screening guidelines for newborns at risk for low blood glucose. Paediatr Child Health. 2004;9(10):723-9.
2   The Royal Children's Hospital Melbourne. Hypoglycaemia. Available at: http://www.rch.org.au/clinicalguide/guideline_index/Hypoglycaemia_Guideline/
3   Hoffman RP. Paediatric Hypoglycaemia. Available at: http://emedicine.medscape.com/article/921936-overview
4   Nottingham University Hospitals NHS Trust. Hypoglycaemia guideline. Available at: https://www.nuh.nhs.uk/handlers/downloads.ashx?id=39628
5   Sunehag A, Haymond MW. Up To Date: Approach to hypoglycemia in infants and children. Available at http://www.uptodate.com/contents/approach-to-hypoglycemia-in-infants-and-children

Growth

1   Cheetham T, Davies JH. Investigation and management of short stature. Arch Dis Child. 2014;99:767–71. doi:10.1136/archdischild-2013-304829
2   Wit JM et al. Idiopathic short stature: definition, epidemiology, and diagnostic evaluation. Growth Horm IGF Res. 2008;18(2):89-110. doi: 10.1016/j.ghir.2007.11.004
3   Ross JL et al. Phenotypes Associated with SHOX Deficiency. J Clin Endocrinol Metab. 2001;86:5674–80. doi: 10.1210/jcem.86.12.8125
4   Brook CGD, Dattani MT. Handbook of Clinical Pediatric Endocrinology. Second edition. Chichester: Wiley-Blackwell; 2012.
5   BMJ Best Practice. Assessment of short stature: Diagnosis. http://bestpractice.bmj.com/best-practice/monograph/749/diagnosis.html

Puberty and Disorders of Sexual Development

1   Hutcheson J. Disorders of Sexual Development. Available at: http://emedicine.medscape.com/article/1015520-overview
2   Wilson TA. Congenital Adrenal Hyperplasia. Available from: http://emedicine.medscape.com/article/919218-overview
3   Ahmed SF et al. UK guidance on the initial evaluation of an infant or an adolescent with a suspected disorder of sex development. Clin Endocrinol. 2011;75(1):12-26. doi:10.1111/j.1365-2265.2011.04076.x.
4   Lee PA et al. Consensus statement on management of intersex disorders. Pediatrics. 2006;118(2):e488-500. doi: 10.1542/peds.2006-0738.

Adrenal Disorders

1   Stratakis CA. Cushing syndrome in pediatrics. Endocrinol Metab Clin North Am. 2012;41(4):793-803. doi:10.1016/j.ecl.2012.08.002.
2   Miller W. The Adrenal Cortex and its Disorders. In: Brook CGD, Clayton P, Brown R (eds.) Brook's Clinical Paediatric

Endocrinology. Fifth edition. Malden MA: Wiley-Blackwell; 2005.

Thyroid Disorders

1   Albert BB, Heather N, Derraik JG, et al. Neurodevelopmental and body composition outcomes in children with congenital hypothyroidism treated with high-dose initial replacement and close monitoring. J Clin Endocrinol Metab. 2013;98(9):3663-70. doi: 10.1210/jc.2013-1903.

Calcium Disorders

1   Jeha GS. Up To Date: Etiology of hypocalcemia in infants and children. Available at: http://www.uptodate.com/contents/etiology-of-hypocalcemia-in-infants-and-children

2   Gupta P, Tomar M, Radhakrishnan S, et al. Hypocalcemic cardiomyopathy presenting as cardiogenic shock. Ann Pediatr Cardiol. 2011;4(2):152–155. doi: 10.4103/0974-2069.84655.

3   Tran JT, Sheth AP. Complications of subcutaneous fat necrosis of the newborn: a case report and review of the literature. Pediatr Dermatol. 2003;20(3):257-61. doi: 10.1046/j.1525-1470.2003.20315.x.

Sodium Disorders

1   Disorders of water balance. In: Brook CGD, Clayton P, Brown R (eds.) Brook's Clinical Paediatric Endocrinology. Fifth edition. Malden MA: Wiley-Blackwell; 2005.

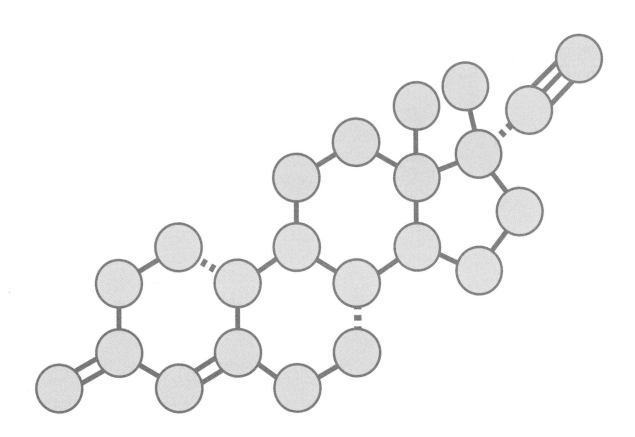

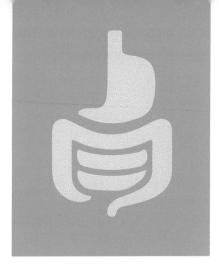

1.07

GASTROENTEROLOGY

MAXINE WILKIE, POOJA PAREKH, AND ZESHAN QURESHI

CONTENTS

MALABSORPTION DISORDERS

Inflammatory Bowel Disease

Inflammatory Bowel Disease (IBD), which includes ulcerative colitis (UC), Crohn's disease (CD) and indeterminate colitis (IC), is a chronic remitting-relapsing disease characterised by inflammation of the gut. IC is diagnosed when the pattern of inflammation is atypical of either UC or CD. In the UK, the prevalence of CD is 55-140 per 100 000 and UC is 160-240 per 100 000 population. Its incidence is increasing, particularly in children.

Aetiology

The aetiology of IBD is complex and involves genetic, environmental and immunological factors.

▷ More than 164 genetic mutations have been associated with CD, UC or both. Mutations of CARD15/NOD2 gene on chromosome 16, amongst others, have been implicated.

▷ The gut microbiota can be seen as a proxy for environmental factors, as several of these factors can alter the gut microbiome. This is increasingly recognised to play a role in IBD.

Other lesser risk factors include family history, use of oral contraceptives and non-steroidal anti-inflammatory drugs (NSAIDs). *Table 1* summarises the key differences between CD and UC. In 10-20% of cases, they cannot be differentiated (indeterminate colitis; IC).

Clinical Features

IBD usually presents in adolescence and early adulthood, though it can also present earlier. IBD in children generally has a more extensive and rapidly progressing course. Children often present acutely, but at presentation patients often report long-standing symptoms.

Relapses may be brought on by emotional and physical stress like acute illness, major school exams and bereavement. With adolescents, poor treatment compliance can be an issue which may also trigger relapses. Often, however, there may be no identifiable trigger.

The symptoms vary depending on whether the underlying illness is CD or UC (*Table 2*).

The severity of disease can be scored using established scales, like Paediatric UC Activity Index (PUCAI) and Paediatric Crohn's Disease Activity Index (PCDAI) (*Table 3-4*). Severe active Crohn's disease is identified by poor general health,

TABLE 1: Key differences between CD and UC		
	Crohn's Disease	**Ulcerative Colitis**
Age of onset.	15–35.	10–40.
Smoking.	Increases risk.	Decreases risk.
Regions of gut affected (*Figure 1*).	Mouth to anus (but most commonly affects the terminal ileum).	Affects the rectum and extends proximally in the colon, (left sided colitis), or potentially the whole colon (pancolitis). It is possible to get a "backwash" ileitis at the site of the ileo-caecal junction.
Diarrhoea.	Half of cases have bloody diarrhoea.	Bloody diarrhoea is almost always seen.
Perianal disease.	Common.	Rare.
Toxic megacolon.	Rare.	More common.
Endoscopic features (*Figure 2*) (Macroscopic).	Skip lesions (discontinuous sites of pathology), and often asymmetrical.	The disease is continuous, with symmetrical areas of pathology.
	The rectum is not always involved.	The rectum is always involved.
	Mucosa has a cobblestone appearance in late disease.	There is formation of crypt abscesses and mucosal ulceration.
	Extramural involvement includes strictures, fissures, fistulae, abscesses, anal skin tags and aphthous ulceration.	Fistulae and strictures are rare.
	Fat wrapping (over 50% of the intestinal surface covered with adipose tissue).	Pseudopolyps are more common.
Biopsy features (Microscopic).	Non-caseating granulomas.	No granulomas.
	Transmural inflammation.	Mucosal and submucosal inflammation.
	Normal glands.	Distorted glands.

93

Crohn's disease **Ulcerative colitis**

FIGURE 1

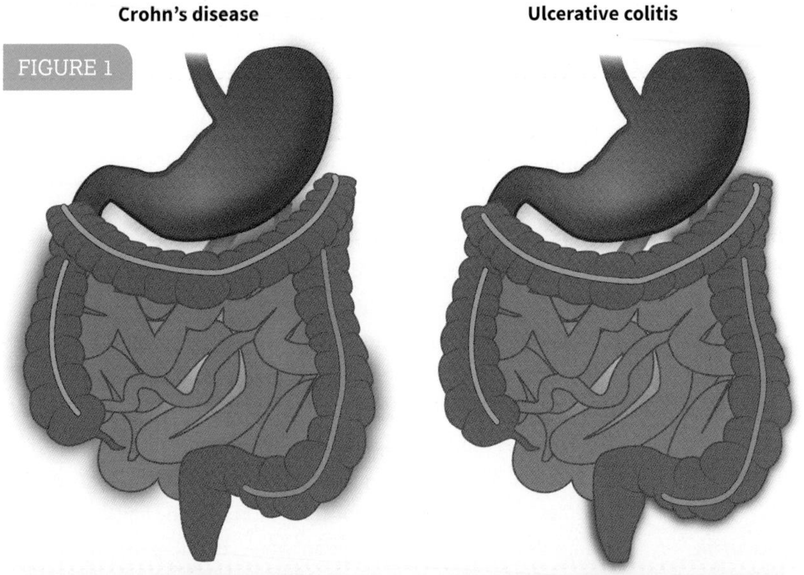

Disease distribution in Crohn's disease (CD) and Ulcerative Colitis (UC). Crohn's disease has "skip lesions", meaning disease segments are found between healthy bowel segments. UC has a pattern of continuous involvement, starting at the rectum, spreading up the left colon, and potentially affecting the whole colon.

TABLE 2: Presenting features of IBD

Both	More Common in Crohn's Disease	More Common in Ulcerative Colitis
• Increased frequency of bowel movements. • Abdominal pain. • Weight loss. • Nausea/vomiting. • Faltered growth. • Delayed puberty. • Reduced appetite. • Malaise/fatigue. • Sweats. • Clinical signs: fever, tachycardia, dehydration and pallor.	• Terminal ileum disease (tenderness or a mass in the right lower quadrant). • Perianal disease (such as anal/perianal skin tags, fistulae and abscesses). • Gallstones due to malabsorption of fat and bile.	• Bloody diarrhoea. • Tenderness in the left lower quadrant.

weight loss, fever, severe abdominal pain and over three diarrhoeal stools daily.

Investigations
Blood Tests
> FBC. An FBC can reveal anaemia, thrombocytosis and leucocytosis (possible infection), all possible complications of IBD.

> Coagulation. If there is rectal bleeding.

> Group and Save. In case a blood transfusion is required.

> ESR and CRP. Inflammatory markers demonstrate degree of inflammation and risk of relapse.

> U&Es. Renal function tests can reveal acute renal failure secondary to dehydration, as well as electrolyte derangement.

> LFTs. Low albumin may suggest malnutrition. Hyperbilirubinaemia and elevated liver enzymes may indicate primary sclerosing cholangitis.

> Coeliac screen. To rule out coeliac disease, which may present similarly.

> H. pylori antigen. To rule out H-Pylori related peptic ulcer disease, if history is suggestive of this. Note that this can also be tested in the stool.

> Amylase. To rule out pancreatitis, if history is suggestive of this.

> Vitamin B_{12}, folate and iron studies. Nutritional deficiencies may co-exist, especially with ileal CD.

Stool and Urine Samples
> Microscopy and culture. Stool samples can rule out infective gastroenteritis, including *campylobacter* and *salmonella* infections.

> Faecal calprotectin. An elevated level serves as an indicator of mucosal inflammation. This may be a result of IBD, but it is also elevated in enteric infection, and in polyps.

> Urine MC&S. To rule out possible UTI.

Imaging and Biopsies
> Abdominal X-ray. A simple radiograph can demonstrate evidence of toxic megacolon (*Figure 3*) and/or intestinal perforation. A chest X-ray may also be requested if perforation is queried.

> Abdominal ultrasound scan. Ultrasonography may assist in assessing liver disease, and identifying bowel changes.

> Upper/lower GI endoscopy and biopsies. Endoscopy and biopsy are required for gold standard diagnosis (*Table 1*). IC is diagnosed when the findings are not typical of either UC or CD. However, endoscopy is contraindicated in toxic megacolon.

> Video capsule endoscopy. This is used to obtain macroscopic images of the small bowel.

> Abdominal CT. CT scan may identify inflammatory masses, or abscesses.

> Barium meal and follow through. This radiological tool can assess small bowel involvement in Crohn's disease, particularly highlighting strictures and fistulae. This is increasingly being replaced by small bowel MRI.

FIGURE 2

Normal

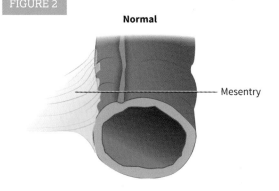

— Mesentry

Crohn's disease

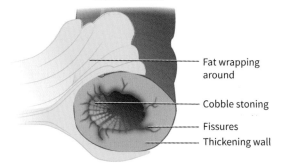

— Fat wrapping around

— Cobble stoning

— Fissures
— Thickening wall

Ulcerative colitis

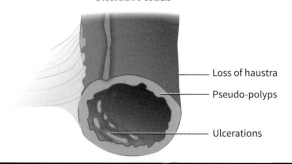

— Loss of haustra
— Pseudo-polyps

— Ulcerations

Macroscopic features of IBD.

TABLE 3: Paediatric Crohn's Disease Activity Index (Severe: >40, Moderate: 37.5-20, Mild: 10-27.5, Remission: <10)	
Feature	**Points**
Abdominal pain.	
• None.	0
• Mild (brief episodes, not interfering with activities).	5
• Moderate/severe (frequent or persistent, affecting activities).	10
Stools.	
• 0-1 liquid stools, no blood.	0
• 2-5 liquid or up to 2 semi-formed with small amounts of blood.	5
• Gross bleeding, >6 liquid stools or nocturnal diarrhoea.	10
Patient functioning, general well-being (Recall, 1 week).	
• No limitation of activities, well.	0
• Occasional difficulties in maintaining age appropriate activities, below par.	5
• Frequent limitation of activities, very poor.	10
Weight.	
• Weight gain or voluntary weight loss.	0
• Involuntary weight loss 1-9%.	5
• Weight loss >10%.	10
Height*.	
• < 1 channel decrease.	0
• 1 to 2 channel decrease.	5
• ≥ 2 channel decrease.	10
Abdomen.	
• No tenderness, no mass.	0
• Tenderness, or mass without tenderness.	5
• Tenderness, involuntary guarding, definite mass.	10
Perianal disease.	
• None, asymptomatic tags.	0
• 1-2 indolent fistula, scant drainage, tenderness of abscess.	5
• Active fistula, drainage, tenderness or abscess.	10
Extra-intestinal manifestations. Fever > 38.5°C x 3 days in week, arthritis, uveitis, erythema nodosum or pyoderma gangrenosum.	
• None.	0
• One.	5
• Two.	10

(*Height channel represents lines crossed on a standard percentile chart)

> Abdominal/Pelvic MRI. MRI provides further evaluation of small bowel and/or pelvic disease, as well as assessment of strictures and fistulae.

Differential Diagnosis

The main differential diagnosis of IBD is infection. However, many conditions can present with diarrhoea (*Table 5*).

Management

Management of IBD involves patient information and support, induction of remission, maintaining remission and preventing complications. This includes discussing medications, smoking, fertility, growth and puberty, cancer risk and surgery.

TABLE 4: Paediatric UC Activity Index (Severe: 65 and above, Moderate: 35-64, Mild: 10-34, Remission: below 10)

Symptom	Points
Abdominal pain.	
• No pain.	0
• Pain can be ignored.	5
• Pain cannot be ignored.	10
Rectal bleeding.	
• None.	0
• Small amount only, in less than 50% of stools.	10
• Small amount with most stools.	20
• Large amount, 50% of stool content.	30
Stool consistency.	
• Formed.	0
• Partially formed.	5
• Completely unformed.	10
Number of stools in 24 hours	
• 0-2.	0
• 3-5.	5
• 6-8.	10
• More than 8.	15
Nocturnal stools	
• No.	0
• Yes.	10
Activity level	
• No limitation of activity.	0
• Occasional limitation of activity.	5
• Severe restricted activity.	10

TABLE 5: Differential diagnoses of IBD

Differential Diagnosis	Acute or Chronic	Common Symptoms (not all may be present)
Gastroenteritis.	Acute.	Fever, malaise, nausea, vomiting, diarrhoea, dehydration.
Irritable bowel syndrome.	Chronic.	Diarrhoea, bloating, flatulence, abdominal pain.
Appendicitis.	Acute.	Abdominal pain, vomiting, fever (if perforation/abscess).
Coeliac disease.	Chronic.	Abdominal pain, diarrhoea, weight loss.

FIGURE 3

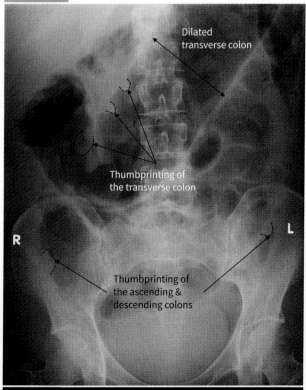

Toxic megacolon, thumbprinting (associated with bowel wall oedema), and loss of haustral markings of the large bowel.

Crohn's Disease

Induction of Remission

The immediate response to a first time presentation or single relapse in a 12-month period of Crohn's disease is enteral nutrition or glucocorticosteroids.

› Enteral nutrition (e.g. Modulen). This is first line treatment in children or young people with CD. Modulen is a liquid feed that contains all required nutrients. It can be taken orally or administered via a nasogastric tube or gastrostomy. This treatment normally takes place over six weeks, and food is then reintroduced gradually after this period. Enteral nutrition is as effective as corticosteroids, although compliance can be an issue. Studies on enteral nutrition show that the feed promotes increased production of anti-inflammatory cytokines and decreased levels of pro-inflammatory cytokines. As this feed is nutritionally complete, it also improves nutritional status of these children, some of whom can be malnourished with faltering growth.

› Glucocorticosteroids. This prevents the breakdown of arachidonic acid into cyclooxygenases and leukotrienes, thereby inducing an anti-inflammatory response. Usually a therapeutic dose is recommended for two weeks to induce remission, followed by a gradual reduction of dose over the following 4-8 weeks. A proton pump inhibitor is usually prescribed alongside the corticosteroids. Adequate dietary intake of vitamins must also be maintained during this treatment.

If glucocorticosteroids cause serious adverse events (e.g. sepsis), another strategy is the use of 5-aminosalicylates (e.g. sulfasalazine), which inhibit prostaglandin and leukotriene production. However, this is less effective than glucocorticosteroids.

If there have been two or more relapses in a 12-month period or if the glucocorticosteroid dose cannot be reduced, immunomodulators (that inhibit DNA synthesis in inflammatory cells) can be considered:

› Azathioprine or mercaptopurine. If thiopurine methyltransferase (TPMT) levels are normal. Patients with low levels are at risk of early profound myelosuppression.

▷ Methotrexate. If the TPMT levels show a deficiency or if azathioprine or mercaptopurine are not tolerated.

Infliximab is a monoclonal antibody that targets tumour necrosis factor (TNF) to reduce inflammation. Consider using infliximab if:

▷ Immunomodulators are not tolerated.
▷ Treatment is still unsuccessful at controlling symptoms.
▷ Severe active Crohn's disease.

In some cases, other treatment strategies may be required when inducing remission. Antibiotics may be used in perianal disease. Parenteral nutrition can be used in severe complicated disease such as CD with strictures. Surgery may be required in localised disease refractory to medical therapy.

Maintenance of Remission

Maintenance of remission usually requires ongoing medical therapy. Medical options for maintenance therapy include:

▷ Azathioprine or Mercaptopurine. For maintenance of steroid-free remission in children at risk of poor outcome.
▷ Methotrexate. If the above were not tolerated, or if methotrexate was required at induction.

If the child required surgery at induction, maintenance options include:

▷ Azathioprine or Mercaptopurine. If the child has had more than one resection, previous complications or if they have debilitating disease.
▷ 5-aminosalicylate. In other cases.

Strictures can be managed with balloon dilation if they are short, straight and accessible by colonoscopy. Children should be monitored for macronutrient and micronutrient deficiencies, growth, and side effects of medications. There is a high risk

of osteoporosis with repeated and/or prolonged glucocorticoid use.

Ulcerative Colitis
Induction of Remission

Patients with UC should be immediately treated and can be initiated on glucocorticosteroids or aminosalicylates.

Acute severe colitis or toxic megacolon is a medical emergency. Children should be admitted immediately to hospital and given intravenous fluids and glucocorticosteroids. If the patient has failed to respond to the intravenous corticosteroids within 72 hours, then cyclosporine (an immunosuppressant acting via calcineurin inhibition) or infliximab and/or a colectomy may be required.

Urgent surgical input is indicated in toxic megacolon. In the event of surgery, the patient and their family need to be educated about the care of stomas, which can be temporary or permanent. If temporary, the patient needs to be counselled on possible future reconnection surgery.

Maintenance of Remission

Maintenance therapy with aminosalicylates should be initiated. Glucocorticosteroids should not be used for maintenance of remission, although azathioprine or mercaptopurine may be required in some cases, particularly those who have presented with acute severe colitis.

Complications

Acute complications:

▷ Toxic megacolon. Dilatation of the colon above 6 cm (or the caecum above 9 cm). It is the most worrying complication of UC, and is usually caused by an acute flare-up. May result in perforation.
▷ Electrolyte imbalances and renal failure. From chronic/acute diarrhoea and inflammation.
▷ Anaemia. From blood loss.
▷ Perianal disease. Fistulae, abscesses and strictures. Strictures occurring

with Crohn's disease can result in life-threatening complications, such as intestinal obstruction and/or perforation.

▷ Infection. At risk of superimposed infection.

Chronic complications:

▷ Psychological effects. The disease is chronic and can have a large impact both at home and at school, with prolonged school absences impacting educational achievement.
▷ Ophthalmological complications. Episcleritis, iritis.
▷ Urinary complications. Renal stones.
▷ Haematological complications. Anaemia, hypercoagulability.
▷ Dermatological complications. Erythema nodosum, pyoderma gangrenosum, aphthous mouth ulcers.
▷ Malignancy. There is increased risk of developing colon cancer, particularly with a family history of bowel cancer, severe disease and inflammation, prolonged duration of disease and associated primary sclerosing cholangitis.
▷ Malnutrition, hypoalbuminaemia, electrolyte imbalance and faltering growth. As a result of malabsorption and chronic disease.
▷ Arthropathy. e.g. ankylosing spondylitis, sacroiliitis and peripheral arthritis.
▷ Liver disease. e.g. hepatitis, pericholangitis, gallstones and primary sclerosing cholangitis (commonly associated with UC).
▷ Steroid toxicity. e.g. osteoporosis.

Prognosis

IBD is a lifelong condition, with unpredictable relapses and a reduced life expectancy compared to the general population.

Coeliac Disease

Coeliac disease is an autoimmune disorder caused by inflammatory responses to gliadin, which is present in gluten. This damages the mucosal lining of the small intestine and results in malabsorption. Gluten is a protein found in wheat, barley and rye. Coeliac disease has a prevalence of 0.8-1.9% in the UK. In children, the peak age of diagnosis is between 6–months-old and 3–years-old. However, about a third of cases are undiagnosed.

Aetiology

In those with the disease, B-lymphocytes from the gut-associated lymphoid tissue (GALT) produce antibodies to gliadin, endomysial cells (the connective tissue around muscle fibres), and tissue transglutaminase.

The disease affects more women than men and is more likely if there is a family history. It can only occur in people with genetic susceptibility, although the mechanism is complex and polygenetic. For example, HLA-DR3-DQ2 and HLA-DR4-DQ8 are found in 95% and 5% of people with coeliac disease, respectively. Rotavirus infection in childhood has been found to increase the chance of developing coeliac disease. Conversely, continuing breastfeeding whilst introducing gluten into the diet, and introducing gluten-containing foods between four and six months of age reduces risk.

Clinical Features

Coeliac disease can present at any age but can also be asymptomatic. The most common symptoms are:

- Unintentional weight loss.
- Fatigue.
- Chronic diarrhoea or constipation.
- Flatulence.
- Pale stools.
- Severe recurrent abdominal pain.
- Anorexia.
- Mouth ulcers.
- Vomiting.

Signs that can be noticed are unexplained anaemia, faltering growth, low impact fractures, motor weakness and vitamin deficiencies. In children, the abdomen may become distended and there may be faltering growth.

Coeliac disease is associated with many other conditions. Routine screening should be offered in those with:

- Dermatitis herpetiformis (an autoimmune blistering skin disorder).
- Autoimmune thyroid disorders.
- Addison's disease.
- Type 1 diabetes mellitus.

Investigations

Because the symptoms of coeliac disease are non-specific, investigations are needed to confirm the diagnosis.

Blood Tests

- FBC. Can demonstrate anaemia due to iron or folate deficiency.
- Iron Studies, Vitamin B_{12}, Folate. To look for nutrient deficiency.
- U&Es, Bone Profile, Magnesium. May show electrolyte derangement such as hypokalaemia, hypocalcaemia or hypomagnesaemia.
- Liver function tests (LFTs). A liver profile can show elevated levels of transaminases, which should revert to normal on changing to a gluten-free diet. However, persistently elevated levels may warrant further investigation to look for autoimmune liver conditions, which are associated with coeliac disease. Low albumin is associated with malnutrition.

- Tissue transglutaminase antibody (tTGA) and IgA endomysial antibodies (EMA). The patient needs to have included gluten-containing foods in their diet over the previous six weeks on a daily basis to increase the likelihood of an immunological response.
  - If there is positive serology, the patient should be referred for endoscopy and intestinal biopsy which will provide a histological diagnosis (with the patient continuing a gluten-containing diet until then).
  - If the serology is negative, an IgA serology should be done to check for IgA deficiency, as this may mask a positive test (an IgA response is unlikely if the patient is IgA deficient, and therefore IgG testing can be done instead). If this is also negative, the patient is unlikely to have coeliac disease.

Endoscopy

Upper gastrointestinal endoscopy can enable biopsies to be taken for histology. Histological findings include atrophic villi (*Figure 4*) and crypt hyperplasia, and this is the gold standard for

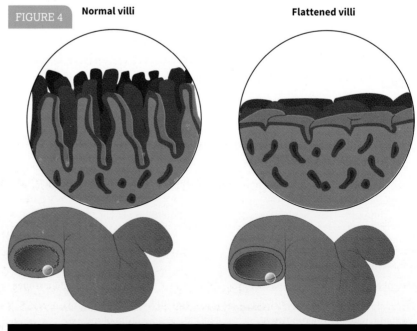

FIGURE 4   **Normal villi**   **Flattened villi**

Normal vs. flattened villi, reducing the effective surface area for intestinal absorption.

diagnosis. However, recent guidelines have suggested that diagnosis can be made without endoscopy if:

- The child is symptomatic.
- tTGA is ten times above normal on two occasions.
- The child is either HLA DR3-DQ2 or DR4-DQ8 positive. This is confirmed on genetic testing.

Differential Diagnosis

Due to its non-specific presentation, coeliac disease can have multiple differential diagnoses which are shown in *Table 6*.

In some situations, refractory coeliac disease is present. This is characterised by persistent or recurrent malabsorption and villous atrophy despite the removal of gluten from the diet after 6–12 months.

Management

The child should be informed of the diagnosis and the implications as soon as they are old enough to understand. Services used by the child, such as nurseries and schools, should also be informed of the diagnosis.

The most effective treatment for coeliac disease is a strict, lifelong gluten-free diet. Gluten-free products can be prescribed. Patients should be referred to a dietician for advice on optimising their diet.

All patients with coeliac disease should have lifelong follow up appointments. Key to follow up is:

- Checking adherence to the gluten-free diet. The levels of tTGA and EMA decrease 6-12 months after a gluten-free diet has been initiated and can be used to monitor adherence to the diet. Generally, adherence is poorest in adolescents, as this is the time when the patient starts to take control of their own diet, increasing the chance of complications.
- Ensuring adequate nutrition and growth.
- Osteoporosis screening with a dual energy X-ray absorptiometry (DEXA) scan should be carried out every three years in patients on a gluten-free diet.

TABLE 6: Differential diagnoses of coeliac disease		
Differential Diagnosis	**Acute or Chronic**	**Common Symptoms**
Gastroenteritis.	Acute.	Diarrhoea, vomiting and abdominal pain.
Inflammatory bowel disease.	Chronic.	Unexplained weight loss, abdominal pain, diarrhoea, constipation, faecal blood and vomiting.
Irritable bowel syndrome.	Chronic.	Bloating, diarrhoea, abdominal pain relieved by defecation and constipation.
Lactose intolerance.	Chronic.	Bloating, abdominal pain, flatulence, loose watery stools and perianal itching.
Anaemia.	Chronic.	Fatigue, shortness of breath, palpitations and failure to thrive.

- As some patients have splenic dysfunction, they should be offered vaccinations against pneumococcus, *Haemophilus influenzae* type B and influenza.
- Assessment of psychosocial wellbeing.

Complications

Untreated coeliac disease can lead to many complications. However, the risk of complications due to malabsorption decreases after 12 months of treatment on a gluten-free diet.

Complications due to malabsorption are:

- Iron-deficiency anaemia.
- Vitamin B_{12} deficiency.
- Folate deficiency.
- Calcium or Vitamin D deficiency.
- Faltering growth.

There is an absolute increase in the risk of some conditions, including:

- Bone fragility, causing fractures.
- Adverse pregnancy outcomes, including miscarriages, low birth weight and intrauterine growth restriction.
- Some cancers, including oesophageal cancer, intestinal cancer, Hodgkin's and non-Hodgkin's lymphoma.
- Splenic dysfunction.

Prognosis

Patients adherent to a gluten-free diet have a normal life expectancy.

OESOPHAGEAL DISORDERS

Gastro-Oesophageal Reflux Disease

Gastro-oesophageal reflux (GOR) is the effortless passage of gastric contents into the oesophagus with or without regurgitation and vomiting. It is a normal physiological occurrence, especially common in infants. Gastro-oesophageal reflux disease (GORD) refers to either the symptomatic regurgitation of gastric contents into the oesophagus or GOR with complications. It is different from vomiting, which requires forceful contraction of the diaphragm and abdominal muscles. GORD commonly presents in infancy, with a prevalence of 4.3% at six-months-old, decreasing to 2% at 18-months-old. In older children, GORD is more likely to become chronic.

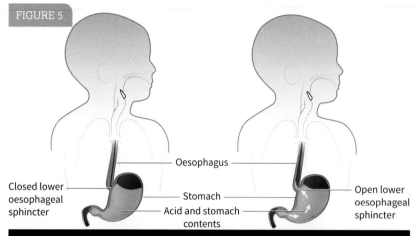

FIGURE 5

Oesophagus

Closed lower oesophageal sphincter

Stomach

Acid and stomach contents

Open lower oesophageal sphincter

Open lower oesophageal sphincter as a mechanism for causing reflux.

Aetiology

GOR is a symptom caused by:

- Laxity of the lower oesophageal sphincter (*Figure 5*). In infants it is partly due to immaturity of the lower oesophageal sphincter. Symptoms improve as the sphincter tone increases, a more solid diet is introduced and the child spends more time in an upright posture.
- Food allergy or intolerance, such as cow's milk protein allergy.
- Foregut intestinal dysmotility associated with gut inflammation or neurological disorder.
- Increased gastric pressure, due to a more distal intestinal obstruction, obesity or chronic respiratory disorders.

Clinical Features

The common symptoms and signs of GORD in children are:

- Persistent/recurrent regurgitation, particularly after meals (which may be reported as vomiting).
- Feeding difficulties, food refusal and/ or crying/irritability post feeds.
- Arching of the back and neck in infants (opisthotonus).
- Respiratory symptoms, such as coughing and wheezing.
- Sore throat or hoarseness.
- Apnoeic/bradycardic episodes (particularly in neonates).
- Heartburn or chest pain.

It is more common in high risk groups such as those with cerebral palsy.

Investigations

GORD in older children may be identified with a typical history and physical examination, making further investigations unnecessary. In challenging or complicated GORD, further investigations can aid understanding the cause and severity of disease. These include:

Blood Tests

- FBC. To identify associated anaemia.
- U&Es. To identify electrolyte imbalances in severe and acute vomiting.
- Arterial Blood Gas. To identify a metabolic acidosis, suggesting a metabolic disorder, or metabolic alkalosis, suggesting pyloric stenosis in the baby up to 6 weeks of age (usually suspected on history).
- Vitamins and Trace Elements. To reveal associated micro-nutrient malnutrition.

pH Studies

- pH Impedance Study. This measures the pH as well as non-acid reflux in the oesophagus (via impedance) by placing a probe into the stomach. This particularly benefits infants on milk feeds, with non-acidic reflux that won't be detected on "pH", but will on "impedance". Parents/carers are asked to note symptoms or signs during the recording. A potential causal relationship between symptoms and reported GOR can then be established.

If cow's milk protein (CMP) allergy is suspected, a 24-hour pH impedance (off CMP diet/feed) can be followed by another 24 hours of monitoring and recording on a CMP-containing diet or feed. Worsening symptoms and GOR on CMP can assist in the diagnosis of cow's milk protein allergy.

- pH Study. This is performed in older children to detect acidic content in the oesophagus. Symptoms are correlated with possible GOR.

Endoscopy

- Upper GI Endoscopy and Biopsies. Can detect oesophagitis such as eosinophilic oesophagitis. Absence of oesophagitis does not exclude GORD. Ulcers and other causes of haematemesis, such as oesophageal varices, can also be found.
- Oesophageal and Antroduodenal Manometry. This can be used to detect gut peristalsis, is a sensitive assessment of gut function and can detect abnormalities such as oesophageal strictures.

Radiology

- Abdominal USS. May identify reflux.
- Barium Contrast Study. This may identify anatomical abnormalities, such as gut malrotation or volvulus.
- Gastric Emptying Scan. This detects delayed or abnormal gastric emptying due to intestinal dysmotility.

Differential Diagnosis

GORD has a wide range of presentations, but a common one, particularly in neonates is with vomiting after feeds. A broad differential for vomiting is shown in *Table 7*.

Management

Conservative Management

As with all other conditions, parental/ carer education and support are essential in the management of GORD. In most infants, GOR is due to laxity of the lower oesophageal sphincter, and will self-resolve as diet becomes more solid, the child starts to sit upright more and the sphincter tone increases. Reassurance

TABLE 7: Differential diagnoses for vomiting

Differential Diagnosis	Acute or Chronic	Common Symptoms
Infection.	Acute.	Diarrhoea, vomiting, and abdominal pain in gastroenteritis. UTIs may present non-specifically with isolated vomiting. If there is altered responsiveness, consider meningitis.
Infantile colic.	Chronic.	Inconsolable crying, drawing knees up and arching back. In first weeks of life and resolved by 4–months-old.
Cow's milk protein intolerance.	Chronic.	Abdominal pain, eczema, flatulence, bloody stools, loose watery stools or constipation.
Pyloric stenosis.	Acute.	Frequent projectile vomiting, poor weight gain, lethargy and distress after feeds. Under 2-months-old.
Intermittent intestinal obstruction, such as malrotation.	Acute on Chronic.	Bilious vomiting.
Raised intracranial pressure.	Chronic.	Associated with other signs of elevated intracranial pressure, such as increasing head circumference and bulging fontanelle, or in older children, early morning headache. May have no accompanying nausea.

and conservative measures are all that is needed:

> Optimise position by raising the cot base (not mattress) at the head end by 30°.
> Avoid over-feeding and consider smaller, more frequent feeds.
> Use feed thickeners which may offer benefit to some infants, e.g. Carobel® or Nestrogel®.
> Ensure adequate nutrition with regular monitoring of weight.

Older children with mild or uncomplicated GOR may benefit from strategies including:

> Weight loss for overweight children.
> Avoiding chocolate, acidic food and drink, peppermint and coffee.
> Avoid eating within three hours of bedtime.
> Raising the head of the bed.
> Avoiding positions where gravity may assist reflux.
> Avoiding smoking.

Medical Therapy

Recommended treatment varies depending on age, symptoms and feeding methods. For babies with suspected GORD:

> If breast fed, a one to two week trial of an antacid (e.g. Gaviscon® Infant should be considered).
> If formula fed, try reduced feed volumes, increased feed frequencies, and thickened feeds (e.g. Instant Carobel®).

If the above aren't effective, a four week trial of ranitidine or omeprazole should be considered. Long-term use of antacids is not recommended, due to effects on calcium absorption. Rarely, nasogastric tube feeding may be required.

For older children, consider a four week trial of ranitidine or omeprazole. Prokinetic agents, such as domperidone and erythromycin, can be beneficial in some patients. However, their side effects, such as abdominal pain and diarrhoea, may worsen symptoms.

Surgical Therapy

Patients with suspected intestinal dysmotility or obstruction require assessment by paediatric specialists in the field. Surgical intervention may be necessary for these patients. Nissen's fundoplication (uses the top of the stomach to strengthen the lower oesophageal sphincter) may be considered in:

> Older infants.
> Children with severe GORD unresponsive to medical therapy.
> Children who have previously suffered or are at increased risk of 'life-threatening' events like aspiration pneumonia and apnoea.

Fundoplication is often performed laparoscopically and can have a high failure rate, especially in the presence of foregut intestinal dysmotility.

Complications

Chronic GORD may lead to complications, such as:

> Reflux oesophagitis. Barrett's oesophagitis in children is unusual. Severe oesophagitis may lead to formation of oesophageal strictures.
> Sandifer syndrome. Reflex associated with abnormal neck movements: spasmodic torticollis/dystonia, with back arching. Resolves with treatment of reflux.
> Dental enamel erosion. Particularly in those with neurodisability.
> Frequent otitis media and aspiration pneumonia. May also have choking episodes, apnoeas, laryngeal/pharyngeal inflammation from regurgitated contents entering the trachea.
> Faltering growth. Associated with nutritional deficiency, anaemia.
> Surgical complications. Adhesions from surgical intervention, recurrence of reflux.

Prognosis

For most children with mild to moderate uncomplicated GOR, the outcome is positive. In most cases, GORD will resolve within a few months to a few years, although it is more persistent in those with neurodisabilities.

Eosinophilic Oesophagitis

Eosinophilic oesophagitis (EO) is a primary oesophageal disorder characterised by an eosinophilic inflammatory infiltrate, secondary to food and/or aeroallergens.

Clinical Features

EO presents with features of oesophageal dysfunction, usually in atopic individuals, with a male preponderance. Oesophageal dysfunction may present as:

> Infants and toddlers. Feeding difficulty/refusal, vomiting, regurgitation.
> Older children. Retrosternal pain, epigastric pain, dysphagia, food impaction.

Investigations

The diagnosis is dependent on an eosinophil-predominant oesophageal inflammation, obtained on endoscopic biopsy. Macroscopic features such as trachealisation of the oesophagus may also be seen. Testing for sensitisation to food and/or aeroallergens can also help establish the diagnosis. The peripheral eosinophil and IgE levels are often elevated as well.

Management

A subset of patients with EO are responsive to proton pump inhibitors (e.g. omeprazole), but if this is ineffective, dietary restriction or topical corticosteroids should be considered:

> Dietary restriction. This is likely to be most effective with an elemental diet, although due to social inconvenience, such a diet may be difficult to maintain. Good effect can also be obtained from a six-food elimination diet [milk, egg, soya, wheat, nuts and seafood]. Milk exclusion plus targeted therapy using allergy testing can also be trialled.
> Topical corticosteroids. Usually involves inhaled steroid therapy, such as beclomethasone. Systemic steroids should only be considered in severe dysphagia, dehydration, weight loss, oesophageal strictures and failure of other treatments.

GASTRIC DISORDERS

Gastritis

Gastritis is inflammation of the stomach lining due to infection, food intolerances or medications.

Aetiology

Gastritis can be erosive or non-erosive, with the latter generally caused by infection with *Helicobacter pylori*. The main symptoms are nausea, vomiting, diarrhoea, upper abdominal pain, loss of appetite, fever, abdominal distension, acidic taste in the mouth and flatulence. Risk factors for developing gastritis include:

> Stress.
> Poor diet.
> Illness.

> NSAIDs.
> Caffeinated drinks.

Management

Mild cases do not require further investigations. Management of gastritis involves dietary modification and medication.

> Dietary modification. Caffeinated drinks and spicy foods should be reduced. Adequate water and milk intake are needed.
> Medication. Antacids may be required (e.g. Gaviscon), or if not effective, a proton pump inhibitor (e.g. omeprazole), which reduces the amount of acid produced by gastric cells, may be needed.

Cases showing greater severity merit endoscopy and investigation. If *Helicobacter pylori* is confirmed, *H. pylori* eradication therapy should be commenced.

Peptic Ulceration

Peptic ulcers are ulcers in the lining of the digestive tract, typically the stomach or duodenum. They are much less common in children than in adults.

Aetiology

Peptic ulcers are a result of a relative excess of gastric acid, which erodes through the muscular layer of the stomach wall, forming ulcers. Risk factors for developing peptic ulcers are:

> *Helicobacter pylori* infection.
> Use of NSAIDs, corticosteroids and immunosuppressants.
> Lifestyle factors, e.g. fatty foods/smoking.
> Physiological stress.
> Hypersecretion states, such as gastrinoma (i.e. Zollinger-Ellison syndrome) or multiple endocrine neoplasia type 1.

Clinical Features

Symptoms of peptic ulceration include:

> Upper abdominal pain which occurs either after eating a meal or on an empty stomach.
> Flatulence.
> Abdominal distension.
> Nausea.
> Vomiting.
> Dyspepsia.
> Heartburn.
> Chest pain.

Black stools and haematemesis are worrying as they show upper gastrointestinal bleeding. Sudden onset of symptoms may imply a perforated peptic ulcer.

Investigations

Diagnosis of peptic ulcers is through endoscopy, and through a blood/stool test for *Helicobacter pylori*. An erect chest X-ray may be useful to identify free air if abdominal perforation is suspected.

Management

Acute presentations of bleeding and abdominal pain should be assessed using an ABCDE approach. Endoscopy can reduce the likelihood of recurrent bleeding and decreases the need for surgery. Under endoscopy, coagulation therapy and haemostatic clips can be used to stop bleeding. Urgent reasons for surgical intervention are failure to stop haemorrhage endoscopically, recurrent bleeding or perforation.

Treatment for ulcers caused by *Helicobacter pylori* involves triple therapy (e.g. omeprazole plus amoxicillin, and clarithromycin) or quadruple therapy (e.g. omeprazole plus metronidazole, amoxicillin and bismuth). Maintenance therapy with anti-secretory medications for up to one year is indicated in patients with recurrent ulcers, particularly if infection with *H. pylori* has not been documented. Precipitating factors (e.g. NSAID use) should be stopped where possible.

Complications

Peptic ulcer disease is associated with a number of complications including:
- Bowel obstruction.
- Bowel perforation.
- Gastrointestinal haemorrhage.
- Gastric malignancy (rare in children).

MOTILITY DISORDERS

Constipation

Constipation is the passing of infrequent and/or hard stools and can be acute or chronic. Chronic constipation is diagnosed in children who have had symptoms over the previous eight weeks.

Aetiology

The cause is not well understood, but it is likely to be multifactorial. Constipation can begin after a precipitating factor, such as infection or change in diet. Fluid and fibre intake are particularly important.

Clinical Features

The most common signs and symptoms are:
- Infrequent bowel activity.
- Excessive foul-smelling flatulence.
- Irregular stool texture.
- Passing occasional large stools or frequently passing small pellets (*Figure 6*).
- Not wanting to go to the toilet to prevent pain on defecation.
- Overflow diarrhoea.
- Abdominal pain and bloating with large volume stool palpated in the left iliac fossa, and the rectal vault being filled with hard stool (although rectal examinations are avoided in children).

- Poor appetite.
- Fatigue.
- Irritable or angry mood.
- Occasional blood in stool (e.g. from anal fissures).

In chronic constipation, encopresis can ensue. Encopresis is involuntary defecation at an age where continence should be present. Faecal matter is retained, causing secondary overflow incontinence. Alternatively, a large bolus of faeces in the rectum can become difficult for the child to pass, leading to rectal dilatation, and loss of the awareness for emptying the rectum.

Investigations

These are usually unnecessary, as typical constipation is a clinical diagnosis.

Differential Diagnosis

Important differentials include:
- Hirschsprung's disease. Look for constipation from the first few weeks after birth, failure to pass meconium in the first 48 hours after birth, and abdominal distension.
- Bowel obstruction. Enquire about vomiting and abdominal pain. Look for abdominal distension, and perform an abdominal X-ray if concerned.
- Spinal cord compression. Look for leg weakness, asymmetry of the gluteal muscles and abnormal reflexes.
- Imperforate anus. Look for abnormal appearance of the anus.
- Hypothyroidism/Coeliac disease. Consider screening for these if constipation doesn't resolve after four weeks of treatment.
- Electrolyte disturbance. Hypokalaemia and hypercalcaemia may cause constipation.

Many other conditions are associated with constipation; for example, Down syndrome, cow's milk intolerance and cerebral palsy. However, they are unlikely to present with constipation in isolation. Check the side effects of any medications as well.

Management

Non-pharmacological management includes:
- Dietary changes. Increasing intake of water and fibre (wholemeal bread, brown rice, fruit and vegetables). This aids the production of softer stools.
- Regular toileting. Children should be encouraged to use the toilet regularly, especially after meals, to help change any avoidance behaviour that the child may have developed.

Children should have an abdominal examination before starting any medications. Medication involves "disimpaction" and "maintenance" therapy.

FIGURE 6

Appearance	Type	Description
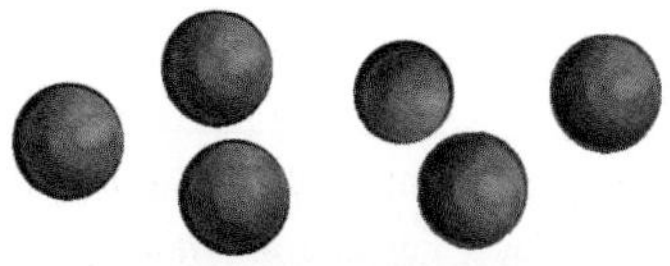	1.	Hard lumps.
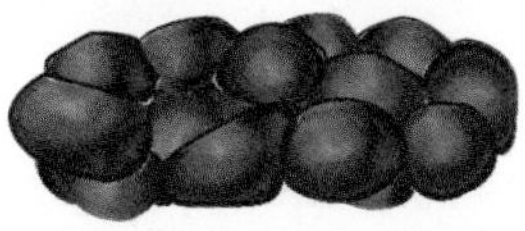	2.	Sausage shaped, but lumpy.
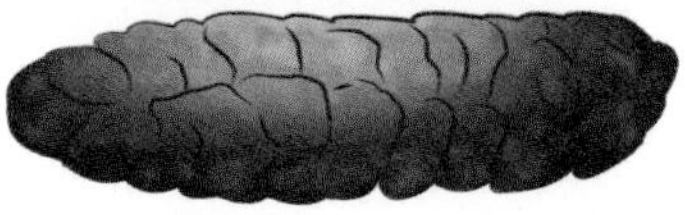	3.	Sausage shaped, with cracks on surface.
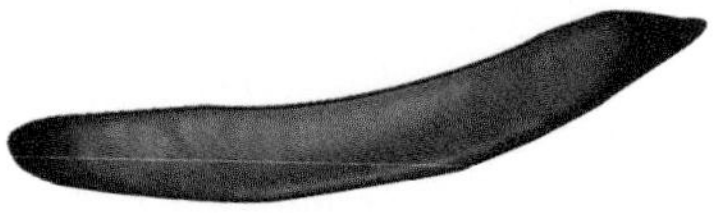	4.	Sausage shaped, with a smooth soft surface.
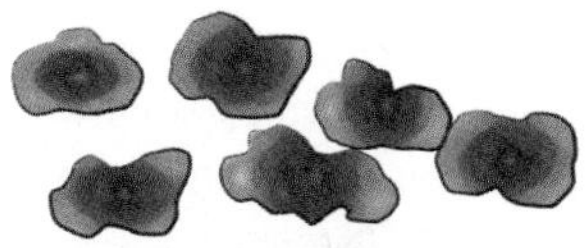	5.	Soft blobs.
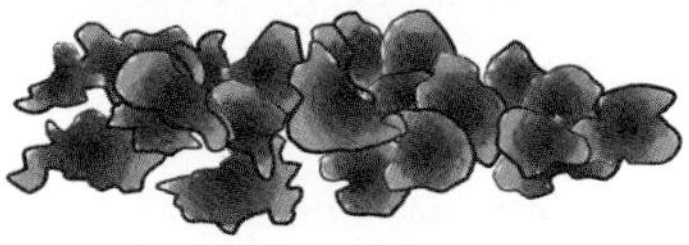	6.	Fluffy pieces, with a mushy texture.
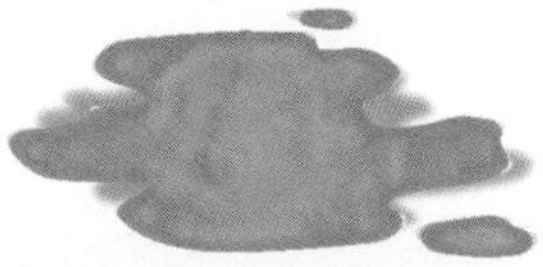	7.	Entirely liquid.

Bristol Stool Chart. Types three and four constitute normal stool. (Adapted from Lewis SJ, Heaton KW. Stool form scale as a useful guide to intestinal transit time. Scandinavian Journal of Gastroenterology 32: 920-4).

The laxatives should be continued for several weeks after a regular bowel habit has been established, alongside conservative measures to promote a healthy bowel regime. Dosage should subsequently be gradually reduced according to symptoms.

Prognosis

Constipation is usually mild and self-limiting, with dietary changes +/- short courses of medication sufficient to resolve symptoms. A minority will require ongoing therapy.

Toddler's Diarrhoea

Toddler's diarrhoea is a common disorder characterised by diarrhoea in young children. The diarrhoea is transient and the child is otherwise well.

Aetiology

The main aetiological factors are nutritional: a low fat diet, excessive fluid intake and poor absorption of sucrose and fructose due to gut immaturity. These dietary factors can increase the amount of water held in the colon, which in children can lead to looser stools.

Clinical Features

Toddler's diarrhoea normally presents in children aged between six months and five years. The main symptoms are diarrhoea that lasts over a number of weeks, followed by a period of normal stools. Stools often contain undigested food particles, hence also being called "peas and carrots" diarrhoea. In some cases, there may be mild abdominal pain. Children are otherwise healthy and growing as expected.

If the child experiences blood or mucus in the stool, faltering growth, fever, severe abdominal pain, vomiting or incontinence, a more serious cause should be investigated.

Management

Parents should be reassured that the condition is self-resolving as the gut lining matures. Treatment with

> Disimpaction. If stools are felt in the left lower quadrant, a "disimpaction regime" should be started using an oral macrogol (e.g. Movicol). A macrogol is an osmotic laxative which softens the stool by increasing the osmotic pressure within the colon, therefore drawing water into the colon. The increased water volume stimulates peristalsis to occur. An oral stimulant laxative (e.g. Senna) can be added if disimpaction doesn't occur within two weeks. Rectal medications (e.g.

sodium picosulfate, a stimulant) should only be used if oral therapy fails.

> Maintenance. Maintenance therapy should be initiated in children without impacted faeces or after a disimpaction regime. Maintenance therapy involves using a macrogol as first-line treatment, the dose of which can then be adjusted according to symptoms. If a macrogol is not tolerated or constipation is resistant to first-line treatment, a stimulant laxative can be added.

medication is rarely required, and often the symptoms can be improved with dietary changes like:

- Limiting fruit juices and carbonated drinks.
- Avoiding excessive fluid intake.
- Increasing the fat content of the diet with full-fat milk and other dairy products.
- Optimising dietary fibre.

Inform parents to be vigilant for the symptoms of more severe disease and return for investigations to discover the cause.

Complications
There are no significant complications of toddler's diarrhoea.

Prognosis
Toddler's diarrhoea normally self-resolves by 5-years-old, regardless of whether dietary changes are made. There are no significant complications of toddler's diarrhoea.

HEPATIC DISORDERS

Hepatitis
Hepatitis is inflammation of the liver. The most common causes in children are infection and autoimmune disease, as summarised in *Table 8*. Investigations into hepatitis should identify the underlying cause of the disease as well as assess liver damage. This involves looking for viral causes [Hepatitis A to E, cytomegalovirus, Epstein-Barr virus, human immunodeficiency virus (HIV)] and autoimmune disorders, as well as performing LFTs and considering liver ultrasound, or in rare cases, a liver biopsy. Hepatitis may present quite non-specifically and can have an insidious onset.

Symptoms may include:

- General features. Fatigue, joint and muscle pain, fever, headache.
- Gastrointestinal features. Nausea, vomiting, right upper quadrant abdominal pain, constipation, diarrhoea.

TABLE 8: Possible causes of hepatitis in children				
	Risk Factors	**Presentation**	**Management**	**Prognosis**
Hepatitis A	Travelling to an area with high prevalence of the disease, clotting disorders, and close contact with someone with hepatitis A.	Acute illness. In children under five-years-old, most infections are asymptomatic.	In a well child, only symptomatic treatment is required. In children where the liver function is deteriorating or they become unwell, admission to hospital is usually required. Hepatitis A is considered a "notifiable disease" and needs to be reported due to its contagiousness. Severe disease may merit liver transplantation.	Hepatitis A is usually self-resolving; however, in a small number of cases, the disease can relapse. Cholestasis and liver failure are complications of severe cases.
Hepatitis B and C	Travelling to areas with a high prevalence, maternal infection and receiving contaminated blood products. Vertical transmission at delivery is an important cause of hepatitis B. There is also a risk of this with hepatitis C at birth, although the disease is less common.	In older children, acute hepatitis B is usually self-resolving. However, in younger children, although the acute infection is usually asymptomatic, it is more likely to result in chronic disease. Hepatitis C causes chronic, slow, progressive liver disease. The acute phase is usually asymptomatic; however, 75% will develop chronic disease.	In Hepatitis B, monitoring of liver function is required. Pharmacological management may reduce the risks of progression to cirrhosis, hepatocellular carcinoma and liver failure. Liver biopsy can be used to assess the need for antiviral treatment e.g. pegylated interferon alfa-2a (blocks viral protein synthesis). Hepatitis C is managed similarly, and both are notifiable diseases.	There is a possibility of chronic infection, resulting in a long-term risk of liver cirrhosis, and hepatocellular carcinoma.
Autoimmune Hepatitis	Autoimmune hepatitis has a multifactorial aetiology with environmental triggers, a failure of immune tolerance and genetic predisposition that lead to hepatocyte inflammation and necrosis.	May present asymptomatically, as acute hepatitis, as chronic hepatitis or as well-established cirrhosis.	Autoimmune hepatitis should be managed pharmacologically if there are signs of active inflammation. Corticosteroids modulate the inflammatory process and can reduce the amount of hepatocyte inflammation. Some children may be considered for liver transplantation if they have acute liver failure or hepatocellular carcinoma.	Autoimmune hepatitis is a lifelong disease that can progress to liver failure and hepatocellular carcinoma.

> Hepatobiliary features. Jaundice, pale stools, dark urine, pruritus, hepatomegaly, splenomegaly.

Prognosis is variable, and dependent on the cause.

ABDOMINAL PAIN-RELATED FUNCTIONAL GASTROINTESTINAL DISORDERS

Irritable Bowel Syndrome

Irritable bowel syndrome (IBS) is a chronic functional disorder with frequent episodic relapses. It is characterised by recurrent abdominal pain or discomfort relieved by defecation, associated with a change in bowel habit and abdominal bloating.

Aetiology

IBS is thought to be multifactorial in nature. Its development may be related to:

> Recent infection.
> Gastrointestinal inflammation.
> Diet.
> Antibiotics.
> Surgery.
> Family history of irritable bowel syndrome.
> Psychosocial factors, such as anxiety or depression.

Clinical Features

IBS tends to affect older children. It is a collection of symptoms which have been occurring over at least two months and primarily include:

> Abdominal pain that is relieved by defecation at least once per week.
> Abdominal bloating.
> Change in bowel habit leading to constipation, diarrhoea or both.
> Passage of mucus in stools.

Other common symptoms associated with IBS are nausea, lethargy, backache and dysuria.

Investigations

Investigations in IBS are not usually needed, particularly if there is a strong suspicion of the diagnosis. Tests aim to assess possible differential diagnoses:

> FBC. Anaemia may be suggestive of malabsorption.
> CRP and ESR. Inflammation may be present in inflammatory bowel disease, gastroenteritis and other autoimmune conditions.
> LFTs and U&Es. To check electrolytes, renal and liver function. Depending on the location of the pain, it may be associated with kidney or liver disease.
> Coeliac antibody screening. To rule out coeliac disease.
> Stool MC&S.
> Urine dipstick/MC&S. To rule out UTI.

> Faecal calprotectin. If concerned about possible IBD.
> H. pylori antigen. Stool/blood test to rule out *H. pylori* related peptic ulcer disease, if history is suggestive of this. Note that this can also be tested in the stool.

Differential Diagnosis

All patients with suspected IBS should also be asked about "red flag" symptoms to rule out a more serious underlying pathology. Faltering growth may be associated with malabsorption disorders such as inflammatory bowel disease and cystic fibrosis. Rectal bleeding may be associated with inflammatory bowel disease, or a Meckel diverticulum.

Management

The aims of management in IBS are not to cure the condition, but to alleviate and control the symptoms experienced. The main focus of management is on the child's diet.

Children may find that large meals increase symptoms, so trial small, regular meals. Certain food and drink products can exacerbate symptoms in some children, including:

> High fat foods.
> Dairy products.
> Caffeinated drinks.
> Artificial sweeteners.
> Foods that cause flatulence, e.g. beans.

Parents and children can identify trigger foods with the help of a food diary to track symptoms against the foods eaten. If one of the main symptoms is constipation or diarrhoea, an adjustment to the amount of dietary fibre can help to improve symptoms. A gluten-free, lactose-free, or FODMAP (Fermentable Oligo-Di-Monosaccharides & Polyols) diet may also be helpful.

In some cases, the child's symptoms may be inadequately controlled with dietary modifications. Medications given to the child do not cure IBS but may control and reduce the symptoms experienced. Children can be given:

> Laxatives. Reduce constipation by increasing gut motility or increasing osmotic pressure in the gut.
> Antidiarrhoeal medications. Reduce diarrhoea by inhibiting excessive gut propulsion and motility, and improve stool consistency.
> Antispasmodics. Reduce muscle spasms to reduce pain experienced during episodes of abdominal muscle spasms.
> Tricyclic antidepressants. Alter pain responses in the gut to provide visceral analgesia. Rarely used.

As psychosocial factors can influence the development of the disease, psychosocial interventions may be needed. In children, cognitive behavioural therapy and counselling reduce symptoms severity and have a positive effect on other aspects of the child's life. Relaxation training also has a role in helping children to control situations that they find stressful and can improve symptoms associated with IBS.

Complications

A large component of IBS morbidity is psychosocial. Dietary avoidance may lead to malnourishment, but if there is significant faltering growth, or other red flag features, alternate diagnoses should be investigated.

Prognosis

IBS is a lifelong condition, and although the condition itself is not associated with increased mortality, it may have a large psychological impact on children.

Functional Abdominal Pain

Functional abdominal pain is intermittent or continuous abdominal pain that cannot be explained by any physical abnormality after examination and investigations, and does not fit with other functional gastrointestinal disorders.

Aetiology

It is thought to be caused by inappropriate nerve signalling from the brain or the gut that increases the sensitivity of nociceptors in the gut.

Risk factors for developing functional abdominal pain are:
- Psychological disorders.
- Physically or emotionally traumatic experiences. For instance, a change in family circumstances, or a new sibling.
- Preceding gastrointestinal infections.

However, it often occurs in otherwise healthy children. It is much more common in children than in adults.

Clinical Features

The most common symptom is mild to moderate peri-umbilical abdominal pain. However, the character and course of the pain can vary between patients. It may also be associated with vomiting, nausea, dyspepsia and poor appetite. Functional abdominal pain syndrome is defined by presence of symptoms more than 25% of the time, associated with somatic symptoms, and some loss of daily function.

Investigations

There is no diagnostic test, but investigations (as with IBS) may be carried out to rule out other causes.

Differential Diagnosis

Functional abdominal pain is a diagnosis of exclusion; consider sinister causes such as appendicitis, UTI, peptic ulcer disease, coeliac disease and inflammatory bowel disease.

Management

If no other sinister cause is found for the child's abdominal pain, reassure the child and their parents. The main aim of management is to improve the child's quality of life with better coping skills. This may involve the community child/adolescent mental health team. Other possible interventions include:
- Dietary changes may be beneficial depending on the history of the child's pain. In some children, lactose intolerance can accompany functional abdominal pain, and excluding lactose from the diet may be useful.
- Anti-spasmodic medications can be used to relieve abdominal cramps by relaxing the abdominal muscles.
- Constipation can be treated with laxatives or dietary changes (increase fibre/water intake).
- Antacids can be given to relieve dyspepsia symptoms.

Complications

In some patients, functional abdominal pain can have a chronic, debilitating course, causing difficulties with sleep or school and have a negative psychological effect.

Prognosis

Functional abdominal pain tends to be self-resolving over a number of months.

Abdominal Migraine

Abdominal migraine is an idiopathic disorder characterised by recurrent episodes of midline abdominal pain lasting 2 to 72 hours.

Clinical Features

The pain is associated with nausea, vomiting, anorexia and/or pallor. The pain can be severe enough to prevent the child from going to school and carrying out normal activities. Between episodes, the condition resolves and there are no apparent symptoms. Triggers can be similar to that for classic migraines, like chocolate or stress.

Investigations

There is no diagnostic test, but investigations (as with IBS) may be carried out to rule out other causes.

Management

Management of abdominal migraine includes advice, analgesia and prophylactic medication. Advice should be offered to help children and their parents recognise and avoid triggers. Sleep can also help relieve pain. Prophylactic medications include beta blockers and tricyclic antidepressants. Beta blockers act by reducing neuronal activity, but the mechanism of tricyclic antidepressants is unclear.

Prognosis

Children who experience abdominal migraines often develop migraine headaches later in life.

ADDITIONAL PATHOLOGY

Gastroenteritis

Gastroenteritis is inflammation of the gastrointestinal tract secondary to an infection.

Aetiology

Gastroenteritis may be caused by bacteria, viruses or protozoa.

> Viral infections, especially rotavirus, are the most common, particularly affecting children under five. The introduction of rotavirus vaccination is decreasing the disease burden, but other viral causes include adenovirus, enterovirus, and norovirus.

> The most common bacterial infection is with *Campylobacter jejuni*. Other bacteria that can cause gastroenteritis are *Escherichia coli*, *Salmonella* and *Shigella*.

> *Yersinia enterocolitica*, *Cryptosporidium*, *Entamoeba histolytica* and *Giardia* are parasites that can cause gastroenteritis.

The causative organism is normally ingested and may be found on raw meats, fish, unpasteurised milk or untreated water. Toxins from bacteria can also cause gastroenteritis. The most common toxins are from *Staphylococcus aureus*, *Bacillus cereus* and *Clostridium perfringens*.

In gastroenteritis, the responsible pathogen damages the villi, leading to malabsorption of intestinal contents and osmotic diarrhoea. Toxins bind to receptors in the intestine, leading to the release of chloride ions and causing secretory diarrhoea.

Clinical Features

Symptoms of gastroenteritis usually start suddenly and include diarrhoea and vomiting. Disease severity tends to depend on the degree of dehydration in the child. Depending on the infective agent, other symptoms include fever, headache, lethargy, abdominal pain, poor feeding, dysuria and weight loss.

Dehydration is more likely in certain groups of people including those:

> Under one, especially those under 6–months-old.
> With a low birth weight.
> Who have stopped breastfeeding.
> Who have not been offered, or not tolerated fluids pre-presentation.
> Who have had more than five episodes of diarrhoea, or two episodes of vomiting in 24 hours.
> Who have signs of malnutrition.

Investigations

The clinical history may identify a possible source of the infection. Ask questions about dietary intake (seafood, unwashed vegetables, unpasteurized milk, contaminated water, uncooked meats, takeaways/unusual foods), recent travel and exposure to other individuals with gastroenteritis.

Most cases of gastroenteritis are mild, with a clear history. In such instances, no investigations are needed.

Stool examination is the primary test for acute gastroenteritis. Stool samples should be sent if:

> There is diagnostic doubt.
> The patient is septic.
> There is blood or mucus in the stool.
> If the child is immunocompromised.
> If an unusual infective organism is suspected.
> The diarrhoea has continued for greater than two weeks.

Other sources of infection should be investigated if a definitive focus cannot be found. This may include urine microscopy, culture and sensitivity, chest X-ray and a lumbar puncture. If the child appears significantly dehydrated, monitor urine output and take blood samples for urea and electrolytes to look for electrolyte disturbances and acute kidney injury. Other useful blood tests in a potentially septic or significantly shocked patient include blood gas, inflammatory markers and blood cultures.

Differential Diagnosis

Many conditions can present with diarrhoea, as detailed in *Table 9*. The hallmark of gastroenteritis compared to the alternative diagnoses is its acute onset.

Management

A clinical assessment of dehydration should be made in all children (*Table 10*). If there are no signs of clinical dehydration, home management is appropriate. Parents should be advised to continue feeding and ensure adequate clear fluid intake. An oral rehydration solution (ORS) can be supplemented to reduce the risk of developing dehydration.

Treating dehydration involves small frequent fluid intake:

> 50ml/kg of ORS should be given over four hours (in addition to maintenance fluids). This can potentially be given by NG feed if not orally tolerated.

After rehydration, the parents should be advised to restart the child's normal diet. In those at risk of dehydration, consider giving 5ml/kg of ORS after large watery stools. Younger children are more likely to need admission to hospital, as are those with no improvement on ORS. Parents should prevent spread by isolating the affected child as far as possible.

Intravenous Fluids

Intravenous (IV) fluids should only be given if:

> Shock is suspected.
> Red flag symptoms and clinical deterioration persist despite oral fluids.
> Persistent vomiting whilst on ORS, given orally or NG.

TABLE 9: Causes of diarrhoea in a child

Differential Diagnosis	Common Symptoms
Irritable bowel syndrome	Diarrhoea, bloating, flatulence.
Inflammatory bowel disease	Blood in stools, diarrhoea, constipation, abdominal pain and weight loss.
Coeliac disease	Abdominal pain, diarrhoea, weight loss.
Toddler's diarrhoea	Diarrhoea, normal weight gain.

TABLE 10: Clinical signs to assess in a patient with possible dehydration. "Red flag" signs are written in red

No Clinical Dehydration	Clinical Dehydration	Clinical Shock
Appears well	Appears to be unwell or deteriorating	
Alert and responsive	Altered responsiveness	Decreased level of consciousness
Normal urine output	Decreased urine output	
Normal skin colour	Normal skin colour	Pale or mottled skin
Warm extremities	Warm extremities	Cold extremities
Eyes not sunken	Sunken eyes	
Moist mucous membranes	Dry mucous membranes	
Normal heart rate	Tachycardia	
Normal breathing rate	Tachypnoea	
Normal peripheral pulses	Normal peripheral pulses	Weak peripheral pulses
Normal capillary refill time	Normal capillary refill time	Prolonged capillary refill time
Normal skin turgor	Reduced skin turgor	
Normal blood pressure	Normal blood pressure	Hypotension (decompensated shock)

Fluid boluses of 20ml/kg of 0.9% sodium chloride should be given, followed by isotonic maintenance fluids (e.g. 0.9% sodium chloride/5% dextrose). The fluid deficit (100ml/kg if initially shocked, 50ml/kg if not initially shocked) should be replaced on top of maintenance therapy. Consider adding potassium once plasma levels are known. If IV fluids are started, regular blood tests should be performed to monitor kidney function, as well as glucose and electrolyte levels. If the child is hypernatraemic at presentation, replace fluids cautiously over 48 hours, with regular monitoring of sodium level, aiming to reduce it at a rate <0.5mmol/L/hour.

Antibiotics

Antibiotics should not routinely be prescribed for gastroenteritis as the majority of cases are viral. Antibiotics should, however, be considered in special circumstances, including:

> *Salmonella* gastroenteritis if either immunocompromised, malnourished, or under six months.
> Suspected septicaemia.
> Extra-intestinal spread of bacterial infection.
> *Clostridium difficile*-associated pseudomembranous colitis, giardiasis, dysenteric shigellosis, dysenteric amoebiasis or cholera.

Complications

Most cases of gastroenteritis are mild, with no significant complications. In more severe cases, gastroenteritis may lead to electrolyte imbalances or acute kidney injury. Other possible complications include:

> Acquired lactose intolerance.
> Persistent diarrhoea.
> Irritable bowel syndrome.
> Systemic infection.
> Haemolytic uraemic syndrome (p308).

Prognosis

Gastroenteritis is a self-limiting illness which rarely causes severe or lasting adverse effects.

Mesenteric Adenitis

Mesenteric adenitis is a common acute condition especially in children under 15-years-old. It is caused by inflammation of the mesenteric lymph nodes in the abdomen, resulting in secondary abdominal pain. Presentation can mimic appendicitis.

Aetiology

Mesenteric adenitis is most likely to be caused by a viral pathogen. However, some bacterial pathogens have been implicated in the disease process, including *Yersinia enterocolitica*, *Helicobacter pylori*, *Campylobacter jejuni*, *Salmonella* and *Shigella*. Infection with these pathogens is thought to trigger an inflammatory response in the mesenteric lymph nodes.

Clinical Features

The main symptom is acute abdominal pain that follows a similar pattern to appendicitis. It can be associated with fever, feeling unwell, anorexia, nausea, diarrhoea, headache, pharyngitis and cervical lymphadenopathy. Sometimes it is preceded by a viral upper respiratory tract infection (URTI).

Investigations

Investigations are used to rule out differential diagnoses, but in a well child the diagnosis is made clinically, as there is no clear-cut investigation to positively diagnose mesenteric adenitis. The most important differential diagnosis is acute appendicitis. Others include intussusception and Meckel's diverticulum.

Blood Tests

> Full blood count (FBC) and C-reactive protein (CRP). To indicate possible infection and/ or inflammation suggestive of appendicitis.

Imaging

> Abdominal X-ray. To reveal possible bowel obstruction (fluid levels) or perforation.
> Abdominal ultrasound. May show signs of appendicitis, swollen lymph nodes, or ovarian pathology.
> Abdominal CT. More sensitive than ultrasound for picking up the above changes.

Additional Tests

> Urine dipstick/MC&S. To rule out a UTI.
> Pregnancy test. In any menstruating girl. If a child is old enough to possibly be pregnant, exclude ectopic pregnancy.
> Diagnostic laparoscopy. To exclude appendicitis, where there is strong clinical suspicion. If a case of abdominal pain has progressed to this level of investigation, it is unlikely to be mesenteric adenitis.

Differential Diagnosis

The signs and symptoms of mesenteric adenitis follow a similar pattern to appendicitis. *Table 11* lists key differences.

Complications

The most common complication is dehydration from both poor oral intake and inflammation. However, mesenteric adenitis can rarely lead to abscess formation and sepsis. Very rarely, the swollen lymph glands in the

TABLE 11: Key features differentiating acute appendicitis and mesenteric adenitis		
Feature	Mesenteric Adenitis	Appendicitis
Abdominal pain.	Common.	Common (but usually more severe and localised to right iliac fossa (RIF)).
Cervical lymphadenopathy.	Common.	Uncommon.
Preceding viral URTI.	Common.	Uncommon.
Tachycardia.	Uncommon.	Possible.
Local/generalised peritonism (Abdominal guarding, percussion tenderness).	Uncommon.	Possible (if perforation).
Vomiting.	Uncommon.	Common.
Elevated inflammatory markers.	Uncommon.	Common.

gut can cause intussusception and bowel obstruction.

Management

Management involves analgesia and hydration. Parents need to be advised that increasing pain or becoming more unwell requires urgent review, as appendicitis (or another diagnosis) may have presented atypically or at the early stages.

Prognosis

Mesenteric adenitis is usually self-limiting and will typically resolve within a few days, but may take up to two weeks.

Infantile Colic

Infantile colic is defined as repeated episodes of excessive and inconsolable crying in an infant who is otherwise healthy. It should be diagnosed in a child whose crying lasts for more than three hours per day, on more than three days in a week, and has persisted for longer than three weeks in the absence of any other cause.

Aetiology

The cause of infantile colic is unknown. However, some research has shown that transient lactase deficiency, excessive intestinal gas and cow's milk intolerance may be implicated. There is also evidence that infants with colic may have higher levels of the gastrointestinal regulatory

peptide, motilin. Additionally, women who smoke during pregnancy have a higher risk of having a child with infantile colic.

Clinical Features

Colic usually begins in the first few weeks after birth, and crying is often worst in the late afternoon or evening. Other symptoms include drawing the knees up to chest and arching of the back (opisthotonus).

Investigations

No specific investigations are required, other than to rule out other differential diagnoses depending on the clinical scenario.

Differential Diagnosis

A detailed history should be obtained including when the child cries, how much they cry, character of the cry and the family's normal daily routine. Other questions and examinations should try to exclude other causes of excessive crying. Children with colic have normal (or accelerated) growth with otherwise normal findings on examination. The differential for crying is wide.

Sudden onset, inconsolable crying may be due to:

> Intussusception.
> Strangulated hernia.
> Testicular torsion.
> Corneal abrasion.
> Non-accidental injury.

Persistent crying may be due to:

- Discomfort.
- Constipation.
- GORD.
- Cow's milk intolerance.
- Seizures.
- Cerebral palsy.
- Chromosomal abnormalities.

Management

Parents should be assured that their child is healthy, and that colic will pass with time. They should also be reminded to look after themselves as infantile colic can often make parents feel guilty. Support groups can be a useful resource for parents.

Holding the infant whilst they are crying may help. Soothing techniques such as gentle movements and a warm bath can also be useful to reduce the extent of crying episodes. If parents are not coping, symptoms may improve by conducting a one week trial of any of the following:

- Excluding cow's milk protein from the diet. If breastfeeding, the mother can exclude cow's milk from her diet (taking calcium supplements if done long-term).
- Simethicone drops. Simethicone joins small gas bubbles in the bowel into larger bubbles that are easily expelled as wind or during burping.
- Lactase drops. Lactase helps the digestive system to digest lactose in the diet.

In children where a trial has improved symptoms, treatment can be stopped after the child is three-months-old, when colic tends to resolve.

Prognosis

Infantile colic is usually self-resolving by 3 or 4-months-old, but can persist in infants up to 6-months-old. It is not known to be associated with long-term morbidity.

Meckel Diverticulum

A Meckel diverticulum is an ileal remnant of the vitelline duct, and is present in two percent of the population. It is usually found 40-60cm proximal to the ileocecal valve, and frequently contains ectopic pancreatic or gastric mucosa.

Clinical Features

These are usually asymptomatic and are discovered as incidental findings during an operation for another reason. However, they can present with:

- Rectal bleeding. This is the most common complication, secondary to haemorrhage from peptic ulceration.
- Ulceration. The gastric mucosa may form a chronic ulcer, which may perforate. Acid secretion can also damage surrounding tissue.

- Intussusception. The diverticulum may form the lead point for an intussusception.
- Volvulus. May occur around vitelline duct remnants.
- Diverticulitis. May mimic appendicitis and can lead to perforation/peritonitis.
- Umbilical abnormalities. Fistulas, sinuses, cysts and fibrous bands between the diverticulum and the umbilicus.
- Neoplasm. Meckel diverticulum may rarely develop benign (e.g. leiomyoma) and malignant (e.g. carcinoid) tumours.

Management

A Meckel scan is excellent at identifying the Meckel diverticulum. This nuclear medicine scan identifies increased uptake of technetium by the gastric mucosa. Definitive treatment of a complication (e.g. bleeding) is surgical excision along with the adjacent ileal segment. Management of an incidental finding of a Meckel diverticulum is controversial, with most advocating for prophylactic excision. If it is a planned procedure (positive history and positive Meckel scan), it is removed laparoscopically.

REFERENCES AND FURTHER READING

Inflammatory Bowel Disease

1 Sandhu BK et al. Guidelines for the management of inflammatory bowel disease in children in the United Kingdom. J Pediatr Gastroenterol Nut. 2010; 50: S1-13.
2 Turner D et al. Management of pediatric ulcerative colitis: joint ECCO and ESPGHAN evidence-based consensus guidelines. J Pediatr Gastroenterol Nutr. 2012; 55:340-61.
3 Ruemmele FM et al. Consensus guidelines of ECCO/ ESPGHAN on the medical management of pediatric Crohn's disease. J Crohns Colitis. 2014; 8:1179-207.
4 NICE Guideline CG152. Crohn's Disease: management. 2012. Available at: https://www.nice.org.uk/guidance/cg152.
5 NICE Guideline CG166. Ulcerative colitis: management. 2013. Available at: https://www.nice.org.uk/guidance/cg166.

Gastro-oesophageal Reflux Disease

1 NICE Guideline NG1. Gastro-oesophageal reflux disease in children and young people: diagnosis and management. 2015. Available at: https://www.nice.org.uk/guidance/ng1.

Coeliac Disease

1 NICE CKS. Coeliac Disease. 2010. Available at: http://cks. nice.org.uk/coeliac-disease
2 NICE Guideline CG86. Coeliac disease: recognition and assessment. 2009. Available at: https://www.nice.org.uk/ guidance/cg86.
3 Murch S et al. Joint BSPGHAN and Coeliac UK guidelines for the diagnosis and management of coeliac disease in children. Arch Dis Child. 2013; 98:806-11.

Gastroenteritis

1 NICE Guideline CG94. Diarrhoea and vomiting in children: Diarrhoea and vomiting caused by gastroenteritis: diagnosis, assessment and management in children younger than 5 years 2009. Available at: https://www.nice.org.uk/guidance/cg84.

Constipation

1 NICE Guideline CG99. Constipation in children and young people: Diagnosis and management of idiopathic childhood constipation in primary and secondary care. 2010. Available at: https://www.nice.org.uk/guidance/cg99.
2 Lewis SJ, Heaton KW. Stool form scale as a useful guide to intestinal transit time. Scandinavian Journal of Gastroenterology. 1997; 32: 920-4.

Mesenteric Adenitis

1 Medscape. Mesenteric lymphadenitis. 2015. Available at: http://emedicine.medscape.com/article/181162-overview.

Irritable Bowel Syndrome

1 NICE CKS. Irritable Bowel Syndrome. 2013. Available at: http://cks.nice.org.uk/irritable-bowel-syndrome.
2 Spiller R et al. Guidelines on the Irritable Bowel Syndrome: Mechanisms and practical management. Gut. 2007; 56:P1770-98.

Functional Abdominal Pain

1 Chiou E, Nurko S. Management of functional abdominal pain and irritable bowel syndrome in children and adolescents. Exp Rev Gastroenterol Hepatol. 2010; 4:293-304.

Infantile Colic

1 NICE CKS. Colic- infantile. 2012. Available at: http://cks.nice.org.uk/colic-infantile.

Eosinophilic Oesophagitis

1 Hansen R, Russell RK, Muhammed R. Recent advances in paediatric gastroenterology. Arch Dis Child. 2015; 100:886-90.

Meckel Diverticulum

1 Medscape. Pediatric Meckel Diverticulum. 2015. Available at: http://emedicine.medscape.com/article/931229-overview.

Peptic Ulcer Disease

1 Medscape. Peptic Ulcer Disease. Available at: http://emedicine.medscape.com/article/181753-overview.

Hepatitis

1 NICE CKS. Hepatitis A. 2014. Available at: http://cks.nice.org.uk/hepatitis-a.
2 NICE CKS Hepatitis B. 2014. Available at: http://cks.nice.org.uk/hepatitis-b.
3 NICE CKS. Hepatitis C. 2010. Available at: http://cks.nice.org.uk/hepatitis-c.
4 Manns MP et al. Diagnosis and management of autoimmune hepatitis. Hepatology. 2010; 51:2193-213.

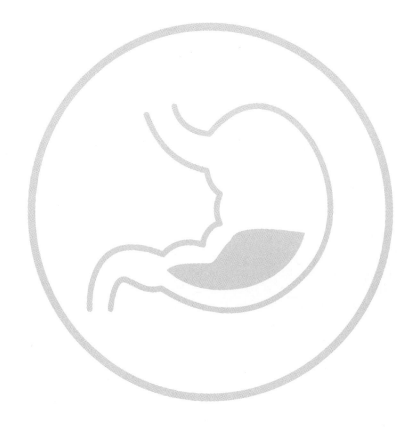

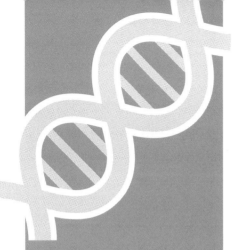

1.08
GENETICS

ISABEL MAWSON, CHRISTOPHER HARRIS, MAXINE WILKIE AND ZESHAN QURESHI

CONTENTS

APPROACHING GENETIC PROBLEMS

All cells in the human body, except gametes, have 46 chromosomes arranged into 23 pairs. Autosomes account for 22 of these pairs. The 23rd pair is made up of two sex chromosomes. In addition, every cell carries DNA within its mitochondria.

Through the processes of transcription and translation, genes enable each cell to build all the required proteins. Errors in an individual's genetic makeup can therefore affect every cell in the body. Genetic syndromes can be caused by problems at the gene or chromosome level or by errors in the packaging of the DNA. Detailed below are some of the mechanisms by which genes cause disease.

Patterns of Genetic Disease

Mendelian Inheritance
This describes a pattern of inheritance caused by mutations on a single gene, as seen in neurofibromatosis and Marfan syndrome.

Multifactorial, Polygenic Disorders
Some genetic mutations increase the risk of a disease, without necessarily causing the disease. For example, a mutation in the NOD2/CARD15 gene (which relates to the immune system) is associated with a slightly increased risk of Crohn's disease, though most people with the mutation remain healthy. This could be due to a certain environmental trigger required to make the genetic defect apparent, or it may be because other genes compensate for any problems related to the mutant gene. Such genes are said to have a low "penetrance", which means a low percentage of those with the defective gene (genotype) express the symptoms of the disease (phenotype).

Chromosomal Disorders
These disorders result from the absence or duplication of entire chromosomes. Examples include Down syndrome (Trisomy 21), Edward syndrome (Trisomy 18), Patau syndrome (Trisomy 13) and Turner syndrome (45,X).

Disorders of Imprinting

Only the maternal or paternal alleles of some genes are expressed. These genes are known as "imprinted" genes. The DNA of the unexpressed allele is bound tightly as chromatin. If the expressed allele is missing from a cell or if a cell has two unexpressed alleles, the gene is non-functional and may result in a genetic syndrome, e.g. Prader-Willi syndrome.

Expanding Trinucleotide Repeat Disorders

These disorders, like myotonic dystrophy, occur when a certain trinucleotide sequence within a gene expands during meiosis, resulting in a longer trinucleotide repeat sequence with each generation. The larger the number of repeats, the more severe the disease. As such, the disease becomes more severe with every subsequent generation.

Identifying a Genetic Problem

Parental Screening

In some circumstances, parents can be tested to assess the risk of their child having a genetic disorder. This is sometimes done with cystic fibrosis, particularly for couples who already have a child with the disease. If neither parent carries the defective gene for cystic fibrosis, the child is extremely unlikely to get the disease, whereas if both parents carry it, the child has a 25% chance of being affected. However, sometimes, a genetic defect that leads to a syndrome arises spontaneously, or "de novo", in a child with no apparent inheritance pattern.

Antenatal Screening

Routine antenatal screening can be a useful tool in the early identification of syndromes. In the UK, combined screening is offered at 12 weeks gestation to identify those at risk of Down syndrome. Abnormalities in these screening tests can also raise suspicion of other genetic syndromes. Ultrasound scans performed after 20 weeks gestation give more in-depth knowledge of anatomical abnormalities which can identify other syndromes and assess for specific organ involvement in the trisomy disorders. Antenatal diagnoses can be confirmed in utero by amniocentesis or chorionic villus sampling. *Table 1* summarises the tests which may be performed during pregnancy. Diagnoses can be made after birth based on identification of congenital defects.

Describing Birth Defects

When describing birth defects, it is important to appreciate the differentiation of several categories, as described below. Dysmorphic features may suggest the need for genetic testing. Important genetic tests to be aware of are karyotyping, array CGH and FISH (*Table 2*).

Syndrome

This is when multiple abnormalities commonly occur together, e.g. Down syndrome. There is usually a specific gene, group of genes, or chromosomal abnormality known

TABLE 1: Tests that may be performed during pregnancy to identify genetic disorders	
Test	**Comments**
Nuchal translucency scan (11–14 weeks).	Ultrasound measurement of the thickness of the subcutaneous fluid beneath the skin on the back of the foetal neck (should be less than 3.5mm), used in the screening for trisomies and Turner syndrome.
Foetal anomaly scans (18–21 weeks).	Foetal anomaly scans enable a more detailed assessment of foetal anatomy and screen for foetal anomalies. Not all anomalies can be detected on ultrasound accurately at approximately 20 weeks, and the sensitivity and specificity vary for detecting each anomaly.
Maternal blood tests.	Screening for chromosomal abnormalities, i.e. trisomies. These are not 100% sensitive so they need to be followed up with amniocentesis or chorionic villus sampling for definitive diagnosis. Tests might include: Combined test (10 to 14 weeks' gestation). • Free beta HCG. • PAPP-A. • Nuchal translucency scan. Quadruple test (14 to 20 weeks' gestation). • Free beta HCG. • Unconjugated oestriol. • AFP. • Inhibin-A.
Chorionic Villus Sampling (CVS) (11-14 weeks).	CVS involves taking a sample of the placenta, which is developed from the same genetic material as the foetus. It is taken either with a needle through the abdomen or by passing a small tube through the cervix under ultrasound guidance. Complications of CVS are infection, heavy bleeding and miscarriage.
Amniocentesis (15-20 weeks).	Amniocentesis involves sampling the amniotic fluid which surrounds the foetus. The sample is obtained by passing a needle through the abdominal wall under ultrasound guidance. Complications of amniocentesis are infection, bleeding and miscarriage.

to cause a syndrome. Another example is CHARGE syndrome (coloboma of the eye, heart defects, atresia of the choanae, retarded growth and development, genital/urinary defects, ear abnormality).

Association

This is a group of defects occurring in association more often than would be expected by chance. An association shows a greater variability in phenotype than a syndrome. An example would be the VACTERL association (vertebral anomalies, anal atresia, cardiac defects, trachea-oesophageal fistula, renal anomalies and limb defects).

Sequence

A sequence refers to a phenotype where all the features occur in an order, triggered by one feature. For example, the Pierre-Robin sequence is characterised by a small, posterior jaw in

TABLE 2: Common methods of genetic testing	
Test	**Comments**
Karyotype.	This is a test used to identify the size, shape and number of chromosomes. It is useful for identification of trisomies (additional chromosomes), e.g. Down syndrome, or the absence of a chromosome, e.g. Turner syndrome.
Array comparative genomic hybridisation (CGH).	Array CGH can identify chromosomal micro-deletions or micro-duplications, and therefore reveals much subtler changes than karyotyping. This is done by comparing the patient's gene sequence against a known "normal" gene sequence. This can be further compared to the parents' sequence if any abnormalities are detected.
Fluorescence In-Situ Hybridisation (FISH).	Used to detect and localise the presence or absence of a specific DNA sequence being investigated. Vectors are targeted to these specific sequences, which become visible if present.

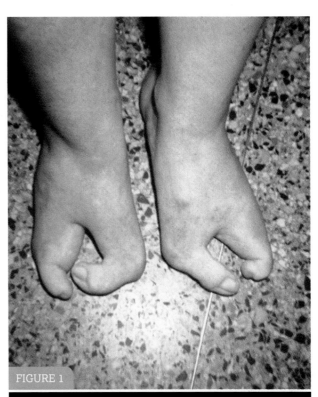

FIGURE 1

Cleft feet, a rare congenital abnormality.

utero, which pushes the tongue back and up in the mouth. This prevents the palate from closing, resulting in a cleft palate. Sequences may be caused by one of several genetic abnormalities, e.g. Potter's sequence, which can be caused by 22q11 deletions.

SYNDROME WITHOUT A NAME

Syndrome without a name (SWAN) is a diagnosis used for children who have a collection of symptoms and signs likely to be genetic in origin, but where the exact genetic cause has not been identified. *Figure 1* shows a rare abnormality picked up on newborn examination: cleft foot. Imagine a baby of consanguineous parents is born with this abnormality in combination with dysmorphic facial features, a ventricular septal defect, single palmar creases and hypothyroidism. It is unlikely for separate pathologies to cause each congenital abnormality, so a genetic aetiology should be suspected. However, such children may have normal chromosome karyotypes/CGH analysis and negative tests for common genetic disorders on FISH testing. This makes a rare or previously undescribed genetic syndrome the most likely diagnosis.

Investigations

Further testing is difficult if no clear specific genetic disorder is available for testing individually. Current estimates indicate that up to 50% of children with learning difficulties and 50% of those in contact with a Regional Genetics Centre never receive a specific diagnosis to explain their disabilities.

Investigating these patients is complicated, and parents understandably suffer significant anxiety. Patients often need exhaustive imaging and blood tests to identify associated defects. Parents and relatives may also be investigated. Increasingly, registries are being developed for the collation of constellations of phenotypic abnormalities, with likely genetic abnormalities then being suggested by a computer algorithm.

Management

Management of SWAN involves active symptom management and multi-disciplinary team support. Dealing with prognostic uncertainty is difficult. It is important to communicate honestly with parents that although the exact nature of the disease is uncertain, their child will be closely followed up to identify any problems early.

As more data becomes available and genetic testing becomes more sophisticated, specific diagnoses may become more likely in the future. Blood samples are stored to facilitate future testing. Parental support groups are also available to help cope with the various challenges associated with having a child with SWAN.

DRAWING A PEDIGREE DIAGRAM

Pedigree diagrams are used for pictorial representation of the family history of a genetic condition and to elucidate the pattern of inheritance. Symbols represent each member of the family, their gender, and disease state, and further information about the person can be written alongside their symbol. Females are represented by circles and males by squares. An affected individual has a closed (filled in) symbol, whereas an unaffected individual has an open (unfilled) symbol, as shown

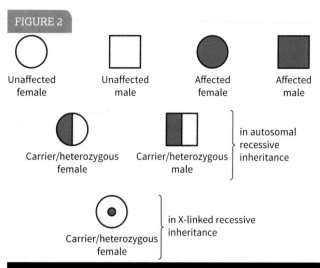

FIGURE 2

Unaffected female

Unaffected male

Affected female

Affected male

Carrier/heterozygous female

Carrier/heterozygous male

in autosomal recessive inheritance

Carrier/heterozygous female

in X-linked recessive inheritance

Symbols used to represent gender and disease status in pedigree diagrams.

in *Figure 2*. Carriers are denoted with a half-filled symbol in autosomal recessive inheritance or with a dot within the symbol if they are a female carrier in X-linked inheritance.

The Affected Individual

The pedigree diagram should be started with the affected individual who presented with symptoms. That person can be identified by adding their age and placing an arrow pointing to their symbol on the diagram, as shown in *Figure 3*.

The Parents

The parents should then be added. To show that the parents are partners, draw a horizontal line between the two symbols, as shown in *Figure 4*. If the individuals are consanguineous, the connection should be shown with two parallel horizontal lines. If the parents are divorced, add two diagonal lines or if separated, one diagonal line through the connecting horizontal line. Add the age of both parents and any known health conditions.

Additional Family Members

After drawing the individual's parents, include any siblings of the individual in age order, with the eldest on the left hand side. Siblings are connected with a horizontal line, which then has vertical branches to which the symbols are added. Add all family members in the same way. All individuals with similar or the same condition should be included in the pedigree diagram. Any family members who have died can be indicated by a diagonal line through their symbol.

For babies who are not yet born, include their estimated date of delivery. Ensure all previous terminations or miscarriages are indicated and whether the baby was affected by the condition or not. In cases of adoption, use brackets and a dotted line to indicate an individual adopted into the family.

Important additional symbols are shown in *Figure 5*.

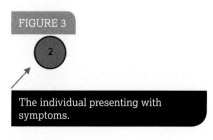

FIGURE 3

2

The individual presenting with symptoms.

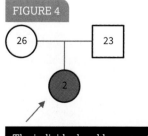

FIGURE 4

26   23

2

The individual and her parents.

MENDELIAN INHERITANCE

Mendelian inheritance patterns describe the inheritance of disorders caused by errors on one specific gene. The types of Mendelian inheritance are described below. The following terms are commonly used in genetics:

> Allele. Every human has two alleles of each gene: one inherited from the mother and one from the father. If both alleles are the same, the patient is described as "homozygous" for the gene. If the alleles are different, the patient is described as "heterozygous" for the gene.

> Autosomal disorders. Disorders caused by a genetic defect on an autosome (one of the 22 non-sex chromosomes).

> X-linked disorders. Disorders caused by genetic defect on the X chromosome.

> Dominant. If the defective gene is "dominant", having one affected allele (being heterozygous) will lead to the disease phenotype, even if the other allele is normal.

> Recessive. If the defective gene is "recessive", two affected alleles (homozygosity) are required for the gene to be phenotypically expressed.

> Carrier. An individual is a carrier if they have one recessive gene but do not phenotypically express it.

Autosomal Dominant

Autosomal dominant inheritance occurs due to a defect on an autosome. Only one abnormal allele (from either the mother or father) is needed for the child to be affected. *Table 3* shows examples of autosomal dominant conditions and *Figure 6* shows a typical pedigree diagram.

Key features include:

> It is very rare for an individual to have two copies of a defective autosomal dominant gene. Those with one copy have a 50% chance of passing the gene on to their child (*Table 4*).

> If a child has the disease, either one parent must have the disease, or the mutation could have arisen "de novo" during gametogenesis. Occasionally, a

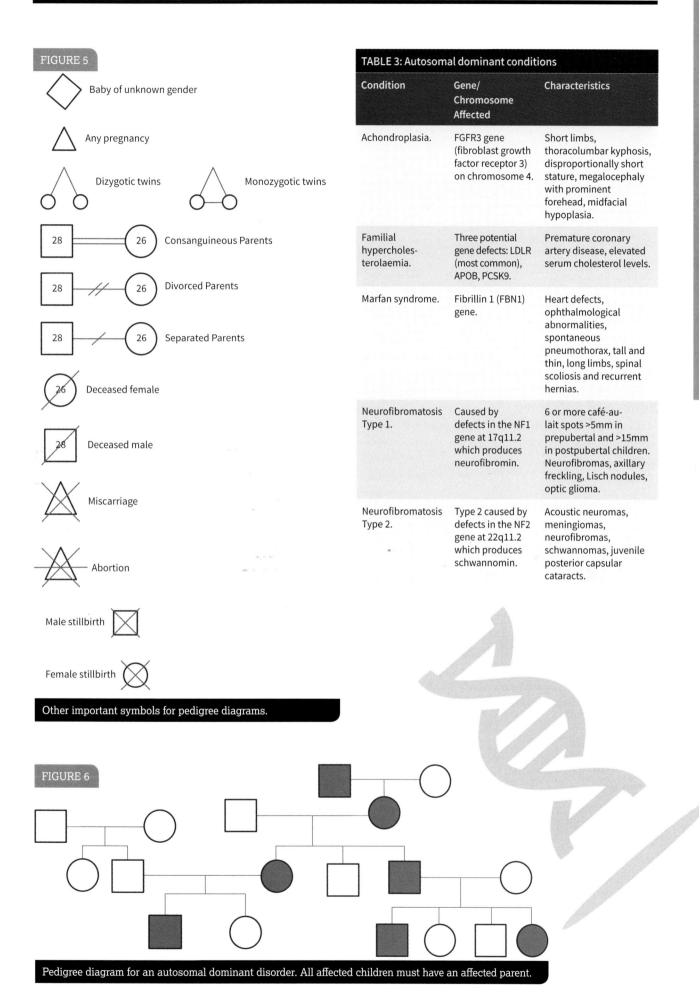

FIGURE 5

Baby of unknown gender

Any pregnancy

Dizygotic twins   Monozygotic twins

28 — 26 Consanguineous Parents

28 —//— 26 Divorced Parents

28 —/— 26 Separated Parents

26 Deceased female

28 Deceased male

Miscarriage

Abortion

Male stillbirth

Female stillbirth

Other important symbols for pedigree diagrams.

TABLE 3: Autosomal dominant conditions

Condition	Gene/ Chromosome Affected	Characteristics
Achondroplasia.	FGFR3 gene (fibroblast growth factor receptor 3) on chromosome 4.	Short limbs, thoracolumbar kyphosis, disproportionally short stature, megalocephaly with prominent forehead, midfacial hypoplasia.
Familial hypercholes-terolaemia.	Three potential gene defects: LDLR (most common), APOB, PCSK9.	Premature coronary artery disease, elevated serum cholesterol levels.
Marfan syndrome.	Fibrillin 1 (FBN1) gene.	Heart defects, ophthalmological abnormalities, spontaneous pneumothorax, tall and thin, long limbs, spinal scoliosis and recurrent hernias.
Neurofibromatosis Type 1.	Caused by defects in the NF1 gene at 17q11.2 which produces neurofibromin.	6 or more café-au-lait spots >5mm in prepubertal and >15mm in postpubertal children. Neurofibromas, axillary freckling, Lisch nodules, optic glioma.
Neurofibromatosis Type 2.	Type 2 caused by defects in the NF2 gene at 22q11.2 which produces schwannomin.	Acoustic neuromas, meningiomas, neurofibromas, schwannomas, juvenile posterior capsular cataracts.

FIGURE 6

Pedigree diagram for an autosomal dominant disorder. All affected children must have an affected parent.

TABLE 4: Likely outcomes for children with regard to autosomal dominant inheritance traits		Mother's Genotype	
		One Mutated Allele	No Mutated Allele
Father's Genotype	One Mutated Allele	75%: Affected 25%: Unaffected	50%: Affected 50%: Unaffected
	No Mutated Allele	50%: Affected 50%: Unaffected	100%: Unaffected

TABLE 5: Autosomal recessive conditions		
Condition	Chromosome/ Gene Affected	Characteristics
Cystic Fibrosis.	Cystic fibrosis transmembrane-conductance regulator (CFTR) gene on chromosome 7.	Thick mucus production from exocrine glands, chronic respiratory infections, faltering growth, diarrhoea, subfertility and meconium ileus.
Sickle Cell Anaemia.	Mutation of the beta globin gene on chromosome 11p15 causing HbS production.	Acute crises (painful/vaso-occlusive, chest, aplastic, splenic sequestration, stroke), chronic haemolytic anaemia and severe infections.
Medium Chain Acyl-CoA Dehydrogenase Deficiency (MCADD).	Mutations of the ACADM gene on chromosome 1p31.	Inability to break down fatty acid chains, resulting in hypoketotic hypoglycaemia after prolonged fasting, lethargy, vomiting and seizures.
Phenylketonuria (PKU).	Mutations of phenylalanine hydroxylase enzyme (PAH) on chromosome 12.	Learning difficulties, seizures, pale skin, blond hair, blue eyes, dietary intolerances and microcephaly.

parent may have "gonadal mosaicism", where a proportion of gametes carry the defective gene.

▸ Equal proportions of males and females are affected.

▸ Altered genes can be passed along any possible familial line, i.e. father to son, father to daughter, mother to daughter and mother to son.

Autosomal Recessive

Autosomal recessive inheritance occurs due to a defect on an autosome. It requires two abnormal alleles (one from each parent) for the child to be affected. However, if just one allele is inherited, the child will be a carrier and not phenotypically affected by the condition. Autosomal recessive conditions are more likely to occur in offspring of consanguineous marriages. *Table 5* shows examples of autosomal recessive conditions and *Figure 7* shows a typical pedigree diagram.

Key features include:

▸ The likelihood of an individual passing on the disease depends on both their own and their partner's genotype, as shown in *Table 6*.

▸ If a child has the disease, both parents must either have the disease or be a carrier. Note that the disease can skip generations.

▸ Equal proportions of males and females are affected.

▸ Recessive alleles can be passed along any possible familial line, i.e. father to son, father to daughter, mother to daughter and mother to son.

X-Linked Dominant Inheritance

X-linked dominant conditions are particularly rare. They occur due to a defect on the X chromosome. These conditions only require one abnormal gene (from either the mother or father) for the child to be affected. *Table 7* shows examples of X-linked dominant conditions and *Figure 8* shows a typical pedigree diagram.

Key features include:

▸ The likelihood of inheritance depends on whether the mother or the father has the disease. With an affected mother, the likelihood of passing on the disorder is 50%. With an affected father, because they always pass their X chromosome

FIGURE 7

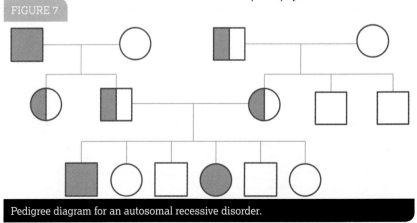

Pedigree diagram for an autosomal recessive disorder.

TABLE 6: Likely outcomes for children with regard to autosomal recessive inheritance traits

		Mother's Genotype		
		Two Recessive Alleles	One Recessive Allele	No Recessive Alleles
Father's Genotype	Two Recessive Alleles	100%: Affected	50%: Affected 50%: Carrier	100%: Carrier
	One Recessive Allele	50%: Affected 50%: Carrier	25%: Affected 50%: Carrier 25%: Unaffected	50%: Carrier 50%: Unaffected
	No Recessive Alleles	100%: Carrier	50%: Carrier 50%: Unaffected	100%: Unaffected

TABLE 7: X-linked dominant conditions

Condition	Gene/Chromosome Affected	Characteristics
X-linked hypophosphataemic rickets.	Phosphate regulating endopeptidase homolog (PHEX) gene.	Reduced phosphate reabsorption in the kidneys leading to hypophosphataemia, short stature and rickets.
Focal dermal hypoplasia.	Porcupine homolog (PORCN) gene.	Variable. Hypoplastic areas of skin present at birth as well as areas of absent skin (cutis aplasia), telangiectasia and papillomas (of skin, larynx and oesophagus). Sparse brittle hair and abnormal teeth with dysmorphic facial features, including cleft lip/palate. Eye deformities (microphthalmia, anophthalmia, coloboma +/- visual impairment). Omphalocoele and horseshoe kidney.

on to their daughters and never to their sons, 100% of daughters will be affected and 0% of sons will be affected.

> If a child has the disease, one parent must have the disease, or the mutation could have arisen "de novo" during gametogenesis.

X-Linked Recessive Inheritance

X-linked recessive inheritance occurs due to a defect on the X chromosome. It requires a defect on both X chromosomes in girls since the gene is recessive. However if a male inherits an affected X chromosome from his mother, he will be affected as males have only one X. Examples of X-linked recessive conditions are shown in *Table 8*, and a typical pedigree diagram is shown in *Figure 9*.

Affected males will pass on their X chromosome to any daughters, who will then become carriers given the other X inherited from their mother is normal. However, sons will receive the Y chromosome and therefore will be unaffected.

Key features include:
> The chance of inheriting the disease depends on the carrier/affected status of both parents and on the sex of the child, as shown in *Table 9*.
> Males are most likely to be affected, since they only need one defective gene to express the disease phenotype. Unless the mutation is "de novo", affected males inherit the abnormal X chromosome from their mother (since they never get an X chromosome from the father).

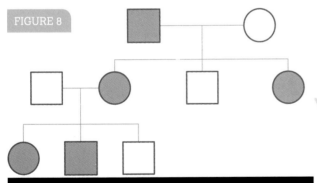

FIGURE 8

Pedigree diagram for an X-linked dominant disorder. Note that the affected father passes on the disease to all daughters.

TABLE 8: Examples of X-Linked recessive conditions

Condition	Gene/Chromosome Affected	Characteristics
Haemophilia.	Type A = factor VIII gene mutation. Type B = factor IX gene mutation.	Prolonged bleeding and easy bruising. Heavy menstrual flow in female carriers.
Duchenne and Becker muscular dystrophy.	Dystrophin gene.	Progressive muscle weakness, starting with proximal muscle groups (usually of lower limbs), delayed motor milestones, calf pseudohypertrophy and Gower's sign (walking hands up one's own legs to assist movement from lying to standing). Becker muscular dystrophy presents at an older age.
Red-green colour blindness.	OPN1LW, OPN1MW on the X chromosome.	Colour blindness due to a fault in the development of L or M retinal cones.

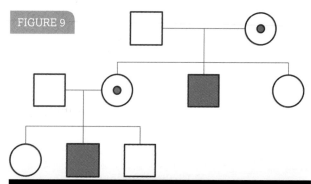

FIGURE 9

Pedigree diagram for an X-Linked recessive disorder. Note that males are disproportionately affected. When initially diagnosing a family with an X-linked recessive condition, the female carriers may not be known. Therefore, their symbols may not initially have the additional dot.

TABLE 9: Outcomes for children with regard to X-linked recessive inheritance traits

Father	Mother	Sons	Daughter
Affected	Unaffected	100% Unaffected	100% Carrier
Affected	Carrier	50% Affected 50% Unaffected	50% Affected 50% Carrier
Affected	Affected	100% Affected	100% Affected
Unaffected	Unaffected	100% Unaffected	100% Unaffected
Unaffected	Carrier	50% Affected 50% Unaffected	50% Carrier 50% Unaffected
Unaffected	Affected	100% Affected	100% Carriers

Note that "lyonisation" or "X-inactivation" can be seen in females. This describes the inactivation of one of the two X chromosomes, meaning it is unable to transcribe any proteins. Rarely, this disproportionately happens to just the maternally- or the paternally-inherited X chromosome. Therefore, by this process, females may phenotypically express an X-linked recessive disease from just one recessive gene.

DISORDERS OF CHROMOSOMAL INHERITANCE

Aneuploidy describes a condition where cells do not have the expected number of chromosomes and where the number of chromosomes is not an exact multiple of the haploid number (23 in humans). The commonest cause of aneuploidy is meiotic nondisjunction during oogenesis or spermatogenesis, leaving a gamete with zero or two copies of a particular chromosome. When this gamete is fertilised, the resulting embryo would have one or three copies of the affected chromosome, instead of the expected two, leading to 47 or 45 chromosomes overall (instead of the normal 46). This process is shown in *Figure 10*. Autosomal chromosome aneuploidy can lead to conditions like Down syndrome (trisomy 21), and less commonly Edward syndrome (trisomy 18) and Patau syndrome (trisomy 13). Sex chromosome aneuploidy may lead to syndromes like Turner syndrome.

Down Syndrome

Down syndrome is the most common chromosomal abnormality in humans occurring in one in 1000 lives births. It is also known as trisomy 21.

Aetiology

Down syndrome can be caused by three possible mechanisms:

> Nondisjunction. Most commonly (approximately 95% of cases) three full copies of chromosome 21 are inherited due to meiotic nondisjunction during gametogenesis (*Figure 10*). Higher incidence is seen in older parents, particularly women.

> Translocation. A chromosomal translocation, as seen in *Figure 11*, can give rise to three copies of chromosome 21 in each cell, with the third copy being attached to a different chromosome (most commonly chromosome 14). It occurs in only three to five percent of children with Down syndrome. This is known as an unbalanced Robertsonian translocation. This often arises if one parent has a balanced Robertsonian translocation.

> Mosaicism. Mosaicism is where nondisjunction occurs after zygote formation, meaning some cells are normal and others have trisomy 21, as seen in *Figure 12*. This also occurs in around one to four percent of the cases.

Clinical Features

Down syndrome is commonly a clinical diagnosis purely made on physical features which prompt confirmatory genetic tests. These may include:

> Low birth weight.
> Hypotonia (which may cause difficulty with feeding and swallowing).
> Upslanting palpebral fissures and epicanthic folds.
> Brachycephaly (flattening of the head), from early fusion of coronal sutures.
> Low set ears.
> Depressed nasal bridge.
> Large protruding tongue.
> Singular palmar creases and clinodactyly (curving of the digit) of the fifth fingers.
> Brushfield spots (small white/greyish/brown spots on the periphery of the iris).
> Enlarged space between the first and second toes (sandal gap).

A baby with Down syndrome is shown in *Figure 13*. Patients with Down syndrome generally have a slower rate of growth. The World Health Organisation (WHO) has produced special growth charts to be used for children with Down syndrome.

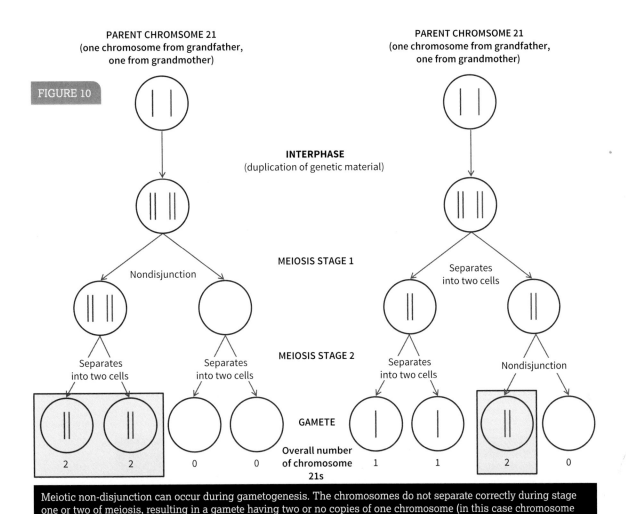

FIGURE 10

Meiotic non-disjunction can occur during gametogenesis. The chromosomes do not separate correctly during stage one or two of meiosis, resulting in a gamete having two or no copies of one chromosome (in this case chromosome 21). Those highlighted in blue have two copies of chromosome 21, and therefore when fertilisation occurs with a normal gamete, the resulting zygote will have three copies of chromosome 21, and 47 chromosomes overall (instead of 46).

Investigations

Antenatal Screening

All women are offered antenatal screening in the United Kingdom for a variety of genetic conditions (p114), including Down syndrome. Most women in the UK are screened between the 11th and 14th week of pregnancy using combined screening known as the "triple test". This is followed by a structural anomaly ultrasound scan at 22 weeks. Combined screening involves an ultrasound to assess nuchal translucency, blood tests for β-hCG (high in affected pregnancies) and PAPP-A (low in affected pregnancies). Later in pregnancy, a "quadruple test" can be performed, based on blood tests alone (AFP, β-hCG, inhibin-A, oestriol). The structural anomaly scan may show features of cardiac disease or duodenal atresia. If the screening test determines a high risk of Down syndrome, parents can be offered pre-natal diagnostic testing using amniocentesis (15–20 weeks) or chorionic villus sampling (<15 weeks).

Postnatal Diagnosis

If Down syndrome is suspected after a baby is born, blood samples are sent to a genetics laboratory for chromosomal tests.

> Fluorescence in-situ hybridisation (FISH). This technique is used to detect the number of chromosomes or chromosome segments through a fluorescent DNA probe which binds to specific sequences. In Down syndrome, it can be performed quickly (within 48 hours) to show the presence of three copies of chromosome 21.

> Chromosomal karyotyping. A sample of blood is taken from the baby to analyse chromosomes. Cells are grown and chromosomes extracted and sorted to show the number and structure of each set of chromosomes. The test can take up to ten days to produce a result, due to the time taken to culture cells.

Neonatal screening should be undertaken to assess any immediate complications. This screening includes:

> Echocardiogram. To exclude structural cardiac abnormalities.

> Full blood count or spun packed cell volume (PCV). To assess for neonatal polycythaemia.

> Thyroid function tests.

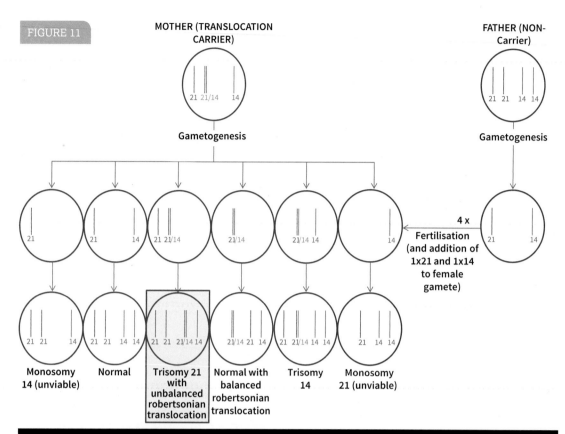

FIGURE 11

Robertsonian translocation, showing all six possible outcomes when a mother with a balanced Robertsonian translocation has a child with a father with normal chromosomes. The trisomy 21 cases are highlighted in blue.

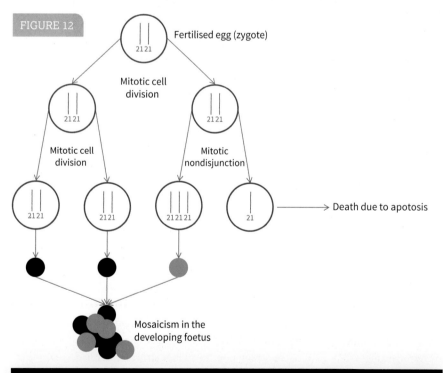

FIGURE 12

Mosaicism caused by mitotic nondisjunction. The red line depicts one chromosome. Patients with mosaic Down syndrome usually have a less severe phenotype, although severity is very variable. Note that offspring will only be affected if gamete-producing cells carry the defect.

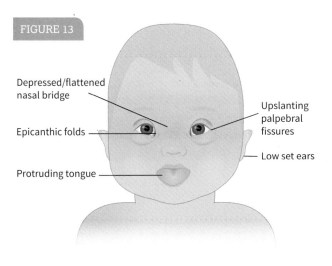

Depressed/flattened nasal bridge

Epicanthic folds

Protruding tongue

Upslanting palpebral fissures

Low set ears

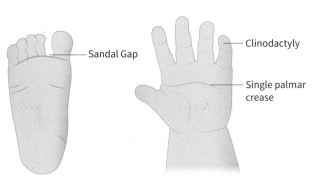

Sandal Gap

Clinodactyly

Single palmar crease

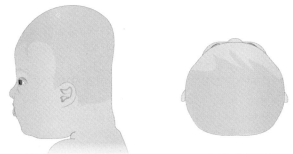

FIGURE 13

A baby with Down syndrome: face, hands and feet, head. Note the increased head height and width, as well as the flattened back of the head (brachycepahaly).

Normal screening throughout infancy should also be undertaken, along with additional checks:

› Hearing screen. At 8-months-old.
› Vision screen. To check for cataracts, nystagmus and squint, throughout childhood.

Management

Parents should be made aware of the clinical suspicion of Down syndrome before genetic investigations are performed. If the diagnosis is confirmed, parents should be informed as soon as possible in a supportive environment. Advice should be offered about aetiology, physical features, medical complications and management of Down syndrome. It is important to mention

that many adults with Down syndrome are active, mobile and able to lead semi-independent lives. However, they are also likely to have special educational needs and therefore require additional, specialised support in school.

In the UK, a multi-disciplinary team will support the family throughout their child's formative years. There are also many support groups available, including the Down Syndrome Association.

After Delivery

In the immediate postnatal period, it is important to screen for any of the congenital complications of Down syndrome, as mentioned above. Babies born with Down syndrome often have low muscle tone, making sucking and swallowing difficult. Parents therefore should be supported with feeding until a regime has been established. A referral to Speech and Language Therapy (SALT) can help parents with initial feeding difficulties and later if there is speech delay. Children will also be referred for physiotherapy if they have any difficulties with mobility or delayed gross motor development.

Ongoing Management

The long-term care of children with Down syndrome is usually managed by a multi-disciplinary team in the community. It may include:

› Dieticians.
› Physiotherapists.
› Occupational therapists.
› A community paediatrician.
› A speech and language therapist.

Depending on complications, other specialists may get involved. Sleep apnoea is common in children with Down syndrome, which may require input from ENT and respiratory specialists. Investigations of sleep apnoea may include a sleep study or trial of continuous positive airway pressure support (CPAP).

If parents are considering having another child, a referral to a genetics team may be helpful to assess the risk of the diagnosis recurring.

Adulthood

After the age of 18 years, all adults with Down syndrome may benefit from an annual health screening programme with their primary care physician. This is done routinely in the UK, where the check involves looking at each body system and asking specific questions that could indicate the development of any of the complications of Down syndrome. The patient is then supplied with a "Personal Health Action Plan" to address any health needs identified, including a review date.

Complications

› Cardiac. Structural cardiac abnormalities can occur (40%), with the commonest being atrioventricular septal defect.

123

- Respiratory. Recurrent respiratory tract infections can occur, especially otitis media. Children with Down syndrome often have enlarged adenoids (and tonsils) and small upper airways due to their face shape, leading to obstructive sleep apnoea. Secretory otitis media can lead to conductive hearing loss.
- Gastrointestinal. There may be gastrointestinal structural abnormalities (6%) including duodenal atresia and Hirschsprung's disease.
- Infection. There is a generalised increased susceptibility to infections.
- Autoimmune. Autoimmune problems, including type 1 diabetes and coeliac disease, are more frequent.
- Neurological. Seizure disorders are more common, and Alzheimer's disease affects the majority by their 5th decade.
- Haematological. Increased frequency of leukaemia, especially of the acute lymphoblastic and acute myeloid subtypes.
- Endocrinological. Hypothyroidism.
- Musculoskeletal. Short stature and atlanto-axial instability.
- Ophthalmological. Cataracts (3%) and visual impairment.
- Developmental delay. Learning difficulties are evident as the child grows up.
- Poor feeding. Sucking and swallowing difficulties may be present.
- Psychological. There is an increased incidence of anxiety, depression and other psychological disorders.

Prognosis

There is marked variability in the prognosis for children with Down syndrome. Some adults with Down syndrome lead active and at least semi-independent lives, including pursuing further education and gaining employment. Life expectancy for children born with Down syndrome has improved greatly over the last 30 years, and today, the majority of children live to be over 60 years old.

Turner Syndrome

Turner syndrome is a relatively common chromosomal abnormality that can only affect females. It occurs in approximately one in 2500 live female infants. A diagnosis of Turner syndrome is not always evident at birth, and some patients pass through adulthood without the diagnosis being formally made.

Aetiology

Turner syndrome is caused by the absence of one set of genes from the short arm of an X chromosome. Most patients with Turner syndrome have a karyotype of 45 chromosomes and only one X chromosome, i.e. 45,X. In these patients, most are missing the paternal X chromosome due to meiotic nondisjunction during gametogenesis. In these cases, the parents are not affected.

Mosaic Turner syndrome occurs when a proportion of cells contain 46 chromosomes (46,XX) and others (45,X) due to mitotic nondisjunction very early in foetal life. The offspring cell containing only one X chromosome does not undergo apoptosis, but instead goes on replicating to form parts of the foetus. Again parents will not have Turner syndrome.

Rarely, children may have a karyotype of 46,XXiq, where the short arm of an X chromosome is missing. These cases can be inherited from parents with Turner syndrome.

Clinical Features

Physical signs classically associated with Turner syndrome include:

- Short stature.
- Broad/webbed neck with a low hairline.
- A shield-shaped chest with widely spaced nipples.
- A wide carrying angle of the arms (cubitus valgus).
- Hypoplastic nails.
- High arched palate.

Lymphoedema of the hands and feet may be the only sign seen in newborn babies. This disappears rapidly after birth and can be easily missed.

The most concerning features associated with Turner syndrome are:

- Cardiovascular abnormalities. Turner syndrome is particularly associated with coarctation of the aorta and less commonly, hypoplastic left heart syndrome, aortic dissection and aortic aneurysms. It is also associated with a bicuspid aortic value and hypertension.
- Gonadal development. Streak ovaries (aplasia of the ovaries), often causing primary ovarian failure and infertility. As these patients age, they usually have short stature and an absent adolescent growth spurt. At puberty, pubic hair develops normally. However, due to ovarian failure, there is usually amenorrhoea and absent breast development.

Other features that may be present include:

- Eye abnormalities e.g. myopia, usually minor and corrected by glasses.
- Ear abnormalities e.g. otitis media in early childhood, which may lead to hearing loss.
- Renal abnormalities e.g. horseshoe kidneys, renal aplasia, duplex kidneys.

Intellectual function is mostly normal in patients with Turner syndrome. A child with Turner syndrome is shown in *Figure 14*.

Investigations

At prenatal ultrasound scans, Turner syndrome may be suggested by the presence of a cystic hygroma, structural renal

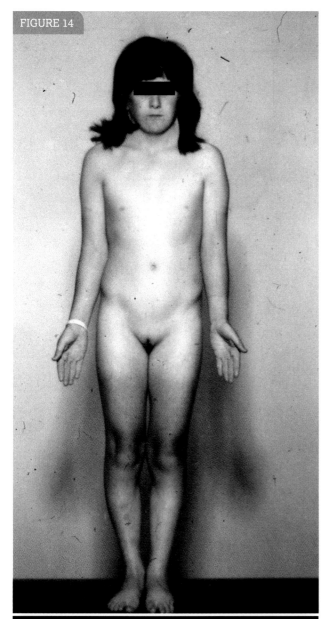

FIGURE 14

Turner syndrome. Note the broad and webbed neck, broad chest, and widely spaced nipples. There is also absent breast development.

of LH and FSH rapidly rise to menopausal levels as they try to stimulate the streak ovaries to produce oestrogen.

› Thyroid function tests. A diagnosis of Turner syndrome is associated with increased prevalence of hypothyroidism. Therefore, baseline tests are required which can be repeated regularly and if symptoms develop.

› Urea and electrolytes. Renal function is assessed because of the association between Turner syndrome and renal disease.

In children older at diagnosis, fasting blood glucose levels and glycated haemoglobin (HbA1c) tests are helpful. Diabetes mellitus is more common in Turner syndrome and regular screening is required.

Imaging studies may include:

› Renal ultrasound. Horseshoe kidneys and abnormalities in the urine collecting system are more common in girls with Turner syndrome.

› Echocardiography or Magnetic Resonance Imaging (MRI) of the heart. In Turner syndrome, coarctation of the aorta is common and hypoplastic left heart syndrome is possible.

A hearing assessment should also be performed after diagnosis, as well as at one-year-old and before starting primary school. Hearing assessments should then be performed every five years, or more frequently if the child suffers with recurrent otitis media.

Complications

Turner syndrome is commonly associated with chronic conditions, including hypertension and hypothyroidism. Almost all patients with Turner syndrome are infertile. Less commonly, Turner syndrome may be associated with an increased risk of type 1 diabetes mellitus, osteoporosis, coeliac disease and inflammatory bowel disease.

Management

As Turner syndrome is associated with chronic conditions, early preventative care and regular screening should be undertaken to reduce the risk of developing untreated complications. Any congenital abnormalities or complications related to Turner syndrome should be managed accordingly and children may have to see multiple specialists as part of the multidisciplinary team.

Hormone Supplementation

Girls with Turner syndrome reach a normal height until puberty. However, as the adolescent growth spurt is absent, growth hormone supplementation may be required to prevent short stature in adulthood. Ovarian failure may lead to lack of breast development and primary amenorrhoea. Oestrogen replacement therapy can be helpful in these cases. It is best initiated when the girl is between 12 and 15-years-old. The replacement can be given transdermally, which is preferred as it reduces the first-pass metabolism effects in the liver.

abnormalities, cardiac abnormalities or non-immune foetal hydrops. If any of these signs are found, Turner syndrome can be diagnosed with amniocentesis or chorionic villus sampling.

Initial blood tests in suspected cases include:

› Karyotype testing. After birth, karyotyping should be performed as soon as possible because the diagnosis is confirmed by the presence of 45,X or cells with deletion of the short arm of an X chromosome.

› Luteinising hormone (LH) and follicle stimulating hormone (FSH). As levels of circulating oestrogen are low, both LH and FSH are abnormally elevated in children under four-years-old. The disease pattern, however, leads to a reduction in LH and FSH levels in children between four and ten-years-old. In children more than 10–years-old, the levels

Osteoporosis Prevention

Prevention of osteoporosis requires, in addition to oestrogen replacement therapy, an adequate intake of vitamin D and calcium. Due to the already increased cardiovascular risks and the increased prevalence of diabetes mellitus, obesity should be avoided. A dietician may need to be involved with the family to ensure that the child has a healthy balanced lifestyle and to reduce avoidable risk factors.

Prognosis

The vast majority of cases of Turner syndrome result in stillbirth or abortion. However, those that survive to birth usually have a good prognosis in terms of life expectancy and cognitive development.

Most female infants born with Turner syndrome reach adulthood. Egg donation and IVF are now making it possible for some women with Turner syndrome to become pregnant as adults. However, a number of complications can affect them at any time during their life. Turner syndrome is associated with an approximately 13-year reduction in life expectancy in comparison to the general population.

Edward Syndrome

Edward syndrome is also known as trisomy 18 and is the second most common trisomy condition after Down syndrome. It affects seven in 10,000 births, but only one in 10,000 live births.

Aetiology

Edward syndrome is most likely to be caused by meiotic nondisjunction during the formation of gametes, leading to three copies of chromosome 18 in each cell. Rarely, it can also be due to an unbalanced translocation of the long arm of chromosome 18, i.e. the cells have two normal copies of chromosome 18 and a third long arm of chromosome 18 attached to another chromosome.

Clinical Features

Dysmorphic features include classic facies with a small jaw, low set ears and prominent occiput as well as flexed overlapping fingers and clenched hands, "rocker-bottom" feet with a short dorsiflexed great toe or "hammer toes" and growth restriction.

Other clinical features can include:
> **Cardiovascular malformations.** e.g. atrial septal defect, ventricular septal defect, coarctation of the aorta.
> **Gastrointestinal malformations.** e.g. omphalocoele, oesophageal atresia, diaphragmatic/umbilical/inguinal hernias.
> **Renal defects.** e.g. cystic kidneys, renal agenesis.
> **Neurological defects.** e.g. choroid plexus cysts, microcephaly.
> **Developmental delay.**

Some features are shown in *Figure 15*.

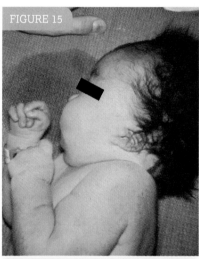
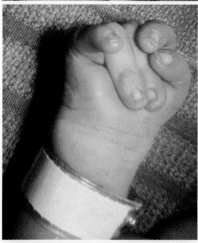

Some features of Edward Syndrome. A. Low set ears. B. Overlapping fingers.

Investigations

At the prenatal ultrasound scans, Edward syndrome may be indicated by the presence of increased nuchal translucency and multiple congenital abnormalities, including diaphragmatic hernias and congenital heart disease, intrauterine growth restriction (IUGR) and choroid plexus cysts. This may be confirmed with chorionic villus sampling or amniocentesis. After birth, the diagnosis should be confirmed using chromosomal karyotyping.

Management

If Edward syndrome is identified antenatally, termination of pregnancy or immediate palliative care post-delivery can be offered. Those that survive require intense medical support from the multidisciplinary team.

Prognosis

Most foetuses are stillborn or miscarry, and only 11% survive until birth. Half of neonates born alive with Edward syndrome will die in the first two weeks of life, and only eight percent will survive to 1-year-old.

Patau Syndrome

Patau syndrome is also known as trisomy 13. It is the third most common trisomy syndrome after Down syndrome and Edward syndrome, affecting one in 25,000 live births.

Aetiology

Three mechanisms can result in trisomy 13:
> **Meiotic nondisjunction.** This results in three copies of chromosome 13 in each cell.
> **Unbalanced chromosomal translocation.** This results in two normal copies of chromosome 13 and an extra segment of chromosome 13 that has attached itself to another chromosome, giving rise to three copies per cell.
> **Mosaicism.** Mitotic nondisjunction can result in some cells having three copies of chromosome 13, whereas the rest have the normal two copies.

Clinical Features

The main clinical features of Patau syndrome are:

- Low birth weight.
- Cardiac malformations. e.g. atrial septal defects, ventricular septal defects, patent ductus arteriosus and dextrocardia.
- Facial defects. e.g. microcephaly, scalp defects (cutis aplasia), ear abnormalities, cleft lip and palate, microphthalmia (small eyes), anophthalmia (no eyes), nasal malformation, hypotelorism (eyes close together), cyclopia (one eye), and proboscis anomaly (blind-ended tube-like structure, commonly located in the midface).
- Nervous system defects. e.g. neural tube defects (meningomyelocoele), holoprosencephaly, severe learning disabilities and seizures.
- Gastrointestinal defects. e.g. omphalocoele, hernias.
- Genitourinary system defects. e.g. renal abnormalities, micropenis, clitoral hypertrophy.
- Limb abnormalities. e.g. polydactyly, "rocker-bottom" feet.

Investigations

Patau syndrome may be suspected on antenatal ultrasound screening due to increased nuchal translucency and organ defects. Holoprosencephaly (the forebrain fails to divide into two hemispheres) and other central nervous system abnormalities, congenital cardiac disease and urogenital abnormalities may be seen.

Prenatally, this syndrome can be confirmed by amniocentesis or chorionic villus sampling. Postnatally, diagnosis is made with karyotyping and FISH studies.

Management

Care is often palliative immediately after birth and investigations kept to a minimum due to the poor outcome.

Prognosis

Children born with Patau syndrome have a high early mortality rate due to multiple congenital defects. Most die in the neonatal period. Mosaic Patau syndrome may have a better prognosis. Approximately half die within one month and only 8-10% live longer than one year. Any children with Patau syndrome usually have profound learning difficulties and developmental delay. Seizures and feeding difficulties are very common.

Other Genetic Mechanisms

Disorders of Imprinting

Most inherited genes have two working copies/alleles, but for some genes, only the allele inherited from either the father or mother is expressed. The other allele carries epigenetic markers which result in it being tightly packaged as chromatin. Once bound as chromatin, transcription and translation cannot occur and the allele is silenced. Genetic syndromes arise if both alleles inherited are silenced i.e. both are inherited from the same parent (uniparental disomy), or the active allele is not present (deletion).

An example of this is seen in Prader-Willi syndrome and Angelman syndrome. Chromosome 15 contains a region (15q11-13) which carries several imprinted genes. Some genes express the paternal allele only, whereas others express the maternal allele only. Prader-Willi syndrome occurs if this region on the paternal chromosome is deleted (can occur "de novo") or uniparental (maternal) disomy occurs, meaning two maternal copies of these genes are inherited. Either of these genetic defects results in a complete lack of active paternal alleles of several genes, as maternal alleles are all silenced and cannot compensate.

When the opposite occurs, maternal 15q11-13 deletion or uniparental (paternal) disomy results in a complete lack of an active maternal allele of UBE3A, causing Angelman syndrome.

More examples of errors of imprinting are given in *Table 10*.

Expanding Trinucleotide Repeat Disorders

"Trinucleotide" describes three consecutive nucleotides and their attached base pairs within the DNA structure. The same trinucleotide repeating consecutively is known as a trinucleotide repeat. Trinucleotide repeats are a normal part of DNA if the number of repeats is below a disease-causing threshold. An increasing numbers of repeats can make a gene unstable, alter the structure of the protein it produces and cause a disease phenotype. As the number of repeats increases, so does the severity of the disease. Interestingly, the number of repeats can increase as the gene is inherited. Therefore, each generation is affected more severely than the last. This phenomenon is known as "genetic anticipation". Examples of such disorders are shown in *Table 11*.

Mutations in Mitochondrial DNA

Mutations in mitochondrial DNA can be inherited or arise spontaneously ("de novo"). They cause disordered mitochondrial function leading to disease. Mitochondrial DNA is only inherited from the maternal ovum, as sperm do not carry mitochondria. Therefore, mitochondrial disorders are always maternally inherited. Examples include Leber's hereditary optic neuropathy and Leigh syndrome. *Figure 16* shows a typical pedigree diagram.

Genetic Counselling

When a child is diagnosed with a genetic disorder, it is important to accurately inform parents and the child (if they are old enough) of the likely effects of the disease. An additional feature with genetic diseases is a discussion of recurrence risk in future pregnancies, which can be explored based on any known inheritance patterns. Consultation may also occur for asymptomatic individuals with a genetic risk of a disease.

TABLE 10: Examples of Imprinting Disorders

Condition	Gene/Chromosome Affected	Characteristics
Prader-Willi syndrome	• Chromosome 15. • 70% paternal deletion. • 30% maternal uniparental disomy.	• Learning difficulties. • Short stature. • Severe hypotonia with poor feeding during the neonatal period. • Later hyperphagia in childhood often resulting in obesity. • Hypogonadism.
Angelman syndrome	• Chromosome 15. • UBE3A gene encoding an E3A ubiquitin protein ligase. • 80% maternal deletion. • 2-3% paternal uniparental disomy.	• "Happy puppet" – unusually happy disposition with inappropriate laughter/clapping. • Characteristic facial appearance. • Severe learning difficulties and developmental delay with microcephaly. • Seizures. • Ataxia.
Beckwith-Wiedemann Syndrome	• Chromosome 11p15. • Paternal uniparental disomy or maternal deletion/rearrangement of this area leads to overexpression of IGF-2 gene (insulin-like growth factor 2 gene).	• Neonatal macrosomia (overgrowth). • Hemihypertrophy. • Neonatal hypoglycaemia. • Macroglossia and external ear abnormalities. • Exomphalos (omphalocoele). • Increased cancer risk in childhood, especially Wilms' tumour.

TABLE 11: Examples of trinucleotide repeat disorders

Condition	Gene/Chromosome Affected	Characteristics
Friedreich's Ataxia	GAA codon in FXN gene on chromosome 9.	• Weakness. • Dysarthria. • Loss of proprioception. • Ataxia. • Hypertrophic cardiomyopathy. • Diabetes mellitus.
Huntington's Disease	CAG codon in HTT gene on chromosome 4.	• Personality changes, e.g. irritability, impulsiveness. • Psychiatric problems, e.g. depression. • Movement disorder, e.g. chorea.
Fragile X Syndrome	CGG codon in FMR1 on X chromosome.	• Learning difficulties. • Prominent ears and jaw. • Stereotypical hand movements. • Seizures and hyperactivity. • Macro-orchidism.
Myotonic Dystrophy	CTG codon in DMPK on chromosome 19.	• Hypotonia. • Breathing difficulties at birth due to diaphragmatic involvement. • Feeding difficulties. • Developmental delay and cardiac conduction defects as a child.

One area to consider is genetic testing for adult-onset disease. Clinical geneticists play an important role in mediating these services. Children of persons with Huntington's disease are born asymptomatic, but have a 50% risk of developing the disease later in life. Parents may ask for their child to be tested, but it is important to wait until the child can consent to having the test done themselves, as there is no immediate health benefit to testing and thus the child's autonomy would be compromised without good cause.

Gene Therapy

Gene therapy involves the therapeutic delivery of genetic material into a patient's cells. It has shown some success in clinical trials but is not yet routinely available. It is often done

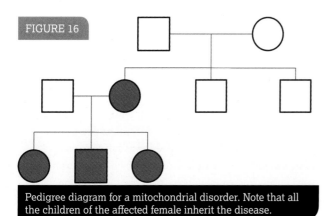

FIGURE 16

Pedigree diagram for a mitochondrial disorder. Note that all the children of the affected female inherit the disease.

using a viral vector, which is used to allow entry into individual cells. The new genetic material may be expressed as a protein, may block the expression of other proteins or may simply correct a genetic mutation. Such therapy has been used in trials to successfully treat diseases such as acute lymphoblastic leukaemia and severe combined immunodeficiency. However, this therapy needs to be approached with extreme caution. Insertion of the gene into the wrong location can have devastating consequences. For example, if the treatment interferes with a tumour suppressor gene, the risk of malignancy will increase.

REFERENCES AND FURTHER READING

SWAN (syndrome without a name)

1   Swan UK (eds.) General Leaflet: Support for families of children with undiagnosed genetic conditions. Genetic Alliance UK. 2014. http://undiagnosed.org.uk/wp-content/uploads/2014/04/SWAN.UK_.general.leaflet.2014.pdf.

Drawing a Pedigree Diagram

1   Kingston H. Ch. 8: Genetics, In: Lissauer T, Clayden G (Eds). Illustrated Textbook of Paediatrics. Third Edition. St. Louis: Mosby Elsevier. 2007. 105-22.

Mendelian Inheritance

1   Genomics Education Programme. Autosomal Dominant Inheritance. National Genetics Education and Development Centre. 2012. https://www.youtube.com/watch?v=dw-raR6E9zU&list=PLpMgTX_sXoj6kA9i-04a126NP7zGSY-hA.

2   Genomics Education Programme. Autosomal Recessive Inheritance. National Genetics Education and Development Centre. 2013. https://www.youtube.com/watch?v=oE9BUuv2pTo&list=PLpMgTX_sXoj6kA9i-04a126NP7zGSY-hA.

Down Syndrome

1   Bull M. Health Supervision for Children with Down syndrome. Pediatrics. 2011; 128:393-406 DOI: 10.1542/peds.2011-1605.

2   Marder L, McCall C, Burton G. Nottingham Guidelines for the Management of Children with Down Syndrome. Nottingham Children's Hospital, Nottingham University Hospitals NHS Trust. 2010. https://www.nuh.nhs.uk/handlers/downloads.ashx?id=34220.

3   Hoghton M. A Step-by-Step Guide for GP Practices: Annual Health Checks for People with a Learning Disability. Royal College of General Practitioners. 2010. http://www.rcgp.org.uk/learningdisabilities/~/media/Files/CIRC/CIRC-76-80/CIRCA%20StepbyStepGuideforPracticesOctober%2010.ashx.

4   Down's Syndrome Association. Down's Syndrome Association: Supporting People with Down's Syndrome throughout their lives. www.downs-syndrome.org.uk.

Edward and Patau Syndrome

1   Springett AL, Morris JK. Antenatal detection of Edwards (Trisomy 18) and Patau (Trisomy 13) syndrome: England and Wales 2005-2012. J Med Screen. 2014 ;21:113-9.

2   NHS National Genetics and Genomics Education Centre. Edwards Syndrome. http://www.geneticseducation.nhs.uk/genetic-conditions-54/651-edwards-syndrome-new

3   NHS National Genetics and Genomics Education Centre. Patau Syndrome. http://www.geneticseducation.nhs.uk/genetic-conditions-54/691-patau-syndrome-new.

Turner Syndrome

1   Health and Social Care Information Centre. NHS Choices: Turner syndrome – Treatment. http://www.nhs.uk/Conditions/Turners-syndrome/Pages/Treatment.aspx.

2   Werther G. Turner Syndrome Management Guidelines. Australasian Paediatric Endocrine Group. 2003. http://www.apeg.org.au/portals/0/documents/turner_posstate.pdf.

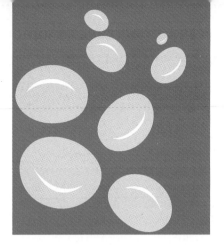

1.09

HAEMATOLOGY

AMY MITCHELL AND ANNA CAPSOMIDIS

CONTENTS

ANAEMIA

Overview of Anaemia

Anaemia is defined as a reduction in haemoglobin, and is due to a variety of possible causes. It is important to interpret the haemoglobin (Hb) level in relation to the age specific normal values (*Table 1*).

Aetiology

Three main processes lead to anaemia:

1. Failure of red cell production. e.g. iron deficiency, aplasia.
2. Ineffective red cells. e.g. haemoglobinopathies, sickle cell anaemia.
3. Increased destruction of red cells. e.g. hereditary spherocytosis.

Haemoglobinopathies are an important cause of anaemia. A haemoglobinopathy results in an abnormality in red cell structure. This may result in impaired oxygen carriage or decreased red cell life expectancy, thus giving rise to anaemia. There are two categories of inherited haemoglobinopathies:

1. Structurally abnormal haemoglobin molecules. e.g. sickle cell anaemia.
2. Impaired production of globin chains. e.g. beta-thalassaemia.

The majority of haemoglobinopathies are autosomal recessive conditions. This means those with only one allele are asymptomatic carriers, i.e. sickle cell trait, beta-thalassaemia trait. Only homozygotes present with clinically detectable disease. These diseases have persisted in endemic areas because the asymptomatic presence of one allele (i.e. being a carrier) offers some protection from malaria.

Investigations

If anaemia is confirmed on a full blood count:

- Check whether it is isolated, or if there are other abnormalities in the blood count, such as associated thrombocytopaenia or neutropaenia. Check the blood film. Abnormalities increase the clinical suspicion of malignancy.
- Consider the size of the red cells by checking the mean cell volume (MCV), as this is suggestive of possible underlying causes (*Table 2*).
- Other tests look to identify a specific cause for anaemia, depending on clinical suspicion; for example, checking B12 and ferritin levels. Haemolysis is made more likely by reduced haptoglobin, elevated bilirubin, elevated reticulocyte count or elevated lactate dehydrogenase (LDH). A positive Coomb's test implies immune mediated haemolysis. A coagulation screen should be considered to rule out a coagulopathy. Haemoglobinopathies may be screened for, depending on ethnicity.
- A group and save sample is needed if transfusion may be required.

Clinical Features

Anaemia may be detected incidentally, or with very minimal symptoms. Classic presentations include:

- Pallor, the most common sign.
- Lethargy/weakness.
- Pale conjunctivae.
- Flow murmur.
- Shortness of breath.
- Tachycardia.

Other presentations include jaundice (haemolytic anaemia), angular cheilitis (iron deficiency anaemia) and occasionally cardiac failure, due to increased cardiac output. In the long-term, it may present with faltering growth or developmental delay. It may also be present in chronic disease, like malabsorption syndromes or malignancy.

Management

Management involves attempting to identify the underlying aetiology and providing symptomatic treatment. Underlying causes are discussed below.

Admission to hospital may be required if:

- The child is unwell.
- A malignancy or infiltrative disorder is suspected.
- Hb <60g/L — for investigation and/or treatment.
- There is concern about ongoing significant haemolysis, as the child may need monitoring.
- An acute blood transfusion is required. Where possible, defer transfusion until a definitive diagnosis is made.

Iron Deficiency Anaemia

The commonest cause of anaemia in children is iron deficiency.

Aetiology

Causes of iron deficiency anaemia can be divided into three categories:

- Insufficient intake. In infants, this may be due to prolonged breastfeeding without supplements and over-reliance on a cow's milk diet. In adolescents, the main cause

is insufficient red meat, fish, chicken, green vegetables or pulses.

- Malabsorption e.g. coeliac disease.
- Chronic blood loss e.g. Meckel diverticulum, *Helicobacter pylori* gastritis or menorrhagia.

Risk factors for iron deficiency include:

- Prematurity.
- Low birth weight.
- Babies exclusively breastfed after six-months-old.
- Older infants who drink cow's milk exclusively.

Note that iron deficiency can lead to reduced cognitive and psychomotor performance even in the absence of anaemia.

Investigations

Diagnosis is through blood tests with:

- Low serum iron.
- Elevated transferrin. This measures iron binding capacity.
- Low serum ferritin. Bear in mind that this is also an acute phase reactant and therefore may rise artificially.

There will be also be low bone marrow haemosiderin (iron tissue stores). Blood film will show hypochromic, microcytic cells (*Figure 1*). There may also be target cells and pencil cells (rod poikilocytes).

Management

Treatment involves addressing any underlying cause, dietary advice, iron replacement therapy and rarely, transfusion in the acute setting. Oral iron supplements need to be continued for at least two to three months after target iron levels are achieved to replenish

TABLE 1: Normal values for haemoglobin (Hb) (g/L)	
Age	Lower limit of normal range of Hb (g/L)
2 months	90
2 - 6 months	95
6 - 24 months	105
2 - 11 years	115
> 12 years	120 (girls) 130 (boys)

TABLE 2: Causes of anaemia based on red cell size		
Microcytic Anaemia (low MCV)	Normocytic Anaemia	Macrocytic Anaemia (high MCV)
• Iron deficiency. • Thalassaemia. • Sickle cell (if associated with thalassaemia trait). • Chronic infection. • Lead poisoning.	• Acute blood loss. • Aplasia. • Sickle cell.	• Chronic haemolysis. • B12 and folic acid deficiency.

iron stores. Milk intake is limited and ferrous salts increased. Within 72–96 hours, reticulocytosis should occur. Haemoglobin will increase over the month following dietary iron. Failure to achieve a rise in haemoglobin of 1g/dL a week may indicate non-compliance, blood loss or malabsorption.

In rare circumstances, intravenous iron may be given (dextran) when the oral route is not possible. However this has been known to cause death due to anaphylaxis and does not result in a faster resolution of iron levels. As such, it is rarely used in the UK in children.

Vitamin B12 and Folate Deficiency

Folic acid and vitamin B12 deficiencies produce the same indistinguishable effects:

> Macrocytic anaemia (*Figure 2*) with megaloblastic changes in the marrow. Megaloblastic anaemia refers to enlargement of red blood cells due to ineffective erythropoiesis.
> Associated thrombocytopaenia +/- leucopenia.

> Elevated serum LDH. This is due to ineffective erythropoiesis.
> Low serum B12/folate.

Children who have chronic conditions causing a severe deficiency, especially of vitamin B12, may present with acute neurology or neuropsychiatric symptoms.

B12 Deficiency

This is usually due to either:

> Insufficient intake. Vitamin B12 is found in animal products including dairy, eggs, meat and fish. A strict vegan diet therefore increases risk.
> Insufficient absorption. Vitamin B12 is absorbed in the terminal ileum, with a requirement for intrinsic factor and transcobalamin to facilitate absorption. Therefore, B12 deficiency can be due to:
>> Inflammatory bowel disease affecting the terminal ileum, blind loop syndrome or gastric surgery.
>> Pernicious anaemia. Autoimmune destruction of intrinsic factor (rare).

>> Congenital deficiency of intrinsic factor (very rare).
>> Inherited transcobalamin II deficiency (very rare).

Treatment is with B12 injections (e.g. hydroxocobalamin).

Folic Acid Deficiency

This is usually due to either:

> Insufficient intake. This is relatively common. Folic acid is found in green leafy vegetables and fruit but is destroyed by prolonged cooking.
> Insufficient absorption. This is usually due to intrinsic small bowel disease, e.g. coeliac disease. Also, several drugs interfere with folate metabolism or absorption (e.g. phenytoin, sodium valproate, methotrexate, trimethoprim).

Treatment is with oral folic acid supplementation.

Haemolytic Anaemia

Haemolytic anaemias occur due to red cell destruction. When red cells are

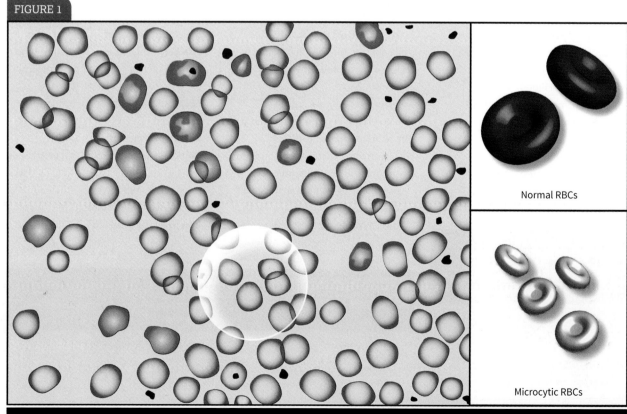

FIGURE 1

Normal RBCs

Microcytic RBCs

Blood film showing microcytic, hypochromic anaemia consistent with iron deficiency.

FIGURE 2

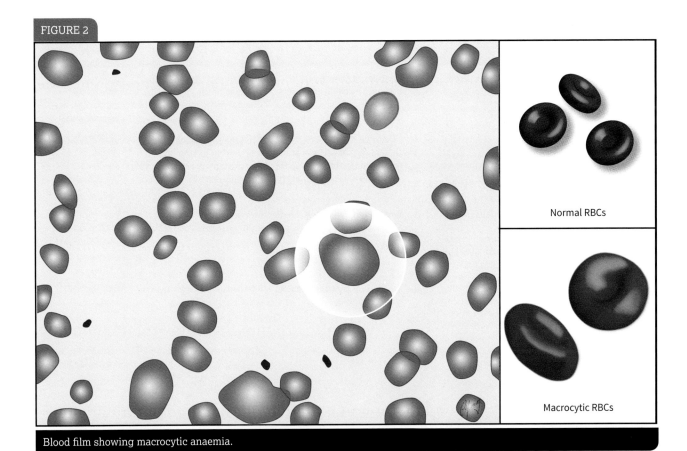

Normal RBCs

Macrocytic RBCs

Blood film showing macrocytic anaemia.

being destroyed, there is a resulting anaemia with increased reticulocytes and an unconjugated hyperbilirubinaemia. Presentation is with pallor (from anaemia) and jaundice/splenomegaly (from red blood cell destruction).

Several laboratory methods can aid in identifying the cause of a haemolytic anaemia. The temperature at which the antibodies react can help to characterise the autoimmune haemolytic anaemias (warm versus cold). The response to the direct antigen test is also helpful, as is the morphology of the cells seen under the microscope and specific enzyme assays. Sickle cell and thalassaemia are discussed separately, but other causes are summarised in *Table 3*. *Figure 3* shows a blood film that might be seen in hereditary spherocytosis.

Sickle Cell Anaemia

About 250,000 people in the UK are carriers of the sickle cell gene and up to 13,500 people have a sickle cell disorder, most commonly in black African and Afro-Caribbean people. Approximately 350

babies are born with sickle cell disease in the UK each year.

Aetiology

In sickle cell disease, the substitution of the amino acid valine for glutamic acid in the DNA coding for haemoglobin results in a functionally impaired ß-globin chain. Such haemoglobin is known as HbS.

This condition causes the red cells to deform when deoxygenated leading to so-called "sickling" of the red blood cells. The severity of the clinical course depends on the amount of HbS present. The deformed red blood cells can get stuck in the small blood vessels of the body which results in the hallmark "sickle cell crisis", a painful vaso-occlusive crisis. Symptoms and severity depend on where the red blood cells are getting stuck and what percentage of the red cells are affected.

Clinical Features

The hallmark of sickle cell disease is the occurrence of painful vaso-occlusive

crises. Microvascular occlusion results in ischaemia in an organ or bone, which is the cause of many of the clinical manifestations of sickle cell disease. Vaso-occlusive crises can be triggered by hypoxia, cold, infection, dehydration, excessive exercise or stress. They often affect the extremities, head, chest, back or abdomen and require opioid analgesia.

Since foetal haemoglobin is not affected by sickle cell disease, the disease does not usually cause problems in utero, or in the first six months of life.

Investigations

Sickle cell disease is diagnosed by haemoglobin electrophoresis. Those with homozygous alleles are HbSS, whereas heterozygous ones are HbSC. The carrier state does not cause significant disease, but is protective, because the sickling morphological change in the red blood cells protects against malaria invasion (*Figure 4*).

133

TABLE 3: Causes of haemolytic anaemia

Name	What causes it?	What is it?	Management	Diagnosis
Glucose-6-phosphate dehydrogenase deficiency (G6PD).	Inherited enzyme defect.	Episodes of haemolysis triggered by oxidising agents.	Avoidance of triggers such as broad beans, moth balls, Chinese medicines and certain drugs.	Glucose-6-phosphate dehydrogenase enzyme assay.
Hereditary spherocytosis.	Inherited red cell membrane defect.	Leads to defective sphere shaped red cells. These are destroyed leading to pigment gallstones and splenomegaly.	Life-long supportive care, folic acid supplementation, transfusions as required and normally elective splenectomy after age of 5 years.	Spherocytes visible on blood film.
Autoimmune haemolytic anaemia (warm).	50% are idiopathic. Other causes include lymphoma, leukaemia, systemic lupus erythematosus (SLE) and ulcerative colitis (UC).	Destruction of red cells due to auto-antibodies.	Steroids first line and immunosuppression second line.	Direct antigen test (DAT) positive.
Autoimmune haemolytic anaemia (cold).	50% are idiopathic. Other causes include mycoplasma, viral pneumonia and rarely cancers.	Destruction of red cells due to auto-antibodies.	Remove underlying cause, avoid cold.	DAT positive.
Pyruvate kinase deficiency.	Rare, autosomal recessive enzyme deficiency.	Causes haemolysis without spherocytes.	May require splenectomy.	Pyruvate kinase enzyme assay.

FIGURE 3

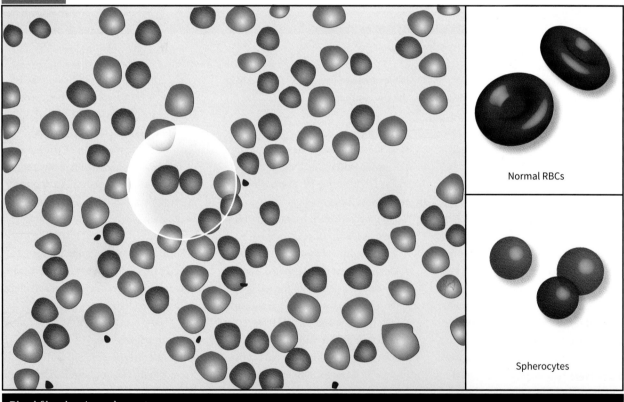

Normal RBCs

Spherocytes

Blood film showing spherocytes.

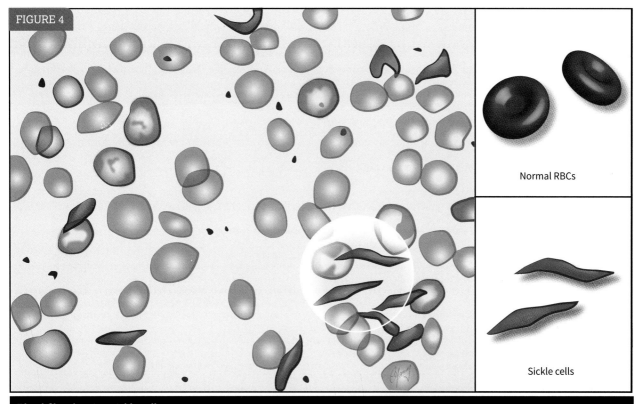

FIGURE 4

Normal RBCs

Sickle cells

Blood film showing sickle cells.

Management

Acute management is focused on identifying the underlying process and involves appropriate analgesia, oxygenation and treatment of associated sepsis, as outlined above.

Long-term outpatient management involves:

▷ Life-long prophylactic penicillin.
▷ Appropriate vaccinations (additional pneumococcal and influenza vaccines on top of routine schedule).
▷ Close monitoring for complications such as acute haemolysis, and painful episodes.

Corticosteroids, blood transfusions and hydroxycarbamide (which increases foetal Hb levels) may be helpful in those with severe episodes.

The requirement for long-term transfusions puts the child at risk of iron overload. This can be monitored by serum ferritin but more often now specialist MRI scanning techniques are being used to identify degree of iron overload. Other than limiting transfusions the other treatment of iron overload is to use an iron chelator such

as desferrioxamine usually via long-term subcutaneous infusion.

Haemopoeitic stem cell transplantation (HSCT) is increasingly being utilised for haemoglobinopathies. The principle is replacement of the child's bone marrow, thereby fixing the underlying haemoglobinopathy. However, HSCT has important side effects, including risk of death during the transplant itself. HSCT is reserved for severe disease (four or more vaso-occlusive crises, acute chest crises despite therapy with hydroxycarbamine and disease in the central nervous system).

Complications

Complications are shown in *Table 4*.

Prognosis

Early identification of affected children in routine post-natal screening in many countries like the UK can be helpful in managing patients from an early age. In the UK, 99% of children with sickle cell survive to 16-years-old, but sickle cell accounts for 16% of all deaths in West African countries.

Thalassaemia

Thalassaemia is a heterogeneous group of inherited conditions with autosomal recessive inheritance in which abnormal haemoglobin is produced in low quantity. As with sickle cell disease, the presence of thalassaemia trait (having one thalassaemia gene and one normal gene) confers some protection from malaria, thus giving carriers a selective survival advantage.

Classification

Thalassaemias are classified according to which chain of the haemoglobin molecule is affected.

▷ In α-thalassaemia, production of the α globin chain is affected.
▷ In β-thalassaemia, production of the β globin chain is affected.

The most common clinical condition is β-thalassaemia major, which is characterised by a total absence of production of adult β-globin chains. β-thalassaemia intermedia is also autosomal recessive, but has milder symptoms. β-thalassaemia trait (with one normal gene) is usually asymptomatic.

135

TABLE 4: Complications of sickle cell disease

Complication	Comments
Infection.	• Functional hyposplenism (from splenic infarction) results in an increased susceptibility to encapsulated organisms such as pneumococcus and haemophilus infections. • Universal prophylaxis with oral penicillin V (double dose if child becomes unwell) is required. • HiB/MenC/Prevenar (pneumococcal) vaccinations are essential. • Advised to seek medical help if high fever, cough, pallor, lethargy. • Sepsis is a medical emergency requiring cultures and urgent antibiotics.
Dactylitis.	• Young children may present with swollen, painful fingers and toes due to a vaso-occlusive crisis affecting the hands and feet: "hand-foot syndrome". Management includes appropriate analgesia, hydration and careful review.
Osteomyelitis/ septic arthritis/ avascular necrosis (usually hips).	• Osteomyelitis requires a high index of suspicion, as children with sickle cell disease may complain of musculoskeletal pain which commonly affects the hips, shoulders and spine. They may present with localised pain and fever. Salmonella osteomyelitis is a particular risk. • MRI imaging and prompt involvement of orthopaedic colleagues is essential. • Management requires a prolonged course of IV antibiotics.
Sequestration crisis (hepatic/splenic).	• Acute splenic or hepatic sequestration is caused by intra-organ trapping of red cells leading to acute hepatomegaly or splenomegaly, causing a precipitous fall in haemoglobin level and the potential for hypovolaemic shock. • Once recognised it needs to be treated by correcting the hypovolaemia with an urgent supportive blood transfusion.
Chest crisis.	• Micro-vascular occlusion of pulmonary vasculature can occur and can lead to infarction of lung segments which presents as pain, shortness of breath, hypoxia, cough and fever. • Severe cases may need non-invasive ventilator support and red cell exchange transfusion to reduce the percentage of sickle cells. • Severe respiratory failure occurs in about two to five percent who require invasive ventilation.
Priapism.	• Priapism is a sustained penile erection in the absence of sexual activity or desire. This is a significant cause of morbidity later on in life. It needs prompt recognition and management, potentially requiring an exchange transfusion. Untreated, it can lead to penile ischaemia and impotence.
Stroke.	• Children with sickle cell disease have 300 times the risk of stroke compared to healthy children. Eleven percent of children with HbSS have a stroke by age 20 (mainly ischaemic). Strokes recur in two out of three patients. • Children with HbSS are regularly screened with transcranial Doppler looking at the blood flow velocity. High velocity is associated with high risk of stroke. Children who have had a stroke or have an abnormal transcranial Doppler scan are put onto a lifelong transfusion programme.
Pigmented gallstones.	• This is a result of chronic haemolysis.

Clinical Features

Thalassaemias present with microcytic anaemias. Clinical features may include:

> Delayed growth, due to anaemia and pubertal delay.

> Congestive heart failure and abnormal heart rhythms.

> Splenomegaly, as destroyed red cells clog up the spleen.

> Bony deformity; marrow expansion occurs as the marrow tries to produce more Hb which can give the characteristic facial bossing appearance.

> Increased risk of infections.

> Iron overload, from the disease itself and from the requirement for frequent transfusions. Iron builds up and causes damage to the heart, liver and endocrine glands.

Management

The majority of children with β-thalassaemia major are treated with regular blood transfusions and careful measurement of iron levels. Iron chelation is often required with desferrioxamine.

In children with thalassaemia using related donors, HSCT can provide a 95% cure rate with a 2% rate of chronic GvHD (graft-versus-host disease). Newer transplant approaches aim to use less toxic conditioning regimens with the goal of preserving fertility.

Prognosis

Thalassaemia minor is usually associated with mild asymptomatic microcytic anaemia, with no effect on life expectancy. In thalassaemia major, prognosis depends on adherence to treatment. HSCT can be curative.

Anaemia of Chronic Disease

Aetiology

Anaemia of chronic disease is better described as anaemia of chronic inflammation. Situations of malignancy, chronic infections or chronic immune activation are accompanied by a marked increase in production of inflammatory cytokines such as interleukin-6. This works in several ways:

> It prevents release of iron from the stores and reduces production of the iron carrier protein ferroportin.

> It also has a direct effect on the bone marrow, suppressing production of haemoglobin by reducing the effect of erythropoietin and by driving the marrow to produce white cells instead of red cells.

Other types of anaemia of chronic disease can now be understood as more separate entities, such as anaemia associated with renal failure due to the poor production of erythropoietin.

Investigations
Patients with anaemia of chronic disease have normal or increased iron stores in the marrow and a normal or increased ferritin level. Because of the block in delivery, serum iron levels fall, as does the total iron binding capacity (TIBC) and the transferrin saturation. This is a normochromic and normocytic type of anaemia in most; however, it can also be mildly microcytic and hypochromic. Reticulocytes are either normal or mildly decreased.

Management
Anaemia of chronic disease is usually mild but can be severe. The severity can be exacerbated if there is concomitant iron deficiency. Treatment includes:
> Identification and treatment of the underlying cause.
> Parenteral iron therapy may be used, but if the underlying cause is infection, it should be used with caution as there appears to be a survival advantage to starving microbes of iron.
> Erythropoietin may be indicated in severe cases but it is costly and can be dangerous.

Aplastic Anaemia
Aetiology
Aplastic anaemia occurs secondary to bone marrow failure. There is concurrent anaemia, thrombocytopaenia and leukopaenia. It is often of unknown aetiology, with a likely infectious or auto-immune trigger.

One important cause of aplastic anaemia or pancytopaenia is Fanconi anaemia. This autosomal recessive condition presents at school age due to bone marrow failure and is associated with short stature, hyperpigmentation, renal malformation, developmental delay and abnormal radii and thumbs. It is important to recognise, as it is a DNA repair disorder and is associated with an increased risk of malignancies, including leukaemia.

Other causes include infection (e.g. EBV/CMV/HIV), malignancy, drug/radiation toxicity and inherited disorders such as Shwachman-Diamond syndrome.

Management
Treatment strategies have changed in recent years due to the improvement in survival and reduction of toxicity related deaths from bone marrow transplant. Now the first line treatment is HSCT in most cases, although it may be appropriate in the first instance to try horse or rabbit anti-thymocyte globulin (ATG), which works as an immunosuppressant.

COAGULATION DISORDERS

Overview of Coagulation Disorders
Maintaining blood flow through the blood vessels requires a fine balance between:
> Factors that promote formation of blood clots (platelets, and clotting factors).
> Natural anti-coagulants and the fibrinolytic system that try to break down clots.

The system relies on careful self-regulation to ensure the optimum amount of clot formation. It is essential to take a careful and detailed bleeding history. This will help determine where the bleeding is coming from, gain an understanding of the severity based on how the child has responded to life's haemostatic challenges, and indicate the likely mode of inheritance by checking for other affected family members.

Key points in a bleeding history include:
1 Nature of bleeding. Bleeding into the skin and mucous membranes is characteristic of disorders of platelets and blood vessels (purpuric disorders) and may be manifested as petechiae and/or bruising. Bleeding into soft tissue, muscle and joints suggests the presence of haemophilia or other disorders of coagulation proteins.
2 Family history. A family history of bleeding problems may identify inherited disorders such as haemophilia, which is X-linked.
3 Previous treatments. How the child has responded to previous haemostatic challenges (neonatal, vaccinations, teething, walking, nursery/school, surgery and other trauma) may give a clue to the diagnosis. Bleeding after vaccinations, for example, suggests a tendency to bleed into muscles and would be suggestive of haemophilia.

Haemophilia
The haemophilias are a group of inherited bleeding disorders caused by factor deficiencies. Haemophilia A is the commonest, occurring in one in 30,000 male births, and will be discussed below. Haemophilia B (Christmas disease) is the next most common haemophilia. It results from factor IX deficiency and is also X-linked. It presents similarly to Haemophilia A, but treatment is aimed at replacing factor IX instead.

Aetiology
Haemophilia A is due to Factor VIII deficiency and is usually an X-linked disease. One third of cases are due to new mutations.

Clinical Features
Haemophilia A presents with easy bruising or excessive bruising/bleeding after trauma or during surgery. It is often associated with bleeding into joints and muscles. This may lead to severe arthritis if left untreated. Expanding haematomas may compress nerves and vessels. There may only be mucosal or soft

tissue bleeding (*Figure 5*). There may also be intra-cranial bleeds.

Investigations
> Coagulation studies identify an isolated prolongation of the activated partial thromboplastin time (APTT).
> Factor VIII assay gives confirmation of the diagnosis.

Management
Care for all children with haemophilia should be delivered with a multi-disciplinary approach in specialist centres. Recombinant factor VIII has revolutionised the treatment of Haemophilia A. Mild haemophilia may respond to desmopressin (DDAVP), which promotes the release of von Willebrand factor (vWF) and increases survival of vWF, thereby reducing bleeding severity. Treatment of an acute bleed depends on bleed severity (aiming for factor levels of 50% for joint/muscle bleeds or 100% for intracranial bleeds) and may need to be repeated for a few days. Rarely, a continuous infusion may be required.

In severe disease, prophylactic factor VIII is given one to three times a week. However, up to 30% of children develop

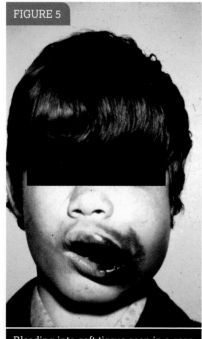

FIGURE 5

Bleeding into soft tissue seen in a case of haemophilia.

antibodies which inhibit the infused factor VIII (inhibitors). In 5–10% of cases where this is clinically significant, factor VIII is stopped because it is ineffective. Instead, bleeding is treated with other agents (such as recombinant factor VIIa).

Prognosis
Intracranial bleeds and bleeding around vital areas like the airway are the most important complications of haemophilia. Severe haemophilia is also associated with impaired cognitive function. Although mortality is significantly higher in haemophilia compared to the general population, much is historically related to blood-borne viruses. This is now largely excluded by improved donor screening and improved methods of factor concentrate purification.

Von Willebrand Disease
Von Willebrand disease (vWD) is the most common inherited bleeding disorder. It is autosomal dominant, with a greater prevalence amongst females. Von Willebrand factor (vWF) is a large multimeric protein which contributes to platelet plug formation and acts as a carrier protein for factor VIII.

Aetiology
VWD occurs when there is a defect in vWF. There are three subtypes (type 1 to 3), with Type 1 the mildest and Type 3 the most severe. It usually presents with mucocutaneous bleeding (nosebleeds, severe menorrhagia, gastrointestinal bleeds), excessive bleeding after trauma or excessive bleeding after surgery.

Investigations
Investigations involve looking at:
> Coagulation profile. If there are associated low levels of factor VIII, then there will be a prolongation of the APTT.
> Quantification of vWF antigen. This helps to determine how much von Willebrand factor is present.
> Functional assay. Platelet ristocetin cofactor (RiCOF) and collagen

binding activity (CBA). These tests evaluate how well vWF works.

Management
Management hinges on elevating the vWF level, particularly to prevent bleeding after surgery, and to secure haemostasis in the event of an acute bleed. Desmopressin (DDAVP) and vWF can achieve this. Treatment varies by subtype:
> Type 1: Responds to DDAVP.
> Type 2: May respond to DDAVP. If not consider vWF plasma concentrate.
> Type 3: Treat with vWF plasma concentrate.

Prognosis
The majority of people with vWD have the mildest type; they often have no major problems with bleeding and can live normal and active lives. In severe cases, patients must avoid contact sports and exercise caution by using protective equipment for activities with a high risk of bleeding or bruising.

Disseminated Intravascular Coagulation
Aetiology
Disseminated intravascular coagulation (DIC) is characterised by widespread, uncontrolled activation of clotting factors and fibrinolytic enzymes throughout the body's small blood vessels. This leads to tissue necrosis, bleeding and ultimately multiple organ damage. Multiple causative triggers have been identified, such as sepsis, malignancy, trauma and shock.

Clinical Features
DIC can present with bleeding from any site, including pulmonary, gastro-intestinal, intracranial, genitourinary and vaginal bleeding. There may also be bleeding from wounds or venepuncture sites.

Investigations
Blood films will likely show a haemolytic anaemia and prominent red cell fragmentation. Haemoglobin and platelet count need to be monitored.

There may be prolongation of the prothrombin time (PT) and APTT, reflecting the underlying consumption and impaired synthesis of the coagulation cascade. Fibrinogen levels are not particularly helpful as it is an acute phase reactant so will be elevated in sepsis, but low levels are characteristic in DIC.

Management

Management involves identifying and treating the underlying cause (e.g. antibiotics for sepsis), plus achieving homeostasis for acute bleeding. Rapidly declining platelet levels may become problematic. In acute DIC particularly, correction of PT, APTT, fibrinogen and platelets may be needed using vitamin K and blood products, such as fresh frozen plasma, cryoprecipitate and platelet transfusion. Conversely, thrombosis may be the problem, and in this case heparin or anticoagulant protein replacement may be needed.

ADDITIONAL PATHOLOGIES

Immune Thrombocytopenic Purpura

Aetiology

Immune thrombocytopenic purpura (ITP) occurs in four in every 100,000 children. It is more common in girls than boys, with peak prevalence in children aged 2 to 4-years-old. For the majority of children, a viral trigger such as an upper respiratory tract infection (URTI) leads to the development of specific platelet membrane glycoprotein antibodies causing an auto-immune destruction of platelets.

Clinical Features

Most cases of ITP present when the platelet count is less than 20×10^9/L (normal 150-400 x 10^9/L). The symptoms present suddenly with (in an otherwise well child):

> A petechial rash.
> Excessive bruising "purpura".
> Unexplained bleeding.

Investigations

The diagnosis is confirmed with a FBC. Other investigations, such as coagulation studies, a blood film and inflammatory markers are used to exclude differentials.

Differential Diagnosis

If the child is unwell, diagnoses which should be excluded include sepsis and malignancy. In infants or children with a positive family history, inherited disorders such as Wiskott-Aldrich syndrome (WAS) should be considered. Other differentials include autoimmune disease, haemolytic uraemic syndrome, viral infection and haemophagocytic syndrome. Haemophagocytic syndrome is rare, but is caused by uncontrolled proliferation of activated lymphocytes and macrophages. Patients are usually unwell, with jaundice and hepatosplenomegaly.

Management

In patients with significant bleeding, intravenous immunoglobulin (IVIG), oral corticosteroids or intravenous anti-D immunoglobulin (in Rhesus positive patients) should be considered. Unless there is life-threatening bleeding, platelet transfusion is not likely to be useful as antiplatelet antibodies rapidly destroy them. If the case is not life-threatening, a bone marrow aspirate to exclude leukaemia is normally performed before a course of oral prednisolone is commenced. This is because corticosteroid treatment may partially treat a malignancy, and therefore mask the underlying diagnosis.

Children diagnosed with ITP are followed up closely with regular platelet counts. Any abnormal features should prompt consideration of bone marrow examination to exclude leukaemia.

Complications

Rarely, the low platelets cause a more significant life threatening problem, such as intracranial haemorrhage (one in 300 cases) or severe gut bleeding (three in 100 cases). Most often, these occur in the first week of ITP in children with pre-existing vascular abnormalities. Treatment in this case combines intensive platelet transfusion support, high dose IVIG, intravenous (IV) methylprednisolone and consideration of emergency splenectomy. The risk of serious bleeds is much lower once platelet counts recover to over 20×10^9/L.

Prognosis

ITP is normally an acute, self-limiting illness, with recovery of the platelet count with no active treatment over four to six weeks. However, 10–20% of children remain thrombocytopenic for over six months due to the continued production of autoantibodies (chronic ITP). Even in these cases, the majority eventually make a spontaneous recovery.

Neutropenia

Neutropenia can be described as mild (neutrophil count =1.0-1.5 $\times 10^9$/L), moderate (0.5-1.0 $\times 10^9$/L) or severe (<0.5$\times 10^9$/L). Mild cases are unlikely to cause any clinical problems, whereas life threatening problems may occur at neutrophil counts of less than 0.2x10^9/L.

Clinical Features

In clinical practice, the main group of children with neutropenia are those on immunosuppressive regimens for treatment of malignancy. They have decreased production of neutrophils and normally develop severe neutropenia. The risk of infection increases with duration of neutropenia.

Neutropenic sepsis is a medical emergency and children known to be at risk for neutropenia who develop a temperature need to be swiftly assessed, have blood cultures taken, and started on empirical antibiotic therapy. Neutropenia is associated with severe bacterial infections, especially the formation of deep abscesses, septicaemia and cellulitis.

Investigations

Unless a clear cause of the neutropenia is evident, such as drug suppression, bone marrow aspiration may be required to ascertain the presence of neutrophil precursors and exclude infiltrative malignancy.

Differential Diagnosis

There are multiple causes of neutropenia:

› Acquired causes of decreased marrow production. This is part of aplastic anaemia (p137).

› Congenital syndromes. Such syndromes result in decreased marrow production, and include Kostmann syndrome and Shwachman-Diamond syndrome.

› Metabolic conditions. Certain metabolic conditions affect export of metabolites, e.g. propionic acidaemia.

› Situations resulting in excessive consumption of neutrophils. This includes fulminant sepsis or the development of auto-immune antibodies.

› Conditions causing sequestration of the neutrophils. This includes viral infections or hypersplenism.

› Conditions of immunodeficiency. There are a broad range of immunodeficiencies, e.g. X-linked hypogammaglobulinaemia.

Management

Management depends on the underlying aetiology, severity and duration of neutropenia. Early recognition of infection and aggressive treatment with antibacterial agents is important. Granulocyte-colony stimulating factor (G-CSF) stimulates the bone marrow to produce neutrophils, and may be required acutely. Other treatments include short courses of corticosteroids or splenectomy in selected cases.

REFERENCES AND FURTHER READING

1 Marks PW, Glader B. Approach to Anemia in the Adult and Child. In: Hoffman F, Benz EJ, Shattil SJ, (Eds). Hematology: Basic Principles and Practice. Fifth edition. Philadelphia: Churchill Livingstone; 2009. 439-46.

2 Hoffbrand AV, Pettit JE, Moss PAH. Essential Haematology. Fourth edition, Oxford: Blakewell Publishing; 2001.

3 McIntosh N, Helms P, Smyth R, Logan S. Forfar & Arneil's Textbook of Paediatrics. Sixth edition. Philadelphia: Churchill Livingstone; 2008.

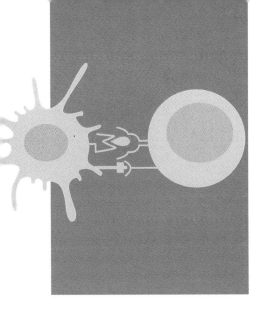

1.10
IMMUNOLOGY AND ALLERGY

MAANASA POLUBOTHU

CONTENTS

OVERVIEW OF THE IMMUNE SYSTEM

The immune system combats the numerous microorganisms the body encounters daily. The body's immune response to infection has both innate and adaptive components. Disorders of the immune system can lead to immunodeficiency, allergy and autoimmune disease.

Innate Immune System

The innate immune system refers to the immune defences that exist in all individuals, regardless of prior pathogen exposure. Therefore, innate immunity can be elicited immediately. It serves as the body's first-line defence. Its key components are detailed below.

Physical Barriers
› Tight junctions. These are found between cells in the skin and mucous membranes.
› Secretions. These include mucus, bile, enzymes and acid.

Cells that Secrete Inflammatory Mediators
› Natural Killer Cells. Cytotoxic lymphocyte cells able to identify foreign cells and trigger cell death.
› Mast Cells. White cells containing toxic granules including histamine which can be triggered to burst or "degranulate" upon activation.
› Macrophages. Large white blood cells capable of phagocytosis, able to engulf and digest cellular debris, microbes and foreign substances.

Cells that Detect Pathogens
› Cells with Toll-like Receptors. Receptors found on the membranes of macrophages and dendritic cells that detect microbes or parts of microbes (Pathogen-associated molecular patterns (PAMPS).
› Antigen Presenting Cells. These cells are capable of engulfing and presenting foreign antigens to T cells to elicit an adaptive immune response. Examples include dendritic cells, some macrophages and some types of B cells.

Phagocytes
> Neutrophils. These are circulating phagocytes which can be recruited to sites of infection or inflammation. They are able to engulf and digest cellular debris, microbes and foreign substances.
> Macrophages. As described earlier.
> Monocytes. These are large circulating white blood cells able to differentiate into macrophages or dendritic cells; they can be recruited to sites of infection or inflammation.

Antimicrobial Proteins
> Defensins. These are small proteins capable of integrating within the membranes of microbes. They create pores that cause efflux of essential ions and nutrients from the microbial cell, leading to their destruction.

Enzymes Capable of Degradation
> Lysosomal enzymes. These are enzymes capable of digesting biomolecules.

Serum Proteins
> Complement. This family of proteins can be activated and are important in immunity. Complement attracts cells of the immune system upon identification of a pathogen, enhances phagocytosis of pathogens, triggers lysis of foreign cells and clusters/binds pathogens.
> Lectins. These proteins have a high binding affinity for carbohydrate molecules. They can be toxic upon binding to microbes. Mannose binding lectin activates the lectin pathway of the complement system.
> Immunoglobulin. IgA forms part of the innate immune system; it is primarily present on mucosal surfaces.

Adaptive Immune System

Adaptive or specific immunity is a learned response which is precisely targeted to the pathogen encountered. It is activated when microorganisms evade first-line innate mechanisms, and although it takes time to mount, it is a highly effective defence strategy. It comprises humoral and cellular branches, both orchestrated by lymphocytes. In humoral immunity, pathogens are targeted by specific antibodies produced by plasma cells derived from B lymphocytes, whereas in cell-mediated immunity, the pathogens are damaged directly by cellular responses.

Table 1 shows the key differences between the innate and adaptive immune systems.

B lymphocytes produce antibodies and additionally act as antigen-presenting cells, signalling the presence of pathogens, in order to activate various components of the immune system.

Antibodies are glycoproteins produced by B lymphocytes in response to an antigen. They are composed of four polypeptide chains: two heavy chains and two light chains. IgM forms part of the innate immune response. Antibodies are also included here as they are primarily associated with the adaptive immune system. There are five classes of antibody: IgE, IgA, IgM, IgG

TABLE 1: Innate vs adaptive immunity	
INNATE IMMUNITY- rapid, non-specific, no memory	**ADAPTIVE IMMUNITY- slow, specific, with memory**
General protection (not antigen-specific).	Highly specific for a particular pathogen (antigen-specific).
Early phase of host response to pathogens without requiring prior exposure.	Late phase response of antigen-specific lymphocytes to antigens.
Immediate maximal response	Lag time between exposure and maximal response
Does not alter on repeated exposure (no immunological memory).	Improves with each successive exposure (immunological memory).

TABLE 2: Immunoglobulins	
IgM.	This exists as a pentamer and is part of the innate immune response to antigens.
IgG.	This exists as a monomer and is the predominant immunoglobulin in the serum, produced as part of the adaptive immune response. IgG can cross the placenta and maternal IgG confers protection to the newborn for the first six months of life.
IgE.	This exists as a monomer and is responsible for defence against parasites and allergic reactions. It is generally found in low quantities in the serum, but levels are greatly increased in atopic individuals and those prone to allergy.
IgA.	This exists as either a monomer or dimer. In its dimeric form, it is known as secretory IgA and forms a first-line of defence in body secretions (e.g. mucus, saliva, tears) as part of the innate immune response.
IgD.	This is a monomer and exists in small quantities in the serum. Little is known about its function, and few clinical signs/symptoms are associated with its absence.

and IgD. They are distinguished by the type of heavy chain found in the molecule, as summarised in *Table 2*.

The two main classes of T lymphocytes are:
> Cytotoxic T cells. Involved in direct cellular attack of pathogens.
> Helper T cells. Have a central role in supporting other components of the immune system.

The pathogen-specific and targeted response elicited by the adaptive immune system can be rapidly mobilised upon subsequent encounters with the same pathogen, owing to the adaptive immune system's capability to form an immunological memory. Exploiting this unique feature has enabled the effective immunisation against, and near eradication of, many common infectious diseases.

TABLE 3: Hypersensitivity reactions			
Type	Onset	Mediation	Example
I.	Immediate in onset (usually occurs within 15-30 minutes of exposure).	This is mediated by IgE antibodies, which are produced in excessive amounts following sensitisation with the offending antigen (allergen). Upon exposure to the allergen and binding to IgE, IgE associated mast cells and basophils degranulate, releasing preformed mediators (e.g. histamine, tryptase, prostaglandins). Up to 20% of people will experience a late phase response, with symptoms recurring within the first 30 hours without repeat exposure to the allergen. The pathogenesis of this is unknown but is thought to be secondary to inflammatory changes initiated by the initial response (*Figure 1*).	• Asthma. • Atopic conditions.
II.	Delayed in onset (occurs within minutes to hours).	This is IgG mediated cell destruction. The complement system also has an important role. Antigens are usually endogenous, but may result from exogenous antigens attaching to the cell membrane (haptens).	• Goodpasture syndrome. • Drug-induced haemolytic anaemia.
III.	Delayed in onset (occurs within three to 10 hours of onset).	This is mediated by soluble immune complexes (mostly IgG but may be IgM). The complement system also has an important role. Antigens can be endogenous (e.g. SLE) or exogenous (e.g. chronic bacterial and parasitic infections).	• Rheumatoid arthritis. • Systemic lupus erythematosus.
IV.	Delayed in onset (peaking at 48–72 hours post exposure).	This is cell-mediated, via T-cells and macrophages.	• Contact dermatitis.
V.	Delayed in onset.	This is endocrine receptor-mediated, resulting in impaired cell signalling.	• Graves' disease. • Myasthenia gravis.

ALLERGY

Hypersensitivity Reactions

An allergic reaction is an exaggerated reaction to an allergen in a normally functioning immune system. It comes under the broader remit of hypersensitivity reactions, which also includes autoimmunity. An allergen is a non-parasitic antigen that can elicit a type I hypersensitivity reaction.

Four types of hypersensitivity reactions are widely recognised. Type V is also included, though its existence is more debatable, as shown in *Table 3*.

Atopic Triad

The atopic triad comprises:

▸ Eczema.
▸ Rhinitis.
▸ Asthma.

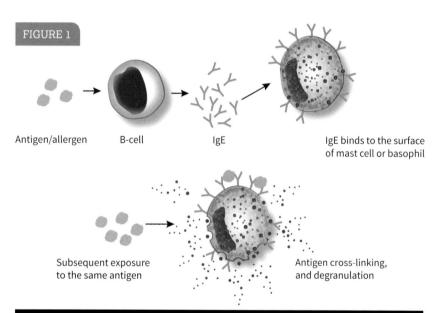

FIGURE 1

Antigen/allergen   B-cell   IgE   IgE binds to the surface of mast cell or basophil

Subsequent exposure to the same antigen   Antigen cross-linking, and degranulation

Simplified scheme for IgE-mediated Type I hypersensitivity reaction. Mast cells/basophils are sensitised with allergen-specific IgE. On subsequent exposure, there is rapid degranulation, leading to the release of inflammatory cytokines and elicitation of a hypersensitivity reaction.

Classically, these develop in a typical sequence, alongside food allergy, and this is referred to as the allergic march (*Figure 2*). Atopic individuals are likely to have a genetic predisposition to Type I hypersensitivity reactions in response to common allergens. Circulating levels of IgE are elevated and immunoassays may reveal a positive response of IgE to a specific allergen. In such tests, the patient's serum is exposed to a specific antigen. If the patient has IgE antibodies that bind to the antigen, they are then visualised by the use of a second antibody that binds specifically to IgE.

Treatment of atopy is largely symptomatic and focuses on dampening the allergic response. Owing to its genetic component, atopy tends to run in families, although environmental exposure to allergens plays a large part in the disease course. The prevalence of atopy is increasing in industrialised areas. The hygiene hypothesis postulates that this increased prevalence is the result of better hygiene, which has decreased human exposure to microbes. This has caused a shift in the immune response from the cells involved in fighting infection to those involved in

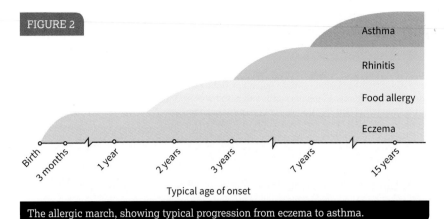

FIGURE 2

Asthma

Rhinitis

Food allergy

Eczema

Birth | 3 months | 1 year | 2 years | 3 years | 7 years | 15 years

Typical age of onset

The allergic march, showing typical progression from eczema to asthma.

allergic pathways. The result has been an increase in allergic disease in most high income countries.

Anaphylaxis

Anaphylaxis represents the most severe end of the allergy spectrum, and can potentially have fatal results.

Clinical Features

Anaphylaxis results in rapid-onset clinical deterioration. Symptoms include:

- Respiratory. Laryngeal oedema, leading to upper airway obstruction and stridor, and bronchospasm, leading to lower airway obstruction and wheeze.
- Gastrointestinal. Abdominal cramping, nausea, vomiting and diarrhoea.
- Cardiovascular. Hypotension, tachycardia and shock.
- Skin. Urticaria and angioedema.

Diagnosis

Anaphylaxis is a life-threatening emergency requiring prompt treatment. Its diagnosis should be made based on the history and clinical presentation. Levels of tryptase, a proteinase contained in mast cells, can support the diagnosis. It is measured as treatment begins and again within one to four hours.

Management
Acute Management

- Resuscitate the patient using an ABCDE approach.
- Remove the offending allergen if possible.

- Adrenaline should be administered immediately and repeated after 5 minutes if no response:
  › Child >12 years old: 500 micrograms IM (0.5mL of a 1:1000).
  › Child 6-12 years old: 300 micrograms IM (0.3mL of 1:1000).
  › Child <6 years old: 150 micrograms IM (0.15mL of 1:1000).
- Following resuscitation, for all established cases of anaphylaxis give:
  › Chlorpheniramine. Anti-histamines are important for ameliorating the rapid release of histamine by mast cells.
  › Hydrocortisone. Use of a corticosteroid will suppress the immune response and may prevent a late-phase response.

Long-term Management

- Allergen avoidance is key in preventing future episodes.
- The patient should undergo skin prick testing and immunoassay testing for IgE to specific allergens if there is doubt over the culprit allergen.
- Prescription of an Epipen (under the supervision of an allergy clinic) will provide some security in case of further anaphylaxis, as will appropriate training of the family/child/school in the management of future reactions.
- Allergen-specific immunotherapy involving gradual administration of increasing amounts of allergen can modify the immune response and

induce protective immunological change. It can be used to prevent an anaphylactic reaction to certain venoms and medications.

Prognosis

Recurrence of a severe anaphylactic reaction is likely upon re-exposure to the offending antigen. Subsequent reactions can be of the same severity, milder or worse than the initial episode. The use of allergen-specific immunotherapy has transformed the prognosis for some allergens.

Adverse Reactions to Foods

Food presents a large antigenic load to the body, but the gut is normally able to discriminate between food and invasive pathogens. However, the immune system of young infants is less able to achieve this discrimination, making this age group susceptible to food hypersensitivity.

Adverse food reactions refer to any adverse reaction following the ingestion of food or a food additive. They are broadly divided into two groups:

- Food intolerances. Adverse physiological reactions.
- Food hypersensitivities. Adverse immunological responses and allergies.

Table 4 shows key differences between these two groups.

Food Hypersensitivity

"Hypersensitivity" broadly describes an immunological reaction to a given food which occurs reproducibly on repeat exposure. These reactions can be classified as either IgE-mediated (type I hypersensitivity) reactions, or non-IgE-mediated reactions.

- IgE-mediated allergies. These develop immediately and result in the classic features of type I hypersensitivity reactions. Common culprits include peanuts, soy, egg, fish and shellfish.
- Non-IgE-mediated food allergies. These tend to present sub-acutely and may be chronic. The pathogenesis is less clear but immune-complex (type

TABLE 4: Differences between hypersensitivity and intolerance

	Hypersensitivity	Intolerance
Possible mechanisms.	• IgE mediated, e.g. anaphylaxis, bronchospasm, urticarial. • IgE and Cell mediated e.g. dermatitis, gastroenteritis, eosinophilic oesophagitis.	• Enzyme deficiency, e.g. lactase deficiency, galactosaemia (deficiency in enzyme breaking down galactose). • Psychological, e.g. food phobia. • Direct effects of foods/additives, e.g. monosodium glutamate additive.
Onset of symptoms.	• May be rapid, particularly IgE mediated reactions.	• Delayed usually by at least a few hours, but potentially longer.
Severity.	• Can be immediately life-threatening.	• Rarely immediately life threatening.
Typical symptoms.	• Anaphylaxis, blood/mucus in stool, reflux, bloating, abdominal pain, diarrhoea, skin rashes, faltering growth.	• Bloating, abdominal pain, diarrhoea, skin rashes.
Ingestion required to trigger response.	• Small amount can trigger severe reaction (e.g. a peanut allergy may be triggered when eating non-peanut based foods that have been prepared by cooks who have handled peanuts).	• Large load usually required.

III) and cell-mediated (type IV) hypersensitivities have been implicated. Non-IgE mediated food allergies usually result in isolated gastrointestinal symptoms such as nausea, vomiting, abdominal pain and diarrhoea.

Diagnosis is based on a careful history and elimination of other causes of the symptom. Testing for IgE-mediated disease can include the use of skin prick testing (injecting a small amount of the suspected allergen into the skin and assessing the reaction) or looking for specific IgE antibodies to the suspected allergen in the blood. If there is diagnostic doubt, or other tests are not available, another option is to perform a food challenge after a period of eliminating the allergen (e.g. exposing the patient to cow's milk after a period of a diet free of cow's milk protein).

Patients with confirmed hypersensitivity should be referred to a dietician for advice on food exclusions.

Cow's Milk Protein Allergy

Cow's milk protein allergy results from ingestion of cow's milk protein, or maternal ingestion of cow's milk protein for breastfed infants, causing an inflammatory response in the rectum and distal sigmoid colon. It can be both IgE-mediated (onset within two hours of exposure) and non-IgE-mediated (onset after two hours of exposure). Infants are typically well but may report blood-tinged stool and occasionally change in frequency of stool, usually presenting at 2 to 8-weeks-old. Dermatological manifestations, e.g. eczema and urticaria, are also common. The IgE-mediated form may also present with cardiorespiratory compromise.

Treatment involves elimination of cow's milk protein from the diet, and use of a protein hydrolysate formula (where the protein is already broken down). In the case of breastfed infants, the mother must avoid consumption of cow's milk protein. Resolution of symptoms is seen quickly following an elimination diet. In the vast majority of infants, cow's milk can be reintroduced with no adverse effects at 9-months-old.

Food Intolerance

True food allergies are rare, whereas non-immunological responses to food are common. These may occur secondary to many processes, including anatomical abnormalities, enzyme deficiencies, gastrointestinal infection and toxins.

Lactose Intolerance

Primary lactose intolerance is most frequently a consequence of lactase deficiency. Lactase is the enzyme required to hydrolyse lactose into its simple sugar components, glucose and galactose. Until 5-years-old, most children will have normal lactase levels. Therefore, primary lactase deficiency is uncommon. Increased incidence is seen with increasing age and with certain ethnicities, most commonly the East Asian population and least commonly Caucasian populations. Secondary lactose malabsorption can result from bacterial overgrowth following gastroenteritis (transiently) and following mucosal injury, e.g. coeliac disease, drug or radiation-induced enteritis or inflammatory bowel disease.

Clinical manifestations are a result of:
- Lactose acting as an osmotic laxative: diarrhoea, abdominal pain.
- Lactose acting as a growth substrate for intestinal bacteria: flatulence, bloating, abdominal distension.

Lactose intolerance may be suspected following a thorough history and can be supported by a food diary and low faecal pH (pH<5) or the presence of reducing substances in the stool. Management centres on lactose restriction, with care to maintain calcium and vitamin D levels. Another possible option is lactase enzyme replacement.

Drug Allergies

Drug allergy is an immunological reaction to a drug and presents with a number of adverse clinical features. Drug allergies can give rise to any of the four main types of hypersensitivity reaction. Type I IgE-mediated hypersensitivity reactions tend to occur within one hour of administration and can be life-threatening. Common culprits include ß-lactam antibiotics, platinum-based chemotherapy (e.g. cisplatin, carboplatin) and foreign proteins (e.g. rituximab, cetuximab). Type II-IV hypersensitivity reactions vary in severity and typically show a delayed onset. Diagnosis for type I hypersensitivity reactions can be confirmed with skin prick testing, although these should be performed in controlled environments due to the risk of anaphylaxis. Type II-IV hypersensitivity drug allergies are diagnosed by a suggestive history, associated with patterns of clinical and laboratory findings. Given the range of possible reactions, it is always important to note the exact reaction when a patient reports a drug allergy. Management focuses on avoidance of the culprit drug and use of alternative therapies where possible.

IMMUNODEFICIENCIES

Primary immunodeficiencies result from an inherited defect of the immune system. This can be an isolated defect in a component of the immune system or a combination of defects and can involve innate and/or acquired branches of the immune system.

Secondary immunodeficiencies are more common, and may be related to systemic disease (SLE, malignancy), malnutrition, splenectomy, drugs and infections (e.g. human immunodeficiency virus [HIV], Epstein Barr virus [EBV], and measles).

Key Features of Immunodeficiencies

Clinical Features

Recurrent infections are the hallmark of an immunodeficiency. However, this presents a diagnostic dilemma as the average child with an intact immune system will have numerous gastrointestinal and respiratory infections every year.

Features that should arouse suspicion include:

> Concurrent infections at multiple sites.
> Persistent and/or recurrent infections resistant to antibiotics.
> Atypical, opportunistic, or unusual organisms causing infection, e.g. *Pneumocystis jirovecii* pneumonia.
> Accompanying faltering growth.
> Recurrent severe infections in sterile sites e.g. pneumonia, meningitis.

Many primary immunodeficiencies result from gene mutations on recessive genes. Thus, be vigilant for:

> X-linked family history (more common in males).
> Family history of early infant deaths.
> Consanguineous family history.
> Infections apparent at around 6-months-old, when

protection from transplacentally acquired maternal immunoglobulins diminishes.

Investigations

> Full blood count with differential white cell count.
>> Lymphopaenia can be a normal finding during infection, but persistent lymphopaenia should raise suspicion about an underlying immune problem.
>> Anaemia and thrombocytopenia are seen in severe, chronic and recurrent infection, secondary to bone marrow suppression.
>> Thrombocytosis may occur in a chronic inflammatory state.
>> Eosinophilia suggests an allergy or parasitic infection.
> Immunoglobulin levels (IgG, IgM and IgA).
>> Maternal IgG confers protection until six months of age, but following this, low levels of immunoglobulin can indicate humoral immune deficiencies.
> Poor response to childhood vaccines.
>> Poor production of antibodies in response to childhood vaccines such as pneumococcus, diphtheria and tetanus can also indicate a humoral immune deficiency.
> HIV testing.
>> Human immunodeficiency virus is a cause of secondary immunodeficiency and can be vertically transmitted at birth. Any child presenting with a T cell deficiency should undergo HIV testing.
> Complement levels.
>> Any patient presenting with recurrent infection or infection with *Neisseria meningitides* (a susceptible infection in complement deficiency) should have their complement levels tested.
> Lymphocyte subsets.
>> Low levels of lymphocytes can indicate a defect in cellular immunity. A lymphocyte test is important in Severe Combined Immunodeficiency (SCID) as classification is based on absence or presence of cytotoxic T cells, T helper cells, B cells and Natural Killer Cells.

Complications

Overwhelming infection and secondary organ damage are the greatest concern. These can be prevented by early and aggressive use of prophylactic antibiotics and immunoglobulin therapy.

Management

The management depends on the specific cause, but it is predominantly supportive. In general, consider:

> Prophylactic antibiotics for opportunistic infections, e.g. *Pneumocystis jirovecii*.
> Aggressive and early antibiotic treatment for infection.
> Avoidance of live vaccines.
> Isolation precautions as deemed necessary.

In specific diseases, consider the following:

▸ Immunoglobulin.
  › Humoral immune deficiency, such as that seen in SCID and X-linked agammaglobulinaemia, may require regular immunoglobulin transfusions to prevent overwhelming infection.
▸ Enzyme replacement.
  › In SCID secondary to adenosine deaminase deficiency (ADA SCID), some patients may respond to frequent enzyme replacement.
▸ Hematopoietic stem cell transplant.
  › Haematopoietic stem cell transplant (HSCT) remains the only definitive cure for many severe immunodeficiencies including SCID, Chronic Granulomatous Disease (CGD), Wiskott-Aldrich syndrome and X-linked hyper IgM syndrome.
▸ Gene therapy.
  › Gene therapy shows promise in some forms of SCID (ADA SCID), Wiskott Aldrich syndrome and has been trialled for CGD. However, long-term prognosis and adverse effects of treatment have yet to be evaluated.

Early diagnosis significantly improves quality of life and genetic counselling is recommended for those conditions with a known hereditary genetic component.

Prognosis

The prognosis of primary immunodeficiencies is highly variable and depends on the nature of the immunodeficiency. Minor impairment in immunity, such as IgA deficiency, may be largely asymptomatic and remain undiagnosed throughout life. By contrast, defects of greater severity, such as SCID, are invariably fatal in the first year without haematopoietic stem cell transplant.

Examples of Immunodeficiencies

Immunodeficiencies take many forms. Therefore, it is important to know when to suspect an immunodeficiency, rather than making a specific diagnosis and management plan, since immunodeficiencies are normally handled by specialists. Below are examples of important primary immunodeficiencies to keep in mind.

IgA Deficiency

This is a deficiency in serum IgA, in the setting of normal IgG and IgM levels. It occurs more commonly in patients with a family history of IgA deficiency (or other immunodeficiencies), and in those with autoimmune disease. Many patients are asymptomatic, but some may present with recurrent infections (most commonly sinopulmonary), which can progress to bronchiectasis in severe cases. This deficiency can potentially progress to common variable immunodeficiency.

Severe Combined Immunodeficiency (SCID)

SCID arises from severe defects in both humoral and cellular immunity. It is due to molecular defects that result in defective development and/or functioning of T and B cells. It is a severe, life-threatening immunodeficiency presenting in early childhood. It is more common in males, and in those with consanguineous parents. Recurrent severe infections typically begin to present at 6-months-old, as maternal IgG persists up to this point. Be aware of candidiasis, opportunistic infections (e.g. *Pneumocystis pneumoniae*), and severe or fatal infection following vaccination with live vaccines or exposure to common viruses (e.g. Epstein-Barr virus, cytomegalovirus, rotavirus, adenovirus, varicella zoster virus). SCID may also be associated with chronic diarrhoea and faltering growth.

The only curative option for most SCID patients is haematopoietic stem cell transplant. Live vaccines are contraindicated, and isolation may be needed to prevent infection. Irradiated, leukodepleted and CMV-negative blood products are required if blood is needed. Without curative or aggressive supportive management, SCID is usually fatal, often in the first year of life.

Chronic Granulomatous Disease (CGD)

This is a primary immunodeficiency characterised by recurrent and severe bacterial and fungal infections, with granuloma formation due to defects in phagocyte NADPH oxidase. It is more common in males and in the offspring of consanguineous parents. The majority of cases are diagnosed in the first five years of life. The diagnosis of CGD is suggested by recurrent and persistent infections, and infections caused by catalase-producing organisms (e.g. *Staphylococcus aureus*). Other organisms include aspergillus, serratia, and burkholderia. Presentation includes skin abscesses and osteomyelitis. Severe complications arise from infection, as well as from inflammatory disease leading to gastrointestinal and urinary tract obstruction (from granuloma formation). Stem cell treatment is the main curative treatment, although gene therapy has shown promise. The inflammatory manifestations may be treated with glucocorticosteroids. HSCT can be curative.

X-linked Agammaglobulinaemia

This is caused by a defect in B cell development due to mutations in Bruton's tyrosine kinase, and has an X-linked recessive inheritance pattern. It characteristically presents with recurrent sinopulmonary infections from 6 to 18-months-old (note maternal IgG is present until six months). Patients also have associated faltering growth.

Common Variable Immunodeficiency (CVID)

This is a diagnosis covering a group of conditions primarily resulting in failure of antibody production (hypogammaglobulinaemia). CVID presents with recurrent respiratory tract infections (particularly encapsulated bacteria, such as *Streptococcus pneumoniae*) and faltering growth. IV immunoglobulin is the mainstay of treatment, but severe cases may require a bone marrow transplant.

Wiskott-Aldrich Syndrome

This is an X-linked disorder caused by mutations in the gene that encodes the Wiskott-Aldrich protein, required for normal T cell function. It presents clinically with the triad of increased susceptibility to infection, microthrombocytopaenia and eczema; these become apparent in the first few years of life. In later life, affected patients are more prone to autoimmune conditions such as vasculitis and haemolytic anaemias. They are also more prone to malignancy in adolescence and adulthood, most commonly B cell lymphomas and leukaemias. Diagnosis is supported by a decreased number and reduced function of T cells, poor antibody response to vaccines and high levels of IgE and IgA. Prophylactic antibiotics and anti-viral drugs can reduce the number of infections. In cases of severe bleeding or prior to surgical procedures, platelet transfusions may be used. Haematopoietic stem cell transplant remains the only curative option and gene therapy trials look promising.

Ataxia Telangiectasia

This is an autosomal recessive disorder characterised by ataxia, telangiectasia and impaired immunity. Most children appear healthy for the first year of life and walk at a normal age. However, they walk with a narrow gait and are notably ataxic. Gross and fine motor skills deteriorate after school age. Most patients are wheelchair bound by the second decade of life and suffer dysarthria and dysphagia. Telangiectasias are visible from 3 to 5-years-old, most notably on the bulbar conjunctivae, pinnae, nose, face and neck. Both cellular and humoral immunity is impaired, resulting in frequent sinopulmonary infections. Diagnosis is based on the clinical presentation but can be further supported by elevated serum alpha foetoprotein, reduced serum IgA and chromosomal fragility. Diagnosis can be confirmed by genetic testing. These patients have a predisposition to malignancy in childhood, most commonly lymphomas and acute leukaemias. Life expectancy is around 25-years-old. Death is secondary to pulmonary causes, following repeat infection or malignancy. No curative treatment exists and management centres on prevention of infections, a multidisciplinary team approach to maximise function, and prompt diagnosis and treatment of malignancy.

DiGeorge Syndrome

This is caused by a deletion on chromosome 22, leading to defective development of the pharyngeal pouch system.

This results in the classic triad of cardiac abnormalities, hypocalcaemia (secondary to parathyroid hypoplasia) and an absent or hypoplastic thymus. A wide spectrum of immunodeficiency is seen in DiGeorge syndrome, ranging from recurrent sinopulmonary infections to severe combined immunodeficiencies. Other features frequently seen include developmental delay, speech and feeding problems, palatal abnormalities and characteristic facies with hypertelorism, posteriorly rotated low set ears and a bulbous nose tip. Prognosis is dependent on the severity of the cardiac defect, hypoparathyroidism and immunodeficiency. Management involves a paediatric cardiologist, paediatric endocrinologist and a large multidisciplinary team to manage speech and feeding problems and ensure optimal development.

REFERENCES AND FURTHER READING

Immunology

1 Jyothi S, Lissauer S, Welch S, Hackett S. Immune deficiencies in children: an overview. Arch Dis Child Educ Pract Ed. 2013; 98:186-96.
2 Wood P et al. Recognition, clinical diagnosis and management of patients with primary antibody deficiencies: a systematic review. Clin Exper Immunol. 2007; 149:410-23.
3 Park MA, Li JT, Hagan JB, Maddox DE, Abraham RS. Common variable immunodeficiency: a new look at an old disease. Lancet. 2008; 372:489-502.
4 Rosen FS, Cooper MD, Wedgwood RJ. The primary immunodeficiencies. New Engl J Med. 1995; 333:431-40.

Allergy

1 NICE. Food allergy in children and young people: Diagnosis and assessment of food allergy in children and young people in primary care and community settings. 2011. https://www.nice.org.uk/guidance/cg116/evidence/full-guideline-136470061.
2 NICE 2011. Anaphylaxis: assessment to confirm an anaphylactic episode and the decision to refer after emergency treatment for a suspected anaphylactic episode. https://www.nice.org.uk/guidance/cg134
3 APLS APLSG. 2010. Anaphylaxis algorithm. Resuscitation Council UK.

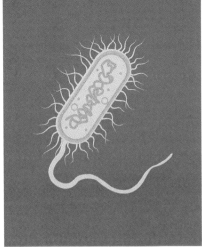

1.11
INFECTION
PHILIPPA KING, ZESHAN QURESHI AND DAVID K K HO

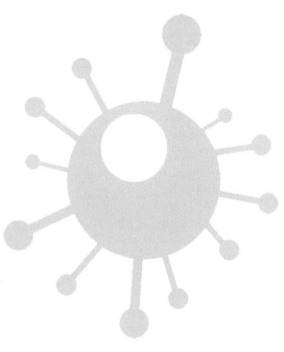

CONTENTS

IMMUNISATION

Introduction

Immunisation refers to the process of creating active or passive immunity in an individual to protect them from acquiring disease. The impact of immunisation on public health is well recognised, and data clearly demonstrate how the prevalence of certain diseases can be reduced by vaccination. For example, smallpox was eradicated as a disease in 1979 after the development of the vaccine, and the fight to eradicate poliomyelitis has advanced with the use of the polio vaccine. The Measles, Mumps, Rubella (MMR) vaccine scare is a good example of how disease rates rise when vaccine uptake falls. The publication of a later discredited paper that claimed a link between the MMR vaccine, autism and inflammatory bowel disease resulted in a sharp decrease in children being vaccinated and a subsequent increase in the MMR diseases.

Vaccines work by stimulating the immune system in a process known as active immunity. This contrasts with passive immunity, which is acquired by administering immunoglobulins.

Successful immunisation programmes rely on the principle of herd immunity. Herd immunity is achieved when uptake of immunisation increases above a certain threshold, leading to decreased transmission. This then lowers the incidence of disease in the overall population, protecting those who might be at risk but remain unvaccinated. The threshold varies for different diseases and depends on the specific disease and its transmission mode, amongst other factors.

Important vaccine rules are shown in *Box 1*.

Different Types of Vaccines

Live Attenuated Vaccines

These contain a weakened (or attenuated) form of the infective organism, and the body responds as it would do to an infection, creating long-lasting antibodies and thus immunity to the disease. The MMR, Bacillus Calmette-Guérin (BCG), varicella, nasal spray influenza vaccine and rotavirus vaccines are live attenuated vaccines. Most live vaccines can now be given at any time before or after each other, with few exceptions. If a patient has recently received immunoglobulin, the live vaccine has a diminished immune response if given shortly before or for a long time afterwards, as immunoglobulin can neutralise vaccine antigens. Therefore, in such cases, one should wait at least three months before giving the vaccine.

Inactivated Vaccines

These are vaccines where the organism has been killed (or inactivated). They usually stimulate a weaker immune response than live vaccines, meaning that several boosters are required. The immune response can be strengthened by conjugation, such as the addition of a protein. Inactivated vaccines include diphtheria, tetanus, pertussis, polio, *Haemophilus influenzae* type b, pneumococcal conjugate, meningococcal conjugate, influenza and hepatitis B.

Subunit Vaccines

Subunit vaccines contain just part of the organism, often the antigens which stimulate the immune response, instead of the whole organism. The human papilloma virus vaccine is a subunit vaccine.

Although some vaccines are single vaccines against one disease, many vaccines are given as a combined injection consisting of several vaccines, e.g. the tetanus/diphtheria/inactivated polio vaccine. The majority of vaccines are injections, with notable exceptions being rotavirus (oral vaccine), live attenuated oral polio vaccine and the live attenuated influenza vaccine (nasal spray).

The Routine Vaccination Schedule

Table 1 shows the current UK immunisation schedule. Childhood vaccination schedules vary throughout the world, depending on the regional prevalence of diseases. The schedule is implemented so that young babies are immunised early in life against serious infectious diseases, and further booster vaccinations are given to ensure adequate protection. A new meningitis B vaccine was introduced to the UK immunisation schedule in September 2015.

Several additional vaccines are available for at-risk groups of children. These include:

› BCG vaccine. This is given to at-risk infants at birth, e.g. born in a high prevalence tuberculosis (TB) area. This includes most urban centres. The BCG vaccine should be avoided in infants with symptomatic Human Immunodeficiency Virus (HIV) and SCID.

› Hepatitis B vaccine. This is given to at-risk infants at birth.

› Influenza vaccine. This is given to at-risk children annually, e.g. those with chronic heart disease, chronic respiratory disease, diabetes and other chronic conditions.

Box 1: Vaccine rules

- Vaccines from different manufacturers can be mixed. However, it is preferable to use the same manufacturer (as the vaccines may have different antigen content or additives).
- Most vaccines can be safely administered simultaneously at separate sites. There are specific rules for certain vaccines, e.g. yellow fever and MMR should be administered at least four weeks apart.
- A lapse in the immunisation schedule does not require starting over.
- Vaccinations must be documented on a formal immunisation record.
- Only give the recommended dose.

TABLE 1: Current UK immunisation schedule (Adapted from www.gov.uk/government/collections/immunisation)

Age at Immunisation	Vaccination
2 months.	• Diphtheria/Tetanus/Pertussis/Polio/ *Haemophilus influenzae* type B (DTaP/IPV/ Hib). • Pneumococcal conjugate (PCV). • Meningococcal group B (MenB). • Rotavirus.
3 months.	• Diphtheria/Tetanus/Pertussis/Polio/ *Haemophilus influenzae* type B (DtaP/IPV/ Hib). • Rotavirus.
4 months.	• Diphtheria/Tetanus/Pertussis/Polio/ *Haemophilus influenzae* type B (DtaP/IPV/ Hib). • Pneumococcal conjugate (PCV). • Meningococcal group B (MenB).
12-13 months.	• *Haemophilus influenzae* type B/ Meningococcal C conjugate (HiB/MenC). • Pneumococcal conjugate (PCV). • Measles/Mumps/Rubella (MMR). • Meningococcal group B (MenB).
2 to 7 years.	• Influenza.
3 years 4 months Preschool booster.	• Diphtheria/Tetanus/Pertussis/Polio (DTaP/ IPV). • Measles/Mumps/Rubella (MMR).
Girls 12-13 years.	• Human Papillomavirus (HPV).
14 years.	• Tetanus/Diphtheria/Polio (Td/IPV). • Meningococcal ACWY.

> ► **RSV vaccine.** Palivizumab is a monoclonal antibody against Respiratory Syncytial Virus (RSV), the commonest cause of bronchiolitis, and is recommended for young children with severe chronic disease such as congenital cardiac disease or chronic lung disease and very premature infants.

Children with asplenia or splenic dysfunction should receive additional pneumococcal, meningococcal ACWY vaccine, *Haemophilus influenzae* type B and influenza vaccines.

Complications

Vaccinations are generally very safe. Complications include:
► Localised side effects such as swelling, redness and discomfort at the injection site.
► Fever.
► Malaise and rash (vaccine may stimulate a mild form of the disease).
► Anaphylaxis (rare).

Contraindications

If the child has an acute febrile illness or a moderate to severe illness, then vaccination should be postponed until they are well. However, a mild infection with or without fever is not a contraindication. A history of personal or family febrile convulsions is not a contraindication.

Immunosuppressed children, such as children with HIV, in general must not receive live vaccines such as BCG (but MMR and rotavirus vaccines can be given to children with HIV). Vaccines are also contraindicated in those with previous anaphylaxis. All live vaccines are contraindicated in pregnancy, but breastfeeding is never a contraindication.

Each vaccine is made of unique constituents, and therefore it is important to check individual contraindications e.g. egg allergy (some influenza vaccines), neomycin/streptomycin anaphylaxis (MMR/IPV/Varicella).

APPROACH TO A CHILD WITH FEVER

Definition

Fever is defined as a temperature of greater than 38°C. The most common cause of fever is infection, although the source of infection may not always be clear.

Temperature Regulation

Temperature is controlled by a thermoregulatory centre in the hypothalamus, which has a set point of around 37°C. Infection, cancer, trauma and inflammation trigger the release of pyrogens and a cascade of events which leads to a rise in the body's temperature set point. This leads to vasoconstriction and muscle contraction which, in turn, generates fever. Body temperature also varies with age of the child and activities. The body temperature is lowest in the morning and highest in the early evening. Rectal temperature measurements are around 0.4°C higher than oral temperature measurements. Taking these into consideration, a low grade fever can be normal.

Fever itself has a broad range of causes, as summarised in *Table 2*.

Assessing a Child with Fever

The assessment of a child with fever involves identifying the severity of the illness and trying to identify the cause of the fever.

Severity of the Illness

Feverish patients can be very sick, and as with all patients, they should be resuscitated using an ABCDE approach. This is usually in the context of severe infection. NICE guidelines recommend the utilisation of the traffic light system for identifying severity, with green being low risk and red being high risk. This is summarised in *Table 3*.

In the patient that appears relatively well, it is important to ensure they are well hydrated. Good urine output is a sensitive marker of this. Also check that ongoing fluid intake is adequate, particularly in a child that is vomiting or has diarrhoea. As a rough guide, even when ill, children should be drinking 50% of their normal fluid volume. It is acceptable for a child to go completely off food during the acute phase of illness.

INFECTION

151

TABLE 2: Differential diagnosis for fever

Infectious Causes.	Common serious bacterial infections.	• Sepsis. • Pneumonia. • Meningitis. • Urinary tract infection. • Osteomyelitis.
	Other common conditions.	• Gastroenteritis. • Pharyngitis. • Tonsillitis. • Otitis media. • Lower respiratory tract infections.
	Conditions depending on geographical area or exposure.	• HIV. • Tuberculosis. • Malaria. • Typhoid. • Cat scratch disease (*Bartonella henselae*). • Brucellosis (*Brucella*). • Leishmaniasis (*Leishmania*). • Yersiniosis (*Yersinia*). • Q fever (*Coxiella burnetii*).
	Viruses that can give rise to a prolonged course of fever.	• Epstein-Barr virus. • Cytomegalovirus.
Non-Infectious Causes.	Autoimmune/ Inflammatory disorders.	• Kawasaki disease. • Juvenile idiopathic arthritis. • Systemic lupus erythematosus. • Haemophagocytic lymphohistiocytosis. • Vasculitides. • Sarcoidosis. • Periodic fever syndromes (e.g. Familial Mediterranean syndrome).
	Malignancy.	• Leukaemia. • Lymphoma.
	Central thermoregulatory disorder.	• Absent corpus callosum. • Dysautonomia (malfunction of autonomic nervous system). • Hypothalamic dysfunction.
Other.	Factitious fever/Munchausen syndrome by proxy.	

Origin of Fever

Infective Causes

Infection is the most common cause of fever. Sometimes the cause is not immediately apparent. Non-specific features of illness include poor appetite, lethargy, lymphadenopathy, and generalised aches and pains. *Table 4* summarises key information in the history and possible examination signs which may help localise the cause of any infection. Height and weight should be plotted on a growth chart, as faltering growth could indicate possible immunodeficiencies. Dysmorphic features should be identified, since, for example, DiGeorge syndrome is associated with immunodeficiency.

Unimmunised children are at risk of infection from measles, pneumococcal disease and meningococcal infections amongst others, so ensure immunisations are up-to-date. Other key questions include history of recent travel, eating undercooked or unpasteurised food, contact with infectious diseases such as TB, or even just attendance at a nursery where children have close contact with lots of other children and can easily pick up infections.

Non- Infective Causes

Non-infective causes of fever are usually identified and managed in a specialist setting. It is usually in the setting of prolonged fever, periodic fever, recurrent fever or fever of unknown origin:

> Prolonged fever. This is when the number of days with fever exceeds what would be expected for a single episode of illness. The number of days would depend on the nature of illness. For example, a fever lasting more than three weeks would be prolonged in infectious mononucleosis, whereas a fever of more than ten days would be considered prolonged in gastroenteritis. In such cases, an alternative cause for the fever should be considered. This could include infection, connective tissue disease or malignancy.

> Recurrent fever. This can be from a single illness or from multiple illnesses occurring at different intervals, usually lasting months or years. This should trigger consideration of further investigations, particularly if there is no obvious infective aetiology. If the fever is a sign of recurrent infection, there may be a possible concern about immunodeficiency.

> Periodic fever. This describes predictable episodes of fever lasting days to weeks, which can recur at regular or sporadic intervals. Crucially, such episodes do not have an infective cause, and the child is well between episodes. Familial Mediterranean fever is the most common periodic fever syndrome, although collectively these are rare.

> Fever of unknown origin (FUO) or pyrexia of unknown origin (PUO). This refers to fever where a focus cannot be found. It usually applies to a fever lasting more than three weeks, with no focus identified despite intensive initial investigations. FUO may last for over a year, particularly if due to inflammatory disorders. Other causes include infection and neoplasm.

A thorough history is required in this regard, since many non-infective causes of fever like systemic lupus erythematosus are multi-system diseases. Any family history of unexplained deaths, specifically in early life, would be important as this may point

TABLE 3: Assessment of child presenting with fever. (Adapted from NICE guidelines Feverish Illness in Children, 2013)

DOMAIN	GREEN	AMBER	RED
Colour (skin/lips/tongue).	• Normal.	• Pallor reported by parent/carer.	• Pale/mottled/ashen/ blue.
Activity.	• Normal response to social cues. • Smiles. • Awake/ awakens quickly. • Strong normal cry/not crying.	• Abnormal response to social cues. • No smile. • Wakes only with prolonged stimulation. • Reduced activity.	• Unresponsive to social cues. • Appears ill to a healthcare professional. • Asleep, or if roused does not stay awake. • Weak/high-pitched/continuous cry/ unresponsive.
Respiratory.	• Normal respiratory rate and breathing pattern.	• Nasal flaring. • Tachypnoea (respiratory rate (RR)>50 breaths/ minute if 6 to 12–months-old, or >40 breaths/ minute if over 12-months-old). • Oxygen saturation ≤95% in air. • Chest crackles.	• Grunting. • Tachypnoea: RR >60 breaths/minute (any age). • Moderate or severe chest recession.
Circulation and hydration.	• Normal cardiovascular parameters. • Well hydrated.	• Tachycardia (heart rate >160 beats/minute if age under 1, or >150 beats/minute if age 1-2, >140 beats/minute if age 2 to 5-years-old). • Capillary refill time ≥3 seconds. • Dry mucous membranes. • Poor feeding/reduced urine output.	• Reduced skin turgor.
Other.	• Absence of amber/red features.	• Age 3 to 6–months-old. • Temperature ≥39°C. • Fever for ≥5 days. • Rigors. • Swelling of a limb or joint. • Non-weight bearing limb/not using an extremity.	• Age <3–months-old. • Non-blanching rash. • Bulging fontanelle. • Neck stiffness. • Status epilepticus. • Focal neurological signs.

TABLE 4: Key symptoms and signs that help localise infection

	History	Examination
Meningitis.	• Headache, neck stiffness, photophobia. • Symptoms are non-specific in infants but more classical in older children.	• Bulging fontanelle/increased head circumference (in infants with open fontanelle). • Neck stiffness, positive Kernig sign, photophobia.
Sepsis.	• Unwell, palpitations, light headed, high temperatures, white/cold peripheries, difficulty breathing.	• Evidence of tachycardia, end organ hypoperfusion. Non-blanching rash of meningococcal septicaemia.
Endocarditis.	• Usually non-specific.	• New or changing murmur. • Splinter haemorrhages. • Clubbing, Osler Nodes, Janeway lesions, splenomegaly, Roth spots.
Upper respiratory tract infection.	• Sore throat, cough, swollen glands.	• Tender sinuses, enlarged/red/pus on tonsils, cervical lymphadenopathy, retracted/red tympanic membrane.
Pneumonia.	• Chest pain, cough, productive sputum, shortness of breath. May present with abdominal pain.	• Tachypnoea, productive sputum, tracheal tug, head bobbing, intercostal recession, subcostal recession, reduced oxygen saturations.
Cellulitis.	• Erythematous, swollen, hot, painful rash.	
Urinary tract infection.	• Increased urinary frequency, nocturia, urinary incontinence, dysuria (pain on urination), urgency, vomiting. Young children and infants often do not have typical urinary symptoms.	• Cloudy or foul smelling urine (both very non-specific).
Gastroenteritis.	• Vomiting, diarrhoea, abdominal pain.	• Abdominal tenderness.
Osteomyelitis/ septic arthritis.	• Bone/joint pain, swelling, reluctance to weight bear.	• Restricted movements, inability to weight bear.

to an immunodeficiency disorder. Ethnic and genetic background can help with rarer diseases like familial Mediterranean fever.

Non-infectious causes of fever are more likely if:

> The fever is prolonged, recurrent, or periodic.
> Red flags are evident, such as weight loss, night sweats, epitrochlear, popliteal and supraclavicular lymphadenopathy, significant hepatomegaly or splenomegaly.

Investigations

In determining investigations for fever, the age of the child is crucial. The highest risk age group is the neonatal period, with sepsis and meningitis being a common concern. This is because both sepsis and meningitis can present with isolated fever or no fever. If not treated at this point, the disease may progress rapidly. Therefore, in the under one month age group, and often extended to under three months, any child with a documented fever will invariably receive a full septic screen (blood tests, urine microscopy culture and sensitivity, chest X-ray, lumbar puncture). They will be treated for presumed sepsis or meningitis until blood and cerebral spinal fluid (CSF) cultures come back negative.

As the child gets older, being systemically well becomes more reassuring, particularly over the age of one year. If there is a clear focus of infection from the history and examination, no further investigation may be needed. Even if there is no clear cause for the fever, it is reasonable to have a period of observation or to arrange follow up before further investigation, particularly if the fever has been present for less than 48 hours.

Infective Causes

Common investigations are presented below:

> **Urine microscopy, culture & sensitivity (MC&S).** This is a simple investigation and is particularly helpful in children who cannot report urinary symptoms. The sensitivity of urine dipstick testing is lower in children younger than 3-years-old; therefore, MC&S is preferred. It also allows identification of the pathogen and antibiotics sensitivity testing. The gold standard is a clean catch or catheter specimen urine with >10^5 organisms on culture.
> Blood tests:
>> **Full blood count (FBC).** Both high white cell count (WCC) and low WCC suggest serious bacterial infections. Neutrophilia can suggest a bacterial infection. Elevated lymphocyte count is generally associated with viral infection but also with whooping cough. A low platelet count can indicate severe sepsis at any stage, but particularly in the newborn. A high platelet count can result from an immune response to infection or inflammation, such as in Kawasaki disease.
>> **C-reactive protein (CRP).** CRP is a protein synthesised in the liver in response to inflammation. CRP rises with infection, although if there is associated severe liver disease, a response might not be seen. The rate at which CRP doubles or halves is a useful marker of infection and its resolution.
>> **Urea & electrolytes (U&E).** U&Es are a good measure of hydration status.
> **Blood gas.** Blood gas is useful if there is respiratory compromise suggesting the need for non-invasive or invasive ventilation. It also provides an indicator of acidosis in children with sepsis or severe dehydration. If sepsis is present, lactate should be measured as an indicator of end organ perfusion.
> **Throat swab.** This can be done in suspected bacterial tonsillitis. If rapid Group A streptococcus antigen testing is available, it can be used as a guide to help make decisions on antibiotic treatment as the result can usually be obtained within 30 minutes.

> **Chest X-ray.** Chest X-ray is indicated if respiratory signs are present in infants less than three-months-old. For infants and children older than three-months-old, a chest X-ray is only indicated if red flag signs or symptoms are present (*Table* 3). Pneumonia does not routinely require a chest X-ray to confirm diagnosis.
> **Blood culture (BC).** Blood culture is the gold standard test for detecting pathogens in the blood and allows antibiotic sensitivity testing. Sensitivity of BC is reduced if an insufficient amount of blood was taken; aim for 1 mL in neonates and 5 mL in older children. Generally speaking, if BCs are taken, a commitment has been made to start intravenous antibiotics for 36-48 hours. BCs should be taken before starting antibiotics.
> **Skin/wound swab.** This may be done in the context of an abscess, infected eczema, wound or cellulitis.
> **Stool culture.** Stool culture may be indicated if diarrhoea is present, particularly if it has lasted more than two weeks, if it is bloody, or if an unusual organism is suspected. Newer faecal multiplex polymerase chain reaction (PCR), if available, can offer a quicker turnaround time and higher sensitivity. However they do not offer an antibiotic susceptibility profile.
> **Lumbar puncture (LP).** An LP is indicated in any child where meningitis is a significant concern. Any neonate with a temperature over 38°C should have an LP regardless of how well they seem. LP should also be considered in this age group with any significant rise in CRP. This approach is usually extended to those under three months as well. If it is possible, an LP is performed before administration of antibiotics. However, it should not delay the administration of antibiotics. Note that there are additional tests for specific suspected organisms, e.g. meningococcal PCR in suspected meningococcal sepsis (which is performed on CSF and whole blood), or viral PCR.

> Line tip culture. If there are any indwelling lines and line sepsis is suspected, the line should be removed and the tip sent for analysis.
> Ultrasound/X-Ray/Magnetic Resonance Imaging (MRI) bone. Radiological investigations are indicated if osteomyelitis is suspected. X-ray may be performed as it can show late changes of the disease, as well as to rule out trauma or malignancy. Ultrasound may identify earlier infective changes, but MRI is the most sensitive for detecting the earliest stages of infection.
> Echocardiography. Echocardiography is indicated if infective endocarditis is suspected.

Non-Infective Causes

Generally, investigation first involves searching for an infective cause, with a thorough history to identify the most likely candidates, which may include malaria, TB or HIV, all of which can be tested for specifically. Blood tests would include FBC (including a blood film), CRP, erythrocyte sedimentation rate (ESR), U&Es, liver function tests (LFTs), thyroid function tests (TFTs), and autoimmune screen (including anti-neutrophil cytoplasmic antibodies (ANCA), anti-neutrophil antibodies (ANA), and Rheumatoid factor) to identify possible connective tissue disorders or malignancies. Imaging may include ultrasound, Computed Tomography (CT) or MRI, and will help identify malignancy and deep seated infections. After initial results, more invasive testing such as lymph node biopsies, bone marrow aspirates or liver biopsies may be needed, depending on the suspected diagnosis.

Management

Management of a child with fever is tailored to the cause, and these are all addressed individually under the relevant specialty within this textbook.

Sepsis

Septic patients crucially require rapid fluid resuscitation and initial broad spectrum antibiotic therapy. These patients are likely to deteriorate quickly, so early intervention gives a markedly improved prognosis. Further to this point, a seemingly well child with an infection may rapidly deteriorate following discharge from the ED. It is therefore vitally important to ensure that a child with abnormal observations is only discharged once an improvement is seen, or when an alternative cause is found for the abnormal results. For example, although sepsis may cause tachycardia, a child may initially be tachycardic because of anxiety, a temperature or pain. Once these are managed, the tachycardia should improve. Otherwise, even in a well child, there should be a low threshold for admission.

'Sepsis six', developed by the United Kingdom Sepsis Trust, is aiming to improve mortality from sepsis by the implementation of six tasks which should be started within one hour. These are oxygen, antibiotics, fluids, blood cultures, checking lactate and urine output monitoring.

Antibiotic Selection

Most hospitals will have an antibiotic guideline covering key infections and suggested antibiotics to prescribe. These will vary between hospitals, mainly due to local patterns of resistance seen. *Table 5* is an example of an antibiotic guideline showing key infections, likely organisms involved in the pathogenesis and suggestions for antibiotic use.

Fever Control

Antipyretic agents such as paracetamol and ibuprofen are commonly used when children are non-specifically unwell. It is not recommended to give both agents simultaneously unless symptoms are not controlled by one agent. Although rare, both paracetamol and ibuprofen can have potentially serious side effects (liver toxicity in paracetamol overdose and acute kidney injury or gastric side effects with ibuprofen). Antipyretic agents do not prevent febrile convulsions, and there is no medical reason to reduce body temperature in children with fever other than for comfort.

Safety Netting

Parents should be educated on spotting signs of dehydration and advised to ensure regular fluid intake. They should also be taught about the importance of identifying any non-blanching rashes, as well as to check on their child during the night. Regarding nursery or schooling, it is important for parents to quarantine their child for the duration of the fever. Children with diarrhoeal illness should be advised to stay at home for 48 hours after the resolution of symptoms and to avoid swimming for two weeks after as well. Written advice should be given where possible.

Finally, many infections have public health implications and may need to be reported if they are on the list of notifiable diseases.

TABLE 5: Example antibiotic selection for common infections

Infection	Organisms implicated in pathogenesis	Example antibiotic regime
Neonatal sepsis – Early onset (<48hrs).	• Group B Streptococcus. • *E.coli.* • *Listeria.* • *H. influenzae.*	Benzylpenicillin IV + Gentamicin IV.
Neonatal sepsis - Late onset (>48hr).	As above and also: • Coagulase Negative Staphylococci (particularly line sepsis). • *Staphylococcus aureus.*	Flucloxacillin IV + Gentamicin IV. OR Vancomycin IV + Cefotaxime IV.
Cellulitis.	• *Staph aureus.* • Group A Strep.	Flucloxacillin IV or PO. Benzylpenicillin IV +/- Clindamycin IV (if severe as inhibits exotoxins).
Pre-septal periorbital cellulitis/ Orbital cellulitis.	• *Staph aureus.* • Streptococci. • *H. influenzae.*	Co-amoxiclav PO (mild periorbital cellulitis). Ceftriaxone IV + Metronidazole IV or PO.
Bone and joint infections.	• *Staph aureus.* • Streptococci. • Gram negative e.g. *E. coli,* esp. in newborn.	Infants <3 months: Cefotaxime IV + amoxicillin IV. >3 months and <5 years: Cefuroxime IV. >5 years: Flucloxacillin IV.
Lower respiratory tract infections.	• *S. pneumoniae.* • *H. influenzae.* • *Mycoplasma.*	Amoxicillin/co-amoxiclav IV or PO +/- Clarithromycin PO
Otitis media.	• *S. pneumoniae.* • *H. influenzae.* • Group A Strep. • *Moraxella catarrhalis.*	Amoxicillin PO or co-amoxiclav PO (although most cases don't require antibiotic treatment).
Tonsillitis.	• Group A Strep.	Penicillin V PO.
Abdominal sepsis.	• *E. coli.* • *Enterococcus.* • Anaerobes e.g. *Bacteroides, Clostridium.*	Amoxicillin IV + gentamicin IV + metronidazole IV or PO.
Lower urinary tract infection.	• *E. coli.* • *Proteus.* • *Klebsiella.*	Trimethoprim PO.
Acute pyelonephritis.	• *E. coli.* • *Proteus.* • *Klebsiella.*	Co-amoxiclav IV/Ceftriaxone IV +/- Gentamicin IV (caution in renal failure).
Neonatal meningitis.	• Group B Strep. • *E.coli.* • *H. influenzae.* • *Listeria.*	Cefotaxime IV + Amoxicillin IV.
Meningitis (infant/child).	• *Neisseria meningitidis.* • *S. pneumoniae.* • *H. influenzae.*	Ceftriaxone IV.

VIRAL INFECTIONS

Human Herpes Virus

Eight different types of herpes virus affect humans. The herpes virus is a linear double-stranded Deoxyribonucleic Acid (DNA) virus that has the ability to establish latency after primary infection. It can therefore reactivate at a later stage to cause further disease. The following are common herpes infections that children can encounter.

Herpes Simplex Virus Type 1 (HSV-1)

Primary infection with HSV-1 typically causes oral infection (also known as cold sores) affecting the facial area around the mouth, lips, tongue, gingiva and palate. The incubation period is variable but generally around eight days. A prodromal period may be experienced, consisting of tingling and soreness where the lesions will appear and occasionally fever. Although most HSV-1 infections are asymptomatic, children can present with fever, distress, reduced oral intake and dehydration. Treatment is supportive, with topical anaesthesia and oral rehydration salts if dehydrated. Rarely, children need to be admitted for intravenous fluids.

Herpes Simplex Virus Type 2 (HSV-2)

Genital herpes infection is typically caused by HSV-2 but can also be caused by HSV-1. Be wary of child sexual abuse presenting with genital herpes. The incubation period is around four days, and again prodromal symptoms include itching and pain prior to the onset of genital lesions. Other symptoms include headache, fever, myalgia and back pain. Other manifestations of herpes include meningoencephalitis, eczema herpeticum and eye infections, for which intravenous antiviral agents may be required.

Maternal Genital Herpes

This can potentially cause congenital herpes infection following intrauterine exposure or vertical transmission after vaginal delivery. Neonatal herpes infection can result in central nervous system infection (meningoencephalitis) and disseminated infection with significant risk of disability and death, even if treated (IV aciclovir).

Human Herpes Virus Type 6 (HHV-6)

This is the most common cause of roseola infantum, with an incubation period of about 10 days. In this condition, a child 6-months-old to 2-years-old presents with two to three days of fever, but then as the fever subsides, a widespread rash emerges. It is also known as "sixth disease", as the rash often emerges on day 6 of the illness. Often, parents get anxious as the child appeared to have been getting better (due to fever subsiding) before the rash emerged, but the condition is benign, requiring no treatment. HHV-6 is also implicated in encephalitis, hepatitis and febrile convulsions.

Varicella Zoster Virus

Varicella-zoster virus (VZV), also known as chickenpox, is a common childhood

infection (*Figure 1*). Children acquire VZV through contact with infected individuals at nurseries, schools or social groups.

The incubation period is 10 to 21 days. Prodromal features include fever, malaise, headache and abdominal pain, usually one to two days before the onset of the rash. The itchy rash is characteristic and begins as macules, progressing to papules and then vesicles which can crust over. These lesions can turn haemorrhagic. The child will be infectious from 48 hours before the onset of the rash until all the lesions have crusted over.

The diagnosis is commonly made clinically, although swabs can be taken and PCR performed if required.

Treatment with antiviral medication is unnecessary in healthy children, as most VZV infections are self-limiting. However, treatment is indicated in asymptomatic neonates (if the mother acquires chickenpox within seven days prior to delivery, or up to four days afterwards), in adolescent children and in immunocompromised children who tend to have more severe disease. Varicella-zoster immunoglobulins are used in certain high risk groups.

If fever persists in children with VZV, complications such as bacterial infections caused by *Staphylococcus aureus* and *Streptococcus pyogenes* need to be considered and treated. Other important complications include cerebellar ataxia, varicella encephalitis, pneumonitis, hepatitis, thrombocytopenia and nephritis.

Shingles

Reactivation of VZV typically occurs in adulthood, causing painful eruptions of vesicles in a dermatomal distribution (*Figure 2*). This is known as herpes zoster or shingles. Antiviral medication such as aciclovir and valaciclovir can shorten the duration of pain and lead to quicker resolution of lesions. A shingles vaccine is also now available and routinely offered to elderly adults.

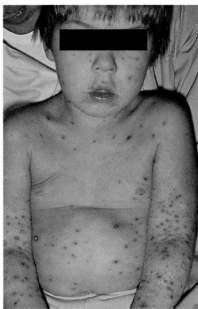

FIGURE 1

Chicken pox (D@nderm).

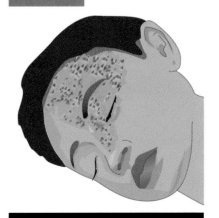

FIGURE 2

Varicella zoster infection of the V$_1$ division of the trigeminal nerve.

Epstein-Barr Virus

Epstein-Barr Virus (EBV) infection, commonly known as "kissing disease" is so-called because of the transfer of infection by oral secretions. It is the major cause of infectious mononucleosis (glandular fever), which can also be caused by cytomegalovirus, toxoplasmosis and HIV.

The incubation period is long, about four to eight weeks, and the prodrome consists of headache and general malaise. The classical triad of symptoms includes fatigue, pharyngitis and lymphadenopathy with other symptoms of fever, hepatosplenomegaly, rash and jaundice. Fever is often high, at 39°C-40°C, and can last for around one week. However fever can sometimes last for more than two weeks. It is hard to distinguish pharyngitis caused by EBV from group A streptococci, as both can present with pustular tonsils and palatal petechiae.

Examination findings include:
> Palpable anterior and posterior cervical nodes, submandibular nodes, as well as epitrochlear nodes.
> Splenomegaly.
> Enlarged and exudative tonsils.

There is a very long period of infectivity, with people continuing to shed the virus for a year and beyond. EBV is an oncovirus, meaning it has the potential to cause malignancies, for example, Burkitt's lymphoma, Hodgkin's disease and nasopharyngeal carcinoma, if unchecked by the immune system.

Diagnosis is often clinical; however, atypical lymphocytes and EBV serology can help with the diagnosis. A classic finding is a rash developing after amoxicillin exposure. Heterophile antibody tests, such as the Paul-Bunnell test or Monospot test, are insensitive in children under 2-years-old, but can be useful in older children.

Treatment is largely supportive. Most of the time, EBV is a self-limiting illness, although some people develop ongoing fatigue and fever. Splenic rupture is rare but potentially life-threatening so patients and parents are advised to avoid contact sports or strenuous activity until recovered. Corticosteroids are given if there are complications such as impending airway obstruction, thrombocytopenia with haemorrhage, autoimmune haemolytic anaemia, Guillain-Barré or Reye's syndrome, interstitial pneumonia, myocarditis or seizures with meningitis.

Influenza

Influenza viruses comprise of seasonal influenza viruses which cause epidemics every winter in temperate climate areas. Seasonal influenza is further divided into groups A, B and C. Type A virus is also named by its two surface proteins haemagglutinin (H) and neuraminidase (N). Current circulating strains of seasonal influenza viruses include H1N1, which caused the 2009 pandemic, and H3N2, as well as influenza B viruses. Birds are the natural host for influenza A. Other species that also harbour influenza A viruses include pigs, dogs, horses, seals, whales and humans. Influenza viruses are transmitted by respiratory droplets.

The incubation period is quite short, usually only one to four days. The prodrome includes fever, myalgia and headache. Symptoms can be quite variable. Infants can present with fever and difficulties with breathing and feeding, similar to a clinical picture of sepsis. Preschool children often have a fever and present with signs and symptoms of upper respiratory tract infections, acute otitis media, croup or pneumonia. Older children have more adult-like symptoms, including fever, chills, headache, myalgia and malaise. Rare manifestations of influenza include myocarditis, encephalitis and encephalopathy. Children are infectious just before the symptoms start and can shed the virus for two weeks after infection.

The gold standard for diagnosis is by culture, where the virus is taken from the nasopharynx. However, PCR, rapid antigen detection test and immunofluorescence assays provide faster and more sensitive results.

Treatment is mainly supportive care. Antiviral medications, such as oseltamivir, reduce the rate of complications, decrease the severity and shorten the duration of symptoms if given within 48 hours of the start of the symptoms. However, benefit needs to be weighed against side effects and resistance. Both the inactivated influenza vaccines and the live-attenuated vaccines have good efficacy against seasonal influenza viruses.

Complications, which tend to occur in the very young, the elderly and the immunocompromised, include:
> Pneumonia.
> Secondary bacterial infection.
> Myocarditis.
> Death.

Parainfluenza

Parainfluenza viruses are a very common cause of respiratory tract infections in children. They are transmitted from person to person and cause syndromes ranging from mild coryzal symptoms to bronchiolitis, croup and pneumonia, which may be severe. Treatment is supportive.

Adenovirus

Adenoviruses comprise seven subgroups, A to G, and many serotypes. They cause a wide variety of clinical syndromes but predominantly affect children between 6-months-old and 5-years-old. Adenoviruses are transmitted by respiratory droplets as well as the faecal-oral route depending on the serotype of the adenovirus. It has no seasonality and can cause sporadic outbreaks.

Commonly, adenoviruses cause febrile respiratory tract infections including tonsillitis, croup, bronchiolitis and pneumonia. Certain serotypes are associated with severe bronchiolitis. A constellation of fever, conjunctivitis, pharyngitis and cervical lymphadenopathy is typical for adenovirus infection. Adenovirus can also cause gastroenteritis, acute haemorrhagic cystitis, pericarditis and myocarditis, aseptic meningitis, encephalitis and transverse myelitis.

Adenovirus is a formidable pathogen in children undergoing haematopoietic stem cell and other transplantation with high mortality.

Diagnosis can be made by culture, PCR and direct antigen detection.

Generally, infections are self-limiting and treatment is supportive. Treatment of immunocompromised or transplanted patients can consist of an antiviral such as cidofovir and/or immunoglobulins.

Parvovirus B19

Parvovirus B19 is a common cause of childhood infection causing a variety of clinical syndromes. It is a very small (parvus in Latin means small) DNA virus that may be transmitted via respiratory droplets as well as through blood transfusion, which was incidentally how it was first discovered.

The incubation period is 4 to 20 days. Most parvovirus B19 infections are asymptomatic or mild, but classically it presents as erythema infectiosum, which is also known as "fifth disease" or "slapped cheek" syndrome. The prodrome is generally very mild, with generalised symptoms such as fever, malaise and coryzal symptoms two to three weeks before the onset of the typical facial rash. The rash of erythema infectiosum is classical, with erythema on the cheeks but sparing the nose, periorbital and perioral regions, hence the name of "slapped cheek disease" (*Figure 3*). After a few days, a secondary lacy rash may occur and spread to the extremities. Generally, symptoms will resolve after a few weeks, but interestingly the rash can recur with stimuli such as heat, exercise and sunlight.

Children are infectious during the prodromal period, but generally not once the rash appears. Parvovirus B19 also infects red blood cell precursors. Therefore, in patients with chronic haemolytic disorders such as sickle cell disease, it can cause a transient aplastic crisis. In the immunocompromised host, parvovirus B19 infection may result in anaemia and red cell aplasia. Other presentations of parvovirus B19 include

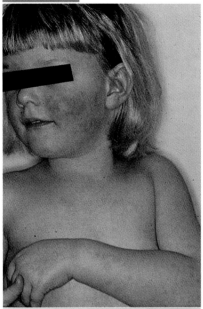

FIGURE 3

Erythema Infectiosum with classic slapped cheek appearance (D@nderm).

polyarthropathy, which is more common in adults. Infection during pregnancy can cause miscarriage, intrauterine foetal death and hydrops fetalis.

Diagnosis is by serology or PCR. No antiviral drug effectively treats parvovirus B19. Immunoglobulins can be given to the immunocompromised patients to clear parvovirus B19 viraemia.

Measles

Measles is a highly infectious viral disease known as the "9-day measles" because of its incubation period of 8 to 12 days. It is caused by the RNA paramyxovirus, which is very contagious. Unimmunised patients and high school or college students are most at risk.

The disease has three stages: incubation, prodrome and then symptomatic illness. The prodrome consists of the 'C' sounds:

> Cough.
> Coryza.
> Conjunctivitis – bilateral.
> Koplik spots – pathognomonic sign of measles, which are white/grey spots inside the buccal mucosa of the mouth, opposite the molars. (*Figure 4*).

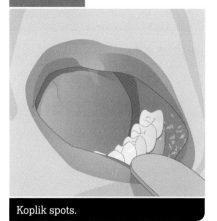

FIGURE 4

Koplik spots.

The main symptoms are simultaneous rash with fever. Typically, the rash starts behind the ears and spreads downwards from head to toe. It may become a confluent rash, which then may desquamate. The rash disappears in the same head to toe order. Children with measles are infectious from four days before the rash onset to four days afterwards.

Diagnosis of measles is primarily clinical, although laboratory tests, such as measles antibody titre and PCR, may be useful.

Treatment is generally supportive. Vitamin A may reduce severity and should be given to children with measles in low income countries to reduce morbidity and mortality, as recommended by the World Health Organisation. To prevent measles, children are vaccinated as part of the MMR vaccination, and globally, the number of deaths from measles has come down by 75% in 2013 compared to 2000. Vaccine coverage needs to be greater than 95% to prevent disease, as seen by the increased number of cases in the UK since the MMR scare. Immunocompromised children without protective antibody levels should receive passive immunisation with immunoglobulin after exposure to measles. Immunoglobulin is recommended for certain groups of immunocompromised patients, such as symptomatic HIV-infected children, even if they have been previously vaccinated.

Measles can be particularly severe in immunocompromised patients and can cause a viral giant cell pneumonia, which can prove fatal.

Complications of measles include:
> Otitis media.
> Pneumonia.
> Encephalitis.
> Diarrhoea.
> Dehydration.
> Devastating complications, including encephalitis and subacute sclerosing panencephalitis (SSPE) (rare).

Measles Encephalitis

Measles encephalitis is rare and typically occurs several days after the onset of illness, with symptoms including headache, irritability and seizures. Neurological sequelae can follow encephalitis and mortality is about 15%. SSPE is a very rare but important complication of measles. It occurs many years (often seven to ten years) after the initial illness and presents with progressive neurological disease leading to death. The cause of SSPE is not clear and is probably due to a combination of persistent viral replication within the central nervous system and host immune responses.

Mumps

Mumps is very contagious and people can transmit the virus in respiratory secretions before symptoms are apparent, and continue to shed the virus whilst parotitis is evident. It occurs usually due to inadequate immunisation. The incubation period of mumps is 14-24 days.

The prodrome is often non-specific and includes:
> Fever.
> Myalgia.
> Earache.
> Headache.

Parotitis develops 24 hours later (*Figure 5*). Parotitis occurs due to both infection and inflammation, and is present in the majority of symptomatic cases of mumps. It often starts unilaterally, but bilateral swelling will commonly occur and may last for longer than a week. However, some people can have mumps with very minor or no symptoms at all.

Diagnosis is essentially clinical. Blood tests may show a leucopaenia and elevated amylase. Specific tests to confirm the diagnosis, such as IgM mumps antibody or isolation of mumps virus, may be required in certain cases, e.g. during outbreaks or in atypical cases where the diagnosis is not clear.

Treatment is symptomatic. Studies of viral shedding indicate that the child should be isolated for five days after the onset of parotitis. Mumps is vaccinated against as part of the MMR vaccine, and as such, cases of mumps have been much less frequently seen.

Mumps Orchitis

Orchitis is the commonest complication of mumps in males, although it is unusual in young children as it tends to affect post pubertal males. Mumps orchitis presents with acute swelling, pain and erythema of the scrotum, accompanied by high fever. Importantly, it may cause testicular atrophy and subsequent reduction in fertility, though this is rare. Mumps can also cause ovarian inflammation in females, which can also reduce fertility.

Meningoencephalomyelitis

Mumps may also cause an aseptic meningitis, which generally has a good prognosis, as well as encephalitis, which may occur without the classical sign of parotitis. Sensorineural deafness,

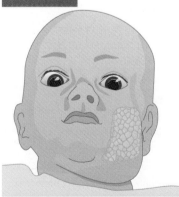

FIGURE 5

Parotid gland swelling.

pancreatitis, myocarditis and arthritis are also potential complications.

Rubella

Rubella, also called the "3-day German measles", is an acute viral infection that usually causes a mild disease in childhood but is important as it can cause severe foetal infection, including death and congenital defects.

The incubation period is 14-21 days. A prodrome is rare, but may include low grade fever. A child may present with a mild fever and maculopapular rash (very similar to the rash of measles) spreading from the face to the rest of the body. Rubella is contagious from two days before the appearance of the rash to five to seven days after. Other symptoms include coryzal symptoms, conjunctivitis and most importantly, lymphadenopathy (classically suboccipital, postauricular and cervical), which distinguishes the condition from measles. Forchheimer spots are seen on the soft palate and this is pathognomonic of the disease.

Diagnosis may be clinical, but is confirmed by PCR testing of saliva or antibody tests on blood or saliva.

Treatment is usually just supportive therapy. Prevention relies on immunisation, and rubella vaccine is part of the MMR vaccination.

Complications are rarely seen, but may include arthritis, thrombocytopenia and encephalitis.

Congenital Rubella

Congenital rubella is the most serious form, as it can result in premature delivery, congenital defects and foetal death, depending on when the foetus is infected. Generally, the earlier the infection, the more severe the results, with the highest risk in the first months of gestation. Congenital defects include cardiac abnormalities (patent ductus arteriosus), cataracts, hearing loss, microcephaly and developmental disorders.

Enterovirus

Enteroviruses include coxsackie viruses and echoviruses as well as polioviruses.

Together, over 100 serotypes are recognised and are responsible for causing many childhood infections.

Most infections are asymptomatic. Non-specific symptoms like fever, rash, malaise, irritability, vomiting, diarrhoea or signs of upper respiratory tract infection are common. Enteroviruses are found throughout the world and infections tend to occur most often in summer and autumn, with most cases occurring in children. The incubation period is normally two to five days. Infection is mainly via the faecal-oral route, and after replicating in the gastrointestinal and respiratory systems, the virus can then spread to other organs. Some of the clinical syndromes caused by enteroviruses are discussed below.

Aseptic Meningitis
A neonate or child may present with non-specific symptoms or the more typical symptoms of meningitis. The CSF shows a predominance of lymphocytes and may show a slight rise in protein with a slight decrease in glucose, and enterovirus can be detected by PCR. Treatment is symptomatic and prognosis is good.

Hand-Foot-and-Mouth Disease
Hand-foot-and-mouth disease is usually caused by Coxsackievirus A16 and Enterovirus 71. Vesicular lesions typically appear on the hands, feet and mouth. Oral lesions can ulcerate, causing pain and refusal of food and drink. This self-limiting illness generally resolves in a week. Enterovirus 71 can cause brainstem encephalitis, and epidemics occur in Southeast Asia. Coxsackievirus is also responsible for viral myocarditis.

Polio
Poliovirus, well known for its devastating effect on the central nervous system, has been eradicated in most parts of the world due to a successful vaccination programme. In 2015, it was endemic in only Afghanistan and Pakistan. The majority of infections caused by poliovirus are asymptomatic, but it can cause a non-specific viral illness, viral meningitis and the classical paralytic polio with asymmetric flaccid paralysis.

Others
Enteroviruses can also cause myositis, myocarditis and pericarditis, herpangina (vesicular lesions on soft palate), pleurodynia (a combination of fever and pleuritic chest pain) and eye infections.

HIV
HIV is a ribonucleic acid (RNA) virus of the Retroviridae family. Like other RNA viruses, HIV RNA undergoes reverse transcription into proviral DNA and is integrated within the host genome. HIV infects lymphocytes, macrophages, monocytes and dendritic cells, causing the majority of these immune cells to die. Over time, this triggers chronic immune activation and a subsequent immunodeficiency state.

The incubation period is two to four weeks, though it can be longer. Most children acquire HIV through vertical transmission, which may occur antenatally, perinatally or postnatally (via breast milk). Other modes of transmission include blood transfusion and sexual practice.

Presentation in newborns can be rapid, occurring in the first few months of life with *Pneumocystis jirovecii* pneumonia, lymphadenopathy, hepatosplenomegaly, encephalopathy, faltering growth, chronic diarrhoea, oral thrush, disseminated TB infection or lymphoid interstitial pneumonitis. Symptoms are often categorised by the CDC classification system shown in *Table 6*. Acquired Immunodeficiency Syndrome (AIDS), which is the final stage of HIV infection, occurs when the immune system becomes exhausted. The patient then becomes susceptible to a wide range of infections and malignancies.

Diagnosis involves first identifying HIV antibodies. HIV viral load and CD4 T lymphocyte count should also be established. Mothers are routinely screened for HIV in many countries, including the UK. Substantial progress has been made in preventing mother-to-child transmission of HIV (PMTCT) by improving coverage of antiretroviral therapy (ART) amongst pregnant women. In developed countries, PMTCT has virtually eliminated HIV in children.

Patients with HIV should commence antiretroviral therapy with at least three drugs from at least two different drug classes (e.g. a protease inhibitor, a non-nucleoside reverse transcriptase inhibitor and a nucleoside reverse transcriptase inhibitor) to maximise the likelihood of successful treatment. With highly active antiretroviral therapy (HAART), prevention of opportunistic infection with co-trimoxazole, immunisation and better nutrition, children are expected to reach adult life but with a slightly shorter life expectancy.

TABLE 6: Examples of symptoms of HIV infection		
CATEGORY A (mild)	CATEGORY B (moderate)	CATEGORY C (severe)
Lymphadenopathy.	Lymphoid interstitial pneumonitis.	Candidiasis.
Parotitis.	Chronic thrush.	Cryptococcosis.
Hepatosplenomegaly.	Chronic diarrhoea.	Cryptosporidiosis.
Dermatitis.	Persistent fever.	Encephalopathy.
Otitis media.	Hepatitis, nephropathy.	Malignancy.
Sinusitis.	Recurrent herpes simplex virus.	Pneumocystis pneumonia.
	Cardiomegaly.	Cerebral toxoplasmosis.

The management of children and adolescents with HIV is particularly challenging and a multi-disciplinary team approach is needed for diagnosis, disclosure to the child, maintaining adherence to ART and sexual health education.

BACTERIAL INFECTIONS

Staphylococcal Infections

Staphylococcus aureus is the main staphylococcal species responsible for causing disease. It commonly causes skin infections such as cellulitis, orbital cellulitis, abscesses and impetigo. As well as skin and soft tissue infections, *Staphylococcus aureus* can also cause invasive disease including osteomyelitis, septic arthritis, pneumonia, septicaemia and endocarditis. The organism can cause disease directly, but it is also capable of producing toxins which then act as superantigens. This causes a massive T-cell activation and cytokine release, which can cause toxic shock syndrome, food poisoning and toxic epidermal necrolysis (scalded skin syndrome).

Treatment depends on the site and severity of infection. Beta-lactam antibiotics, such as flucloxacillin, are the main treatment for methicillin-sensitive *Staphylococcus aureus* infections. Macrolides such as erythromycin, can be used if penicillin allergic. Glycopeptides, such as vancomycin, are effective against methicillin-resistant *Staphylococcus aureus* (MRSA).

Methicillin-Resistant
Staphylococcus Aureus

Healthcare-associated methicillin-resistant *Staphylococcus aureus* (MRSA) is a multi-resistant form of the organism. It is more common in patients in hospital or in a healthcare institution. Community-associated MRSA (CA-MRSA) tends to be found in young healthy people, who may be colonised with the organism rather than having active infection. CA-MRSA is usually not multi-drug resistant.

Streptococcal Infections

Many types of streptococcal organisms are known and they cause a wide range of infections. Like *Staphylococcus*, they can cause skin and soft tissue infections. However, they can also cause serious invasive diseases, including meningitis, toxic shock syndrome, and septicaemia.

Treatment depends on the disease, but will often be a penicillin. Pneumococcal vaccines are effective in reducing mortality and morbidity from pneumococcal infections and are being rolled out to developing countries with the help of an international organisation, Global Alliance for Vaccines and Immunization (GAVI).

Streptococcus pneumoniae

Streptococcus pneumoniae can cause mild infections such as otitis media, pharyngitis, conjunctivitis and sinusitis, but it can also cause very serious invasive disease including pneumonia, meningitis and sepsis. Although it is commonly carried as a commensal organism in the nasopharynx of healthy children, it can be spread to those at risk by respiratory droplet transmission. It is an encapsulated organism, and those at high risk include young infants, as well as children with hyposplenism, such as in sickle cell disease.

Group A β-haemolytic streptococcus

Group A β-haemolytic streptococcus, also known as *Streptococcus pyogenes*, most commonly causes pharyngitis (diagnosed through a throat swab), but can also cause severe invasive disease including necrotising fasciitis, toxic shock syndrome and bacteraemia. It also causes puerperal sepsis, scarlet fever and longer term effects post infection, such as rheumatic fever, post-streptococcal glomerulonephritis and paediatric autoimmune neuropsychiatric disorders associated with streptococcal infections (PANDAS).

Group B streptococcus (GBS)

Group B streptococcus (GBS) is a common commensal in the genital tract of women but can result in neonatal sepsis. Women who are known to be GBS positive should receive intrapartum antibiotics to decrease the risk of neonatal GBS disease.

Viridans streptococci

Viridans streptococci are commensal organisms that colonise oral, upper respiratory, gastrointestinal and female reproductive tracts, but can cause endocarditis, bacteraemia and meningitis. Treatment will depend on the disease and organism isolated, but will generally be with a penicillin.

Meningococcal Infections

Neisseria meningitidis is a gram negative diplococcus capable of causing severe infections such as meningitis and meningococcal septicaemia. It can cause infection very quickly so prompt diagnosis and treatment are imperative. The main serogroups are A, B, C, W and Y.

Meningococcus is carried in the nasopharynx of about 10% of healthy people, and is transmitted from person to person. It can then spread to the bloodstream and meninges. It causes infection most commonly in younger children, especially those under the age of 3 years.

Children may present with the classical signs of meningitis or septicaemia, with the characteristic non-blanching purpuric rash. Meningitis can occur with or without septicaemia and so the rash may not be present.

Diagnosis is made by blood culture, or CSF if meningitis is suspected. Blood may also be sent for meningococcal PCR. Treatment should be started empirically if septicaemia or meningitis are suspected, without waiting for results, and should be with a broad spectrum third generation cephalosporin such as IV ceftriaxone. Intensive care may be required. Meningococcal disease is a notifiable disease and Public Health should be informed and contact tracing undertaken.

Mortality is highest for meningococcal septicaemia whilst meningococcal meningitis alone has a better prognosis.

Vaccinations for serogroups A, B, C, W and Y are available and incorporated into the childhood immunisation schedule.

Lyme Disease

Lyme disease is caused by *Borrelia burgdorferi* and is acquired by tick bites. Ticks spread the infection by feeding on infected animals such as deer, and then pass on the infection to humans by a tick bite. There may be a history of camping or walking in a forest, although the actual tick bite may not have been noticed.

The typical lesion of erythema migrans (target lesion) can occur around the tick bite (*Figure 6*), along with fatigue, lymphadenopathy, myalgia, headache and fever. Neurological features, such as meningitis, facial palsy and cerebellar ataxia, can occur from 2 to 10 weeks after the tick bite. Arthritis, usually affecting the knee, can occur from one month to one year after the tick bite.

Diagnosis is confirmed via antibody testing. Treatment is started on suspicion of disease, without waiting for test results, as antibodies which are tested for may not be positive until six weeks after the tick bite. Lyme disease is usually treated with amoxicillin (or doxycycline in children over 12) for two to three weeks.

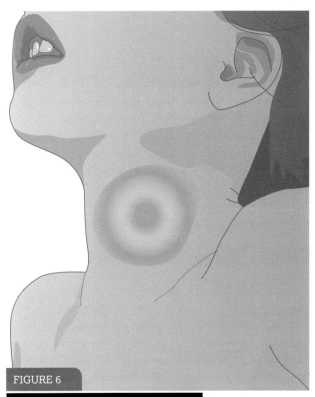

FIGURE 6

Target lesion in Lyme disease.

Typhoid

Typhoid is caused by *Salmonella typhi* and is a form of enteric fever. It initially manifests as abdominal symptoms, including pain and bloody diarrhoea, alongside constitutional symptoms such as fatigue and dizziness. Fever classically rises throughout the day and drops by the following morning. Spread is generally by consumption of faecally contaminated food or water. *Salmonella paratyphi* causes a similar but usually less severe disease called paratyphoid.

Diagnosis is by culturing the organism from faeces, blood or urine.

Treatment with a quinolone, such as ciprofloxacin, has been used for many years. However, increasing antibiotic resistance is being seen, and third generation cephalosporins such as ceftriaxone are now first line. Prevention is with improved sanitation and clean water, as well as vaccines.

Escherichia Coli (E. coli)

E. coli are gram-negative motile bacilli that can cause urinary tract infections (UTIs), enteric infections and disseminated infections, such as meningitis, sepsis and pneumonia. Enterohaemorrhagic *E. coli* (EHEC), usually serotype 0157, is also associated with haemolytic uraemic syndrome (HUS) (p308).

Diagnosis is by microscopy and culture. *E. coli* urine infections are usually treated with trimethoprim or amoxicillin, but severe infections will require IV antibiotics tailored to the antibiotic susceptibility pattern of the organism. However, for diarrhoea caused by *E. coli* 0157, antibiotics should be avoided as they may increase the risk of HUS by increasing the amount of toxin released.

Tuberculosis

Tuberculosis (TB) is caused by *Mycobacterium tuberculosis*. An important concept that can help understand the disease process of TB is exposure, infection and disease, which can be seen as a continuum. High risk reservoirs include immigrants, the poor, HIV-infected individuals and the elderly. One-third to two-thirds of children acquire TB after exposure to household contacts who have pulmonary TB as diagnosed by positive sputum. This can then lead to latent infection, which can be diagnosed by a reactive tuberculin skin test. However, children are more likely to develop active infection than adults.

Most patients are asymptomatic, although infants are more likely to have symptoms. Occasionally, low grade fever, mild cough and malaise can be seen that resolves in a week. Local infection in the lung occurs with hilar adenopathy. Most children develop pulmonary disease (p324). Extrapulmonary disease is often seen with erosion into the blood or lymph, causing miliary tuberculosis in the lungs, spleen, liver, bone marrow and brain. TB meningitis is the most deadly complication. Younger children with poor nutritional status who have not received the BCG vaccine are most at risk. A compromised immunological state, such as HIV infection, increases the risk of TB.

A variety of tests can be used for diagnosis (p324). Rapid tuberculosis diagnostic tests, based on nucleic acid amplification, are increasingly recognised as the gold standard, with newer tests able to pick up isoniazid and rifampicin resistance.

Similarly to adults, drug sensitive primary pulmonary TB in children is usually treated with a combination of rifampicin and isoniazid for 6 months, with the addition of pyrazinamide and ethambutol for the first 2 months. The treatment course for TB meningitis, disseminated TB or TB osteomyelitis usually lasts one year, while latent TB is treated with isoniazid for 9 months.

Chlamydia

Chlamydia trachomatis

Chlamydia trachomatis is probably best known for causing sexually transmitted infections (STIs), and can lead to pelvic inflammatory disease and subsequent infertility. However, it is also an important cause of neonatal pneumonia acquired from the maternal genital tract during delivery. It may also cause neonatal and adult conjunctivitis. Lymphogranuloma Venereum (LGV) describes small ulcers on the genitalia, followed by development of tender, enlarged inguinal lymph nodes called buboes. The last stage of LGV is characterized by rectovaginal fistula formation and strictures. It can also cause ocular trachoma, which is a chronic keratoconjunctivitis and commonly causes blindness in the developing world, where it may be endemic.

Diagnosis is via PCR on a *Chlamydia* conjunctival swab (eye infection) and/or urine nucleic acid amplification test (if genital infection is suspected in either the child or the parent).

Treatment is usually with doxycycline (for children over 12), azithromycin or erythromycin for trachoma and sexually transmitted infections. Neonatal infections, including conjunctivitis, require oral therapy, usually with erythromycin for two weeks.

Chlamydophila psittaci

Chlamydophila psittaci is a bacterium that infects birds and can be passed from unwell birds to humans, such as zoo and pet shop workers or those who keep birds as pets. It can present as fever, fatigue, cough, shortness of breath and headache. Treatment is with erythromycin in children or doxycycline in adults.

Chlamydophila pneumoniae

Chlamydophila pneumoniae is a cause of community acquired pneumonia, though most infections are mild. As above, it is treated with doxycycline or erythromycin.

Gonorrhoea

Gonorrhoea, an STI, is caused by *Neisseria gonorrhoeae*, a gram-negative diplococcus. Infection is transmitted to neonates as they pass through the birth canal during delivery. It most commonly causes eye infections with purulent discharge. If untreated, corneal ulceration and blindness can follow. Disseminated disease, such as meningitis or septic arthritis, occurs rarely. Diagnosis is by microscopy and swab culture and/or urine testing. Infection can be treated with a third generation cephalosporin.

PARASITIC INFECTIONS

Threadworm

Threadworm, also known as pinworm, is the colloquial term for *Enterobius vermicularis*, a form of parasitic worm that infects the large intestine. They are small white worms, 2 to 12 mm long, and as their name suggests, they look like small pieces of thread. They are common throughout the world, especially in young children. They live in the intestine and the pregnant female lays her eggs around the perianal and perineum region, generally at night. This causes the typical symptom of perianal itching at night, with restless sleep. The eggs can be transferred to bedding or clothes, or as the child scratches, the eggs can get under their fingernails and be transmitted to the mouth, resulting in auto-infection. Some children may remain asymptomatic.

Diagnosis is by collecting the worms from the perianal area using a cellotape slide and identification of the eggs by microscopy.

Treatment is with mebendazole or alternatively albendazole, and implementing strict hygiene measures. The whole family is likely to need treatment with a single dose to prevent ongoing infection.

Malaria

Malaria is caused by a protozoan called *Plasmodium* and is transmitted by the female *Anopheles* mosquito when taking a blood meal from humans. There are four types of the infection; *Plasmodium vivax, ovale, malariae* and *falciparum*.

Plasmodium falciparum often presents with severe disease and is responsible for most malaria-related deaths. Children typically present with fever, vomiting, headache, muscle aches and anorexia. In severe malaria, extensive infection of red blood cells can lead to multi-organ failure, which results in a clinical picture of impaired consciousness and respiratory distress.

Diagnosis is via thick and thin blood film assessment under a microscope. Thick film allows identification of malaria infection, whilst thin film allows more specific species identification. Antigen testing can be used if available.

Treatment for severe malaria often involves intensive care support. Artemisinin-based combination therapy has improved the outcome of children with uncomplicated or severe malaria, compared with older drugs such as chloroquine, sulfadoxine-pyrimethamine and quinine.

REFERENCES AND FURTHER READING

Immunisations

1   Demicheli V, Rivetti, A, Debalini MG, Di Pietrantonj, C. Vaccines for measles, mumps and rubella in children. Cochrane Database Syst Rev. 2012;2:CD004407.

2   Public Health England. MenB Vaccination: Introduction from September 2015. https://www.gov.uk/government/publications/menb-vaccination-introduction-from-1-september-2015.

3   Public Health England. Immunisation. 2015. www.gov.uk/government/collections/immunisation.

4   Glezen WP. Universal influenza vaccination and live attenuated influenza vaccination of children. Pediatr Infect Dis J. 2008;27(10 Suppl):S104-9.

5   WHO. Estimated Hib and pneumococcal deaths for children under 5 years of age. 2013. http://www.who.int/immunization/monitoring_surveillance/burden/estimates/Pneumo_hib/en.

6   WHO. Immunization, Vaccines and Biologicals. http://www.who.int/immunization/en.

Infection

1   NICE CG160. Feverish Illness in Children. 2013. https://www.nice.org.uk/guidance/cg160.

2   Perry RT, Halsey NA. The clinical significance of measles: a review. JInfectDis. 2004; 189 Suppl 1:S4-16.

3   Measles pneumonitis following measles-mumps-rubella vaccination of a patient with HIV infection. 1993. MMWR Wkly Rep. 1996; 45:603-6.

4   Centers for Disease Control and Prevention. 1993. Revised classification system for HIV infection and expanded surveillance case definition for AIDS among adolescents and adults. MMWR Recomm Rep. 1992; 41(RR-17):1-19.

5   Affronti M et al. Low-grade fever: how to distinguish organic from non-organic forms. Int J Clin Pract. 2010; 64:316-21.

6   Bleeker-Rovers CP, Vos FJ, de Kleijn EM, et al. A prospective multicenter study on fever of unknown origin: the yield of a structured diagnostic protocol. Medicine. 2007; 86:26-38.

7   Chow A, Robinson JL. Fever of unknown origin in children: a systematic review. World J Pediatr. 2011; 7:5-10.

8   Cohen JI. Herpes Zoster. New Engl J Med. 2013; 369:255-63.

9   Smith JG, Wiethoff CM, Stewart PL, Nemerow GR. Adenovirus. Curr Top Microbiol Immunol. 2010; 343:195-224.

10   WHO. HIV/AIDS Programmes. 2014. http://www.who.int/entity/hiv/data/en.

11   Young NS, Brown KE. Parvovirus B19. New Engl J Med. 2004; 350:586-97.

12   Kotzbauer D, Andresen D, Doelling N, Shore S. Clinical and laboratory characteristics of central nervous system herpes simplex virus infection in neonates and young infants. Pediatr Infect Dis J. 2014; 33:1187-9.

13   WHO. Global tuberculosis report. Tuberculosis. 2014. http://apps.who.int/iris/bitstream/10665/137094/1/9789241564809_eng.pdf?ua=1.

14   WHO. World Malaria Report. Malaria. 2014. http://apps.who.int/iris/bitstream/10665/144852/2/9789241564830_eng.pdf?ua=1.

15   Centers for Disease Control and Prevention. www.cdc.gov.

16   Public Health England. Guidance on infection control in schools and other childcare settings. 2014. https://www.gov.uk/government/publications/infection-control-in-schools-poster.

17   Servey JT, Reamy BV, Hodge J. Clinical presentations of parvovirus B19 infection. American Family Physician. 2007; 75:373-376.

18   Biesbroeck L, Sidbury R. Viral exanthems: an update. Dermatol Ther. 2013; 26:433-8.

19   WHO. Measles. 2015. http://www.who.int/mediacentre/factsheets/fs286/en.

20   Public Health England. Immunisation against infectious disease. 2014. https://www.gov.uk/government/collections/immunisation-against-infectious-disease-the-green-book.

21   Alter SJ, Vidwan NK, Sobande PO, Omoloja A, Bennett, JS. Common childhood bacterial infections. Curr Probl Pediatr Adolesc Health Care. 2011. 41:256-83.

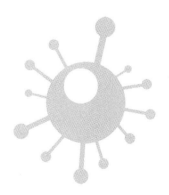

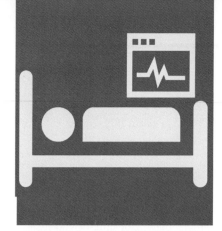

1.12
INTENSIVE CARE
KUNAL BABLA AND SAM THENABADU

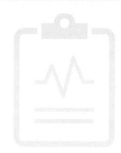

CONTENTS

INTRODUCTION

Intensive care is suitable for patients with potentially recoverable life-threatening conditions who would benefit from more detailed observation, treatment and technological support than is available in general wards or high dependency facilities. Complex monitoring equipment is available (*Table 1*), as well as more advanced interventions. It is also recognised that end-of-life management, including potential organ donation and family bereavement care are integral to caring for critically ill children.

The paediatric intensive care unit serves the most unwell children, who present with a range of both common and rare clinical conditions. The caseload varies throughout the year but will include a mix of emergency medical, surgical and trauma cases from both within the designated paediatrics hospital and the paediatric transfer team from the regional hospitals it supports. Certain planned surgeries may require a high level of airway support or monitoring post-operatively and may also command the need for ICU beds.

The clinician's priorities, at the bare minimum, involve:
› Regimented airway management and ventilator support.
› Cardiovascular monitoring, invasive circulatory support, with renal assessment and close fluid management.

In addition, assessment of the child's nutrition, microbiology, radiology, and invasive lines and resuscitation status are all carefully considered on a daily basis.

It is important for the paediatric intensive care unit (PICU) team to remember that as well as delivering high-quality medical care, the team must involve the child's family in the care plan. This places heavy emphasis on clear and effective communication on all aspects of their child's care. This can often involve difficult conversations about how unwell a child is or even when it might be appropriate to consider palliative care. The PICU clinician should be sensitive to a family's wishes and views on their child's care.

TABLE 1: Monitoring equipment that is commonly used in the PICU setting

Central venous line.	• Allows venous access to large, central veins. Allows measurement of central venous pressure. Also allows measurement of central venous saturation, which can be useful in monitoring balance between oxygen delivery and consumption at a tissue level.
Cerebral function monitoring.	• Monitors electrical activity in the brain, and can give indications about seizure activity over a period of hours to days.
End-tidal CO_2 monitoring.	• Measures the amount of expired CO_2, and gives an indication of the efficacy of ventilation.
Heart monitor.	• Gives information such as heart rate, and morphology of ECG in one lead (e.g. lead II).
Invasive blood pressure (Arterial line).	• Makes beat-to-beat blood pressure readings. The arterial line also allows repeated blood sampling.
Non-Invasive blood pressure.	• Makes "spot-check" blood pressure measurements with a cuff.
Pulse oximetry.	• Gives information about oxygen saturation.
Urinary catheter.	• Allows accurate measurement of urine output.

ADMISSION TO PICU

Early escalation of concerns to paediatric seniors is important in any setting, and involvement of the PICU and retrieval teams at an early juncture is crucial. Retrieval teams provide mobile intensive care to allow safe transfer of the acutely unwell child. Transfer to PICU can be from a local general hospital (ED or ward) or from tertiary units dealing with children with more complex pathology.

Definitive referral criteria to PICU does not exist and specific features for referral are often pathology-dependent. Common pathologies are shown in *Table 2*. Discussion with the PICU team can provide forewarning for them of the sick patient and thus put them on "their radar", as well as allowing the treating clinicians some early specialist advice on management.

Some generic areas should be considered for all sick children when considering referral:

➤ Does this child's condition have the potential for acute deterioration?
➤ Can the resources locally support the acuity of the child's illness?
➤ Are there physiological observations that are not responding to treatments that now need high dependency/intensive care level monitoring and interventions?

TABLE 2: Common pathologies in PICU

System	Case examples
Cardiac.	Post cardiac arrest, severe shock, dysrhythmias.
Respiratory.	Bronchiolitis, asthma, sepsis.
Neurological.	Seizures, head trauma, meningitis, post-operative.
Renal.	Acute kidney injury, electrolyte imbalance.
Metabolic.	Diabetic ketoacidosis, severe electrolyte imbalance, inborn errors of metabolism.
Haematology / Oncology.	Sickle crises complications (acute chest crisis), tumour lysis syndrome, compressive tumours, neutropenic sepsis.
Surgical.	Post-operative, e.g. cardiac, ENT and spinal surgeries.
Multi system.	Multi-organ failure, toxicology related, e.g. tricyclic antidepressant overdose.
Trauma.	Polytrauma.

The PICU team will always make the following four decisions:

1 Is review or retrieval necessary?
2 How urgent is this review?
3 What priority does this child take?
4 What advice should be given in regards to immediate interventions and treatments by the referring team?

Decisions to admit and retrieve patients should involve the PICU consultant.

AIRWAY

The deteriorating patient must be managed in a systematic ABCDE approach, and the airway is the starting point for this.

A child's airway can be managed using several methods. These range from basic to more advanced methods for critically ill children and include:

➤ **Airway opening manoeuvres.** Head tilt, chin lift and jaw thrust.
➤ **Oropharyngeal airway (Guedel).** This stops the tongue from occluding the airway and allows non-invasive (bag-valve-mask) ventilation to be performed.
➤ **Nasopharyngeal airway.** This is similar to an oropharyngeal airway in purpose but is inserted via the nose not mouth.
➤ **Laryngeal mask airway.** This sits above the vocal cords and allows provision of positive pressure ventilation (with a ventilator or bag-valve). This is **not** an alternative to endotracheal intubation, as it does not protect the airway below the vocal cords.
➤ **Endotracheal tube.** This offers definitive airway protection, allowing for a range of invasive ventilation techniques to be performed.
➤ **Tracheostomy.** This facilitates long-term ventilation. It is usually (but not always) an elective procedure. The tube is placed through the anterior wall of the trachea and sits below the cords, providing a definitive airway.

167

BREATHING

It is important to remember basic principles when trying to understand the concepts of ventilation. Ventilation has two basic aims: to deliver oxygen and to remove carbon dioxide.

It is useful to understand that mechanical ventilation is different from normal breathing, as it is positive pressure ventilation. This means oxygen is pushed into the lungs by the ventilator rather than pulled in by the negative intrathoracic pressure generated in normal inspiration. Expiration is still largely dependent on elastic recoil or patient effort.

A number of parameters can be adjusted on a ventilator to manipulate oxygen delivery and carbon dioxide clearance. These are summarised in *Table 3* and *Figure 1*.

Oxygenation

Oxygen delivery is controlled by the Mean Airway Pressure (MAP), which is indicative of how hard oxygen is being pushed in, and the Fraction of Inspired Oxygen (FiO_2). Oxygen delivery is directly related to the mean airway pressure and FiO_2. The mean airway pressure can be manipulated by changing:

1 Positive End Expiratory Pressure (PEEP). What is the pressure at the end of expiration? The higher this value is, the greater the MAP.
2 Peak Inspiratory Pressure (PIP). What is the peak pressure during inspiration? The higher this value is, the greater the MAP.
3 Inspiration Time (Ti). How long is each inspiration? The longer this is, the shorter the relative expiratory phase (which is lower pressure), and therefore the greater the MAP.

Ventilation (carbon dioxide clearance)

Carbon dioxide clearance is governed by minute volume. This is the amount of air entering (and exiting) the lungs each minute. It is a product of the tidal volume and respiratory rate:

Minute volume = tidal volume x respiratory rate.

Therefore, the higher the tidal volume and the higher the respiratory rate, the greater the carbon dioxide clearance. Tidal volume is most sensitive to increasing the PIP, but can also be increased by increasing the Ti, or decreasing the PEEP.

Non-Invasive Ventilation

Non-invasive ventilation allows ventilator support, but in a patient that is able to breathe spontaneously, without airway support. Therefore the patient does not require intubation, and support can be delivered through a facemask.

The two most commonly used types are:

> CPAP (Continuous Positive Airway Pressure). PEEP is delivered to the patient continuously, through both inspiration and expiration, with the respiratory rate and Ti being fully patient dependent.
> BiPAP (Biphasic Positive Airway Pressure). The ventilator delivers PIP and PEEP at set levels dependent on the patient's efforts.

Invasive Ventilation

In the more unwell child, invasive ventilation may be required. This allows control of more than just the PIP and PEEP, meaning a much greater degree of respiratory support can be offered. For all forms of invasive ventilation, intubation is mandatory. A tracheostomy is required for long-term invasive ventilation.

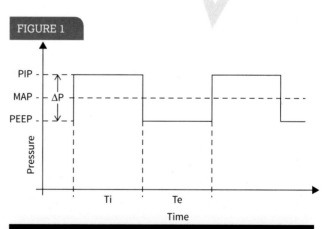

FIGURE 1

The basic parameters of ventilation. Ti=inspiratory time, Te=expiratory time, PIP=Peak Inspiratory Pressure, PEEP=Positive End Expiratory Pressure, MAP= Mean Airway Pressure, ΔP=Change in pressure with each breath.

TABLE 3: Key parameters that are defined by ventilators			
Parameter	Definition	Effect of increasing parameter	
PIP.	Peak Inspiratory Pressure: Highest pressure achieved during inspiration	⇑⇑⇑ oxygenation.	⇑⇑⇑ CO_2 clearance.
PEEP.	Positive End-Expiratory Pressure: Minimal pressure achieved during expiration	⇑⇑⇑ oxygenation.	↓CO_2 clearance.
MAP.	Mean Airway Pressure: Average pressure in airway	⇑⇑⇑ oxygenation.	⇑⇑ CO_2 clearance.
Ti.	Inspiratory time	⇑⇑⇑ oxygenation.	Little effect.
FiO_2.	Fraction of inspired oxygen	⇑⇑⇑ oxygenation.	No effect.
Rate.	Respiratory Rate	Little effect.	⇑⇑⇑ CO_2 clearance.

Examples of invasive ventilation options include:

> **Controlled mandatory ventilation.** This involves the ventilator completely taking over the child's breathing. It controls when the patient breathes, how fast they breathe, and how they breathe. Often the child is sedated and/or paralysed during this to stop them fighting the machine.

> **Patient triggered ventilation.** This involves the ventilator attempting to synchronise with the patient's own breathing, meaning it supports breaths already happening, rather than taking over breathing completely. It is therefore more physiological than controlled mandatory ventilation. The safety net in this mode is that a minimum breathing rate is set: if the child doesn't breathe enough times, extra breaths are given by the machine.

CIRCULATION

Circulatory compromise is a common feature of the patients on PICU. This can be due to a range of pathologies such as dehydration and blood loss, through to septic, cardiogenic, anaphylactic or neurogenic shock. Circulatory compromise due to most of these aetiologies can present with classic signs and symptoms of oliguria, confusion, cool clammy peripheries, tachycardia, tachypnoea and a metabolic acidosis. A failure to address these issues will lead to tissue hypoperfusion, hypoxia and eventually cell death. The use of fluid boluses and vasoactive drugs can support circulation and achieve tissue perfusion.

The management of the circulation can be best understood by briefly considering the physiology of preload, afterload and contractility, and from there, the vasoactive drugs that act on these factors.

> **Preload.** The tension in the ventricular wall at the end of diastole—the "stretch" (Frank-Starling mechanism).

> **Afterload.** The tension in the left ventricular wall required to push blood into the aorta—the "squeeze".

> **Contractility.** The intrinsic ability for the heart to adapt to the pre- and afterload. Acidosis, hypoxaemia and electrolyte imbalance all affect this.

Adequate fluid resuscitation should always be initiated before vasoactive drugs are considered. The common vasopressors and inotropes are catecholamines. Dopamine, noradrenaline and adrenaline are naturally occurring, but synthetic drugs such as dobutamine are also available (*Table 4*). It is important to remember that each of these agents has a varying effect upon alpha-1, beta-1 and beta-2 receptors, so the area that requires most focus needs identifying to deploy the correct treatments (*Figure 2*).

Establishing Vascular Access

Circulatory support will require good intravenous access. Two functioning venous access points are essential in the first instance. Dopamine can be started peripherally without the need to wait for central access. This can allow circulatory support and control to be achieved and buy time for PICU retrieval teams to arrive and transfer to PICU to be arranged. Central lines and arterial lines are useful but should not delay starting therapies.

TABLE 4: Vasoactive drugs			
Drug	**Receptors**	**Actions**	**Major Side Effects**
Noradrenaline.	• Predominantly alpha 1 and, to a lesser extent, beta 1 and 2.	• Increases perfusion pressure (by increasing systemic vascular resistance).	• Reduces renal perfusion. • Cardiac ischaemia. • Arrhythmias. • Digital ischaemia.
Adrenaline.	• Predominantly alpha 1, but greater affinity to beta 1/2 receptors than noradrenaline.	• Increases heart rate, stroke volume and cardiac output. • Increases perfusion pressure (by increasing systemic vascular resistance).	• Arrhythmias. • Cardiac ischaemia. • Sudden cardiac death.
Dopamine.	• Predominantly alpha 1 (higher doses), and dopamine receptor D_1 (lower doses).	• Increases perfusion pressure (by increasing systemic vascular resistance). • D_1 receptor stimulation results in selective vasodilation in renal, mesenteric, cerebral and coronary beds.	• Arrhythmias.
Dobutamine.	• Beta 1 and 2 activity. Has some alpha 1 activity, particularly at higher doses.	• Increases heart rate and cardiac output. • Vasodilation and reduces systemic vascular resistance (at lower doses).	• Tachycardia. • Arrhythmias. • Cardiac ischaemia.
Milrinone.	• Inhibits breakdown of cAMP in cardiac/vascular smooth muscle.	• Increases cardiac output and reduces systemic vascular resistance.	• Hypotension. • Arrhythmia. • Cardiac ischaemia.
Vasopressin.	• V1 receptor (vascular smooth muscle), V2 receptor (renal collecting ducts).	• Increases systemic vascular resistance by reducing fluid loss via the kidneys, and by vasoconstriction.	• Arrhythmia. • Hypertension. • Cardiac ischaemia. • Peripheral ischaemia.

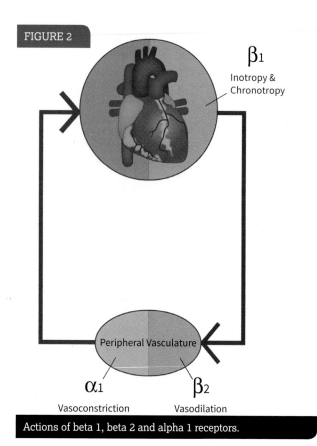

FIGURE 2

β_1

Inotropy & Chronotropy

Peripheral Vasculature

α_1

Vasoconstriction

β_2

Vasodilation

Actions of beta 1, beta 2 and alpha 1 receptors.

TABLE 5: Indicators of abnormal fluid balance	
Dehydration	**Fluid Overload**
• Tachypnoea/Increasing oxygen requirements. • Tachycardia. • Hypotension. • Reduced skin turgor. • Sunken eyes / fontanelle. • Increased capillary refill time. • Weak pulses. • Cool peripheries. • Reduced urine output.	• Tachypnoea/Increasing oxygen requirements. • Oedema. • Crackles on auscultation of chest. • Disproportionate weight gain.

> A raised urea or creatinine can indicate dehydration.

> Often, in younger children and babies, raised serum sodium can be a sensitive marker for dehydration.

> It is useful to consider the child's nutritional status and monitor protein and albumin levels. Hypoalbuminaemia can contribute significantly to oedema due to loss of the intravascular oncotic pressure.

Fluid imbalances may require a change to the amount/type of fluid being given to the child, and in some cases, a fluid bolus (5–20 mL/kg of fluid, usually 0.9% sodium chloride, given rapidly), or a diuretic agent may be required to regain some balance.

FLUID MANAGEMENT

It is important to keep tight control of fluid management in the critically ill child. A combination of maintenance fluids and boluses are used. Infusions of medication can contribute significantly to the daily fluid input for a child on PICU. In addition, tight control of electrolytes, particularly sodium, potassium, calcium and magnesium is necessary. This can be controlled by manipulating the content of parenteral nutrition, by adding electrolytes into the maintenance fluid or by giving oral supplements. Maintaining appropriate blood glucose levels in children is essential. For this reason, most maintenance fluids will contain dextrose, with the most common choice being 0.9% sodium chloride with 5% dextrose. The dextrose content can be increased if required.

Monitoring Fluid Balance

When managing fluids for a critically ill child, it is important to assess the potential fluid requirements before deciding on how much fluid to give. This should be done using both bedside clinical assessment and blood tests (*Table 5*).

Potential sources of loss of fluid in the dehydrated patient are important to consider. For example, there may be vomiting, or increased stoma losses in the surgical patient, or increased losses via a nasogastric tube in an ileus. Significant insensible losses can be made in patients with significant respiratory distress who are tachypnoeic.

Blood tests can also be useful when considering a child's fluid balance:

RENAL REPLACEMENT THERAPY

In some children with poor renal function, poor biochemical markers, persistent poor urine output or difficulties in maintaining adequate fluid balance, renal replacement therapy may be required. This is often to provide two functions:

> Filtration and removal of the waste products or toxins from the bloodstream that a normally functioning kidney would filter.

> Fluid and electrolyte balance control of the child.

Two main methods are available for providing renal replacement therapy: peritoneal dialysis and haemofiltration.

Peritoneal Dialysis

Peritoneal dialysis is a commonly used method of renal replacement therapy in babies, as it does not require invasive vascular access. It also does not result in the removal of large volumes of blood required with a haemofiltration circuit.

A catheter is inserted into the abdomen, with one lumen being used to instil dialysis fluid into the abdomen and the other to remove the used fluid containing the waste products.

Once the dialysis fluid is instilled, it is left for a time to allow molecules to diffuse across the peritoneum, which acts as a partially permeable membrane. The fluid is then drained and replaced for the next "cycle". The dialysis effect can be manipulated by adjusting the content of the dialysis fluid, in order to modify the diffusion gradients, or by changing the time ("dwell time") the fluid remains in the abdomen.

A strict record of fluid input and output is kept in order to monitor the efficacy of the dialysis. Blood tests are regularly performed to monitor the electrolyte balance and renal function.

Haemofiltration

This method of renal replacement therapy is used more commonly in older children, as well as in adults. It relies on blood flow through a machine that filters waste products and toxins before returning the blood to the patient. It requires invasive vascular access.

ANALGESIA AND SEDATION

The classic triad of anaesthesia—analgesia, sedation and muscle relaxation—is also essential in the PICU setting. Medications are often similar to those used in an adult setting; however, the duration, quantity and pharmacokinetic effects upon the child pose different challenges. Drug tolerance, toxicity and withdrawal remain key issues that the PICU clinician must consider in all children. Beyond the theatre, continuation of muscle relaxation and paralysis may also be required to prevent children fighting against the ventilators.

Certain medications, such as morphine, will be primarily administered for analgesic qualities but will also have an effect upon sedation. Ketamine is a good example of a drug that has sedative as well as analgesic and, to an extent, muscle relaxant qualities. These examples highlight the attention required to ensure an effective balance of treatments.

Analgesia

All unwell children require accurate pain score assessment. Analgesia can be both pharmacological and non-pharmacological (*Table 6*). A pain ladder approach should still be used and a range of analgesic options, from simple analgesia to complex mixes of patient controlled analgesia, are possible. Equally important is the reassessment of pain using subjective patient responses, and objective physiological parameters such as heart rate and respiratory rate, where possible.

Sedation

The level can vary from conscious sedation, where a child can obey commands, and deep sedation, where the child will not respond to commands, to general anaesthesia where airway patency is lost. Intravenous sedation can be delivered incrementally to optimise the level of sedation required. Unlike the adult ICU setting, propofol is not routinely used in children as it is associated with metabolic acidosis, cardiac failure and rhabdomyolysis.

A range of sedation agents are available and oral sedatives such as chloral hydrate and trimerazine (Vallergan) are used for procedures both on wards and the PICU (*Table 7*).

PICU patients on longer periods of sedation are at risk of developing tolerance and subsequent withdrawal effects. Midazolam remains a commonly used maintenance sedative, but withdrawal symptoms can develop in one-third of patients,

TABLE 6: Analgesia	
Non Pharmacological	
Parents.	To offer familiarity and comfort.
Touch.	Therapeutic touch – passive and active massage.
Music.	Familiar rhymes, classical music.
Play.	Play therapists.
Pharmacological	
Simple Analgesia.	NSAIDs.
	Paracetamol.
Opioids.	Morphine.
	Fentanyl – 100 times more potent than morphine.
	Remifentanil – short acting.
Patient Controlled Analgesia.	Maintenance with bolus doses. Children > 7yrs.
Regional Anaesthesia.	Local anaesthetic.

TABLE 7: Sedative agents	
Sedative agents	**Comments**
Chloral and triclofos.	Purely sedative drug that is enterally absorbed.
Antihistamines, e.g. trimeprazine and promethazine.	Antihistamines with sedating properties.
Benzodiazepines, e.g. midazolam.	Sedative, anticonvulsant and anxiolytic but with no analgesic qualities.
Barbiturates, e.g. thiopentone.	Older drugs that caused global CNS depression; now largely replaced by benzodiazepines.
Ketamine.	Dissociative anaesthesia (giving a sense of detachment from the body/personal world).

e.g. agitation, vomiting, tachycardia, tremor. Strategies to reduce withdrawal include alternating the type of drug used, sedation "holidays" and looking to switch to oral agents where possible.

NUTRITION

Enteral Nutrition

Enteral nutrition remains the preferred method of feeding as long as the gut is functioning. Early commencement of feeds within 24 hours has benefits, such as:

> Maintenance of gut integrity.
> Decreased infection rates.
> Enhanced immune function.
> Reduced length of stay on PICU.

171

Contraindications to initiating feeds would include a bowel obstruction, confirmed necrotising enterocolitis (NEC) and an ischaemic gut.

Assessing gastric residual volumes at set time intervals can determine ongoing success. A system of bolus feeds can be utilised (i.e. giving a bolus every X hours) unless high volume aspirates are seen. At that point, a change to a slower continuous infusion may be better tolerated.

Parenteral Nutrition

If enteral feeds are not possible, parenteral nutrition should be started. Close communication with the dietician and pharmacists is required and a dedicated intravenous central line is mandatory. Close monitoring of thiamine levels and electrolytes, including potassium, magnesium and phosphate, is needed. If significant abnormalities are found, feeds should be stopped and parameters corrected before restarting, as "refeeding syndrome" can occur.

DISCHARGE CRITERIA

There are no set discharge criteria and each patient is assessed individually. Key areas to consider are the following:
1 Stable objective haemodynamic parameters.
2 Stable respiratory status (patient extubated with stable arterial blood gases) and ongoing airway patency.
3 Minimal oxygen requirements.
4 No further requirement for inotropic support, vasodilators and antiarrhythmic drugs.
5 Cardiac arrhythmias are controlled.
6 Neurological stability with control of seizures.
7 All haemodynamic monitoring catheters are removed.

The majority of children will step down to ward-level care. Some units within themselves will have intensive care and high dependency unit level beds and this interim step can be utilised. A few children may be discharged to outpatient ambulatory care, but this depends upon geographical provision.

WITHDRAWING OR WITHHOLDING CARE

Sometimes difficult decisions must be made about limiting or withdrawing life-sustaining treatment. These decisions should be made sensitively, in partnership with the child's family. Conversations about withdrawal or limiting care will remain in the parents' memories for many years. As such, it is imperative that they are held in a sensitive and professional manner. Discussions on withholding care are best done in a clinic setting whilst a child is stable, so that a clear plan for a ceiling of care is in place before any acute deterioration. Withdrawal of care is a much more delicate subject, as the initiation of therapy implied that there was initially some hope of progress.

The Royal College of Paediatrics and Child Health has produced guidance on when withdrawing or withholding care is appropriate:

1 When life is limited in quantity. If treatment is unlikely or unable to prolong life.
2 When life is limited in quality. If treatment may prolong life, but prove too much of a burden, or not improve symptoms.
3 Informed competent refusal of treatment. An older child with an understanding of their illness and treatments may repeatedly and competently consent to withdrawal or withholding of treatment. In these circumstances, with the support of parents, there is no obligation on the medical team to provide treatment.

There may be situations that do not fit into any of the above headings. Nonetheless, a discussion with the child and their family is important to help make a decision about the child's care. There may also be situations where the medical team and the child's family disagree about what is in the best interest of the child. These are always extremely difficult situations, which should be managed sensitively. Ethical and legal guidance may be required in order for a clear decision to be reached. It is important to remember that any decision made about a child's care should always be in their best interest, and where possible, to include the child in that process. Finally, with withdrawal of care, it is important to incorporate palliative treatment to ensure maximisation of quality of life.

REFERENCES AND FURTHER READING

Airway and Ventilation
1 Barry P, Morris K, Ali T. Oxford Specialist Handbooks in Paediatrics: Paediatric Intensive Care. First Edition. Oxford: Oxford University Press; 2010.

Inotropes
1 Garg S, Singhal S, Sharma P, Jha AA. Inotropes and Vasopressors Review of Physiology and Clinical Use. J Pulmon Resp Med. 2012; 2:128.

Fluid Management and Renal Replacement Therapy
1 Great Ormond Street Hospital. Peritoneal dialysis: Information for families. 2013 http://www.gosh.nhs.uk/medical-information-0/procedures-and-treatments/peritoneal-dialysis.

Withdrawing or Withholding Care
1 Larcher, V. et al., 2015. Making decisions to limit treatment in life-limiting and life-threatening conditions in children: a framework for practice. Archives of Disease in Childhood, 100(Suppl 2), pp.s1–s23. Available at: http://adc.bmj.com/cgi/doi/10.1136/archdischild-2014-306666.

Retrieval
1 South Thames Retrieval Service PICU guidelines. http://www.strs.nhs.uk/homepage.aspx.

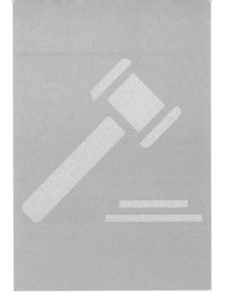

1.13
CHILDREN AND THE LAW

ZESHAN QURESHI

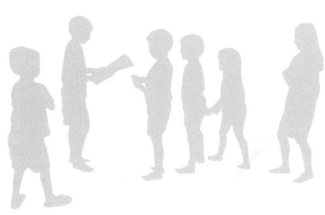

INTRODUCTION

Children are a vulnerable group and may not be able to represent their own wishes. Governments therefore place significant emphasis on making sure children's rights are protected and that their needs are adequately represented. This section will predominantly reflect law in England and Wales, but the underlying principles are more universal.

Children's rights are enshrined in the United Nations Convention on the Rights of the Child, which states:

> Actions taken concerning a child must have their best interests as a primary consideration.

> If the child can voice their opinion, they should be able to express it freely.

> The child's view should be given due weight (based on age and maturity).

In the UK, the Children Act 2004 states that the welfare of the child is paramount, and all professionals dealing with children have the duty to put the child at the centre of their actions. Similar legislation exists across the world.

Incorporating Multiple Viewpoints

In making decisions for children, one should try to incorporate the views of:

> The child. This includes both previously expressed beliefs and current wishes. Someone under 16-years-old may be deemed to have capacity, but even if they do not, their wishes and beliefs must be taken into account, as far as it is in their interests to do so.

> The child's parents. They may provide valuable insight into their child's wishes, beliefs and normal behaviour. Looking at the cultural background of the child and speaking to friends and other relatives may help as well in this regard.

> The multidisciplinary team. This will include nurses, physiotherapists, school teachers and any other professionals involved in the child's care.

Other sources of information include:

> Legally appointed representatives. Child independent advocates may be appointed to represent the child's best interests; in England and Wales, the Child and Family Court Advisory and Support Service (CAFCASS) provides guardians and advocates to represent the child in court.

> Specialist doctors. Many hospitals will have a lead named professional for safeguarding (child protection doctor).

These sources of information should be used where appropriate when making a clinical decision in the interests of the child. However, difficulties arise on a number of levels. Which sources of information are relevant in each case? How is weight apportioned between different sources of information when they conflict?

It is also important to make a decision only if necessary, and any decision should be the least restrictive in the long term. If the decision can be put off until the child has capacity, without significant harm (for example, if a child did not want to be circumcised), then deferral should be considered.

Making the Final Decision

The clinician should take into account what is in the best interests of the child, considering the physical, social, emotional and psychological benefits, and weighing up:

> The patient's wishes and ability to understand.
> The patient's physical and emotional needs.
> The risk of harm or suffering for the patient.
> The effectiveness of treatment, alternative options, risks and benefits.
> The implications for the family.
> Religious and cultural issues.

CONSENT

Consent can be obtained from:

> The child, if they have capacity.
> Someone with parental responsibility.
> A court.

In England and Wales, children who are 16 to 17-years-old (young people) are presumed to have capacity. By contrast, preschool age children, apart from making the most basic decisions, are unlikely to have the ability to truly understand the implications of medical decision making. In the group in between, up to their 16th birthday, a child with capacity is referred to as being "Gillick Competent" and, although parental involvement is still encouraged, the child can legitimately say "yes" to medical treatment without parental involvement. However, in contrast to the law for adults, children of any age, with or without capacity, are almost always prevented from refusing life-saving therapy (e.g. a blood transfusion after a large bleed); in these circumstances, if there is time, a legal opinion from a court is needed. Generally, competent children are allowed to refuse non-life-saving elective treatment

(e.g. circumcision), and they do so very frequently. The law varies from country to country, but the broad principles are similar.

Assessing Capacity

When assessing capacity, the assessment should be decision specific. If an individual is unable to consent to an appendicectomy, that does not necessarily mean that they cannot consent to taking the necessary accompanying pain relief. They may understand the risks and benefits of medication, but not those of surgery.

To establish their capacity, children should be able to:

1 Understand and retain the information given to them. It is useful to ask the patient to repeat back the information given to them. The patient could also be asked to explain what they believe the consequences of their decision will be.

2 Show evidence of reason and deliberation, acting on a set of consistent and clear values. An individual may legitimately refuse to give consent to a particular treatment, even though refusal might seem unwise or irrational to their doctor.

3 Act free of coercion. A patient's expressed opinion may differ when family members are in the same room, or after speaking to a relative. Coercion may also occur from medical staff. The occurrence of coercion may be difficult to assess. If an individual fully understands the facts and provides a logical argument for what they have proposed, it can be difficult to tell if it is not their true desire.

4 Communicate the decision they have made. This is relevant in the case of patients with learning difficulties, including language or sensory problems.

If the child meets the criteria above, they have proved that they are Gillick Competent.

Treating Children and Young People without Parental Knowledge

Trying to involve parents in medical decisions affecting their children is important, even if the child has capacity. Children will usually present to the primary care physician with the parents; however, for some issues, such as asking for an abortion or for contraception, the competent young person may not want their parents to know about their visit. In England and Wales, although the clinician should try to persuade the child or young person to inform their parents, such treatment is lawful based on the child's sole consent.

The Fraser guidelines (which were formulated in the context of reproductive decision making) stated that contraception could be prescribed without informing the parents providing that the child meets all the criteria below:

1 The child is competent to provide consent.

2 The child cannot be persuaded to inform their parents.

3 The child is likely to have sex regardless of whether they are given contraceptive treatment.

4 It is in the child's best interests to receive contraception, and if they do not receive it, their physical or mental health are likely to suffer.

PARENTAL RESPONSIBILITY

When children lack capacity, decisions have to be made on their behalf. In England and Wales, those with parental responsibility have the duty to make these decisions. Parental responsibility (or its equivalent) will be conferred in a variety of ways in different jurisdictions, but in England and Wales, it is acquired by:

▷ Mother and married father, or an unmarried father if he is on the birth certificate (since December 2003).

▷ Those that have entered into a "Parental Responsibility Agreement" with the mother of the child.

▷ Those that have been granted a "Parental Responsibility Order" (PRO) from the courts.

▷ Legal guardians of the child.

▷ Local authorities (in some circumstances).

A parent surrenders their parental responsibility if their child is adopted, and loses it automatically when their child reaches adulthood. It is shared with local authority if the child is taken into local authority care. People who care for a child (e.g. step parents/ grandparents) may consent if they share parental responsibility with the parents. However, doctors should make sure treatment is in line with parental wishes, especially if it involves a controversial/ important decision.

CHILDREN AND PARENTS REFUSING TREATMENT

It is important to remember that, in exceptional circumstances, treatment can be given without consent.

Consider the following:

▷ Does the child need treatment now? Possibly, there is no immediate need to act and no significant harm is associated with delaying treatment whilst resolving a disagreement with the child or parents. Administering a whooping cough vaccine would be an example.

▷ If the child is under 16-years-old and lacks Gillick competence, and treatment is immediately necessary, consent should first be sought from an individual with parental responsibility. However, if this fails, treatment may proceed in the child's best interests if serious harm would otherwise arise.

▷ If time permits, authorisation for treatment should be sought from the courts, but only after all attempts to resolve the disagreement over treatment have failed. For instance, if the family is refusing to allow their child to have a blood transfusion, can the child be treated in another manner? Can consent be obtained with further discussion? Is there someone else with parental responsibility that can be contacted? Failing this, a clinician may apply for a court order (In England and Wales, a "Specific Issue Order").

▷ If restraint is required to treat an unwilling child, such restraint must be necessary, proportionate, and the least restrictive possible to enable administration of the treatment. If parents (or clinicians) disagree with the proposal of restraint, a legal opinion should be sought, providing that time permits.

CONFIDENTIALITY

As with adults, the right to confidentiality of the child should be respected. A patient has the right to allow or disallow sharing of personal information. This is recognised in both national and international law. Disclosure of data should always be kept to a minimum, and research data should be anonymised.

Confidentiality is particularly important in clinical genetics. For example, the clinician must consider if obtaining genetic information on one person has implications for the health or disease risks of others. In some cases, testing one person can reveal the genetic status of others. Further, can the information from one individual be accessed or divulged to another without the first individual's permission? Such questions will require assessments of (i) the harm/ benefit of sharing information and (ii) the reasons for information not being shared. The potential to avoid serious harm to third parties needs carefully balancing with the potential harms arising from breaching patient confidentiality.

Breaking Confidentiality

Consent from the patient should be sought before information is disclosed to a third party. However, if a patient withholds consent, disclosures are permissible if they are:

▷ Required by law.

▷ In the public interest.

▷ Necessary to prevent serious harm to the individual.

Only the minimum data required should be shared, and it should be anonymised if possible.

Legal requirements for notification of patient identifiable data:

▷ All abortions, deaths and births must be registered.

▷ The government must be informed of "notifiable diseases" for which a list exists (on Public Health England's website in England). It is deemed in the public interest to know about new cases of these diseases. For example, information on the incidence of contagious diseases like tuberculosis may help contain their spread.

Breaching of confidentiality is also allowable if it is considered in the public interest to do so. This usually means that significant harm is likely to occur to an identifiable third party without disclosure. Judgements about "public interest" can be difficult to make. It is not enough for information to be in the public interest; it must also be sufficiently important to override an individual's confidentiality. Child protection concern is one realm in which confidentiality may be broken, if considered in the child's best interest.

Consent should be gained, if at all possible. If not possible, the person whose confidence will be breached should be notified of the intention to do so. The exception to this is where communicating the decision to share information without the patient's consent undermines the purpose of doing so. This may be the case where information is shared in the public interest in the context of a criminal investigation. If information is shared with a third party, it is important to ensure the party understands that the information is given in confidence.

REFERENCES AND FURTHER READING

1   British and Irish Legal Information Institute. Gillick v West Norfolk & Wisbech Area Health Authority 1985 UKHL7. https://www.bailii.org/uk/cases/UKHL/1985/7.html.

2   Royal College and Paediatrics and Child Health et al. 2014. Safeguarding children and young people: roles and competences for healthcare staff. http://www.rcpch.ac.uk/sites/default/files/page/Safeguarding%20Children%20-%20Roles%20and%20Competences%20for%20Healthcare%20Staff%20%2002%200%20%20%20%20(3)_0.pdf.

3   General Medical Council. 2013. Good Medical Practice. http://www.gmc-uk.org/guidance/good_medical_practice.asp.

4   General Medical Council. 2008. Consent: patients and doctors making decisions together. http://www.gmc-uk.org/guidance/ethical_guidance/consent_guidance_index.asp.

5   General Medical Council. 2009. Confidentiality. http://www.gmc-uk.org/static/documents/content/Confidentiality_core_2009.pdf.

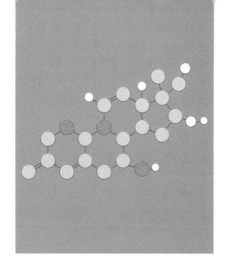

1.14

METABOLIC MEDICINE

ZESHAN QURESHI, STEPHANIE CONNAIRE AND ZAINAB KAZMI

WHAT IS METABOLIC DISEASE?

Metabolic disease results from defects in enzymes involved in metabolic pathways of the body leading to accumulation of toxic metabolites, deficiency of essential metabolites or both. Principles of management therefore focus on reversing catabolism, replacing the deficiency and chelating or excreting toxic metabolites. Symptoms and signs as well as clinical course relate to which pathway is involved.

The term "inborn error of metabolism" refers to metabolic disorders that are inherited, usually as a result of a single gene defect affecting a significant enzyme in a metabolic pathway. Hundreds of different metabolic disorders have been described. Although each metabolic disorder is individually rare, collectively, they are not uncommon, with around 1 in every 2500 children in the UK born with an inherited metabolic disease.

Metabolic medicine is becoming increasingly important, particularly in the context of newborn screening, where these diseases can be detected at the pre-symptomatic stage. In the UK today, the diagnosis of medium-chain acyl-CoA dehydrogenase deficiency (MCADD) is given via a phone call to the parents of a well baby with a positive screening test, rather than when the child presents with hypoglycaemia and its complications.

This chapter will give a brief introduction regarding when to suspect metabolic disease and an overview of a few common forms of these diseases.

WHEN SHOULD METABOLIC DISEASE BE SUSPECTED?

The wide variation and non-specific presentation of metabolic disease means that a high index of suspicion is required to make the diagnosis. Affected children who are not diagnosed through neonatal screening may present as acutely unwell, with an undiagnosed metabolic disorder. Metabolic disorders tend to present at times of metabolic stress, for example, during the neonatal period (when presentation can be easily mistaken as sepsis), at times of dietary change or with intercurrent illness. Clues can be found in the history, examination and investigations.

Newborn Screening

The neonatal heel prick or Guthrie test is a screening test performed on newborn babies at day five to day eight of life.

CONTENTS

All babies in the UK are screened for a number of different inherited metabolic diseases, including:

- Medium-chain acyl-CoA dehydrogenase deficiency (MCADD). 1 in 8 000 UK livebirths.
- Phenylketonuria (PKU). 1 in 15 000 UK livebirths.
- Glutaric aciduria type 1 (GA1). 1 in 109 000 UK livebirths.
- Maple syrup urine disease (MSUD). 1 in 116 000 UK livebirths.
- Isovaleric acidaemia (IVA). 1 in 155 000 UK live births.
- Homocystinuria. 1 in 344 000 live births worldwide, but 1 in 65 000 in Ireland.

History

- Family history of metabolic disease. Inheritance is most often autosomal recessive.
- Consanguineous parents. Children with consanguineous parents are at a higher risk of an autosomal recessive disorder.
- History of sudden infant death.
- Neonatal presentation. Neonates may present with difficulty feeding, as well as vomiting, hypotonia, hypoglycaemia, seizures and encephalopathy.
- Older child presentation. Older children may present with recurrent vomiting, lethargy, encephalopathy and seizures. They may also develop liver or renal failure or cardiomyopathy. A more insidious onset may present with developmental delay or regression.

Examination

Examination findings that may lead to a suspicion of metabolic disease include:

- Dysmorphic features. e.g. Marfanoid features in homocystinuria, coarse facial features in mucopolysaccharidoses.
- Eyes. e.g. cataracts in galactosaemia, corneal clouding in mucopolysaccharidoses and cherry-red spot in Tay-Sachs disease.

- Hepatosplenomegaly. e.g. storage diseases.
- Unusual odours. e.g. sweet smell of nappies in MSUD.

Investigations

- An initial metabolic screen may involve a blood gas, ammonia, lactate, glucose level, ketones, plasma amino acids, urine organic acids and acylcarnitines.

Common findings in metabolic disorders include:

- Metabolic acidosis. Acidosis from the presence of abnormal metabolites, such as lactate, organic acids and keto acids (giving an increased anion gap).
- Lactic acidosis. Lactate is elevated in certain metabolic conditions; e.g. pyruvate dehydrogenase deficiency, organic acidaemias and disorders of the mitochondrial electron transport chain.
- Hypoglycaemia. This occurs when glucose as a substrate is depleted. It may occur due to disorders of carbohydrate metabolism or fatty acid oxidation disorders. Hypoglycaemia is covered in detail on p66. Some key tests in differentiating metabolic causes of hypoglycaemia are shown in *Table 1-2*. Free fatty acids and beta-hydroxybutyrate should be raised during hypoglycaemia, since these are mobilised as an alternative energy source. If there is a defect in fatty acid metabolism, intermediate products of fatty acid metabolism (between free fatty acids at the start and beta-hydroxybutyrate at the end) will increase (e.g. acylcarnitines) as they cannot be processed further along the metabolic pathway.
- Ketosis or ketonuria. Ketosis occurs when fats are being utilised as an energy substrate.
- Hyperammonaemia. This is particularly common in urea cycle defects, where ammonia cannot be broken down. It is also seen in organic acid disorders, fatty acid oxidation disorders and severe liver failure.

TABLE 1: Interpretation of hypoglycaemia screen

Free fatty acids	• Raised.	• Raised.	• Raised.
Acylcarnitine	• Raised.	• Normal.	• Normal.
Lactate	• Normal/raised.	• Raised.	• Normal.
Beta-hydroxybutyrate	• Normal.	• Raised.	• Raised.
Pathophysiology	• Fatty acid oxidation disorder.	• Defective glycogen metabolism/gluconeogenesis.	• Normal fatty acid oxidation, gluconeogenesis and glycogen metabolism.
Differential diagnoses	• Medium-chain acyl-CoA dehydrogenase deficiency. • Very long-chain acyl-CoA dehydrogenase deficiency.	• Glycogen storage disease.	• Prolonged fast. • Ketotic hypoglycaemia. • Growth hormone/cortisol deficiency. • Glycogen storage disease.

TABLE 2: Ketotic vs. non-ketotic hypoglycaemia

Ketotic	Non-ketotic
• Glycogen storage disease. • Cortisol deficiency. • Growth hormone deficiency. • Hypothyroidism. • Starvation. • Idiopathic ketotic hypoglycaemia.	• Fatty acid oxidation defects (although some can be ketotic). • Hyperinsulinism. • Medication. e.g. insulin.

COMMON METABOLIC DISORDERS

Galactosaemia

Aetiology
Lactase breaks down dietary lactose to glucose and galactose. Galactose can then be mobilised for energy, via the pathway described in *Figure 1*. Galactosaemia can result from deficiency in any of the three enzymes: galactokinase, galactose-1-phosphate uridyl transferase (GALT) and UDP galactose-4-epimerase. Enzyme defects lead to an elevated blood galactose level. The most common and severe form is from GALT deficiency.

Clinical Features
Affected infants will often present in the neonatal period with jaundice, hepatomegaly, coagulopathy and cataracts. Older children may present with faltering growth or renal pathology. Galactosaemia is associated with *E.coli* sepsis.

Investigations
Diagnosis is made by testing urinary reducing substances and a Gal-1-PUT (galactose-1-phosphate uridyltransferase) assay. Liver function tests may be deranged, with prolonged jaundice and possible coagulopathy. Affected children should have an eye examination.

Management
Management of galactosaemia is through a lactose/galactose free diet (soya based formula and then dairy-free diet) and ensuring adequate calcium and Vitamin D intake.

Prognosis
The immediate prognosis is good with early diagnosis and appropriate treatment. Death from liver failure or sepsis is possible if appropriate dietary changes are not made.

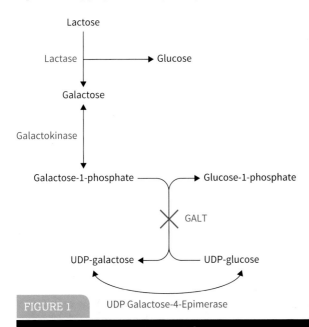

FIGURE 1 UDP Galactose-4-Epimerase

Galactose metabolism and GALT deficiency.

Hypogonadotrophic hypogonadism is common in women, with a high risk of ovarian failure. There may also be developmental delay.

Glycogen Storage Disease (GSDs)
This section will mainly focus on GSD type 1, with a general overview of other types.

Aetiology
Glucose is stored as glycogen in the liver and muscles, with specific enzymes involved in glycogenolysis (*Figure 2*). Individuals affected by GSDs have a defect in one of these enzymes, leading to glycogen build-up (and intermediate compounds), plus difficulty maintaining normoglycaemia. GSDs are categorised according to the enzyme defect involved (*Table 3*). Type 1 GSD is the most common.

Clinical Features
Some disorders affect the liver, some affect the muscles and some affect both (*Table 3*). The main role of glycogen in the liver is to maintain glucose homeostasis; therefore, GSDs affecting the liver may lead to hypoglycaemia and hepatomegaly. GSDs affecting the muscles cause weakness and fatigue.

Investigations
Investigations include checking glucose, lactate, uric acid and lipids. Confirmation of the diagnosis is via enzymology assays or genotyping, depending on the subtype. Liver biopsy may be needed in some cases.

Management
For most types of GSD, no specific treatment is available and therefore symptomatic management is important. Hypoglycaemia may occur frequently, particularly during periods of starvation. In the long term, liver transplantation may be necessary.

In GSD 1a, regular feeding during the day is essential, including continuous feeding overnight, with slow release carbohydrates (e.g. uncooked corn starch in those over two) to facilitate longer gaps between feeds. As there is a risk of gout from hyperuricemia, allopurinol should be given. GSD 1b requires the addition of septrin or granulocyte colony-stimulating factor in view of neutrophil dysfunction.

Prognosis
The prognosis for GSD type 1 depends on glucose control. Complications include short stature, renal disease, osteoporosis and liver adenomas (which may become malignant).

Homocystinuria
Aetiology
Homocysteine is an amino acid formed by converting methionine to cysteine. Homocystinuria is a rare inherited metabolic disorder characterised by high concentrations of

TABLE 3: Sub-types of glycogen storage disease		
GSD	Aetiology	Clinical Features
GSD Ia (Glucose-6-phosphatase deficiency, Von Gierke's disease)	Deficiency in glucose-6-phosphatase results in failure to remove phosphate from glucose-6-phosphate and a consequent inability to export glucose from the liver. Glucose homeostasis cannot be maintained after a prolonged fast; therefore, presentation usually occurs when an infant begins having feeds spaced out. Note that GSD 1b also exists: this is caused by glucose-6-phosphate translocase deficiency. It is similar to GSD Ia but with added neutrophil dysfunction.	Presents with massive hepatomegaly, enlarged kidneys, abnormal fat distribution, hypoglycaemia, faltered growth and bruising (platelet dysfunction). Liver adenoma is a risk and may become malignant. Neutrophil dysfunction in GSD 1b occurs in conjunction with associated skin sepsis, mouth ulcers and inflammatory bowel disease.
GSD II (Lysosomal acid maltase deficiency, Pompe disease)	Deficiency in the lysosomal enzyme acid maltase leads to impaired breakdown of glycogen to glucose. This results in accumulation of glycogen in lysosomes.	Essentially a lysosomal storage disorder, and the infantile form presents with cardiomyopathy, severe hypotonia, weakness, reduced reflexes, feeding difficulties, respiratory distress, and tongue enlargement. The late form is more insidious and has a slower progression, with relative lack of cardiac involvement.
GSD III (Debranching enzyme deficiency, Cori disease)	Non-functional glycogen debranching enzyme or debranching enzyme with reduced function leads to cellular accumulation of partially broken down glycogen. Type IIIa affects liver and muscle; type IIIb is purely hepatic.	Can present similarly to GSD 1, although enlarged kidneys are not a feature, and liver adenomas are rare.
GSD IV (Branching enzyme deficiency, Andersen's disease)	Deficiency of glycogen branching enzyme leads to the production of abnormal glycogen molecules called polyglucosan bodies, which accumulate in cells and cause cell damage.	Presents with hepatomegaly and liver disease.
GSD V (Myophosphorylase deficiency, McArdle's disease)	Myophosphorylase (which breaks down glycogen to glucose-1-phosphate) is deficient, resulting in impaired energy production in the muscle cells.	Presents with weakness, fatigue and post exercise stiffness.

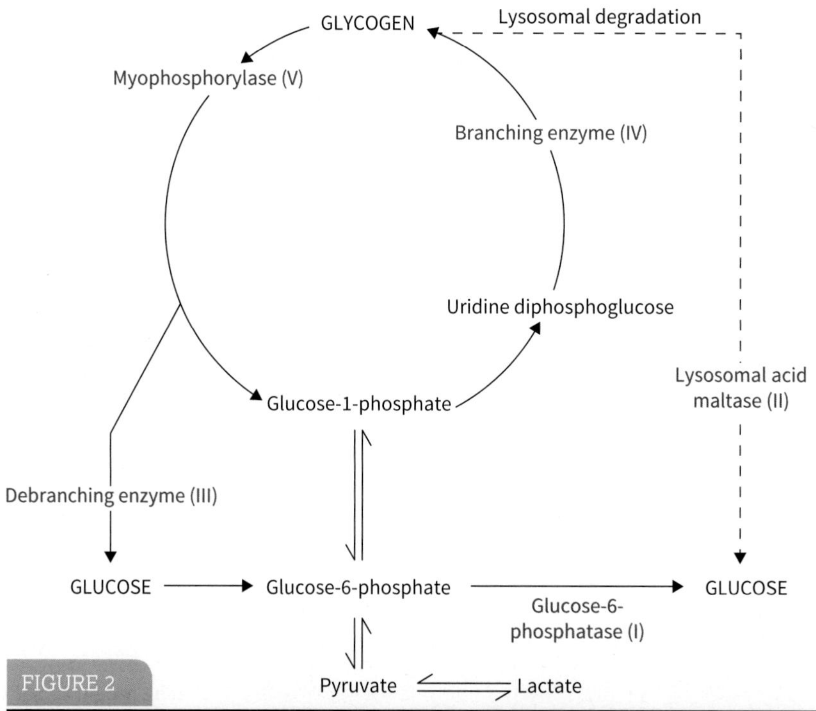

homocysteine in the blood and the urine. A number of types are recognised, but deficiency in cystathionine β synthase (CBS) results in "classical homocystinuria" (*Figure 3*).

Clinical Features

> Marfanoid habitus. Body span greater than height, arachnodactyly, high arched palate, pectus excavatum and pectus carinatum.
> Restricted joint movement.
> Ectopia lentis. Displacement of the lens of the eye, classically downwards.
> Developmental delay/ intellectual impairment.
> Thrombosis. DVT/PE.
> Osteoporosis.

Investigations

Diagnosis is based on raised homocysteine, raised methionine and enzymology assays.

Management

Treatment includes restriction of methionine and supplementation with vitamins. Around half of affected patients respond to pyridoxine (vitamin B6), as this is involved in activation of key enzymes in the homocysteine metabolism pathway. Folate supplementation is also recommended. Betaine may be used to lower homocysteine levels through remethylation, in those who do not respond to pyridoxine.

FIGURE 2

Glycogen metabolism. Enzyme deficiency in subtypes of GSD are labelled.

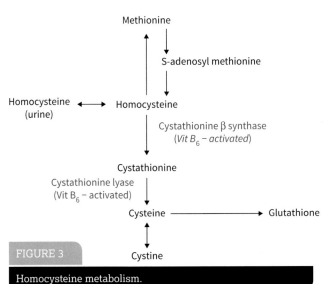

FIGURE 3

Homocysteine metabolism.

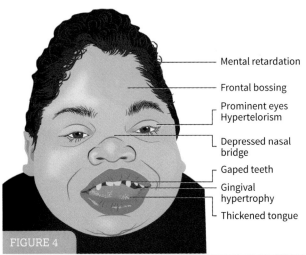

FIGURE 4

Facial features associated with Hurler syndrome.

Prognosis

If picked up on screening, then long term outcome is excellent. However, reducing homocysteine levels at any age improves outlook, including thrombotic risk and neurological features.

Hurler's Syndrome

Aetiology

Mucopolysaccharidoses (MPS) are lysosomal storage disorders caused by deficiency in the enzymes required to break down mucopolysaccharides, also known as glycosaminoglycans (GAGs). GAGs can be found in the cells of bones, cartilage, synovial fluid, skin and connective tissues. Lysosomes are cytoplasmic organelles containing enzymes. There are many different types of MPS, but Hurler's syndrome is a classic example, caused by a deficiency in alpha-L-Iduronidase. Others include Sanfilipo syndrome and Hunter syndrome.

Clinical Features

Affected individuals tend to appear normal at birth but then develop the following clinical features (*Figure 4*):

> Coarse facial features. Frontal bossing, prominent eyes, hypertelorism, depressed nasal bridge, macroglossia leading to airway problems.
> Hepatosplenomegaly.
> Hernias. Umbilical, inguinal, femoral.
> Dysostosis multiplex. Typical skeletal abnormalities.
> Developmental delay and intellectual impairment.
> Infection. Recurrent respiratory infections, secretory otitis media.
> Corneal clouding.
> Cardiac problems. Cardiomyopathy, valvular regurgitation, heart failure.

Investigations

Diagnosis is via urinary screen for glycosaminoglycans and enzymology assay.

Management

Enzyme replacement therapy is available, as well as haematopoietic stem cell transplantation. Supportive care is the mainstay of management, particularly in untransplanted patients.

Prognosis

Prognosis is poor, with severe neurodevelopmental deterioration and death in childhood. Bone morrow transplantation may alter neurological symptomatology, but other features, particularly skeletal complications, do not appear to be altered.

Medium-Chain Acyl-CoA Dehydrogenase Deficiency (MCADD)

Aetiology

Fatty acid oxidation is particularly important in the production of energy during periods of fasting.

The process of mitochondrial fatty acid β-oxidation is shown in *Figure 5*. Fatty acyl-CoA is gradually cleaved, releasing acetyl-CoA to enter into the TCA cycle each time it goes through the reaction circle.

Four reactions occur, performed by chain length specific enzymes.

1. Dehydrogenation of the fatty acyl-CoA by very long chain (VLCAD), medium chain (MCAD) or short chain (SCAD) acyl-CoA dehydrogenases to create enoyl-CoA,
2. Hydration by the enoyl-CoA hydratase activity of the MTP or ECHS1 to add water to enoyl-CoA to form 3-hydroxyacyl-CoA,
3. A second dehydrogenation by MTP or HADH to generate 3-ketoacyl-CoA.
4. Thiolysis by the thiolase activity of the MTP or KAT to produce a shortened fatty acyl-CoA and acetyl-CoA.

Acetyl-CoA then enters the TCA cycle, and the shortened fatty acyl-CoA re-enters the fatty acid β-oxidation pathway to be cleaved again.

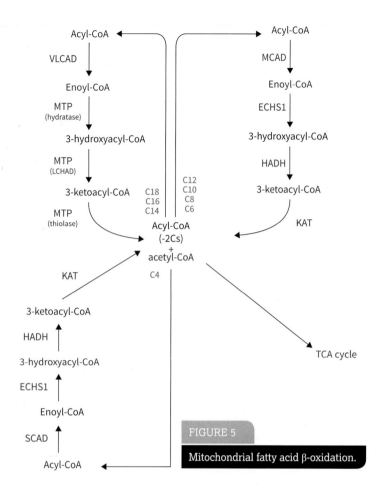

FIGURE 5

Mitochondrial fatty acid β-oxidation.

MCADD is an autosomal recessive disorder caused by mutations in the ACADM gene (commonly G985 mutation). Mutations in the ACADM gene lead to a deficiency in the MCAD enzyme needed to metabolise medium chain fatty acids (6 to 12 carbons) as part of the mitochondrial fatty acid β-oxidation spiral. MCADD is the most common fatty acid oxidation disorder in the UK and is included in the neonatal screening programme.

MCADD results in reduced acetyl-CoA production and therefore an inability to mobilise fat stores for energy. Other defects can arise from VLCAD and SCAD defects. Long chain defects are more severe, as the block occurs earlier in the β-oxidation spiral.

Clinical Features
Clinical features of MCADD arise during periods of fasting or intercurrent illness, e.g. vomiting, and include:

> Drowsiness and lethargy.
> Hypoketotic hypoglycaemia.
> Encephalopathy.

> Hepatomegaly and liver dysfunction.
> Sudden infant death (particularly in over six month olds).

Investigations
Diagnosis is by identifying hypoglycaemia with low/absent ketones, raised octanoyl carnitine (C8 carnitine), raised hexanoylglycine in urinary organic acids, and genotyping.

Management
Children with MCADD must eat regularly and avoid prolonged periods of time without food. In times of decompensation, children should take oral emergency regimen drinks. If these are not tolerated or ineffective, hospital admission for IV dextrose and electrolyte replacement is required.

Prognosis
Neonatal screening has transformed the outcome for these patients, with those picked up through screening having an excellent outlook. Previously, MCADD presented symptomatically, often with

profound brain injury secondary to hypoglycaemia and with high mortality.

Organic Acidaemias
Aetiology
Organic acidaemias are a result of defects in the catabolism of amino acids, resulting in organic acid generation as a by-product (which can be detected in the urine).

Maple syrup urine disease (MSUD) is one type of organic acidaemia. It is a disorder affecting the branched-chain amino acids leucine, isoleucine and valine. It is caused by a deficiency in the branched-chain alpha-keto acid dehydrogenase complex responsible for breakdown of these amino acids (*Figure 6*). Leucine accumulation in particular results in neurological symptoms.

Other examples of organic acidaemias are shown in *Table 4*.

Clinical Features
Maple syrup urine disease
MSUD presents with seizures, encephalopathy, feeding difficulty and psychomotor retardation. It gets its name from the sweet odour of the urine (secondary to isoleucine accumulation). Intermittent forms, with the child appearing entirely symptom free between bouts, may appear later on in childhood.

Propionic, methylmalonic and isovaleric acidaemias

> Vomiting, dehydration and poor feeding.
> Acute neonatal encephalopathy (or chronic intermittent).
> Progressive extrapyramidal syndrome/basal ganglia necrosis (PA, MMA).
> Renal insufficiency (PA).
> Cardiomyopathy (PA, MMA).
> Lethargy.
> Hypotonia.

Glutaric aciduria type 1
In the asymptomatic stage, macrocephaly/frontal bossing may be the only feature. However, on decompensation (e.g. triggered by an infection), encephalopathy, dystonia, irritability and feeding difficulties may ensue.

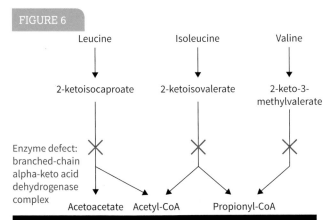

FIGURE 6

Leucine   Isoleucine   Valine

2-ketoisocaproate   2-ketoisovalerate   2-keto-3-methylvalerate

Enzyme defect: branched-chain alpha-keto acid dehydrogenase complex

Acetoacetate   Acetyl-CoA   Propionyl-CoA

Maple syrup disease metabolic pathway.

TABLE 4: Organic acidaemias

Organic acidaemia	Amino acid pathway affected
Methylmalonic acidaemia (MMA).	Branched-chain amino acid.
Propionic acidaemia (PA).	Branched chain amino acid.
Isovaleric acidaemia.	Leucine.
3-hydroxy-3-methyl-CoA lyase deficiency.	Leucine.
Glutaric aciduria type 1.	Lysine and tryptophan.

Investigations

Depending on the subtype, diagnosis involves identification of increased anion gap metabolic acidosis, ketosis (although ketone production is prevented in 3-hydroxy-3-methyl-CoA lyase deficiency), raised lactate, raised ammonia, glucose changes (low or high or normal) and neutropenia/thrombocytopenia (bone marrow suppression).

More definitive diagnosis is on measuring urinary organic acids, genotyping and enzymology assays. Maple syrup urine disease diagnosis is based on elevated branched chain amino acids (plus alloisoleucine) and elevated branched-chain oxoacids in the urine. An MRI head should be performed in suspected glutaric aciduria type 1: it may show frontal atrophy, subdural haematomas and decreased basal ganglia signal.

Management

Management during episodes of decompensation includes IV fluids and correction of biochemical derangements such as metabolic acidosis, hypoglycaemia and hyperammonaemia.

More broadly the specific management of the individual organic acidaemias varies but aspects to be aware of include:

> Dietary protein restriction. In MSUD, dietary therapy involves carefully controlling the levels of leucine, isoleucine and valine in order to prevent toxic metabolites and neurological damage. Valine and isoleucine may require supplementation as levels may fall dangerously low while controlling leucine.

> Carnitine to facilitate renal excretion of organic acids.

> Metronidazole. (PA, MMA), as propionate is partly produced by gut organisms and metronidazole reduces this, as well as altering the gut flora.

> Vitamin B12. May be helpful in some cases of MMA.

> Liver transplant. Can be considered in select cases.

> Thiamine. In maple syrup urine disease a trial of thiamine may be helpful (as this is an enzyme cofactor).

Prognosis

MMA and PA can lead to death in the neonatal period, or during an episode of metabolic compensation. Cardiomyopathy is associated with high mortality. Undiagnosed and untreated glutaric aciduria type 1 leads to cerebral atrophy, developmental delay and pyramidal tract signs.

With maple syrup urine disease, the best outcome occurs in those who begin treatment before becoming symptomatic. Cognitive outcome correlates with leucine concentration. Acute metabolic compensation can result in brain injury and death.

Phenylketonuria (PKU)

Aetiology

PKU is the most common inborn error of metabolism in the UK. The body is unable to convert the amino acid phenylalanine (from dietary protein) into tyrosine due to phenylalanine hydroxylase deficiency (*Figure 7*). Phenylalanine build-up is neurotoxic.

Clinical Features

In cases that are not detected by neonatal screening, children usually present with progressive developmental delay. Other clinical features include learning difficulties, behavioural problems, dry/hypopigmented skin and a musty odour.

Investigations

Testing for PKU is included in the UK neonatal screening programme, meaning that raised phenylalanine levels are detected at birth. Molecular testing is also available.

Management

Management is through dietary restriction of phenylalanine and supplementation of other amino acids (including tyrosine). Some cases of PKU result from defects in biopterin (an essential cofactor for phenylalanine hydroxylase and

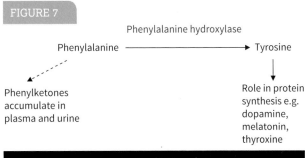

FIGURE 7

Phenylalanine hydroxylase

Phenylalanine   →   Tyrosine

Phenylketones accumulate in plasma and urine

Role in protein synthesis e.g. dopamine, melatonin, thyroxine

Metabolic pathway involved in PKU.

neurotransmitter synthesis). These cases require additional neurotransmitter replacement.

Prognosis

The prognosis is excellent with early treatment. Compliance with diet during pregnancy is particularly important to avoid neonatal complications.

Tyrosinaemia (type 1)

Aetiology

Tyrosinaemia results from a defect in the pathway that breaks down the amino acid tyrosine. Three types of tyrosinaemia are recognised, but type 1 is the commonest and most severe form. It is due to deficiency in fumarylacetoacetase and leads to a build-up of succinylacetone, which is nephrotoxic and hepatotoxic (*Figure 8*).

Clinical Features

Tyrosinaemia type 1 tends to present in the first few months of life. Initial features may purely be faltering growth, vomiting and diarrhoea. Early onset liver disease is present, with jaundice and coagulopathy. A "cabbage like" odour may be noted. Renal tubular disease may result in Fanconi syndrome. Other features include rickets and developmental delay. The risk of hepatocellular carcinoma is increased.

Investigations

Diagnosis is via raised tyrosine levels, raised succinylacetone levels and enzymology (fumarylacetoacetase). Liver and renal function may be deranged, with electrolyte disturbance.

Management

Management includes tyrosine restriction and amino acid supplementation (apart from tyrosine and phenylalanine). Nitisinone can be used as an adjunct to dietary modification. It blocks the catabolic pathway proximal to the production of succinylacetone, thereby reducing the build-up of toxic metabolites. Liver transplantation is reserved as a last resort for those not responding to nitisinone or those who have developed serious complications, such as hepatocellular carcinoma.

Prognosis

In the absence of liver disease, the prognosis is usually excellent.

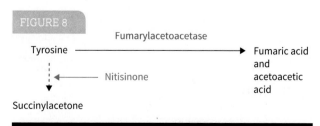

FIGURE 8

Tyrosine metabolism.

Urea Cycle Defects

Aetiology

The urea cycle involves the conversion of nitrogen to urea for excretion. Several different enzymes in the cycle can be defective, resulting in different patterns of intermediate amino acid build up.

Clinical Features

Typically, patients present with vomiting, encephalopathy and tachypnoea. These defects may also lead to progressive spastic diplegia and developmental delay. Tachypnoea is driven by a build-up of ammonia and may result in a respiratory alkalosis.

Investigations

Diagnostic confirmation requires enzymology, but measuring plasma amino acids and urinary organic acids can give an indication of the level of the enzymatic block in the urea cycle.

Management

Acutely, a patient with hyperammonaemia requires normal feeds to be stopped and intravenous dextrose to be commenced to reduce catabolism.

Long term management involves:

➢ Protein restriction and use of specialised formulas.
➢ Sodium benzoate and sodium phenylbutyrate — these conjugate glycine and glutamate, facilitating kidney excretion and avoiding the urea cycle.
➢ Arginine supplementation — an essential amino acid although it should not be given in arginase deficiency.
➢ Multivitamin and fluoride supplementation.

Liver transplants may be required if medical management fails.

Prognosis

Patients that present with severe, prolonged hyperammonaemic crisis in the neonatal period have very poor outcomes, particularly if associated with severe encephalopathy, which may lead to death or neurodevelopmental delay. Late presentations, with milder disease, have better outcomes.

REFERENCES AND FURTHER READING

1   Baynes J, Dominiczak M. Medical Biochemistry. United States: Saunders. 2014.
2   Fletcher J. Metabolic emergencies and the emergency physician. Journal of Paediatrics and Child Health 2016; 52: 227-230.
3   Beattie M, Champion M. Metabolic Medicine. In: Essential Revision Notes in Paediatrics for the MRCPCH. Third edition. Cheshire: PasTest. 2012.
4   Strobel S, Spitz L, Marks S. Metabolic Diseases. In: Great Ormond Street Handbook of Paediatrics. Second Edition. New York: CRC Press. 2016.
5   British Inherited Metabolic Disease Group. 2016. http://www.bimdg.org.uk/site/index.asp

6   Public Health England. Health Professional Handbook: a guide to newborn blood spot screening for healthcare professionals. 2012. https://www.gov.uk/government /uploads/system/uploads/attachment_data/file/390977 /Health_Professional_Handbook_2012_v1.0_December _2012.pdf

7   The Association for Glycogen Storage Disease UK. 2016. https://www.agsd.org.uk/tabid/1134/Default.aspx

8   The National Society for Phenylketonuria. 2016. http:// www.nspku.org/information/whatispku

9   Genetics Home Reference. Tyrosinaemia. 2016. https://ghr .nlm.nih.gov/condition/tyrosinemia

10 Valayannopoulos V, Wijburg FA. Therapy for the mucopolysaccharidoses. Rheumatology 2011; 50: 49-59.

11 MPS Society. http://mpssociety.org/mps-diseases/

12 National Organization for Rare Disorders. Mucopolysaccharidoses. 2016. http://rarediseases.org /rare-diseases/mucopolysaccharidoses/

13 NHS Choices. MCADD. 2016. http://www.nhs.uk /conditions/mcadd/Pages/Introduction.aspx

14 Up to Date. Mitochondrial Myopathies: Treatment. 2016. http://www.uptodate.com/contents/mitochondrial-myopathies-treatment?source=search _result&search=mitochondrial+disease&selectedTitle =2%7E150

15 UCSF Children's Hospital. Inborn Errors of Metabolism. 2004. https://www.ucsfbenioffchildrens.org/pdf/manuals /53_Metabolism.pdf

16 The University of Chicago. Hypoglycaemia. 2013. https:// pedclerk.bsd.uchicago.edu/page/hypoglycemia

17 Paediatrics Clerkship. Hypoglycaemia. 2016. https:// pedclerk.bsd.uchicago.edu/page/hypoglycemia

18 Sunehag A, Haymond M. Approach to hypoglycaemia in infants and children. 2015. UpToDate. https://www .uptodate.com/contents/approach-to-hypoglycemia -in-infants-and-children?source=search_result& search=algorithm+hypoglycaemia&selectedTitle=1%7E150

19 The Association for Glycogen Storage Disease UK. 2016. https://www.agsd.org.uk/tabid/1134/Default.aspx

20 Reid Sutton V. Galactosaemia: Clinical features and diagnosis. UpToDate. 2015. https://www.uptodate.com/contents /galactosemia-clinical-features-and-diagnosis?source=search _result&search=galactosaemia&selectedTitle=1%7E46

21 Genetics Home Reference. Maple syrup urine disease. 2016. https://ghr.nlm.nih.gov/condition/maple-syrup -urine-disease

22 British Inherited Metabolic Diseases Group. HCU clinical management guidelines. http://www.bimdg.org.uk/site /guidelines-enbs.asp?t=3

23 National MPS Society. MPS Diseases. 2011. http:// mpssociety.org/mps-diseases/

24 O'Ferrall E. Mitochondrial Myopathies: Treatment. 2016. UpToDate. http://www.uptodate.com/contents /mitochondrial-myopathies-treatment?source=search _result&search=mitochondrial+disease&selectedTitle =2%7E150

METABOLIC MEDICINE

185

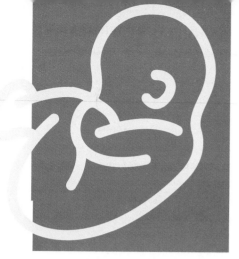

1.15
NEONATOLOGY

CHRISTOPHER HARRIS AND
ZESHAN QURESHI

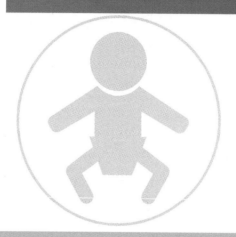

CONTENTS

THE NEWBORN EXAMINATION

Introduction

All newborn babies should have a neonatal examination performed within 72 hours of birth, regardless of whether they are born in hospital or at home. In the UK, this is governed according to the National Newborn and Infant Physical Examination (NIPE) screening programme. This screening may be carried out by trained midwifes or by paediatricians. The aim of the examination is to diagnose health problems soon after birth. Fortunately, most babies will have a normal examination. The examiner should have understanding of both normal variants and causes of concern in a routine baby check (*Figure 1*).

Neonatal Observations

Table 1 shows the normal neonatal observation ranges. Notably, the heart rate and respiratory rate are much higher than those seen in adults or older children, and the blood pressure also differs. Temperature is much more difficult to maintain in neonates, partly due to the large surface area of a baby compared to their internal volume, but also due to limited ability to shiver and their poor metabolic reserves. It is important that immediately after delivery and resuscitation, the baby is kept warm and dry. In a well baby, drying and wrapping them in a towel can achieve this.

TABLE 1: Normal neonatal observations	
Heart Rate.	120-160 bpm.
Systolic Blood Pressure.	50-70 mmHg.
Respiratory Rate.	40-60 breaths/minute.
Temperature.	36.5°C–37.5°C.

Physiological Changes at Birth

During foetal life, the lungs are filled with fluid and the maternal placenta provides the foetus with oxygen. Blood from the right side of the heart bypasses the lungs, flowing through the ductus arteriosus and foramen ovale to the left side of the heart. The baby only takes its first breath after delivery. This results in a fall in pulmonary vascular resistance, an increase in blood flow through the lungs and a subsequent oxygenation of the blood. These pressure changes, combined with the increasingly oxygenated blood, trigger closure of the umbilical vessels and the ductus arteriosus. Furthermore, the return of oxygenated blood into the left atrium (via the pulmonary veins) increases left atrial pressure, resulting in closure of the foramen ovale. *Figure 2* summarises the key differences between the foetal and neonatal circulation.

Head

During birth, the foetal head experiences pressure from the vaginal wall, and potentially from instruments used in delivery e.g. forceps. This can lead to swelling and an apparent misshaping of the head. The suture lines and fontanelles should be palpable, as shown in *Figure 3*. Fontanelles should normally be soft and flat.

Skull Shapes

> Moulding. This refers to overlapping skull bones resulting from passage through the birth canal. It usually resolves within two to three days.

FIGURE 1

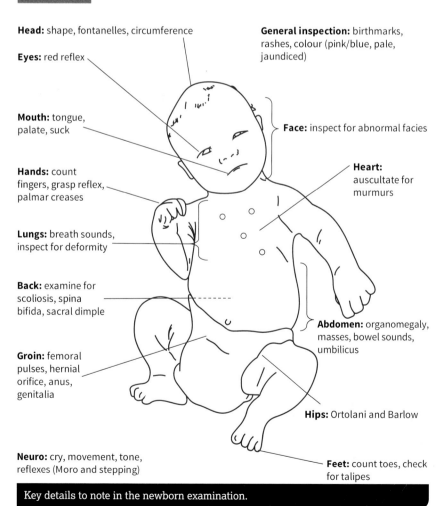

Head: shape, fontanelles, circumference

Eyes: red reflex

Mouth: tongue, palate, suck

Hands: count fingers, grasp reflex, palmar creases

Lungs: breath sounds, inspect for deformity

Back: examine for scoliosis, spina bifida, sacral dimple

Groin: femoral pulses, hernial orifice, anus, genitalia

Neuro: cry, movement, tone, reflexes (Moro and stepping)

General inspection: birthmarks, rashes, colour (pink/blue, pale, jaundiced)

Face: inspect for abnormal facies

Heart: auscultate for murmurs

Abdomen: organomegaly, masses, bowel sounds, umbilicus

Hips: Ortolani and Barlow

Feet: count toes, check for talipes

Key details to note in the newborn examination.

Capillary Haemangioma

Commonly referred to as strawberry naevi, capillary haemangiomas are benign tumours of the vascular endothelium (*Figure 8*). They occur within the first few months after birth and grow rapidly in the first year of life (due to the rapid proliferation of blood vessels) and then gradually regress. Involution occurs in around half by 5-years-old and in the majority by 9-years-old. Intervention is not usually required, although it may be needed in periorbital haemangiomas that may compromise visual development or haemangiomas that affect function, e.g. haemangiomas of the airway, oral cavity or auditory canal. Most haemangiomas are asymptomatic, but lesions can ulcerate, potentially leading to pain, blood loss and secondary bacterial infection. Where treatment is indicated, oral propranolol (a beta blocker) can restrict growth and induce involution. Excisional surgery may also be required to treat haemangiomas affecting function and those refractory to medical treatment. It is important to note that haemangiomas of the skin, particularly when in large numbers, may be associated with haemangiomas elsewhere, such as the liver, gut, brain and lungs.

Erythema Toxicum Neonatorum

This consists of a migratory, raised erythematous rash with overlying papules or pustules (*Figure 9*). It normally appears on day two to three of life. The exact pathogenesis is unclear but it resolves spontaneously after three to five days.

Milia

Milia, sometimes referred to as "milk spots" are white papules present at birth and found most commonly on the nose and cheeks (*Figure 10*). They are caused by build-up of keratin and sebaceous material in skin follicles. They are benign skin lesions and resolve in the first few weeks of life.

Mongolian Blue Spot

These blue pigmented macules that present at birth most commonly occur in the sacral gluteal region (*Figure 11*). Lesions can be large and have a higher incidence in darker pigmented skin. They are benign lesions and tend to fade within the first two years of life. Most resolve by 10-years-old, although a small number persist into adulthood. It is vital to document these at the baby check as in an older child they may be confused for bruises.

Naevus Simplex

This describes a benign pink, blanching macule present in newborns, also known as "salmon patch" or "stork's bite/mark." They are typically found on the glabella, eyelid or nape of the neck and the majority fade within the first two years of life,

FIGURE 8

Capillary haemangiomas.

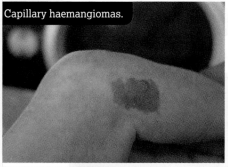
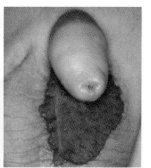
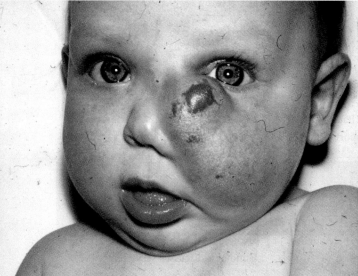

FIGURE 9

Erythema toxicum neonatorum.

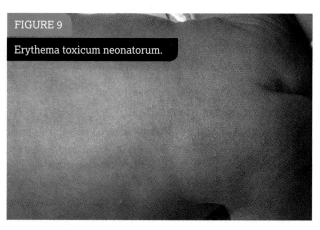

FIGURE 10

Milia.

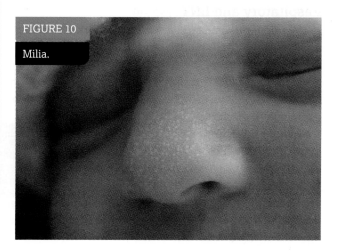

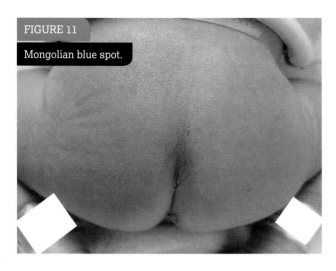

FIGURE 11

Mongolian blue spot.

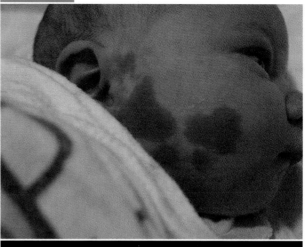

FIGURE 12

Port wine strain.

although lesions found on the nape of the neck may persist into adulthood.

Port Wine Stain

Port wine stains (also known as naevus flammeus) result from low-flow vascular malformations of the dermal capillaries and post-capillary venules (*Figure 12*). These flat, blanching, pink-red lesions are present from birth. They can be found anywhere on the body, but tend to be unilateral with midline demarcation. These lesions do not regress and may become darker and thicker with age. Complications include thickening, nodularity and bleeding. The majority of these lesions occur as isolated lesions but they may occur as part of a syndrome (e.g. Sturge-Weber syndrome: facial port wine stain, ipsilateral venous malformation in the meninges and ocular abnormalities). Glaucoma is associated with periocular port wine stains; therefore, neonates with port wine stains in the distribution of the ophthalmic or maxillary branches of the trigeminal nerve should be referred for ophthalmology review. The presence of a facial port wine stain and glaucoma or neurological symptoms should rouse suspicion of Sturge-Weber syndrome and a neurological review and brain imaging should be sought. Treatment aims are improvement of the aesthetic appearance and prevention of complications. This may involve repeated treatments with pulsed dye laser therapy.

Benign Pustular Melanosis

This consists of superficial pustules, present at birth, which rupture easily without any actual pus content, leaving a spot of hyperpigmentation (*Figure 13*). Pustules usually last for one or two days, although the hyperpigmentation may persist.

Melanocytic Naevi

Melanocytic naevi represent benign proliferations of a subtype of melanocyte cell known as the naevus cell (*Figure 14*). They can be classified as congenital (occurring from birth) or as acquired. Congenital melanocytic naevi tend to grow rapidly in infancy, starting as flat lesions with even pigment,

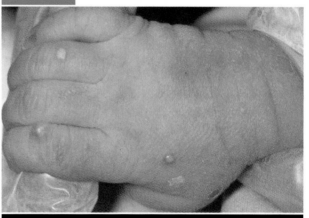

FIGURE 13

Benign pustular melanosis.

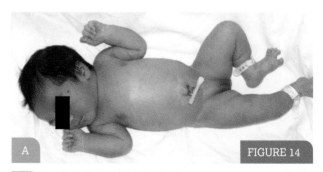

A

FIGURE 14

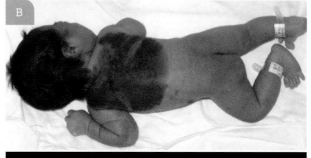

B

A) Small naevus on the face B) Giant naevus.

but the surface later becomes uneven, developing a pebbled appearance. Proliferative nodules are sometimes seen within large congenital melanocytic naevi. Additionally, large congenital melanocytic naevi predispose to a significantly increased risk of developing melanoma or neurocutaneous melanosis, and therefore must be placed under close surveillance. Acquired melanocytic naevi begin to occur after the first six months of life and increase in number during childhood and adolescence. An increased number is seen in those of light pigmentation, a family history of a large number of melanocytic naevi and secondary to increased sun exposure. Most melanocytic naevi remain benign but all have malignant potential. Lifelong self-evaluation should be encouraged to identify early changes.

Collodion Baby

A group of disorders present at birth with a collodian membrane, describing a shiny cellophane-like membrane covering the entire body. These babies have an increased risk of fluid and heat loss through this abnormal layer of skin and may need to be nursed in a humidified incubator. This outer layer of skin is normally shed in the first few days of life, which may reveal normal skin or a range of rare disorders known as the ichthyoses, in which the skin has abnormal scaling. All such children require referral to a paediatric dermatologist.

Napkin Rash

Napkin rash is predominantly irritant in aetiology and appears as erythema in the perineal area. It may have painful scaling papules or skin erosions in severe cases. Napkin rash can be complicated by secondary infection with *Candida albicans*, which appears as red plaques, satellite papules and superficial pustules. Fungal infection is more common following a course of broad-spectrum antibiotics. Secondary bacterial infections are less common but can be due to *Staphylococcus aureus* infection,

presenting with fragile pustules and crusting. Treatment involves exposure of the affected area and use of topical barrier creams to prevent skin irritation from urine and faeces. Secondary fungal and bacterial infections require treatment with topical or oral anti-fungals and antibacterials, respectively. A rare cause of severe napkin rash is lactose intolerance, which presents with frothy, explosive diarrhoea.

Breast Enlargement

This is most often a normal finding and is associated with milky discharge. It is secondary to maternal oestrogens, and may occur in both boys and girls. However, persistence of this finding beyond one to two months may indicate a pituitary tumour.

Cardiovascular

Not all neonates with congenital heart disease will have a detectable murmur at birth and not all those with murmurs will have congenital heart disease.

Reassuring signs in babies with murmurs are:

> Pink baby, no cyanosis, with normal pre and post ductal oxygen saturations.
> No respiratory distress.
> Quiet, intermittent, positional murmur.
> Baby feeding well.
> Normal four limb blood pressures.

The femoral pulses should be examined as they may be absent or reduced in coarctation of the aorta. Common causes of pathological murmurs in the neonatal period are a patent ductus arteriosus (PDA) and ventricular septal defects (VSD). A senior opinion should be sought if a murmur is picked up on routine newborn examination and echocardiography performed if the murmur persists for more than 24 hours.

Abdomen and Genitalia
Umbilical Hernia

This is a herniation at the site of the umbilicus (*Figure 15*). It is usually

benign but can be associated with genetic syndromes such as Beckwith-Wiedemann Syndrome. They do not typically obstruct or strangulate.

Ambiguous Genitalia

In cases where the genitalia cannot be clearly identified as either male or female (ambiguous genitalia), an urgent senior review should be sought (p78). The causes may include congenital adrenal hyperplasia or another endocrine abnormality. Genetic, biochemical and endocrine work ups are required to ascertain the cause and aid decisions regarding the sex of the baby. Informing parents as soon as concerns arise reduces the emotional trauma associated with these complex cases.

Hypospadias

Hypospadias may be glandular (on the glans penis), distal (on the penile shaft) or proximal (on the scrotum) (*Figure 16*). It is always important to ensure there is a good urinary stream, educate the parents to not circumcise their baby (as

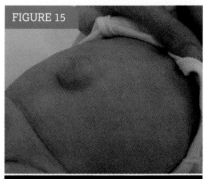

FIGURE 15

Umbilical hernia.

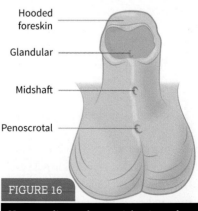

Hooded foreskin

Glandular

Midshaft

Penoscrotal

FIGURE 16

Hypospadias and potential points of urethral opening.

the foreskin is often used in the repair), and to ensure paediatric surgical follow up. In the case of proximal hypospadias, it may be necessary to complete the chromosomal and endocrine work up as detailed above, as severe hypospadias (p350) may be difficult to differentiate from ambiguous genitalia (p78).

Undescended Testes

Palpable but undescended testes need routine follow-up. If not descended at 2-years-old, they will likely require surgical correction to reduce the chance of later malignancy (p348). If a testis is impalpable just on one side, laparoscopy is required to identify its position. Bilateral undescended, impalpable testes require investigation as for ambiguous genitalia.

Scrotal and Groin Swellings

Hydrocoeles (scrotal swellings which transilluminate) normally resolve spontaneously but may be followed up for parental reassurance (*Figure 17*). Care should be taken not to miss an inguinal hernia. These require surgical referral. If there is doubt about whether the lump is an inguinal hernia or a hydrocoele (p348), ultrasound investigation is helpful.

Anorectal Malformation

It is important to examine the anus even if meconium has been passed as the

passage of meconium does not always equate to a patent anus, or an anus in the correct place. Anorectal malformations are commonly associated with urogenital malformations (p358).

Withdrawal Bleeds

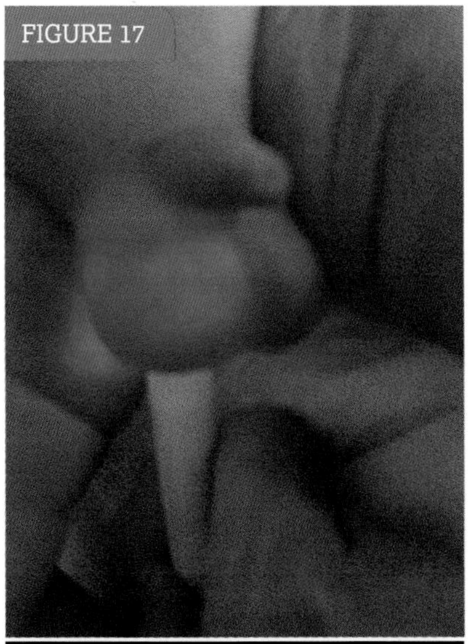

Female babies may have a small amount of bleeding from the vagina, normally on day two to four. This is a result of the withdrawal from maternal oestrogens. This requires no treatment and resolves spontaneously.

Palpable Bladder

A palpable bladder requires prompt evaluation as it may be a sign of urinary obstruction (for example due to posterior urethral valves in males).

Musculoskeletal and Spine

Midline Abnormalities

Sacral dimples may be normal (*Figure 18*). Dimples that are deep, discharging, or associated with abnormal neurology or skin discolouration are more likely to indicate spinal cord tethering and should be investigated with MRI or ultrasound. Hairy tufts may also be associated with spina bifida occulta (*Figure 19*).

Talipes Equinovarus

Talipes equinovarus refers to inversion of the feet which cannot be manually corrected with dorsiflexion (*Figure 20*). This requires referral to physiotherapy. Positional talipes, which can be brought to a normal position with very little pressure, may not need any treatment beyond just gentle straightening exercises, which can be done by the parents with each nappy change.

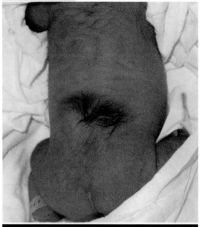
FIGURE 19
Hairy tuft.

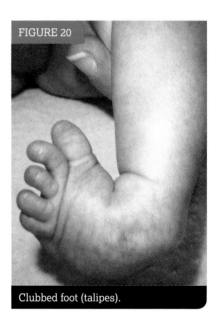
FIGURE 20
Clubbed foot (talipes).

Polydactyly

This refers to additional fingers, or parts of fingers. Polydactyly often runs in families and is most commonly an isolated finding. Whole, functional fingers may be kept but finger segments (*Figure 21*) are removed by paediatric or plastic surgeons.

Congenital Dislocation of the Hip

Congenital dislocation of the hip is tested using two tests:

› **Barlow's test** (*Figure 22*).
› **Ortolani's test** (*Figure 23*).

Infants with a positive test should have a hip ultrasound, and urgent review in

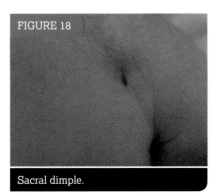
FIGURE 17
Hydrocoele.

FIGURE 18
Sacral dimple.

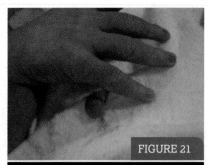

FIGURE 21

Polydactyly: finger segment pre surgical removal.

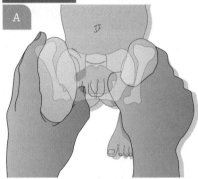

FIGURE 22

A

B

Barlow's test. Stabilise the non-test hip (A). For the side being tested, adduct the hip, and push the femur into the acetabulum (B). This will dislocate a dislocatable hip, giving a "click" and moving the hip posteriorly.

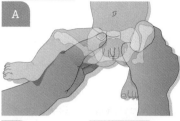

FIGURE 23

A

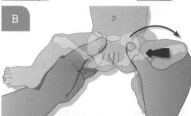

B

Ortolani's test. This starts in the position where a hip has been dislocated (A). Stabilise the pelvis by firmly holding the symphysis pubis and coccyx between the thumb and middle finger. Then, with the baby's hips and knees flexed, and the index finger of the examiner's other hand on the greater trochanter, abduct the baby's hip (B). A palpable "clunk" signifies relocation of a posteriorly dislocated hip.

> › Erb's Palsy (*Figure 24*). This results from injury to C5-6 peripheral nerves (resulting in weakness in elbow flexion, and arm supination).
> › Klumpke's Palsy (*Figure 25*). This results from injury to C8-T1 (resulting in weakness of the extensors in the arm and of the intrinsic muscles of the hand). It may be associated with Horner syndrome.
> › Facial nerve palsy. This can be a result of forceps injury or birth trauma and often manifests with an asymmetrical facial expression when crying. Care must be taken to ensure the infant can completely close the eye of the affected side.
> › Clavicular fracture (*Figure 26*). This may be a complication of assisted delivery (e.g. in shoulder dystocia).
> › Long bone fracture. (*Figure 27*) Rarely, the humerus or femur may fracture during delivery. This is more likely in breech and shoulder dystocia deliveries.

a neonatal or specialist hip clinic for follow-up. Treatment in the first instance is with a Pavlik harness.

Birth Injuries

Possible injuries occurring at the time of birth are described below. These are often picked up during the newborn examination.

> › Brachial plexus palsy. This is more common in breech deliveries and shoulder dystocia. There are two common subtypes:

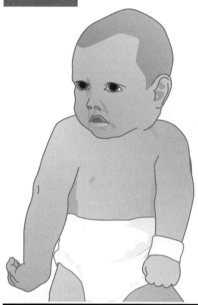

FIGURE 24

Erb's Palsy of the right arm. Note the arm is pronated, and that the elbow is extended.

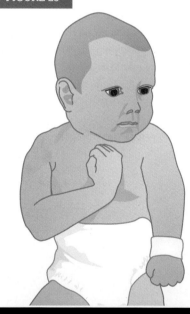

FIGURE 25

Klumpke's Palsy. Note flexion of the elbow, wrist and fingers.

FIGURE 26

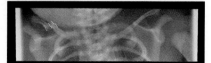

Right clavicular fracture after a traumatic delivery.

FIGURE 27

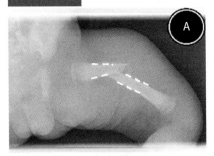

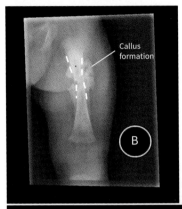

Callus formation

Femur fracture: immediate X-Ray (A) and several weeks later, with realignment of the bone, and callus formation (B)

> Traumatic cyanosis. This can result from a tightly wrapped cord around part of the baby. It causes petechiae and cyanosis around that part (without central cyanosis).

> Bruising. This is common and can occur anywhere, secondary to birth trauma. Pre-term infants are more vulnerable. Ventouse deliveries can cause "chignon" oedema and bruising at the site of application. Similarly, forceps can leave marks on the baby's head.

Many possible abnormalities might be discovered for the first time in a newborn examination. *Table 2* summarises some particularly important findings in apparently well babies.

NEONATAL LIFE SUPPORT

Basic Life Support

Neonatal Basic Life Support is specific to the newborn infant. It usually takes place in the context of a newborn infant who is yet to have taken their first breath. This section describes the

key aspects of neonatal resuscitation. Paediatricians and midwives who are expected to perform resuscitation should undergo the appropriate training.

The majority of newborn infants require no intervention. Some require very minimal intervention, for example, drying with a towel, stimulation, and warming under a heater.

A minority will require help to adapt to extra-uterine life with airway manoeuvres, inflation breaths, intermittent positive pressure ventilation and, rarely, chest compressions with drugs.

Interventions

The airway is vital in the resuscitation of the newborn. A conscious, crying baby will invariably be able to maintain their airway. A floppy baby will need help to counter the effects of their relatively large occiput, which acts to push the chin forward, away from the neutral position. A jaw thrust, airway adjuncts and, finally, intubation can secure the airway.

The initial breaths during a newborn resuscitation event are long breaths lasting three seconds and are designed to inflate the chest. If the chest is not seen to rise, the breaths should be repeated after repositioning the airway.

If breathing does not spontaneously return despite adequate airway opening

and delivery of inflation breaths, ventilation breaths can be delivered at a rate of 30 per minute. If the heart rate remains slow or absent despite the above actions, chest compressions should begin at a rate of three compressions to every breath. Drugs and fluids used in newborn resuscitation include adrenaline, 10% dextrose, sodium bicarbonate, 0.9% sodium chloride and, where there is a clear history of blood loss, packed red cells.

The neonatal life support algorithm is summarised in *Figure 28*.

APGAR Scoring

APGAR scoring is a system used to objectively assess a baby's wellbeing immediately after birth. The score is from 0-10, and is calculated at 1, 5 and 10 minutes after delivery, as shown in *Table 3*. Many babies have a low APGAR score at one or even five minutes, but are then able to fully recover. However, a poor APGAR score at 10 minutes is a predictor of adverse outcome.

TABLE 2: Some key examination findings that may be missed in a well baby		
Examination Finding	**Possible diagnosis**	**Urgent action required**
Absent femoral pulses.	Coarctation of the aorta.	Echocardiogram, four limb blood pressures/ saturations and referral to paediatric cardiac surgeons.
Absent red reflex.	Retinoblastoma. Congenital cataracts.	Ophthalmology review.
Absent/misplaced anus.	Anorectal malformation.	Nasogastric tube, intravenous fluids and urgent surgical review.
Lump in the groin.	Inguinal hernia.	Urgent surgical referral.
Ambiguous genitalia.	Congenital Adrenal Hyperplasia.	Check sodium, potassium and glucose. Urgent karyotyping should be done to aid sex determination.
Murmur.	Undiagnosed cardiac condition (e.g. ventral septal defect).	Echocardiogram, four limb saturations/blood pressures.

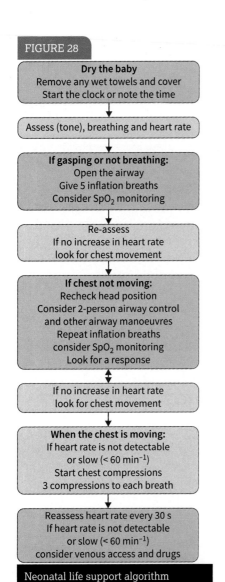

FIGURE 28

Dry the baby
Remove any wet towels and cover
Start the clock or note the time

↓

Assess (tone), breathing and heart rate

↓

If gasping or not breathing:
Open the airway
Give 5 inflation breaths
Consider SpO₂ monitoring

↓

Re-assess
If no increase in heart rate
look for chest movement

↓

If chest not moving:
Recheck head position
Consider 2-person airway control
and other airway manoeuvres
Repeat inflation breaths
consider SpO₂ monitoring
Look for a response

↓

If no increase in heart rate
look for chest movement

↓

When the chest is moving:
If heart rate is not detectable
or slow (< 60 min⁻¹)
Start chest compressions
3 compressions to each breath

↓

Reassess heart rate every 30 s
If heart rate is not detectable
or slow (< 60 min⁻¹)
consider venous access and drugs

Neonatal life support algorithm
(adapted from the UK Resuscitation
Council guidelines, UK)

TABLE 3: Calculating APGAR scores			
Score	0	1	2
Appearance.	White / Pale.	Blue peripherally.	Pink.
Pulse.	Absent.	<100 bpm.	>100 bpm.
Grimace (reflex irritability).	Unresponsive.	Grimace/feeble cry when stimulated.	Pulls away/cries when stimulated.
Activity (tone).	None.	Some flexion.	Flexed arms and legs that resist extension.
Respiration.	Absent.	Weak and irregular.	Strong cry.

PREMATURITY

Key definitions are summarised in *Table 4*.

Risk Factors

It is important to look for risk factors that may indicate a baby will be born prematurely or with a low birth weight (*Table 5*). These babies will often need urgent medical attention and admission onto a suitable neonatal unit. Parents can be counselled regarding the potential outcomes, clinical course and treatment options before the baby is delivered. It is also important to consider where is best to care for the baby. For example, extremely premature babies are likely to require intensive support that is best delivered in specialist units. In these cases, it is preferable to arrange for the pregnant mother to be transported to one of these units before delivery, if it is safe to do so.

Management

Management varies dramatically, depending on the individual baby. A baby born at 36+5 weeks gestation, with a birth weight of 2.4 kg, may require little in the way of medical support. In contrast, a baby born at 24 weeks gestation with a birth weight of 500 g, requires resuscitation at birth, followed by intensive therapy on a dedicated neonatal unit for six months or more. Even with the best medical care in the world, the baby may not survive or may survive with profound disability needing ongoing lifelong support from a variety of specialist and therapists. *Table 6* summarises the general issues associated with prematurity and how they might be managed.

TABLE 4: Definitions relating to premature and low birth weight infants	
Category	Definition
Premature infant.	Born before 37 weeks gestation.
Extremely premature infant.	Born before 28 weeks gestation.
Very low birth weight.	Born with a weight less than 1.5 kg.
Extremely low birth weight.	Born with a weight less than 1 kg.
Small for gestational age (SGA).	Born with a weight below the 10th centile for gestation.
Intrauterine growth restriction (IUGR).	When growth velocity falls during the pregnancy causing the foetal weight to cross gestation related weight centiles on serial scans.

TABLE 5: Risk factors for prematurity and low birth weight		
Placental Factors.	**Uterine Factors.**	**Other Factors.**
• Placenta previa.	• Uterine malformation.	• Premature rupture of membranes.
• Placental abruption.	• Cervical incompetence.	• Trauma.
• Placental insufficiency.		• Iatrogenic.
Maternal Factors.		**Foetal Factors.**
• Pre-eclampsia.		• Foetal distress.
• Chronic medical illness (e.g. chronic kidney disease).		• Multiple pregnancy.
• Maternal infection.		• Chromosomal abnormality.
• Maternal smoking and drug abuse.		• Foetal/neonatal infection.

TABLE 6: Management of issues related to prematurity		
Respiratory.	Surfactant deficiency.	Mothers may be given corticosteroids to enhance the maturation of type II alveolar cells in the foetal lungs. These cells produce surfactant. The baby may also have artificial surfactant given through an endotracheal tube post-delivery.
	Pneumothoraces.	These are more common in premature infants with their "stiff" surfactant deficient lungs. Artificial surfactant has reduced the incidence of pneumothorax in preterm babies.
	Apnoea of prematurity.	This is a result of poor central respiratory drive. The risk can be reduced by administration of caffeine to stimulate respiratory drive.
	Broncho-pulmonary dysplasia.	Lung disease, often acquired in early periods of premature life, resulting in an oxygen requirement at 28 days or 36 weeks corrected gestation is classified as broncho-pulmonary dysplasia.
Cardiovascular.	Patent ductus arteriosus (PDA).	A persistence of the ductus arteriosus after delivery can cause respiratory distress due to left to right shunting through the duct. Treatment can be with prostaglandin inhibitors, surgical ligation or percutaneous placement of a device in the PDA to close it.
	Hypotension.	The immature cardiovascular system is less able to compensate for changes in intravascular volume. This is exacerbated by increased fluid loss from the skin and immature kidneys. Treatment can include giving more volume and inotropic support.
Haematological.	Anaemia of prematurity.	An immature bone marrow may lead to repeated transfusions throughout the neonatal period.
Gastrointestinal.	Jaundice.	All babies have a higher bilirubin than expected in the adult population. Preterm babies have a weaker blood brain barrier and so have a lower threshold for when treatment should be started.
	Necrotising enterocolitis (NEC)	The exact pathophysiology of NEC is yet to be fully explained. It is more common in preterm babies and those with intrauterine growth restriction (IUGR). The risk is further exacerbated if enteral feeding is delayed or rapidly increased. Treatment involves antibiotics and surgery if the bowel becomes necrotic or perforated.
	Inguinal hernia.	This is common in preterm infants. Inguinal hernias should always be repaired if seen, as they have a high incidence of strangulation.
	Feeding difficulties and long-term faltering growth.	Due to the myriad of problems faced by preterm and low birthweight babies, feeding and weight gain can be difficult issues with complex management plans required.
Endocrine/ metabolic.	Hypothermia.	Babies have a large surface area, less muscle mass and immature skin. They need incubator support, often to a weight of 1.4-1.6kg.
	Hypocalcaemia, hyponatraemia, hyperglycaemia, hypoglycaemia, metabolic bone disease.	Renal salt losses associated with immature kidneys, poor absorption of enteral feeds and immature insulin secreting pathways mean that premature babies often require supplements of many vitamins and minerals. Fractures are commonly seen in this population.
Developmental and nervous system.	Intraventricular haemorrhage (IVH).	Many premature babies are found to have blood in the ventricles within the first 72 hours of life. Small amounts of blood are not predictive of future problems but larger amounts can indicate an increased risk of cerebral palsy, post-haemorrhagic hydrocephalus and developmental delay.
	Periventricular leukomalacia (PVL).	The finding of small cysts in the periventricular regions is highly suggestive of long-term developmental delay. Babies who have a stormy neonatal course are more likely to develop PVL.
	Developmental delay, cerebral palsy, social skills deficit.	Premature babies, particularly if admitted to the neonatal unit, require long-term follow up.
Eyes.	Retinopathy of prematurity.	The abnormal proliferation of retinal blood vessels can be mitigated by carefully targeting oxygen saturations in preterm infants to reduce their exposure to oxygen. Routine surveillance has greatly reduced blindness associated with this condition in the UK. Treatment is with laser therapy.
Ears.	Hearing deficit.	All premature infants require a hearing check pre-discharge as part of routine child health surveillance.
Infection.	Early onset and hospital acquired infection.	This group of patients have weaker immune systems, have various venous lines and other inserted medical devices. All of these factors increase the likelihood and the potential severity of sepsis. Early recognition and prompt treatment are vital.

On discharge, premature babies requiring admission to the neonatal unit should be followed up by specialist neonatal doctors. It is particularly important to monitor growth and development. Babies are at an increased risk of hospitalisation, particularly for chest infections and bronchiolitis. Prophylactic vaccinations are now available against RSV bronchiolitis, which should be considered in this group. However, this is tightly regulated due to the high cost of these vaccines.

Prognosis

A baby's chance of survival without disability increases with increasing gestational age. Survival under 23 weeks gestation is very rare and those that do survive have the severest of disabilities. Although recent evidence suggests that more preterm babies are surviving, little progress is apparently being made in reducing moderate and severe disability in these groups.

MULTIPLE BIRTHS

Key definitions are summarised in *Table 7*. Twin pregnancy is usually confirmed antenatally on ultrasound. All twin pregnancies should be considered at a higher risk of developing complications and requiring close observation during labour and in the immediate neonatal period. Monochorionic and monozygotic twins are at an even higher risk.

Twin pregnancy may be associated with:

› Hyperemesis gravidarum.
› Pre-eclampsia.
› Polyhydramnios.
› Premature rupture of membranes (PROM).
› Prematurity.
› Abnormal foetal presentations.
› Intrauterine growth restriction (IUGR).
› Congenital abnormalities.

The second delivered twin is at a greater risk than the first twin for respiratory distress and an acute intrapartum event. The more foetuses in a pregnancy, the greater the risk. Some countries offer "selective foetal reduction" to improve outcomes when a large number of foetuses are identified in utero. This can be particularly problematic with in vitro fertilisation, when several fertilised eggs are placed in the uterus.

Twin-to-Twin Transfusion Syndrome

This is a rare complication of monochorionic twinning. It usually results in transfusion of blood from an artery in one twin to a vein in the other twin via abnormal vascular connections (*Figure 29*). This results in one twin becoming plethoric and large (the recipient of extra blood) and the other becoming anaemic and small (the donor of excess blood). Management in the postnatal period can

TABLE 7: Definitions relating to twins	
Category	**Definition**
Monozygotic twins.	Derived from the same ovum; identical twins
Dizygotic twins.	Derived from two separate ova; non-identical twins
Monochorionic twins.	Twins sharing the same placenta
Dichorionic twins.	Twins with two separate placentas

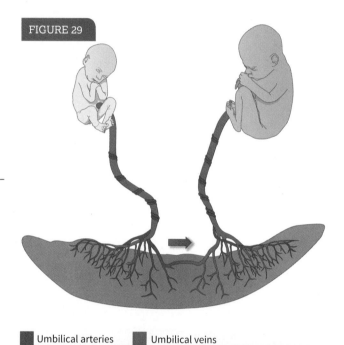

FIGURE 29

■ Umbilical arteries   ■ Umbilical veins

Twin-to-twin transfusion syndrome: Blood from the umbilical artery of the donor twin communicates with the umbilical vein of the recipient twin, and there is a net flow of blood away from the donor.

be challenging, as infants affected by this are often very unwell. In utero treatments are also now possible, with laser therapy applied to the vascular connection in the placenta to stop communication. Despite these advances, mortality remains high.

JAUNDICE

Jaundice is due to bilirubin being deposited in the skin. Bilirubin is a protein derived from the breakdown of red blood cells, specifically haemoglobin. It is conjugated in the liver and excreted in the stool and urine. All babies will have a higher bilirubin level than is expected in the adult population. This is because foetal haemoglobin gives the red blood cells a shorter life span of 90 days versus 120 days for an adult red blood cell. Babies have immature livers and reduced elimination of bilirubin due to the low volume colostrum babies receive in the first 24 to 48 hours of life. Once bilirubin saturates the liver, it begins to be deposited in the skin.

Several causes of further increased levels of bilirubin are detailed below. The effects of hyperbilirubinaemia on the neonate depend on the gestational age, the chronological age and on the general health of the baby.

Aetiology
Jaundice can be categorised in terms of time of presentation:

Jaundice Presenting within 24 hours
Haemolytic Disease
- Rhesus incompatibility. This is a result of the mother being rhesus negative, and the baby being rhesus positive.
- ABO incompatibility. This is a result of the baby having either A group or B group antigens (either being A+, B+ or AB+), and the mother being negative to that same group. Group O mothers are most at risk of this.
- G6PD deficiency. This is an X-linked recessive condition that affects red cell function and predisposes to haemolysis.
- Hereditary spherocytosis. This is an autosomal dominant condition that affects the shape of red blood cells, making them more fragile. As a result, the cells are more likely to haemolyse.

Infection
This is an important cause of jaundice in the first 24 hours of life and should be suspected in all cases of early jaundice, unless there is a clear alternative diagnosis.

Jaundice Presenting between 24 hours and 2 weeks
- Breastfeeding jaundice. The exact aetiology is unclear but it resolves without treatment or complication. Mothers should be encouraged to continue to breastfeed.
- Physiological jaundice. This usually presents at day two or three of life. It is related to immature liver function and the high red cell turnover in babies.
- Polycythaemia. Babies have a naturally high packed cell volume (PCV). The higher red cell number means greater red cell breakdown, and therefore more bilirubin generation.
- Resolving cephalohaematoma.

Prolonged Jaundice (jaundice present at 2 weeks or beyond)
- Bile duct obstruction (e.g. biliary atresia). This is the most important condition to exclude and requires urgent surgical assessment. There will be a conjugated hyperbilirubinaemia. The presence of pale stools and dark urine implies limited or no passage of bile into the gut, and is a worrying sign. Delay in diagnosis leads to a worse prognosis.
- Hypothyroidism. This is a possible presentation, although it should usually be picked up earlier as it is part of neonatal screening programmes.
- Urinary tract infection. An undiagnosed urinary tract infection may present with prolonged jaundice as the only symptom.

- Neonatal hepatitis. Inflammation in the liver causes biliary flow disruption.
- Physiological/breast feeding jaundice is the most common cause of prolonged jaundice, but it is a diagnosis of exclusion.

Clinical Features
Jaundice commonly presents in a well, asymptomatic baby with a yellow tinge (*Figure 30*). This is easiest to detect in the sclera of the eye.

Investigations
All jaundiced babies require a bilirubin check. Trying to judge the bilirubin by sight is highly inaccurate. Transcutaneous bilirubinometers, in select cases, allow measurement of bilirubin levels without a blood test.

Other investigations of jaundice presenting before two-weeks-old depend on clinical suspicion. Tests may be needed to assess the severity of any dehydration and possible causes of the jaundice. It is useful to consider:
- Blood film and full blood count (FBC). This is to look for any red cell abnormalities, anaemia and inflammatory markers.

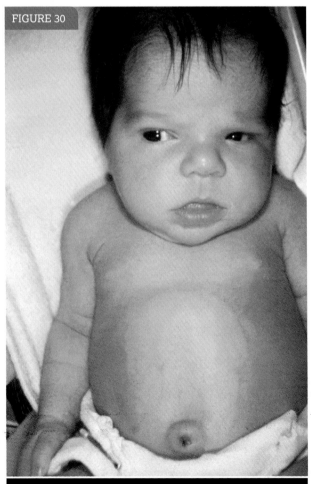

FIGURE 30

A jaundiced baby with congenital hypothyroidism.

- Direct antibody test (DAT or Coombs test). This is to look for evidence of haemolysis.
- C-reactive protein (CRP). As a marker of possible infection although this can be normal in the neonatal population in spite of overwhelming sepsis.
- Blood cultures. If treating for infection, a blood culture should be taken before starting antibiotics.

In a prolonged jaundice screen, it is helpful to assess thyroid function, liver function (including conjugated bilirubin) and a clean catch or catheter urine sample for bacteria.

Management
In a baby under 2-weeks -old, the bilirubin level can be plotted onto a treatment threshold graph, which can indicate the need for observation, treatment with ultraviolet phototherapy (*Figure 31*) or, in severe cases, exchange transfusion. Some early jaundice requires specialist treatment, such as the use of immunoglobulin in haemolytic disease.

Phototherapy is the most common treatment. Whilst under phototherapy, good feeding should be ensured, as well as regular monitoring of bilirubin. A rebound bilirubin should be checked, after phototherapy is stopped, to ensure that the bilirubin has not increased significantly post treatment.

Complications
Babies with significant unconjugated hyperbilirubinaemia are prone to kernicterus. Kernicterus occurs when unconjugated bilirubin crosses the blood-brain barrier. Bilirubin binds irreversibly to neuroreceptors in the basal ganglia of the brain, resulting in permanent neurological effects. Its occurrence is rare in developed countries, as neonatal jaundice tends

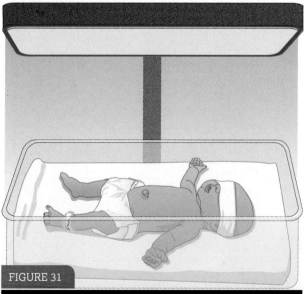

Phototherapy: an ultraviolet light is shone over the baby, with maximal skin exposed. The baby's eyes are covered to prevent damage.

to get identified and treated early. Mild cases present with poor feeding and lethargy, whilst more severe cases are associated with irritability, hypertonia, seizures and coma. The long-term effects of kernicterus mimic a parkinsonian picture due to the effects on the basal ganglia and severe developmental delay.

Prognosis
Babies with neonatal jaundice that has been well treated generally have a good prognosis, with no long-term ill effects. Kernicterus is, in theory, completely avoidable with early detection and treatment of jaundice

HAEMATOLOGICAL DISORDERS

Vitamin K Deficiency Bleeding
Aetiology
Vitamin K deficiency bleeding results from a relative deficiency in vitamin K-dependant clotting factors (II, VII, IX and X), and is more prevalent in breastfed babies. It also may be more likely in mothers taking medications that interfere with vitamin K metabolism, such as certain anticonvulsants or anticoagulants.

Clinical Features
The classic presentation is bleeding from the umbilical stump. The disease may also present with bruising, haematemesis or melaena. In severe cases, presentation may be an intracranial bleed.

Management
Vitamin K prophylaxis is recommended for all children in the UK and elsewhere. This is routinely given as an intramuscular injection. It can also be given orally, although this route is not recommended as absorption is variable and three doses are required over a four week period. There have, in the past, been some safety concerns about the use of IM vitamin K (e.g. link between the intramuscular vaccine and leukaemia) but these have now been discredited in larger studies.

NEONATAL INFECTION
Sepsis is still a leading cause of neonatal mortality worldwide. It is important to have a high index of suspicion regarding sepsis and to start treatment early when it is suspected. The use of blood inflammatory markers is highly unreliable in the neonatal population, particularly in the early stages of sepsis.

Early-Onset Infection (within 48 hours)
Early-onset infection is usually acquired via vertical transmission from the mother. These infections can be devastating. Therefore, babies are often started on antibiotics purely on the basis of risk factors identified pre-delivery.

NEONATAL INFECTION

Risk Factors for Infection

> Invasive group B streptococcal infection in a previous pregnancy.
> Maternal group B streptococcal colonisation, bacteriuria or infection in current pregnancy.
> Prolonged rupture of membranes.
> Preterm birth.
> Intrapartum fever or suspected chorioamnionitis.
> Suspected or confirmed infection in another baby in the case of a multiple pregnancy.
> Suspected or confirmed invasive bacterial infection in the mother.

Clinical Features

Infection may present non-specifically, but possible signs include temperature instability, poor feeding, vomiting, respiratory distress, apnoeas, bradycardia, tachycardia, shock, hypo/hyperglycaemia, irritability, lethargy/drowsiness, seizures, jaundice (particularly in the first 24 hours of life) and poor urine output.

Aetiology

Likely microbes include group B *streptococci* (and other strep species) and coliforms. Rarer microbes include *Listeria*, *Klebsiella* and *Pseudomonas* species.

Investigations

Blood cultures and baseline inflammatory markers should be taken. High inflammatory markers or worrying clinical signs warrant further assessment, with consideration of a lumbar puncture. If any respiratory signs are present, a chest X-ray should be performed.

Management

In cases of possible infection, broad-spectrum antibiotics (e.g. benzylpenicillin and gentamicin) are usually started.

Duration of treatment with antibiotics depends on bacteria isolated from the baby or mother, whether any rise occurs in inflammatory markers and whether any symptoms were present at the onset or during treatment. Treatment should be for a minimum of 36-48 hours, pending blood culture results.

Late-Onset Infection (after 48 hours)

Late-onset infection is more likely to be contracted from the baby's environment, particularly if they are an inpatient. This may be from staff/visitors, or it may arise due to indwelling lines and poor aseptic technique in performing neonatal procedures.

Aetiology

Group B streptococcal infection can present after the first 48 hours, including those babies discharged to the community. Staphylococcal infections, including *Staphylococcus aureus,* are found with increasing frequency in this population. Coagulase-negative *Staphylococcus* is the most common infecting organism on the neonatal unit, particularly in infants with long lying venous catheters, although it is also part of normal skin flora. Coliforms and pseudomonal species are also causes of late-onset infections.

Management

Management strategies should consider the wide variability of infections found in this vulnerable group. Treatment is likely to include broad spectrum antibiotics to cover both gram positive and negative bacteria (e.g. flucloxacillin and gentamicin). It is important to target antibiotic therapy based on sensitivity data, which may vary from population to population.

Congenital Infections

Table 8 summarises some common congenital infections.

TABLE 8: Congenital neonatal infections	
Herpes Simplex	This is usually transmitted via the birth canal. If the mother has primary active vaginal herpes, the baby should be delivered by caesarean section. Neonatal infection may present with skin lesions (*Figure 32*), encephalitis or disseminating disease. Treatment is with aciclovir; however, mortality is high.
Syphilis	All mothers in the UK are screened antenatally for syphilis. Syphilis may present in the newborn with fever, irritability, a saddle nose (no bridge), and rashes or ulceration. Babies born to mothers with active syphilis should be treated with penicillin, even in the absence of symptomatic infection.
Listeria	Listeria can be transmitted to the mother through foods such as soft cheeses and unpasteurised milk. It is characteristically associated with a preterm delivery complicated by meconium passage. Treatment is with amoxicillin.
Hepatitis B	Hepatitis B can be vertically transmitted; therefore, all infants of mothers that are hepatitis B surface antigen (HBsAg) positive should receive the hepatitis B vaccination. In some countries where the prevalence of hepatitis B is high, hepatitis B vaccine is offered to all infants. Certain mothers are more high risk. These include those with active hepatitis B in pregnancy and those that are "e" antigen positive, or "e" antibody negative. Their babies should also receive hepatitis B immunoglobulin.

(Continued)

TABLE 8: *Continued*

Hepatitis C	The rate of maternal to child transmission is linked to the maternal viral RNA load. No treatment for either the mother or the neonate has proven to reduce the risk of transmission. Neonatal hepatitis C infection is diagnosed by measuring HCV RNA using PCR techniques. An infant may be assumed to have an active infection if the HCV PCR remains positive for six months. Treatment should be coordinated with paediatric liver and infectious disease specialists. Options include interferon treatment and antiretroviral medications.
HIV	HIV testing is routinely done during the antenatal period in most countries. If detected, a viral load is useful for predicting the risk to the neonate. Low viral loads in mothers are associated with low vertical transmission rates. Initial tests on neonates can be inaccurate and serial tests over several months are required to confirm that a baby is HIV negative. The use of zidovudine immediately after birth reduces the risk of infection. HIV can be transmitted via breast milk. Care should be taken regarding advice to stop breast feeding in the developing world, where formulas, sterilising equipment and clean water may not be readily available.
Maternal Varicella (Chicken pox)	If the mother contracts chicken pox during pregnancy, there is a risk of transmission to the baby. However, if it is greater than seven days before birth, antibodies are likely to have been transmitted to the baby via the placenta, and additional treatment is not required for the baby. If the mother develops chicken pox within seven days of delivery (or up to four days after delivery), then varicella zoster immunoglobulin should be administered to the baby, and the mother and baby should be isolated. Vesicular lesions should be treated with intravenous aciclovir.
Cytomegalovirus (CMV)	Antenatal infection with CMV is associated with microcephaly, hepatosplenomegaly, IUGR, cardiac defects and jaundice. Congenital CMV has a high mortality rate. Postnatal (acquired) infections can result in neurological deficit, feed intolerance, hepato-renal failure and eye disease. Postnatally, CMV can be treated with ganciclovir.
Rubella	Congenital infection with rubella is associated with cataracts, deafness and congenital heart disease. Babies may be born with a rash.
Toxoplasmosis	Congenital toxoplasmosis infection is associated with microcephaly, hepatosplenomegaly, IUGR, hepatitis, chorioretinitis and thrombocytopenia.
Parvovirus	Maternal infection with parvovirus can lead to foetal hydrops (excess fluid, e.g. ascites or pleural effusion), hydrocephalus and foetal anaemia.
Conjunctivitis	Most "sticky" eyes in the neonatal period are not bacterial in origin and often represent blocked tear ducts that resolve with simple cleaning. Persistent discharge or signs of inflammation should be swabbed for microbiological examination. Chlamydia should be suspected in the presence of maternal history or ulceration of the corneas.

FIGURE 32

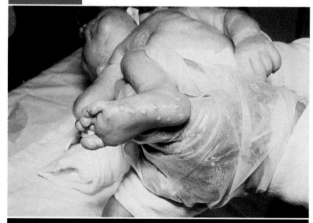

Herpes blistering rashes on the foot.

RESPIRATORY DISORDERS

Respiratory Distress Syndrome

Respiratory distress syndrome (RDS) is the result of surfactant deficiency.

Aetiology

Respiratory distress syndrome is more common in premature infants and in infants of diabetic mothers. Surfactant deficiency leads to alveolar collapse and consequent impairment of gas exchange. Without artificial surfactant therapy, respiratory distress worsens over the first three days of life, but is followed by gradual improvement should the baby survive.

X-Ray Appearance

The X-ray appearance of respiratory distress syndrome is typically described as having a ground glass appearance (*Figure 33*).

Management

Mothers expected to deliver prematurely may be given corticosteroids antenatally to promote the maturity of type 2 alveolar cells, which produce surfactant in the lungs. Additionally, artificial surfactant can be given through an endotracheal tube immediately after delivery or at a later stage when the condition is recognised. Otherwise, supportive therapy is given. In premature infants, in particular, this may involve intubation and ventilation. Giving steroids to the baby after delivery does not promote surfactant production and has no effect on morbidity or mortality with respect to lung disease.

Broncho-Pulmonary Dysplasia (Chronic Lung Disease)

This refers to babies who have a persistent oxygen requirement from birth up until 28-days-old or 36 weeks corrected gestation.

FIGURE 33

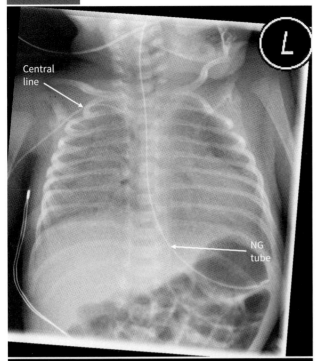

Respiratory Distress Syndrome. Note the interstitial shadowing bilaterally, giving a ground-glass appearance. An NG tube is present in the stomach and a central line is present, entering from the right arm.

FIGURE 34

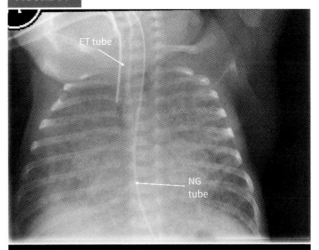

Diffuse interstitial shadowing in evolving bronchopulmonary dysplasia. Note also there is an NG tube in situ and an endotracheal (ET) tube sitting at the level of T3.

FIGURE 35

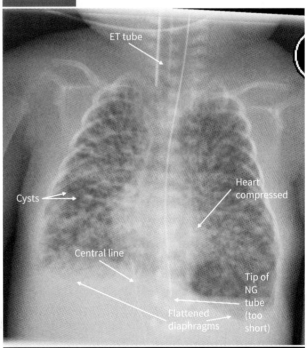

Broncho-pulmonary dysplasia. There is diffuse interstitial shadowing throughout the lung fields. There is hyperexpansion of the lungs, due to air trapping, resulting in flattening of the diaphragms. Cysts are visible in both lung fields. The heart also appears smaller, as the elevated intrathoracic pressure reduces venous return. Note also the ET tube present at the level of T1 and the central line at approximately T11. The nasogastric tube is short, only just crossing the diaphragm.

Aetiology

Those most likely to be affected are extremely premature neonates. Other risk factors include infection and postnatal lung injury from ventilator support.

X-Ray Appearance

The appearance on X-ray begins with that of RDS (*Figure 34*), but then can evolve into that of pulmonary interstitial emphysema (*Figure 35*).

Management

Management involves nutrition optimisation, oxygen supplementation and ventilation support as required. Corticosteroid therapy and/or diuretic therapy may be helpful in improving lung function. Many babies with chronic lung disease will get better as they grow; some go home on oxygen and perhaps remain ventilator-dependent or die subsequently of the disease.

Transient Tachypnoea of the Newborn

This is the most common cause of respiratory distress in term babies, and is due to a delay in clearance of foetal lung fluid.

Aetiology

It is more common following delivery by caesarean section. The exact pathophysiology is unclear, but it is likely due to a lack of exposure of the infant to hormones and stresses involved during labour.

X-Ray Appearance

Radiological features may include cardiomegaly, pleural effusions, fluid in the horizontal fissure and prominent perihilar interstitial markings (*Figure 36*).

FIGURE 36

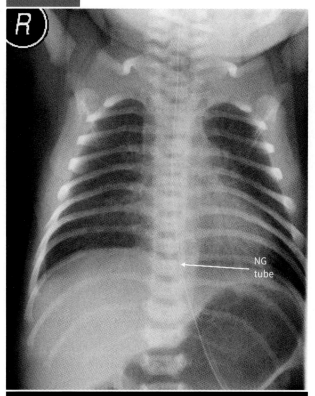

NG tube

Illustration of some features of transient tachypnoea of the newborn, with prominent perihilar interstitial markings.

FIGURE 37

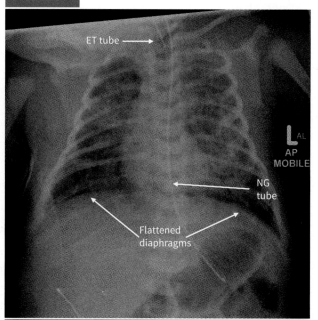

ET tube

NG tube

Flattened diaphragms

Meconium Aspiration Syndrome. Bilateral diffuse heterogeneous opacification. There is also hyperinflation of the lungs. The ET tube is sitting at T1.

Management

Transient tachypnoea of the newborn begins immediately at birth and usually resolves within the first four hours of life. Supportive therapy may be briefly required.

Meconium Aspiration Syndrome

Aetiology

Meconium may be passed in utero or at the time of birth and is a response to foetal distress in utero. Meconium in the lungs causes initial mechanical obstructive disease, which in itself can be fatal. After some hours, the meconium draws inflammatory cells into the lungs, causing a chemical pneumonitis and further preventing gas exchange. This may result in pulmonary hypertension. Symptoms of meconium aspiration normally present in the first four hours of life.

X-Ray Appearance

Chest X-rays show classical areas of over-inflation and heterogeneous opacification, representing collapse and consolidation (*Figure 37*).

Management

Treatment is supportive and may include intubation and ventilation, surfactant therapy, inotropic support of blood pressure and inhaled nitric oxide.

Pneumothorax

Aetiology

This may occur spontaneously, or secondary to respiratory distress syndrome, meconium aspiration or mechanical ventilation. It may be asymptomatic, but may require aspiration or chest drain insertion.

X-Ray Appearance

A pneumothorax may be classed as simple (*Figure 38*) or tension (*Figure 39*).

Management

Infants with a pneumothorax should be nursed in higher concentrations of oxygen, as this can aid in spontaneous resolution of pneumothorax. Larger pneumothoraces or those under tension will require aspiration and/or chest drain insertion.

Pneumonia

Aetiology

This can be congenital or acquired after birth (*Figure 40*). It is more common in babies with risk factors for infection, such as prolonged rupture of membranes or chorioamnionitis. The causative pathogen is usually bacterial, most commonly Gram-negative bacilli (e.g. *E. coli, Klebsiella, Pseudomonas*), group B streptococcus and staphylococcus.

X-Ray Appearance

Chest X-ray appearance characteristically shows a heterogeneous opacity.

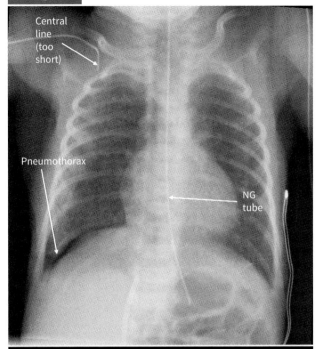

FIGURE 38

Central line (too short)

Pneumothorax

NG tube

Small pneumothorax at the base of the right lung. An NG tube is also in situ, and a too short central line (inserted into the right arm) is sitting at the shoulder.

Management

Management involves supportive care with oxygen and ventilatory support as needed. IV fluids and/or an NG tube may reduce respiratory distress. Broad spectrum antibiotics should be commenced.

Persistent Pulmonary Hypertension of the Newborn (PPHN)

PPHN is an acute neonatal emergency resulting from the failure of high pulmonary vascular resistance to fall at birth and the subsequent persistence of foetal intracardiac shunts. It primarily affects infants close to term and shortly after birth with almost all cases diagnosed within the first 72 hours of life.

Aetiology

PPHN is most often secondary to parenchymal lung disease, such as meconium aspiration syndrome and RDS. The lungs are designed to redirect blood flow to the most oxygen rich parts of the lungs by causing vasoconstriction in low oxygen environments. If a baby is affected by homogeneous lung disease, such as meconium aspiration syndrome or RDS, the lung vasculature constricts globally across both lungs. The resulting high pulmonary pressures cause right-to-left shunting of blood through the foramen ovale and ductus arteriosus. This leads to the typical presentation of worsening cyanosis, tachypnoea and hypoxia, despite increasing oxygen and ventilator support. The spectrum of severity ranges from mild and transient respiratory distress to severe hypoxia and cardiopulmonary instability.

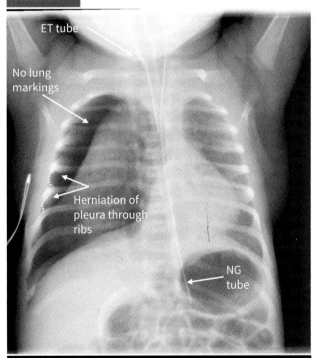

FIGURE 39

ET tube

No lung markings

Herniation of pleura through ribs

NG tube

Tension pneumothorax on the right. Note the shift of both the upper and lower mediastinum to the left, and the herniation of the pleura to the right side of the thorax. An ET tube is at level T3/4, and an NG tube is in situ.

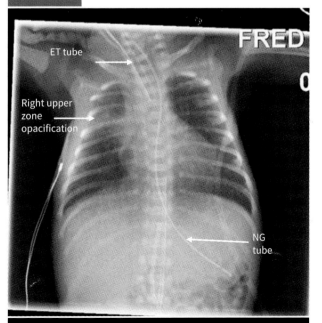

FIGURE 40

ET tube

FRED

Right upper zone opacification

NG tube

Congenital right upper zone pneumonia. An ET tube is at T2, and an NG tube is present in the stomach.

Management

The aim of management is to cause pulmonary vasodilation and reverse the cycle explained above. The most potent pulmonary vasodilator is oxygen, so babies are normally intubated and ventilated in high oxygen concentrations. Inhaled nitric oxide also causes pulmonary vasodilatation and can be delivered directly to the lungs via an endotracheal tube. Systemic blood pressure must be kept higher than the pulmonary pressures to avoid right to left shunting across a ductal cardiovascular circulation. In extreme cases, extracorporeal membrane oxygenation (ECMO) can be used to bypass the lungs and oxygenate the blood outside the body. The complications can be serious and relate to the placement of the large vascular catheters and heparinisation of the blood flow to prevent clotting in the ECMO circuit. Preterm babies are not suitable for ECMO due to their increased risk of haemorrhage and their small size, making it difficult to place the vascular catheters.

Congenital Pulmonary Airway Malformations

Also known as congenital cystic adenomatoid malformations (CCAMs), this rare congenital condition involves an error in lung development, leaving part of the lung as non-functional cystic tissue. Paediatric surgeons usually remove these malformations if large or symptomatic. The timing of surgery depends on the symptoms present in the infant at the time of birth versus the anaesthetic risk, which reduces with the age of the infant. Severe cases may require urgent surgery (*Figure 41*).

Broncho-Pulmonary Sequestration

This rare condition comprises normal lung tissue which is supplied with blood vessels from the systemic circulation rather than the pulmonary circulation. It is also not attached to the bronchial tree. It is usually surgically removed.

NEUROLOGICAL DISORDERS

Neonatal Seizures

Seizures in the neonatal period are repetitive, rhythmic movements that, if isolated to a limb, continue even when that body part is restrained.

Aetiology

Causes of neonatal seizures include infection (particularly meningitis), hypoglycaemia, intraventricular haemorrhage, neonatal cerebrovascular events, cerebral malformation, hypoxic ischaemic encephalopathy, withdrawal from maternally ingested drugs, and electrolyte imbalances. Pyridoxine deficiency is a rare but treatable cause of intractable neonatal seizures.

Differential Diagnosis

Jitteriness in a baby can be a normal finding, but it may be associated with hypoglycaemia, hypocalcaemia or neonatal abstinence syndrome (physiological withdrawal experienced by an infant exposed to opiate drugs antenatally by maternal ingestion). These can be diagnosed or excluded by careful history taking, examination and investigation.

Myoclonic jerks can occur during sleep and periods before waking. These are a normal finding and need no treatment.

Management

Any baby with seizures requires admission to the neonatal intensive care unit. A cranial ultrasound should be performed, as well as electrode monitoring of cerebral activity (using a Cerebral Function Analysing Monitor [CFAM] if available). The baby should be treated for meningoencephalitis, with broad spectrum antibiotics and antiviral agents. If the seizures persist, antiepileptic medication may be required, e.g. phenobarbitone.

Cerebral Infarction

This is a rare event in neonates, but may occur secondary to thrombosis. The middle cerebral artery is most commonly implicated. Babies do not usually develop encephalopathy, instead presenting with seizures in isolation. The diagnosis is confirmed on an MRI scan. The prognosis is often good, demonstrating the plasticity of the neonatal brain.

Acute Intrapartum Events and Hypoxic Ischaemic Encephalopathy

Aetiology

Acute intrapartum events are a significant cause of neonatal mortality worldwide, particularly in settings with poor emergency obstetrics care. It can often be difficult to pinpoint the seminal event causing the hypoxic insult. Events may include an antepartum haemorrhage, cord prolapse/

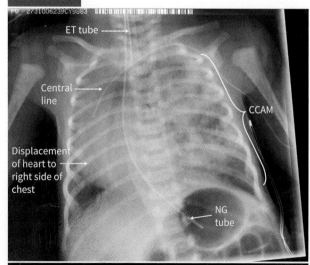

FIGURE 41

Large CCAM on the left, causing displacement of the heart to the right. Note the NG tube in situ, and the central line. The ET tube is sitting at approximately T2.

obstruction, or shoulder dystocia. All of these events lead to a rapid and sustained drop in blood flow to the foetus causing hypoxia.

Clinical Features

Clinically, foetal monitoring may give an indication of foetal distress. The babies are often born floppy with little or no respiratory effort. Breathing may need to be supported as the baby may remain encephalopathic following delivery. Later in the natural course of hypoxic-ischaemic encephalopathy (HIE), babies may become irritable with hypertonia and develop seizures. Multi-organ failure may ensue due to the hypoxic damage to other organs in the body. Long-term neurodisability may result in the moderate to severe cases. HIE can be graded as mild, moderate or severe, which can help to decide the course of treatment (*Table 9*).

Management

Treatment is supportive in the first instance, including adequate ventilation, and seizure control. Fluid restriction is advised if there has been a significant insult (due to associated renal impairment). Evidence now shows that total body cooling following HIE can improve long-term outcomes by reducing swelling and reperfusion injury to the recovering brain. An MRI conducted once the baby is more stable may help to predict outcome.

Intraventricular Haemorrhage

This is particularly common in low birth weight or premature infants, normally within the first three days of life. Other risk factors include severe respiratory distress syndrome, and perinatal asphyxia. Four grades are recognised, as summarised in *Table 10*.

Cranial Ultrasound

Cranial ultrasound is used to identify intraventricular haemorrhages, with MRI then sometimes used to confirm more concerning pathology. *Figure 42* shows a normal

TABLE 9: Classification of Hypoxic Ischaemic Encephalopathy (HIE)	
Degree of Encephalopathy	**Characteristics**
Mild.	Increased tone and reflexes. Transient behavioural changes, but resolves with 24 hours.
Moderate.	Lethargic, hypotonic, sluggish/absent reflexes and occasional apnoeas. Seizures. May recover within 1-2 weeks, but full recovery is unlikely if symptoms persist beyond the neonatal period.
Severe.	Stupor, coma, hypotonia, sluggish/absent reflexes and irregular breathing. Fixed and dilated pupils, irregular heart rate/blood pressure. Seizures subside as the injury progresses.

TABLE 10: Grades of intraventricular haemorrhage		
Grade	**Description**	**Prognosis**
I.	Bleeding into germinal matrix (this is the highly vascular and cellular region of the brain out of which cells migrate during brain development).	Usually associated with resolution and good prognosis.
II.	Bleeding into germinal matrix and ventricles.	
III.	Bleeding into ventricles causing enlargement due to blood accumulation.	Long-term neurological deficit more likely. May lead to hydrocephalus (from obstruction) or cerebral palsy.
IV.	Bleeding extending to tissue beyond ventricles.	

cranial ultrasound, with examples of a grade II, III and IV intraventricular haemorrhage shown in *Figures 43-5*. Coronal and sagittal images are taken to view as wide a spectrum of the brain as possible. The ultrasound probe is placed on the anterior fontanelle.

Two images are shown for each picture:
1 **Coronal.** This involves taking a picture as if dividing the front of the brain from the back of the brain. Normally, five

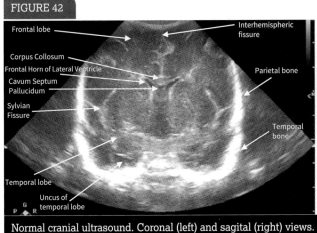
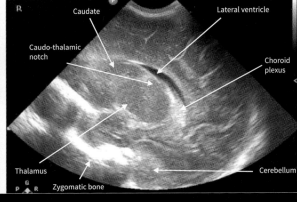

Normal cranial ultrasound. Coronal (left) and sagital (right) views.

FIGURE 43

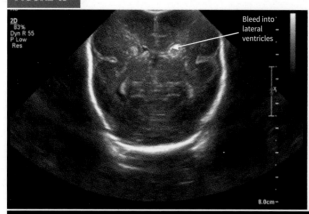
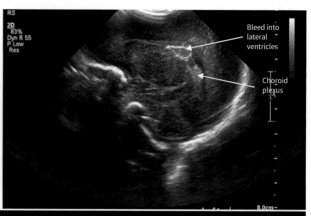

Grade II IVH. Bleed into both lateral ventricles, with no associated dilatation of the ventricle. Coronal (left), parasagittal (right).

FIGURE 44

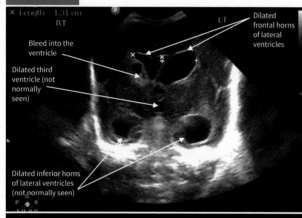
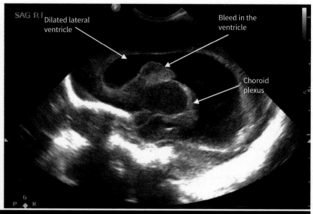

Grade III IVH. Bleed into the lateral ventricles with associated dilatation of the ventricles. Coronal (left), parasagittal (right).

FIGURE 45

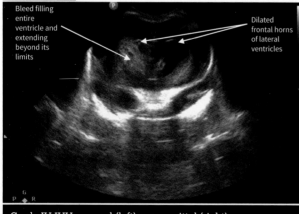
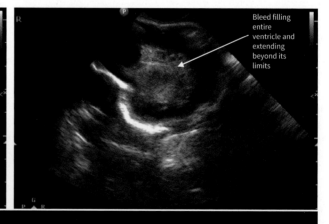

Grade IV IVH: coronal (left), parasagittal (right).

such images are taken, with the probe angled forwards and backwards from the fontanelle to get different angles of the brain. In the example pictures, for simplicity, just the image looking directly downwards is shown.

2 Sagittal. This involves taking a picture as if dividing the left and the right sides of the brain. Normally, one image is taken right down the middle, and two with the probe angled out either side. The example images are "para sagittal" views, i.e. the probe is angled out slightly to get a good view of the lateral ventricles.

Periventricular Leukomalacia

Periventricular leukomalacia (PVL) is a form of white matter brain injury. This may be secondary to ischaemia, or inflammation. Mild white matter injuries are difficult to detect acutely, but over time the characteristic periventricular cystic changes emerge on imaging such as ultrasound or MRI. The presence of PVL has a high association with cerebral palsy and learning difficulties.

HYPOGLYCAEMIA

Aetiology

Neonates are able to tolerate far lower blood sugars than the adult population. The accepted normal blood glucose in the immediate neonatal period is 2.6mmol/L. Term infants have brown fat, which generates energy and heat. However, in the presence of maternal and neonatal risk factors for hypoglycaemia (*Table 11*), the neonate may be unable to metabolise glycogen effectively or absorb enough milk enterally to sustain a normal blood glucose. Babies with known risk factors for hypoglycaemia should have their blood sugars monitored after birth. Hypoglycaemia may also be a sign of sepsis in the newborn infant. Babies with hypoglycaemia may present with lethargy, poor feeding, jitteriness, seizures or apnoea.

Management

Ensuring good feeding is normally sufficient to treat hypoglycaemia. Intravenous dextrose infusions may be needed and, rarely, diazoxide may be used to suppress insulin secretion. The majority of unstable blood sugars resolve within one to three days of good feeding.

TABLE 11: Risk factors for hypoglycaemia in the neonate.
• Infant of diabetic mother.
• IUGR/SGA.
• Prematurity.
• Macrosomia.
• Maternal beta blocker treatment.
• Sepsis.

Prognosis

The prognosis for mild hypoglycaemia without symptoms is excellent. The effect of hypoglycaemia on the newborn brain is uncertain but prolonged exposure to low blood sugars, particularly if the infant is symptomatic, has been shown to have a detrimental effect on development. Severe symptomatic hypoglycaemia is associated with developmental delay and MRI brain changes, particularly in the occipital regions.

ADDITIONAL PATHOLOGY

Cleft Palate and Lip

Cleft palate is the failure of fusion of the palatine processes and the nasal septum. Cleft lip is failure of fusion of the fronto-nasal and maxillary processes (*Figure 46*).

Clinical Features

During the routine baby check, the palate should be examined closely. The hard and soft palate should be felt and visualised to ensure a subtle cleft is not missed. An abnormally shaped or absent uvula may be indicative of a sub-mucous cleft that may not otherwise be visible.

Cleft palate and lip usually occur in isolation, but they may be part of a chromosomal abnormality or sequence. They may also occur secondary to anticonvulsant therapy. Large abnormalities are often picked up on antenatal ultrasound scanning, however smaller defects may be missed.

Management

Management is via a multidisciplinary team, involving paediatric surgeons (ENT, maxillofacial, and plastic), orthodontists, audiologists and speech therapists. The biggest immediate concern with cleft palate is feeding. Most babies can breast feed normally, but special teats may be helpful, particularly in more severe cases. Surgery for cleft lip can take place early, although repair of the palate is usually delayed until the infant is several months old.

FIGURE 46

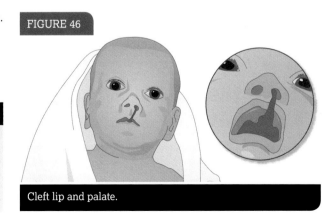

Cleft lip and palate.

Pierre Robin Sequence

This is a congenital disorder comprising:

> Micrognathia.
> Posterior tongue displacement.
> Cleft palate.

It is a clinical diagnosis and may present with feeding difficulties or difficulty breathing, particularly in the supine position. Management involves managing the airway and optimising nutrition. The supine position and a nasopharyngeal airway may help. In some cases, feeding assistance with a nasogastric tube may be required. The cleft palate can later be repaired surgically.

Foetal Alcohol Syndrome

Alcohol is a teratogen that passes into the foetal circulation, causing disruption to normal foetal development and permanent damage to the foetus. The incidence in the developed world may be as high as two in 1000 live births. The diagnosis can be challenging and may not be identified (*Table 12*). Foetal alcohol syndrome has no cure, but early intervention may increase functional outcomes of neonates that are affected. Input may be required from physiotherapists, occupational therapists, school assistance, social services support, community paediatricians and paediatric neurologists.

NEWBORN SCREENING

Newborn screening is not just limited to the physical examination at birth and six weeks, but also comprises a biochemical screening. *Table 13* summarises the diseases assessed in the UK by the NHS Newborn Blood Spot Screening programme (done in the first week of life). In all likelihood, more diseases will be tested in this way as laboratory tests improve and costs decline. Neonates also have a hearing screening in the first month of life with an Automated Otoacoustic Emission test.

TABLE 13: Diseases detected on neonatal biochemical screening in the UK

Disease Being Screened	Comments
Neonatal hypothyroidism.	Assesses TSH levels to identify neonatal hypothyroidism. It has been very successful, and has largely eliminated cretinism from the UK.
Cystic fibrosis.	Assesses immunoreactive trypsin levels, and has significantly reduced the age of diagnosis for cystic fibrosis.
Sickle cell disease.	A haemoglobinopathy particularly prevalent in those from Afro-Caribbean descent.
Phenylketonuria.	A defect in amino acid (phenylalanine) breakdown. Early detection allows early implementation of a restricted diet, thereby reducing the risk of neurological associated complications.
Medium-chain acyl-CoA dehydrogenase deficiency.	This is an abnormality in the breakdown of fats. Early diagnosis improves outcome by ensuring the child is treated actively during episodes of illness or fasting. Specialised diets may be required.
Homocystinuria.	A metabolic condition with a defect in amino acid (homocysteine) breakdown.
Maple syrup urine disease.	A metabolic condition with a defect in amino acid (leucine, isoleucine, valine) breakdown.
Isovaleric acidaemia.	A metabolic condition with a defect in amino acid (leucine) breakdown.
Glutaric aciduria type 1.	Defect in amino acid (lysine, hydroxylysine, tryptophan) breakdown.

TABLE 12: Features of foetal alcohol syndrome

Criteria	Comments
Growth Restriction.	• Pre- and post-natal growth restrictions affect both height and weight.
Facial Features.	• Smooth philtrum. • Thin vermilion (upper lip). • Small palpebral fissures.
Central Nervous System Involvement.	• Structural: epilepsy, neurosensory hearing loss, dyspraxia. • Functional: developmental delay, behavioural problems, learning difficulties, cognitive deficit.
Alcohol consumption during pregnancy.	• Either confirmed or unknown.

REFERENCES AND FURTHER READING

Newborn Resuscitation

1   Murthy V et al. The first five inflations during resuscitation of prematurely born infants. Arch Dis Child Fetal Neonatal Ed. 2012; 97:F249-53.

2   Murthy V et al. End tidal carbon dioxide levels during the resuscitation of prematurely born infants. Early Hum Dev. 2012; 88:783-7.

3   UK Resuscitation Council. New Born Life Support. Third edition. UK:Resuscitation Council. 2010.

Neonatal Respiratory Medicine

1   Nouraeyan N, Lambrinakos-Raymond A, Leone M, Sant'Anna G. Surfactant administration in neonates: A review of delivery methods. Can J Respir Ther. 2014; 50:91-5.

2   Polin RA et al. Surfactant replacement therapy for preterm and term neonates with respiratory distress. Pediatrics. 2014; 133:156-63.

3   Bassler D. Inhalation or instillation of steroids for the prevention of bronchopulmonary dysplasia. Neonatology. 2015;107:358-9.

4   Reuter S, Moser C, Baack M. Respiratory distress in the newborn. Pediatr Rev. 2014; 35:417-28.

Neonatal Neurology

1   Azzopardi D et al. The TOBY Study. Whole body hypothermia for the treatment of perinatal asphyxial encephalopathy: a randomised controlled trial. BMC Pediatr. 2008; 8:17.

2   Milani WR, Antibas PL, Prado GF. Cooling for cerebral protection during brain surgery. The Cochrane database of systematic reviews. 2011(10):CD006638.

Prematurity

1   Welsh L et al. The EPICure study: maximal exercise and physical activity in school children born extremely preterm. Thorax. 2010; 65:165-72.

Jaundice

1   NICE Guideline. Neonatal Jaundice (CG98). https://www.nice.org.uk/guidance/cg98.

Miscellaneous

1   Roman E et al. Vitamin K and childhood cancer: analysis of individual patient data from six case-control studies. Br J Cancer. 2002; 86:63-9.

2   White R, Blasier RD. Clubfoot: nature and treatment. Today's OR Nurse. 1994; 16:29-35.

3   Choices N. Newborn Blood Spot Test - Pregnancy and Newborn Guide. http://www.nhs.uk/Conditions/pregnancy-and-baby/Pages/newborn-blood-spot-test.aspx2015.

NEONATOLOGY

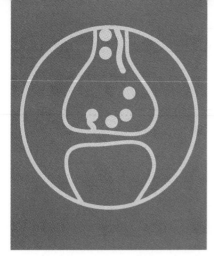

1.16
NEUROLOGY

JOHN JUNGPA PARK, ZESHAN QURESHI AND DEBASREE DAS

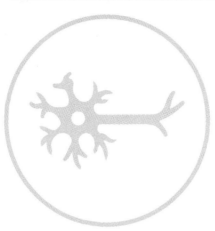

CONTENTS

SEIZURES

Introduction
Aetiology
A seizure is a disruption of normal neurological electrical activity that usually (but not always) is associated with either a change in behaviour, abnormal movements, or other changes in neurological function. Seizures can present in a myriad ways depending on where they originate in the brain. A diagnosis of epilepsy is made after two separate seizures, at least one day apart, where both are thought to originate from abnormal electrical activity in the brain. Epileptic seizures can be further sub-categorised as generalised or focal (partial), or as part of an epilepsy syndrome. Non-epileptic seizures can be organic (due to a pathological cause) or non-organic (psychogenic cause). *Figure 1* summarises seizure classifications.

FIGURE 1

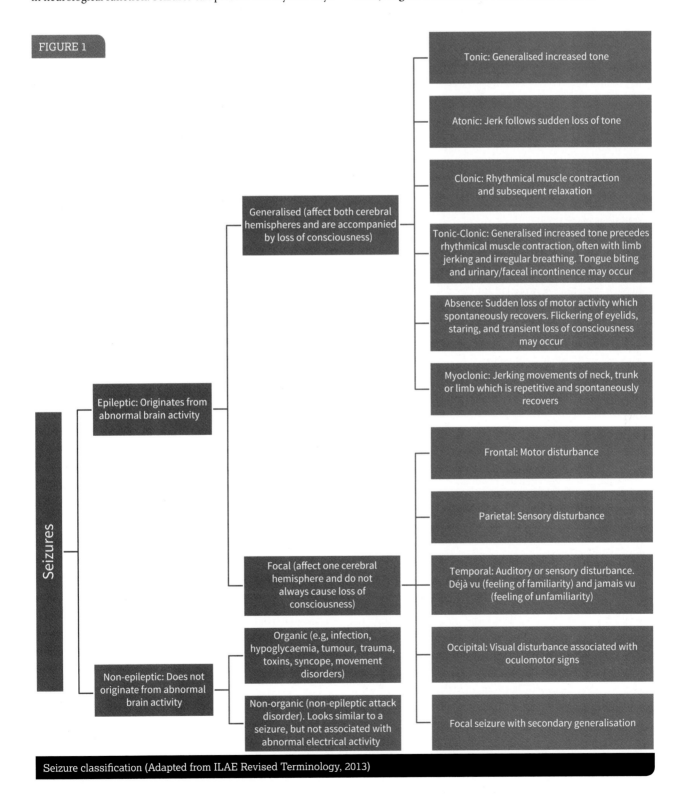

Seizure classification (Adapted from ILAE Revised Terminology, 2013)

Differential Diagnosis

Seizures

Though often idiopathic, seizures have a wide range of causes:

> Febrile convulsion. Febrile seizures are the most common cause of seizures in children. They present as a single episode, without a prior history of seizures, but can be recurrent.

> Non-epileptic attack disorder. These are also referred to as psychogenic non-epileptic seizures, or pseudoseizures, and are psychological in origin. They are notoriously difficult to diagnose and appear externally as seizures. Video telemetry, a specialised EEG synchronized with video recording, and observed admission may aid diagnosis. Features include dramatic flapping of limbs that do not follow a tonic or clonic pattern, tightly shut eyes which resist forced opening and distractibility out of episodes. Note that epilepsy may coexist.

> Epilepsy. See page 216.

> Meningoencephalitis. Seizures may occur secondary to infections in the CNS.

> Infection. Sepsis, cerebral abscesses, and subdural empyemas can all lead to seizures.

> Tumour. Seizures may occur secondary to an intracranial mass. A focal mass may present with focal signs or signs of increased ICP.

> Toxins. Toxins such as drugs can cause disturbance of neuronal activity and trigger seizures.

> Metabolic. Metabolic disturbances such as electrolyte imbalance or hypoglycaemia can lead to neuronal dysfunction and trigger seizures. In the infant, inborn errors of metabolism should be considered e.g. urea cycle defects.

> Head injury. Trauma is an important cause of seizures. In the infant, this is much more likely to be related to non-accidental injury than in older children.

Loss of Consciousness

Loss of consciousness may occur in the context of a seizure. Differentiating between the two requires a careful history. Common causes of loss of consciousness include:

> Breath-Holding Attacks or Spasms. Children usually three–years-old or younger (provoked by temper or frustration), on getting upset, may hold their breath, go blue (cyanotic) and then go limp, leading to loss and then regaining of consciousness. The episodes resolve spontaneously and no intervention is required.

> Reflex Anoxic Seizures. These can occur at any age, with a peak incidence from 6-months-old to 2-years-old They are usually triggered by an event (e.g. pain, minor head trauma, cold or fever) causing the child to have a vagal-induced brief cardiac asystole or bradycardia, resulting in a syncopal episode where they turn pale and fall to the floor. The subsequent hypoxia may lead to a seizure, which resolves spontaneously. Children often have a first degree relative with a history of fainting.

> Vasovagal Syncope. Inadequate cardiac output to the brain may lead to a brief loss of consciousness. This often occurs in warm environments or after standing for long periods. A seizure can also occur as part of the syncope.

> Cardiac arrhythmias. Arrhythmias may cause collapse or cardiac syncope. Prolonged QT may be present on the resting ECG, predisposing to ventricular arrhythmia.

Febrile Convulsion

Febrile convulsions occur in children between 6-months-old and 6-years-old. They are associated with a temperature of 38°C or above, in the absence of CNS infection, metabolic imbalance or a neurological condition.

Febrile convulsions can be classified as:

> Simple. Generalized tonic-clonic seizure lasting up to 15 minutes and not recurring within 24 hours.

> Complex/atypical. Lasting over 15 minutes, focal, or recurring within the same febrile illness.

> Status. Lasting over 30 minutes.

Aetiology

The aetiology of febrile convulsions is not completely understood. The two factors considered most important are genetic and infection:

> Genetic. A familial predisposition exists.

> Infection. Febrile seizures are believed to occur due to viral infections. However, bacterial infection should always be considered. Febrile seizures often occur with infections such as tonsillitis, otitis media, herpes simplex virus, shigella or rotavirus gastroenteritis, or roseola.

Clinical Features

They are the most common presentation of seizures (~5% of pre-school children) in the emergency department (ED). They are usually less than five minutes in duration and children with a simple febrile seizure have rapid and full neurological recovery. Nevertheless, serious conditions such as meningitis should always be considered in the differential diagnosis.

Investigations

The diagnosis of febrile convulsion is clinical and as such no specific investigations are needed. Initial investigations to rule out hypoglycaemia or urinary tract infections (UTIs) in infants should be taken as general precautions.

Differential Diagnosis

> Meningoencephalitis. Meningoencephalitis should always be considered in a child with fever and seizures, because it is a potentially life-threatening condition.

> Epilepsy. This may be the first presentation of epilepsy, particularly if there is no clear infective focus.

Management

Most children presenting with a febrile convulsion are well by the time they attend the ED, and have a clear focus. In such cases, management involves:

▸ Antipyretics. Paracetamol and ibuprofen are effective in decreasing the discomfort of the child but not in preventing further convulsions.

▸ Education and reassurance of relatives. Parents should be educated about the risks of recurrence and how to manage future febrile seizures. This includes recognition and reduction of fever by undressing and administration of antipyretics. They should also know how to keep the child safe during a seizure, to seek medical advice if it lasts for less than five minutes and to call an ambulance if it lasts longer.

Admission should be considered in the following scenarios:

▸ First febrile seizure.
▸ Seizure lasting >15 minutes.
▸ Focal seizure.
▸ Seizure recurring within same febrile illness within 24hrs.
▸ Incomplete recovery after one hour.
▸ Child <18-months-old.
▸ Parental anxiety.
▸ Suspected serious cause for infection (e.g. pneumonia).
▸ No apparent focus of infection.

Benzodiazepines (e.g. buccal midazolam, PR diazepam) can be effective treatments if episodes last for longer than five minutes. Prophylactic anti-epileptics are not routinely recommended, even if seizures are recurrent.

Prognosis

The overall risk of recurrence after a febrile convulsion is approximately 1 in 6. Febrile seizures are associated with a good neurological outcome and there is a two percent risk of developing epilepsy (compared to a one percent risk in those who do not have a history of febrile seizures). Complex febrile seizures have a higher risk of epilepsy.

Afebrile Seizure

Afebrile seizures are a common cause of admission to ED, accounting for one to two percent of attendances. The history is an important part of deciding what investigations are required and the differential diagnosis.

Clinical Features

It is important to obtain an accurate history of the event from first-hand witnesses and the child. Some parents may take a video of the child having an episode, especially in those with recurrent episodes. Key features to consider in the history include:

▸ Before. What was the child doing just before and at the time of the seizure?

▸ During. What happened to the child during the seizure (awareness, responsiveness, staring, facial twitching, eyelid flutter, jerking, pallor, cyanosis or autonomic features)?

▸ After. What was the child like after the seizure and how long was the duration of recovery?

▸ Timing. The frequency and duration of the episode(s) and any previous seizures.

▸ Additional systemic features. This includes persistent headaches, change in behaviour, change in academic performance, relevant past medical history and history of trauma.

Investigations

Check a full set of observations, including BP. Children under 2-years-old are more likely to require further investigation. The differential diagnosis for a 2-month-old with an afebrile seizure is different to a 6-year-old, and the management is therefore different. For example, a baby is more likely to have a metabolic cause for seizures.

▸ Blood tests. A child presenting after a first afebrile seizure should have a blood glucose test as soon as possible. Further laboratory investigations may be indicated if clinical features point towards an underlying cause. These include a full blood count (FBC) (concurrent illness or infection), urea and electrolytes (U&Es), Ca and Mg (electrolyte imbalance), vitamin D, metabolic work-up (ammonia, lactate, glucose, urinary ketones and blood gas, particularly if there are also feeding or growth issues) and toxicology (accidental ingestion of toxin). If the child is already on medication for seizures, it may be appropriate to check drug levels to ensure a therapeutic effect.

▸ ECG. Children may have cardiogenic syncope due to prolonged QT syndrome or cardiac arrhythmia. A standard 12 lead ECG is useful to diagnose cardiac arrhythmia or prolonged QT. A 24-hour ECG and loop recording may be requested if a cardiac abnormality is still suspected (despite an initial ECG being normal).

▸ EEG. An electroencephalogram (EEG) is obtained:
  › Acutely, if encephalopathy or subclinical status epilepticus is suspected.
  › If a diagnosis of epilepsy is suspected (after a second seizure or after one seizure typical of an epileptic syndrome).
Background rhythms are useful and the EEG may support a diagnosis of epilepsy. In some cases, it can define the epilepsy syndrome (for example, "hypsarrhythmia" in infantile spasms). EEG changes during tonic-clonic seizures show a generalised, symmetrical waveform. An inter-ictal EEG may be normal in up to 50-60% of cases with underlying epilepsy, but the EEG will usually be abnormal during a seizure. Non-specific electrophysiological abnormalities can be found in two to three percent of children with no clinical symptoms.

▸ Imaging. Head computed tomography (CT head) is required in the critically ill child if there is trauma, evolving focal neurology, reduced GCS, elevated intracranial pressure or ongoing seizures. Magnetic resonance imaging (MRI) is the imaging modality of choice since it is more sensitive in looking at more subtle structural changes such as temporal lobe sclerosis which is a common finding in idiopathic epilepsy. However, MRI is less readily available in the acute setting than a CT.

> Lumbar puncture (LP). LP is performed in stabilised children with suspected meningoencephalitis or an intracranial bleed if no evidence of abnormality is found on CT head. The cerebrospinal fluid (CSF) can be sent for xanthocromia testing (intracranial bleed) and culture (infection).

Management

The majority of seizures terminate without medication. If actively seizing, an emergency alarm should be triggered to draw attention to the patient. It is worth having an anaesthetist present early in case of deterioration. History, examination and investigations help guide management for specific conditions (e.g. meningitis, encephalitis, neoplasms, intracranial haematomas or cerebral abscess).

First Afebrile Seizure

Depending on the age of the child (>1-year-old), it is appropriate to allow the parents to take the child home provided there are no other criteria present requiring admission (*Table 1*).

Child with Known Seizures

Termination of seizures may require benzodiazepines or phenytoin. Note that if a child is already on phenytoin, they should be given phenobarbitone instead. Paraldehyde is another adjuvant therapy that may be used if a seizure is prolonged. However, often the seizures are brief, and are both managed and discharged from the ED. If the seizure is typical for a child with a pre-existing diagnosis of epilepsy, they may be discharged after they are stabilised. It may be worth updating the patient's neurologist, as more frequent seizures may require changes in regular medication.

TABLE 1: Criteria for admission after a seizure (SIGN, 2005)	
Category	**Criteria**
Age.	<1-year-old.
Neurology.	GCS <15 one hour after seizure.
Raised ICP.	Papilloedema, tense fontanelle.
Generally unwell.	Irritable, disinterested, vomiting.
Meningism.	Kernig's sign positive, photophobia, neck stiffness.
Signs of respiratory aspiration.	Respiratory distress, need for oxygen.
High parent anxiety.	Parents unhappy to take child home.
Complex seizure.	Prolonged (>15 minutes), focal or recurrent.

Status Epilepticus

Status epilepticus is a medical emergency, and is discussed on p218.

Epilepsy

Epilepsy refers to recurrent (at least two unprovoked episodes, 24 hours apart) seizures which are thought to be of electrical origin in the brain. The term describes a predisposition to have epileptic seizures. It is also possible for children who do not have epilepsy to have such seizures. The incidence of epilepsy is 0.05% and the prevalence is 0.5%.

Aetiology

There are six main causes of epilepsy.

> Idiopathic. The majority of cases of epilepsy are idiopathic (70%).
> Genetic. Genetic defect directly contributes to epilepsy and seizures (e.g. channelopathies).
> Structural. Structural disorder of the brain (e.g. tuberous sclerosis, cortical malformation, mesial temporal lobe epilepsy with hippocampal sclerosis).
> Metabolic. Metabolic disorder of the brain (e.g. pyridoxine deficiency).
> Immune. Autoimmune mediated CNS inflammation (e.g. NMDA receptor antibody encephalitis or voltage gated potassium channel antibody encephalitis).
> Infectious. Infectious aetiology causing seizures often have a structural correlate (e.g. HIV, TB, cerebral malaria or cerebral toxoplasmosis).

Seizure Types

> Tonic-clonic seizures. Previously known as grand mal seizures, these are the commonest type of generalized seizures. Tonic seizures involve sudden rigidity, stiffening and muscle contraction. Clonic seizures involve rhythmic twitching or muscle jerking. Tonic-clonic seizures are a combination of these two seizure forms, in a specific pattern. Usually, tonic-clonic seizures last for one minute. EEG changes during tonic-clonic seizures show a generalised, symmetrical waveform.
> Myoclonic seizures. Myoclonic seizures comprise one or several brief arrhythmic muscle jerks, often localised to one body part. Sometimes, visible movement of the affected region is not seen, but the child can feel a shock-like sensation in their muscles.
> Focal seizures. Also known as simple partial seizures, these can be motor, sensory, autonomic or psychic in symptomology. The symptomology varies depending on the part of the brain affected. Motor symptoms include jerking or twitching. Sensory symptoms include altered sensation, such as tingling or numbness in the affected region, or altered vision or hearing. Autonomic symptoms indicate altered autonomic balance, causing sweating or nausea. Other symptoms include déjà vu and altered mood.

> Complex partial seizures. Also known as temporal lobe epilepsy, this type of seizure starts in one region of the brain but also affects other regions controlling consciousness. As such, complex partial seizures are characterized by reduced consciousness. These seizures are often preceded by an aura, including automatisms, e.g. lip smacking.

Epilepsy Syndromes

Epilepsy syndromes are epilepsies which present with an "electro-clinical" pattern of clinical features and characteristic EEGs. Two syndromes are described below:

> Infantile spasms (West Syndrome). This uncommon, but serious, form of epilepsy typically presents between 3 and 8-months of age. The seizures are described as "salaam attacks", characterised by sudden flexor spasms, bending at the waist and nodding of the head, and subsequent extension of the arms. The movements last one or two seconds, but often occur in clusters. The EEG displays hypsarrhythmia which is diagnostic: chaotic, irregular, high amplitude waves and spikes, with a background of disorganised and chaotic electric activity. Developmental delay or even regression are often associated. It is also associated with tuberous sclerosis. Treatment options include corticosteroids, ACTH and vigabatrin.

> Childhood Absence Epilepsy. This type of epilepsy usually presents at 4-9 years of age, with girls more likely to be affected. A typical seizure last between 5 and 20 seconds and usually involves an arrest of movement and awareness, whilst staring into space blankly without loss of tone. These seizures can occur multiple times a day and are sometimes associated with purposeless movements of the mouth and eyes, such as eyelid flickering and lip smacking, called automatisms. Although development is usually normal, learning may be impaired due to the episodes. The ictal EEG typically shows generalised and bilaterally synchronous three-per-second spike and wave discharges. Spontaneous remission often occurs in adolescence.

Investigations

The diagnosis of epilepsy is made clinically and is based primarily upon a detailed history from the patient and eyewitnesses. In addition to the investigations described previously for seizures, the following may support a diagnosis of epilepsy:

> Home Video Recording. Home video camera recordings can be useful to identify information not elicited in the history and aid in the investigation of seizures.

> EEG. Changes may support a diagnosis of epilepsy and define the epilepsy syndrome. A sleep deprived EEG or telemetry may be indicated to increase the sensitivity of picking up EEG changes in those with a high clinical suspicion of generalised or focal epilepsies. Intracranial EEG (where electrodes are placed directly on the brain) is the gold standard for identifying neuronal activity, and if surgery is being considered, this can be used to localise the exact epileptogenic zone.

> Imaging. MRI is the imaging of choice recommended for children who have epilepsy before the age of 2 years and for focal epilepsy, myoclonic epilepsy, intractable seizures, loss of previous good control, seizures continuing despite first line medication, associated neurological deficits/ evolving neurological signs, developmental regression or infantile spasms. CT imaging can be used to identify a focal structural defect if focal neurological signs are identified. Functional scans [functional MRI (fMRI), positron emission tomography (PET) and single-photon emission computed tomography (SPECT)] are not used except in specialist cases and identify areas of hyperactivity and metabolism in the brain. They are used to assess brain involvement and to plan neurosurgical resections.

> Genetic Tests. Genetic studies are used to identify known epilepsy syndromes (e.g. gene deletions related to ion channels).

Management

> Education. It is important to share the diagnosis, action and emergency plan with relatives and school so they know how to recognise and deal with a seizure. Advice should be given on supervision, such as when bathing, swimming and doing outdoor activities. A discussion about driving and future careers is important with adolescents.

> MDT. Each child with complex epilepsy with or without developmental needs has multidisciplinary team involvement. This may include an epilepsy specialist nurse, consultant neurologist, local paediatrician, educational psychologist, physiotherapist and occupational therapist. Establishing successful therapeutic relationships is important. Adherence is often an issue, especially with adolescent patients.

> Medications. Children are likely to be initiated on antiepileptic drugs (AEDs) by a specialist after the second epileptic seizure (*Table* 2). The choice of medications depends upon:
>   › The type of epilepsy (*Table 3*).
>   › The tolerability of side effects.
>   › The treatment goal (seizure elimination vs seizure reduction).

In complex or intractable epilepsy, further management may be considered at tertiary centres:

> Surgical intervention. Surgery has the potential to benefit selected patients. Patients who may benefit include children with a clearly identified focus of seizure activity, a mass triggering the seizure, or recurrent seizures causing significant morbidity despite maximal medication therapy. Potential types of epilepsy surgery include:
>   › Resection. Remove epileptogenic focus.
>   › Multiple subpial transection. Involves cutting nerves in the outer layers of the brain, theoretically preserving vital function concentrated in the deeper layers of the brain.

217

TABLE 2: Common seizure medications and their side effects

Name	Main mechanism of action	Common side effects
Phenytoin.	Sodium channel inhibition.	Reduced coordination and tremors. Slurred speech. Insomnia. Uncontrolled eye movements.
Carbamazepine.	Sodium channel inhibition.	Diplopia. Blurred vision.
Lamotrigine.	Sodium channel inhibition.	Changes in vision. Skin rash.
Oxcarbazepine.	Sodium channel inhibition (derivative of carbamazepine).	Changes in vision. Reduced coordination. Altered mood.
Sodium valproate.	Sodium channel inhibition. Increasing GABA activity.	Hepatotoxic (particularly in children under two-years-old and in those with mitochondrial disease). Pancreatitis.
Ethosuximide.	Calcium channel inhibition.	Dizziness/drowsiness. Irritable or unusual behaviour.
Levetiracetam.	Calcium channel inhibition.	Drowsiness/dizziness. Easy bruising. Altered mood. Increased seizures.
Vigabatrin.	Inhibits the deactivation of GABA.	Altered vision. Hyperactivity and restlessness. Weight gain.
Midazolam.	Benzodiazepine receptor-increasing GABA activity.	Respiratory depression. Fatigue.
Corticosteroids.	Hormonal action altering immune and inflammatory activity.	Thin skin/easy bruising. Weight gain. Immunosuppression. Poor growth.

TABLE 3: Recommended AED by Epilepsy Type (Adapted from NICE guidelines on the epilepsies in adults and children, 2013)

Focal	First line is carbamazepine or lamotrigine. Adjunctive treatment includes levetiracetam, oxcarbazepine or sodium valproate.
Absence	First line is ethosuximide or sodium valproate. Second line is lamotrigine.
Tonic or Atonic	First line is sodium valproate. Adjunctive treatment is lamotrigine.
Generalised tonic-clonic	First line is sodium valproate. Second line is lamotrigine.
Myoclonic	First line is sodium valproate. Second line is levetiracetam or topiramate.
Infantile Spasms	Refer to tertiary paediatric specialist. First line is corticosteroid or vigabatrin.

> › Corpus callosotomy. Surgery to the corpus callosum to contain any seizure in one half of the brain.
> › Ketogenic diet. A specialised diet higher in fats and lower in carbohydrates may be used in children with intractable epilepsy, although the mechanism of action is unclear. Such a diet is initiated under careful supervision of a Consultant Paediatric Neurologist and dietician. It can be difficult for children to be adherent.
> › Vagus nerve stimulation. A device called a generator is implanted under the skin below the collar bone. This is connected to a thin wire which stimulates the vagus nerve at regular intervals to help prevent seizures.
> › Deep brain stimulation. Involves fitting a device with a neurostimulator that stimulates the part of the brain where the seizures originate.

Complications
Acute Seizure
A prolonged, uncontrolled seizure is a medical emergency because it can lead to cardiac or respiratory arrest. As the seizure becomes more prolonged, there is an increased risk of cerebral damage. Seizures also put a child at risk of physical injury from trauma, such as haematomas, bruising, abrasions, and burns.

Long-term
There is a small increased risk in mortality, usually related to impaired consciousness. Sudden unexpected death in epilepsy (SUDEP) is a risk, particularly in the context of uncontrolled seizures or poor medical compliance. The exact mechanism is unclear, but it may relate to cardiac arrhythmias, respiratory arrests or neurogenic pulmonary oedema. Anti-epileptic medications come with significant side effects (*Table 2*), and school absences may be frequent.

Prognosis
Prognosis can depend on the type of epilepsy, underlying medical conditions and structural brain abnormalities. Whilst most children have well-controlled seizures and attend mainstream school, some have more complex needs. They may require involvement from the epilepsy nurse specialist, educational support and support from the extended multidisciplinary team. Some childhood epilepsies abate by adulthood.

Status Epilepticus
Status epilepticus is defined as a seizure or repeated seizures which lasts more than 30 minutes without the regaining of consciousness. The risk of serious brain injury and respiratory arrest are very high. Senior assistance should be sought immediately and treatment should be escalated (*Figure 2*).

FIGURE 2

Initial actions
- High flow oxygen.
- Check glucose.
- Ensure patent airway.

Seizure treatment
- Lorazepam if IV access present (can give a second dose after 10 minutes).
- Buccal midazolam or rectal diazepam if no IV access (can also give a second dose after 10 minutes).

Seizure persists
- IV phenytoin (or phenobarbitone if already on phenytoin). Paraldehyde can be given whilst preparing phenytoin if available.

Seziure still persists
- Rapid sequence induction with thiopentone and intubation.

Management of Status Epilepticus (Adapted from APLS guidelines, 2010).

INFECTIONS OF THE CENTRAL NERVOUS SYSTEM

Meningitis

Meningitis is an acute inflammation of the meninges (the protective covering of the CNS). It is an important neurological emergency as it can rapidly kill within hours, and even when treated can have a high morbidity.

Aetiology
Infectious Causes

Infection may occur spontaneously but risk factors include:
› **Immunosuppression.** Cancer, chemotherapy, HIV/AIDS, congenital T-cell deficiency or splenic disease.
› **Intracranial foreign bodies.** Cochlear implants, CSF shunts.
› **Trauma.** This may lead to a basal skull fracture.

Common causes of infection include:
› **Viral.** Viruses account for two-thirds of all cases of meningitis.
  › Most are caused by enteroviruses, which are self-limiting. Other viral causes include Epstein Barr virus (EBV), adenovirus, varicella zoster virus (VZV), cytomegalovirus (CMV), measles and mumps.
  › Herpes simplex virus is a rare but devastating cause of meningoencephalitis. In neonates, it is usually acquired from the mother, usually during delivery when the baby comes into contact with maternal secretions. Hallmarks of the disease include seizures and liver dysfunction.
› **Bacterial.** Common causes by age group are shown in *Table 4*. The epidemiology of bacterial meningitis in the UK

TABLE 4: Causes of bacterial meningitis in children in the UK		
Age Group	Under 3 months	3 months to 16 years
Causes	Group B streptococcus. Escherichia coli. Listeria.	Streptococcus pneumoniae Neisseria meningitides (meningococcus) Haemophilus influenzae type b (Hib)

has dramatically changed due to the introduction of the haemophilus influenzae B (HiB), meningococcal C (Men C) and pneumococcal vaccines.
› Group B streptococcus. This is the most common cause of bacterial meningitis, septicaemia and infectious cause of death in children three-months-old or less in the UK. It is usually vertically transmitted and can occur up to six months of age. If the mother is colonised with Group B streptococcus, there is a low threshold to treat the baby with antibiotics prophylactically to prevent this complication.
› *Streptococcus pneumoniae.* This can affect any age but is usually found in children under 5-years-old. It is associated with a higher mortality and neurological sequelae.
› *Meningococcus.* This usually spreads from mucosal surfaces of the nasopharynx via the bloodstream to the CNS. If meningococcal septicaemia is also present, this disease is associated with a typical non-blanching rash, which can consist of petechiae and/or purpura.
› Tuberculosis (TB) meningitis. This is rare in countries with a low incidence of TB and good Bacillus Calmette-Guérin (BCG) vaccine uptake, although there is a higher risk of TB in some inner city areas in the UK.

219

It can be difficult to diagnose as children often present with vague non-specific symptoms such as feeling generally unwell, aches/pains and a low grade fever for up to eight weeks. It usually has a poorer prognosis because of late diagnosis.

› Fungal. Rare, but more common in the immunocompromised. The most common cause is *Cryptococcus*.

Non-Infective Causes

Non-infective causes are rare but often missed and can result in significant morbidity. Symptoms tend to be milder, develop more slowly and fail to respond to antimicrobial treatment. Causes include malignancies (e.g. leukaemia, lymphoma and CNS tumours), chemotherapy and autoimmune diseases (e.g. Kawasaki disease, systemic lupus erythematosus, vasculitis and connective tissue disease).

Clinical Features

The classic triad of meningitis is:

› Fever.
› Headache.
› Neck stiffness.

However, younger children, particularly neonates, usually present with non-specific signs and symptoms, such as lethargy, irritability, high-pitched cry, poor feeding and high temperature. Symptoms and signs are summarised in *Table 5*.

Investigations
Blood Tests

› FBC. Elevated white cell count and altered platelet levels in infection.
› U&E. Renal function may be compromised from shock with associated electrolyte disturbance. A low sodium may be secondary to SiADH.
› LFTs. May have hypoxic injury from shock or may be directly infected as classically seen with HSV infection.
› CRP, blood culture, viral PCR, meningococcal PCR. Elevated CRP gives indication of infection. CRP may not immediately rise, and can also be low as a result of liver dysfunction. Enterovirus can be isolated from stool.
› Lactate. If elevated (greater than 2), this can indicate compromised end organ perfusion (although note that sepsis and meningitis can occur both separately and concurrently).
› Glucose. Sepsis may be associated with hypoglycaemia or hyperglycaemia. Aids interpretation of CSF glucose.
› Blood gas. Decreased arterial blood pH with low bicarbonate levels may show a metabolic acidosis.

Imaging

› CT Scan. Should always be performed if there are focal neurological signs or if there is evidence of raised ICP. It may be performed in a child with closed fontanelles before an LP. A normal CT scan does not exclude raised ICP. It is not necessary to exclude raised ICP in neonates, as raised ICP is generally prevented by the sutures and fontanelles being open.
› Cranial USS. This should be considered in neonates as it may identify any intracranial bleeds. As the fontanelles are open, USS can access the brain.

Lumbar Puncture

An LP is indicated in suspected meningitis to:

a Confirm the diagnosis.
b Determine antibiotic sensitivities to any bacteria cultured.
c Determine the length of treatment according to the organism.

The white cell count, protein level, glucose level and opening pressure via manometer can give an indication of the aetiology (*Table 6*). As well as bacterial culture, CSF samples can be sent for meningococcal and viral PCR. Paired glucose from serum and CSF are necessary to help accurately interpret the results.

The absolute contraindications to an LP include:

› Signs of raised ICP (relative hypertension and bradycardia, focal neurological signs, papilloedema, doll's eyes or fluctuating level of consciousness).
› Cardiopulmonary compromise.
› Infection overlying the skin.
› Coagulopathy or thrombocytopenia.

Additional Tests

› Throat swabs. Throat swabs may be taken for bacterial and viral cultures to help identify a causative organism.
› Urine culture. UTIs can present very non-specifically, particularly in the neonatal age group.
› Sputum culture. If there is a possible respiratory focus.
› Stool culture. If there is a possible gastrointestinal focus.
› Chest X-ray. If there are any signs of respiratory distress.
› ECG. Not done as frequently in children as adults. It may be helpful if there is a suspected arrhythmia (e.g.

TABLE 5: Signs and symptoms of meningitis			
	Children under 1	All age groups	Older children
Symptoms	• High-pitched cry.	• Seizures. • Lethargy. • Irritability. • Poor feeding/off food. • Poor urine output. • Vomiting/diarrhoea. • Respiratory distress.	• Headache. • Neck stiffness. • Photophobia. • Confusion. • Muscle aches/pains.
Signs	• Tense fontanelle. • Reduced tone. • Apnoeas. • Bradycardias. • Temperature instability.	• Fever. • Non-blanching rash. • Seizures. • Focal neurological signs.	• Positive Kernig sign (when the thigh is bent at 90 degrees at both the knee and hip, extension of the knee is painful).

TABLE 6: CSF features in different causes of meningitis. (Adapted from Kliegman RM, Stanton BF, Geme JW, Schor NF, Behram RE. Nelon Textbook of Paediatrics. 19th Edition. New York: Elsevier Inc.; 2011. 2088)

Meningitis.	Appearance	Pressure (mm H$_2$0)	Leukocytes (cells per mm³)	Protein (mg/dL)	Glucose (mg/dL)
None.	Clear.	50-80.	<5 (75% lymphocytes).	20-45.	>50 (or 75% serum glucose).
Bacterial.	Turbid.	Elevated.	100-10,000. Predominately neutrophils.	100-500.	<40 (or 50% serum glucose).
Bacterial (partially treated).	Turbid/ Clearing.	Normal/Elevated.	5-10,000. Predominately neutrophils (although if prolonged treatment already, lymphocytes may predominate).	100-500.	Normal/ decreased.
Viral.	Clear.	Normal/Slightly elevated.	Usually <1,000. Predominately neutrophils in early stages, then predominately lymphocytes.	50-200.	Usually normal. Decreased in some viral disease e.g. mumps.
TB.	Fibrinous.	Elevated.	10-500. Predominately neutrophils in early stages, then predominately lymphocytes.	100-3000.	<50.
Fungal.	Clear or Cloudy.	Elevated.	5-500. Predominately neutrophils in early stages, then predominately lymphocytes.	25-500.	<50.

an irregular heart rhythm or persistent tachycardia not responding to fluid resuscitation).

› EEG. If there are associated seizures.

Management

› Resuscitation. As in all resuscitation scenarios, start with airway, breathing and circulation. In a child with signs of shock, seizures or raised ICP an anaesthetist and senior clinician should be present. Children with meningococcal sepsis are likely to require multiple fluid boluses (p162).

› Antibiotics. Children with suspected meningitis should be treated immediately with IV antibiotics as soon as access is gained. One treatment regimen would be to use a third generation cephalosporin (e.g. cefotaxime) with amoxicillin added if the patient is under 3-months-old (to cover *Listeria*). A macrolide antibiotic may be considered to broaden cover (e.g. suspected mycoplasma infection). The duration of the treatment should be guided by clinical response, cultures and microbiology advice. This is typically 7 to 10 days.

› Antivirals. Antivirals should be added if HSV encephalitis is suspected. This should be considered in:

› Recent contact with HSV.
› Altered behaviour, cognition or consciousness.
› Seizures.
› Deranged liver function tests.
› Severely unwell.

› Corticosteroids. These are not indicated in those less than 3-months-old. In older children, some evidence suggests that these drugs may reduce pneumococcal meningitis related hearing loss, but as the evidence of benefit in meningitis generally is unclear, routine administration remains controversial. When it is given, it is usually a one-off dose prior to antibiotics.

› Report to public health authorities. Household contacts of the index case should be given prophylactic antibiotics.

Complications
Acute Complications
Children with meningitis can present with immediate complications. Even with appropriate treatment, children can die within hours. They may develop:

› Septic shock. Co-existing septicaemia presents as tachycardia, respiratory distress, reduced Glasgow coma scale (GCS) score, pale/cold peripheries and poor urine output.

› Disseminated intravascular coagulation. This is due to sepsis, leading to a coagulopathy and widespread bleeding.

› Raised intracranial pressure. This results from cerebral oedema and is a very poor prognostic sign. The classic symptoms are hypertension, bradycardia, reduced GCS and irregular respiration (Cushing's Triad).

› SiADH. The elevated concentration of serum antidiuretic hormone (ADH) is a host response to infection, and leads to fluid retention and hyponatraemia.

› Hydrocephalus. This results from obstruction due to cerebral oedema or infection. Permanent post-infectious scarring may result in long-term hydrocephalus, necessitating a ventriculoperitoneal (VP) shunt.

› Cerebral abscess/encephalitis/ subdural empyema. This is caused by infection spreading to the brain.

Long-term Complications
› Hearing loss. This is the most common complication of bacterial meningitis. It is caused by cochlear infection and occurs in 5-30% of children with meningitis. Children

should undergo hearing assessment after discharge from hospital within six weeks. If hearing is impaired, the earlier a cochlear implant is inserted, the better the prognosis.

› Subdural effusion. This is more common in infants, affecting 10-30% of children with meningitis. Most are asymptomatic, but it may result in a bulging fontanelle, enlarging head size and/or seizures.

› Neurological complications. Learning difficulties, motor and neurodevelopmental deficits.

› Renal complications. Acute and chronic renal impairment, secondary to septic shock (if there is associated sepsis).

› Orthopaedic complications (rare). Amputation, growth plate damage and arthritis due to nerve damage, secondary to septic shock.

› Skin complications (rare). May occur secondary to septic shock. Reconstructive surgery may be indicated.

Prognosis
Most children recover fully from viral meningitis. Bacterial meningitis has a 5 to 10% mortality, and 10% of survivors suffer long-term complications. Herpes simplex virus (HSV) meningoencephalitis has an association with significant morbidity and mortality (70% progress to coma and death if left untreated). Group B streptococcus meningitis has a poor prognosis, with up to 50% mortality and a high morbidity.

Encephalitis
Encephalitis is inflammation of the brain parenchyma. Due to their close anatomical proximity, meningitis and encephalitis often occur simultaneously. Consider encephalitis if there is altered consciousness or behaviour, confusion or seizures. The most common infectious causes are herpes simplex virus 1 and 2, enteroviruses and varicella.

Herpes simplex encephalitis may be diagnosed based on serum and CSF viral PCR. It also has characteristic MRI and EEG findings. It carries significant morbidity and mortality and if suspected aciclovir should be given.

Chronic encephalitis may occur with HIV or following measles (subacute sclerosing panencephalitis or SSPE). SSPE can have a latent period of six to eight years and is a progressive condition.

Other Causes of Encephalitis
Acute disseminated encephalomyelitis (ADEM) is an autoimmune mediated inflammatory demyelinating neurological condition, which has symptoms similar to multiple sclerosis and presents at 5 to 8-years-old. It presents as an acute onset encephalopathy with poly-focal neurological deficits often with a preceding infectious illness or history of immunisation. It is relatively uncommon, with about three to six cases each year in UK regional centres.

Other less common causes of encephalitis are autoimmune and include:

› NMDA-Receptor antibody encephalitis. This can be associated with malignancy particularly in females.

› Voltage-gated potassium channel-complex antibody-associated limbic encephalitis.

› Rasmussen Encephalitis. This is associated with autoimmune antibodies, e.g. anti-GluR3 antibodies.

Cerebral Abscess
A cerebral abscess refers to an infection encapsulated within one region of the brain. This can affect the function of the brain and spinal cord.

Aetiology
The cause is most often bacterial, but can also be viral or fungal in nature. Predisposition to infection includes:

› Spread of local infection. Middle ear/sinus/dental/face/scalp/meninges infection.

› Head injury/skull fracture. This allows direct entry of pathogens.

› Spread of systemic infection. The source could be anywhere, and spread via the bloodstream.

› Congenital heart disease. Right to left shunting means blood bypasses the lungs, a site where phagocytosis normally occurs.

› Intracranial shunts (for hydrocephalus). Such shunts may get infected.

Clinical Features
The clinical features of cerebral abscesses relate to infection, neurological disturbance, and raised intracranial pressure. Babies may present non-specifically with sleepiness, irritability, and poor feeding. Features include:

› Fever. Particularly if it is prolonged, and not responding to initial antibiotics. This may occur if an ear infection has subsequently spread to the brain.

› Neurological features. Raised intracranial pressure may precipitate vomiting (often without associated nausea), headache (particularly early morning), drowsiness, and seizures. Babies may have a bulging fontanelle, or a high pitched cry. Older children may have neck stiffness, abnormal movements/muscle tone and changes in personality/speech.

Investigations
The presenting features of a cerebral abscess are often difficult to distinguish from other pathology such as an intracranial bleed, malignancy or meningoencephalitis. Investigations seek to narrow the differential, and identify a possible focus of initial infection. Investigations are similar to that for meningitis. However:

› Lumbar punctures should generally be avoided as there may be raised intracranial pressure. If performed, viral PCR, fungal cultures and acid-fast bacilli (TB) testing should be considered in addition to standard investigations.

› MRI scans are more helpful than a CT scan, and contrast is used as this highlights abscesses more clearly. Classically, a ring enhancing lesion is seen. Any associated cerebral oedema, mass effect, or bleeding can also be seen. The sinuses and mastoid are also imaged, as they are possible primary sources of infection.

Management
Management involves excision of the abscess, or drainage/aspiration of the pus, followed by a prolonged antibiotic course. If there is associated sinusitis/middle ear infection, a combined ENT and neurosurgical approach may be needed. Patients with a small abscess, or patients with confirmed bacteriology from another focus, may respond to medical therapy alone.

Complications
Long-term complications include delayed-onset seizures, focal neurological deficits and cognitive dysfunction.

Prognosis
Overall cure rate is approximately 90%. Poor prognostic factors include delayed diagnosis, rapid progression, neurological impairment, multiple/deep abscesses, being immunocompromised and specific organisms e.g. *Aspergillus*.

NEURODEVELOPMENTAL DISORDERS

Cerebral Palsy
Cerebral Palsy (CP) is a fixed neurological disorder primarily affecting motor movement and posture. The incidence in the UK is two to three in 1000 and males are 1.5 times more likely to develop CP than females. It is caused by non-progressive injury in the developing brain in the first two years of life. After two years, any new insult is termed an "acquired brain injury". CP is frequently accompanied by changes in sensation, communication, behaviour, perception and cognition. It may also be linked to seizures and musculoskeletal difficulties. All of these problems as a constellation may cause significant disability.

Aetiology
The aetiology of CP is complex and includes developmental, genetic, metabolic, ischaemic and infectious causes. Risk factors include antenatal infection, multiple pregnancy and low/high birth weight. It is important to note that although both prematurity and acute intrapartum events are risk factors, the majority of children with cerebral palsy are term babies with uncomplicated labour and delivery.

CP can be classified into three broad categories:
- 80% are due to antenatal factors which result in abnormal brain development (e.g. maternal infection, radiation exposure, intraventricular haemorrhage, periventricular leukomalacia or congenital malformations).
- 10% are due to hypoxic-ischaemic injury during delivery.

- 10% are due to postnatal factors. There is overlap, but it is helpful to consider different age groups:
  - Neonatal. Intraventricular haemorrhage, hyperbilirubinaemia, hypoglycaemia, cerebral infarcts, meconium aspiration syndrome.
  - Infant. Hydrocephalus, hypoglycaemia, head injury secondary to non-accidental injury, CNS infections.
  - Child. Hypoxic events (e.g. drowning), head trauma, lead poisoning, CNS infections.

Clinical Features
CP is primarily a motor disability, but other neurological function may also be affected. Non-motor symptoms include:
- Hearing and visual problems (e.g. strabismus/squint).
- Feeding difficulties/gastro-oesophageal reflux/faltering growth.
- Aspiration pneumonia.
- Dental caries.
- Behavioural/emotional difficulties.
- Communication difficulties (which may or may not be associated with intellectual impairment).
- Bladder and bowel dysfunction.
- Skeletal deformities, e.g. scoliosis, hip dislocation, contractures.
- Intellectual impairment.
- Seizures.

It is important to note that although the brain injury is "non-progressive", symptoms may only appear at a later stage of life (e.g. a perinatal insult may result in a child presenting with delayed walking at 18 months).

There are three main clinical subtypes: spastic cerebral palsy, extrapyramidal cerebral palsy and ataxic cerebral palsy (*Figure 3*).

FIGURE 3

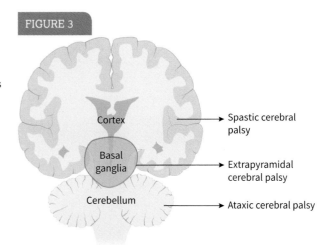

Subtypes of cerebral palsy.

Spastic Cerebral Palsy

Spastic cerebral palsy results from upper motor neurone injury and thus manifests with classic signs of upper motor neuron injury, including:

› Muscle weakness (particularly antigravity muscles e.g. dorsiflexion of the feet).
› Increased muscle tone.
› Brisk tendon reflex.
› Sustained clonus.

Depending on the location of the insult different parts of the body are affected. Three subtypes of spastic CP are recognised: spastic hemiplegia, spastic diplegia and spastic quadriplegia (*Table 7*).

Extrapyramidal Cerebral Palsy

Extrapyramidal cerebral palsy (also known as athetoid, choreoathetoid or dyskinetic cerebral palsy) arises in response to damage to the extra-pyramidal tracts in the brain (particularly the basal ganglia). Therefore, upper motor neurone signs are absent (*Figure 4*). Causes include hypoxic-ischaemic injury during delivery and kernicterus.

Infants are initially hypotonic, with poor head control, but show increased tone and dyskinetic movements as they develop. Dyskinetic movements include:

› **Dystonia.** A broad term describing involuntary, sustained contractions of opposing muscle groups. This leads to abnormal posture, twisting movements and repetitive movements.
› **Athetosis.** Slow, involuntary, writhing movements.
› **Chorea.** Brief, irregular movements that are non-repetitive/rhythmic. They appear to flow smoothly, giving them the appearance of dance-like movements.

TABLE 7: 3 Subtypes of Spastic Cerebral Palsy			
	Affected body parts	Presentation	Additional Features
Spastic Hemiplegia.	The arm and leg on one side, with arms affected more, and sparing of the face. Spasticity greatest in antigravity muscles.	Affected arm: • Flexed, pronated arm, with fisting of the hand. • Hand preference before 12 months. • Difficulty in hand manipulation. Affected Leg: • Circumduction gait on affected side (stiff leg, not flexed at knee/ankle, rotated away and then towards the body with each step). • Toe-heel (tip toe) gait on affected side. • Delayed walking.	• May have growth arrest in the extremities (particularly if parietal lobe affected). • Moderate incidence of seizure disorders, and intellectual impairment.
Spastic Diplegia.	Lower limbs (with some involvement of upper limbs). Referred to as paraplegia if no involvement of upper limbs.	• Commando crawl (dragging legs while crawling). • Scissoring of the lower legs. • Severely delayed walking. • Toe-heel (tip toe) gait, with feet held in equinovarus position. • Legs may be significantly underdeveloped compared to the arms.	• May have disuse atrophy, and impaired growth of the lower extremities compared to upper extremities. • Usually have normal intellectual development. May have learning difficulties and deficits in other neurological pathways (e.g. hearing). • Minimal risk of seizures.

TABLE 7: *Continued*

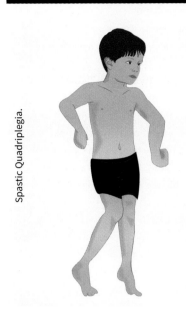

Spastic Quadriplegia.

All four limbs.	Have features as above in all four limbs, with increased tone throughout, and decreased spontaneous movements.	• Swallowing difficulties (bulbar palsy). Weak suck. Tonic bite (bites down and unable to release). Tongue thrust (tongue protrudes through the incisors). • High incidence of seizure disorders. • Significant intellectual impairment. • Associated developmental abnormalities common (e.g. speech/vision).

FIGURE 4

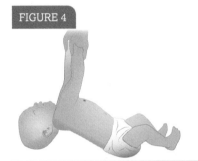

Poor head control and reduced tone in dyskinetic cerebral palsy.

Oropharyngeal muscles are affected, leading to speech and feeding problems. Seizures are uncommon and intellect is usually preserved.

Ataxic Cerebral Palsy

This is due to damage to the cerebellum. Symptoms include hypotonia, an intention tremor, poor coordination (e.g. dysdiadochokinesia, past pointing on finger nose testing), a broad-based unsteady gait (*Figure 5*) and delayed motor development.

Investigations

Cerebral palsy is primarily a clinical diagnosis. However, investigations are important to identify the possible aetiology and to predict the extent of any neurological insult.

FIGURE 5

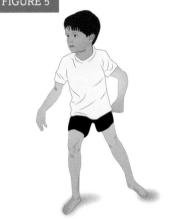

Wide based gait in ataxic cerebral palsy.

> Imaging. MRI of the brain will determine the nature of any structural abnormalities. The spine may also be imaged if there are any concerns about spinal pathology.

> Chromosomal testing. Particularly if any congenital abnormalities are identified.

> Metabolic work up. Organic acids, amino acids and magnetic resonance spectroscopy (which measures biochemical changes in the brain). Disorders such as glutamate decarboxylase-1 deficiency, arginase deficiency or sulphite oxidase deficiency may be considered.

> Hearing and visual testing. Both can be impaired.

Differential Diagnosis

The key element in diagnosing cerebral palsy is to ensure there is no progressive neurological deficit, and that a reversible condition is not missed:

> Muscular dystrophies. Duchenne muscular dystrophy, Becker muscular dystrophy or myotonic dystrophy.

> Spinal disorders. Spinal muscular atrophy, vascular malformations of the cord.

> Ataxic disorders. Ataxia telangiectasia, Niemann-Pick disease.

> Metabolic disease. Glutaric aciduria type 1, urea cycle disorders.

> Endocrine disease. Hypothyroidism.

> CNS tumours.

In patients with a normal MRI but prominent dystonia, consider the rare condition dihydroxyphenylalanine (DOPA)-responsive dystonia. This is very similar to Parkinson's disease. It can be tested using CSF neurotransmitter analysis and by giving a test dose of DOPA.

Management

CP can range from mild cases with a normal life expectancy to severe cases whereby children are incapacitated and bedridden. There is no cure for CP, as the brain damage cannot be reversed. However, with a multidisciplinary team, patients can be supported to reach their full potential.

Non-Pharmacological

› **Adequate nutrition.** Children with CP are at risk of malnutrition and faltering growth. They may require nasogastric (NG) or percutaneous endoscopic gastrostomy (PEG) feeding.

› **Speech and language therapy.** This promotes the use of language and improves swallowing. Communication can be aided by electronic devices and tablet computers that produce speech.

› **Occupational therapy and physiotherapy.** This is important to promote mobility and physical activity for normal daily living.

› **Adaptive and communicative equipment.** Walkers, poles, frames, braces, splints and wheelchairs/special seats can be useful aids to improve mobility.

› **Education.** Children may require special needs education. Vocational training can help young adults prepare for jobs.

› **Psychologist/counsellor.** These will address the emotional needs of child/family.

Pharmacological

› **Anti-muscarinics** (e.g. glycopyrronium bromide). Anti-muscarinic agents prevent drooling. Hyoscine patches may also be of benefit, as can botulinum injection into the salivary gland.

› **Anti-reflux medication** (e.g. domperidone, ranitidine). Reflux is commonly seen in conjunction with CP.

› **Bisphosphonates** (e.g. pamidronate). These prevent osteoporosis.

› **Anti-spasmodics** (e.g. benzodiazepines, baclofen, dantrolene, botulinum toxin). Anti-spasmodics help to relieve

spasticity. Baclofen can be delivered intrathecally.

› **Reserpine.** This drug is a vesicular monoamine transporter (VMAT) blocker affecting neurotransmitter levels. It can be useful for hyperkinetic movements (e.g. chorea/athetosis).

Some evidence now points to benefits of prenatal treatment with magnesium sulphate to reduce the incidence of cerebral palsy in high risk mothers, particularly women at risk of preterm delivery before 34 weeks gestation or with low birth weight babies.

Surgical

Surgery can be performed to release joint contractures (e.g. achilles tendon), reduce muscle spasms (e.g. around the hip girdle), and correct bony abnormalities (e.g. scoliosis). More complex procedures may be considered to relieve muscle tightness, improve posture, and the ability to stand, sit and walk (e.g. selective posterior rhizotomy, where nerves are selectively severed to decrease contractures).

Prognosis

Morbidity and mortality are related to both the severity of the condition, and to respiratory/gastrointestinal complications. Life expectancy varies from mild cases with only a slightly reduced life expectancy, to the more severe forms with significantly increased mortality and morbidity.

HEADACHE IN CHILDHOOD

Headache is one of the most common reasons for adolescent and older children to seek medical advice. Primary headaches (e.g. migraines, tension type headaches and, less frequently, cluster headaches) should be differentiated from secondary headaches, which are as a symptom of another underlying disorder.

Possible causes of secondary headache include:

› Intracranial mass.

› Intracranial bleed, e.g. subarachnoid haemorrhage, subdural haematoma.

› Infection, e.g. meningitis, sinusitis, encephalitis.

› Ischaemic stroke.

› Benign intracranial hypertension.

The majority of headaches are primary and self-limiting. Since secondary headaches can have significant causes, there should be a low threshold for imaging, particularly in children under 5-years-old. Indications for brain imaging are shown in *Box 1*.

Migraine

Migraine is a complex disorder, defined as shown in *Table 8*.

Aetiology

Migraine is the most common type of recurrent headache. It may be associated with an aura, nausea, vomiting, photophobia and phonophobia. The mechanism remains incompletely understood, but it is likely to be neurovascular in origin. Risk factors include:

› **Family history.** Ninety percent of children have a first or second degree

---

Box 1: Indications for considering CT or MRI brain scans in headaches

- Focal neurological features.
- Signs of raised intracranial pressure.
- Headaches which are worse on lying down.
- Confusion.
- Altered consciousness.
- Change in personality.
- Abnormal gait.
- Growth failure.
- Diplopia.
- Facial nerve palsy.
- Visual field effects.
- Seizures.
- Atypical auras.
- Thunderclap headaches.
- Known existing secondary cause such as intracranial mass.

TABLE 8: Migraine Diagnostic Criteria (Adapted from International Headache Society, ICHD-III Beta The International Classification of Headache Disorders, 2013)

Migraine without aura	Migraine with aura

1. Headaches are defined as at least two of:
  a. Unilateral location.
  b. Pulsating.
  c. Moderate to severe pain.
  d. Aggravated by or causing avoidance of normal physical activity.
2. At least five attacks.
3. Headaches lasting 4 to 72 hours.
4. Headaches with at least one of the following:
  a. Nausea or vomiting.
  b. Photophobia and phonophobia.
5. Not attributed to another disorder.
	1. At least two attacks.
	2. Aura lasting 5 to 60 minutes of either:
	  a. Fully reversible visual symptom.
	  b. Fully reversible sensory symptom.
	  c. Fully reversible dysphasic speech disturbance.
	3. At least two of:
	  a. Homonymous visual symptoms or unilateral sensory symptoms.
	  b. Aura symptoms for over five minutes or different aura symptoms occurring in succession over five minutes.
	  c. Each symptom lasting over 5 minutes and less than 60 minutes.
	4. Headache criteria (migraine without aura, as above) occurs during aura or follows within 60 minutes.
	5. Not attributed to another disorder.

family member with recurrent headaches.

▸ **Triggers.** Stress, menstruation, not eating food at regular intervals, irregular or inadequate sleep, dehydration, exercise and weather changes.

Clinical Features

▸ Migraine without aura ("common migraine") is the most common type of migraine, accounting for 90% of cases. It is characterised by a focal, throbbing headache.

▸ Migraine with aura ("classical migraine") occurs in 10% of cases.
  › Photopsia (bright flashes of light) is the most common type of aura which children have before migraine. Going to a dark room can be helpful and sleeping can relieve the episode.
  › Rare auras include dysphasic auras (inability to speak) and hemiplegic aura (transient unilateral weakness), which can last for several hours to days.

The recurrence and episodic character of the headache can help distinguish it from tension type headaches and secondary headaches. For patients with migraine with aura, consider more rarely transient ischaemic attack (TIA) or stroke. Some features which can help to distinguish between them is the onset of symptoms (migraine aura is more gradual in onset,

as opposed to the sudden onset of visual disturbance in TIA and stroke); duration (TIA and migraine are fully reversible); and imaging. Additionally, migraines are rare in young children, so it is important to have a low index of suspicion for a brain tumour. If the headache lasts over 72 hours, it is termed status migrainosus.

Management

▸ **Conservative management.** This includes avoiding triggers and selecting strategies for dealing with an attack (such as lying still in a dark room).

▸ **Drugs.**
  › **Acute episodes.** Combination therapy of triptans (e.g. sumatriptan) and NSAIDs/paracetamol. Antiemetics can be given to relieve nausea and vomiting.
  › **Prophylaxis.** β Blocker (e.g. propranolol), topiramate (targets voltage gated ion channels and neurotransmitter activity), or pizotifen (a serotonin antagonist).

Prognosis

Generally, migraines improve with age. However, around half of children will continue to have migraines in adulthood. There is a small increased risk of ischaemic stroke and a very small increased risk of mental health problems such as depression.

Tension Type Headaches

Tension type headaches are usually associated with stress. At least ten headaches with durations of 30 minutes to seven hours are required for formal diagnosis. Both muscular and psychogenic factors are implicated in causing the pain.

Clinical Features

Classically, the headaches are described as:

▸ Symmetrical.
▸ Gradual onset.
▸ Non-throbbing.
▸ Feel like a band of pressure/tightness.
▸ Unaffected by physical activity.

Management

Paracetamol or NSAIDs should be considered for acute treatment.

Cluster Headaches

Cluster headaches are recurrent bouts of acute, unilateral pain, centred over the eye, temple or forehead. The pain is very severe and tends to be relieved by physical activity. Autonomic features often accompany the headache (e.g. nasal congestion, watering/redness of the eye).

Cluster headaches can be classified as:

▸ **Episodic.** Headache free periods > one month (90%)
▸ **Chronic.** Headache free periods < one month (10%)

Management

Providing oxygen and subcutaneous/nasal triptan may be beneficial in acute attacks. Verapamil can be effective prophylactically.

HEAD INJURY IN CHILDHOOD

Head Injury

Head injury is a common cause of presentation to ED in the child population. The vast majority are minor. However, major head injury is the commonest cause of death and disability in the population of 1 to 40-years-old in the UK. 25-30% of head injuries in children aged less than two-years-old admitted to hospital are estimated to be due to abusive head injury. Head injury often occurs in the context of polytrauma, and therefore all injuries must be considered together (e.g. transfer to a neurosurgical centre for a small bleed into the brain is a not a priority if the same patient is exsanguinating into their pelvis from a fractured hip). It is important to identify:

1   **What led to the head injury?** It is often assumed that head injuries occur accidentally in previously well children. However, in some cases it may be due to non-accidental injury, or alternatively, it may have been precipitated by a medical condition (e.g. syncope or a seizure). With regard to non-accidental injury, it is important to get a clear story of what happened and ensure that there is a full and believable account of all injuries sustained.

2   **How significant has the injury been?** Superficial cuts or bruises are usually the first thing identified by parents/ children. This may require staples, steristrips or sutures. There may potentially be an underlying skull fracture, although this is rare. More significant is any intracranial bleed. This is the most worrying acute problem and therefore needs to be actively considered in any case of head injury. This can be suspected from the following:
    › Reduced consciousness, confusion or drowsiness.
    › Focal neurological deficit.
    › Signs of a basal skull fracture. Panda eyes (dark rings around the eyes; *Figure 6*), haemotympanum (blood in the ear; *Figure 7*), Battle's sign (bruising over the mastoid process; *Figure 7*) or CSF leakage from ear/nose.
    › An open fracture.
    › Significant bruising or swelling on the head. This indicates significant trauma.
    › Persistent vomiting. This may be a sign of raised intracranial pressure.

Investigations

The most important investigation to consider is a CT scan to look for intracranial bleeding. The criteria to determine whether CT scans are required in head injury, as reported by the NICE guidelines for head trauma, include:

› Any one of:
    › On initial emergency department assessment GCS <14 (if older than 1-year–old), or GCS <15 (if less than 1-year–old).
    › GCS <15, more than two hours post-injury.
    › Post-trauma seizure but no history of epilepsy.
    › Suspected non-accidental injury.
    › Suspected open or depressed skull fracture or tense fontanelle.
    › Sign of basal skull fracture such as panda eyes, Battle's sign, haemotympanum or CSF leakage from ears or nose.
    › Child aged less than 1-year-old with a bruise, swelling or laceration on head measuring ≥five centimetres.
    › Focal neurology deficit.
› Any two of:
    › Witnessed loss of consciousness (more than five minutes).
    › Three discrete episodes of vomiting (>30 minutes apart).
    › Abnormal drowsiness.

FIGURE 6

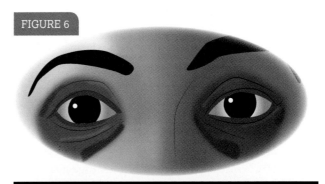

Panda eyes.

FIGURE 7

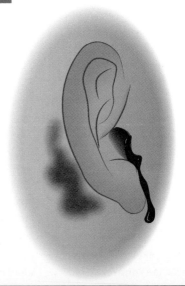

Battle's sign and haemotympanum.

› Amnesia (more than five minutes).
› Dangerous mechanism of injury (e.g. high speed collision).

CT scans may still be indicated without the above features present. For example, a patient may be persistently tachycardic after a head injury with no other clear explanation.

If there is a suspected cervical spinal injury, the C-spine should be imaged as well. X-rays may be sufficient if the head is not being scanned. Criteria for a CT of the C-spine include:

› Plain X-rays are technically difficult or inadequate or identify a significant bony injury.
› There is strong clinical suspicion of injury despite normal X-rays.
› GCS less than 13 on initial assessment.
› Focal peripheral neurological signs.
› A definitive diagnosis of cervical spine injury is needed urgently (e.g. before surgery).
› The patient is having other body areas scanned for head injury or multi-region trauma.
› The patient has been intubated.

Management

Initial management of any child with a head injury involves:

▸ **Resuscitation and stabilisation.** Any child with a significant intracranial bleed will be unstable and will require adequate resuscitation. Early involvement of an anaesthetist is required if the GCS is reduced or if the child is very unwell.
▸ **C-spine immobilisation.** This should be performed until any suspicion of a C-spine injury/spinal cord compression is cleared.
▸ **Analgesia.** This should be given early and is particularly helpful if there is raised intracranial pressure. Pain aggravates raised ICP.
▸ **Treatment of any superficial wounds.** This may require simple cleaning, steristrips, staples or sutures.

Children with minor head injury who are well can be discharged home with appropriate advice about signs of raised intracranial pressure and when to return. Those with possible signs of an intracranial bleed, but not warranting a CT head, should be observed for at least four hours. Note also that even if the CT scan is normal, it may still be necessary to discuss with a neurosurgical unit if there is a strong suspicion of a bleed.

Skull fractures usually require observation for 12–24 hours and discussion with the neurosurgical team, but no specific treatment is needed if there is no underlying bleed.

Those with intracranial bleeds should be transferred early to a neurosurgical centre. They may require neurosurgical intervention (e.g. burr hole for subdural haematoma).

Raised Intracranial Pressure

Elevated intracranial pressure (ICP) is a life threatening condition. It can present acutely or chronically. Causes include:

▸ Traumatic brain injury.
▸ Hydrocephalus.
▸ Brain tumours.
▸ Intracranial infections.
▸ Metabolic, e.g. diabetic ketoacidosis.
▸ Idiopathic intracranial hypertension (IIH).

Aetiology

The intracranial component has a fixed volume in which there is brain (80%), CSF (10%) and blood (10%). Homeostatic mechanisms can protect the brain against pressure changes of up to 15 mmHg. Beyond this, intracranial pressure will rise or intracranial components will be displaced (e.g. coning of the cerebellar tonsils). Raised ICP compresses brain structures, including vasculature, leading to hypoxia and compromised neurological function.

Clinical Features

Any child with raised ICP will appear unwell. Important symptoms and signs are summarised below.

Symptoms

▸ **Headache.** It is classically an early morning headache associated with cough, micturition or defecation. In chronic conditions, the headache gradually increases in frequency and severity over time.
▸ **Vomiting.** Usually without nausea in the early stages, and vomiting early in the morning.
▸ **Other neurological symptoms.** This may help localise the site of any mass or represent increased pressure globally. Symptoms include ptosis, hemiparesis and double vision, but could potentially include any focal neurological sign.
▸ **Changes in mental state.** This presents in late stages as reduced consciousness, drowsiness and irritability.

Signs

▸ **Papilloedema.** This normally takes several days to appear but is indicative of raised ICP.
▸ **Sunset sign.** This is seen in infants and young children. It is due to an up-gaze paresis, thereby resulting in downward looking pupils. The pupil may be covered by the lower eyelid.
▸ **Retinal haemorrhage.** This should raise the suspicion of head trauma and NAI.
▸ **Pupillary abnormalities.** Cranial nerve abnormalities affecting the eye include:
  › III (*Figure 8*). Superior/inferior/medial rectus, and inferior oblique palsy gives a "down and out" position of the pupil. If the pupillary pathways are involved, it will be fixed and dilated. Levator palpebrae palsy gives a droopy eyelid.

› IV (*Figure 9*). Superior oblique palsy, resulting in head tilt to the unaffected side.
› VI (*Figure 10*). Lateral rectus palsy, resulting in a medial position of the pupil.

› Cushing's sign. Usually a pre-terminal event. Bradycardia, hypertension, fluctuating consciousness and irregular respiration.

Investigations

Raised ICP should be identified from the clinical history, examination and initial observations. In cases where there is impending herniation, treatment should be started before any further investigations. GCS and vital signs need to be monitored closely. Tests that may be helpful include:

› Brain imaging. CT or MRI head imaging should be considered to find an underlying cause (e.g. mass lesion) or findings consistent with raised ICP (e.g. midline shift). However a normal scan does not exclude the diagnosis of raised ICP.

› CO_2 monitoring. CO_2 levels should be optimised to low/normal levels as this affects vascular dilatation and therefore ICP and oxygenation.

› Monitor glucose. Hypoglycaemia is an easily correctable cause of acute deterioration.

› Correct electrolytes. Any electrolyte imbalance should be corrected taking care to correct abnormal sodium levels slowly.

Management

Advice should be taken from neurosurgeons and intensive care. The purpose of management is to maintain adequate pressure for brain perfusion:

› Elevation of the head of the bed (30 degrees). This improves jugular venous flow and therefore lowers ICP.

› Maintain airway patency. If there is an acute rise in ICP, it may cause a reduced GCS, loss of airway protective reflexes and acute herniation. If this is the case, a definitive airway

FIGURE 8

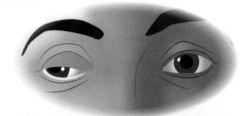

Right sided CN III palsy. Pupils are fixed, dilated, looking down and out. Ptosis of the eyelid is present.

FIGURE 10

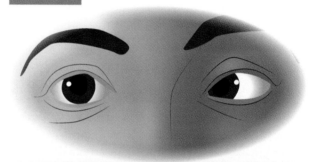

Left sided CN VI palsy. Medial rectus acts unopposed, meaning that the eye cannot move laterally.

FIGURE 9

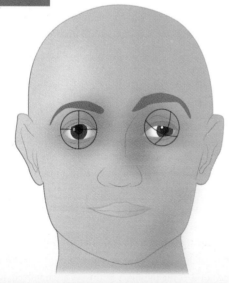
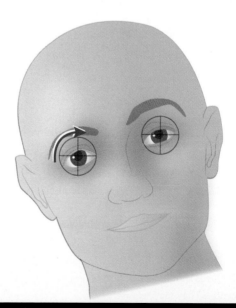

Left sided CN IV palsy. Inferior oblique acting unopposed. At rest, this results in the eye being extorted (rotated outwards), abducted and looking up. Note the inferior oblique also elevates the eye whilst in abduction. Head flexion, and being tilted to unaffected side minimises diplopia as it compensates for the extorsion and increases the size of the visual field.

must be established. Intubation also reduces the energy expenditure of the body by taking over the management of respiration.

▸ **Maintain adequate ventilation and circulation.** Ventilation should be controlled and hyperventilation is preferred as hypocapnia leads to vasoconstriction and therefore reduces ICP. However, this must be done carefully as excessive vasoconstriction may exacerbate cerebral ischaemia. The optimal pCO_2 is around 4.5 kPa.

▸ **Antipyretics.** Fever should be treated aggressively by antipyretics and cooling blankets, since fever worsens outcomes.

▸ **Analgesia, sedation +/- neuromuscular blockage.** To reduce pain as well as ICP. Sedation also reduces oxygen consumption.

▸ **Anti-seizure prophylaxis.** This should be given to children at high risk of seizures. Seizures following traumatic brain injury can increase ICP and lead to secondary brain damage.

▸ **Hyperosmolar therapy.** A bolus of 3% sodium chloride can decrease ICP and increase cerebral perfusion pressure. Mannitol is an alternative, but hypertonic sodium chloride is preferred.

▸ **Fluid restriction.** Restrict fluid to 1mL/kg/hr. Fluid boluses/ inotropes may be needed on top of this to maintain blood pressure. These should be giving carefully at 10ml/kg.

▸ **Surgical decompression.** Surgery should be the last intervention to be considered. CSF drainage via an intracranial drain can be placed to remove CSF and monitor ICP in uncontrolled intracranial hypertension. Decompressive craniectomy (where part of the skull

is removed) may be useful when all other treatments have failed.

Definitive treatment depends on the underlying causes, but may, for example, involve resection of a mass lesion.

Prognosis

Prognosis depends on the underlying cause, severity at presentation and the quality of initial management. In idiopathic cases (IIH), the most common complication is partial or complete vision loss.

Intracranial Bleeds

Intracranial bleeds are rare in children. However extradural, subdural and subarachnoid haemorrhage can occur, particularly in the context of trauma (*Table 9*).

NEUROCUTANEOUS SYNDROMES

Neurofibromatosis

Neurofibromatosis (NF) is an autosomal dominant disorder causing tumours to grow on nerves. It classically causes skin and bone deformities, but potentially involves any organ.

Aetiology

Half of all cases are sporadic, accountable to *de novo* mutations (not inherited). NF1 and NF2 are genetically and clinically distinct conditions. They do, however, have some clinical overlap, and are both associated with phaeochromocytoma, pulmonary hypertension, renal artery stenosis and gliomatous

TABLE 9: Intracranial bleeds

Bleeds	Cause	Clinical Features	Radiological Features	Treatment
Extradural haemorrhage.	This usually occurs due to bleeding from the middle meningeal artery, secondary to trauma.	Focal neurological signs may be present and consciousness levels may deteriorate. Seizures, hemiparesis, nerve paresis, anaemia and shock may be present.	Imaging by CT confirms the diagnosis by demonstrating a lenticular convex shaped lesion.	Neurosurgery to evacuate the haematoma and stop the bleeding may be necessary.

CT showing extradural haemorrhage (reproduced with kind permission from Radiopedia).

(Continued)

TABLE 9: *Continued*

Subdural haemorrhage.	This occurs due to stretching of bridging veins (which puncture the dura and drain underlying neural tissue). It typically occurs secondarily to falls, shaking or traumatic injuries in children.	Retinal haemorrhages may be present. The diagnosis may be delayed until the fluid volume expands, producing bulging fontanelle and seizures.	CT imaging confirms the diagnosis by demonstrating a crescent shaped lesion. 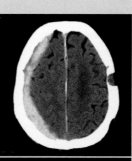 CT showing subdural haemorrhage (reproduced with kind permission from Radiopedia).	Neurosurgery to evacuate the haematoma and stop the bleeding may be necessary.
Subarachnoid haemorrhage.	The cause of a subarachnoid haemorrhage is usually aneurysms or arterio-venous malformations.	Clinical presentation is typically silent. However, symptoms include headache, neck stiffness and fever. Retinal haemorrhage, seizures and coma may develop.	CT imaging is diagnostic, but lumbar puncture 12 hours post-onset of symptoms should be performed if the CT is negative and there is still a strong clinical suspicion of a bleed. 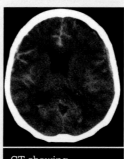 CT showing subarachnoid haemorrhage (reproduced with kind permission from Radiopedia).	Treatment is neurosurgical or by interventional radiology with clipping/coiling of aneurysms.

change. Features can be present at birth, but presentation may be delayed.

Clinical Features

NF1, also known as Von Recklinghausen disease, involves chromosome 17 and has an incidence of one in 3000. Two or more of the features below are diagnostic.

1　Café-au-lait spots. Flat pigmented macules (*Figure 11*). 6+ in number, >5mm pre-puberty or >15mm post-puberty is required to meet diagnostic criteria.
2　Axillary/inguinal freckling (*Figure 12*).
3　Bony lesions. e.g. sphenoid dysplasia or osteoarthritis.

4　More than two neurofibroma tumours (*Figure 13*) or one plexiform neurofibroma (larger more extensive tumours). These are cutaneous tumours.
5　First degree relative with NF1.
6　Two or more iris hamartomas (also known as Lisch nodules). These are only visible on slit lamp examination. Hamartomas are benign tumours.
7　Optic nerve glioma.

NF2 involves chromosome 22, and has an incidence of one in 25,000. Café-au-lait macules and skin neurofibromas are common in NF1 but are rarely found in NF2. NF2 typically presents with hearing loss or CNS tumours. Bilateral acoustic neuroma is pathognomonic of the condition. Those with

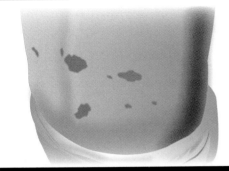

Café-au-lait spots.

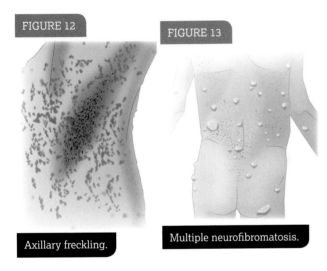

Axillary freckling.

Multiple neurofibromatosis.

a probable diagnosis must have a family history of NF2 and either:

i One unilateral acoustic neuroma.

ii Any two of: meningioma, glioma schwannoma, juvenile posterior subcapsular lenticular opacities/ juvenile cortical cataracts.

Investigations and Management

This is no cure for NF. However, many patients have such mild symptoms that they do not present for medical attention. The key to management is identifying complications early. Management includes:

> Imaging. MRI scans help to determine the site and delineate the invasion of tumours in the eyes, bones, nerve or brain.

> Eye tests. Annual ophthalmology examinations are important to detect eye signs early.

> BP monitoring. May develop hypertension secondary to renal artery stenosis or phaeochromocytoma.

> Genetic testing. Genetic testing and counselling may be necessary.

> Removal of neurofibromas. Either with laser technology or surgical resection. Medical treatment may be considered in unresectable or metastatic lesions.

Prognosis

NF1 is associated with a reduced mortality of approximately eight years, mainly due to hypertension, spinal cord lesions and malignancy. NF2 is also associated with significant rates of mortality and morbidity.

Tuberous Sclerosis Complex

Tuberous sclerosis complex is an autosomal dominant inherited disorder which causes non-malignant tumours to form in multiple organs, primarily in the skin, brain, heart, kidney, eye or bone. It has a prevalence of one in 9000 births. A wide range of manifestations are seen in the same family. Spontaneous mutations account for two thirds of cases. A younger presentation accounts for a higher risk of intellectual disability.

Clinical Features

The skin and the brain are the most frequently included organs. The classic features are:

> Skin lesions.
  > Ash leaf macules (*Figure 14*). Depigmented patches of skin which fluoresce under UV light (Wood light).
  > Angiofibromata (*Figure 15*). A sebaceous adenoma in a butterfly distribution over the nose and cheeks after 3 years of age.
  > Shagreen patches (*Figure 16*). Roughened skin patches over lumbar spine.
  > Subungual fibromata (*Figure 17*). Fibromata beneath nails.
  > Fibrous plaques. On forehead/temple.

> Brain lesions.
  > Epilepsy. 85% develop this, 70% in the first year of life. Infantile spasms occur in 33%.
  > Cognitive impairment.
  > Autism.
  > Neuropsychiatric issues. e.g. severe anxiety.

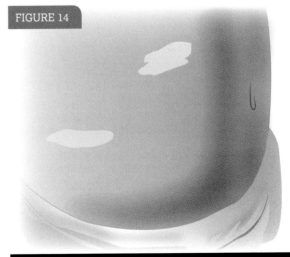

Ash leaf macules.

FIGURE 15

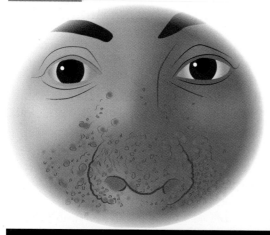

Angiofibromata.

FIGURE 16

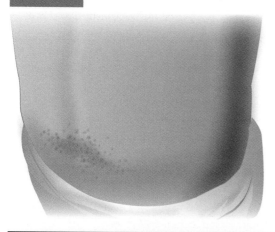

Shagreen patch.

Additional features may include brain tumours, rhabdomyoma of the heart, cystic/fibrous changes in the lungs and polycystic kidney disease.

Investigations

> Brain Imaging. MRI (or CT) is performed to assess for cortical/subcortical tubers, subependymal nodules, neuronal migration defects, and subependymal giant cell astrocytomas.
> EEG. This is used to assess for seizures.
> Abdominal imaging. Ideally MRI would be used to look for renal involvement, particularly angiomyolipoma, and renal cysts.
> Echocardiogram. This is used to identify atrial myxoma.
> ECG. This is used to look for cardiac arrhythmia.
> Blood pressure. This is used to assess for hypertension.
> Ophthalmological examination. This is used to look for retinal hamartomas.
> Dental and skin examination. This is used to look for defects such as facial angiofibroma and tooth enamel defects.

FIGURE 17

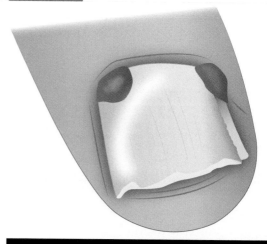

Subungual fibromata.

> Genetic testing. The TSC1 or TSC2 pathogenic gene mutations are sufficient to make the diagnosis.

Management

> Laser therapy. This can be used to remove angiofibromas.
> Seizures. Seizures can be difficult to manage, particularly in the context of infantile spasms. Vigabatrin, corticosteroids, ACTH, a ketogenic diet or vagus nerve stimulation may be helpful. Recurrent seizures and raised intracranial pressure due to an intracranial mass may require urgent surgical intervention. Epilepsy is the most common cause of death.
> Blood pressure control.
> Dialysis. Patients may require dialysis for renal failure.
> Lung monitoring. Women over 18-years-old may develop lymphangioleiomyomatosis of the lungs, which involves cyst formation in the lungs; therefore, CT lung scans should be used to identify lung pathology early.
> mTOR inhibitors. mTOR is a protein kinase that controls cell growth and proliferation; therefore, inhibiting it can reduce non-malignant tumour growth. mTOR inhibitors may be used in individuals with subependymal giant cell astrocytomas, renal angiomyolipomas and lymphangioleiomyomatosis.

Sturge-Weber Syndrome

Sturge-Weber Syndrome (SWS) is a sporadic vascular disease which occurs in one in 50,000 live births. It is characterised by abnormal blood vessels in:

> Skin. A port-wine stain (*Figure 18*). This is a facial capillary lesion, present at birth, covering at least the ophthalmic division of the trigeminal nerve. It can also cover the lower face, the trunk and the mucosal surface of the mouth.
> Brain. Leptomeningeal angiomas are abnormal blood vessels in the brain. Leptomeninges refers to both the pia and the arachnoid mater. Angiomas are benign vascular tumours

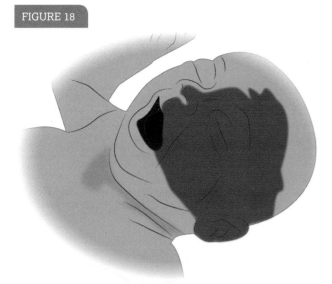

FIGURE 18

Characteristic port wine stain.

but can lead to seizures, which are typically focal and on the opposite side to the port-wine stain. Other neurological abnormalities include cognitive impairment, hemiparesis, headache and developmental delay.
▸ Eye. Abnormal blood vessels here can lead to glaucoma and buphthalmos (enlargement of the eyeball).

Investigations

Cranial contrast MRI will demonstrate white matter abnormalities, cerebral atrophy and leptomeningeal angiomatosis. Calcification of the gyri may also be noted, but this is more apparent on CT scanning.

Management

Management involves control of seizures, and in intractable cases, hemispherectomy or lobectomy. Monitoring for complications (e.g. glaucoma) and consideration of laser therapy for port-wine stains may be useful.

Von Hippel-Lindau Disease

Von Hippel–Lindau (VHL) disease is a multi-organ autosomal dominant disease affecting a tumour suppressor gene. The incidence is approximately one in 30,000. It causes cerebellar haemangiomas and retinal angiomas. Cystic lesions in the kidney, pancreas and epididymis are also associated with the condition. Renal carcinoma is the most common cause of death. Regular renal and brain imaging are required for early identification of cysts or masses. Dialysis may be required for kidney failure. Pancreatic enzyme supplementation for severe pancreatic disease may be necessary.

STROKE

Ischaemic strokes will be described below. Intracranial bleeds are described on p231.

Ischaemic Stroke

Stroke is the leading cause of acquired brain injury in children. The perinatal period carries the greatest risk. Hemiparesis is the most common presentation but visual, speech, sensory and balance dysfunction may also be seen.

Aetiology

Stroke in children is classified as either neonatal or childhood stroke.

In neonates, the stroke typically occurs in the middle cerebral artery, with or without seizure in the first hours of life after a normal delivery. It is either thrombotic from placental vessels or secondary to thrombophilia. The diagnosis is best confirmed on MRI.

In the post neonatal period, stroke has three main aetiologies:
▸ **Cardiac.** Congenital heart diseases account for the majority of acute strokes in children. Other causes include arrhythmias, cardiomyopathy and infective endocarditis.
▸ **Thromboembolic.** Arteriopathy, vasculitis, arterial infection and post varicella angiopathy.
▸ **Haematological.** Sickle cell anaemia and coagulation disorders.

Other causes include infections, inflammatory disease (e.g. systemic lupus erythematosus; SLE), drugs and toxins.

The majority of strokes affect the middle cerebral artery involving the anterior circulation and leading to hemiparesis with or without dysarthria. Damage to the posterior circulation is associated with visual or cerebellar dysfunction.

Investigations

Investigations aim to: i) identify aetiology, ii) direct treatment, and iii) identify how to prevent further episodes. This may include:
▸ Blood tests. Thrombophilia, infection, vasculitis and haemoglobinopathy screen may identify a treatable underlying condition.
▸ ECG. This is used to look for any underlying cardiac arrhythmia.
▸ CT/MRI of the brain and Magnetic Resonance Angiography (MRA) of cerebral arteries. This will identify the ischaemic lesion and any thrombus in the vessels.
▸ Carotid doppler. USS imaging can visualise the carotid arteries for dissection or thrombus.
▸ Echocardiogram. Echocardiogram can exclude structural lesions and cardiac thrombi which can form emboli.

Management

Management centres on good neurorehabilitation, with identification of important complications. Aspirin therapy is recommended.

Complications

Complications of ischaemic stroke include death, long-term neurodisability (including cerebral palsy) and epilepsy.

Prognosis

Often children recover faster and more completely than adults, due to neuroplasticity at younger ages. However, although changes in physical ability may be apparent immediately, cognitive and behavioural deficits may not be discovered until later on, e.g. difficulties with reading or concentration.

MOTOR DISORDERS

Facial Nerve Palsy

Aetiology

Idiopathic (Bell's palsy) aetiology is the most likely aetiology. This may be associated with herpes simplex infection.

Other causes include:

›   Trauma. Fracture of temporal bone is particularly associated with facial nerve palsy as is forceps delivery.
›   Infective. Otitis media, Lyme disease.
›   Ramsay Hunt syndrome. Reactivation of latent herpes zoster in the dorsal route ganglion of the facial nerve can give rise to facial nerve palsy.
›   Tumour. Acoustic neuroma, parotid gland neoplasm.
›   Moebius syndrome. This is a congenital defect affecting cranial nerve VI and VII.
›   Sarcoidosis.

The majority of facial nerve palsies are unilateral, lower motor neurone lesions. If the facial nerve palsy is bilateral, recurrent or if an upper motor neurone lesion is suspected then this is more concerning (e.g. stroke or tumour). The hallmark feature of an upper motor neurone lesion is sparing of the muscles of the forehead as the frontalis muscle has bilateral cortical representation.

Clinical Features

Symptoms include:

›   Inability to close eye (which may lead to dry eyes/conjunctivitis).
›   Mouth droop.
›   Loss of nasolabial fold.
›   Loss of taste on the anterior two thirds of tongue on affected side (50%).
›   Inability to raise eyebrows (in lower motor neurone lesions).

Management

Although there is limited evidence for early use of corticosteroids, they may speed recovery if given within 48 hours of the onset of symptoms. Additional antiviral therapy (e.g. aciclovir) may be added if herpes simplex virus or varicella zoster virus are suspected. Physiotherapy may also be of benefit.

Prognosis

Bell's palsy has a good prognosis and recovery should be expected although may take as long as six to eight weeks for full resolution.

Guillain-Barré Syndrome

Guillain-Barré syndrome is a post-infectious autoimmune demyelinating symmetrical polyneuropathy. It is the most common cause of flaccid paralysis. Symptoms occur typically around ten days after a non-specific viral or bacterial infection of the gut or upper airways. Causative organisms include EBV, *Campylobacter jejuni* or *Mycoplasma pneumoniae*.

Clinical Features

It typically affects motor function, but can also have sensory features (e.g. pain) and autonomic features (e.g. urinary retention, or bradycardia). Guillain-Barré presents with ascending weakness, gradually rising from the lower limbs and affecting the trunk, lungs, upper limbs and bulbar muscles/eyes symmetrically. Typically reflexes are reduced in the affected limbs. Symptoms last for two to three weeks and resolve spontaneously.

Investigations

Nerve conduction studies and CSF analysis (elevated protein) support the diagnosis. It is important to monitor lung function and cardiac function as they can both deteriorate rapidly. In severe cases, ventilation and cardiac pacing may be needed.

Management

Management is generally supportive in a high dependency or intensive care setting. Physiotherapy is helpful to aid mobilisation. In rapidly progressing cases, IV immunoglobulin (IVIG) or plasmapheresis may be required along with immunosuppressive therapy.

Spinal Muscular Atrophy

Spinal muscular atrophy (SMA) is an autosomal recessive disease causing degeneration of the lower motor neurones (anterior horn cells) leading to progressive denervation and weakness of skeletal muscles. It is due to a defect in the Survival Motor Neuron (SMN) gene, and is classified into type 1 to 4, with type 1 being the most severe.

SMA Type 1 (Werdnig-Hoffman disease)

Onset of SMA type 1 is normally between birth and 6-months-old. The characteristic features are a result of rapid motor neurone dysfunction:

›   Severe progressive hypotonia.
›   Generalised weakness including the tongue, face and jaw resulting in "floppy baby" with difficulty feeding.
›   Respiratory insufficiency.
›   Absent deep tendon reflexes.
›   Tongue and finger fasciculations (classic in LMN lesions).

The most effective test is finding the molecular genetic marker in blood for the SMN gene. Electromyography (EMG) shows fibrillation potentials and other nonspecific signs of denervation. Muscle biopsy shows muscle atrophy and muscle denervation. Life expectancy is between one and two years.

SMA Type 2-4

> Type 2. This normally appears between 6 and 18 months of age. It describes children who may be able to sit in a position without support but who tend to be unable to walk. The weakness progresses over time. However, feeding and swallowing problems are not as common and most patients live into adulthood.

> Type 3. This appears between 18-months-old and early adolescence. Children initially can walk without support, but eventually become wheelchair bound as the weakness develops.

> Type 4. This appears in adulthood. It normally manifests in the 4th decade of life and causes gradual weakening of the proximal muscles. Life expectancy is unaffected.

Myasthenia Gravis
Aetiology
Myasthenia Gravis (MG) is a chronic neuromuscular junction disease which presents as muscle fatigability. Juvenile MG is similar to the adult form of MG and is most commonly caused by immune mediated blockade of the acetylcholine receptor (AChR) at the neuromuscular junction. Transient neonatal MG is a type that occurs in neonates due to maternal antibodies crossing the placenta. Several syndromes cause a congenital MG (e.g. slow channel syndrome).

Clinical Features
These tend to worsen with muscle fatigue/as the day progresses, and include:

> Ptosis and extraocular muscle weakness.
> Dysphagia and facial weakness with early feeding problems.
> Generalised weakness.
> Respiratory muscle involvement causing difficulty breathing, chest infection or apnoea.

Investigations

> Blood tests. Anti-AChR antibody test is the most commonly used serological test. Anti-MuSK (muscle-specific kinase) and anti-striated muscle antibodies can also be used to support the diagnosis.

> EMG. This shows a decreasing response to repetitive nerve stimulation that is reversed after cholinesterase inhibitor (edrophonium) with improvement within seconds.

> Edrophonium test. Involves administration of a short acting anticholinesterase (increasing the amount of effective acetylcholine (ACh)), with rapid improvement in symptoms (e.g. improved peak flow, improved strength and improved ptosis). It is now less commonly used due to the risk of cardio-respiratory compromise.

Management
If the MG is mild, there may be no need for medications. However, treatment options include:

> Anticholinesterase. Neostigmine or pyridostigmine are the mainstay of treatment, acting by interfering with the breakdown of ACh, and thus increasing levels.

> Thymectomy. This should be considered in patients who have high levels of anti-AChR antibodies, those with thymomas and those with no response to medical therapy. Twenty-five percent achieve remission. It is ineffective in those with congenital or familial forms.

> Immunosuppressive therapy. In severe cases, prednisolone or azathioprine can be given for long-term therapy due to the autoimmune basis of the condition.

> Intravenous immunoglobulin or plasmapheresis. This may be required for acute, severe exacerbations.

Prognosis
Most patients with MG and optimal management have a near normal lifespan. Morbidity results from impaired muscle strength, leading to aspiration, falls and respiratory failure.

MUSCLE DISORDERS

Duchenne Muscular Dystrophy
Duchenne muscular dystrophy (DMD) is an inherited primary myopathy. It is an X-linked recessive disease which causes a lack of dystrophin, leading to progressive muscle necrosis and weakness. It is the most common inherited neuromuscular disease, affecting one in 3,600 male children.

Clinical Features
Children first present with:

> Delayed walking.
> Frequent falls.
> Developmental delay (e.g. language delay).

Weakness leads to a waddling gait or a Trendelenburg gait (both due to proximal muscle weakness). Muscle pseudo-hypertrophy (particularly in the calves) is also seen, where the muscle enlarges due to fat deposition rather than muscle (*Figure 19*). Gower's sign typically starts as early as the age of three and develops by five to six years of age. It refers to the motion of using the hands to climb over their body in order to stand (*Figure 20*). Muscle weakness in the back can also lead to kyphoscoliosis.

Other possible features include cardiomyopathy, respiratory failure, gastro-oesophageal reflux, intellectual impairment and seizures.

Investigations
The diagnosis is supported by an elevated creatine kinase. Definitive diagnosis is obtained by testing for the dystrophin

FIGURE 19

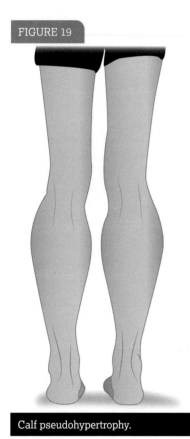

Calf pseudohypertrophy.

gene mutation, but if this is negative and there is still a high clinical suspicion, a muscle biopsy specimen can be tested, looking for the presence of dystrophin.

Management

Management involves:

> Optimising nutrition. Monitor diet, swallowing, bowel function and weight gain. Antireflux medication may be required, and in some cases gastrostomy feeding.
> Promptly treating infections.
> Close cardiac monitoring. Early identification and treatment of heart failure is important. Cardiomyopathy is treated with ACE inhibitors and B Blockers.

> Respiratory support. Non-invasive positive pressure ventilation may be needed. Tracheostomy and cough-assist devices may be helpful for airway clearance.
> Musculoskeletal. Physiotherapy and occupational therapy may delay/prevent contractures. Orthotic devices improve function and mobility. Calcium, vitamin D and bisphosphonate therapy may be helpful. Bone density scans are useful for monitoring.
> Corticosteroids. Steroids can reduce the rate of muscle necrosis, but have side effects of increased risk of infection, osteoporosis and weight gain.
> Surgery. Contractures can be treated surgically. Procedures to lengthen the Achilles tendon can be helpful for ambulation. Scoliosis management.

New therapies are emerging that may treat the underlying genetic cause. Ataluren is a small molecular compound which increases expression of dystrophin which was recently approved in the UK for a subgroup of patients.

Prognosis

Prognosis is generally poor and life expectancy is typically around 20 years of age.

Becker's Muscular Dystrophy

Becker's muscular dystrophy (BMD) is a similar disease to DMD and is caused by a similar genetic defect in the same locus on the X chromosome. The clinical presentation is milder because dystrophin is still produced in small amounts. Its age of onset is delayed, typically at around 10-years-old. Patients are usually able to walk until they are 20 to 30-years-old. Management is similar to DMD, but life expectancy is far greater, at around 40-years-old. Key differences between DMD and BMD are shown in *Table 10*.

Myotonic Dystrophy

Myotonic dystrophy is an autosomal dominant disease which causes muscle wasting in both striated and smooth muscle. It is

FIGURE 20

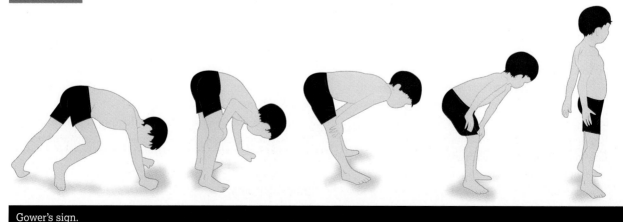

Gower's sign.

TABLE 10: Duchenne and Becker's muscular dystrophy		
	DMD	**BMD**
Dystrophin function.	Non-functional.	Partially functional.
Frequency.	More common.	Less common.
Severity.	More severe.	Less severe.
Age of onset.	Around 3-years-old.	Around 10-years-old.
Life expectancy.	Around 20-years-old.	Around 40-years-old.

the second most common cause of muscular dystrophy, with an incidence of approximately one in 50,000 births.

Clinical Features
Neonates typically present with:
› Hypotonia.
› Facial muscle wasting (particularly temporalis).
› Breathing difficulties.
› Feeding problems.

Congenital myotonic dystrophy is a severe form of the disease but in some cases babies may be normal at delivery. Other problems include dysarthria, arrhythmias including heart block, hypothyroidism, adrenal insufficiency, immunological deficiency, cataracts and intellectual impairment. Death is most commonly associated with cardiomyopathy.

Investigations
Diagnosis is via genetic testing as the widely scattered degenerative muscle fibres may be missed on muscle biopsy.

Management
There is no cure, but complications can be treated. Physiotherapy and exercise training to improve muscle weakness and mobility may be beneficial. Respiratory complications due to weakness, and sleep related problems such as apnoea, can be managed with non-invasive positive pressure ventilation. Speech and language therapy and gastroenterology support are important in patients with increased risk of aspiration due to dysphagia. Myotonia may be improved by drugs such as phenytoin and carbamazepine that increase the depolarisation threshold of muscle cells.

Dermatomyositis
Juvenile dermatomyositis is the most common inflammatory myositis in children. It occurs in children 4 to 10-years-old and its incidence is three per million births.

Clinical Features
Children often present with a rash (first symptom in 50% of cases) and weakness of the proximal muscles. There is a characteristic rash on the eyelids (heliotrope), face (nasolabial

folds) and on the extensor surfaces of the elbows and knees. Other classical features include:
› Lipodystrophy. Loss of subcutaneous and visceral fat.
› Calcinosis. Calcium deposits in the skin.
› Gottron's papules. Bright pale atrophied plaques located on distal and proximal interphalangeal joints that are classic of the disease.

Respiratory muscles, neck muscles and smooth muscle in the gut can be affected, leading to respiratory failure, dysphagia and reflux. Note that adult dermatomyositis is associated with malignancies, but there is no strong evidence for this in the juvenile form.

Investigations
Diagnosis is supported by elevated creatine kinase (CK), EMG changes and/or muscle biopsy changes.

Management
Corticosteroids are the mainstay of treatment. Methotrexate and cyclosporine can be used as steroid sparing agents. Physiotherapy is an important part of management to prevent contractures and sustain mobility and strength. Mortality is less than 5%.

EMBRYOLOGICAL DISORDERS

Neural Tube Defects
Neural tube defects (NTD) are the major cause of congenital abnormalities of the CNS. They result from the failure of neural tube closure during the first four weeks of in-utero development. The prevalence is one in 10,000 births in the UK. Risk factors include:
› Previous child with NTD.
› Poor maternal nutrition.
› Lack of folic acid intake during pregnancy.

There are four main categories of NTDs, as described below (*Figure 21* and *22*).

Spina Bifida Occulta
Spina bifida occulta is the mildest NTD. There are variable definitions of spina bifida occulta. Some consider it to purely refer to an isolated posterior body fusion defect with no spinal abnormalities. By this definition, it is completely asymptomatic.

Closed spinal cord malformations associated with a posterior body fusion defect are correctly termed "occult spinal dysraphism", rather than spina bifida occulta. In most cases, such defects are associated with skin lesions such as a lipoma, dimple, a tuft of hair, birth-mark or a dermal sinus. Closed spinal cord malformations include tethering of the cord. This may lead to neurological dysfunction and requires surgical correction.

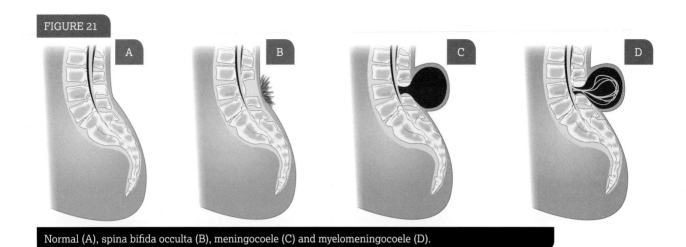

Normal (A), spina bifida occulta (B), meningocoele (C) and myelomeningocoele (D).

FIGURE 22

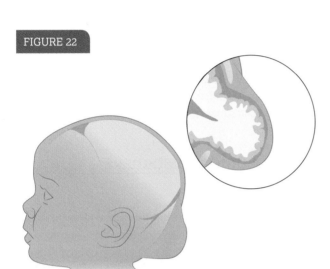

Encephalocoele.

Meningocoele

Meningocoele is the protrusion of the meninges through the skull, posterior arches of the vertebra or the sacrum. The spinal cord is normally positioned but there is a midline and fluctuant mass in the back covered with thin skin. It is associated with CSF leak and hydrocephalus. Abdominal/sacral USS is initially used to diagnose meningocoele and differentiate it from other pelvic cystic lesions, and CT or MRI provides more definitive imaging. Brain CT or cranial USS is indicated if hydrocephalus is suspected. Bladder and bowel dysfunction are common. Corrective surgery reduces the likelihood of complications.

Myelomeningocoele

Myelomeningocoele is the protrusion of the meninges and spinal cord through the vertebra, most commonly in the lumbosacral region. Nerves below the point of protrusion do not develop properly. Depending on the location, myelomeningocoele is associated with bladder and bowel incontinence, CSF leak, muscle wasting/paralysis, hydrocephalus, sensory loss, cranial nerve palsies and scoliosis. Hydrocephalus develops in 85% of cases. This is because a myelomeningocoele is associated with an Arnold Chiari malformation (downward herniation of the brainstem and fourth ventricle through the foramen magnum) resulting in CSF obstruction.

Surgery is used to treat the initial defect and a shunt may be required for the hydrocephalus. Patients require multidisciplinary input for associated problems. Urology input is vital, as renal failure can be prevented by intermittent catheterisation of a neurogenic bladder. Other input includes physiotherapy, occupational therapy, educational support, orthopaedics and seizure medications.

Encephalocoele

Encephalocoele is the protrusion of the brain and meninges through a midline skull defect. It most often involves the occipital brain. USS, MRI or CT is most useful to determine the lesion, and surgery can correct some defects. These patients are at greater risk of cerebral abnormalities, hydrocephalus, visual defects, microcephaly, cognitive loss and seizures. Definitive treatment is surgical.

Microcephaly

Microcephaly is defined by a head circumference which is three standard deviations below the mean for age and sex. It is often associated with developmental delay and lower cognitive function. It can be classified into primary or secondary causes.

Primary causes include:

> **Isolated microcephaly.** Autosomal recessive or autosomal dominant microcephaly.
> **Part of a syndrome.** Down Syndrome, Edward's Syndrome.

Secondary causes include:

> **Congenital Infection.** Rubella, CMV, toxoplasmosis, Zika.
> **Maternal drug use.** Foetal alcohol syndrome.
> **Vascular.** Ischaemic/haemorrhagic stroke.

Treatment is directed at the underlying cause, although for many conditions management may purely be supportive through the multidisciplinary team.

Anencephaly

Anencephaly is failure of the development of parts of the brain and skull. Often there is no cerebral hemisphere and cerebellum, and the pyramidal tracts in the spinal cord are missing. Those born are stillborn or die shortly after birth. It can be detected during USS screening at antenatal clinic and termination of pregnancy is usually offered. The incidence is one in 1000 live births. There is a strong association (50% of cases) with polyhydramnios.

CEREBELLAR DISORDERS

Cerebellar disorders in childhood are most often characterised by ataxia. Ataxia is a movement disorder characterised by the inability to make smooth, accurate and coordinated movements due to cerebellar dysfunction. The most common primary causes of ataxia are Friedreich ataxia and ataxia telangiectasia. There are several secondary causes of ataxia, such as infection, alcohol, brain tumours, Arnold-Chiari malformations and trauma.

Friedreich Ataxia

Friedreich ataxia is an autosomal recessive inherited condition of the frataxin gene. It causes progressive disease of the spinocerebellar tracts. It presents before 10-years-old with ataxia and wasting of the legs, absence of leg reflexes, with preserved extensor plantar responses, pes cavus (high arched feet), optic atrophy and dysarthria. There is also degeneration of the posterior columns of the spinal cord causing impaired joint position and vibration sense with skeletal abnormalities like kyphoscoliosis. Hypertrophic cardiomyopathy can cause congestive cardiac failure and become the major cause of death at 40 to 50 years-old. Patients have normal intellect, although they may appear apathetic. Genetic testing provides a definitive diagnosis. Management is supportive therapy. It is associated with diabetes.

Ataxia Telangiectasia

Ataxia telangiectasia is an autosomal recessive inherited degenerative ataxia which occurs in children at around 5-years-old and leads to difficulty in balance and coordination. Telangiectasia forms in the conjunctiva, nose, ears, neck and shoulders. There is an increased risk of infection (particularly sinopulmonary) and malignancy. Patients are also very sensitive to ionising radiation. Blood tests reveal an elevated alpha fetoprotein (AFP), elevated CA125, lymphopenia, eosinophilia, immunodeficiency (IgA, IgG, CD4+), and white cell sensitivity to irradiation. The A-T gene can be identified on genetic testing. Management is supportive therapy.

HYDROCEPHALUS

Hydrocephalus is an abnormal accumulation of cerebrospinal fluid in the brain and can result in macrocephaly (*Figure 23*).

Aetiology

Hydrocephalus may be due to:

> Overproduction of CSF. This is rare, but it may occur with a choroid plexus papilloma.
> Decreased absorption of CSF in the subarachnoid granules/superior sagittal sinus. This occurs with infection/haemorrhage.
> Obstruction to the outflow (e.g. haemorrhage, tumour, trauma or infection). The most common congenital cause of blockage is stenosis of the cerebral aqueduct, whilst the commonest acquired cause is ventricular haemorrhage.

Clinical Features

Hydrocephalus may be picked up on routine antenatal USS or as an incidental finding of child's head circumference crossing centile lines on growth chart monitoring.

In symptomatic infants, it may present with:

> Bulging anterior fontanelle.
> Broadening of forehead.
> Enlarged head circumference (see centile chart).
> 'Sun-setting' of the eye, with the sclera visible above the iris and the pupil disappearing below the lower eyelid.
> Irritability, lethargy or drowsiness.
> Muscle spasticity with brisk reflexes.
> Dilated scalp veins.

In addition to the above, older children may present with headache, signs of raised intracranial pressure, confusion, blurred vision or urinary/faecal incontinence.

Investigations

The ventricular system should be imaged by cranial USS in the neonate, as there is an open anterior fontanelle. MRI is the gold standard imaging technique, as it visualises the CSF pathways most effectively.

Management

Treatments may initially include acetazolamide and furosemide to temporarily reduce the rate of CSF production. Ventriculo-peritoneal (VP) shunts, which are narrow tubes that divert the passage of CSF, relieve the pressure caused by fluid accumulation and are the mainstay of treatment.

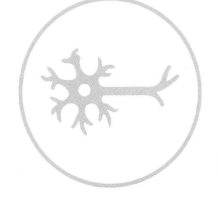

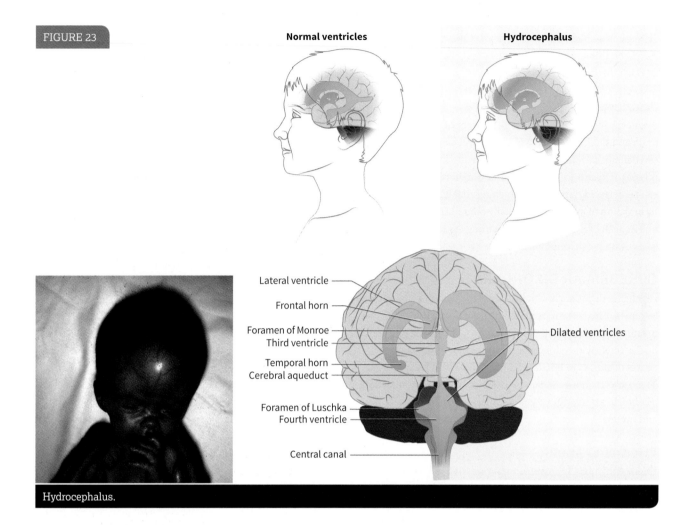

FIGURE 23

Normal ventricles   Hydrocephalus

Lateral ventricle
Frontal horn
Foramen of Monroe
Third ventricle
Temporal horn
Cerebral aqueduct
Foramen of Luschka
Fourth ventricle
Central canal

Dilated ventricles

Hydrocephalus.

REFERENCES AND FURTHER READING

Seizures/Epilepsy

1 Berg, et al. Revised terminology and concepts for organization of seizures and epilepsies: Report of the ILAE Commission on Classification and Terminology, 2005–2009. Epilepsia. 2010; 51:676–85.

2 International League Against Epilepsy. ILAE Revised Terminology for Organization of Seizures and Epilepsies 2011-2013. Connecticut:ILAE; 2013. http://www.ilae.org/Visitors/Centre/documents/OrganizationEpilepsy-overview.pdf.

3 Advanced Paediatric Life Support (APLS) Fifth Edition, Advanced Life Support Group (ALSG).London: Blackwell Publishing, 2010.

4 National Institute of Health and Care Excellence. The epilepsies: the diagnosis and management of the epilepsies in adults and children in primary and secondary care. NICE clinical guideline 137. London:NICE; 2012. http://www.nice.org.uk/guidance/cg137/resources/guidance-the-epilepsies-the-diagnosis-and-management-of-the-epilepsies-in-adults-and-children-in-primary-and-secondary-care-pdf.

5 Scottish Intercollegiate Guidelines Network. Diagnosis and management of epilepsies in children and young people. A national clinical guideline. Edinburgh:SIGN; 2005. http://www.sign.ac.uk/pdf/sign81.pdf.

Intracranial Infections

1 Kneen R, Michael BD, Menson E, Mehta B, Easton A, Hemingway C, Klapper PE, Vincent A, Lim M, Carrol E, Solomon T. On behalf of the National Encephalitis Guidelines Development and Stakeholder Groups. Management of suspected viral Encephalitis in children: Association of British Neurologists and British Paediatric Allergy, Immunology and Infectious Diseases Group National Guidelines. J Infect. 2012; 64(5): 449-77.

2 Meningitis Research Foundation. Meningococcal Meningitis and Septicaemia Guidance Notes. London: Meningitis Research Foundation; 2014. http://www.meningitis.org/assets/x/50631.

3 Ministry of Health, New South Wales, Australia. NSW Kids and Families Infants and Children: Acute Management of Bacterial Meningitis: Clinical Practice Guideline. North Sydney:Ministry of Health New South Wales; 2014.

http://www0.health.nsw.gov.au/policies/gl/2014/pdf/GL2014_013.pdf.

4   National Institute of Health and Care Excellence. Bacterial meningitis and meningococcal septicaemia: Management of bacterial meningitis and meningococcal septicaemia in children and young people younger than 16 years in primary and secondary care. NICE clinical guideline 102. London:NICE; 2010. http://www.nice.org.uk/guidance/cg102.

5   Medscape Paediatrics.. Management of Brain Abscesses. http://www.medscape.com/viewarticle/581536_1.

6   Kliegman RM, Stanton BF, Geme JW, Schor NF, Behram RE. Nelon Textbook of Paediatrics. 19th Edition. New York: Elsevier Inc.; 2011. 2088.

Cerebral Palsy

1   Up To Date. Clinical Features of Cerebral Palsy. http://www.uptodate.com/contents/clinical-features-of-cerebral-palsy.

2   Up To Date. Diagnosis and Classification of Cerebral Palsy. http://www.uptodate.com/contents/diagnosis-and-classification-of-cerebral-palsy.

3   Up To Date. Management and Prognosis of Cerebral Palsy. http://www.uptodate.com/contents/management-and-prognosis-of-cerebral-palsy.

Headache Disorders

1   Headache Classification Committee of the International Headache Society (IHS). The International Classification of Headache Disorders, 3rd edition (beta version). *Cephalalgia*. 2013;33:629-808. http://www.ihs-classification.org/_downloads/mixed/International-Headache-Classification-III-ICHD-III-2013-Beta.pdf

2   National Institute of Health and Care Excellence. Headaches: Diagnosis and management of headaches in young people and adults. NICE clinical guideline 150. London:NICE; 2012. http://www.nice.org.uk/guidance/cg150/resources/guidance-headaches-pdf.

3   Up to Date. Elevated intracranial pressure (ICP) in children. http://www.uptodate.com/contents/elevated-intracranial-pressure-icp-in-children?source=search_result&search=raised+icp&selectedTitle=3~150.

Head Injury

1   National Institute of Health and Care Excellence. Head injury: Triage, assessment, investigation and early management of head injury in children, young people and adults. NICE clinical guideline 176. London: NICE; 2014. https://www.nice.org.uk/guidance/cg176.

Cerebrovascular Disorders

1   Radiopaedia. Extradural Haemorrhage Teaching. http://radiopaedia.org/cases/extradural-haemorrhage-teaching.

Radiopaedia. Subdural Haemorrhage. http://radiopaedia.org/cases/subdural-haemorrhage-1.

2   Radiopaedia. Subarachnoid Haemorrhage. http://radiopaedia.org/articles/subarachnoid-haemorrhage.

3   The Clinical Effectiveness and Evaluation Unit (CEEU), Royal College of Physicians. Stroke in childhood: Clinical guidelines for diagnosis, management and rehabilitation. London:RCP; 2004. https://www.rcplondon.ac.uk/sites/default/files/documents/stroke-in-childhood-guideline.pdf.

Spinal Muscular Atrophy

1   Up To Date. Spinal Muscular Atrophy. http://www.uptodate.com/contents/spinal-muscular-atrophy.

2   The SMA Trust. About SMA. http://www.smatrust.org/what-is-sma/about-sma.

Guillain-Barré Syndrome

1   Up To Date. Epidemiology, clinical features, and diagnosis of Guillain-Barre Syndrome in Children. http://www.uptodate.com/contents/epidemiology-clinical-features-and-diagnosis-of-guillain-barre-syndrome-in-children.

Myasthenia Gravis

1   Myasthenia Gravis Foundation of America. Clinical Overview of Myasthenia Gravis. http://www.myasthenia.org/HealthProfessionals/ClinicalOverviewofMG.aspx.

Facial Nerve Palsy

1   Up To Date. Facial Nerve Palsy in Children. http://www.uptodate.com/contents/facial-nerve-palsy-in-children.

Duchenne/Becker's Muscular Dystrophy

1   Up To Date. Clinical Features and diagnosis of Duchenne and Becker muscular dystrophy. http://www.uptodate.com/contents/clinical-features-and-diagnosis-of-duchenne-and-becker-muscular-dystrophy.

2   Up To Date. Treatment of Duchenne and Becker muscular dystrophy. http://www.uptodate.com/contents/treatment-of-duchenne-and-becker-muscular-dystrophy.

3   NICE. NICE recommends ataluren for treating Duchenne muscular dystrophy caused by a nonsense mutation. https://www.nice.org.uk/news/press-and-media/nice-recommends-ataluren-for-treating-duchenne-muscular-dystrophy-caused-by-a-nonsense-mutation.

Myotonic Dystrophy

1   Up To Date. Myotonic Dystrophy: Etiology, clinical features, and diagnosis. http://www.uptodate.com/contents/myotonic-dystrophy-etiology-clinical-features-and-diagnosis.

Dermatomyositis

1   Up To Date. Pathogenesis and clinical manifestations of juvenile dermatomyositis and polymyositis.

http://www.uptodate.com/contents/pathogenesis-and-clinical-manifestations-of-juvenile-dermatomyositis-and-polymyositis.

Neural Tube Defects

1   Up To Date. Prenatal screening and diagnosis of neural tube defects. http://www.uptodate.com/contents /prenatal-screening-and-diagnosis-of-neural-tube -defects.

2   Up To Date. Pathophysiology and clinical manifestations of myelomeningocele spina bifida. http://www.uptodate.com/ contents/pathophysiology-and-clinical-manifestations-of-myelomeningocele-spina-bifida.

Hydrocephalus

1   Up To Date. Hydrocephalus. http://www.uptodate.com/ contents/hydrocephalus.

Microcephaly

1   Up To Date. Microcephaly in infants and children: Etiology and evaluation. http://www.uptodate.com/contents/ microcephaly-in-infants-and-children-etiology-and-evaluation.

Ataxia

1   Up To Date. Acute cerebellar ataxia in children. http://www.uptodate.com/contents/acute-cerebellar-ataxia-in-children.

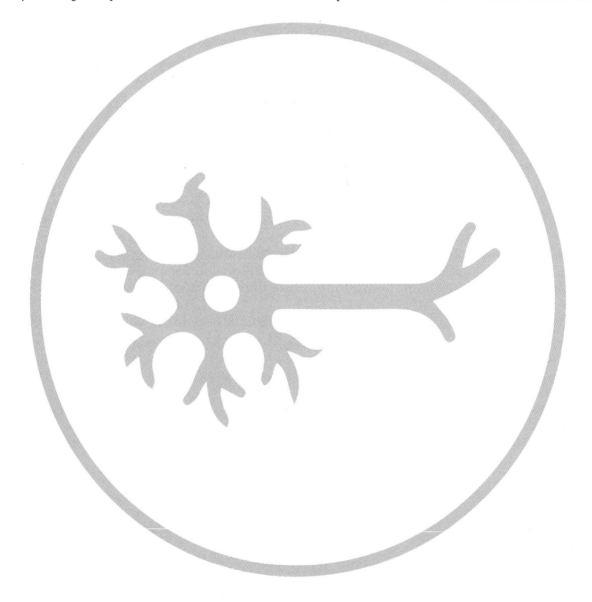

1.17 NUTRITION

CHI HAU TAN

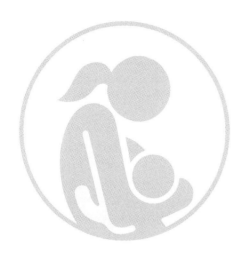

CONTENTS

FEEDING

Breastfeeding

Breastfeeding has many advantages and breast milk is considered the ideal food for infants (*Table 1*). The World Health Organization (WHO) has recommended exclusive breastfeeding (i.e. no other fluids or solids) until an infant is 6–months-old. Breastfeeding is encouraged until the baby is at least 12-months-old, as long as both the mother and child desire it. *Box 1* lists some contraindications.

Jaundice and Breastfeeding

Breastfed babies are more likely to become jaundiced in the neonatal period. This may be for two reasons:

> If breastfeeding is slow to establish, a baby may lose significant weight in the first week of life. Dehydration due to insufficient intake exacerbates jaundice.

> Breast milk innately inhibits certain liver enzymes involved in bilirubin excretion (glucuronyl transferase), making jaundice more prominent.

TABLE 1: Benefits of breastfeeding	
For infants	**For mothers**
• Provides the right composition of nutrients for healthy growth and development. • Readily absorbed by the body. • Not complicated by infections associated with formula milk preparation. • Contains antibodies. • Numerous long-term health benefits, including improved visual acuity and cognitive development, and reduced risk of developing allergies, inflammatory bowel disease, cardiovascular diseases, diabetes and obesity.	• Stimulates release of oxytocin that helps with uterine contraction and reduces postpartum haemorrhage. • Facilitates postpartum weight loss. • Contraceptive effect through prolongation of lactational amenorrhoea (if used exclusively). • Lowers the risk of breast cancer, ovarian cancer and osteoporosis. • Saves the time and expenses associated with preparation of formula milk. • Provides opportunity for infant-mother bonding.

Jaundice related to breastfeeding is usually mild, and does not represent a reason to stop breastfeeding. If mum is not producing breast milk, but still wants to exclusively breastfeed, donor breast milk may be an option.

Formula Feeding

For mothers who are unable to breastfeed or who have made an informed decision not to breastfeed, infant formula milk is used as an alternative. Cow milk-based formula is also suitable for infants under 12 months of age unless medically contraindicated. *Table 2* shows key differences between breastfeeding and formula feeding.

Weaning

By 6-months-old, a baby can no longer obtain all the essential nutrients for normal growth and development from breast milk alone. At this stage, the child can be slowly introduced to solid foods of appropriate texture (puréed at first), along with breast milk. Infants who have been breastfed may find it easier to accommodate to this change as they have previously been exposed to the food consumed in the family through

the mother's breast milk. Due to the declined store of iron in breast milk by six months of age, iron-rich nutritious foods, such as iron-enriched rice-based cereals, are recommended as the first foods to be introduced. Iron is critical in cognitive development. A wide variety of solid foods can be introduced in any order so that the child is consuming a broad range of food by 12-months-old. Different types of food, however, should be introduced one at a time to help identify potential allergies. Pasteurised full cream cow's milk (instead of low fat milk), rich in calcium and protein, can be introduced to the diet at 12-months-old. Constant supervision must be provided during feeding and small particles of food such as nuts should be avoided to reduce risk of choking. Growth and weight gain should be monitored closely in the first year of life to ensure adequate dietary intake. *Box 2* shows a suggested timetable for introducing foods.

Maintaining a Healthy Diet

Dietary requirements vary as the child grows, to accommodate the various developmental stages, including the rapid growth spurt during adolescence. Young children can sometimes be picky eaters due to new textures or tastes. Foods high in energy but lacking in nutrients, such as cakes, biscuits, confectionaries

TABLE 2: Comparison of breastfeeding and formula milk		
	Breastfeeding	Formula milk
Absorption.	Readily absorbed by the body.	Some babies may have difficulty tolerating certain nutrients in formula milk.
Content.	Content varies according to changing nutritional requirement of the infant.	Adjustment (including type of formula milk and volume provided at each feed) to be made by carer.
Antibodies.	Presence of antibodies provides protection against infections during infancy.	Lack of antibodies.
Preparation.	Always at the right temperature, minimal preparation required.	Optimal preparation required to ensure right temperature and to reduce risk of contamination.
Cost.	Free.	Considerable cost involved.
Feeding duties.	Mother must be present or have expressed milk beforehand if absent.	Feeding duties can be shared with the partner.
Maternal physical health.	Ability to breastfeed may be affected by medical conditions and medications used, e.g. statins. May also cause pain.	The child can be fed at all times, regardless of the mother's health and medications.

and sugary drinks, should be limited to avoid the negative impacts of weight gain and tooth decay. Healthy foods such as vegetables, fruits, whole grains, nuts, fish and lean meats should be prioritised. Family meal times in a relaxed environment, without television viewing, should also be encouraged.

Faltering Growth

Faltering growth (also referred to as "failure to thrive") is defined as a significant interruption in the expected rate of growth compared with other children of the same gender, and of similar age. How to track height and weight is discussed on p68, along with the assessment of short stature. As a rough guide, the expected average weight gain per week for a child are:

› 0 to 3-months-old: 180g per week
› 3 to 6-months-old: 120g per week
› 6 to 9-months-old: 80g per week
› 9 to 12-months-old: 70g per week

Aetiology

The fundamental mechanism of faltering growth is inadequate nutrition relative to metabolic needs. This can be secondary to nutritional, medical or psychosocial issues. Causes are classified as organic and non-organic, although they often coexist (*Table 3*).

Management

As the potential causes of faltering growth are diverse, a thorough history and examination is essential. Laboratory investigations are not necessary for an otherwise healthy child with a clear non-concerning cause. Possible investigations and more detailed assessment are described on p71.

Multidisciplinary input from a primary care physician, paediatrician, dietician, speech and language therapist, and in cases of suspected abuse, children's social care is beneficial. Hospitalisation of a child is considered when there is a failure of outpatient management, suspicion of abuse or neglect, or severe psychosocial impairment.

The primary goal of therapy is to achieve catch-up growth through provision of sufficient nutritional intake and treatment of any underlying disorder. The child will initially demonstrate an accelerated growth rate, followed by deceleration towards normal growth rate. Children with severe nutritional deficiency should be monitored cautiously during the treatment due to the risk of refeeding syndrome—a metabolic complication that occurs due to increased cellular uptake of potassium, phosphate and magnesium. The resultant electrolyte disturbance can cause arrhythmias.

Children with faltering growth should be followed up closely until catch-up growth is demonstrated.

Malnutrition

Malnutrition contributes to approximately one-third of child deaths worldwide. It develops when the body does not get adequate energy and nutrients to maintain organ function. Malnutrition results in the disturbance of childhood physical and mental growth, and particularly growth stunting. Growth stunting affects more than 147 million children under five in low income countries.

Severe acute malnutrition in 6 to 59-month-old children has been defined as:

› Weight-for-height of less than -3 standard deviations from the mean.
› Mid-upper arm circumference of less than 11.5 cm.
› Presence of bilateral pitting oedema.

Severe acute malnutrition is associated with wasting, whilst chronic malnutrition results in stunted growth. As the body tries to adapt to malnourishment, a child is particularly prone to hypoglycaemia, electrolyte disturbances, hypothermia, dehydration and infection. A child's weight should be monitored for adequate growth from birth until two years of age.

TABLE 3: Causes of faltering growth		
Organic	Inadequate intake.	• Anatomical anomalies, such as cleft lip and/or palate. • Oromotor dysfunction from conditions such as cranial nerve palsy or neuromuscular disease. • Prolonged exclusive breastfeeding.
	Surgical.	• Intestinal obstruction (e.g. pyloric stenosis).
	Inadequate absorption.	• Coeliac disease. • Chronic liver disease. • Cystic fibrosis. • Chronic diarrhoea or vomiting.
	Excessive metabolic requirement.	• Recurrent infections. • Congenital heart disease. • Chronic pulmonary disease. • Endocrine disorders, such as diabetes mellitus and hyperthyroidism.
	Perinatal factors.	• Teratogenic exposures. • Intrauterine growth restriction. • Prematurity and low birth weight.
	Other.	• Genetic syndromes, e.g. Russell Silver syndrome. • Inborn errors of metabolism. • Anaemia.
Non-organic		• Poverty. • Inappropriate diet for age (e.g. excessive consumption of fruit juice). • Coercive feeding. • Distraction at meal times. • Social isolation. • Life stresses. • Poor parenting skills. • Child abuse or neglect. • Parental mental health issues (e.g. postpartum depression). • Parental eating disorders (e.g. anorexia nervosa).

This period is described as the critical "window of opportunity" for early interventions to prevent the development of irreversible damages secondary to malnutrition. Possible causes of malnutrition are shown in *Table 4*. In high income countries, malnutrition is more commonly caused by chronic medical illness, with associated malabsorption and increased metabolic requirements. Malnutrition can also occur secondary to overeating, when large quantities of high-energy food with minimal nutrients are consumed.

Severe protein-energy malnutrition is associated with the clinical pictures of marasmus, and then in more severe cases, kwashiorkor. The transition from marasmus to kwashiorkor is associated with high risks of morbidity and mortality due to acute infection. The characteristics of the two conditions are summarised in *Table 5* (although there may be overlap).

Clinical Assessment

Clinical assessment involves trying to ascertain both the cause of malnutrition and its severity.

History

> Clarify exact date of birth and birth weight.
> Feeding practices.
>> Duration of breastfeeding.
>> Age when solid foods were introduced.
>> Quantity and type of food.
>> Food preparation, e.g. milk preparation with contaminated water resulting in infections or infestations.
>> Behavioural issues around mealtimes and selective food intake.
>> Parental dietary history as parents may also be malnourished.
> Parental height and weight.
> Concurrent illnesses or symptoms suggestive of the following:
>> Recurrent infections and infestations.
>> Chronic diarrhoea and malabsorption.

TABLE 4: Causes of malnutrition

Causes	Examples
Lack of access to nutritious food.	Poverty, rising food prices.
Poor feeding practices/eating habits.	Inadequate breastfeeding, inappropriate food for age, preparation of food with contaminated water. Fast food, overeating.
Poor hygiene and infections.	Worm infestations.
Diseases resulting in malabsorption.	Persistent diarrhoea, coeliac disease, Crohn's, preparation of food with contaminated water.
Diseases resulting in increased energy requirements.	Congenital heart diseases, childhood cancer, HIV.
Eating disorders.	Anorexia nervosa, bulimia.
Children with disabilities.	Cerebral palsy.

TABLE 5: Differences between marasmus and kwashiorkor

Marasmus	Kwashiorkor

Marasmus figure labels: Thin sparse hair, Prominent ribs, Redundant skin folds

Kwashiorkor figure labels: Swollen abdomen, Hyperpigmentation, Oedema

Marasmus	Kwashiorkor
Deficiency in caloric intake.	Deficiency in protein intake.
Emaciated with prominent ribs.	Bilateral pitting oedema, begins in the feet and progresses to anasarca (generalised oedema).
Alert and irritable.	Apathetic, irritable and lethargic.
Loss of muscle mass and subcutaneous fat stores.	Weight loss, secondary to muscle and fat tissue loss, masked by excessive oedema.
Redundant skin folds hanging over arms, thighs and gluteal areas due to loss of subcutaneous fat.	Atrophic and fragile, dry, peeling skin with areas of hyperkeratosis and hyperpigmentation, ulceration and weeping lesions prone to infection.
Thin, sparse hair.	Dry and sparse hypopigmented hair which can be plucked easily.
Huge appetite once feeding is in progress.	Universally anorexic.

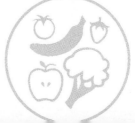

› Coeliac disease.
› Chronic diseases with increased energy requirements, e.g. hyperthyroidism, HIV, endocrine disturbances, chronic heart/lung disease.
› Psychosocial factors.
  › Poverty.
  › Financial and housing stresses.
  › Mental health issues.
  › Parenting.

Examination

› Assessment of growth parameters (weight, height and head circumference) and progression over time.
› Mid-upper arm circumference.
› Presence of oedema or muscle wasting, especially buttock wasting.
› Dehydration: thirst, sunken eyes, poor urine output, weak peripheral pulses and cold peripheries.
› Signs of sepsis.
› Signs of micronutrient deficiencies (see below).

Management

Early intervention and promotion of healthy eating habits are essential to prevent the irreversible physical and mental health consequences associated with malnutrition. Treatment involves close liaison with dieticians, and depends on the severity and underlying aetiology.

Admission to Hospital

Feeding supplements may be needed. Although most children can be managed in the community, some cases will need hospital admission, including:

› Failed appetite test (which assesses whether the child will eat a minimum amount of food).
› Medical complications.
› Severe oedema.

Therapeutic Food

Inpatient management of severe acute malnutrition has two phases:

› Initial stabilisation. This is when life-threatening complications are treated. A low-protein, milk based formula diet is recommended, e.g. F-75. If intensive refeeding is initiated before metabolic and electrolyte abnormalities are corrected, mortality rate is high.
› Nutritional rehabilitation. At this stage, electrolyte abnormalities, metabolic abnormalities, and any infection have been treated. Appetite has usually returned. It is in this phase that catch-up growth occurs. A milk formula with a higher protein and energy content can be used as the therapeutic food in this phase, e.g. F-100 or Ready-to-Use Therapeutic Food (RUTF). RUTFs are lipid-based pastes containing milk powder, electrolytes, iron and micronutrients. Transition should be gradual, as too rapid a transition is associated with diarrhoea, weight loss and refeeding syndrome.

Fluid Management

In children who are clinically dehydrated, slow oral or NG rehydration is preferred. A modified oral rehydration solution for malnourished children (ReSoMaL) with higher potassium and lower sodium concentrations compared to the traditional oral rehydration solution (ORS) should be commenced, especially in children with severe diarrhoea, to overcome the potassium depletion. It also contains zinc, vitamin A and other vitamins, electrolytes, and trace elements. Note that ReSoMaL is contraindicated in children with cholera, or with profuse watery diarrhoea (standard ORS should be given instead).

In children with signs of severely impaired circulation, severe dehydration, or who fail oral and nasogastric (NG) rehydration, intravenous therapy should be instigated, although still slowly, unless there is diarrhoea.

Infants Under 6-Months-Old

For infants under 6-months-old, it is important to prioritise establishing or re-establishing effective exclusive breastfeeding. F-100 should be avoided in this group due to the high renal solute load and the risk of hypernatraemic dehydration. As this group is at high risk of infection, all children should receive broad spectrum intravenous (inpatient) or oral (outpatient) antibiotics.

Monitoring and Discharge

Patients need monitoring for refeeding syndrome. Hypoglycaemia, hypothermia, dehydration and infections should also be identified and treated. Patients should only be discharged from hospital after significant improvement, with a plan for community management. Regular follow up after this is essential to avoid relapse.

VITAMIN DEFICIENCIES

Overview

Vitamins are a group of essential nutrients that must be obtained through external sources to maintain normal metabolism in the human body. They can be classified as either water-soluble or fat-soluble. The fat soluble vitamins, A, D, E and K are stored in liver and adipose tissues. They are eliminated from the body more slowly than water-soluble vitamins and thus pose a greater risk of toxicity if consumed in excess. Absorption of fat-soluble vitamins can be impaired in patients with pancreatic insufficiency or cholestatic liver disease, due to secondary fat malabsorption. Vitamin A and D deficiency are described below, and other important vitamin deficiencies are summarised in *Table 6*.

Vitamin A Deficiency

Vitamin A (retinol) is a group of lipid-soluble organic substances essential for the functioning of the immune system, formation of rhodopsin (photoreceptor pigments in the retina) and maintenance of epithelial tissues. It is found in green leafy and orange/yellow vegetables and fruits. Vitamin A is mainly stored in the liver. Serum retinol levels and retinol binding protein ratios can be used to identify deficiency.

249

TABLE 6: Summary of vitamin deficiencies

Vitamin	Description
Vitamin B1 (thiamine)	Thiamine plays an important role in protein and carbohydrate metabolism. Due to its relatively short half-life, continuous supplementation of thiamine is required to avoid depletion of storage in those that are deficient. Wholemeal cereal grains, legumes, nuts and yeast are excellent sources of thiamine. In the paediatric population, thiamine deficiency can be observed in starved children or in areas where the staple diet is deficient in thiamine. Beriberi is the classical medical condition caused by thiamine deficiency. There are two subtypes: • **Dry beriberi.** This involves the development of symmetrical peripheral neuropathy characterised by paraesthesia in extremities, weakness and poor coordination. • **Wet beriberi.** This manifests as cardiovascular symptoms such as cardiomegaly, heart failure, peripheral oedema and cardiomyopathy. Wernicke-Korsakoff syndrome is associated with thiamine deficiency, but is rarely seen in children.
Vitamin B2 (riboflavin)	Riboflavin is available from many foods, including vegetables, meat, eggs and milk. It is primarily involved in energy production. Riboflavin deficiency is commonly seen along with other vitamin B deficiencies. Pure riboflavin deficiency is rare. Features of deficiency include glossitis, cheilitis, oedema of mucous membranes and seborrhoeic dermatitis.
Vitamin B3 (niacin)	Niacin is essential for the metabolism of carbohydrate, fatty acids and protein for energy production. It is available from many animal and plant products. Niacin deficiency is characterised by the triad of dementia, dermatitis and diarrhoea. This condition is known as pellagra and if untreated, it can lead to death. Pellagra dermatitis is a symmetrical erythematous, blistering rash on sun-exposed areas including neck, arms and hands.
Vitamin B5 (pantothenic acid)	Good sources of pantothenic acid are eggs, liver and milk. It is important for the metabolism of essential molecules in the human body. Pantothenic acid deficiency is extremely rare. Clinical manifestations include paraesthesia in the extremities.
Vitamin B6 (pyridoxine)	Pyridoxine is vital for protein and carbohydrate metabolism, brain development, immune function and steroid hormone activity. It can be obtained from vegetables, meats, nuts and whole grains. Symptoms of pyridoxine deficiency include glossitis, cheilitis, depression, irritability, seizures and confusion. Isoniazid used in the treatment of tuberculosis is associated with the development of peripheral neuropathy due to depletion of pyridoxine. Hence, it is important to always supplement the use of isoniazid with pyridoxine.
Vitamin B7 (biotin)	Biotin is a cofactor for the carboxylase enzyme and plays an important role in metabolism. Chronic deficiency can lead to dermatological conditions such as hair loss, dry scaly skin, cheilitis, glossitis and seborrhoeic dermatitis.
Vitamin B9 (folate)	Folate is necessary for the synthesis of erythrocytes and development of the foetal nervous system. Folic acid supplementation is recommended in pregnancy to reduce the risk of neural tube defects such as spina bifida. Green leafy vegetables and legumes are excellent sources of folate. Apart from neural tube defects, folate deficiency can result in megaloblastic anaemia.
Vitamin B12 (cobalamin)	Similar to folate, cobalamin plays a significant part in erythropoiesis. Apart from that, it helps to maintain the integrity of myelin in the nervous system. Deficiency in cobalamin is common among vegans and breastfed babies of vegan mothers because it is only found in food from animal sources. In addition to dietary insufficiency, it can be caused by pernicious anaemia due to the autoimmune destruction of gastric parietal cells which secrete intrinsic factor to aid the absorption of vitamin B12 from the ileum. Deficiency of vitamin B12 results in megaloblastic anaemia, amnesia, irritability and subacute combined degeneration of the spinal cord, leading to peripheral neuropathy. Presence of hypersegmented neutrophils can be observed in both folate and cobalamin deficiency.
Vitamin C (ascorbic acid)	Vitamin C functions as a cofactor in many biological processes, including collagen synthesis and neurotransmission. Citrus fruits, berries and vegetables are rich in vitamin C. Chronic vitamin C deficiency results in scurvy. Clinical manifestations include easy bruising, spontaneous bleeding from the gums, follicular hyperkeratosis, perifollicular haemorrhage, impaired wound healing, weakness, arthralgia and neuropathy. The condition is reversible with vitamin C supplementation.
Vitamin E	Vitamin E has an antioxidant property. Its deficiency is rare but when present, can cause non-specific neurological deficits and haemolytic anaemia due to the reduced lifespan of erythrocytes.
Vitamin K	Vitamin K is found in green vegetables and plays an important part in the coagulation pathways. Vitamin K deficiency, thus, results in easy bruising and bleeding. This deficiency is common in newborn babies due to minimal transfer across the placenta and through breast milk. Newborns in many countries are given an injection of vitamin K at birth to prevent the development of haemorrhagic disease of the newborn (vitamin K deficiency bleeding, p200).

Aetiology

Vitamin A deficiency can be divided into primary and secondary deficiency:

› Primary Vitamin A deficiency. This is due to prolonged dietary deficiency. It is prevalent in Southeast Asia and Africa.

› Secondary Vitamin A deficiency. This is due to either problems converting carotene to Vitamin A, or problems absorbing, storing or transporting Vitamin A. Examples include:

  › Fat malabsorption, e.g. cystic fibrosis, coeliac disease, pancreatic insufficiency, chronic diarrhoea.

  › Liver disorders, e.g. cholestatic liver disease.

Clinical Features

Vitamin A deficiency can result in:

- **Eye symptoms**
  - Xerophthalmia. Failure to produce tears as a result of keratinisation of the eyes.
  - Dryness, fragility and clouding of the cornea.
  - Bitot's spots. Areas of abnormal squamous cell proliferation, keratinisation of the conjunctiva.
  - Corneal keratomalacia. Thinning and softening of the cornea.
  - Corneal ulceration and scarring.
  - Night blindness, severe visual impairment and complete blindness.
- **Dermatological conditions.** Keratinisation of the skin resulting in dry, scaly skin. Dry hair. Broken finger nails.
- **Impaired immunity.** Increased risks of common childhood infections such as diarrhoea and measles.

Prevention

Preventing Vitamin A deficiency involves ensuring adequate intake. Exclusive breastfeeding provides sufficient Vitamin A for the first six months of life. Fortification of food products with vitamin A has been successful in high income countries and is currently being implemented in the low and middle income countries. The WHO recommends prophylactic vitamin A supplements for children in areas of endemic Vitamin A deficiency. This has translated to a reduction in the mortality of infections such as measles.

Vitamin D Deficiency

Vitamin D is an essential fat-soluble nutrient that plays a vital role in calcium and phosphorus homeostasis and general bone health.

Aetiology

Sunlight is an important source of vitamin D. It is estimated that 90% of vitamin D in humans comes from exposure to sunlight, with less than 10% from dietary sources in the absence of food fortification or supplements. Vitamin D3 (cholecalciferol) is produced through the action of ultraviolet radiation on the skin and is also found in animal products and supplements. Vitamin D2 (ergocalciferol) is found mainly in plants and supplements. In the liver, vitamin D is converted to 25-hydroxyvitamin D (calcidiol) through 25-hydroxylation. Following that, calcidiol undergoes 1-alpha-hydroxylation in the kidneys to become the active form, 1, 25-dihydroxyvitamin D (calcitriol) (*Figure 1*). Risk factors for Vitamin D deficiency are shown in *Table 7*.

Clinical Features

Vitamin D deficiency is often asymptomatic and thus detected incidentally. In high income countries, vitamin D deficiency is frequently diagnosed very early, with other nutritional deficiencies, when a child presents with faltering growth.

Presentation varies depending on age:

- **Infants.** Hypocalcaemia, resulting in seizures. Cardiomyopathy (rare).
- **Children.** Poor growth. Delayed walking. Tooth decay/enamel hypoplasia.
- **Older children.** Bone pain. Osteomalacia.

If left untreated, children with severe vitamin D deficiency may present with rickets from 6-months-old. This condition is characterised by poor

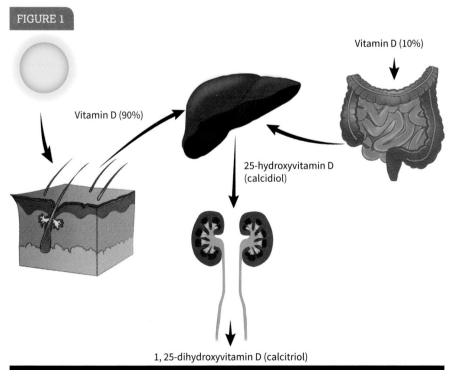

FIGURE 1

Vitamin D (10%)

Vitamin D (90%)

25-hydroxyvitamin D (calcidiol)

1, 25-dihydroxyvitamin D (calcitriol)

Vitamin D metabolism.

TABLE 7: Risk factors for Vitamin D deficiency			
Decreased Synthesis due to Lack of Sun Exposure	**Decreased Nutritional Intake**	**Perinatal Factors**	**Others**
• Dark skin pigmentation. • High latitudes. • Winter season. • Excessive use of sunblock and protective clothing. • Staying indoors.	• Being exclusively breastfed beyond 3 to 6-months-old due to low vitamin D content in breast milk. • Inadequate consumption of natural dietary sources or fortified products.	• Maternal vitamin D deficiency during pregnancy. • Prematurity.	• Medications such as anticonvulsants, antiretrovirals and glucocorticoids. • Impaired intestinal absorption. • Liver and kidney disease.

osteoid mineralisation of bones prior to closure of epiphyseal plates. Normal vascular invasion of the epiphyseal plate is delayed or prevented and results in accumulation of growth plate cartilage, leading to disorganisation of the chondrocytes and abnormalities of the involved skeletal sites. The distal forearm, knee and costochondral junctions are the initial sites of manifestations due to the underlying rapid bone growth. This is associated with an increased tendency to fracture, and delayed motor development.

Typical findings of advanced rickets are:

Skull:
➤ Delayed closure of fontanelles.
➤ Frontal bossing.
➤ Craniotabes (soft, deformable skull bones which depress on indentation).

Chest:
➤ Rachitic rosary (enlarged costochondral junctions visible as beading along anterolateral aspects of chest).
➤ Harrison's sulcus (also known as Harrison's groove) due to the muscular pull of diaphragmatic attachments to the lower ribs.

Limbs:
➤ Widening of wrists.
➤ Bowing of distal radius and ulna (more common in ulna due to the faster growth rate of distal ulnar epiphysis compared to that of radial).
➤ Progressive genu varum (bow legs) and genu valgum (knock knees) (*Figure 2*).

FIGURE 2

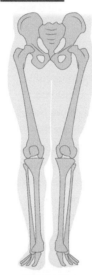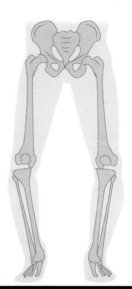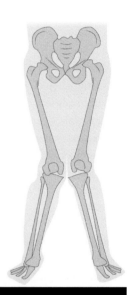

Normal (left), genu varum (middle), genu valgum (right).

➤ Windswept deformity (valgus deformity of one leg and varus deformity of another leg).

Investigations
The stored form of vitamin D, 25-hydroxyvitamin D, is the best indicator of vitamin D status. This is because it is the main circulating form, has a long half-life and is not susceptible to fluctuations. Biochemical changes related to vitamin D deficiency include:
➤ Decreased intestinal calcium and phosphorus absorption.
➤ Increased alkaline phosphatase (ALP) level.
➤ Increase in parathyroid hormone to mobilise calcium from bones.
➤ 1,25-dihydroxyvitamin D level may rise initially in response to parathyroid hormone but decrease subsequently due to limited 25-hydroxyvitamin D.

Management
Children presenting with vitamin D deficiency or clinical features consistent with rickets should be started on replacement therapy. Dosage depends on the patient's age and co-morbidities, such as malabsorption. Calcium supplements should be given with vitamin D as hypocalcaemia can be precipitated by normalisation of parathyroid hormone through vitamin D replacement. The patients should be followed up to ensure compliance with treatment, biochemical improvement and radiographic healing in patients with rickets.

Prevention
In the UK, Vitamin D supplements are recommended for all children between six-months-old and five-years-old. It is also recommended that exclusively breastfed infants receive vitamin D supplementation soon after birth.

WEIGHT-RELATED DISORDERS

Obesity

Childhood obesity is becoming an alarming public health issue, not only in high income countries, but also in urban regions of low and middle income countries. Unlike adults, the paediatric populations grow exponentially in both height and weight. Therefore, the accepted body mass index (BMI) in children varies according to age and sex. For children aged between 2 and 18-months-old, the current definition of overweight is a BMI of between the 85th and 95th percentile for age and sex, whilst obesity is described as a BMI of above the 95th percentile for age and gender. Being overweight or obese as a child is likely to persist into adulthood. The risk of persistence depends on many factors, including severity of obesity and parental obesity.

Aetiology

The gain of excessive fat is as a result of imbalance between caloric consumption and energy expenditure. Environmental factors are mainly held accountable for the rise in prevalence of obesity. These include:
- Availability of high-fat foods and sugary beverages.
- Larger food portion sizes.
- Increasing use of television and computers.
- Decreasing physical activities.
- Use of automated vehicles for commuting.

The interaction of genetic vulnerability with unfavourable environmental factors increases the risk of obesity. Perinatal factors are suggested to be related to obesity in children and in later life, and may be mediated through epigenetics. These include prematurity, large for gestational age babies, poor maternal weight prior to and during pregnancy, gestational diabetes and pre-eclampsia. Obesity also disproportionately affects certain ethnic groups and is particularly associated with low socioeconomic status.

Common endocrine disturbances, including hypothyroidism and Cushing's syndrome secondary to use of corticosteroid medications (for asthma or autoimmune conditions), are identified as causes of obesity in a small population of children. Childhood obesity is also linked to some rare genetic syndromes, such as Prader-Willi syndrome, in which excessive appetite results in uncontrollable weight gain.

Clinical Assessment

Children with BMI above the 85th percentile should be assessed for the underlying causes of excess weight gain. Careful evaluations need be performed to look for medical and behavioural risk factors and obesity-related health complications.

History
- Onset of weight gain.
- Dietary history and eating practices, e.g. high-calorie food, television viewing during meals.
- Assessment of physical activity and use of electronics, e.g. television, computer, phone.
- Current medications, especially corticosteroids and neuropsychiatric medications, e.g. valproate, olanzapine.
- Family history of obesity, cardiovascular disease and diabetes mellitus.
- Psychosocial history, including socioeconomic status, school performance, commuting, availability of facilities for physical activities.

Examination
- BMI measurement and progression over time.
- Fat distribution may provide further information regarding differential diagnoses, e.g. truncal obesity suggests Cushing's syndrome as a cause and may be associated with obstructive sleep apnoea.
- Short stature and dysmorphic features suggesting genetic syndromes.
- Obesity-related health complications.

Laboratory investigations are not usually necessary but are considered in severe obesity. Tests may include fasting lipid profile, blood glucose/oral glucose tolerance tests and liver function test. This is a screen for hyperlipidaemia, type 2 diabetes mellitus and non-alcoholic fatty liver disease. Endocrine investigations (e.g. Cushing's syndrome/ hypothyroidism) should be considered depending on the presentation.

Complications

Obesity can have multisystem complications, particularly if it is long-term:
- **Cardiovascular.** Hypertension, hyperlipidaemia, atherosclerosis.
- **Endocrine.** Insulin resistance, impaired glucose tolerance, diabetes mellitus.
- **Gastrointestinal.** Non-alcoholic fatty liver disease, gallstones (especially following rapid weight loss).
- **Respiratory.** Obstructive sleep apnoea, obesity hypoventilation syndrome.
- **Orthopaedic.** Slipped capital femoral epiphysis, fractures.
- **Dermatological.** Acanthosis nigricans due to insulin resistance, infections in skin folds.
- **Psychological.** Anxiety, depression, poor self-esteem.

Management

Management of childhood obesity aims to encourage healthy lifestyle habits to reduce the risks of obesity in adulthood and its associated co-morbidities. The family should be encouraged to reduce consumption of calorie-rich foods and opt for a healthier diet. Physical exercise can be increased by involving children in sports that they enjoy and by reducing duration of sedentary television and computer use. Aim for 60 minutes of moderate or greater intensity physical activity a day.

It is vital to involve the whole family, and parents should be encouraged to take the main responsibility for lifestyle changes, particularly in children under 12-years-old. Behavioural interventions increase the likelihood of changes being maintained, including goal setting, self-monitoring and rewards for achieving goals.

In more severe cases, a primary care physician can work alongside counsellors experienced in childhood obesity, dieticians and exercise therapists to maximise improvement. More radical approaches include:

› Appetite-suppressing medications. Orlistat is a pancreatic/gastric lipase inhibitor, preventing absorption of dietary fats. Drug treatment is generally not recommended in children under 12-years-old, and only in exceptional circumstances for those over 12-years-old.

› Weight-control surgeries. This can be considered in those with a BMI >40kg/m^2 and severe comorbidities, or a BMI >50kg/m^2 and milder comorbidities. Procedures include:

  › Roux-en-Y gastric bypass. A small part of the stomach is used to create a new stomach pouch, which is connected directly to the jejunum, bypassing the rest of the stomach.

  › Sleeve gastrectomy. The stomach is reduced in size by removing a large portion of it along the greater curvature.

  › Laparoscopic adjustable gastric band. A band is placed around the upper part of the stomach, creating a smaller pouch, slowing transition of food, and giving the sensation of satiety faster.

Prognosis

Childhood obesity is associated with numerous complications as outlined earlier. It is also a predictor of adult obesity. Emotional and psychological morbidity is widespread.

Anorexia Nervosa, Bulimia Nervosa, and Binge-Eating Disorder

These are a group of psychological conditions that can cause severe physical and psychosocial impairments. There are three major types of eating disorders: anorexia nervosa, bulimia nervosa and binge eating disorder. These are summarised in *Table 8*. Other eating disorders also exist:

› Rumination disorder. Persistent regurgitation of food.

› Avoidant/restrictive food intake disorder. Persistent failure to meet nutritional/energy demands, leading to weight loss, nutritional deficiency, dependency on supplements or impaired psychosocial functioning.

Those with feeding or eating behaviours that cause clinically significant distress and impaired functioning, but do not meet specific criteria are labelled as "other specified feeding or eating disorder".

Aetiology

Eating disorders are frequently a result of multiple factors, including genetic, biological, social, cultural and psychological. Risk factors include:

› Adolescents and young adults, with increasing prevalence in young children.

› Female gender, although males are also affected.

› History of mood disorder, personality disorder or substance abuse.

› Perfectionist personality or being a high achiever.

› Poor self-esteem.

› History of being bullied or sexually abused.

› Poor coping to life stresses.

› Body image pressure due to media and cultural influence.

› Positive family history, such as having a sibling with an eating disorder.

TABLE 8: Differences between anorexia nervosa, bulimia nervosa and binge eating disorder			
	Anorexia nervosa	**Bulimia nervosa**	**Binge-eating disorder**
Prevalence in Adolescence.	0.3%	0.9%	1.6%
Eating behaviour.	Restriction of energy intake leading to significantly low body weight. There are two types: restrictive and binge eating/purging.	Eating an excessive amount of food in a discrete period of time, associated with a sense of lack of control over eating. Recurrent inappropriate compensatory behaviours to prevent weight gain, e.g. self-induced vomiting, misuse of laxatives/diuretics, fasting, excessive exercise. On average, episodes occur at least once a week for three months.	Eating an excessive amount of food in a discrete period, associated with a sense of lack of control over eating. It is associated with marked distress. The eating may be excessively rapid, eating until uncomfortably full, eating large amounts of food when not feeling hungry, eating alone due to embarrassment. On average, episodes occur at least once a week for three months. There is no compensatory behaviour, like self-induced vomiting.
Perception of body.	Distorted perception of body weight and shape. Intense fear of weight gain despite the low body weight.	Excessive concern about body weight and shape.	Feeling disgusted with oneself, depressed or guilty after binge eating.

> Participation in certain activities or occupations such as athletes, models, dancers, actors.

Clinical Assessment

Taking a history from these patients may be challenging due to the sensitive nature of these conditions and potential denial of the condition. Collateral histories are critical to get a full insight into the impact of the disease. It is vital to reassure the patients about the confidentiality and privacy of the information that they have provided so they may feel confident speaking up about their condition.

History

> Rapid weight loss or weight gain.
> Persistent calorie counting, meal skipping, fasting and avoidance of high-calorie foods.
> Excessive physical activity.
> Preoccupation with body weight and shape.
> Frequent self-weighing.

> Unusual eating behaviours, such as cutting food into small pieces or refusing to mix certain types of food.
> Obsessive interest in food preparation and recipes.
> Menstrual irregularity, e.g. oligomenorrhoea, amenorrhoea.
> Sensitivity to cold, lethargy, fainting, dizziness, irritability.
> Social withdrawal and avoidance of eating in public.
> Comorbid psychopathology, e.g. depression, personality disorder, suicidal ideation.

Examination findings are summarised in *Table 9*. Investigations are not usually necessary in mild cases, but ones to consider are shown in *Table 10*.

Management

Management of patients with eating disorders includes treatment of medical complications, nutritional rehabilitation and behavioural management. Ideally, this should be in an

---

TABLE 9: Physical findings in anorexia nervosa, bulimia nervosa and binge-eating disorder

Anorexia nervosa	Bulimia nervosa	Binge-eating disorder
• Low body mass index. • Bradycardia, hypotension. • Hypothermia. • Dry scaly skin, brittle hair/nails, hair loss. • Reduced muscle power (sit up-squat-stand test). • Lanugo hair.	• May be overweight/obese. • Bradycardia, tachycardia, hypotension. • Hypothermia. • Dry scaly skin. • Parotid gland hypertrophy. • Erosion of dental enamel. • Russell sign (scarring and calluses on dorsum of hand due to recurrent self-induced vomiting). • Oedema. May be related to diuretic abuse, or protein malnutrition.	• Obesity and associated complications.

TABLE 10: Laboratory tests and findings in eating disorders

Laboratory tests	Findings
Full blood count.	Anaemia secondary to lack of iron, vitamin B12 and folate in the diet. Elevated white cell count secondary to poor immune system due to poor diet.
Blood glucose level.	To assess for hypoglycaemia or hyperglycaemia.
Serum electrolytes including calcium, phosphorus, magnesium.	Particularly looking for hypokalaemia, hypochloraemia and metabolic alkalosis associated with recurrent self-induced vomiting and misuse of laxatives or diuretics. To monitor patients for refeeding syndrome once feeding is started.
Urea and creatinine.	Impaired renal function secondary to recurrent purging and dehydration.
Liver function test.	Reduced total protein and albumin level due to malnutrition. Elevated liver enzymes may indicate liver damage from the poor nutrition.
Amylase.	Patients with eating disorders may develop acute or chronic pancreatitis due to the chronic vomiting and protein energy depletion.
Thyroid function test.	Some of the clinical features described above such as sensitivity to cold and brittle hair can mimic thyroid disturbance, hence it is important to assess thyroid function.
Urinalysis.	High specific gravity can indicate dehydration. Presence of ketones secondary to starvation or low-carbohydrate diet. Elevated urinary protein with strenuous exercise, which is often seen in anorexia nervosa and bulimia nervosa.
Electrocardiogram (ECG).	To assess for cardiac arrhythmias. This is associated with electrolyte disturbances. An ECG in anorexia nervosa may show bradycardia, prolonged QT interval, non-specific T wave changes and, depending on complications, ischaemic or hypokalaemic changes.

outpatient setting. Indications for inpatient therapy are shown in *Box 3*. Ideally this should be on a specialist eating disorders unit (SEDU), but if the patient is less stable, it may have to be on a paediatric ward. Some of the patients may have a high risk of absconding and may need to be treated as involuntary patients.

Therapies

Cognitive behavioural therapy is useful to change distorted perceptions of body weight and shape, and to reverse the food restriction or binge eating/purging behaviour. Consultation with dieticians and a psychiatrist is essential to ensure successful implementation of healthy eating habits. Family-based therapy, also known as the Maudsley method, is useful for treatment in the community. Through this method, the family is used as a resource to ensure that the adolescents eat a healthy amount of food. The parents are initially in charge of the appropriate diet and eating behaviours, in consultation with the therapists, and the control over eating is subsequently transferred back to the patients when they improve.

Medications

Vitamin and mineral supplements may include multivitamins, vitamin B compound-strong/thiamine, vitamin D/calcium, phosphate and potassium. Anxiety and depression may rarely require pharmacological therapy. Anti-depressants such as selective serotonin reuptake inhibitors (SSRIs; e.g. fluoxetine) may be helpful. Antipsychotic agents, and mood stabilisers also have a potential role in selected cases.

Re-feeding in Anorexia Nervosa

Oral feeding is preferred, but NG feeding may be required if oral feeding is ineffective, or if the patient is non-compliant. Refeeding syndrome is an important condition to consider during the initiation of refeeding due to the potential risk of developing cardiac arrhythmias due to electrolyte disturbances, particularly phosphate, magnesium, calcium and potassium.

The risk is reduced by gradual increase in caloric intake. Starting rates of calorific intake can be 5–20 kcal/kg/day, with the lowest rate being used in those at highest risk of refeeding syndrome. Fluid intake should remain below 35ml/kg/day, as refeeding oedema is a recognised complication.

Prognosis

Only 50% of those with anorexia nervosa make a complete recovery. Anorexia nervosa is associated with depression, anxiety, substance abuse, and personality disorders. Death may occur from medical complications or suicide. Death rate is higher in anorexia nervosa than bulimia.

Pica

Pica is characterised by repeated or chronic ingestion of non-nutritive substances. Some predisposing factors have been identified and include iron deficiency anaemia, learning difficulties, neglect and a lack of familial cohesion. Pica is also associated with autism, low socioeconomic status and a number of neuropsychiatric conditions.

Clinical Features

Feeding behaviours can lead to:

- Eating lead-containing paint stripped from the walls of old houses, causing lead toxicity.
- Eating soil, leading to parasitic infection.
- Ingesting foreign bodies, including, for example, foam from sofas.
- Excessive eating of hair can lead to a hair bezoar in the stomach and present with vomiting and possibly bowel obstruction.

Management

Treatment involves a multidisciplinary approach. Nutritional deficiencies are common and need to be treated. Behavioural strategies are key to management. This may involve strategies such as training in discriminating between edible and nonedible items, and self-protection devices that prohibit putting objects in the mouth. Toxic substances, e.g. lead-based paint, should be removed from the environment. Dental input may also be necessary. Pica in children often remits spontaneously.

REFERENCES AND FURTHER READING

Infant Feeding

1. World Health Organization. Global strategy for infant and young child feeding. Geneva; 2001 May 1.
2. National Health and Medical Research Council. Infant Feeding Guidelines. Canberra; 2012.

Faltering Growth

1. ClinicalKey. Failure To Thrive. ClinicalKey; 2012.
2. Cole S, Lanham J. Failure to thrive: an update. Am Fam Physician. 2011; 83: 829-34.

3   Kirkland R, Motil K. Failure to thrive (undernutrition) in children younger than two years: Etiology and evaluation. UpToDate. 2014; Mar 13.

4   Royal Children's Hospital. 2014. Clinical Practice Guidelines: Failure to thrive - initial management. Available from: http://www.rch.org.au/clinicalguide/guideline_index/Poor_Growth.

Malnutrition

1   World Food Programme. What is malnutrition? Rome; 2014.

2   World Health Organization. Guidelines: Updates on the Management of Severe Acute Malnutrition in Infants and Children. Geneva; 2013.

3   World Health Organization. Malnutrition. Geneva; 2014.

4   UNICEF, WHO, UNESCO, UNFPA, UNDP, UNAIDS, WFP and the World Bank. Facts for Life: Nutrition and Growth. New York; 2010.

5   Royal Children's Hospital. 2014. Growth and nutrition. Available from: http://www.rch.org.au/immigranthealth/clinical/Growth_and_nutrition.

6   Nichols B. Malnutrition in children in developing countries: Clinical assessment. UpToDate; 2014. Available from: http://www.uptodate.com/contents/malnutrition-in-children-in-resource-limited-countries-clinical-assessment.

7   United Nations Children's Fund. Clinical Forms of Acute Malnutrition: Marasmus and Kwashiorkor. New York; 2014.

8   Klish W, Nichols B. Severe malnutrition in children in developing countries: Treatment. UpToDate; 2014. Available from: http://www.uptodate.com/contents/severe-malnutrition-in-children-in-resource-limited-countries-treatment.

Vitamin A Deficiency

1   Pazirandeh S, Burns D. Overview of vitamin A. UpToDate; 2014. Available from: http://www.uptodate.com/contents/overview-of-vitamin-a.

2   Johnson L. Vitamin A. New Jersey: Merck Manuals; 2013.

3   World Health Organization. Micronutrient deficiencies: Vitamin A deficiency. Geneva; 2014.

Vitamin D Deficiency

1   Department of Health and Human Services. Vitamin D deficiency for neonates. Melbourne; 2014 Jul 16.

2   Royal Children's Hospital. 2014. Low vitamin D. Available from: http://www.rch.org.au/immigranthealth/clinical/Low_Vitamin_D.

3   Misra M. Vitamin D deficiency and insufficiency in children and adolescents. UpToDate; 2015. Available from: http://stage0www.uptodate.com/contents/vitamin-d-insufficiency-and-deficiency-in-children-and-adolescents.

Other Vitamin Deficiencies

1   Pazirandeh S, Lo C, Burns D. Overview of water-soluble vitamins. UpToDate; 2014. Available from: http://stage0www.uptodate.com/contents/overview-of-water-soluble-vitamins.

2   Better Health Channel. 2014. Vitamin B. Available from: https://www.betterhealth.vic.gov.au/health/healthyliving/vitamin-b.

3   Merck Manuals. Vitamin C. New Jersey: Merck Manuals; 2014.

Obesity

1   Klish W. Definition; epidemiology; and etiology of obesity in children and adolescents. UpToDate; 2014. Available from: http://www.uptodate.com/contents/definition-epidemiology-and-etiology-of-obesity-in-children-and-adolescents.

2   Barlow S. Expert Committee Recommendations Regarding the Prevention, Assessment, and Treatment of Child and Adolescent Overweight and Obesity: Summary Report. Pediatrics. 2007 Aug 31; 120 (Supp 4).

3   Klish W. Clinical evaluation of the obese child and adolescent. UpToDate; 2014. Available from: http://www.uptodate.com/contents/clinical-evaluation-of-the-obese-child-and-adolescent.

4   Klish W. Comorbidities and complications of obesity in children and adolescents. UpToDate; 2012. Available from: http://www.uptodate.com/contents/comorbidities-and-complications-of-obesity-in-children-and-adolescents.

5   NICE guideline CG189. Obesity: identification, assessment, and management. 2014. Available from: http://www.nice.org.uk/guidance/cg189.

Eating Disorders

1   Black D, Grant J. DSM-5 Guidebook: The Essential Companion to the Diagnostic and Statistical Manual of Mental Disorders, Fifth Edition. Arlington: American Psychiatric Publishing; 2013. 224-9.

2   Forman S. Eating disorders: Overview of epidemiology, diagnosis, and course of illness. UpToDate; 2014. Available from: http://www.uptodate.com/contents/eating-disorders-overview-of-epidemiology-clinical-features-and-diagnosis.

3   Better Health Channel. 2014. Eating disorders. Available from https://www.betterhealth.vic.gov.au/health/healthyliving/eating-disorders-adolescents.

4   Royal Children's Hospital 2010. Eating disorders. Available from: http://www.rch.org.au/kidsinfo/fact_sheets/Eating_disorders_types_and_treatment.

5   Mehler P. Anorexia nervosa in adults: Evaluation for medical complications and criteria for hospitalization to manage these complications. UpToDate; 2014. Available from: http://www.uptodate.com/contents/anorexia-nervosa-in-adults-evaluation-for-medical-complications-and-criteria-for-hospitalization-to-manage-these-complications.

6   Mitchell J, Zunker C. Bulimia nervosa and binge eating disorders in adults: Medical complications and their management. UpToDate; 2014. Available from: http://www.uptodate.com/contents/bulimia-nervosa-and-binge-eating-disorder-in-adults-medical-complications-and-their-management.

7   Forman S. Eating disorders: Overview of treatment. UpToDate; 2014. Available from: http://www.uptodate.com/contents/eating-disorders-overview-of-treatment.

8   Royal College of Psychiatrists, Physicians, and Pathologists. MARSIPAN: Management of Really Sick Patients with Anorexia Nervoisa. 2014. Available from: http://www.rcpsych.ac.uk/files/pdfversion/CR189.pdf.

9   Emedicine. Anorexia Nervosa. Available from: http://emedicine.medscape.com/article/912187-overview#a6.

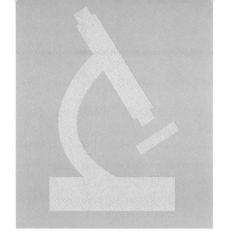

1.18
ONCOLOGY
ANNA CAPSOMIDIS AND AMY MITCHELL

PRINCIPLES OF ONCOLOGICAL CARE

Presentation

Leukaemia, lymphoma and brain tumours are the most common cancers affecting children. As childhood malignancy is rare, there can be a delay in diagnosis after presenting symptoms first emerge. Timely diagnosis and specialist referral can improve outcome. Children referred to paediatric oncology centres for suspected cancer require many investigations to make a histological diagnosis and to assess for metastatic spread before treatment starts.

Management of childhood malignancy depends on:

> Cancer type.
> Metastasis.
> Child's age.
> Co-morbidities.

Whilst the mainstay of treatment for haematological malignancies is chemotherapy, treatment of solid tumours usually requires a combination of chemotherapy, surgery and radiotherapy.

History

> Persistent unexplained fever, lethargy or weight loss: after excluding common infections (such as upper respiratory tract infection [URTI], urinary tract infection [UTI] or pneumonia), consider malignancy, atypical infections, inflammatory bowel disease (IBD), and human immunodeficiency virus (HIV).
> Unexplained bleeding from mouth, gums or nose.
> Unexplained bruises.
> Persistent bone pain or back pain (including nocturnal, which may wake the child from sleep).
> New onset limp, or a child who has stopped weight bearing.
> New lump or mass.
> Headaches for more than two weeks severe enough to wake the child from sleep in the morning, or associated nausea and vomiting.
> Shortness of breath (especially when associated with suspicious lymphadenopathy).
> Unexplained new onset seizures.
> Persistent, unexplained vomitting.
> Parental anxiety with no clear diagnosis.
> Behavioral change.
> Visual loss, new onset squint (can be paralytic e.g. due to a 6th nerve palsy, or non-paralytic e.g. brainstem lesion).
> Rapid head growth in under 2-year-olds.

CONTENTS

Examination
- Pallor, petechiae, unexplained bruises.
- Persistent (>two weeks on antibiotics), localised, unexplained enlarged lymph nodes >two centimetres (cervical, axillary or inguinal) or supraclavicular nodes of any size.
- Generalised lymphadenopathy and hepatosplenomegaly.
- Unexplained lumps or masses (especially abdomen, testes, skull, limbs).
- Repeated episodes of inspiratory stridor or acute wheeze implying extratracheal compression.
- New onset neurological signs including: ataxia at any age, worsening handwriting, focal convulsions, cranial nerve abnormalities, motor or sensory signs, reduced level of consciousness, bulging fontanelle, macrocephaly in an infant, abnormal eye movements or nystagmus.
- Behavioural change in a school-age child or irritability in an infant.
- White pupillary reflex (no red reflex in an infant – often noticed in photographs), new onset squint, loss of or change in vision, proptosis.
- Precocious puberty.

Investigations
Investigation of suspected malignancy will depend on the presenting symptoms and examination findings. Baseline blood tests including full blood count (FBC), blood film, and bone/liver/renal profile, should be ordered in children with pallor, unexplained bruising, persistent fever, bone pain or generalised lymphadenopathy.

Imaging tests are also often required. More specialist tests will be dependent on cancer type and are usually carried out in specialist paediatric oncology centres. Tumour markers, immunophenotyping (cancer cell surface markers) and genetic tests also play an important role in the diagnosis and monitoring of certain cancers.

Imaging
- X-Ray. Plain X-rays can be useful for identifying some tumours (e.g. bone tumours) and metastases (although uncommon in children). Chest X-ray is routinely indicated at diagnosis, especially in leukaemia and lymphoma. This is to exclude a mediastinal mass, which can be an emergency due to airway obstruction.
- Ultrasound. An ultrasound scan (USS) is a useful first-line investigation for suspected soft tissue and abdominal masses.
- CT & MRI. Computed tomography (CT) and magnetic resonance imaging (MRI) are useful diagnostic imaging tests to assess for metastatic spread. Some tumours can be diagnosed on imaging alone without the need for an invasive biopsy. There has been a move towards reducing exposure to radiation associated with CT scans, but they are still required to look particularly for lung metastases.
- MIBG scan. Metaiodobenzylguanidine (MIBG) is a radioisotope given by injection and taken up by neuroblastomas. Neuroblastoma tumours can then be detected by a radiation scanner.
- Bone scan. This is a nuclear imaging method used to identify and characterise bone tumours and bony metastases.

Additional Specialist Tests
- VMA (vanillylmandelic acid) and HVA (homovanillic acid). These can be detected in the urine of neuroblastoma patients.
- AFP (alpha foetoprotein) and HCG (human chorionic gonadotropin). These tumour markers can be detected in the blood of children with germ cell tumours. AFP is also elevated in hepatoblastoma.
- Immunophenotyping. This method identifies cancer cells based on the markers they express on their cell surface.
- Cytogenetics. This can be used to identify genetic mutations common to specific cancers.
- Bone marrow aspirate (BMA) and biopsy (*Figure 1*). Bone marrow is examined for cell morphology, immunophenotype and cytogenetic mutations. Bone marrow is "aspirated" from the iliac crest, and in some cases, a small "core" biopsy is taken using a specialised piece of equipment called a trephine. Young children will require a general anaesthetic for the procedure. All children with leukaemia require BMA and children with certain solid tumours also need a BMA and biopsy as part of their diagnostic workup.
- Tumour biopsy. This involves obtaining a small sample of the tumour to be evaluated for diagnostic purposes by histopathologists.

Chemotherapy
Chemotherapy is administered according to specific protocols. Chemotherapy can be:
- Curative or palliative.
- Given in isolation (e.g. in acute lymphoblastic leukaemia) or in combination with another treatment.

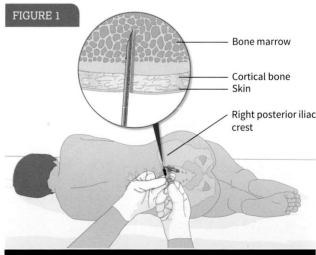

FIGURE 1

Bone marrow
Cortical bone
Skin
Right posterior iliac crest

Bone marrow biopsy being taken from the right posterior iliac crest.

> Given before surgery (neo-adjuvant) to shrink the tumour or afterwards (adjuvant) to treat residual disease or metastasis.

Side Effects

Chemotherapy causes many troublesome side effects, therefore treatment regimens require a careful balance between reducing iatrogenic effects whilst maximising tumour toxicity. Children receiving chemotherapy, depending on the combination of drugs given, will require regular monitoring, including full blood count (FBC), urea & electrolytes (U&Es), glomerular filtration rate (GFR), liver function test (LFT), hearing tests and echocardiograms.

Side effects include:

> Immune suppression.
>> Febrile neutropenia (also known as neutropenic sepsis).
>> Opportunistic infections, e.g. fungal (aspergillosis), *Pneumocystis carinii (jirovecii)* pneumonia (PCP), coagulase negative staphylococcus infection, e.g. *Staphylococcus epidermidis*, a normal skin commensal.
>> Increased susceptibility to viral infections, e.g. varicella exposure, which can be especially dangerous.
> Damage to rapidly dividing cells.
>> Bone marrow suppression causes anaemia, thrombocytopenia and neutropenia. Children will often require blood and platelet transfusions.
>> Gut mucosal damage and mucositis often requiring significant pain relief (i.e. morphine infusions) and nutritional support (i.e. with nasogastric tube feeding).
>> Diarrhoea.
>> Alopecia.
> Drug specific side effects.
>> Doxorubicin (anthracycline-based) ⇒ cardiac toxicity.
>> Cisplatin (platinum-based) ⇒ renal failure and deafness.
>> Cyclophosphamide ⇒ haemorrhagic cystitis.
> Nausea and vomiting.
> Anorexia and weight loss.
> Late effects.
>> These may occur months or years after treatment. It includes reduction in fertility, hormonal imbalances and risk of secondary malignancies.

Surgery

Surgery has multiple roles in the management of childhood cancers:

> Aiding diagnosis (through biopsy).
> Enabling the administration of medication and blood sampling (central venous lines).
> Resection of a malignancy.

Most children require surgery for insertion of a tunnelled central venous line (CVL) or implantable port (also known as a "Hickman®" line or "Portacath®" (*Figure 2-3*) respectively, although there are many different types). These can be used long-term for giving chemotherapy, antibiotics, blood products, and for easy, pain-free blood sampling. A tunnelled CVL or

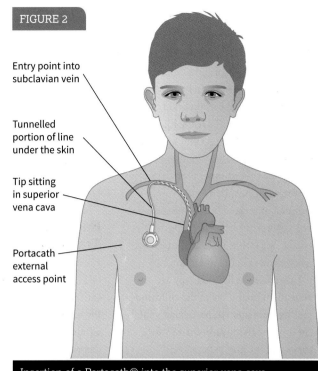

FIGURE 2

Entry point into subclavian vein

Tunnelled portion of line under the skin

Tip sitting in superior vena cava

Portacath external access point

Insertion of a Portacath® into the superior vena cava.

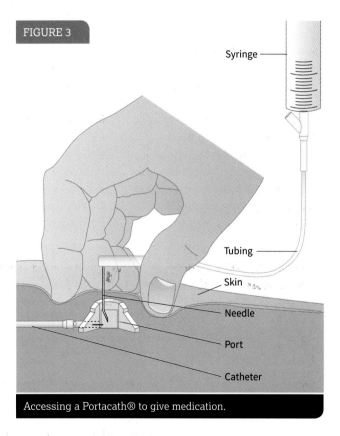

FIGURE 3

Syringe

Tubing

Skin

Needle

Port

Catheter

Accessing a Portacath® to give medication.

implantable port has the advantage of not requiring a needle every time intravenous access is required, and can stay in for many weeks, if not months or years. The disadvantage is risk of blockage or infection, but this risk is reduced by keeping the port clean and covered, with regular flushes and dressing changes.

Radiotherapy

Radiotherapy is important in the treatment of many solid tumours, including Wilms' tumour, neuroblastoma, Hodgkin lymphoma, bone tumours and certain brain tumours. Radiotherapy involves using high energy X-rays to directly target and kill tumour cells. Children must be motionless during the procedure to protect the surrounding healthy tissues. Young children may therefore require sedation or a general anaesthetic. Radiotherapy causes side effects including tiredness, nausea and skin inflammation.

Late effects of radiotherapy are dependent on the age of the child and the site irradiated. In particular, young children receiving radiotherapy for a brain tumour may experience:

> Cognitive delay.
> Growth problems.
> Endocrine impairment (see late effects).

Conventional radiotherapy uses photon beams and advances have been made with specialised planning and technology allowing highly focused and targeted beams. There have been many changes in the delivery of radiotherapy with regards to frequency of doses, with the overall aim to reduce the total amount of radiation exposure and thus reducing unwanted side effects.

Proton therapy is a specialised form of radiotherapy delivered using proton beams. These beams effectively give off less scatter beyond the point that requires treatment. Using protons allows reduction of the effect on surrounding tissues. This is particularly useful for some types of tumour, like those located close to vital structures. It does, however, require very expensive and specialised equipment. and there is relatively little long term follow up data available.

Haemopoietic Stem Cell Transplantation

Haemopoietic stem cell transplantation (HSCT) can treat certain haematological cancers and solid tumours. It involves the infusion of stem cells after the administration of extremely high doses of chemotherapy or total body irradiation. The doses of chemotherapy or radiation would ordinarily be lethal due to the degree of myelosuppression. However, the patient is "rescued" by the infusion of stem cells that will later repopulate the bone marrow. Stem cells for HSCT can either be harvested from the patient before treatment (autologous) or can be donated by a matched donor (allogenic). Stem cells are harvested directly from the bone marrow or from peripheral blood. If stem cells are collected from the bloodstream, the donor will require a short course of a growth factor (called G-CSF) to mobilise the stem cells into the systemic circulation beforehand.

HSCT carries a high risk of morbidity and mortality. This may be related to failure of the new stem cells to populate the bone marrow ("engraftment failure"), life-threatening infection due to prolonged immunosuppression, or graft-versus-host disease (GvHD; when the donor immune system attacks the host).

Late Effects of Cancer Treatments

All survivors of childhood cancer require long-term follow-up and monitoring for late effects of treatment. Children are seen regularly in "late effects" clinics for many years after completion of their cancer treatment. There are many sequelae following cancer treatment, and early identification and treatment may improve outcome. Key late effects are summarised in *Table 1*.

Palliative Care

Palliative care is defined by the World Health Organisation (WHO) as: active and holistic care that incorporates the physical, psychosocial and spiritual needs of the child and their family. It aims to enhance quality of life for children with life-limiting disease through the management of distressing symptoms such as pain, nausea, vomiting and dyspnoea. The paediatric palliative care team consists of specialist nurses, doctors, psychologists, social workers and play specialists. Palliative care

TABLE 1: Late effects of cancer treatment	
Secondary malignancies.	• Increased risk following radiotherapy and some chemotherapy. • Most common secondary malignancies are leukaemia and lymphoma.
Cardiac.	• Heart failure secondary to anthracycline-based chemotherapy (e.g. doxorubicin).
Pulmonary.	• Pulmonary fibrosis (e.g. following chemotherapy with bleomycin).
Renal.	• Renal impairment caused by chemotherapy with platinum based drugs (e.g. cisplatin).
Endocrine/Growth.	• Growth hormone deficiency, early or delayed puberty and hypopituitarism can occur following cranial irradiation. • Bone growth failure at site of irradiation.
Infertility.	• Caused by certain chemotherapy drugs and gonadal radiotherapy. • Consider sperm banking in pubescent males. • Experimental methods of ovarian cortical strip preservation are available for females.
Neurocognitive impairment.	• Caused by cranial irradiation and neurosurgery.
Hearing impairment.	• Resulting from platinum-based chemotherapy drugs (e.g. cisplatin).

can be delivered in the child's own home, in hospital, or in a children's hospice. Traditionally, children were referred to the paediatric palliative care team when their disease was no longer curable. However, more recently a "parallel planning" approach has become more popular. The aim of this approach is for much earlier involvement and collaborative working to enable appropriate symptomatic management alongside curative treatment.

Making end-of-life decisions is extremely challenging for children, their families and the healthcare professionals involved. Communication is essential to respect the best interests of the child. Children and young people should be involved in end-of-life discussions as much as possible, unless this is deemed harmful to the child.

COMMON MALIGNANCIES

Leukaemia

Leukaemia is the most common childhood cancer, with approximately 400 new cases in the UK each year.

Aetiology

Leukaemia is a haematological malignancy caused by abnormal cellular division of immature blood cells (lymphoblasts or myeloblasts) in the bone marrow. Clinical presentation reflects the infiltration of leukaemic cells into normal tissues including the bone marrow, lymph nodes, liver, spleen, brain and testes:

> Bone marrow failure leads to anaemia (pallor), thrombocytopenia (bleeding, bruising and petechiae) and neutropenia (infections).
> Tissue infiltration leads to features such as bone pain, hepatosplenomegaly and lymphadenopathy.

Leukaemia is classified into acute or chronic, as well as into myeloid or lymphoid, according to the cell of origin (*Figure 4*). Various genetic and inherited factors have been shown to play a role in the development of leukaemia (*Box 1*).

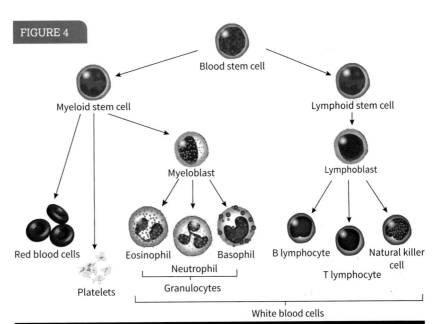

FIGURE 4

Normal haematopoiesis showing the lymphoid and myeloid cell lines.

Siblings of those affected also have a higher risk of developing the disease.

Approximately 80% of childhood leukaemias are acute lymphoblastic leukaemias (ALL) and 15% acute myeloid leukaemias (AML). Key differences between ALL and AML

Box 1: Genetic Syndromes associated with increased risk of childhood leukaemia

- Down Syndrome.
- Fanconi anaemia.
- Ataxia telangiectasia.
- Neurofibromatosis type 1.
- Wiskott-Aldrich syndrome.
- Noonan syndrome.

are summarised in *Table 2*, but they generally present with similar symptoms. Chronic lymphocytic leukaemia (CLL) and chronic myeloid leukaemia (CML), although common in adults, are extremely rare in children.

Clinical Features

Children with ALL usually present with a short history over days or weeks, whereas the symptoms and signs of AML may develop more slowly. Initially, symptoms may appear very non-specific and mimic a viral infection.

Common presenting symptoms and signs include:
> Fever.
> Pallor.
> Petechiae and bruising.
> Tiredness or lethargy.

TABLE 2: Acute lymphoblastic leukaemia vs. Acute myeloid leukaemia		
	ALL	AML
Cell line affected.	Lymphoid.	Myeloid.
Percentage of leukaemia in children.	80%.	15%.
Peak age incidence.	2 to 3-years-old.	Under 2-years-old.
Sex predominance.	Boys > Girls.	Boys = Girls.
Auer rods.	Auer rods not present.	Auer rods usually present.
Prognosis (children <14-years-old).	Approximately 90% five-year survival rate.	Approximately 60-70% five-year survival rate.

- Poor appetite or weight loss.
- Bone pain or limp.
- Recurrent infections.
- Lymphadenopathy.
- Hepatosplenomegaly.
- Unilaterally or bilaterally enlarged testes.
- Soft tissue lumps (so called myeloid sarcoma or leukaemia cutis).

Investigations

Leukaemia is diagnosed using a combination of different tests as outlined below. Definitive diagnosis is by the detection of leukaemic blast cells on either blood film, or on bone marrow aspiration.

- Full blood count (FBC). This most commonly shows anaemia, thrombocytopenia and lymphocytosis.
- Blood film. This looks for the presence of immature blast cells. Auer rods are seen in myeloid blast cells, but not lymphoid blast cells (*Figure 5*).
- Chest X-ray (CXR). A CXR assesses the presence of a mediastinal mass representing enlarged lymphatic tissue. It is essential prior to any anaesthetic, as it is very dangerous to anaesthetise a child with a mediastinal mass as it could result in respiratory arrest.
- Clotting screen. Some rarer leukaemias (such as acute pro-myelocytic leukaemia) can cause coagulopathy.

Specialist Investigations

- Bone Marrow Aspirate (BMA). The samples are then analysed for:
  - Morphology (showing the appearance of blast cells).
  - Immunophenotyping (can detect which type of lymphocyte (T-cell or B-cell), or myelocyte is causing the leukaemia by expression of specific cell-surface markers).
  - Cytogenetic analysis (studies specific genetic mutations that are found in some leukaemias).
- Lumbar puncture. This is to look for immature blast cells in the cerebrospinal fluid (CSF).

Differential Diagnosis

- Other paediatric cancers which cause bone marrow failure through infiltration can have similar presentations e.g. neuroblastoma, rhabdomyosarcoma and Ewing's sarcoma.
- Infections.
  - Epstein-Barr Virus (EBV).
  - Cytomegalovirus (CMV).
  - Parvovirus B19.
  - Mycobacteria.
- Non-infectious.
  - Aplastic anaemia.
  - Juvenile idiopathic arthritis (JIA).
  - Idiopathic thrombocytopenic purpura (ITP).
  - Other congenital or acquired causes of anaemia/neutropenia.
- Haemophagocytic lymphohistiocytosis (HLH).
- Langerhans cell histiocytosis (LCH).

Management

Chemotherapy is the mainstay of treatment for ALL. International collaboration has led to the development of standardised treatment protocols. Those over 10-years-old, with T cell disease, or with a white cell count (WCC) >50 x 10^9/L, have a poorer prognosis and are therefore treated with more intensive chemotherapy.

Standard treatment protocols include several "blocks" of chemotherapy, which occur in a specific order. They proceed as follows: "induction", "consolidation", "interim maintenance", "delayed

FIGURE 5

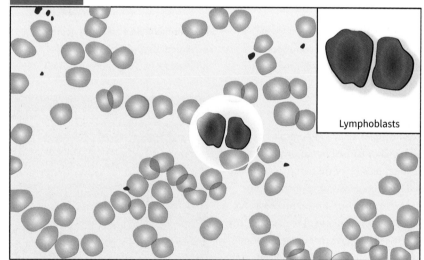

Lymphoblasts

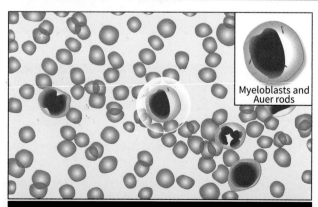

Myeloblasts and Auer rods

Blood film showing lymphoblasts (above), and myeloblasts, with Auer rods (below). Their appearance is very similar, with large nuclei. Presence of Auer rods morphologically distinguishes AML from ALL. However, immunophenotyping is frequently required to differentiate the two.

intensification" and "maintenance" (*Figure 6*).

The overall treatment plan for ALL lasts for up to three years in boys and two years in girls. Chemotherapy may be given intrathecally (i.e. directly into the cerebrospinal fluid) for central nervous system prophylaxis. Occasionally, bone marrow transplantation is required for children who do not enter remission or later relapse. Radiotherapy is reserved for central nervous system disease or when the testes are affected, and is rarely required.

In contrast to ALL, the treatment for AML is shorter in duration but much more intensive and highly myelosuppressive. It consists of four courses of chemotherapy and lasts approximately six months. Children with high risk cytogenetics or poor response to treatment will require a HSCT for cure.

Complications

> Febrile neutropenia (neutropenic sepsis). This is a potentially life-threatening condition if not immediately recognised and treated. It is defined as a neutrophil count of <0.5 x 10⁹/L and fever >38°C. Investigations must include FBC, CRP, lactate and blood culture. Treatment with intravenous broad-spectrum antibiotics should not be delayed as overwhelming bacterial infection can be fatal within hours.

> Opportunistic infections. Bone marrow suppression results in high risk of acquiring opportunistic infections. Common infections include fungal infections (e.g. aspergillosis), *Pneumocystis carinii* (*jirovecii*) pneumonia (PCP) and coagulase-negative staphylococcus central venous line infections. Fungal or PCP prophylaxis may be indicated depending on the type of cancer and treatment regime.

> Anaemia/thrombocytopenia. Children often require blood product support (including red cells and platelets) due to anaemia and thrombocytopenia caused by either the cancer itself or chemotherapy.

> Tumour lysis syndrome (TLS). This is a life-threatening complication caused by the rapid break down of blast cells leading to release of large quantities of intracellular contents into the bloodstream. TLS is commonly associated with "high white cell count" leukaemia and can occur either spontaneously or soon after starting treatment. It is characterised biochemically by hyperkalaemia, hyperphosphataemia, hyperuricaemia and hypocalcaemia.

> Hyperviscosity syndrome/leucostasis. This is caused by increased blood viscosity resulting from a very high WCC. This can lead to stroke.

> Superior vena cava obstruction (SVCO). This results from a mediastinal mass compressing the superior vena cava. Partial airway obstruction may occur, which makes lying flat or giving a general anaesthetic or sedation extremely dangerous. Additional symptoms include chest pain, dyspnoea, cough, facial swelling and plethora (redness).

FIGURE 6

Induction therapy

The aim of 'induction' therapy is to destroy the leukaemia cells and induce remission. This phase lasts 29 days.

Consolidation

This is further treatment to destroy any remaining leukaemic cells. This phase lasts 4-8 weeks, depending on the treatment regimen.

Interim maintenance

This is further treatment to destroy any remaining leukaemic cells. This phase lasts 8 weeks.

Delayed intensification

This is the final intensive block of chemotherapy to ensure maximal destruction of leukaemic cells. This phase lasts 8 weeks.

Maintenance

This consists mainly of oral chemotherapy, and intends to maintain remission. The child is normally well throughout maintenance and is able to return to school. This phases lasts 2-3 years.

Treatment schedule for acute lymphoblastic leukaemia.

Prognosis

The cure rate for childhood ALL has improved dramatically over the last few decades. Currently almost 90% of children with ALL survive and approximately two-thirds with AML. Adverse prognostic indicators are shown in *Box 2*.

Lymphoma

Lymphoma is a malignancy of the cells of the lymphatic system. Lymphoma can be divided into two distinct subtypes: Hodgkin disease (HD) and non-Hodgkin lymphoma (NHL) as shown in *Table 2*. Both diseases have very different characteristics, presentation and management. NHL typically has a rapid onset of symptoms whereas HD presents more insidiously. Definitive diagnosis is on lymph node biopsy.

Lymphadenopathy is common and, although usually benign, urgent paediatric referral is required if possible malignancy is suspected (*Box 3*). These red flags should be taken in the context of the clinical situations, e.g. a local infection may explain transient lymphadenopathy.

Brain Tumours

Brain and central nervous system (CNS) tumours are the most common cause of mortality from cancer in children. They are almost always primary, unlike in adults, and rarely metastasise outside the CNS.

Classification

Paediatric brain tumours can be classified according to either their site (cerebral hemisphere, central brain, posterior fossa or brain stem), or by histological subtype. Symptoms and signs may point to the possible tumour location within the CNS (*Figure 7*).

The most common brain tumours affecting children are:

> Astrocytoma (43%). The most common type of low-grade glioma. These tumours are generally slow growing and rarely metastasise.

> Embryonal tumours (19%). These are mostly primitive neuroectodermal tumours (PNET) including medulloblastoma. Medulloblastoma characteristically arises in the posterior fossa of the brain and often presents with ataxia and signs of elevated intracranial pressure. In approximately 15% of cases, tumour cells have spread via the CSF by the time of diagnosis.

> Ependymoma (10%). Tumours arising from the ependyma. The ependyma is the lining of the ventricular system of the brain. Its cells are involved in CSF production.

Clinical Features

There is often a significant time delay between symptom onset and diagnosis.

Box 2: Adverse prognostic indicators in leukaemia

- Males have a slightly lower chance of being cured than females.
- Age of the child less than 1-years-old or over 10-years-old is considered high risk.
- Initial high WCC (>50 x10^9/L).
- Type of leukaemia; AML has a poorer prognosis than ALL, and T-cell leukaemia has a poorer prognosis than B-cell leukaemia.
- Certain genetic mutations, e.g. Philadelphia chromosome t(9;22) or rearrangements of the MLL gene (chromosome 11q23) have a less favourable prognosis.
- CNS or testicular involvement.
- Failure to enter remission following "induction" treatment.

Box 3: Lymphadenopathy "red flags"

- Non-tender, firm or hard lymph nodes.
- Lymph nodes >2 cm.
- Lymph nodes progressively enlarging.
- Axillary lymph nodes.
- Supraclavicular lymph nodes.
- Systemic symptoms including persistent fever and weight loss.
- Hepatosplenomegaly.
- Shortness of breath (may indicate mediastinal mass).

TABLE 2: Hodgkin disease and non-Hodgkin lymphoma		
	Hodgkin Disease	**Non-Hodgkin Lymphoma**
Presenting Features	HD affects older children and teenagers. It often presents as a painless neck lump, usually cervical or supraclavicular. Systemic symptoms including night sweats, pruritus, weight loss and fever may also be present (known as "B-symptoms").	Lymphadenopathy, a palpable abdominal mass or respiratory symptoms due to mediastinal mass. Pancytopenia may result from bone marrow infiltration. B-symptoms are less common.
Pathology	Reed-Sternberg cells are pathognomonic.	NHL can be classified histologically into "lymphoblastic" (T- or B-cell acute lymphoblastic lymphoma), "mature forms" (mature B-cell or Burkitt's lymphoma) or "large cell" (e.g. anaplastic large cell lymphoma).
Investigations	Bone marrow aspiration, lumbar puncture, lymph node biopsy and staging CT.	
Treatment	Chemotherapy, radiotherapy and/or surgery.	Chemotherapy is the mainstay of treatment.
Prognosis	Approximately 80% of children survive.	Over 70% of children survive.

FIGURE 7

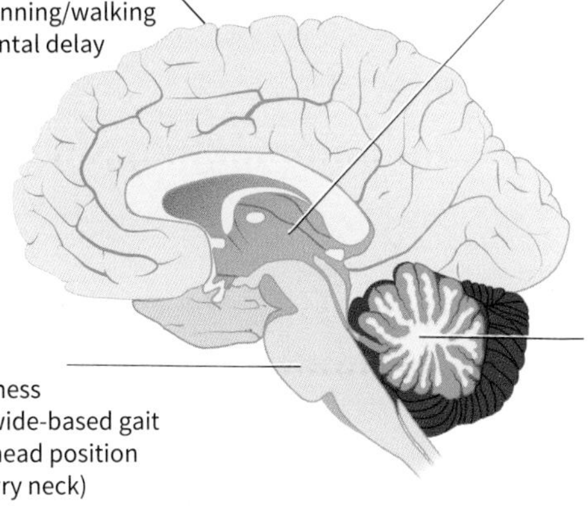

Cerebral Hemisphere
- Limb weakness
- Difficulty running/walking
- Developmental delay
- Seizures

Central brain
- Nystagmus
- Poor vision
- Abnormal growth/puberty
- Weight loss
- Drinking excess water/ passing excess urine

Brain Stem
- Limb weakness
- Unsteady/wide-based gait
- Abnormal head position (head tilt/wry neck)
- Squint
- Dysphagia
- Facial nerve palsy
- Parinaud's syndrome (dysconugate eye movements and loss of upward gaze)

Cerebellar Hemisphere
- Poor co-ordination
- Abnormal head position (head tilt/wry neck)
- Nystagmus
- Unsteady/wide-based gait
- Developmental delay

Location of brain tumour, and correlation with symptoms and signs (adapted from www.headsmart.org.uk).

This is because brain tumours often initially present with non-specific symptoms that mimic other common childhood conditions, such as migraine or a vomiting illness. Children may also present with symptoms and signs of elevated intracranial pressure.

> Headache. This is classically progressive and worse in the mornings.
> Vomiting. This is often in the morning and with no accompanying nausea.
> Visual symptoms and signs. This may include papilloedema, nystagmus, double vision, head tilt and squint.
> Motor symptoms and signs. Features may include ataxia, weakness, swallowing difficulties, speech disturbance and cranial nerve palsies.
> Behavioural change or drowsiness.
> Seizures.
> Bulging fontanelles (infants).

The presentation may also be more subtle, with developmental delay or regression. Endocrine changes such as hypothyroidism, diabetes insipidus and precocious puberty may also occur. Red flag features of headache that should warrant concern about malignancy are shown in *Box 4*. Brain tumours can be the presenting feature of genetic conditions or may develop in children identified through screening programmes. 10-20% of children with neurofibromatosis type 1 have optic pathway gliomas and children with tuberous sclerosis complex may develop sub-ependymal giant cell astrocytomas.

Investigations

Children with a suspected brain tumour need urgent imaging (either CT or MRI). If elevated intracranial pressure is suspected, an emergency CT brain and referral to a paediatric neurosurgeon is required. Lumbar puncture is contraindicated in the presence of elevated intracranial pressure as it may cause herniation of the brainstem though the foramen magnum.

Management

Multidisciplinary team management is essential as children may suffer from chronic growth, endocrine, motor, cognitive and neuropsychological problems. Treatment will depend on the type of tumour and age of the child. Some children have inoperable tumours based on their large size or location (e.g. close to the brainstem). Radiotherapy is contraindicated in very young children and infants due to unacceptable neurodevelopmental outcomes. Only some CNS tumours are responsive to chemotherapy.

Box 4: "Red Flags" for children presenting with headaches

- Headaches that wake a child at night.
- Headaches that occur first thing in the morning.
- Headaches that occur at any time in a child under four-years-old.
- Confusion or disorientation.

Prognosis

Prognosis is dependent on many factors including tumour site and size, age of the child, histological grade and presence of metastasis. Of the children that survive, 60% have long-term disability.

Other Important Malignancies

In *Table 3*, the key features of neuroblastoma, Wilms' tumour, bone tumours and rhabdomyosarcoma are shown. *Figure 8* shows the features of a likely bone tumour on X-ray. Other rarer malignancies are detailed in *Table 4*.

Cancer (% all childhood cancers)	Primary Tumour Site	Clinical Features	Outcome
Neuroblastoma (7%).	• Anywhere along the sympathetic chain from neck to pelvis. • Adrenal glands.	• Most common in children less than 5-years-old. • Pallor, weight loss, malaise. • Abdominal mass. • Bone pain, limp. • Lymphadenopathy. • Spinal cord compression. • Bone marrow suppression. • Diarrhoea. • Hypertension.	• Dependent on stage and adverse prognostic indicators. • 30-40% survival for high-risk disease and 90% for low risk disease.
Wilms' tumour (nephroblastoma) (6%).	• Kidney.	• Most common in children less than 4-years-old. • Palpable abdominal mass. • Haematuria. • Hypertension.	• 70-95% cure rate depending on stage.
Bone tumours (Ewing's Sarcoma and Osteosarcoma) (4%).	• Long bones (osteosarcoma). • Central skeleton (Ewing's).	• Teenagers and young adults. • Pain. • Swelling. • Pathological fracture.	• Overall survival 60%.
Rhabdomyosarcoma (6%).	• Bladder. • Pelvis. • Nasopharynx. • Parameningeal. • Paratestis.	• Most common in children <10-years-old. • Varied presentation dependent on tumour site. • Palpable abdominal mass. • Pain. • Urinary obstruction. • Nasal obstruction.	• Overall survival 65%. • Poor prognosis for children with bony metastatic disease.

TABLE 3: Neuroblastoma, Wilms' tumour, bone tumours and rhabdomyosarcoma

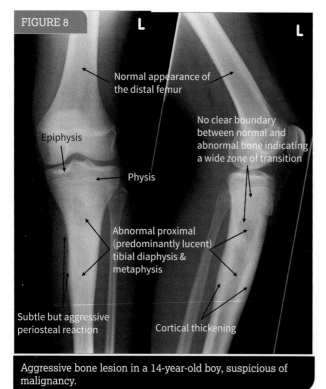

FIGURE 8

L   L

Normal appearance of the distal femur

No clear boundary between normal and abnormal bone indicating a wide zone of transition

Epiphysis

Physis

Abnormal proximal (predominantly lucent) tibial diaphysis & metaphysis

Subtle but aggressive periosteal reaction

Cortical thickening

Aggressive bone lesion in a 14-year-old boy, suspicious of malignancy.

REFERENCES AND FURTHER READING

Common Presentations, Investigation and Management

1   NICE CG21. Referral for Suspected cancer: recognition and referral. June 2015. https://www.nice.org.uk/guidance/cg27.
2   NICE QS55. Children and Young People with Cancer. February 2014. https://www.nice.org.uk/guidance/qs55.
3   NICE CG151. Neutropenic sepsis: prevention and management of neutropenic sepsis in cancer patients. September 2012. https://www.nice.org.uk/guidance/cg151.
4   Dang-Tan T, Franco EL. Diagnosis lays in childhood cancer: a review. Cancer. 2007;110(4):703-13.
5   National Registry of Childhood Tumours/Childhood Cancer Research Group University of Oxford. 2006-2008. http://www.ccrg.ox.ac.uk/datasets/registrations.shtml.
6   Childhood Cancer Research Group (CCRG). National Registry of Childhood Tumours (NRCT). March 2014.

Haematopoietic Stem Cell Transplant

1   Copelan EA. Hematopoietic stem-cell transplantation. New Engl J Med. 2006;354(17):1813-26.

Late Effects of Cancer Treatment

1   Landier W, Wallace WH, Hudson MM. Long-term follow-up of pediatric cancer survivors: education, surveillance, and screening. Pediatr Blood Cancer. 2006;46(2):149-58.

TABLE 4: Rarer malignancies		
Cancer	% Childhood Cancers	Key Features
Germ cell tumours.	3%.	• Tumours derived from primitive germ cells. • May be benign or malignant. • Tumour site may be gonadal or extragonadal. • AFP and HCG tumour markers may be elevated.
Retinoblastoma.	3%.	• Presents with a white pupillary reflex or squint. • 40% autosomal dominant inheritance. • Retinoblastoma susceptibility gene – Chromosome 13q14. • Most common in children less than 3-years-old.
Hepatic tumours.	1%.	• Hepatoblastoma most common. • Most common in children less than 2-years-old. • Increased incidence in children with Beckwith-Wiedemann syndrome or Familial Adenomatous Polyposis. • Elevated AFP.
Langerhans cell histiocytosis.	Very rare.	• Caused by abnormal proliferation of Langerhans cells. • Affects children of any age. • Presents with pain, swelling or pathological fracture on X-ray. • Disease may be localised (e.g. bone, skin) or multisystemic.
Phaeochromocytoma.	Very rare.	• Presents with features of catecholamine excess, e.g. hypertension, headache, sweating, palpitation and tremor. • Diagnosed by measuring catecholamine levels. • Treatment is usually surgical.

2   SIGN. Long-term Follow-up Care of Survivors of Childhood Cancer. January 2004. http://www.rcpch.ac.uk /sites/default/files/asset_library/Research/Clinical%20 Effectiveness/Endorsed%20guidelines/Survivors%20of%20 Childhood%20Cancer%20(SIGN)/Guideline%2076.pdf.

Palliative Care

1   GMC. End of life treatment and care: Good practice in decision-making. 2009.
2   WHO Definition of Palliative Care. Available from: http:// www.who.int/cancer/palliative/definition/en/.
3   David Widdas KM, Francis Edwards. A Core Care Pathway for Children with Life-limiting and Life-threatening Conditions Third Edition, Together for Short Lives. February 2013.

Leukaemia and Lymphoma

1   UK ALL 2011. https://http://www.ctsu.ox.ac.uk/research /mega-trials/leukaemia-trials/ukall-2003/interim-guidelines.
2   ALL Treatment Protocol. http://www.ctsu.ox.ac.uk /research/mega-trials/leukaemia-trials/ukall-2003 /interim-guidelines.

Brain Tumours

1   Wilne S, Koller K, Collier J, Kennedy C, Grundy R, Walker D. The diagnosis of brain tumours in children: a guideline to assist healthcare professionals in the assessment of children who may have a brain tumour. Arch Dis Chile. 2010;95(7):534-9
2   Eaton BR, Yock T. The use of proton therapy in the treatment of benign or low-grade pediatric brain tumors. Cancer J. 2014;20(6):403-8.

Useful Websites

1   Children's Cancer and Leukaemia Group: www.cclg.org.uk.
2   HeadSmart educational resources for healthcare professionals: www.headsmart.org.uk.
3   Children's Cancer Statistics: http://www.cancerresearchuk .org/health-professional/cancer-statistics/childrens-cancers.
4   Cancer Research UK: www.cancerresearchuk.org.
5   MacMillan Cancer Support: www.macmillan.org.uk.
6   Anthony Nolan Trust: www.anthonynolan.org.

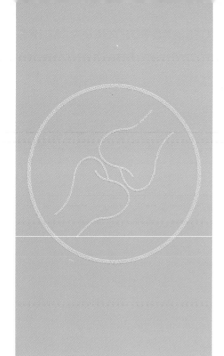

1.19

ORTHOPAEDIC AND RHEUMATOLOGICAL DISORDERS

ANAND GOOMANY AND ALEXANDER YOUNG

CONTENTS

TRAUMA

A fracture is a break in the structural continuity of bone. The anatomy and biomechanics of children's bones are different to those of the adult, resulting in unique fracture patterns, healing mechanisms and management. The immature skeleton has more bony mass per unit area, greater vascularity and thicker periosteum than adult bone. This means that compared to adults, children's fractures have:

› Quicker healing time.
› Significantly reduced rates of non-union.
› A higher degree of energy required to fracture the bone compared to adults.

Paediatric Bone Anatomy

Children's bones can be divided into four main anatomical regions (*Figure 1*):

1 Epiphysis. The expanded articular end of a long bone associated with joint cartilage.
2 Physis (growth plate). Cartilaginous cells between the secondary ossification centre and the metaphysis. This region is responsible for longitudinal bone growth.
3 Metaphysis. The wide area below the physis.
4 Diaphysis. The shaft of the bone.

Fracture Patterns in Children

1 Greenstick fracture. This is a transverse fracture of the cortex which extends into the midportion of the bone, while the opposite side remains intact (*Figure 2*).
2 Buckle (torus) fracture. This is common after axial loading on a limb e.g. falling on an outstretched hand. A buckle fracture is an incomplete fracture of the diaphysis of a long bone resulting in bulging of the cortex (*Figure 3*).
3 Plastic deformation. This is caused by several microfractures on the concave surface of the bone with an intact cortex on the convex surface. Plastic deformations commonly affect the ulna (and the radius). It is associated

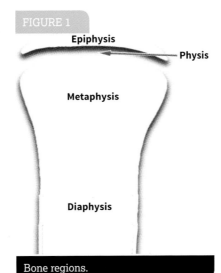

FIGURE 1

Epiphysis

Physis

Metaphysis

Diaphysis

Bone regions.

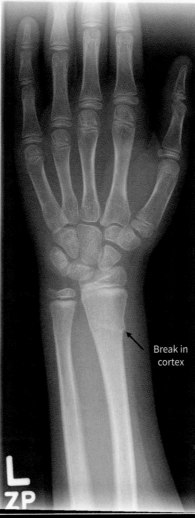

FIGURE 2

Break in cortex

L ZP

Greenstick fracture, indicated by break in the cortex on the ulna.

with axial loading. This leads to bowing of the affected bone (*Figure 4*).
4 Complete fracture. This fracture completely propagates through the bone. Complete fractures are classified as spiral, transverse or oblique depending on the direction of the fracture line (*Figure 4*).
5 Physeal fractures. These are fractures through the growth plate (*Figure 5*).

Physeal Fractures

Physeal injuries are unique to childhood. They usually occur secondary to a fall or traction injury. The physis (growth plate) is a relatively weak portion of the bone making it prone to fracture, with over 10% of childhood fractures occurring through the physis.

Classification

The Salter-Harris classification is used to describe the pattern of growth plate fracture and is useful in estimating prognosis. It is summarised in *Table 1*, and an example of a fracture is shown in *Figure 5*.

Clinical Features

Children present with localised pain and swelling over the physis. Lower limb growth plate fractures may affect the child's ability to weight-bear, whereas upper limb injuries cause impaired function and reduced range of motion. Deformity is usually minimal.

Investigations

Most children presenting with severe limb pain following trauma require X-ray. Despite this, physeal injuries are difficult to identify on plain X-ray as the physis is radiolucent and the epiphysis may be incompletely ossified. Features suggestive of physeal injury include:

› Widening of the physeal "gap".
› Incongruity of the joint.

Marked displacement makes diagnosis easy, but even Salter-Harris type IV growth plate fractures may only exhibit minor displacement. To further delineate

FIGURE 3

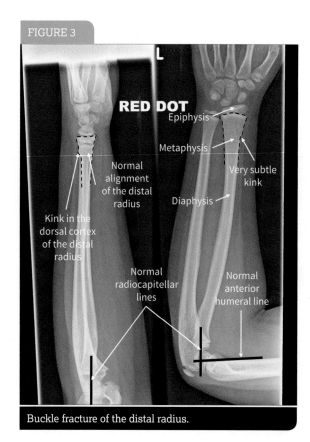

Buckle fracture of the distal radius.

FIGURE 4

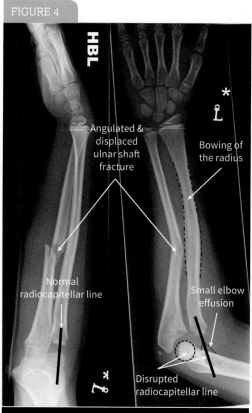

Complete fracture of the ulnar (transverse), and bowing of the radius, in keeping with a plastic deformity.

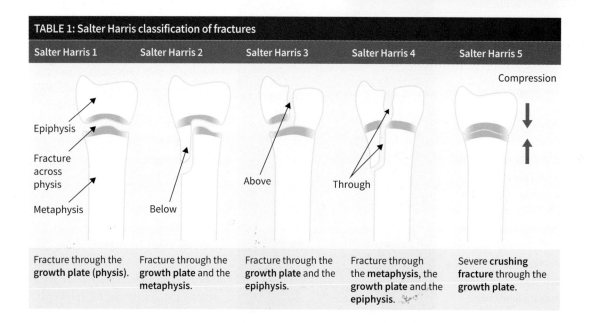

TABLE 1: Salter Harris classification of fractures

Salter Harris 1	Salter Harris 2	Salter Harris 3	Salter Harris 4	Salter Harris 5
Fracture through the **growth plate (physis)**.	Fracture through the **growth plate** and the **metaphysis**.	Fracture through the **growth plate** and the **epiphysis**.	Fracture through the **metaphysis**, the **growth plate** and the **epiphysis**.	Severe **crushing fracture** through the **growth plate**.

the injury, at least two radiographic views are required (anteroposterior and lateral). Even if there is the smallest chance of a physeal fracture, a second X-ray after four or five days is essential. For this reason, many children with a history of trauma but normal initial radiographs are brought to fracture clinic at one week to ensure resolution of symptoms. If there is ongoing discomfort, further radiographs can be ordered.

Management

Specific treatment depends upon the bone fractured, the Salter-Harris fracture type and the degree of fracture displacement and angulation:

> Undisplaced fractures. Conservative management with cast immobilisation. Type III and IV fractures will require follow up X-rays after one week to detect late displacement.

> Displaced fractures. Urgent reduction is required. Closed reduction techniques followed by splinting can be used for type I and II fractures. Type III and IV fractures may be amenable to closed reduction but will require open reduction and internal fixation if accurate reduction is not achieved.

Prognosis

These fractures must be carefully reduced to minimise the risk of premature ossification of the affected part, causing serious growth arrest and deformity. Salter-Harris type I and II fractures rarely result in growth arrest or deformity, in contrast to types III-V where the risk of growth arrest is far greater.

Supracondylar Fractures

Ossification centres are present in children. These are the sites of new bone formation. The presence of six ossification centres around the elbow can make interpreting a child's X-ray difficult (*Figure 6*). These ossification centres appear in a fairly constant order and can be remembered by the acronym CRITOE:

> Capitellum - age 1.
> Radial head - age 3.
> Internal epicondyle - age 5.
> Trochlea - age 7.
> Olecranon - age 9.
> External epicondyle - age 11.

Knowing the order of ossification is helpful. The most important reason is that the site of an ossification centre may be mistaken for a fracture. An example is shown in *Figure 7*.

Clinical Features

Supracondylar fractures are common fractures in children. Classic features include:

> Arm extension injuries.
> They commonly occur following a fall onto an outstretched hand.
> Tenderness and swelling over the elbow.

There is an associated forearm injury in 10%, and compartment syndrome may ensue. There is also a risk of injury to the brachial artery and the radial, ulnar and median nerves.

Management

Management may be conservative, using plaster immobilisation, or surgical, depending upon the degree of displacement and associated neurovascular injury.

Clavicle Fracture

This is the most common paediatric bone to be fractured (*Figure 8*).

FIGURE 5

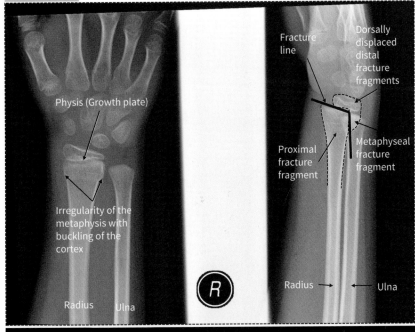

Physis (Growth plate)

Irregularity of the metaphysis with buckling of the cortex

Radius   Ulna

Fracture line

Dorsally displaced distal fracture fragments

Proximal fracture fragment

Metaphyseal fracture fragment

Radius   Ulna

Salter Harris Type 2 fracture.

FIGURE 6

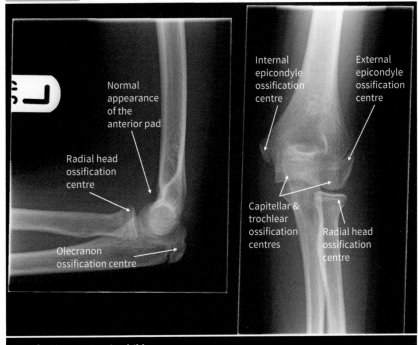

Normal appearance of the anterior pad

Radial head ossification centre

Olecranon ossification centre

Internal epicondyle ossification centre

External epicondyle ossification centre

Capitellar & trochlear ossification centres

Radial head ossification centre

Ossification centres in children.

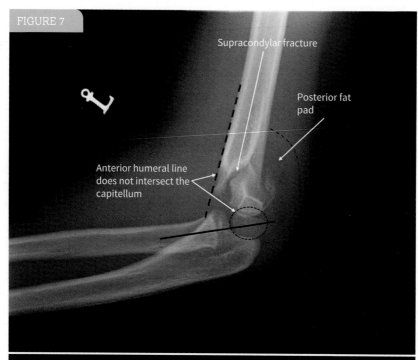

FIGURE 7

Supracondylar fracture

Posterior fat pad

Anterior humeral line does not intersect the capitellum

Supracondylar fracture. Note that the anterior humeral line does not intersect with the capitellum and that a posterior fat pad is visible (which is always pathological).

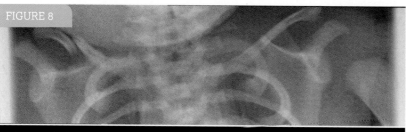

FIGURE 8

Right clavicular fracture secondary to a traumatic delivery.

Clinical Features

> The usual mechanism is a fall onto an outstretched hand.
> Most fractures occur in middle-third of the bone.
> The distal fragment is pulled down by the weight of the arm whilst the proximal fragment is pulled up by the sternocleidomastoid muscle.
> Clinically, tenderness with any shoulder movements and arm is held to chest.
> An associated pneumothorax or brachial plexus injury may occur.

Management

> Clavicular fractures are usually treated in a broad arm sling for two to four weeks. Open fractures, severely displaced fractures or fractures

causing tenting of the overlying skin require open reduction and internal fixation.
> The clavicle is the last bone in the body to ossify. Thus, paediatric clavicle fractures have an excellent chance of union, even with displacement, and are invariably treated conservatively.

Toddler's Fracture

> This is an undisplaced spiral fracture of the tibial shaft only (with no associated fibular fracture).
> It commonly occurs in children less than 3-years-old.
> It is caused by low energy trauma with a rotational component, which might relate to falling awkwardly.

> It is not always visible on plain radiographs and should be suspected when a child fails to weight-bear following trauma.
> Treatment involves a short-term immobilisation to protect the limb and relieve pain.

Pathological Fracture

A pathological fracture is one occurring in a bone affected by another disease process. Such fractures often follow minimal trauma. Causes of childhood pathological fractures include:

> Rickets.
> Bone tumours.
> Osteomyelitis.
> Osteogenesis imperfecta.
> Copper deficiency.

ORTHOPAEDIC HIP DISORDERS

Developmental Dysplasia of the Hip

Previously known as congenital hip dislocation, Developmental Dysplasia of the Hip (DDH) describes a spectrum of hip abnormalities, ranging from dysplasia (underdevelopment of the joint) to subluxation (partial dislocation), through to frank dislocation. Early recognition is vital as DDH usually responds well to conservative treatment at an early stage, whereas late diagnosis is associated with hip dysplasia requiring complex, and often surgical treatment.

The incidence is approximately 1.5 per 1000 live births, with girls being affected seven times more commonly than boys. The left hip is more often affected than the right and 20% of cases are bilateral.

Aetiology

The true aetiology is unclear and is thought to be multifactorial:

> Genetic factors. DDH tends to run in families. Inheritable features contributing to hip instability are generalised joint laxity and a shallow acetabulum.
> Hormonal changes. Changes occurring in late pregnancy may

aggravate ligamentous laxity in the infant.

> Post-natal factors. Neonatal positioning of the child may contribute to DDH. This may explain the high incidence of DDH in Native Americans who swaddle their babies with the legs held in full extension.

Risk Factors

> Female.
> First born.
> Positive family history.
> Breech presentation at delivery.
> Maternal oligohydramnios (due to restriction of intrauterine foetal movement).
> Associated neuromuscular disorders such as cerebral palsy and myelomeningocoele.

Clinical Features

Neonates

The ideal is to diagnose every case of DDH at birth. Screening forms part of the examination of the newborn and 6 to 8-week-old babies. Screening takes the form of Barlow and Ortolani tests (p193). The above tests can detect almost all unstable hips if performed by an experienced clinician. However, sometimes DDH is missed in the neonatal period. This may be due to examiner inexperience, if the hip is irreducible at birth or in the minority of cases in which the femoral head slips slowly out of the acetabulum during the first year of life.

Older Children

If diagnosis is missed in the neonatal period, DDH may present in several ways, including:

> Asymmetry of the skin folds around the hip (unless DDH is bilateral).
> Painless limp.
> Limited abduction of the hip.
> The child may walk on their toes on the affected side.
> Leg length discrepancy.

Investigations

Any neonate with suspected hip instability should undergo ultrasound scanning of the hip. Ultrasound is superior to plain radiography in children up to three months of age as the cartilaginous skeletal structure does not show on the latter.

Suspected DDH in older infants and children should be imaged with plain radiography. Sometimes arthrography, magnetic resonance imaging (MRI) and computed tomography (CT) are required to further delineate the extent of the disease.

Differential Diagnosis

In the neonatal period, screening usually picks up DDH before there are any obvious symptoms. In older children, a limp has a wide differential, including transient synovitis, septic arthritis, malignancy, rheumatological disorders, and other congenital malformations e.g. clubfoot.

Management

Treatment depends upon the age at which the diagnosis is made.

> In the newborn. If DDH is diagnosed at birth, it can be corrected conservatively by putting the baby in double nappies or by using a harness that holds the hips abducted and flexed. A padded Von Rosen splint can be used for babies up to 3-months-old, but a Pavlik harness should be used for older infants who would otherwise be able to crawl out of a Von Rosen splint. If worn correctly for approximately 12 weeks, a stable hip will be achieved. Following removal of the splint, the hip is examined radiologically or with ultrasound to ensure that the hip is reduced.
> 6-months-old to 6-years-old. The hip must be reduced and held in this position until acetabular development is adequate. Closed reduction is performed gradually over three weeks as manipulation under anaesthesia carries a high risk of avascular necrosis. Traction is applied to both legs and abduction increased until the legs are widely separated. If reduction is achieved, the legs are splinted in a plaster cast in the flexed, abducted and slightly internally rotated position. If closed reduction is unsuccessful, formal open reduction in theatre may be required.
> After 6-years-old. Unilateral DDH is usually managed with open reduction, sometimes combined with a corrective osteotomy of the femur. Bilateral disease results in symmetrical deformity and therefore is less noticeable. Surgical management carries greater risk as failure on one side results in asymmetrical deformity. Therefore, surgery is avoided unless pain or deformity is severe.

Complications

> Early secondary osteoarthritis.
> Subluxation of the hip may follow inadequately treated DDH.
> Spinal changes such as scoliosis, exaggeration of the normal lumbar lordosis and chronic low back pain.

Prognosis

Without treatment, DDH results in progressive deformity and disability associated with an increased risk of secondary osteoarthritis. The earlier the treatment begins, the more likely the child will develop a normal (or near normal) hip. The best outcomes occur in children treated within one to two weeks of birth; however, favourable outcomes are also achieved by measures between six months and six years. Presentation after this period is likely to require surgical intervention.

Slipped Upper Femoral Epiphysis

Slipped upper femoral epiphysis (SUFE) is a relatively rare condition of the adolescent hip joint. It describes the postero-inferior displacement of the upper femoral epiphysis through the epiphyseal plate. It is the anatomical equivalent of an intracapsular femoral neck fracture in the adult population.

Aetiology

The aetiology is not well understood, although it is thought to be multifactorial. The slip may be secondary to a Salter-Harris Type I fracture following minor

275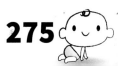

trauma, or it may occur more insidiously as a protracted event. Thirty percent of cases affect bilateral hip joints.

Risk Factors
- Boys are more commonly affected than girls (3:2).
- Obesity (single greatest risk factor).
- Pubertal growth surge.
- Afro-Caribbean ethnicity.
- Delayed skeletal maturity.
- Endocrine disorders.
  - Related disorders include hypothyroidism, growth hormone supplementation, hypogonadism and panhypopituitarism.
  - In patients with unusual presentations (e.g. patients who are younger than eight years, older than 15 years, or underweight), an endocrine disorder should be considered.

Classification
SUFE may be classified as stable or unstable according to the ability of the child to weight bear on the affected leg:
- Stable. The child is able to ambulate with or without the assistance of crutches. Stable disease accounts for 90% of cases and has a more favourable prognosis when compared with unstable disease.
- Unstable. The child is unable to ambulate even with the assistance of crutches.

Clinical Features
The typical patient is an overweight boy aged 10 to 15-years-old. Presentation can be vague and accounts for the delay in diagnosis in many cases. SUFE frequently causes referred pain to the ipsilateral knee and should be considered in any adolescent child presenting with knee pain with an absence of knee signs on examination.

The following features suggest a diagnosis of SUFE:
- Limping.
- Hip, thigh or knee pain.
- Pain on movement in all directions.
- Reduced range of movement with a progressive loss of abduction and internal rotation as the slip progresses.
- Affected leg is shortened and externally rotated.

Investigations
Plain radiographs of the pelvis and hip are the mainstay of diagnosis. Even in the early stages of the disease, changes can be seen. Stable slips require antero-posterior (AP) and frog leg lateral views of both hips. Frog leg lateral views should be avoided in unstable slips as it may worsen the slip. Instead, cross table lateral views should be requested in these circumstances. In cases where SUFE is suspected but radiological angles appear normal MRI scanning may be employed to diagnose so-called "pre-slip" conditions or subtle slips.

The radiological features of SUFE include (*Figure 9*):
- Steel sign. Double density at the metaphysis on the AP view.
- Widening of the ipsilateral growth plate. This is compared to the unaffected side.
- Decreased epiphysis height.
- Klein's line. A line drawn along the superior edge of the femoral neck should pass through the edge of the epiphysis. In SUFE the epiphysis falls below this line.

Differential Diagnosis
- Hip fracture. This is more likely following significant trauma.
- Transient synovitis. Self-limiting condition.
- Perthes disease. This occurs more commonly in children aged between 4 and 8 years of short stature.
- Osteomyelitis/septic arthritis. Elevated inflammatory markers in a potentially systemically unwell child.

Management
The treatment of SUFE is surgical. However, conservative treatment of SUFE is an emerging concept and involves a combination of spica casts and skin traction to prevent progressive displacement.

The aim of management is to prevent slip progression and avoid complications. Analgesia should be given, with the patient maintained in a non-weight-bearing position. Urgent orthopaedic referral should be arranged. Any attempt to manipulate the head back onto the femoral neck is dangerous and will disrupt the blood supply, potentially leading to avascular necrosis. Degree of displacement determines management:
- Mild to moderate displacement. This is treated by fixing the epiphysis with one or two cannulated screws under X-ray guidance.

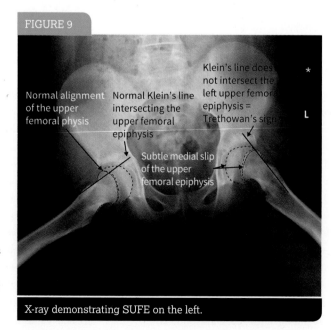

FIGURE 9

Normal alignment of the upper femoral physis

Normal Klein's line intersecting the upper femoral epiphysis

Klein's line does not intersect the left upper femoral epiphysis = Trethowan's sign

Subtle medial slip of the upper femoral epiphysis

X-ray demonstrating SUFE on the left.

> Severe displacement. This may require corrective osteotomy (where the bone is cut) and pinning if displacement is more than one half of the epiphyseal width.

Prophylactic fixing of the contralateral epiphysis may be indicated if there is the slightest suspicion of contralateral disease, those with a low likelihood of follow-up and in patients at high risk of subsequent slips e.g. obese patients or those with endocrine disorders.

Complications

> Avascular necrosis. This is seen almost exclusively in unstable slips after the slip has been reduced or pinned. This serious complication is relatively untreatable at present.
> Coxa vara. The angle between the head and shaft of the femur is reduced to less than 120 degrees. This deformity may occur secondary to failure to reduce/inadequate reduction of the displacement and fusion of the epiphysis in the deformed position. Results in a painless deformity.
> Secondary osteoarthritis. This results from avascular necrosis or failure to reduce the displacement.
> Contralateral SUFE. Thirty percent of cases are bilateral.
> Chondrolysis. This is loss of articular cartilage, and results in joint stiffness and pain.

Prognosis

Prognosis depends on the initial degree of epiphyseal slippage. Patients with stable slips invariably have better outcomes than those with unstable slips. The end result is good-to-excellent in 94–96% of cases, if displacement is less than one-third of the diameter of the epiphysis. With increasing displacement, the complication rate increases.

Perthes Disease

Perthes disease is an idiopathic disorder of the childhood hip characterised by segmental osteonecrosis of the femoral head.

The paediatric hip joint has a complex vascular supply. By adolescence, blood supply to the hip joint is formed by anastomoses between the medial and lateral circumflex femoral arteries, which usually arise from the profunda femoris artery. The acetabular artery traversing the ligamentum teres also contributes. However, before childhood is reached, blood supply to the hip is dynamic, variable and potentially at risk.

Aetiology

The cause of the avascular necrosis seen in Perthes disease remains unknown although several factors may play a role including repetitive microtrauma, growth plate disruption and vascular insufficiency. The highest incidence is found amongst the Caucasian population of the United Kingdom and Norway.

> Perthes disease usually affects children between 4 and 8-years-old.
> It is more common in boys with a male:female ratio of 4:1.
> Fifteen percent of cases are bilateral.

Risk Factors

> Family history (12% of cases).
> Low birth weight.
> Low socio-economic status.
> Delayed skeletal age.

Clinical Features

> Limp. This is in the absence of trauma, classically following physical exertion.
> Groin pain. The limp may be associated with groin pain and in 25% of cases the pain radiates to the ipsilateral thigh or knee.

Clinically the hip may appear deceptively normal. However, the following signs may be present depending upon the disease severity and stage:

> Antalgic gait. Pain on walking.
> Trendelenburg sign. This is found in children with weak hip abductors or pain limiting movement of the hip abductors. When standing on one leg, the pelvis drops on the opposite side (rather than staying in the same position). The hip abductors on the side of the standing leg are not able keep the pelvis straight, because of pain. This is a positive test.
> Limited range of movement of the hip. Specifically abduction and internal rotation are limited.
> Muscle wasting. This occurs from disuse of the limb.
> Leg length discrepancy. This occurs in severe Perthes disease.

Investigations

Blood Tests

Basic blood tests including a full blood count and inflammatory markers should be obtained to help exclude septic arthritis (these tests are usually within normal reference ranges in Perthes disease).

Imaging

Plain anterior-posterior (AP) and lateral radiographs are the mainstay of diagnosis and allow for classification, prognosis estimation and disease progression monitoring. Radiological findings vary with age of the child, the extent of the ischaemia and the stage of the disease.

Features of Perthes disease on plain radiographs include (*Figure 10*):

> Collapse and flattening of the femoral head.
> Sclerosis resulting from reduced resorption and relative osteopaenia of the rest of the bone.
> Widening of the joint space.
> Subchondral fractures, partial collapse and femoral head fragmentation.
> Coxa magna (spherical enlargement of the femoral head due to increased vascularity).
> Subluxation.

Magnetic resonance imaging (MRI) and radioisotope bone scanning also have a role to play in the diagnosis of Perthes disease in the early stages or if the diagnosis is in doubt.

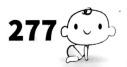

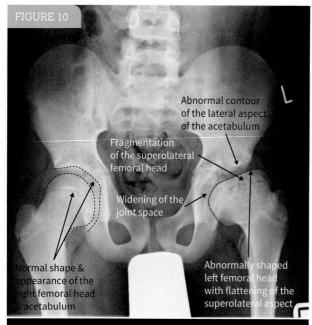

FIGURE 10

Abnormal contour of the lateral aspect of the acetabulum

Fragmentation of the superolateral femoral head

Widening of the joint space

Normal shape & appearance of the right femoral head & acetabulum

Abnormally shaped left femoral head with flattening of the superolateral aspect

X-ray demonstrating classic features of Perthes Disease.

Differential Diagnosis

> Transient synovitis. This is a self-limiting condition in an otherwise well child.
> Juvenile idiopathic arthritis. This commonly affects more than one joint with extra-articular features.
> Septic arthritis/Proximal femoral osteomyelitis. Elevated inflammatory markers.
> Proximal femoral fracture. This follows significant trauma.
> Acute or chronic slipped upper femoral epiphysis. This is more likely in older, overweight children.

Management

The aims of treatment are to relieve the symptoms, improve mobility, reduce mechanical stress and to contain the femoral head in the acetabulum until it reforms (containment). Treatment can be conservative or surgical and is governed by:

> The radiological severity of the disease.
> The degree of reduced hip motion.
> The age of the patient.

Conservative Management

Mild to moderate disease (less than 50% involvement of the femoral head with preservation of joint space) is generally managed conservatively.

> The patient is initially kept non-weight bearing.
> Non-steroidal anti-inflammatory medications are used until pain subsides.
> Regular program of physiotherapy (once pain under control).
> If an adductor muscle contracture is present, botulinum toxin injections together with physiotherapy may help to improve containment by increasing the range of movement in abduction.

Surgical Management

Surgical treatment may be required if there is severe disease, the patient is older than six, or when conservative management fails. If immobilisation in plaster cast is indicated, the majority of orthopaedic surgeons would recommend surgical management since immobilisation is heavily restrictive. Options include a varus osteotomy of the femur or innominate osteotomy of the pelvis. Both approaches aim to increase the containment of the femoral head in the acetabulum. A total hip replacement at skeletal maturity can be performed for patients with severe functional impairment.

Complications

> Joint stiffness.
> Limb length discrepancy.
> Coxa magna. Broadening of the head and neck of the femur.
> Osteoarthritis. This is secondary to abnormal weight bearing.
> Premature fusion of the growth plates leading to overgrowth of the trochanter.
> Hinged abduction.

Prognosis

In patients less than 6-years-old, the outcome is good, irrespective of treatment. Children more than 6-years-old with severe Perthes disease have significantly better outcomes with surgical treatment than those with conservative treatment. However, half of all patients require joint arthroplasty after a median of 50 years.

Indices for poor prognosis include:

> Girls (earlier skeletal maturity).
> Onset beyond the age of 6–years-old (lower remodelling potential).
> >50% involvement of the femoral head.
> Lateral displacement of the femoral head impinging on the acetabular margin.
> Subluxation.

BONE AND JOINT INFECTIONS

Septic Arthritis

Septic arthritis is a serious infection of the joint space and an important cause of joint swelling in children. The most commonly affected joint in the paediatric population is the hip joint, although almost any joint can be affected. Monoarticular septic arthritis is classical, although infants may present with multiple joint involvement. Prompt diagnosis and treatment of septic arthritis is paramount to prevent rapid destruction of the articular cartilage and joint space.

Aetiology

Infection can spread to the joint in three ways:

1 Direct invasion from an adjacent focus of infection, e.g. acute osteomyelitis.

2 Direct inoculation from a penetrating wound.

3 Haematogenous spread from a distant infection/septicaemia.

Risk Factors
- Prematurity.
- Penetrating injury.
- Diabetes mellitus.
- Joint surgery.
- Hip or knee prosthesis.
- Skin infection, e.g. chickenpox, cellulitis.
- Immunocompromise.
- Sickle cell disease.

Causative Organisms
- Streptococci. This predominates in the neonatal period.
- Staphylococcus aureus. This is the most common infecting agent beyond the neonatal period.
- Haemophilus influenzae. This is largely eradicated in developed countries due to the Hib immunisation but remains an important cause in young children (especially those less than 3 years old) from developing countries.
- Neisseria gonorrhoeae. More common in sexually active teenagers.
- Pseudomonas. This is more common in drug users, and the immunocompromised.
- E. coli. This may affect any age group but is more common in teenagers and young adults.

Clinical Features
Septic arthritis is easily overlooked in children because the classic signs may be absent. The condition may also mimic common, benign conditions, such as transient synovitis. Classic features of septic arthritis are:
- Acute pain and swelling of a joint with overlying erythema of the skin.
- Severely restricted joint movement. Any attempt at active or passive movement of the affected joint is exquisitely tender. For this reason children often hold the limb still (pseudoparalysis).
- Joint effusion.
- Posture. With hip involvement the leg is held flexed and abducted.
- Systemic features. This includes fever, rigors and tachycardia (however their absence does not exclude septic arthritis).

Differential Diagnosis
The main differential diagnosis to consider is transient synovitis, and key differences between the two conditions are shown in *Table 2*. Other causes of hip pain, such as SUFE, Perthes disease, reactive arthritis and haemarthrosis should all be considered.

TABLE 2: Septic arthritis and transient synovitis

	Transient synovitis	Septic arthritis
Incidence.	More common.	Less common.
Weight bearing.	May be able to weight bare.	Unable to weight bare.
Pain.	None/mild, particularly when at rest.	Moderate-severe even at rest.
Temperature.	Normal, or low grade temperature.	Elevated.
Inflammatory markers.	Normal, or minimally elevated.	Elevated.
Fluid in the joint capsule.	No pus, negative cultures.	Pus, bacteria identified on culture.
Treatments.	Anti-inflammatory medications.	IV antibiotics.

Investigations
Laboratory Tests
- Full blood count. White cell count will be elevated.
- CRP and ESR. Both acute phase reactants which will also be elevated in septic arthritis.
- Blood cultures. These should be taken before the commencement of antibiotic therapy.

Elevation of the above blood tests (with or without positive blood cultures) provide supportive evidence of bacterial infection and help to exclude other common conditions such as transient synovitis. Kocher's modified criteria can also be a helpful guide (*Box 1*).

Imaging
Laboratory tests should be followed by radiological imaging. An ultrasound scan of deep joints such as the hip is useful to identify a joint effusion. Plain radiographs are helpful to exclude trauma or other bony lesions. However, the radiographic appearance of a septic joint is often normal in the early stages of septic arthritis, so a normal appearance of the joint does not exclude the disease. As the disease progresses,

Box 1: Kocher's modified criteria for assessment of the painful hip in children

- Temperature > 38.5°.
- CRP > 20mg/dL.
- ESR > 40mm/h.
- Non-weight bearing.
- WCC > 12 x 10⁹/litre.

5 criteria met = 97.5% chance of septic arthritis; 4= 93%; 3= 82%; 2= 62%; 1= 36%; 0= 16%

joint space narrowing due to effusion and soft tissue swelling precede the appearance of a narrowed joint space secondary to articular cartilage destruction.

Joint Aspiration

This is the definitive investigation. Joint aspiration should be carried out under aseptic conditions (to reduce the risk of contamination of a sterile joint) by an orthopaedic surgeon. The aspirate should be sent to the lab for urgent gram staining and microscopy, culture and sensitivity.

Management

Treatment should be started without delay, to minimise joint damage. After joint aspiration and blood cultures, the joint should be splinted and empirical broad-spectrum intravenous antibiotics should be started whilst arranging urgent surgical drainage and irrigation of the affected joint.

A prolonged course of broad spectrum antibiotics are required after drainage and the choice of antimicrobial agent should be tailored according to culture results.

Complications

> Joint stiffness. This may occur secondary to cartilage damage.
> Septic dislocation. This is due to damage to the joint capsule and bone.
> Osteonecrosis. This is due to ischaemia.
> Shortening of the limb. This is due to dislocation and osteonecrosis.
> Secondary osteoarthritis. This is from damage to the joint capsule.

Prognosis

With prompt recognition and management, the prognosis is usually good. However, delayed diagnosis may result in joint destruction. This is most likely to occur in the neonates, due to the difficulties with diagnosis.

Osteomyelitis

Osteomyelitis is an infection of the metaphysis of long bones.

Aetiology

The metaphysis is prone to infection because the area is supplied by the terminal branches of the nutrient arteries. Osteomyelitis can be acute or chronic. Similar to septic arthritis, bacteria can seed in the bone via three portals of entry:

1 Penetration from trauma.
2 Contiguous spread from a nearby soft tissue infection.
3 Haematogenous spread from a distant focus of infection.

Common sources of the bacteraemia in children include an infected umbilical cord, a septic tooth, boils and abscesses.

Risk Factors

> Penetrating injury.
> Diabetes mellitus.
> Skin infection, e.g. chickenpox, cellulitis.
> Immunosuppression.
> Sickle cell disease.
> Chronic steroid use.

Causative Organisms

> *Staphylococcus aureus.* This is the most common causative organism affecting children of all ages.
> *Streptococcus pyogenes* and *Streptococcus pneumoniae.* These are less common than *S. aureus* and also affect all age groups.
> *Haemophilus influenzae.* This is uncommon in developed countries due to the Hib immunisation.
> *E. coli* and *Bacteroides* spp. This commonly causes neonatal osteomyelitis as a result of umbilical sepsis.
> *Salmonella.* Children with sickle cell anaemia are at higher risk of *Salmonella* osteomyelitis.

Clinical Features

The presentation of acute osteomyelitis is usually:

> A markedly painful, immobile limb. Even the slightest touch or manipulation of the affected limb is acutely painful.
> Febrile illness.
> Occasionally, a history of a preceding sore throat, skin lesion or injury may be present.
> Skin changes. The skin overlying the affected site may be swollen, warm and erythematous.
> Toxaemia. If there is a delay in presentation, the child may exhibit features of toxaemia, for example, tachycardia.

Untreated acute osteomyelitis may result in the formation of a subperiosteal abscess due to the infection eroding into the cortex allowing pus to strip the periosteum off the bone. This bone abscess will eventually discharge through a sinus onto the skin surface. At this point, the child is said to have chronic osteomyelitis.

Vertebral osteomyelitis (uncommon in the paediatric population) may present with chronic, unremitting back pain, which is worse at rest.

Differential Diagnosis

> Cellulitis. The infection is limited to the skin only.
> Septic arthritis. This may be difficult to differentiate clinically although septic arthritis is associated with an acutely hot, swollen, tender joint.
> Rheumatic fever. Musculoskeletal involvement is usually a polyarthritis. Cardiac, dermatological or abdominal signs and symptoms often co-exist.
> Sickle-cell crisis. This may be suspected in cases of known sickle cell disease.

Investigations

- Blood tests. The full blood count may demonstrate a leucocytosis. Acute phase reactants such as ESR and CRP are also likely to be elevated in acute osteomyelitis. Blood cultures prior to antibiotic therapy are mandatory and are positive in approximately 50% of cases.
- Plain radiographs. These do not demonstrate any abnormality in the early stages of the disease, but should be obtained to exclude any other bony lesions and to provide a baseline to monitor disease progression. After approximately 10 days, subperiosteal new bone formation and localised bone rarefaction may become visible.
- Magnetic resonance imaging (MRI). This may be useful to distinguish between bone and soft tissue infection. MRI can also detect acute osteomyelitis at an earlier stage by detecting bone changes caused by altered blood supply secondary to acute infection. This imaging modality is the most useful to delineate the degree of soft tissue and medullary involvement.
- Bone biopsy. This is performed percutaneously through non-infected tissue if the diagnosis remains in doubt or to obtain tissue samples to direct antibiotic therapy.

Management

In the acute phase, analgesics should be administered generously and the affected limb should be splinted. Prompt intravenous antibiotic therapy is mandatory. Therapy should begin with 'best guess' antibiotics guided by microbiology advice. A prolonged course of antibiotics is required, and the regimen can be changed from intravenous to oral antibiotics as the inflammatory markers begin to settle and the child's clinical condition improves. If the condition does not begin to respond to antibiotic therapy within 36 hours, or investigations demonstrate an abscess/subperiosteal collection, surgical exploration and drainage is required.

Complications

- Bone abscess. This may occur if treatment is not early or aggressive.
- Bacteraemia. The infection may spread to the systemic circulation, as the bone is very vascular.
- Chronic osteomyelitis. This may occur if inadequately treated.
- Altered bone growth. This may occur if there is damage to the growth plate.
- Fracture. A pathological fracture may occur as a result of increased susceptibility from infection.
- Septic arthritis. This is due to spread of the infection to the joint.

Prognosis

Prognosis is variable depending on the number of risk factors and the child's general condition. Prompt diagnosis and treatment in an otherwise well child results in a full recovery in 90-95% of cases. However, the disease can recur at any point as walled off nests of bacteria can reactivate. For this reason, long-term follow-up is required to monitor for relapse.

RHEUMATOLOGICAL DISORDERS

Transient Synovitis

Transient synovitis is a common cause of benign hip pain affecting children between 2 and 12-years-old.

Aetiology

The aetiology is unclear, but infection and trauma are thought to be precipitating factors. However, prospective studies have shown infection (usually an upper respiratory tract infection) and trauma to be associated only in 30% and 5% of cases, respectively.

Clinical Features

- Sudden onset limp with hip and/or knee pain.
- Absence of rest pain.
- Decreased range of hip movement, especially internal rotation.
- The limb is held in the position of greatest comfort, typically flexed, abducted and slightly externally rotated.
- There may be a preceding or accompanying upper respiratory tract infection.
- The child is systemically well.

Differential Diagnosis

- Septic arthritis and osteomyelitis. There is evidence of infection, with significant pain and elevated inflammatory markers.
- Perthes disease. There is persistent pain with radiographic changes.
- Slipped upper femoral epiphysis. There are characteristic radiographic changes.

Investigations

The diagnostic workup should include tests to exclude alternative diagnoses and demonstrate confirmatory features. Transient synovitis is a diagnosis of exclusion and septic arthritis should always be considered.

- Blood tests. White cell count, C-reactive protein and erythrocyte sedimentation rate are usually normal in transient synovitis (but elevated in septic arthritis).
- Plain radiographs and ultrasound scanning. Plain radiographs do not usually demonstrate any joint abnormality, however a small joint effusion may be seen on ultrasound scanning. If an effusion is noted, it should be aspirated and the fluid sent to the laboratory for microscopy, culture and sensitivity to exclude an infective cause.

The modified Kocher criteria (*Box 1*, p279) can help to differentiate between septic arthritis and transient synovitis.

Treatment

Transient synovitis is a benign, self-limiting condition and is managed conservatively. The mainstay of treatment is rest and simple analgesia.

Prognosis

Symptoms usually resolve within two weeks and there do not appear to be any long-term complications.

Reactive Arthritis

Reactive arthritis is the most common form of childhood arthritis.

Aetiology

It is an autoimmune condition characterised by transient joint swelling (usually less than six weeks) following an extra-articular infection. There is a strong association with the major histocompatibility antigen HLA B27 and seronegative arthropathies.

Classification

Two broad subgroups are recognised:

1 Post enteric form. This is related to gastrointestinal infection with microorganisms such as *Salmonella*, *Campylobacter*, *Yersinia* and *Shigella*.
2 Post venereal form. This is related to sexual activity and infection with chlamydia and gonorrhoea (rare in children).

Clinical Features

Signs and symptoms of reactive arthritis usually develop two to four weeks after gastrointestinal or genitourinary infection. Onset is often acute with malaise, fever and fatigue. Other signs and symptoms are outlined in *Table 3*.

Investigations

> Blood tests. Inflammatory markers (CRP, ESR) will be elevated during the active phase of the disease. Full blood count may demonstrate a leucocytosis, thrombocytosis

or mild normochromic normocytic anaemia. HLA B27 is positive in 65-96% of cases.

> Microbiology. Culture of urethral fluids, faeces or throat swabs may identify the causative organism.
> Joint aspiration. This may be required in the presence of a joint effusion to exclude septic arthritis.
> Plain joint radiographs. These will be normal in early disease. Later, a periosteal reaction may be evident.

Management

The arthritis should be treated with:

> Rest.
> Joint immobilisation.
> Physiotherapy.
> Non-steroidal anti-inflammatory drugs.

Intra-articular steroid injections are beneficial and systemic steroids may be used in refractory disease. Antibiotics are only used when a causative organism has been identified.

Prognosis

Reactive arthritis is a self-limiting condition. The majority of patients see complete resolution of symptoms within 12 months. One-third will develop recurrent or chronic disease and one-third of these will be functionally limited due to destructive arthritis.

Juvenile Idiopathic Arthritis

Juvenile idiopathic arthritis (JIA) is the term used to describe joint inflammation presenting before 16-years-old and persisting for at least six weeks in the absence of infection or other defined cause. It affects one in 1000 children in the United Kingdom.

Classification

There are at least seven different forms of the disease as outlined in *Table 4*.

Investigations

JIA is a clinical diagnosis. Investigations are required to aid diagnosis and detect complications.

> Blood tests. Full blood count may show anaemia, leukocytosis or thrombocytosis in systemic JIA. Erythrocyte sedimentation rate is generally elevated in most forms of JIA.
> Autoantibodies. Antinuclear antibody (ANA), Rheumatoid Factor (RF) and HLA B27 may be positive in subtypes outlined in *Table 4*. ANA positivity predicts risk of uveitis.
> Imaging. Plain radiographs are usually normal in early JIA but are useful to help exclude osteomyelitis, trauma or tumours. Magnetic resonance imaging is most useful to delineate the extent of joint damage and synovitis.

Management

Treatment is aimed at improving the quality of life and preserving joint function.

TABLE 3: Clinical features of reactive arthritis	
Articular	• Mono or polyarthritis affecting the knees, ankles, feet or hands. • Sacroiliitis. • Heel pain due to calcaneal spur enthesopathy. • Plantar fasciitis.
Urethral	• Urethritis (if related to sexual activity).
Ocular	• Conjunctivitis.
Dermatological	• Keratoderma blennorrhagica. • Circinate balanitis. • Macules. • Pustules.
Systemic	• Fever. • Malaise.

Subtype	Clinical features	Blood test abnormalities
Oligoarticular JIA.	• Affects one to four joints. • Joint pain (minimal), stiffness and reduced range of motion. • Five times more common in girls.	ANA positive.
Polyarthritis (RF negative).	• Affects five or more joints. • Can be symmetrical with large and small joint swelling. • Pain and stiffness with minimal swelling.	RF negative.
Polyarthritis (RF positive).	• Symmetrical large and small joint swelling with finger joint involvement.	RF positive.
Systemic JIA.	• Oligoarthritis or polyarthritis with daily spiking of temperature for at least 2 weeks. • Rash, lymphadenopathy, hepatomegaly/splenomegaly or serositis must be present. • More common in girls aged 1 to 10–years-old.	Anaemia, leukocytosis, thrombocytosis and elevated inflammatory markers.
Psoriatic arthritis.	• Asymmetrical arthritis with psoriasis. • Dactylitis or nail pitting is common.	No specific markers.
Enthesitis related arthritis.	• Initially large joint lower limb arthritis and enthesitis (inflammation at the insertion of tendons/ligaments to bone, especially the Achilles tendon), then lumbar or sacroiliac joint involvement. • In addition, for diagnosis to be made, children must have one of; anterior uveitis, HLA B27 positive or family history of HLA B27 related disease.	HLA B27 positive.
Undifferentiated arthritis.	• Arthritis that does not meet the criteria for other forms of JIA.	No specific markers.

TABLE 4: Subtypes, features and blood test abnormalities of JIA

> Physiotherapy is required to maintain joint mobility.
> NSAIDs are effective analgesics and can be combined with intra-articular corticosteroid injections.
> Oral corticosteroids and disease modifying anti-rheumatic drugs (DMARDs) are used in severe/resistant disease.

Complications

Complications depend on the subtype, but may include growth failure, anterior uveitis, amyloidosis and osteoporosis.

Prognosis

The usual course of oligoarticular disease is permanent remission, whilst this is less common in polyarticular disease. Positive rheumatoid factor is associated with worse outcome.

Ankylosing Spondylitis

Ankylosing spondylitis (AS) is a chronic seronegative spondyloarthropathy predominantly affecting the spine and sacroiliac joints. The disease is characterised by progressive ankylosis (stiffening) of affected joints, with initial fibrosis followed by joint ossification. It has a male to female ratio of 3:1 and peak onset is between 15 and 25-years-old.

Aetiology

The aetiology is unknown but is thought to be due to a combination of genetic and environmental factors including:

> A positive family history.
> Strong association with the major histocompatibility complex antigen HLA B27.

> Genitourinary or gastrointestinal infection may trigger the onset of ankylosing spondylitis in genetically susceptible people.

Clinical Features

Disease onset is insidious with a course characterised by flares and remissions. Signs and symptoms can be divided into articular and extra-articular features:

Articular Features

> In children, lower limb oligoarthritis usually precedes spinal involvement.
> Inflammatory back pain and stiffness worse in the morning and after inactivity.
> Reduction in all back movements. Schober's test demonstrates reduced lumbar flexion when the patient is asked to touch their toes from a standing position.
> Sacroiliac joint ankylosis may be felt as diffuse buttock pain.
> Achilles tendonitis.

Extra-articular Features

> Aortic valve insufficiency and cardiac conduction defects.
> Pulmonary fibrosis.
> Anterior uveitis.
> Amyloidosis.
> Cauda equina syndrome.
> Osteoporosis.

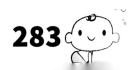

Investigations

Blood Tests

- ▸ FBC. This may show a normochromic normocytic anaemia and/or leucocytosis.
- ▸ ESR, CRP. These may be elevated in the context of inflammation.
- ▸ HLA B27. This is strongly associated with ankylosing spondylitis.

Imaging

Radiological changes include (*Figure 11*):

- ▸ Erosions.
- ▸ Sclerosis and ankylosis of the sacroiliac joints.
- ▸ Bony bridges between adjacent vertebrae (syndesmophytes) produce the characteristic "bamboo spine" appearance.
- ▸ Peripheral joint involvement demonstrates radiographic changes similar to rheumatoid arthritis.

The mnemonic "LOSS" can be helpful: loss of joint space, osteophyte formation, subchondral sclerosis and subchondral cysts.

Management

Physiotherapy is the mainstay of treatment and is aimed at maintaining flexibility. No drugs have been shown to modify the course of the disease but NSAIDs are a useful analgesic for symptom control. Surgery is reserved for complications such as fixation of spinal fractures, correction of severe spinal deformity and hip fractures.

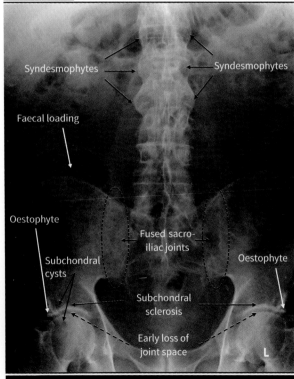

FIGURE 11

Features of ankylosing spondylitis.

Prognosis

Outcomes are generally good in ankylosing spondylitis, with cardiac and neurological complications being the most worrying. Poor prognostic indicators include peripheral joint involvement, early onset, elevated ESR and poor response to NSAIDs.

Systemic Lupus Erythematosus (SLE)

SLE is rare in children but may occur in adolescent girls.

Aetiology

SLE is a chronic, inflammatory autoimmune disease characterised by antinuclear antibodies and vasculitis. The cause is unknown but it is thought to be multifactorial involving genetic and environmental elements. SLE runs in families but no specific causative gene has been identified. It has a female preponderance and occurs more commonly in the South-Asian population, associated with the HLA-DR2 and HLA-DR3 alleles. Environmental influences include Epstein-Barr virus and ultraviolet light.

Clinical Features

Systemic symptoms such as fever, malaise, anorexia and weight loss are common. Other features of SLE are outlined in *Table 5*. A malar rash is characteristic (*Figure 12*).

Investigations

FBC may identify anaemia, thrombocytopenia, or lymphopenia. Renal and liver function should be checked. ESR and CRP may be raised. Complement (C3/4) may be low in active disease. In myositis, creatine kinase may be raised.

Autoantibody tests include ANA, anti-dsDNA, anti-Smith, anti-Ro, anti-La, anti-ribosomal P, Anti-RNP, anticardiolipin, anti-histone, and lupus anticoagulant.

Management

Management of SLE is largely symptomatic. Medical treatment includes supportive care, lifestyle changes, analgesics and NSAIDs. Management of patients with mild to moderate organ involvement includes oral corticosteroids or steroid-sparing agents such as azathioprine and methotrexate. Major organ involvement requires intravenous steroids and biological therapy.

Prognosis

SLE follows a relapsing-remitting course with a five-year survival of 90%. Mortality is often related to cardiovascular and renal disease.

Dermatomyositis

Aetiology

Dermatomyositis is a systemic connective tissue disorder causing acute and chronic inflammation of striated muscle. It is an ischaemic myopathy resulting in muscle infarction.

Clinical Features

Usual onset is between 5 and 10-years-old. Children present with symmetrical proximal muscle tenderness and weakness, arthritis and fever. Occasionally pharyngeal muscle involvement results in dysphagia.

TABLE 5: Features of SLE

Skin.	• Malar rash (classic "butterfly" rash over cheeks and nasal bridge). • Photosensitivity. • Alopecia (hair loss). • Livedo reticularis (lace-like purple discolouration of skin due to thrombi in capillaries. • Vasculitis. • Raynaud phenomenon. • Mucosal ulceration – usually affecting the palate. • Sjögren's syndrome.
Musculoskeletal.	• Myalgia. • Arthralgia. • Myositis.
Renal.	• Painless haematuria and proteinuria. • Glomerulonephritis. • Hypertension.
Pulmonary.	• Pleurisy. • Pulmonary embolism. • Dyspnoea. • Pneumonitis. • Fibrosing alveolitis. • Pulmonary haemorrhage.
Cardiovascular.	• Accelerated atherosclerosis. • Pericarditis/endocarditis/myocarditis. • Recurrent venous/arterial thrombosis.
Neurological.	• Peripheral neuropathy. • Headaches. • Transient ischaemic attacks (TIAs).
Gastrointestinal.	• Nausea and vomiting. • Abdominal pain. • Oral ulceration. • Jaundice. • Hepatomegaly.
Haematological.	• Normochromic normocytic anaemia. • Thrombocytopenia. • Leukopenia. • Splenomegaly.

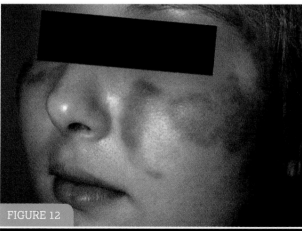

Two cutaneous manifestations are associated with juvenile dermatomyositis, both of which can precede or occur simultaneously with onset of muscular weakness:

▸ The "heliotrope" rash describes a red/purple rash across the upper eyelids. It is associated with periorbital and upper lid oedema and telangiectasia of the eyelid capillaries.

▸ Gottron's papules describe red papules seen classically over the knuckles but can also be seen on the extensor surfaces of the elbows and knees.

Investigations

Inflammatory markers (CRP, ESR) and serum creatine kinase may be elevated and muscle biopsy demonstrates inflammatory cell infiltration and atrophy. Several auto-antibody tests have been identified that may be helpful in prognosis and subtyping (e.g. ANA, Anti–Mi-2, Anti-Jo-1, Anti-SRP), but they are not typically needed for routine diagnosis.

Management

Standard treatment is with oral corticosteroids, with the dose being tailored over a two year period. Other immunosuppressant agents such as methotrexate and cyclosporin may be required in severe disease. Physiotherapy is helpful to prevent joint contractures.

Sarcoidosis

Aetiology

Sarcoidosis is a multisystem inflammatory disorder characterised by the development of non-caseating granulomas in affected organs. The aetiology is unknown but it is thought that certain environmental, occupational or infective agents trigger the disease in genetically susceptible individuals.

Clinical Features

Sarcoidosis is a rare disorder in children and most childhood cases have occurred in children between 13 and 15-years-old. Sarcoidosis can affect any organ, but frequently manifests in the lungs, skin, lymph nodes, eyes, liver and spleen in children. Accompanying constitutional symptoms such as fever, fatigue and weight loss are common. Children below the age of five years often present with a triad of arthritis, rash and uveitis, without the typical hilar lymphadenopathy and lung involvement seen in adult cases.

Investigations

Diagnostic work-up includes serum angiotensin converting enzyme (ACE) levels (elevated in 50% of children with late onset disease) and a chest X-ray to detect hilar lymphadenopathy (*Figure 13*). FBC, renal function, LFTs, and electrolytes including calcium should all be checked as they may be deranged. The diagnosis can be confirmed by the detection of non-caseating granulomas on biopsy specimen.

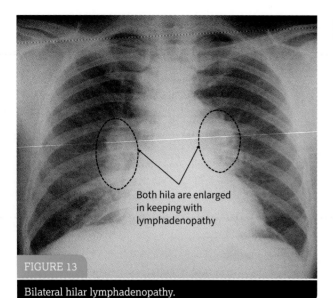

FIGURE 13

Bilateral hilar lymphadenopathy.

Both hila are enlarged in keeping with lymphadenopathy

TABLE 6: Manifestations of Marfan syndrome

Musculoskeletal.	• Arachnodactyly (long fingers). • Tall stature with disproportionately long legs and arms – the span of the arms is greater than the height. • Pectus excavatum (sunken appearance of chest). • Spinal abnormalities – spondylolisthesis, scoliosis. • Generalised joint laxity. • Flat feet. • Mandibular retrognathia (abnormal posterior positioning of mandible). • High arched palate.
Cardiovascular.	• Dilatation of the ascending aorta. • Mitral and aortic regurgitation. • Dissecting aortic aneurysm.
Ocular.	• Lens dislocation. • Retinal detachment.
Skin.	• Striae.
Dural.	• Dural ectasia (enlargement of the dura). • Meningocoele (protrusion of the meninges through a spinal/cranial defect).

Management

Corticosteroids are the mainstay of treatment. Other immunosuppressive drugs (e.g. methotrexate) may be required in steroid resistant cases.

Prognosis

Long-term prognosis is good, with most children demonstrating significant improvement in symptoms and lung function over time.

Marfan Syndrome

Aetiology

Marfan syndrome is an autosomal dominant connective tissue disease with characteristic skeletal, dermatological, cardiac, aortic, ocular and dural malformations. It is thought to be due to a defect in the cross-linkage of collagen and elastin secondary to a mutation in the fibrillin-1 gene.

Clinical Features

Common features of Marfan syndrome are outlined in *Table 6*. More formal diagnosis is with the Ghent Nosology.

Management

Management should involve a multidisciplinary team including geneticists, ophthalmologists, cardiologists and orthopaedic surgeons. Prophylactic beta-blockers have been used with limited efficacy to reduce the rate of aortic dilatation (by reducing the mean arterial pressure and heart rate). Surgical management is indicated with progressive aortic disease, significant valvular disease, or certain orthopaedic problems such as severe scoliosis or flat feet.

Prognosis

Patients with Marfan syndrome can develop severe orthopaedic, cardiovascular and ocular complications, but as treatment and early recognition of complications has advanced, so has life expectancy. The main cause of death is cardiovascular disease and vascular complications.

SKELETAL DISORDERS

Achondroplasia

Achondroplasia is the most commonly occurring form of short-limb dwarfism. It affects one in 30,000 births and the incidence increases as paternal age increases. Inheritance is autosomal dominant, although 80% of cases arise due to sporadic mutation.

Aetiology

Virtually all cases are caused by a G380R mutation in fibroblast growth factor receptor 3 (FGFR3). FGFR3 is also important in craniofacial, vertebral and neurological development, therefore this mutation has multiple effects in affected individuals.

Clinical Features

> The characteristic feature is a normal length trunk with disproportionately short limbs, especially proximally.
> Broad limbs with deep creases.
> Short fingers.
> Small face and flat nasal bridge.
> Enlarged skull vault and frontal bossing.
> Marked lumbar lordosis when standing.
> Increased joint laxity.

Differential Diagnosis

Other forms of short limb skeletal dysplasia include:

> Hypochondroplasia. There is less pronounced skeletal disproportion and spinal abnormalities, with the face and skull appearing normal.

▷ Morquio syndrome. The shortening affects the distal limb segments more than the proximal segments. There are widespread associated defects.

▷ Epiphyseal dysplasias. The head and face are normal but the epiphyses show characteristic changes on plain radiographs.

▷ Proportionate dwarfism. The limbs and trunk are equally affected.

Investigations

Diagnosis is based on the typical features of the condition and characteristic radiographic appearances. If there is clinical suspicion of skeletal dysplasia, a full skeletal survey should be performed. Radiographic features of achondroplasia include:

▷ Short bones.

▷ Metaphyseal irregularity.

▷ Small iliac wings.

▷ Narrow pelvic anteroposterior diameter.

▷ Translucent proximal femur.

▷ Progressive narrowing of the spinal inter-pedicular distance from top to bottom.

It may be possible to diagnose short limb skeletal dysplasia in the prenatal period by ultrasonography. If short limb skeletal dysplasia is diagnosed prenatally, plasma can be analysed for the FGFR3 mutation in the mother.

Management

Achondroplasia is managed symptomatically. It is recommended that children with achondroplasia are followed up at regular intervals to detect any significant complications. These occur in approximately 10% of children, and may require operative treatment.

Complications

▷ Hydrocephalus. There is rapid head growth during the first year of life which needs close monitoring because two percent of children with achondroplasia develop hydrocephalus requiring treatment.

▷ Lower limb deformities. Genu varum is common.

▷ Progressive thoracolumbar kyphosis.

The average final adult height is 131 cm in males and 124 cm in females.

Prognosis

Life expectancy is normal in the majority of affected children. However, because of the large head and short limbs, early motor development is often delayed. Intellectual development is normal.

Osteogenesis Imperfecta

Aetiology

Osteogenesis imperfecta is one of the most common inheritable bone disorders, affecting one in 20,000 children. It is characterised by defective synthesis of collagen type 1, resulting in generalised fragility of bones, teeth, ligaments, sclera and skin.

Clinical Features

There are four subtypes of osteogenesis imperfecta, showing variations in phenotype. However, common features irrespective of subtype include:

▷ Osteopenia.

▷ Bone fragility with proneness to fracture with minimal trauma.

▷ Laxity of ligaments.

Subtypes of osteogenesis imperfecta and their features are outlined in *Table 7*.

In almost all cases, the mode of inheritance is dominant or involves a new dominant mutation irrespective of the phenotypic subtype.

Investigations

▷ Severe variants can be diagnosed prenatally by ultrasound scanning.

▷ In the postnatal period, diagnosis is made on the basis of the clinical features. In mild cases, non-accidental injury is an important differential diagnosis.

▷ Plain radiographs, bone densitometry and genetic testing may all be useful aids to diagnosis. Wormian bones are seen in type 1 disease on skull X-ray.

TABLE 7: Subtypes and features of osteogenesis imperfecta			
Type I (mild)	**Type II (perinatal lethal)**	**Type III (severe deforming)**	**Type IV (moderately severe)**
• Blue sclera. • Hypermobile joints. • Little or no deformity. • Fractures occur throughout life. • Hearing loss in adulthood. • Skull shows multiple Wormian bones (extra bone pieces in the sutures of the skull).	• Multiple fractures in utero. • May be stillborn.	• Blue then white sclera. • Progressively deforming long bones and spine due to fractures. • Short stature. • Dental problems.	• Similar to type I and differentiated on the basis of having white sclera. • Variable short stature.

Management

Treatment involves physiotherapy, rehabilitation and surgery. Gentle nursing of infants is paramount to prevent fractures and prompt splinting of fractures is required to limit deformity. Bisphosphonates may reduce bone pain and fracture rate in severe disease. Surgery may be needed for fracture fixation or to correct deformities.

Prognosis

Life expectancy is normal in type I disease and only slightly reduced in type IV. When there is severe deformity as in type III, the patient may become wheelchair bound.

Osteopetrosis

Aetiology

Osteopetrosis, also known as marble bone disease, is a metabolic bone disease characterised by failure of osteoclast bone resorption secondary to carbonic anhydrase deficiency. This leads to a diffuse increase in bone density and obliteration of the marrow spaces. The end result is skeletal fragility despite an increase in bone mass. The autosomal recessive form presents in children and is more severe than the autosomal dominant form of the disease.

Investigations

X-rays are usually diagnostic. They usually show generalised osteosclerosis, although there may be areas of alternating sclerotic and lucent bands. Fractures and osteomyolytic changes may also be seen.

Clinical Features

Children with autosomal recessive osteopetrosis present with faltering growth, recurrent infections, anaemia and thrombocytopenia (due to bone marrow infiltration). It is often fatal due to overwhelming infection or severe/repeated haemorrhage. The autosomal dominant form usually presents later in childhood with pathological fractures.

Management

Treatment of severe disease is with bone marrow transplant, high dose vitamin D and gamma-interferon. Internal fixation of pathological fractures is extremely difficult as the dense bone makes fixation and drilling challenging.

Idiopathic Scoliosis

Scoliosis is lateral curvature in the frontal plane of the spine. For thoracic scoliosis, characteristic "humps" can be seen on examining the child's back when they are bent forward. This is reflective of rotation of the thoracic ribs, from the scoliosis.

Clinical Features

Although often asymptomatic, scoliosis may cause cosmetic problems, cardiopulmonary compromise, loss of balance when mobilising and pain from spinal degenerative changes. The

TABLE 8: Neurological causes of pes cavus	
Static neurological disorders	Progressive neurological disorders
• Stroke. • Cerebral palsy. • Polio. • Spinal nerve root injury. • Peroneal nerve injury.	• Charcot-Marie-Tooth disease. • Friedreich ataxia. • Spinal/brain tumour. • Spinal trauma. • Muscular dystrophy. • Syringomyelia.

severity of the lateral curvature can be determined by measuring the angle of the curvature on a plain spine radiograph.

Management

Mild curvature does not require treatment. Braces are utilised for 23 hours daily for moderate curvature. Severe scoliosis (>40°) requires internal fixation or fusion.

Pes Cavus

Aetiology

Pes cavus can be a normal variant, or due to a congenital bony abnormality or secondary to neurological disorders where the intrinsic foot muscles are weak or paralysed. Detailed family history helps identify any underlying neurological disorder (*Table 8*).

Clinical Features

In pes cavus, the longitudinal foot arch is higher than normal. Often, there is an associated clawing of the toes as the weight is taken on the metatarsal heads when walking.

Management

Treatment depends on the cause and severity of the deformity. Often no treatment is required. Conservative measures include physiotherapy to loosen tight muscles, orthotic shoes and splints. Surgery is reserved for severe deformity or pain that limits normal activities and is unresponsive to conservative treatments.

ADDITIONAL PATHOLOGIES

Torticollis

Torticollis is a symptom rather than a diagnosis. It describes the tilting of the head in one direction, with rotation of the head in the opposite direction. It can be congenital or acquired (*Table 9*). If it is acquired, it is very important to identify any possible trauma in the history: a C-spine X-ray should be obtained if any doubts, as torticollis may relate to atlanto-occipital subluxation.

The most common cause is congenital muscular torticollis. It presents within the first few months of life, although if present in newborns, it is also important to consider a clavicular fracture as a possible cause. Congenital muscular torticollis is due to a contracture of the sternocleidomastoid muscle and there is often a fibrotic mass palpable within the substance of the muscle. It is thought to be a result of in utero stretching/compression of

TABLE 9: Causes of torticollis	
Congenital	**Acquired**
• Cervical hemivertebrae. • Soft tissue abnormalities, e.g. unilateral absence of sternocleidomastoid. • Congenital muscular torticollis. • CNS malformations.	• Atlanto-occipital subluxation. • Bone/soft tissue tumour. • Cervical lymphadenitis. • Sandifer syndrome (from gastro-oesophageal reflux). • Retropharyngeal abscess. • Ocular disorders.

the muscle. It is managed conservatively by passive stretching, stimulation and positioning. In resistant cases, botulinum toxin injection or surgical release of the sternocleidomastoid muscle should be considered.

In other cases, the underlying cause needs to be treated (e.g. reflux medication in Sandifer syndrome). Otherwise, a trial of analgesia and a soft collar may be used, with consideration of muscle relaxants and traction in those who have persistent symptoms.

Osgood-Schlatter Disease

Aetiology

This is an overuse syndrome characterised by small avulsion fractures within the tibial tuberosity due to traction from the patella tendon during forceful contraction of the quadriceps muscles. It usually occurs around the pubertal growth spurt and is associated with physical exertion before skeletal maturation. It is often seen in children who participate in sports such as football and gymnastics and is more common in boys.

Clinical Features

Children report gradual onset pain and swelling below the knee, exacerbated by physical activity and relieved by rest. Diagnosis is clinical. Examination of the hip is important as SUFE may present similarly.

Management

Osgood-Schlatter disease is self-limiting and resolves with skeletal maturation. Avoidance of strenuous physical exertion, ice packs, analgesia and quadriceps stretching and strengthening are advised.

Chondromalacia Patellae

Aetiology

Chondromalacia patellae is softening of the articular cartilage of the patella. It is a significant cause of anterior knee pain in teenage girls.

Clinical Features

Chondromalacia patellae presents with anterior knee or retropatellar pain exacerbated by standing up from a sitting position (patella becomes tightly apposed to the femoral condyles) or walking down stairs. There may be a knee effusion present. Diagnosis is clinical.

Management

Treatment is with rest, analgesia and physiotherapy for quadriceps muscle strengthening. Rarely there is misalignment of the patella requiring surgical intervention. The majority of cases resolve by 30 years of age.

Osteochondritis Dissecans

Aetiology

Osteochrondritis dissecans is the separation of a small fragment of avascular bone and overlying cartilage from one of the femoral condyles and appears as a loose body in the joint. The disorder is frequently idiopathic but it may result secondary to trauma (microtrauma or repeated minor trauma) or ischaemia.

Clinical Features

Osteochondritis dissecans usually presents in the teenage years with intermittent aching or swelling, worsened by activity. Locking, catching and giving way may occur, especially with an intra-articular loose body.

Investigations

Plain radiographs may demonstrate a loose body or subchondral crescent sign. CT or MRI can further delineate the pathology and guide management.

Management

Physiotherapy and rest is all that is required for small stable lesions. Unstable or large lesions may warrant arthroscopic removal or fixation with pins/screws.

Genu Varum

Genu varum describes bow legs.

Aetiology

Children up to the age of two years may have physiological genu varum, secondary to a tight posterior hip capsule. Pathological genu varum (or genu valgum) should be considered in:

> Any severe and progressive deformity.
> Asymmetrical knees.
> Short stature.
> Family history of skeletal problems.

Causes include rickets and skeletal dysplasias such as achondroplasia. Untreated, the condition may worsen and result in impaired mobility, knee osteoarthritis, meniscal tears and tibiofemoral subluxation.

Clinical Features

Genu varum is characterised by painless, symmetrical bowing of the legs, with a tendency for recurrent falls.

Investigation

Diagnosis is by plain radiography of the lower limbs and is often the only imaging modality required.

Management

Management of genu varum involves medical treatment of any underlying disease. This condition resolves spontaneously as the child grows and does not usually require any treatment. Corrective surgery is required when medical therapy fails or if deformity is severe.

Genu Valgum

Genu valgum describes knock knees.

Aetiology

Children between 2 and 6-years-old may have a physiological genu valgum. Typically, these children have ligamentous laxity but the condition does not cause any functional impairment.

Pathological genu valgum should be considered if:
› The deformity is severe and progressive.
› The lower limbs are asymmetrical.
› There is a family history of skeletal disorders.

Causes of pathological genu valgum include rickets and scurvy. If left untreated, knee instability and osteoarthritis may develop, with a limitation of function.

Clinical Features

It is characterised by painless, symmetrical knock knees.

Investigations

Like the genu varum deformity, genu valgum can be diagnosed with plain radiography of the lower limbs.

Management

For physiological genu valgum, parental reassurance is all that is required as the condition spontaneously resolves around 7-years-old. Although medical control of underlying disease is important, surgery is the only effective treatment for pathological genu valgum.

REFERENCES AND FURTHER READING

Trauma/Fractures

1   Soloman L, Warick D, Nayagam, S. Apley's concise system of orthopaedics and fractures. Fourth Edition. Florida: CRC Press; 2014.
2   Patterson J M. Children's fractures 'not to be missed'. Hosp Med. 2002; 63: 426-8.

Developmental Dysplasia of the Hip

1   Loder T, Skopelja E. The epidemiology and demographics of hip dysplasia. ISRN Orthopedics. 2011; 2011: 1-146.
2   Sewell MD, Rosendahl K, Eastwood DM. Developmental dysplasia of the hip. BMJ. 2009; 24;339:b4454. Available from: DOI: 10.1136/bmj.b4454.
3   Storer S, Skaggs D. Developmental dysplasia of the hip. Am Fam Physician. 2006; 74: 1310-6.

SUFE

1   Water A, Helms P, Platt M. Paediatrics: A Core Text on Child Health. Second Edition. Oxford: Oxford University Press; 2006.
2   Alshryda S et al. Intervention for treating slipped upper femoral epiphysis. The Cochrane Collaboration. 2013. www.cochrane-handbook.org.
3   Peck D. Slipped Capital Femoral Epiphysis: diagnosis and management. Am Fam Physician. 2010; 82: 258-62.
4   Uglow M, Clarke N. The management of slipped capital femoral epiphysis. J Bone Joint Br. 2004; 84: 631-5.

Perthes Disease

1   Kim H, Herring J. Pathophysiology, classifications, and natural history of Perthes disease. Orthop Clin North Am. 2011; 42: 285-95.
2   Shah, H. Perthes disease: evaluation and management. Orthop Clin North Am. 2014; 45: 87-97.
3   Perry D, Bruce C. Evaluating the child who presents with an acute limp. BMJ. 2010; 341:c4250.
4   Kim H, Herring J. Pathophysiology, classifications, and natural history of Perthes disease. Orthop Clin North Am. 2011; 42: 285-95.

Septic Arthritis

1   McCarthy J, Dormans J, Kozin S, Pizzutillo P. Musculoskeletal infections in children. J Bone Joint Surg Am. 2004; 86: 850-63.
2   Kocher M, Zurakowski D, Kasser J. Differentiating between septic arthritis and transient synovitis of the hip in children: an evidence-based clinical prediction algorithm. J Bone Joint Surg Am. 1999; 81: 1662-70.
3   Caird M et al. Factors distinguishing septic arthritis from transient synovitis of the hip in children. A prospective study. J Bone Joint Surg Am. 2006; 88: 1251-7.

Osteomyelitis

1   Lazzarini L, Mader T, Calhorn J. Osteomyelitis in long bone. J Bone Joint Surg Am. 2004; 86: 2305-18.
2   Yeo A, Ramachandran M . Acute haematogenous osteomyelitis in children. BMJ. 2014; 348:g66.

Transient Synovitis

1   Nouri A, Walmsley D, Pruszczynski B, Synder M. Transient synovitis of the hip: a comprehensive review. J Pediatr Orthop B. 2014; 23:32-6.
2   Hart, J. Transient synovitis of the hip in children. Am Fam Physician. 1996; 54: 1587-91.
3   Do T. Transient synovitis as a cause of painful limps in children. Curr Opin Pediatr. 2000; 12: 48-51.

Reactive Arthritis

1   Taylor-Robinson D (ed.). Clinical Problems in Sexually Transmitted Diseases (New Perspectives in

Clinical Microbiology). Dordrecht: Martinus Nijhoff Publishers; 1985.

2   Kvien T et al. Reactive arthritis: incidence, triggering agents and clinical presentation. J Rheumatol. 1994; 21: 115-22.

3   Palazzi C, D'Amico E, Pennese E, Petricca A. Management of reactive arthritis. Expert Opin Pharmacother. 2004; 5: 61-70.

4   Selmi C, Gershwin M. Diagnosis and classification of reactive arthritis. Autoimmun Rev. 2014; 13: 546-9.

Juvenile Idiopathic Arthritis

1   Ravelli A, Martini A. Juvenile idiopathic arthritis. Lancet. 2007; 369: 767-78.

2   Adib N, Silman A, Thomson W. Outcome following onset of juvenile idiopathic inflammatory arthritis: I. frequency of different outcomes. Rheumatology (Oxford). 2005; 44: 995-1001.

3   Oen K et al. Disease course and outcome of juvenile rheumatoid arthritis in a multicenter cohort. J Rheumatol. 2002; 29: 1989-99.

Ankylosing Spondylitis

1   McVeigh, C., Cairns, A. Diagnosis and management of ankylosing spondylitis. BMJ. 2006; 333:581.

2   Zochling J, van der Heijde D, Dougados M, Braun J. Current evidence for the management of ankylosing spondylitis: a systematic literature review for the ASAS/EULAR management recommendations in ankylosing spondylitis. Ann Rheum Dis. 2006; 65: 423-32.

SLE

1   D'Cruz DP. Systemic lupus erythematosus. BMJ. 2006; 332: 890-4.

Dermatomyositis

1   Callen J, Wortmann R. Dermatomyositis. Clin Dermatol. 2006; 24: 363-73.

2   Martin N, Li C, Wedderburn L. Juvenile dermatomyositis: new insights and new treatment strategies. Ther Adv Musculoskelet Dis. 2012; 4: 41–50.

Sarcoidosis

1   Shetty A, Gedalia A. Childhood sarcoidosis: a rare but fascinating disorder. Paediatr Rheumatol. 2008; 6: 16.

Marfan's Syndrome

1   Online Mendelian Inheritance in Man (OMIM). Marfan's Syndrome; MFS. [Online] http://omim.org/entry/154700.

2   Tierney E, Feingold B, Printz B. Beta-blocker therapy does not alter the rate of aortic root dilation in pediatric patients with Marfan syndrome. J Pediatr. 2007; 150: 77-82.

3   Matt P et al. Recent advances in understanding Marfan syndrome: should we now treat surgical patients with losartan? J Thorac Cardiovasc Surg. 2008; 135: 389-94.

4   Williams A et al. Medical treatment of Marfan syndrome: a time for change. Heart. 2008; 94: 414-21.

Achondroplasia

1   Nahar R et al. Molecular studies of achondroplasia. Indian J Orthop. 2009; 43: 194-6.

2   Wright M, Irving M. Clinical management of achondroplasia. Arch Dis Child. 2012; 97: 129-34.

Osteogenesis Imperfecta

1   Rush E, Plotkin H. Genetics of Osteogenesis Imperfecta. Medscape 2012. http://emedicine.medscape.com/article/947588-overview.

Osteopetrosis

1   Wilson C, Vellodi A. Autosomal recessive osteopetrosis: diagnosis, management, and outcome. Arch Disease Child. 2000; 83(5): 449–52.

Scoliosis

1   Altaf F, Gibson A, Dannawi Z. Adolescent idiopathic scoliosis. BMJ. 2013; 346:f2508.

Pes Cavus

1   Marks R. Midfoot and forefoot issues cavovarus foot: assessment and treatment issues. Foot Ankle Clin. 2008; 13: 229-41.

2   Wicart P. Cavus foot, from neonates to adolescents. Orthop Traumatol Surg Res. 2012; 98: 813-28.

Torticollis

1   Tomczak K, Rosman N. Torticollis. J Child Neurol. 2013; 28(3): 365-78.

Osgood-Schlatter Disease

1   Weiler R, Ingram M, Wolman R. 10-Minute Consultation. Osgood-Schlatter disease. BMJ. 2011; 343:d4534.

Chondromalacia Patellae

1   Hong E, Kraft M. Evaluating anterior knee pain. Med Clin North Am. 2014; 98: 697-717.

Osteochondritis Dissecans

1   Pascual-Garrido C, Moran C, Green D, Cole B. Osteochondritis dissecans of the knee in children and adolescents. Curr Opin Pediatr. 2013; 25: 46-51.

2   Hixon A, Gibbs L. Osteochondritis dissecans: a diagnosis not to miss. Am Fam Physician. 2000; 61: 151-6.

Genu Varum and Genu Valgum

1   Soloman L, Warick D, Nayagam, S. Apley's Concise System of Orthopaedics and Fractures. Fourth Edition. Florida: CRC Press; 2014.

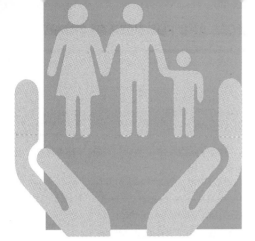

1.20
PUBLIC HEALTH
CHRISTOPHER HARRIS

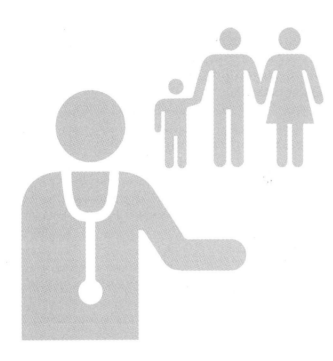

CONTENTS

INTRODUCTION

Calculations for worldwide childhood morbidity and mortality are integral to healthcare planning and political direction. A 2013 article in the *Lancet* reported that 6.3 million children were estimated to die before the age of five, with 51.8% dying of infectious causes and 44% dying in the neonatal period. When compared to mortality rates in 2000, advances in treating pneumonia, diarrhoea and measles were collectively responsible for a reduction of approximately 1.8 million deaths. Projected estimates from this data predict 4.4 million children dying under five years in 2030. Part of the global health agenda is to identify and reduce preventable deaths.

Today, mortality is falling, but morbidity is increasing. For example, of the estimated 1.15 million babies with neonatal encephalopathy in 2010, 287,000 died, but a further 412,000 were estimated to survive with neurological impairment. With the provision of modern medicine and suitable intensive care, more babies are surviving, but the resultant medical complications continue throughout their childhood and into adulthood. These complications can reduce quality of life, and even if well managed, represent a major financial cost. More generally, children who would have died from acute infections or due to complications of a medical condition are surviving longer with chronic health concerns.

A summary of key causes of mortality, and morbidity are shown in *Table 1-2.*

The cost of providing healthcare worldwide is increasing. Ill health and disease have financial, social and potentially health implications that go beyond the single patient who seeks medical attention. Through public health, it is possible to reduce these burdens of healthcare and better manage the finite resources of individual regions, countries and the world as a whole. Forward planning, health promotion and service provision must evolve to meet the growing and ever changing demands of our diverse populations.

As we entered the new millennium, it was recognised that a common framework was needed to provide measurable improvements in health and wellbeing across the developing world. In September 2000, world leaders signed up to the United Nations Millennium Development Goals (MDGs). These were goals designed to focus efforts on a national and international level until 2015. Both progress and solutions

TABLE 1: Causes of mortality in the UK and world (1) – ONS UK 2012, (2)- WHO 2004-14			
UK		**Worldwide**	
Leading causes of mortality in under 5-year-olds	Leading causes of mortality in 5 to 19-year-olds	Leading causes of mortality in under 5-year-olds	Leading causes of mortality in 5 to 15-year-olds
1 Birth complications and prematurity. 2 Congenital abnormalities. 3 Neoplasm. 4 Trauma. 5 Infections. 6 Metabolic and endocrine disorders.	1 Trauma and accidents. 2 Neoplasm. 3 Congenital abnormalities. 4 Infections.	1 Birth complications and prematurity. 2 Pneumonia. 3 Diarrhoea. 4 Malaria. 5 Measles. 6 HIV/AIDs.	1 Trauma and accidents. 2 Infections. 3 Nutritional deficiencies. 4 Congenital abnormalities. 5 Neurological causes. 6 Metabolic and endocrine diseases.

varied dramatically between nations, however, overall the goals were reported as a major success in improving equality across a wide range of issues. In 2015, the MDGs were replaced by the Sustainable Development Goals (*Table 3*). These are far more wide ranging and took note of concerns levelled at the original goals; that they did not go far enough and they were not specific enough. There continues to be a large focus on paediatric health in these goals, recognising that children are a vulnerable group in the developing world with no voice of their own.

Public health officials must work closely with governments and investors to ensure the decisions made have the highest impact at the lowest cost (financial and otherwise) to the public. It is clear that with good public health planning and implementation, the long-term cost to individual countries will be reduced and economic growth strengthened. Public health initiatives are not restricted to medical interventions.

TABLE 2: Causes of morbidity in the UK and world (1) – ONS UK 2012, (2)- WHO 2002-14	
UK Causes of childhood morbidity	Worldwide causes of childhood morbidity
1 Disability relating to birth/ congenital abnormality. 2 Disability relating to trauma. 3 Disability relating to acute illness. 4 Asthma. 5 Diabetes. 6 Obesity.	1 Disability relating to birth/ congenital abnormality. 2 Disability relating to trauma. 3 Disability relating to acute illness. 4 HIV/AIDS. 5 Chronic infection. 6 Malnutrition.

They also include:

> Education.
> Healthy living.
> Accident prevention.
> Reducing health inequality.
> Healthcare provision.

TABLE 3: Millennium and Sustainable Development Goals	
Millennium Development Goals	Sustainable Development Goals
1 Eradicate extreme poverty and hunger. 2 Achieve universal primary education. 3 Promote gender equality and empower women. 4 Reduce child mortality. 5 Improve maternal health. 6 Combat HIV/Aids and other diseases. 7 Ensure environmental sustainability. 8 Global partnership for development.	1 End poverty in all its forms everywhere. 2 End hunger, achieve food security and improved nutrition, and promote sustainable agriculture. 3 Ensure healthy lives and promote wellbeing for all at all ages. 4 Ensure inclusive and equitable quality education and promote lifelong learning opportunities for all. 5 Achieve gender equality and empower all women and girls. 6 Ensure availability and sustainable management of water and sanitation for all. 7 Ensure access to affordable, reliable, sustainable and modern energy for all. 8 Promote inclusive and sustainable economic growth, full and productive employment and decent work for all. 9 Build resilient infrastructure, promote inclusive and sustainable industrialisation and foster innovation. 10 Reduce inequality within and among countries. 11 Make cities and human settlements inclusive, safe, resilient and sustainable. 12 Ensure sustainable consumption and production patterns. 13 Take urgent action to combat climate change. 14 Conserve and sustainably use the oceans, seas and marine resources for sustainable development. 15 Protect, restore and promote sustainable use of terrestrial ecosystems, sustainably manage forests, combat desertification, halt and reverse land degradation and halt biodiversity loss. 16 Promote peaceful and inclusive societies for sustainable development, provide access to justice for all and build effective, accountable and inclusive institutions at all levels. 17 Strengthen the means of implementation and revitalise the global partnership for sustainable development.

Local councils, schools, healthcare workers, national governments, international groups and charities work towards achieving the core aims of public health through a variety of measures. The objectives of these groups vary to reflect the differences in global, national and local causes of morbidity and mortality.

However, the core aims of public health are:

- Promoting and protecting health and well-being.
- Preventing ill health.
- Prolonging life.

PROVIDERS OF HEALTH CARE SERVICES FOR CHILDREN

Primary Care Facilities

Primary care physicians and related services form a vital part of the National Childhood Surveillance Service in the UK through set appointments for:

1 Health visitor visits post birth.
2 Baby checks at six weeks.
3 School medical care (school nurses).

Unwell children are primarily brought to primary care settings, (either primary care physicians or paediatric specialists in a community setting) who can provide diagnosis, treatment and advice in the majority of cases they see. They can also offer medical care for complex groups of patients, such as migrant children and those with social concerns. These patients often have complex medical and psychosocial needs that require special attention. Therefore, other experts are often involved, such as social services and the community paediatric team.

Primary care physicians are able to refer any child, if needed, to a wide range of specialist services such as:

- Physiotherapy.
- Occupational therapy.
- Speech and Language Therapy (SALT).
- Hearing screening.
- Parent support groups.
- Health visitors.
- Community paediatrics.

TABLE 4: Specialist paediatric care	
Secondary and Tertiary Care Facility	**Role in Child Health**
Midwives.	Monitor newborn infants up to 14 to 28–days-old. Ensure good feeding, growth and development.
Emergency Services.	Provide urgent care for sick children. Important role in identifying child protection concerns.
Paediatric Inpatient Wards.	Specialist paediatric care. Provide on-going care for sick children who require admission. Can provide a place of safety for a child.
Paediatric Outpatient Services.	Specialist paediatric care. Children requiring on-going specialist care. Monitoring of illness and development.
Subspecialist Care (e.g. cardiology, endocrinology, surgery and oncology).	Satellite clinics run from a central location. Access to specialised testing, diagnostics and treatment.
Community Paediatric Services.	Developmental assessment. Behaviour assessment. Autism diagnosis and care. Coordinate vaccination strategy. Regular check-ups for looked after children. Assess medical needs for children who require educational support in schools. Child protection.

TABLE 5: Professional groups involved in childcare	
Service Provider	**Role in Child Health**
Schools.	Child surveillance. Identify learning and developmental difficulties. Integrate children with health needs into education. Child protection.
Social Services.	Investigate child protection issues. Care for children when parents are not able or safe to do so, through fostering and adoption placements. Acquire funding to meet health needs of a child (e.g. home alterations).
Local Councils and Governments.	Provide funding for health initiatives and services. Promote healthy living. Provide parks and other leisure activities. Support children's centres. Road safety and accident prevention.
Charities and Interest Groups.	Promote specific agendas to improve child health, some examples: • Barnardo's (homeless children). • NSPCC and Childline. • Sporting groups. • Save the Children. • Oxfam.

- Secondary/tertiary paediatric care.
- Community and Adolescent Mental Health Services (CAMHS).

Secondary and Tertiary Care

Parents and children may access secondary care services directly or by referral from another healthcare professional. Schools, police and social services may also seek specialist paediatric advice or referral. Secondary and tertiary care services work closely with primary care services to ensure good patient centred care.

Examples of professional groups in secondary and tertiary care are listed in *Table 4*.

Other Service Providers

It has been recognised that the health and development of infants and children is affected by a number of factors outside of primary or secondary care. Professionals, charities and other groups can work to improve child health, both directly and indirectly. Some examples are summarised in *Table 5*.

HEALTH PROMOTION FOR CHILDREN

Evidence shows that choices made during a child's development affect health and well-being during adulthood. A key role of public health workers is to promote healthy choices and support a broader agenda for health improvement.

Some key initiatives affecting children have been:

> Promoting breastfeeding through the World Health Organisation (WHO).
> Smoking cessation support for both parents and children.
> Encouraging healthy eating and micronutrient recommendations.
> Increasing the provision and uptake of antenatal and maternity care.
> Increasing public awareness of mental health issues in children and adolescents.
> Free healthy school meals.
> Vitamin D supplementation.

All health workers should recognise issues that may precipitate or worsen medical illness. For example, a health professional that sees a child with worsening asthma can support a family trying to resolve damp in their home. Public health officials may promote the benefits of having greater numbers of open spaces and parks for combating obesity in children.

PROTECTING CHILDREN'S HEALTH

Some diseases, illnesses or injuries can be prevented or their effects mitigated by good planning, preventative measures or early identification.

Immunisation

Since Edward Jenner first discovered the role of cowpox in protecting individuals from smallpox, immunisation has been a key part of global health care. Immunisations are available for a large number of conditions that previously had a high mortality or morbidity rate. They may be given routinely (diphtheria, polio, pertussis, tetanus, meningitis C, pneumococcus, measles, mumps and rubella), in response to increased exposure or outbreak (BCG, measles booster, hepatitis B), or to protect children travelling to an "at risk" area (hepatitis A, typhoid, yellow fever, rabies). In the future, it is hoped that there will be vaccines available for HIV, malaria and many other important diseases. See p150.

Notifiable Diseases

Some infectious diseases must be reported to the relevant public health authority to ensure that there is a prompt investigation, urgent risk assessment and rapid response to the illness. This has been shown to prevent epidemics and pandemics. It is not necessary to confirm the diagnosis, as this may take days with laboratory testing. If a clinician suspects a notifiable disease, the health protection agency should be informed. They will help with contact tracing and provide prophylaxis medication to any deemed at risk of infection. Examples of notifiable diseases are shown in *Table 6*. *Table 7* lists the differences between endemic, epidemic and pandemic diseases.

Accident Prevention

The police, fire brigade and medical profession all have a role in accident prevention. Identifying patterns and geographical locations of injuries presenting to an ED might highlight an on-going safety concern. In addition, some countries review all paediatric deaths such as in the UK (Child Death Review Panel) to identify broader risk to the population. The responsible body can then act on these concerns to reduce or remove the risk. Risks identified this way could be:

> An unsafe piece of equipment in a school playground.
> Poor visibility at pedestrian crossings.
> Lack of supervision at a play centre.
> Lack of a barrier around deep water.

Vulnerable Children

In every society, there are high-risk children for health problems,

TABLE 6: Some notifiable diseases in the UK
Notifiable diseases
Meningitis.
Poliomyelitis.
Anthrax.
Cholera.
Food poisoning (e.g. salmonella).
Hepatitis A and B.
E Coli 0157.
Malaria.
Measles.
Mumps.
Rubella.
Viral haemorrhagic fever (Ebola).
Pertussis.

TABLE 7: Useful definitions in public health		
Word	Definition	Example
Endemic.	A disease regularly found in a population.	Obesity is endemic in the UK.
Epidemic.	A disease that spreads to a large number of people in a population rapidly over a short period.	The measles epidemic in Wales 2013.
Pandemic.	A disease that spreads across different populations.	The HIV pandemic has spread to affect people from all continents.

TABLE 8: Examples of vulnerable children in the UK		
Group of Vulnerable Children	Professionals commonly involved	Specific health needs
Children at risk of neglect, emotional, physical or sexual abuse and children who are removed from their parents.	• Community Paediatrician. • Social Services. • Family Courts.	• Emotional support. • Child protection medicals. • Ensuring normal development. • Behavioural support.
Children with disabilities.	• Community Paediatrician. • General Paediatrician. • Speciality Paediatrician. • Physiotherapist. • Occupational therapist. • Speech and language therapist. • Social services.	• Complex and varied needs. • Coordination of and communication between multiple professionals.
Children seeking or granted asylum.	• Community Paediatrician. • Social Services. • Immigration Services.	• Exposure to tropical diseases. • Emotional support. • Integration.
Children with special educational needs.	• Community Paediatrician. • Social Services. • School teachers and nurse.	• Assess needs in school. • Input support required.

faltering growth or abuse. In the UK, every effort is made to identify these children, anticipate their needs and ensure they receive appropriate care (*Table 8*).

REFERENCES AND FURTHER READING

Mortality and Morbidity

1 Office for National Statistics. Childhood, Infant and Perinatal Mortality in England and Wales, 2013. http://www.ons.gov.uk/ons/rel/vsob1/child-mortality-statistics--childhood--infant-and-perinatal/2013/stb-child-mortality-stats-2013.html.
2 Countdown to 2015. 2010 Countdown to 2010 Decade Report (2000-2010). http://www.countdown2015mnch.org/reports-and-articles/previous-reports/2010-decade-report.
3 The Millennium Development Goals Report 2015. United Nations, Department of Economic and Social Affairs of the United Nations Secretariat; 2015. http://www.un.org/millenniumgoals/2015_MDG_Report/pdf/MDG%202015%20rev%20(July%201).pdf.
4 Wang H et al. Global, regional, and national levels of neonatal, infant, and under-5 mortality during 1990-2013: a systematic analysis for the Global Burden of Disease Study 2013. Lancet. 2014;384:957-79.

Services for Children

1 NHS Choices. 2015. Newborn and Infant Physical Exam. http://cpd.screening.nhs.uk/nipe.
2 Knowles RL et al. Surveillance of rare diseases: a public health evaluation of the British Paediatric Surveillance Unit. J Pub Health. 2012;34:279-86.

Health Promotion

1 Piernas C et al. The double burden of under- and overnutrition and nutrient adequacy among Chinese preschool and school-aged children in 2009-2011. Eur. J. Clin Nutr. 2015;69:1323-9.
2 Liu H, Umberson D. Gender, stress in childhood and adulthood, and trajectories of change in body mass. Soc Sci Med. 2015;139:61-9.

Infectious Diseases

1 Public Health England. 2014. Immunisation against Infectious Disease. https://www.gov.uk/government/collections/immunisation-against-infectious-disease-the-green-book
2 Public Health England. 2014. Notifications of Infectious diseases (NOIDs). https://www.gov.uk/government/collections/notifications-of-infectious-diseases-noids

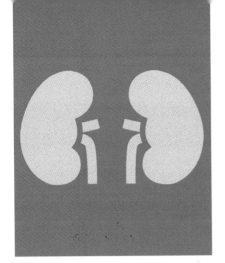

1.21
RENAL MEDICINE

ZESHAN QURESHI, RACHAEL MITCHELL AND STEPHEN D MARKS

CLINICAL MANIFESTATIONS OF RENAL DISEASE

Acute Kidney Injury

Acute Kidney Injury (AKI) can be defined as a sudden decrease in renal function; elevated urea is followed by an elevated creatinine and a resulting decreasing glomerular filtration rate (GFR). There are often associated difficulties in fluid and electrolyte regulation as well as with blood pressure control.

There are numerous definitions for AKI, but one which is widely used is the paediatric RIFLE (pRIFLE) which uses change in creatinine clearance and/or urine output for the definition (*Table 1*). Note that creatinine clearance is an approximation for the GFR, but is an overestimate (as creatinine is both filtered by the glomerulus, and secreted by the proximal tubule).

Aetiology

The causes of acute kidney injury can be pre-renal, renal or post-renal and are summarised in *Table 2*.

Clinical Features

Acute kidney injury can present nonspecifically, particularly in neonates with symptoms such as unexplained crying, restlessness, lethargy, vomiting, or poor feeding. Other features may include reduced urine output and pallor. Most commonly acute kidney injury is related to sepsis or hypovolaemia, in which signs of the cause would be apparent.

TABLE 1: Acute Kidney Injury definitions (pRIFLE)		
Acute Kidney Injury	**Creatinine clearance**	**Urine Output**
Risk.	• Decrease by <25%.	• < 0.5ml/kg/hour for 8 hours.
Injury.	• Decrease by <50%.	• < 0.5ml/kg/hour for 16 hours.
Failure.	• Decrease by <75% (or <35mL/min/1.73m²).	• < 0.3ml/kg/hour for 24 hours, or anuric > 12 hours.
Loss of function.	Prolonged loss of function (> 4 weeks).	
End stage.	Prolonged loss of function (>3 months).	

TABLE 2: Causes and management of acute kidney injury

	Cause	Management
Pre-renal (hypoperfusion of kidney).	• Hypovolaemic shock (e.g. gastroenteritis, burns, haemorrhage, nephrotic syndrome). • Septic shock. • Cardiogenic shock.	• Replacement of intravascular fluid, but if severe it may require more specialist input.
Renal (intrinsic renal pathology).	• Renal disease (e.g. glomerulonephritis, acute tubular necrosis, pyelonephritis, renal vein or venous thrombosis, vasculitis).	• Management is complex, requiring specialist input. Fluid restriction may be necessary if there is circulatory overload. A low-protein high-calorie diet may also be required. A percutaneous renal biopsy may be required to confirm a diagnosis, as some disorders such as rapidly progressive glomerulonephritis require immediate specific treatment.
Post-renal (obstruction of outflow tract).	• Obstruction, which may be congenital (e.g. posterior urethral valves), or acquired (e.g. an abdominal mass obstructing the ureter).	• Treatment requires identification of the site of the obstruction and targeted therapy. This may mean a urinary catheter is needed, or a nephrostomy.

More severe acute kidney injury may present with features such as:

> Haematuria.
> Rash. This may be a purpuric rash as found in HUS and HSP.
> Bloody diarrhoea. This is usually only found if AKI is caused by HUS.
> Confusion. This is usually due to uraemia.
> Abdominal pain.
> Oliguria, or conversely, high urine output.
> Oedema. This is particularly seen in the periorbital region.
> Abdominal mass. This may be due to polycystic kidney disease (PKD) or urinary retention.
> Hypertension.
> Arrhythmia. This is usually secondary to hyperkalaemia.

Investigations

A variety of investigations can be carried out for children with acute kidney injury, depending on the likely cause, severity and duration of the kidney insult. In those who have very mild AKI with a known cause, such as sepsis or dehydration, minimal investigations are needed:

Blood Tests

> U&Es. This is to quantify renal dysfunction and identify electrolyte disturbance.
> Venous blood gas. This is to allow rapid assessment of acid-base balance (pH and bicarbonate).

Urine Tests

> Dipstick. This is to identify proteinuria and haematuria.
> MC&S. This is to exclude infection, and to look for red cell casts in the context of glomerulonephritis.

In those with more severe AKI, or where the cause is unknown, additional investigations are needed:

> FBC and blood film. There may be evidence of anaemia if renal dysregulation is more longstanding. Anaemia is part of HUS, and if this is suspected, the rest of the HUS work up should also be sent.

> Early morning urine protein:creatinine (or albumin:creatinine ratio). This is to look for proteinuria more sensitively.
> Urinary sodium. This is to look for intravascular fluid depletion, which can be challenging to identify in an oedematous patient.
> Blood and stool culture. This is to identify infective causes.
> Throat swab, ASOT/antiDNase B. This is performed to identify possible post-streptococcal glomerulonephritis.
> Complement, anti-dsDNA, anti-GBM antibody, ANCA. This is looking for autoimmune causes of renal injury. Complement is also reduced in post-streptococcal glomerulonephritis.
> Urate. This is to identify urate nephropathy.
> Liver function tests (LFTs) and albumin. Low albumin is seen in nephrotic syndrome.
> Chest X-Ray. There may be pulmonary oedema secondary to AKI.
> Renal ultrasound scan (USS). This may identify a cause for renal failure e.g. hydronephrosis.
> Renal biopsy. If it is not resolving, and there is no clear cause, a biopsy may be indicated.

Management

All children in renal failure require careful fluid management. Dialysis may be required in:

> Failure to respond to conservative management.
> Severe complications from the acute kidney injury.
> > Hyperkalaemia.
> > Hypo/hypernatraemia.
> > Pulmonary oedema/hypertension.
> > Severe acidosis.
> > Severe uraemia.
> > Multisystem failure.

Additional management is shown in *Table 2*.

Complications

In the acute phase, important complications of kidney injury are:

- Metabolic acidosis. This may require fluid boluses, or bicarbonate therapy.
- Electrolyte imbalances. Hyperkalaemia is particularly important to consider. This can be significant, and resistant to standard treatments. It may require dialysis. Hypo/hypernatraemia can also be difficult to manage.
- Uraemia. This may require dialysis if severe. Can result in seizures, coma, loss of consciousness, and pericarditis.
- Pulmonary oedema. This is from fluid overload.

Long-term complications, such as hypertension and/or chronic kidney disease may also emerge.

Prognosis
Generally acute kidney injury has a good prognosis in children, although this is very dependent on the underlying cause.

Chronic Kidney Disease
The National Kidney Foundation (NKF) Kidney Disease Outcomes Quality Initiative (KDOQI) has defined Chronic Kidney Disease (CKD) as any one of the below persisting for more than three months:
- Structural abnormalities of the kidney seen on imaging.
- Functional abnormalities within the kidney (e.g. elevated creatinine and urea).
- Abnormal GFR (<60 mL/min/1.73m^2).

It has been further classified into five stages by KDOQI, as shown in *Table 3*.

GFR values for CKD staging are only accurate for children older than 2 years of age. This can be calculated via the modified Schwartz formula, as shown in *Box 1*.

TABLE 3: Stages of chronic kidney disease

Stage	Definition
1.	Kidney damage with a normal or increased GFR (>90 mL/min per 1.73 m^2).
2.	Mild reduction in the GFR (60 to 89 mL/min per 1.73 m^2).
3.	Moderate reduction in the GFR (30 to 59 mL/min per 1.73 m^2).
4.	Severe reduction in the GFR (15 to 29 mL/min per 1.73 m^2).
5.	Kidney failure (GFR <15 mL/min per 1.73 m^2 or dialysis).

Box 1: Modified Schwartz formula

$$GFR = \frac{K \times height\ (cm)}{Serum\ creatinine\ (\mu mol/L)}$$

(k is a constant coefficient [33])

For those who are age 2 or less, the creatinine clearance can be used as an approximation, as shown in *Box 2*:

Box 2: Creatinine Clearance

$$Creatinine\ Clearance = \frac{Urine\ Creatinine \times Urine\ Volume}{Serum\ Creatinine}$$

Aetiology
- Acute kidney injury due to sepsis or other insult, progressing to chronic kidney disease.
- Congenital Abnormality of the Kidney and Urinary Tract (CAKUT) with or without associated vesico-ureteric reflux.
- Chronic kidney disease secondary to glomerulonephritis.
- Multisystem disease with associated renal failure.
- Inherited conditions with renal involvement.
  - Alport syndrome.
  - Polycystic kidney disease.

Clinical Features
Chronic kidney disease is usually diagnosed late, due to its non-specific symptoms such as anorexia, lethargy or failure to thrive. It may also be identified through screening programmes (antenatally or sibling screening), or as the progression of acute kidney injury. Presentation can be extremely late, at the point of complications, or at the point of an acute kidney injury on already diseased kidneys.

Investigations
Investigations are guided by the clinical history, but all those listed for acute renal failure are potentially helpful in evaluating chronic kidney disease as well. With regard to chronic kidney disease:
- Blood Tests. Fasting lipids are useful to check, due to the association of dyslipidaemia with chronic kidney disease. As renal osteodystrophy is more likely with chronic kidney disease, check calcium, phosphate, vitamin D and parathyroid hormone levels.
- Renal Imaging. USS can identify structural abnormalities and the size of kidneys. Small kidneys may indicate renal hypoplasia. A DMSA scan will identify any scarring. Micturating cystourethrograms will look for any reflux. Other tests, such as mercaptoacetyltriglycine (MAG3) scans, can assess kidney function.

Management
Children with chronic kidney disease are managed in specialist renal centres involving paediatric nephrologists, pharmacists, dieticians and nurses.
Management may include:
- Nutrition. This is due to changes in appetite and increased metabolic requirements. Dietetic input is required, usually with gastrostomy (occasional nasogastric) tube feeding which

ensures adequate calorie and protein intake, so that it is enough to facilitate growth. This may be further manipulated to reduce sodium, potassium and phosphate intake, although some children with salt-losing dysplastic kidneys may require supplementation.

›   Vitamin D supplementation and phosphate binding. Renal failure results in reduced vitamin D activation, leading to secondary hyperparathyroidism, and subsequent hyperphosphataemia.

›   Bicarbonate therapy. To treat acidosis.

›   Iron supplementation and erythropoietin therapy. In children with anaemia.

›   Growth hormone therapy. Growth hormone therapy is helpful if there is no improved growth after dietetic input with enteral feeding. In reality few children require this.

›   Renal dialysis or renal transplantation. May be required in severe cases.

Complications

Complications of chronic kidney disease include that of acute renal injury, plus:

›   Hypertension. This may require long-term medication.

›   Renal osteodystrophy. This is due to secondary hyperparathyroidism, resulting in low calcium and elevated phosphate. Vitamin D levels are also low from reduced renal activation. Renal osteodystrophy is a result of bone mineralisation deficiency, leading to bone deformation, fractures and pain.

›   Anaemia. This occurs secondary to chronic disease, and erythropoietin deficiency.

›   Failure to thrive. This is present due to chronic disease, and anaemia.

›   Dyslipidaemia. Commonly associated with chronic kidney disease, dyslipidaemia increases the risk of cardiovascular disease in later life.

›   Endocrine dysregulation. Chronic kidney disease is associated with gonadal hormone abnormalities, with associated pubertal delay. There is also an effect on the growth hormone and insulin like growth factor axis, contributing to the poor growth seen in chronic kidney disease.

›   Fatigue and sleep disorder. This is common, and worsens with severity of disease.

›   Neurological complications. This is associated with uraemia, and may include intellectual impairment, developmental delay and seizures.

Prognosis

Chronic kidney disease is associated with a significant increase in morbidity and mortality, particularly if it has progressed to stage 5 disease. Cardiovascular disease and infection are the commonest cause of death.

Hypertension

Aetiology

›   Essential hypertension. Primary hypertension which may be associated with obesity.

›   Renal causes. Malignancy, parenchymal disease, renal artery stenosis.

›   Endocrine causes. Neuroblastoma, phaeochromocytoma, congenital adrenal hyperplasia, Cushing's syndrome.

›   Medication. Corticosteroids.

›   Cardiac conditions. Coarctation of the aorta is the most common in those presenting under one.

Clinical Features

Children may have hypertension detected incidentally during routine medical review, for example when registering with a new doctor, during screening (as part of association with a syndrome) or intra-operatively.

Symptomatic hypertension is concerning and may present with headache, vomiting and, in more severe cases, convulsions, with evidence of target organ damage such as left ventricular hypertrophy and hypertensive retinopathy.

Management

Treatment of the underlying condition should be sought, but antihypertensive therapy may be necessary in the long-term. The antihypertensive agent of choice will depend on the aetiology; for example if the cause is fluid overload due to corticosteroids, a diuretic like furosemide would be used. In older children, where long-acting anti-hypertensives are needed, agents such as calcium channel blockers or ACE inhibitors would be used.

Complications

Hypertension predisposes to myocardial infarction, ventricular dysfunction, kidney dysfunction and stroke in later life.

Nephritic Syndrome

The hallmark of nephritic syndrome is microscopic haematuria, but there may also be proteinuria, oedema and hypertension caused by fluid retention due to oliguria. Nephritic syndrome is not a diagnosis, but a clinical syndrome with several underlying causes.

Aetiology

Macroscopic and/or microscopic haematuria has a wide range of differential diagnoses, and the clinical history may help in delineating the cause:

›   Infection. Cystitis, tuberculosis, infective endocarditis, schistosomiasis.

›   Tumours. Renal or bladder.

›   Trauma. This can be anywhere from the kidney to the urethra.

- **Inflammation.** Glomerulonephritis, Immunoglobin A (IgA) vasculitis, IgA nephropathy, Goodpasture syndrome, Alport syndrome.
- **Structural lesions.** Nephrolithiasis, polycystic kidney disease.
- **Haematological.** Sickle cell anaemia, coagulopathies, renal vein and venous thromboses.
- **Medications.** Nonsteroidal anti-inflammatory drugs (NSAIDs), sulphonamides.

Post-infectious Glomerulonephritis

Post-infectious glomerulonephritis is the commonest cause of nephritic syndrome and a mixed nephritic-nephrotic syndrome. It is often caused by Group A *Streptococcus*, and typically presents one to two weeks after a streptococcal throat infection. Diagnosis is based on clinical history, positive anti-streptolysin O antibody titre (ASOT) and Anti-DNase B titres, plus reduced complement C3 and C4 levels. Other infections can also cause a post-infective glomerulonephritis.

IgA Nephropathy

This usually presents as macroscopic haematuria in association with an upper respiratory tract infection (URTI) when IgA levels may be elevated. The only definite way to diagnose this is via percutaneous renal biopsy, but this is rarely required, unless there are recurrent episodes of macroscopic haematuria. The prognosis in children is better than that in adults.

Investigations

Clinical investigations for haematuria may not be necessary if there is a clear superficial site of trauma, which could also cause macroscopic haematuria. If there is a strong clinical suspicion of a urinary tract infection (UTI), and microscopic haematuria, sending a urine specimen for MC&S may be all that is necessary.

More generally, investigations to consider include the following:

Urine Tests

- **Dipstick.** This is to quantify any blood, protein, leucocytes or nitrites.
- **MC&S.** This is to look for infection or red cell casts (associated with glomerulonephritis).
- **Early morning urine albumin:creatinine ratio (and/or protein:creatine ratio).** This is to look for possible nephrotic syndrome, and assess kidney dysfunction.

Basic Blood Tests

- **Renal function, electrolytes, LFTs and albumin.** To identify any acute kidney injury, electrolyte disturbances, and hypoalbuminaemia.
- **ASOT (anti-streptolysin O antibody titres) and Anti-DNase B titres.** This is specific for streptococcal exposure, and helps support a diagnosis of post-infectious glomerulonephritis if there is clinical evidence of previous infection.
- **Full blood count.** This is to look for anaemia from blood loss, and thrombocytopenia.
- **Coagulation screen.** This is to look for bleeding disorders.
- **Complement levels.** Low C3 and/or C4 may be associated with post infectious GN.
- **Erythrocyte sedimentation rate (ESR).** This is associated with autoimmune diseases such as SLE, and with infection.
- **Auto-antibody tests.** Elevated ANA and dsDNA may suggest an autoimmune disorder such as SLE. Anti-glomerular basement membrane (GBM) antibodies are positive in Goodpasture syndrome.
- **Sickle cell screen.** This may be considered in those of Afro-Caribbean descent.

Additional Tests

- **Throat swab.** This is to look for streptococcal infection.
- **Renal USS.** This will identify any parenchymal abnormalities in the kidney, including any masses.
- **Percutaneous renal biopsy.** This may be necessary for persistent haematuria with no obvious cause.
- **Audiology referral.** Alport syndrome is a rare hereditary nephritis characterised by loss of renal function and associated hearing loss. Testing the child's hearing and performing a urine dipstick of the mother's urine may be helpful if this is suspected.
- **Abdominal X-ray.** Kidney-Ureter-Bladder (KUB) X-ray is not routinely used but may be helpful for visualising renal calculi at the vesico-ureteric junction which may be more difficult to identify on ultrasound.

Management

Management should be tailored to the likely cause, but is generally supportive therapy, including fluid and electrolyte monitoring. Renal function may deteriorate, both acutely and long-term, so it needs to be monitored.

Note that the course of nephritic syndrome may be rapidly progressive glomerulonephritis. This is not a diagnosis in itself; rather, it a description of disease progression. It is characterised by rapid deterioration of glomerular filtration rate and usually associated with crescent formation (fibrin deposition in the shape of crescents) on percutaneous renal biopsy. This requires treatment with immunosuppression, usually initially with pulses of corticosteroids with intravenous methylprednisolone (and further immunosuppression). It may also require dialysis and/or plasmapheresis. There is an associated mortality and it may progress from acute kidney injury to chronic kidney disease and the requirement for chronic dialysis and/or renal transplantation.

Prognosis

Outlook is related to underlying aetiology. Children have better outcomes than adults, and usually recover completely.

Nephrotic Syndrome

Nephrotic syndrome is a syndrome of:

- **Nephrotic range proteinuria** (>1g/m^2/day or 3+ of protein on dipstick).

> Hypoalbuminaemia (<25g/L).
> Oedema. May be a later sign or may not be present.

It is also usually associated with hyperlipidaemia.

Aetiology

Eighty percent of cases in children are due to minimal change disease (*Figure 1*), which has normal light microscopy appearance, but a typical electron microscopy appearance with podocyte foot process effacement. Children usually present between 2 and 6-years-old. Rarely, children under 12-months-old can present with infantile nephrotic syndrome, or over 10-years-old with congenital nephrotic syndrome. These have a poorer prognosis.

Other less common causes are as follows:

> Focal and segmental glomerulosclerosis. Scarring in scattered regions of the kidney is seen on histopathology. "Focal" means that only some of the glomeruli become scarred. "Segmental" means damage affects only part of an individual glomerulus.
> Membranous nephropathy. There is thickening of blood vessels in the glomeruli resulting in proteinuria and nephrotic syndrome.
> Membranoproliferative glomerulonephritis. This is a group of disorders. Some of them involve deposition of antibodies in the glomeruli, causing thickening and damage, which usually has a nephritic picture.

Risk factors include:

> Asian ethnicity.
> Male gender.
> Previous infections. Upper respiratory tract infections (URTIs) or hepatitis.
> Medications. e.g. NSAIDs (nonsteroidal anti-inflammatory drugs).
> Systemic lupus erythematosus.

> Diabetes mellitus.
> Human immunodeficiency virus.
> Family history of nephrotic syndrome.
> Previous nephrotic syndrome.

Clinical Features

Symptoms vary depending on the underlying aetiology and the severity of the condition. It may simply present with mild oedema. Periorbital oedema is often the earliest sign (*Figure 2*) and may be initially misdiagnosed as an allergic reaction.

Other possible symptoms include:

> Discomfort relating to swelling or skin breakdown.
> Weight gain.
> Abdominal distension.
> Tiredness.
> Foamy urine.
> Increased infections. This is particularly from encapsulated organisms like pneumococcal or *Haemophilus* infection.
> Poor growth and development.

FIGURE 1

Normal

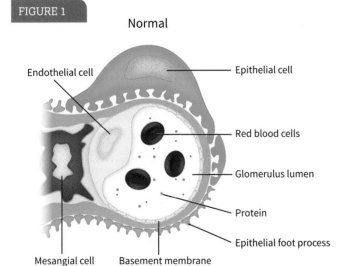

Endothelial cell
Epithelial cell
Red blood cells
Glomerulus lumen
Protein
Epithelial foot process
Mesangial cell   Basement membrane

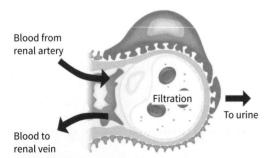

Blood from renal artery
Filtration
To urine
Blood to renal vein

Minimal change disease

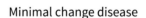
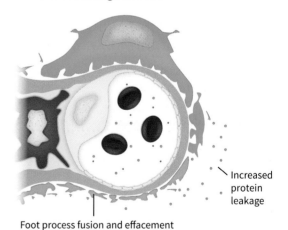

Increased protein leakage

Foot process fusion and effacement

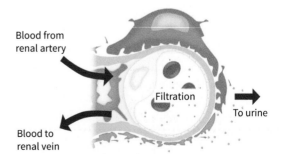

Blood from renal artery
Filtration
To urine
Blood to renal vein

Minimal change disease.

FIGURE 2

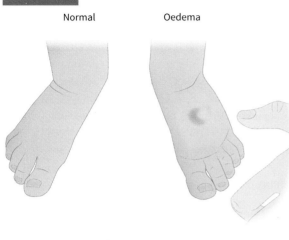

Normal   Oedema

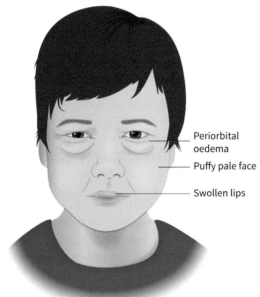

Periorbital oedema

Puffy pale face

Swollen lips

Oedema. Test for the presence by showing indentation of the skin (top). The presence of periorbital oedema (bottom) is often an early sign.

Investigations
Investigations involve confirming the diagnosis and the severity of the condition, and trying to assess the likely underlying pathology.

➤ Assess degree of proteinuria. Multiple tests can be done for this (*Table* 4). Early morning urine protein:creatinine or albumin:creatinine ratios are increasingly being used. These are used as the amount of creatinine excreted is relatively constant; changes in protein or albumin in relation to creatinine can therefore be a good guide to overall proteinuria.

➤ Lipid profile. Nephrotic syndrome is associated with hypercholesterolaemia.

➤ Renal function and urinary sodium. This will guide fluid balance. High urinary sodium indicates intravascular fluid depletion (which may otherwise be difficult to identify in oedematous patients).

TABLE 4: Protein tests	
Test	**Nephrotic syndrome**
Plasma albumin.	<25g/L
Urine dipstick.	3+ of protein
Spot early morning protein:creatinine ratio.	>100 mg/mmol
Spot early morning albumin:creatinine ratio.	>70 mg/mmol
24 hour total urinary protein.	>1g/m^2/day

➤ Thyroid function tests. Hypothyroidism may result from loss of thyroxine-binding globulin.
➤ Full blood count (FBC). This is to look for associated anaemia.

Investigating possible causes of nephrotic syndrome should be guided by the history. Secondary causes include infection, autoimmune disorders and diabetes mellitus. Investigations may include:

➤ Complement level. Hypocomplementaemia with low C3 +/- C4 is consistent with post-infectious GN or SLE.
➤ Autoantibodies. A positive antinuclear antibody (ANA) and double stranded DNA (dsDNA) points towards systemic lupus erythematosus (SLE).
➤ Glucose/glycated haemoglobin (HBA1c). This is to look for evidence of diabetes.
➤ Infection markers. This involves looking for evidence of hepatitis, Epstein-Barr virus (EBV), *Varicella* and human immunodeficiency virus (HIV).

Percutaneous renal biopsies are required in those with atypical features, who are less likely to have minimal change disease. Such features include:
➤ Age <1 or >12-years-old.
➤ Gradual onset of oedema.
➤ Macroscopic haematuria.
➤ Rash or any features of other systemic disease.
➤ Hypocomplementaemia.
➤ Renal dysfunction.
➤ Steroid resistance with failure to respond to steroids by four weeks.
➤ Significant hypertension.
➤ Confirmation of calcineurin nephrotoxicity.

To diagnose a relapse of nephrotic syndrome there must be at least 3+ of proteinuria on urine dipstick testing for three consecutive mornings. To diagnose remission of nephrotic syndrome, urine dipstick must be clear of proteinuria for three consecutive mornings.

Differential Diagnosis
Hypoalbuminaemia has a variety of causes and could be due to:
➤ Poor intake. Malnutrition.

303

> Liver disease. There is loss of synthetic function, and therefore reduced albumin production.

> Excess protein loss. This can be from burns or gastro-intestinal losses.

> Redistributive states (e.g. pregnancy). In such cases, there may be expansion of plasma volume which may also result in relative hypoalbuminaemia.

Intermittent swelling may also point to another diagnosis, such as allergy or infection, particularly if it is very localised. Additionally, cardiac failure may present with oedema.

Proteinuria is the excess of protein in the urine, usually due to leakage from the kidney, but can be due to excess proteins in the serum, or due to reduced reabsorption at the proximal convoluted tubule.

Specific causes include:

> Orthostatic proteinuria.
> Glomerular disease.
> Tubular disease.
> Renal mass.
> Chronic kidney disease (with hypertension).
> Infection.

Complications

> Infection. Increased leakage through the glomeruli results in loss of regulatory proteins important in the immune system. This results in an increased predisposition to infections, particularly pneumococcal and *Haemophilus* infections. Pneumococcal peritonitis is a potentially devastating complication. Cellulitis is also more common, particularly if the child is markedly oedematous.

> Intravascular hypovolaemia. It is important to appreciate that patients can be oedematous, yet simultaneously intravascularly depleted. This is because the fluid is in the interstitial space, not the intravascular space.

> Hypercoagulability. Patients are more vulnerable to thrombosis, because of factors such as a) loss of anti-clotting factors, b) hyperlipidaemia and c) hyperaggregable platelets.

Management

Generally, children are treated with high dose corticosteroids for four weeks, which are subsequently weaned. The length of weaning depends on the risk of side-effects versus the chance of relapse. Most cases of minimal change disease respond within four weeks. Careful monitoring of blood pressure is needed; 25% of children with minimal change nephrotic syndrome have an elevated blood pressure, which may be due to corticosteroids. Other aspects of treatment include:

> Dietary sodium restriction. This is to reduce fluid retention. High sodium can lead to hypertension and fluid overload. A no added salt diet is recommended. Note that fluid restriction can increase thrombosis risk.

> Prophylactic penicillin. This is to reduce infection risk.

> Fluid management. This can be challenging, particularly if oedema is severe. Fluid restrictions should generally be avoided as it may lead to significant intravascular fluid depletion. Diuretic therapy and/or intravenous albumin infusions may be necessary and should be discussed with a specialist.

> Vaccination. Pneumococcal vaccination and varicella immunisation should be considered if the child is not already immune, as there is increased risk of infection secondary to immunoglobulin loss.

Children with nephrotic syndrome unresponsive to corticosteroids, who have frequent relapses, or have features suspecting more serious pathology, usually require a percutaneous renal biopsy before further treatment. Immunomodulatory agents, such as mycophenolate mofetil, tacrolimus, cyclosporine and intravenous rituximab, may be considered in such cases.

Prognosis

Most children who have corticosteroid-sensitive disease will go on to have more than one episode and some will have frequent relapses. However, the majority of patients go into permanent remission around puberty. Children with non-steroid responsive disease have a less satisfactory response to treatment and a worse prognosis.

Renal Masses

Renal masses are uncommon, and when identified should promptly be investigated. Possible causes are shown in *Table 5*.

TABLE 5: Causes of renal masses	
Unilateral	**Bilateral**
• Hydronephrosis. • Renal cysts. • Renal tumour (e.g. Wilms' tumour, which is usually unilateral). • Renal vein or venous thrombosis.	• Renal tumour. • Hydronephrosis. • Renal vein or venous thromboses. • Renal cysts. • Polycystic kidney disease. • Tuberous sclerosis.

RENAL DISORDERS

Urinary Tract Infections

A urinary tract infection (UTI) is defined as an infection of one or more structures in the urinary system, confirmed on urine culture. However, cases are very often treated before confirmation of a positive culture growth, if there are suggestive symptoms or positive urine dipstick results.

In children, UTIs may involve upper structures (pyelonephritis) or lower structures (cystitis). Around one in 10 girls and one in 30 boys will have had a UTI before 16–years-old. UTI is more common in girls, except for in the first six months of life. The most common bacterial cause is *Escherichia coli*. However, *Proteus, Klebsiella, Enterococcus* and coagulase-negative *Staphylococci* are other well-known causes.

Aetiology

Atypical UTIs (*Box 3*) and recurrent UTIs (*Box 4*) are more likely to result from an underlying abnormality. Upper UTIs are generally more serious than lower UTIs, particularly in the very young.

Risk factors include:

> Constipation. A full rectum can cause pressure on the bladder and prevent emptying. Stasis of urine in the bladder increases risk of bacterial growth and predisposes to infection.

> Female gender. Structural abnormalities of the urinary tract are more common in boys; therefore, UTIs are more common in males in the first six months of life. Following this, UTIs are more common in females as their urethra is shorter, reducing the distance that bacteria need to travel to reach the bladder.

> Vesico-ureteric reflux (VUR). VUR is the backflow of urine from the bladder to the upper urinary tract through the ureter to the kidneys. It is usually due to a problem with the valve mechanism in the ureter, which usually prevents abnormal flow. The risk of UTI is increased if the urine in the bladder becomes infected as this can then track backwards. There is a risk that the infected urine may reach the kidney and thus cause pyelonephritis.

> Congenital anomalies of the kidney and urinary tract (CAKUT). May predispose to infection, for example by causing reflux, or obstruction, and urinary stasis.

> Previous UTIs.

Box 3: Atypical UTIs

- Serious illness.
- Poor urine flow.
- Abdominal or bladder mass or spinal lesion.
- Renal dysfunction (with elevated plasma creatinine and reduced glomerular filtration rate).
- Septicaemia.
- Failure to respond to treatment with suitable antibiotics within 48 hours.
- Infection with non-*E. coli* organisms.

Box 4: Recurrent UTIs

- Two or more episodes of UTI with pyelonephritis.
- One episode of UTI with acute pyelonephritis plus one or more episodes of UTI with cystitis.
- Three or more episodes of UTI with cystitis.

> Encopresis. If a child is incontinent of faeces, bacteria from stools can contaminate the perineal area, predisposing to UTI.

> Nephrolithiasis. Obstruction of urinary flow can cause stasis of urine therefore increasing the risk of UTI.

> Uncircumcised boys. There is more likely to be bacteria living under the foreskin of the penis, predisposing to UTI.

Clinical Features

UTIs can present non-specifically, particularly in neonates. The following features increase the likelihood of a UTI being present:

> Changes to the urine such as being bloody (macroscopic haematuria), foul smelling, or cloudy.

> Increased urinary frequency, including urinary incontinence, especially at night.

> Pain or burning with micturition (dysuria).

> Abdominal pain (either flank pain with pyelonephritis, or suprapubic pain with cystitis).

> Fever and rigors.

> Nausea and vomiting.

> Poor growth.

> Non-specific features in neonates (poor feeding, irritability, sleepiness, jaundice or difficulty breathing).

Investigations

Urine Tests

A urine culture is the gold standard investigation to confirm a microbiological diagnosis of UTI.

There are several methods of urine collection:

> Clean catch into a pot. This involves a parent or a nurse patiently waiting for a urine sample by a baby's side. The baby's genitals are exposed, and a urine pot is held in prime position to catch urine when it emerges (*Figure 3*).

> Mid-stream urine. This is the ideal way to catch urine and is done in older children/adults. The patient is instructed to go to the toilet, start passing urine, and then in the middle of the stream, catch urine in a sterile sample pot.

> Catheter (either transurethral or ultrasound guided suprapubic). This has the advantage of being able to instantly get a urine sample, to help make a diagnosis. It is also a pragmatic way of obtaining urine if a catheter is being inserted anyway. However, it is invasive, requires expertise to perform, and has the potential to introduce infection.

> Urine bag. This is rarely used, but involves putting a bag over the genitalia, so that urine is automatically caught when the baby passes it. There is a high risk of a contaminated sample due to skin commensals.

White cells and nitrites on dipstick are consistent with an infection. *E coli* is the most commonly isolated organism, and this will be seen as gram negative rods on urine microscopy (*Figure 4*). Ideally, it is necessary to get a pure growth of one organism from two urine samples, but this should not delay

FIGURE 3

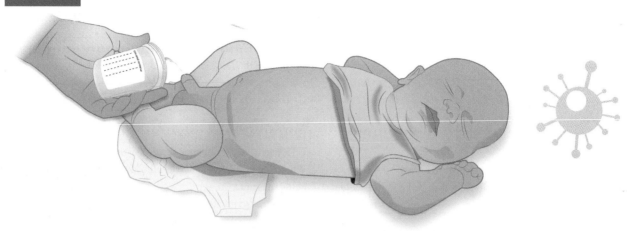

Method of clean catch urine collection.

FIGURE 4

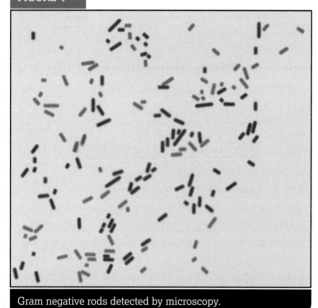

Gram negative rods detected by microscopy.

treatment, especially if a patient clinically has pyelonephritis.

Blood Tests

An elevated white cell count and CRP may suggest infection, but blood tests are not necessary in a well child who does not have atypical features. Blood pressure and renal function should be checked if there are concerns regarding renal damage.

Renal Imaging

Further imaging depends on the clinical suspicion of possible renal tract abnormalities or renal complications from the UTI. Non-recurrent typical UTIs that respond well to antibiotics do not require further investigation, unless the child is under 6-months-old. If the child is less than 6–months-old, a renal USS should be performed, especially if the antenatal USS was

abnormal or if there was no third trimester USS. USS should also be considered during the acute illness in any child with a severe or an atypical UTI.

Two additional tests are useful in selected cases:
- MCUG (micturating cystourethrogram). This demonstrates evidence of posterior urethral valves in boys and/or VUR, which increase the risk of a UTI.
- DMSA (^{99m}Tc-dimercaptosuccinic acid) scan. This assesses presence of renal scarring, but should only be performed three to six months after a UTI. This is because acute infection changes can be misinterpreted for renal scarring (as they both appear as photopaenic areas).

Management

Treatment in the acute setting is oral or intravenous antibiotics, depending on the age and severity of UTI. These may have to be adjusted based on urine culture and antibiotic sensitivity results. In children less than three-months-old, in the acutely unwell patient, or those who are persistently vomiting, intravenous antibiotic therapy should be used, along with additional supportive therapy.

Complications

Generally, UTIs are easily identified, treated with oral antibiotics and leave no long-term complications.

However, potential complications include:
- Sepsis.
- Renal abscess.
- Pyelonephritis.
- Acute kidney injury or chronic kidney disease.
- Hypertension.
- Hydronephrosis.

Prognosis

The majority of children are unlikely to get recurrent UTIs after their first episode. However, recurrence is more likely in:

- Children less than 6-months-old.
- Female gender.
- Evidence of underlying renal tract abnormalities [e.g. vesicoureteric junction obstruction, congenital anomalies of the kidney and urinary tract (CAKUT)].
- Uncorrected predisposing factors (e.g. constipation).
- Renal abscess.
- Hydronephrosis.

Enuresis

Key definitions include:

- Nocturnal enuresis or bedwetting. This describes involuntary bedwetting occurring during sleep.
- Daytime enuresis. This specifically refers to those who have reached an age where bladder control would typically have been achieved (around 5-years-old).
- Secondary enuresis. This is where a previously continent child becomes incontinent. This is always concerning and an organic cause should be excluded.

Aetiology

Most affected children are physically and psychologically completely normal, particularly in younger children with nocturnal enuresis. Enuresis is more common in those with a family history.

Causes of enuresis include the following:

- Bladder instability.
- Bladder neck muscle weakness.
- Neurogenic bladder.
- Anatomical abnormalities such as an ectopic ureter.

For those with polyuria, there may be a urinary concentration defect. This may be due to an osmotic diuresis from diabetes mellitus or insipidus or a primary renal disorder. Other possible triggers include UTIs and constipation. The commonest cause of secondary enuresis is emotional upset.

More generally, enuresis may be due to a child not responding appropriately to bladder sensation. This could be a result of maltreatment or other forms

of stress. However, it could also be due to developmental delay, or a primary neurological disorder such as spina bifida or a spinal cord abnormality.

Investigations

Extensive investigations are not generally required, as the diagnosis is mainly clinical. A diary of fluid intake, bedwetting, and toileting may help clarify the history. A urine MC&S may be performed if there is a concern about a UTI, and similarly diabetes mellitus and insipidus may need to be excluded.

Further renal and bladder investigations are rarely required, but may include bladder ultrasound (to look for a neurogenic bladder/incomplete emptying), spinal MRI (to look for neurological causes), and urodynamic studies (to look for obstructive/neurological causes).

Management

- General advice. General advice should be given as to how common it is, alongside advice about fluid intake and toileting patterns.
- Reward system. A positive reward system is usually helpful, not for dry nights, but for regular toileting (especially before bed), drinking recommended amounts of fluids during the daytime (and avoiding large volumes before going to bed), and engaging in the management of the condition.
- Pelvic floor exercises. This helps to improve bladder control.
- Bell-pad alarms. These are a first line intervention. The key is that the child has to wake up to go to the toilet when the alarm goes off, not with the parents lifting their children. This may not be suitable for all families, but has excellent success rates. Sensors are placed in the bed and in the underwear of the child so that when the child starts to micturate, the alarm goes off and wakes the child.
- Desmopressin. This can be used in those in whom alarm treatment is not suitable, or for an emergency situation. This is a synthetic vasopressin, which

acts to reduce the amount of water that is excreted in urine. It should be taken one hour before bed and fluid restriction should occur from one hour before until eight hours after taking it. This may be useful when children are going away on school trips or staying over at a friend's house, as a short term solution.

- Alternative medications. Failure of desmopressin may warrant tricyclic agents, anticholinergic agents or other specialist medications.

Prognosis

Most children outgrow bedwetting, but some do not, even with treatment. If a patient is still bedwetting at 18-years-old, they may still outgrow it with support from an experienced clinic.

IgA Vasculitis [also known as Henoch Schönlein Purpura (HSP)]

Aetiology

IgA vasculitis is an IgA mediated autoimmune disease known to be precipitated by infections and vaccinations, although the pathophysiology is not completely understood. It classically affects children 3 to 10–years-old and is more common in boys.

Clinical Features

The most common features of IgA vasculitis are:

- Purpuric rash. A characteristic raised purpuric rash, over the buttocks and extensor surfaces of the limbs (*Figure 5*). The child is usually clinically very well (unlike with meningococcal disease).
- Arthralgia. Pain, which is particularly in the knees and ankles, and which is occasionally associated with periarticular oedema. It usually responds well to simple analgesia.
- Abdominal pain. Note that this can also be due to intussusception, which is a complication of the disease.

The rash is pathognomonic of the disease, but very rarely, a skin biopsy is required to confirm the diagnosis.

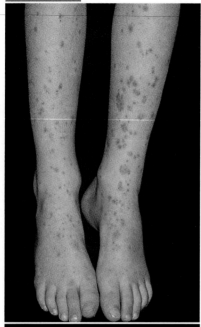

FIGURE 5

The classical rash of IgA vasculitis (D@nderm).

Differential Diagnosis

Other differentials for a purpuric rash are shown in *Table 6*.

Investigations

All children should have the following checked:

› Blood pressure. Hypertension associated with renal impairment.
› Urine dipstick. To look for haematuria/proteinuria.
› Renal function. To identify renal dysfunction.
› Albumin. Hypoalbuminaemia associated with renal dysfunction/nephrotic syndrome.

These should be monitored in primary care until resolution.

Further investigations in atypical cases include:

› FBC. This is to look for anaemia.

› Clotting. This is to ensure there is not a coagulopathy.
› ASOT/anti DNase B. This would be elevated in post infectious glomerulonephritis.
› Early morning urine protein:creatinine ratio. This is to look for evidence of renal dysfunction.
› Complement levels. This will help, for example, in a diagnosis of post infectious glomerulonephritis.
› Immunoglobulins. These will be important to exclude an immunodeficiency.
› Autoimmune profile. This will help for example in a diagnosis of SLE.

Children with evidence of significant renal compromise (e.g. acute nephritic syndrome, acute renal failure, persistent nephrotic syndrome) may require percutaneous renal biopsy to identify HSP nephritis.

Management

Management is generally symptomatic with simple analgesia for pain (avoiding NSAIDs if renal involvement).

Children should be discussed with a paediatric nephrologist if there is:

› Nephrotic range proteinuria ($>1g/m^2$/day).
› Renal dysfunction.
› Hypertension.
› Macroscopic haematuria.

Children with significant renal compromise may require immunosuppression for HSP nephritis.

Complications

› Glomerulonephritis. This is the commonest complication. It is important to check blood pressure, urine dipstick and renal function.

› GI involvement. Intussusception, protein-losing enteropathy, ileus, haemorrhage.
› Central nervous system involvement. This can range from self-limiting headaches and mild behavioural changes to CNS vasculitis.
› Orchitis.
› Pulmonary vasculitis.

Prognosis

Initial attacks of IgA vasculitis can last several months and children may have recurrences. IgA vasculitis generally has a benign course, particularly in those that present at a young age, but renal involvement can be a serious long-term complication. Therefore all patients need to have follow up, and repeat renal function tests.

Haemolytic Uraemic Syndrome

Haemolytic Uraemic Syndrome (HUS) is a triad of:

› Microangiopathic non-immune (Coombs –ve) haemolytic anaemia.
› Thrombocytopaenia.
› Acute kidney injury.

Aetiology

Typical diarrhoea-associated HUS is caused by exposure to *E. coli 0157*, also known as Shiga Toxin Producing *E. coli* (STEC). Shiga toxin binds to glomerular endothelial cells, making them thrombogenic, and activating an inflammatory cascade. This can cause platelet activation, and increased von Willebrand Factor (vWF) activity, which results in microthrombi formation, and a consumptive thrombocytopaenia.

The microthrombi lodge in arterioles and capillaries, with two important effects:

› Ischaemia. The kidneys and brain are most dependent on high blood flow, and therefore are most likely to be damaged.
› Microangiopathic haemolytic anaemia. The microthrombus destroys the red blood cells in its path as it becomes lodged in the smaller vessels.

TABLE 6: Differential diagnosis for a purpuric rash		
	Platelets Normal	**Platelets Low**
Child Well.	• HSP. • Viral infection. • Non-accidental injury.	• Immune Thrombocytopaenic Purpura.
Child Unwell.	• Meningococcal septicaemia. • Non-accidental injury.	• Acute lymphoblastic leukaemia.

Beyond STEC, other pathogens, such as *Shigella,* have been known to cause a similar picture. HUS due to the Thomsen-Friedenreich antigen is usually associated with pneumococcal infection.

There is increasing recognition of genetic predisposition to atypical HUS variants. Atypical HUS is thought to relate to chronic, uncontrolled activation of complement, leading to platelet activation, leukocyte activation and endothelial cell damage. Generally, it has a worse prognosis. Other causes include drugs (e.g. calcineurin inhibitors), malignancy, SLE and glomerulonephritis.

Clinical Features

Diarrhoea associated (or typical) HUS is the most well recognised variant. Presentation is with bloody diarrhoea, severe abdominal pain and vomiting. Other features may include pallor, lethargy, jaundice, petechiae, convulsions, pneumonia and signs of renal injury (e.g. oliguria, fluid overload).

Investigations
Haematological Tests

›   FBC and reticulocyte count. Haemoglobin level will guide need for transfusion. Reticulocyte count is elevated in haemolysis. Thrombocytopaenia may be identified.

›   Blood film. This is primarily to look for fragmented red cells from haemolysis.

›   Group and Save/Coomb's test. There is a high probability of transfusion being needed. A positive Coomb's test implies possible immune-mediated haemolytic disease, whereas a negative test is consistent with HUS.

›   Lactate dehydrogenase (LDH). Elevated due to increased cell turnover secondary to haemolysis.

›   Haptoglobins. This is reduced in haemolytic anaemia.

›   Coagulation screen. This is required to rule out a coagulopathy. In HUS, the fibrinogen, D-Dimer, international normalised ratio (INR) and activated

partial thromboplastin time (APTT) are generally normal, as coagulation factors are not consumed.

Biochemistry Tests

›   Renal function and electrolytes. Renal dysfunction is an important feature. Urea may also be elevated from haemolysis.

›   Renal USS +/- percutaneous renal biopsy. This is to identify any renal damage, and particularly in diarrhoea negative disease, biopsy may be needed to confirm diagnosis.

›   LFTs. This is to check for liver damage.

›   Amylase/lipase. This is to check for pancreatic damage.

›   Glucose. There may be hyperglycaemia (from pancreatic involvement) or hypoglycaemia (from infection, or liver disease).

›   CRP. This is elevated from generalised inflammation and the predisposing infection.

›   Urinalysis. Proteinuria and haematuria may be present.

Infection

›   Stool culture. This is to look for possible initial infective cause, if diarrhoea is present.

›   ASOT titres/anti-DNase B. This is to demonstrate previous streptococcal infection.

›   Thomsen-Friedenreich antigen. This is to demonstrate previous pneumococcal infection.

›   HIV serology. This is if HIV is suspected.

Management

Management is supportive. Antibiotics should be avoided unless the patient appears clinically septic. In many countries, including the UK, HUS is a notifiable disease. Management includes:

›   Renal support. Fluid resuscitation and electrolyte replacement are required. If there is significant renal dysfunction, dialysis may be necessary. Renal monitoring needs to be regular because of the risk of

deterioration. Those that progress to end-stage renal failure may require renal transplantation.

›   Neurological support. Seizure prophylaxis is required if neurological signs are present.

›   Haematological support. Some children may require red blood cell and/or platelet transfusion.

Historically, severe cases of HUS were treated with plasmapheresis, but intravenous eculizimab (a monoclonal antibody that inhibits complement) is beginning to prove beneficial in early clinical trials for atypical HUS.

Complications

Complications are wide ranging, but may include acute or chronic renal failure, seizures, stroke, cardiac problems, hypertension and haematological abnormalities.

Prognosis

Although patients can present very unwell, complete renal recovery is usual in diarrhoea associated HUS, although all forms of HUS can be associated with chronic kidney disease. HUS is rarely associated with neurological sequelae (cerebral vasculitis, cerebrovascular accidents and seizures), and these are the greatest cause of mortality.

Polycystic Kidney Disease

Polycystic renal disease is inherited, either in the autosomal recessive or autosomal dominant form.

Autosomal Recessive Polycystic Kidney Disease

The autosomal recessive form is often diagnosed on antenatal USS, associated with oligohydramnios and pulmonary hypoplasia (Potter sequence). The kidneys are enlarged, cystic (*Figure* 6), and easily palpable in the abdomen. Many infants do not survive the neonatal period due to pulmonary complications. For those that survive, renal failure, with or without hepatic failure, is inevitable in early childhood. Management is

FIGURE 6

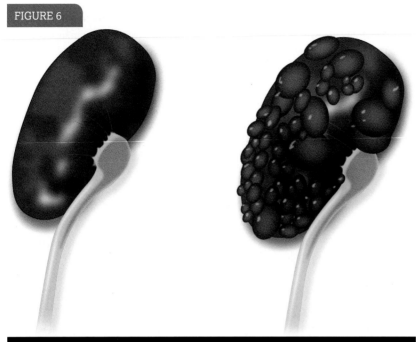

Normal kidney (left) compared to polycystic kidney (right).

supportive, with aggressive control of hypertension and renal function. Renal transplant, with or without liver transplant, may be required in childhood.

Autosomal Dominant Polycystic Kidney Disease

The autosomal dominant form of polycystic kidney disease can be detected antenatally or in childhood but more commonly presents in adulthood. The earlier the presentation, the more severe the disease. There may be multi-organ involvement, with the development of intracranial aneurysms, hepatic cysts and mitral valve prolapse. Aggressive management of hypertension and other cardiovascular risk factors is a key factor influencing disease progression. In view of the inheritance pattern, there are often difficult discussions to be had with asymptomatic family members about screening.

Nephrolithiasis

Aetiology

The most common reasons for renal stones are infection, metabolic, genetic and medication (*Table 7*). The commonest stones seen in children are those containing calcium-phosphate.

As renal calculi are rare, all children presenting with them should have a work-up to exclude urinary tract or metabolic abnormalities.

Clinical Features

Renal calculi are uncommon in children, but should be considered in those presenting with abdominal pain, loin pain or haematuria. Renal calculi may also present with passage of the stone itself, or as a UTI.

Investigations

Imaging is essential to determine if there is a renal calculus and its location.

Further blood and urine tests are vital to further investigate to find the cause.

Imaging

- ▸ Renal USS. This is the first investigation of choice, and will identify the majority of renal stones, particularly if they are large.
- ▸ Abdominal X-ray. These may help identify radiopaque stones and stones at the PUJ. The radiopacity of a stone on X-Ray can be an indicator of its aetiology (*Table 7*).
- ▸ Low dose CT-DMSA. As CT is much more sensitive to tissue attenuation, almost all stones are radiopaque, although based on composition, the density varies considerably.

Blood Tests

- ▸ Urea & electrolytes (U&Es). It is important to know if there is any associated renal dysfunction.
- ▸ Calcium, phosphate, magnesium, oxalate, urate, parathyroid hormone (PTH) and alkaline phosphatase (ALP). These can be an indicator for the likely type of stone present (*Table 7*). Note oxalate can also be measured in blood.
- ▸ Full blood count (FBC) and coagulation. These are important to ensure it is safe to carry out any form of surgical procedure.

Urine Tests

- ▸ Urine dipstick. This will identify the presence of any red or white

TABLE 7: Aetiology of stones and their appearance on X-Ray		
Stone Type	**Likely Aetiology**	**Appearance on X-ray**
• Magnesium ammonium phosphate.	• Infection.	• Poor radio-opacity.
• Ammonium urate.	• Infection.	• Radiolucent.
• Calcium oxalate.	• Non-infective.	• Radio-opaque.
• Calcium Phosphate.	• Non-infective.	• Radio-opaque.
• Uric Acid.	• Non-infective.	• Radiolucent.
• Cystine.	• Genetic.	• Poor radio-opacity.
• Xanthine.	• Genetic.	• Radiolucent.
• Stones caused by drugs.	• Drug related, e.g. ciprofloxacin, loop diuretics.	• Radiolucent.

blood cells, and demonstrate the urinary pH, which is important to determine which type of stone is likely to be present. The presence of nitrites with leucocytes is suggestive of infection.

> Urine microscopy, culture & sensitivity (MC&S). All urine should be sent for culture to look for the presence of a UTI.
> Stone analysis. If a stone is passed, the urine and stone itself should be sent for analysis.

Management

Simple

In such cases, the stone is small. Supportive measures include analgesia and increased fluid intake to help the stone to pass more quickly. Antibiotics may be given if passage of the stone takes longer or is associated with a UTI. Long-term, optimal fluid intake is recommended to prevent recurrence. There is limited evidence to suggest that any other dietary changes are of benefit.

Complicated

A child with a larger stone, or one that blocks urine flow and causes great pain, may need to be hospitalised for more urgent treatment. Early referral for intervention is needed to prevent hydroureteronephrosis. These treatments include:

> Extracorporeal shock wave lithotripsy (ESWL). Shock waves are delivered to the kidney to break down the stone into smaller pieces which can be passed more easily, as shown in (*Figure 7*).
> Ureteroscopy. Surgical removal or lithotripsy can occur via a ureteroscope, a tube like structure which inserts into the child's urethra and slides into the ureter via the bladder.
> Percutaneous nephrolithotomy. Surgical removal of the stone may be necessary through a small incision in the back. Occasionally lithotripsy is needed first, to break the stone down into smaller pieces that can be more readily removed.

Complications

Complete obstruction will eventually lead to hydronephrosis and renal failure. Stones may also become infected and lead to sepsis.

Prognosis

Most stones are small and pass without complications.

REFERENCES AND FURTHER READING

Urinary Tract Infection

1   Craig JC et al. Effect of circumcision on incidence of urinary tract infection in preschool boys. J Pediatr. 1996; 128:23–7.
2   Jodal U. Ten-year results of randomized treatment of children with severe vesicoureteral reflux. Final report of the International Reflux Study in Children. Pediatr Nephrol. 2006; 21:785–92.
3   McGillivray D et al. A head-to-head comparison: "clean-void" bag versus catheter urinalysis in the diagnosis of urinary tract infection in young children. J Pediatr. 2005; 147:451–6.
4   NICE guideline 47. Feverish illness in children: assessment and initial management in children younger than 5 years. 2007. http://www.nice.org.uk/guidance/cg47/
5   NICE guideline 54. Urinary tract infections in children. 2007. http://www.nice.org.uk/guidance/cg54/
6   Zorc J et al. Clinical and demographic factors associated with urinary tract infection in young febrile infants. J Pediatr. 2005; 116:644–8.

Chronic Kidney Disease

1   Hodson E et al. Growth hormone for children with chronic kidney disease. Cochrane Database of Systematic Reviews. 2012; Issue 2. http://onlinelibrary.wiley.com/doi/10.1002/14651858.CD003264.pub3/pdf.
2   Levey AS et al. A simplified equation to predict glomerular filtration rate from serum creatinine. J Am Soc Nephrol. 2011;A0828, 2000.

Polycystic Kidney Disease

1   Mayo Clinic. Normal and Polycystic Kidneys. 1998-2015. http://www.mayoclinic.org/diseases-conditions/polycystickidneydisease/multimedia/normal-and-polycystic-kidneys/img-20006896.

Glomerulonephritis

1   Infokid Website. Glomerulonephritis. 2013. http://www.infokid.org.uk/glomerulonephritis
2   UNC Kidney Center. Glomerular disease. 2012. http://unckidneycenter.org/kidneyhealthlibrary/glomerular-disease

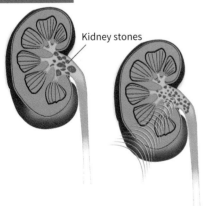
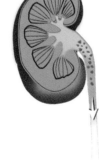

FIGURE 7

Kidney stones

Mechanism of action of lithotripsy.

Kidney Stones

1 National Institute of Health. Medline Plus: Lithotripsy Procedure. 2011. http://www.nlm.nih.gov/medlineplus /ency/imagepages/19246.htm
2 European Association of Urology. Guidelines on Urolithiasis. , 2014. http://uroweb.org/wp-content /uploads/22-Urolithiasis_LR.pdf.

Enuresis

1 NICE Quality Standard 70. Nocturnal enuresis (bedwetting) in children and young people. 2014. http://www.nice.org .uk/guidance/qs70

HUS

1 The Health Protection Agency. The management of acute bloody diarrhoea in children potentially caused by vero-cytotoxin producing *Escherichia coli* in children. 2012. http://webarchive.nationalarchives.gov.uk/20140714084352 /http://www.hpa.org.uk/webc/HPAwebFile/HPAweb _C/1309968515827.
2 Medscape. Paediatric HUS. http://emedicine.medscape .com/article/982025-overview.

Miscellaneous

1 National Kidney Foundation. KDOQI Guidelines. 2002. http://www2.kidney.org/professionals/KDOQI/guidelines _ckd/toc.htm.

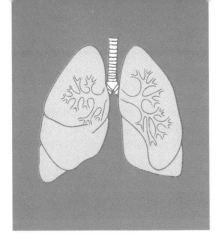

1.22
RESPIRATORY MEDICINE
CHRISTOPHER GRIME

CONTENTS

RESPIRATORY DISORDERS

Asthma

Asthma is a clinical diagnosis characterised by reversible airflow limitation.

Aetiology

Three main features give rise to the asthmatic phenotype:

> Airway hyperresponsiveness. This is an exaggerated bronchial smooth muscle contraction to a wide range of stimuli. The triggers vary according to the individual, but may include cold air, house dust mites or smoke.

> Bronchial inflammation. There is widespread inflammation in the bronchioles, with infiltration by eosinophils, T lymphocytes and mast cells. This is associated with oedema, smooth muscle hypertrophy, mucus plugging and epithelial damage. Some of these changes may be chronic but they are more pronounced during an asthma exacerbation.

> Airflow limitation. This is usually reversible, either spontaneously or with treatment, but there may be some underlying chronic changes.

Asthma is generally characterised by classical helper T cell type 2 (Th2) pathology with increased cytokines such as interleukin 4, 5 and 13 (IL-4, IL-5 and IL-13), which are thought to drive symptoms. The pathology of asthma is characterised by goblet cell hyperplasia and infiltration of inflammatory cells such as CD4$^+$ T cells, eosinophils and mast cells.

Clinical Features

As with most conditions, a clear clinical history is often all that is needed, particularly with young children. Symptoms are induced by weather changes, ill health and exercise. Nocturnal symptoms and improvement on bronchodilation are even more suggestive of the disease.

> Wheeze. Classically, in asthma, the wheeze is an expiratory airflow sound resulting from narrowed and inflamed airways. It can be heard at the bedside or require auscultation. However, the volume of the sound can be misleading. A

quieter wheeze may be suggestive of severely narrowed airways. Paradoxically, in this setting, the volume of the wheeze would increase in response to bronchodilation.

▸ **Coughing.** Bronchoconstriction is often accompanied by severe bouts of coughing. For some children, this can be the main symptom, particularly at night.

▸ **Shortness of breath.** Poorly controlled asthma in a child may present with shortness of breath, showing increased respiratory effort on minimal exertion.

▸ **Exercise induced symptoms.** Children will often have exacerbations while exerting themselves. It is good practice to have a reliever inhaler nearby during sport and for some children, to administer bronchodilators before exercising.

▸ **Atopic nature.** Most childhood asthma is associated with an element of atopic disease such as eczema, rhinitis, hay fever or a family history of atopy. Managing these diseases will often improve asthma symptoms.

▸ **Chest wall remodelling.** Rarely, in severe disease, children can develop pectus carinatum (protrusion of sternum and ribs, also known as pigeon chest). Harrison's sulcus (a horizontal groove along the costal margin) may also be seen in chronic disease.

Examination findings include:

▸ **Wheeze.** Be aware that this may be absent in severe disease, where there is insufficient air flow to generate wheeze.

▸ **Reduced air entry.**

▸ **Hyperexpanded chest.**

▸ **Use of accessory muscles/increased work of breathing.**

Investigations

The combination of classic symptoms with demonstrable variable airflow obstruction make the diagnosis.

▸ **Obstructive pattern to lung function.** Asthma is an obstructive lung disease demonstrated on lung function by showing a reduced forced expiratory volume in one second (FEV_1) with relatively preserved forced vital capacity (FVC) and a reduced FEV_1/FVC (<70%) (*Figure 1*).

▸ **Bronchodilator reversibility.** If a child is able to produce a 12% or greater improvement in lung function or peak flow following bronchodilator administration, this may be diagnostic of asthma. This is only useful in children over 5-years-old, when lung function can be measured.

▸ **Allergy test.** Skin prick test to aeroallergens or specific IgE to allergens suggests an atopic nature, which could be useful when considering aggravating factors in the environment.

If very severe and referred to a tertiary centre, a child may undergo further tests such as a bronchoscopy, formal lung function test and exhaled nitric oxide test (found to be increased with inflammatory conditions) before more novel therapies are considered.

Differential Diagnosis

Many children with underlying bronchiectasis, immunodeficiencies, ciliary diseases and even cystic fibrosis are misdiagnosed as difficult asthma until further investigations are performed. In children under 5-years-old, viral-induced wheeze, or multi-trigger wheeze should be considered as described in *Table 1*. Gastro-oesophageal reflux should be considered and such patients may benefit from a trial of treatment. Disordered swallowing resulting in aspiration should also be considered.

FIGURE 1

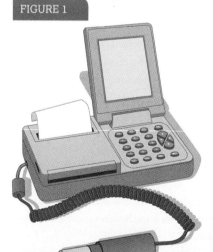
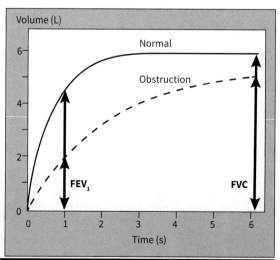

Spirometer (left), and typical inspiratory pattern in normal lungs and obstructive disease. The FEV_1 and FVC are both markedly reduced, with the FEV_1 more dramatically affected.

TABLE 1: Differences between viral induced wheeze and asthma

	Viral induced wheeze	Asthma
Ages.	• More common in preschool age group.	• Can affect all ages.
Infections.	• Symptoms only associated with chest infection.	• More prone to infection and exacerbated by them, but may have other triggers.
Interval symptoms.	• Symptom-free between infections.	• Symptoms associated with exercise, air pollutants, emotions. Still present between infections.
Nocturnal symptoms.	• Absent (unless unwell).	• Cough at night and wheeze, resulting in fragmented sleep. Suggestive of poorly controlled disease.
Inhaled therapies.	• Intermittent benefit during exacerbations. No requirement between illnesses.	• Clear improvement with inhaled bronchodilators and continued need when stable.
Oral steroids in acute exacerbations.	• No benefit.	• Reduces exacerbation severity and duration.

Management

Chronic Asthma

Treatment of chronic asthma should involve a stepwise systematic approach allowing treatment to be escalated and reduced guided by response. One example of this would be the British Thoracic Society and Scottish Intercollegiate Guidelines Network (BTS/ SIGN) guidelines (*Figure 2*).

Corticosteroids

Note that if a child has been receiving high dose corticosteroids for prolonged periods, the adrenal gland can stop producing glucocorticoids. These children then need corticosteroid replacement in the form of hydrocortisone with a plan to increase the dose during periods of ill health and careful monitoring if vomiting or unable to tolerate oral intake to avoid an Addinsonian crisis.

Achieving Complete Control

Focus on trying to reduce treatment once control has been achieved. For the atopic patient, interventions around the home such as damp wiping surfaces to reduce floating dust particles and house dust mite protective bedding can have significant effect on reducing morbidity. It is very important to encourage the parents of an asthmatic child to stop smoking. Even those that smoke outside still exhale smoke and still carry it on their clothing.

Complete control of asthma necessitates:
- No daytime symptoms.
- No need for reliever medications with the exception of during exercise.
- No asthma exacerbation.
- No limitation on daily activity.
- Normal lung function.
- Minimal side effects from medication.

In practice, complete control is difficult to achieve, but it should remain the aim. If control is still a challenge after combination inhaled therapy (i.e. Step 3), a child should be referred to a paediatrician who specialises in respiratory medicine. Children who are referred and deemed as difficult, or who are severe therapy-resistant asthmatics, may be treated with more novel therapies such as:
- Omalizumab which is a humanised antibody used for atopic children.
- Monthly corticosteroid injections.
- Beta-2-agonist subcutaneous infusions.
- Methotrexate.

Acute Asthma

This is the phenomenon when a child has an "asthma attack" resulting in bronchoconstriction and respiratory distress. It can occur in known asthmatics or as a first presentation of asthma. There can be several or multiple reasons why an individual may suffer an exacerbation, although there may be no obvious trigger. Some of the commonest reasons are:
- Viral upper and lower respiratory tract infections. Asthmatics are more prone to chest infections and may experience more severe symptoms and complications.

Step 1. Short acting, relieving bronchodilator used as required, i.e. salbutamol (usually a blue inhaler).

Step 2. Inhaled corticosteroids used daily as a preventative measure.

Step 3. For the under 5 years age group, a leukotriene receptor antagonist (such as montelukast) and for those over 5 years, a long-acting bronchodilator (such as salmeterol)

Step 4. Addition of leukotriene receptor antagonist, increased inhaled corticosteroid dose or use of slow release theophylline.

Step 5. Use of oral corticosteroids as maintenance therapy.

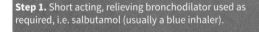

FIGURE 2

Management of chronic asthma.

> Changes in environment. Moving from a cold environment to a warm one, warm to cold, wet to dry and vice versa. Sudden changes can exacerbate a child.
> Environmental allergen. Particularly aero-allergens such as animal dander, grass pollen, tree pollen, house dust mites, mould. Cigarette smoke, either primary or secondary, is particularly irritant.
> Exercise. The classic picture is of a child developing bronchospasm after or during exercise.
> Strong emotional triggers.

Assessment

The severity of the exacerbation will need to be assessed. It is important to note that a peak expiratory flow (PEF) is reliable only if the child is more than 5-years-old and is usually unachievable in a severe exacerbation. *Table 2* gives some guidance as to how this might be categorised. The mnemonic "33, 92 CHEST" can be used to remember life threatening exacerbation:

> **33**: PEFR <33% predicted.
> **92**: oxygen sats <92%.

> Cyanosis.
> Hypotension.
> Exhaustion.
> Silent chest.
> Tachycardia.

If the patient has symptoms and/ or signs which cross categories, always treat them as the worst category they meet.

Treatment

The key to the initial treatment of an acute asthma exacerbation is rapid reversal of bronchoconstriction with bronchodilators. For initial therapy, if oxygen is required, bronchodilators are administered via an oxygen-driven nebuliser, but otherwise bronchodilators administered via an appropriate spacer device are as effective as a nebuliser. Management is summarised in *Table 3*.

When discharging a patient after an exacerbation, careful steps should be put into place to prevent further exacerbations. Inhaler technique should be checked and an asthma management plan should be provided.

Delivery of Asthma Medication

Close consideration should be paid to which device will suit a child best. Inhaler devices include:

> Metered dose Inhaler (MDI). These contain a pressurised inactive gas that propels one dose of medication each time the dose is released by pressing the top of the inhaler (*Figure 3*). They should be used with a spacer device to maximise drug deposition.
> Breath-activated Inhaler. A dose of medication is triggered by breathing in at the mouthpiece (*Figure 4*).

Choice depends primarily on the age of the child as breath-actuated devices require the ability to take a controlled effective self-directed breath. It also depends on the medication prescribed as not all drugs are produced in a range of different devices.

Spacers

These are used with MDIs to improve drug deposition and prevent the majority of the drug remaining in the oral cavity. Every child should be using a spacer device with an MDI. A face mask should

TABLE 2: Symptom guide for assessing severity of clinical signs			
	Moderate Exacerbation	Severe Exacerbation	Life-threatening Exacerbation
Oxygen saturations.	SpO_2 ≥92%.	SpO_2 <92%.	SpO_2 <92% or any of the following:-
Peak Expiratory Flow Rate (PEFR).	PEFR >50% of best/predicted.	PEFR 33-50% of best/predicted.	PEFR <33% of best/predicted.
Other features.	No clinical features of severe respiratory distress.	Too breathless to talk/eat. Use of accessory neck muscles.	Poor respiratory effort. Altered consciousness. Hypotension/tachycardia. Exhaustion. Cyanosis. Silent chest on auscultation.

TABLE 3: Treatment guide for inhaled therapies, steroids and reassessment intervals based on whether the child requires oxygen		
	Mild exacerbation	Moderate–severe exacerbation
Inhaled therapy.	2 to 10 puffs of salbutamol; titrated to response.	10 puffs of salbutamol (nebulised if requiring oxygen).
Corticosteroids.	Not necessary.	Oral prednisolone, but in life threatening exacerbation, use IV hydrocortisone.
Reassessment.	Monitor for four hours. If the patient is stable, they could be sent home with a weaning regime of salbutamol. This means that the dose given in the ED is gradually titrated over a number of days. If they have not managed four hours, they will require more frequent bronchodilator administration and therefore monitoring in hospital.	Reassess after 20 minutes. If further treatment is required, add ipratropium bromide to the nebulisers and keep monitoring response. Repeat nebulisers if required up to three further times 'back-to-back'. An oxygen requirement already necessitates an admission. If no sustained improvement is seen after three nebulisers, start to consider (if not already) intravenous access and IV salbutamol, magnesium sulphate or aminophylline therapy.

be attached to the spacer until the child is old enough or capable of holding the mouthpiece in their mouth and forming a seal around it (*Figure 5 and 6*).

Complications

Complications relate both to the disease itself, and to treatments. Chronic asthma may be associated with mild effects on growth. Medication side effects include:

- Long-term oral steroid therapy can result in adrenal suppression.
- Inhaled steroids have more mild side effects such as oral thrush.
- Leukotriene receptor antagonists may cause disturbed sleep.

Prognosis

About one-third of all children will wheeze at some point in childhood, many of which will grow out of it before formal lung assessment can take place. In general, asthma is a mild condition which, if well managed, has a minimal impact on life, with symptoms disappearing with age. However, there are still a significant number of child and adult deaths due to asthma exacerbations every year.

Preschool Wheezing Disorders

These children should be considered separately to asthmatics, as they may not respond to conventional treatment methods. There is much confusion over the terminology used here. The diagnosis generally refers to those under 5-years-old who wheeze, but do not have an underlying diagnosis of asthma. Two categories have been differentiated:

- Viral-induced (episodic) wheeze. Children who wheeze intermittently, but are well between episodes.
- Multi-trigger wheeze: Children who wheeze both during and between discrete episodes.

Viral induced wheeze may be difficult to differentiate from a viral exacerbation of asthma. *Table 1* highlights the key differences between the two pathologies.

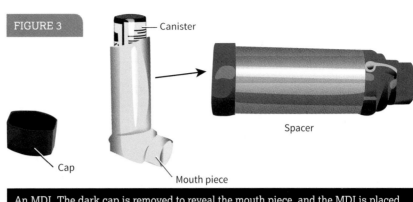

FIGURE 3

Canister

Spacer

Cap

Mouth piece

An MDI. The dark cap is removed to reveal the mouth piece, and the MDI is placed into the back of the spacer.

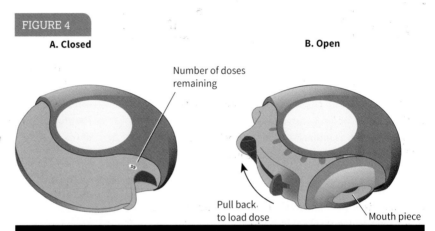

FIGURE 4

A. Closed   **B. Open**

Number of doses remaining

Pull back to load dose

Mouth piece

A breath-activated inhaler. The patient rotates the light purple component anticlockwise, while keeping the dark purple part firmly in place. This reveals a mouthpiece, and as the patient breathes in here, a dose of medication is released.

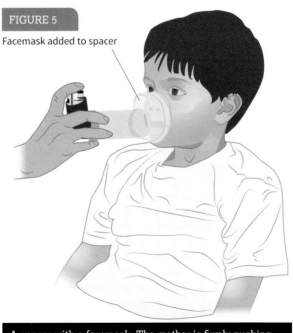

FIGURE 5

Facemask added to spacer

A spacer with a facemask. The mother is firmly pushing the facemask against the child's face, as he inhales.

FIGURE 6

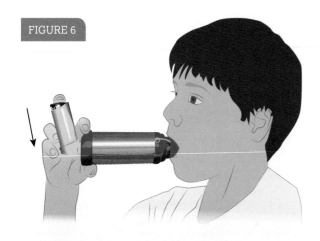

A spacer without a facemask. This is operated independently by the child. After the canister is pushed down, the child takes five breaths in and out.

Management

Bronchodilators can be effective and the frequency of exacerbations should be considered before starting inhaled corticosteroids for long-term control. Leukotriene receptor antagonists such as montelukast may be of benefit. There is no evidence for the use of corticosteroids in acute exacerbations.

Bronchiolitis

Bronchiolitis is inflammation of the bronchioles. It affects approximately one-third of all children in the first two years of life, with three percent admitted to hospital.

Aetiology

Bronchiolitis is most commonly caused by respiratory syncytial virus (RSV) infections but can also be the result of many other infections including adenovirus, human metapneumovirus and rhinovirus. These viruses are more prevalent in the winter months leading to the term "bronchiolitis season". The small airways (bronchioles) become inflamed and obstructed with mucus compromising ventilation (*Figure 7*).

Clinical Features

- Cough. Parents will often describe a dry cough, episodic and often resulting in vomiting. There may be preceding signs of an upper respiratory tract infection.
- Respiratory distress. The signs to look out for are tachypnoea, head bobbing (when the head rocks forward with each respiration), tracheal tug (although it is difficult to clearly visualise the neck in very young infants), and sub-costal/intercostal recession. Dramatic abdominal movements can be seen attempting to aid ventilation.
- Pyrexia. A low-grade fever is common with bronchiolitis due to the viral illness underlying the presentation.
- Poor feeding. Affecting predominantly infants, this is a major consideration as to whether a child needs admission or further intervention. For a non-ambulatory infant, feeding is the most energetic activity of their daily routine. If they are already tired from breathing alone, often they have no energy to feed.

FIGURE 7

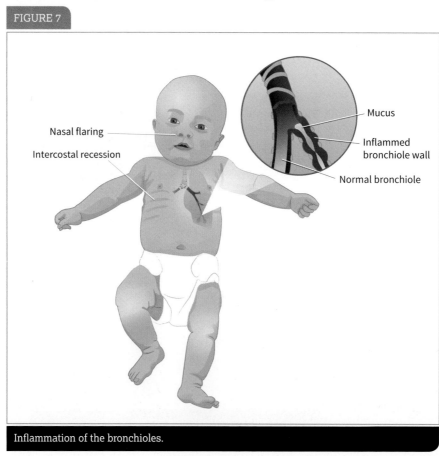

Nasal flaring

Intercostal recession

Mucus

Inflammed bronchiole wall

Normal bronchiole

Inflammation of the bronchioles.

> Apnoea. Parents often describe breathing pauses particularly when sleeping. This is a serious complication of bronchiolitis.

Examination findings include:
> Wheeze. This is a result of airway narrowing.
> Reduced air entry. Suggestive of consolidation or collapse.
> Crepitations/crackles. These can be heard throughout the chest.

Investigations

Bronchiolitis is a clinical diagnosis, and in the majority of cases requires no investigations. Investigations that may be considered are:

> Nasopharyngeal aspirates. Collection of fluid from the nasal passage can be used to identify the viral pathogen. This rarely influences immediate management but can be useful in 'bronchiolitis season' so that children with similar pathogens can be nursed in the same environment to minimise the risk of cross-infection.
> Blood gas. This can be helpful in assessing ventilation, particularly if the child is requiring respiratory support. However, it should be done sparingly, as disturbing the child is likely to exacerbate respiratory distress.
> Chest X-ray. This is rarely required in bronchiolitis unless asymmetric chest sounds are heard and therefore a different or concurrent pathology is suspected. There may be associated lobar collapse, a pneumothorax or a superimposed pneumonia.
> Blood tests. White cell count and C-reactive protein (CRP) may be elevated but are unlikely to influence the management. In a neonate, a high CRP might trigger a lumbar puncture to rule out meningitis. Elevated lymphocyte count may suggest whooping cough if other features are present. Electrolytes and renal function can help identify hydration status.

Differential Diagnosis

An unwell infant with respiratory distress could be suggestive of a bacterial infection. Bronchiolitis, however, can leave a child susceptible to opportunistic bacteria. Therefore, pneumonia is a recognised comorbidity. Broader causes of respiratory distress should also be considered as well as bacterial pneumonia, including gastro-oesophageal reflux with aspiration, heart failure, pneumothorax and collapsed lung.

Prevention

While no direct preventions are available, Palivizumab is a monoclonal antibody against RSV and is recommended for young children with severe chronic diagnoses such as congenital cardiac disease or chronic lung disease.

Management

Despite a significant amount of medical research on the subject, very few treatment options have shown any benefit. The main focus of management is supportive.

> Minimal handling. This is one of the most important aspects of management. Any distress caused to the baby may exacerbate respiratory distress. This is partly the reason why blood gasses and other blood tests should be performed sparingly.
> Oxygen and ventilation. Usually the main indicator of whether a child needs admission is whether they can maintain their oxygen saturations in room air. Some babies will require more invasive support such as high-flow nasal cannula oxygen, continuous positive airway pressure ventilation (CPAP), or intubation and conventional ventilation.
> Hydration support. Once the demand of ventilation is significant, feeding may become compromised. Maintaining hydration is vital. Support can be offered by either a nasogastric tube or if not tolerated, intravenous fluids.

> Inhaled therapies. Controversy remains over the use of nebulised sodium chloride (0.9% isotonic or 3% hypertonic), salbutamol or ipratropium bromide. Bronchodilators such as salbutamol are unlikely to be of benefit as most children under six months do not possess β_2 receptors for the drug to act upon. The wheeze is also more likely due to mucus build up. Inhaled therapy may be more effective in those (i) with a family history of atopic conditions (ii) with co-existent eczema and (iii) that are over six months.

Complications

Acutely, bronchiolitis can lead to lung collapse, superadded pneumonia and respiratory failure. Rarely, those with severe infection develop chronic non-reversible obstructive lung disease called bronchiolitis obliterans due to scarring and fibrosis of the small airways. These children need careful follow up and active management by a respiratory paediatrician.

Prognosis

The natural history of the condition is a peak of symptoms at three to five days before the symptoms start to improve. The vast majority of children will not require any medical intervention at all, and are cared for at home. Often a dry persistent cough will be present for several weeks. Some will require admission to a paediatric unit for supportive measures during the acute phase of the illness. A very small number will go on to need ventilator support.

Pneumonia

Pneumonia is an inflammatory condition affecting the small airways. It is a leading cause of childhood death worldwide, particularly in low income countries.

Aetiology

Pneumonia is the result of an invading pathogen that is usually

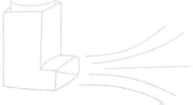

either bacterial or viral. The commonest bacterial pathogens are:

- *Streptococcus pneumoniae.*
- *Staphylococcus aureus.*
- *Haemophilus influenzae.*
- Mycoplasma.

Viral causes include:

- Adenovirus.
- Rhinovirus.
- RSV.

Mycobacteria (tuberculous and non-tuberculous) should also be considered in high risk areas and populations.

Underlying immune problems can present as repeated infections. Any post-immunisation child who acquires pneumonia secondary to a pathogen covered by the vaccination programme should be considered suspect. A long-standing history of coughing and respiratory distress when feeding could suggest that pneumonia is secondary to aspiration.

Clinical Features

- **Cough.** The cough may be associated with vomiting in younger children and sputum production in older children. The cough can be episodic or constant.
- **Respiratory distress.** The blocked, inflamed airways will result in respiratory compromise and a child who needs to use accessory muscles to achieve adequate gas exchange. Look for tachypnoea, tracheal tug and use of subcostal and intercostal recession. Infants may have apnoeas due to poorer central respiratory control. With severe enough hypoxia, any child may be cyanotic. Grunting may also be heard (forced expiration against a closed glottis), and is another sign of respiratory distress.
- **Pyrexia.** The absence of an elevated temperature on the background of a significant consolidation on chest X-ray is suspicious and both tuberculosis (TB) and malignancy should be considered.
- **Poor feeding.** For the very young child, poor feeding is a symptom of ill health and should be taken seriously. The inability to take feeds either due to coughing or general exhaustion is a common reason for hospital admission. The vomiting that can be associated with pneumonia can result in poor oral intake and dehydration.
- **Abdominal pain.** Pleuritic pain can present as abdominal pain in some children, often with very few signs of respiratory distress.

Examination findings include:

- **Crepitations.** A crunching sound of inflamed tissue rubbing against each other, or the opening and collapsing of small airways under the pressures of inspiration and expiration due to secretions.
- **Asymmetrical chest wall movement.**
- **Dull percussive note.**
- **Bronchial breathing.**
- **Reduced air entry.**
- **Increased vocal fremitus.**

Investigations

In a well child with community-acquired pneumonia, with a clear diagnosis, no investigations (including chest X-ray) are needed. However, consider the following in moderate-severe cases, or when there is diagnostic doubt:

- **Chest X-ray.** This may show focal consolidation or bilateral changes (*Figure 8*). Always pay attention to the cardiac border and behind the heart. A chest X-ray cannot differentiate between bacterial or viral pathogens effectively.
- **White cell count.** An elevated white cell count and neutrophilia may be seen, particularly in bacterial pneumonia. A normal white cell count in the presence of a consolidation or effusion may suggest malignancy.
- **C-reactive protein (CRP).** A non-specific marker of inflammation. The CRP will often not peak until 24 hours into the illness so do not rely on this if the child presents early into the illness. In very severe infection, the CRP may not rise. CRP is a synthetic protein produced by the liver, and therefore cannot be produced if the liver shuts down.
- **Sputum culture.** In a sputum-producing child, this is the best indication of the pathogens causing the infection. Bacterial culture, mycobacterial culture (can take up to 8 weeks) or viral Polymerase Chain Reaction (PCR) can result in a positive finding and direct treatment although the latter two tend only to be performed in severe or unusual cases. If sputum is difficult to obtain (e.g. in younger children) techniques such as sputum induction using hypertonic sodium chloride nebuliser can be utilised and in some cases, a bronchoscopy for lavage samples, although these are rarely needed.

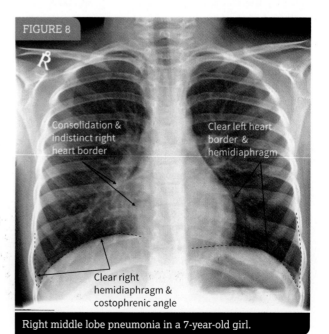

FIGURE 8

Consolidation & indistinct right heart border

Clear left heart border & hemidiaphragm

Clear right hemidiaphragm & costophrenic angle

Right middle lobe pneumonia in a 7-year-old girl.

- Blood culture. This is important to obtain in an unwell febrile child. There may be septicaemia if the bacterial pathogen has crossed over to the blood stream. Viral serology can also be obtained, as can specific tests for legionella (urinary antigen test) and mycoplasma (blood PCR).
- Chest ultrasound. If the chest X-ray suggests an effusion, then ultrasound should be performed to confirm the presence, measure the depth and describe whether it contains debris or is loculated. Collections deeper than 2 cm may require drainage, depending on the context.

Further investigation in more severe cases may include:
- Computed Tomography (CT) scans. May be useful to exclude malignancy.
- Bronchoscopy. This can be used to obtain induced sputum samples, to look for any suspected malignancy, or in recurrent infection to help exclude an inhaled foreign body.
- Baseline immune function. Immunoglobulin levels, functional antibody responses to immunisations, and lymphocyte subsets may be tested if there are concerns about an underlying immunodeficiency. This concern may arise due to unusual infecting pathogens or due to unusually frequent or severe infections.
- Pleural aspiration. If there is a pleural effusion, this may be done

therapeutically to drain the effusion, or diagnostically to identify the cause of the effusion.

Differential Diagnosis

Children can be breathless for many reasons, although in younger children, infection is the most likely cause. Without signs of infection or inflammation, an undiagnosed cardiac lesion should be considered. Respiratory distress and consolidation without supporting inflammation is suggestive of malignancy. These are both rare in children.

Management

This is dependent on the severity and age of the child (*Table 4*). There are two aspects to management:

Treatment of the Infection

Antibiotics are invariably prescribed in almost all cases of pneumonia. It is extremely difficult, however, to differentiate between viral and bacterial causes. The decision as to whether to use oral or intravenous antibiotics is controversial, and there is variability in clinical practice. There has generally been a move in preference to using oral antibiotics where possible. Oral antibiotics are safe and effective for even severe community-acquired pneumonia. However, intravenous antibiotics are given in cases of suspected septicaemia, those with complications, severe hospital acquired infections, and in those unable to take oral medications.

- Oral antibiotics. For younger children with a community-acquired pneumonia, penicillin (e.g. amoxicillin) is usually appropriate as first-line treatment. For older children in whom mycoplasma infections are more common, a macrolide (e.g. erythromycin/clarithromycin) may be more appropriate on its own or in conjunction with a penicillin.
- Intravenous antibiotics. First-line treatment is usually a penicillin or a second/third generation cephalosporin with consideration of additional macrolide cover for atypical infection (e.g. mycoplasma).

Supportive Measures

Compromise to respiratory function can lead to an oxygen requirement. Children may also need support to keep hydrated or with nutrition.

Those with a background of a chronic disease (e.g. cystic fibrosis, immunodeficiency, bronchiectasis) will often be treated more aggressively for the same presentation, as they are more vulnerable to opportunistic infections, and may also decompensate more rapidly due to poorer baseline respiratory function.

Complications

Complications may include parapneumonic effusions, empyema, lung abscesses, septicaemia, respiratory failure and dehydration.

Prognosis

Most children will make a full recovery. However, repeated infections can lead to bronchiectasis. This is scarring resulting in permanent enlargement of the airways (best seen on CT scan). Such patients are vulnerable to long-term, repeated infections.

Cystic Fibrosis

Cystic Fibrosis (CF) is one of the commonest genetically inherited disorders. It is inherited in an autosomal recessive fashion with a carrier rate of 1 in 25. Over 10,000 people currently

	Mild-moderate	Severe
Infant.	• Temperature <38.5°C. • Respiratory rate (RR)<50, with mild recession. • Feeding well.	• Temperature >38.5°C. • RR>70, with severe difficulty in breathing. • Cyanosis and apnoeas. • Poor feeding. • Tachycardia and delayed capillary refill.
Older child.	• Temperature <38.5°C. • RR<50, with mild breathlessness. • No vomiting.	• Temperature >38.5°C. • RR>50, with severe difficulty in breathing. • Cyanosis. • Signs of dehydration. • Tachycardia and delayed capillary refill.

TABLE 4: Signs of mild-moderate and severe pneumonia (adapted from BTS Guidelines; British Thoracic Society guidelines for the management of community acquired pneumonia in children. 2011)

321

live with CF in the UK, with an incidence of 1:2000 people.

Aetiology

The result of the defective gene is a defective cystic fibrosis trans-membrane conductance regulator (CFTR). This receptor is responsible for the transfer of chloride ions out of the cell and inhibition of the adjacent epithelial sodium channel (ENaC). Because no chloride is pumped out of the cell and sodium floods into the cell uninhibited, the cell content becomes very concentrated, with a high osmolality that draws water in from the outside. The result is thick, dehydrated mucus, which builds up in lumens throughout the body.

Thousands of gene mutations are known, with p.Phe508del (previously known as ΔF508) identified as the commonest mutation in the UK Caucasian population, accounting for approximately 85% of cases.

Clinical Features

- Chest infections. The thick mucus that builds up in the airways not only obstructs, but also prevents clearance of bacteria, leading to infection. Recurrent infections lead to scarring or bronchiectasis and if untreated, ultimately respiratory failure. Pseudomonas is a common infection seen in CF.
- Faltering growth. Pancreatic insufficiency leads to failure to digest fat resulting in offensive fat-laden stool. Salt depletion can also cause dehydration. There is higher energy expenditure due to an elevated metabolic rate and higher requirement to fight infection and support an elevated respiratory effort.
- Nasal obstruction/nasal polyps. This occurs in approximately 10-40% of cases but it is uncommon in those under 5-years-old. The enlarged polyps can obstruct the nasal passage affecting the sense of smell and taste. CF should be ruled out in any child with nasal polyps.
- Bowel obstruction. The same effect on dehydrated mucous in the lungs can occur with faecal matter in the bowel. This can present in the neonatal period as meconium ileus or later in childhood as distal intestinal obstruction syndrome (DIOS). The pressure from trying to push this matter out can also result in rectal prolapse.

Investigations

Confirming the Diagnosis

- Immune-reactive trypsinogen. The newborn screening programme tests all babies born in the UK on day five of life for levels of immune-reactive trypsinogen (IRT).
- Sweat test. If the IRT is elevated, the child is referred to a centre for a sweat test and counselling. The gold standard diagnostic investigation is still a sweat test. If the chloride content of the sweat is over 60 nmol/L, the diagnosis is confirmed. Between 40-60 nmol/L, further investigation is required.
- Genetic tests. Genetic tests look for the presence of gene mutations, which may direct therapy.

Pancreatic Function

- Pancreatic function needs to be established as the next priority, and this involves testing faecal elastase. The absence of elastase in the faecal matter would suggest pancreatic insufficiency.

Long-Term Monitoring

- Serial chest X-rays. These have a low sensitivity for early changes in cystic fibrosis. However, they may show hyperinflation, lobar collapse or bronchiectasis.
- Ultrasound scans. Sonography can assess the abdomen for signs of liver disease.
- Bone scans. Bone scans assess bone density.

Methods for monitoring insulin function are also required, e.g. performing a glucose tolerance test.

Additional Assessments

- High resolution CT scans (HRCT). This has a much greater sensitivity for picking up cystic fibrosis changes. Examples include: bronchial wall and/or peri-bronchial interstitial thickening, and mucus plugging, as well as features of bronchiectasis.
- Bronchoscopy. This can be used to obtain sputum samples to look for infection.

Differential Diagnosis

Once the diagnosis of CF has been ruled out, the investigation of a child with recurrent chest infections should include an assessment of their immune system. Other suppurative lung diseases including primary ciliary dyskinesia (PCD) should also be considered.

The poor weight gain and nutritional elements could be the result of coeliac disease, thyroid diseases or indeed any chronic childhood illness.

Management

Acute Infections

Acute infective exacerbations need to be treated aggressively. Supplementary oxygen may be required. Positive sputum cultures allow antibiotics to be tailored to exacerbations. Typically, if treating pseudomonas infections, dual therapy is used with a broad spectrum β-lactam or cephalosporin, and an aminoglycoside. Treatment is usually continued until the symptoms of the exacerbation (for example increased sputum production) are resolved.

Long-Term Treatment

Since CF was first discovered, all available therapies have been focused on treating the effects of the gene defects, rather than the gene defect itself.

Children need careful monitoring of their nutritional status. Some children require regular admission to hospital for scheduled intravenous antibiotics to maintain health. The mainstay of treatment is regular physiotherapy several times a day. The long-term medication load on the average CF child is significantly large. There is variation in what medication might be needed, but the following may all need to be considered.

Prophylactic Anti-Microbial Therapy

‣ Oral antibiotics, e.g. flucloxacillin. For *Staphylococcus aureus* prevention.
‣ Nebulised antibiotics, e.g. colomycin. For *Pseudomonas aeruginosa* prevention.
‣ Oral antifungals. For *Aspergillus* prevention.

Clearance Medication

‣ Nebulised hypertonic sodium chloride. This may help clear respiratory secretions.
‣ Nebulised DNase (e.g. dornase alfa). This aids in the breakdown of respiratory secretions.

Airway Treatment

‣ Bronchodilators, e.g. salbutamol. This results in airway dilatation, aiding clearance of respiratory secretions. It is particularly effective in those with concurrent asthma.
‣ Inhaled corticosteroids. This may have a prophylactic role in those with concurrent asthma.

Nutritional Support

‣ Pancreatic enzyme supplementation, e.g. Creon. Oral enzyme replacement for pancreatic exocrine function.
‣ Micronutrient supplementations, e.g. Vitamin A, D, E and K. Replacement of fat soluble vitamins is particularly important due to fat malabsorption in CF.
‣ Histamine receptor antagonist, e.g. ranitidine, and proton pump inhibitors, e.g. omeprazole. A lower stomach pH reduces the risk of Creon becoming denatured, and therefore increases absorption.
‣ Insulin. Treatment of CF-related diabetes.

A strict daily routine is needed to include all the nutritional requirements and considerations along with the physiotherapy. The psychological

impact of the disease burden is huge and particularly difficult around teenage years.

Small Molecule Therapy

There is now medication for treating the defective protein itself. The first small molecule therapy, Ivacaftor, is licenced for individuals with gating mutations such as the p.Gly551Asp (formally known as G551D) mutation where the CFTR molecule is made and inserted into the cell surface but does not work. Ivacaftor can induce a degree of normal function of the protein. This effect translates to improving weight gain, reducing exacerbation rates and returning sweat chlorides to a normal level. This is only suitable for approximately five percent of the CF population but other therapies are now in development.

Complications

‣ CF-related diabetes. The exocrine function of the pancreas is insufficient resulting in the need for enzyme replacement. The endocrine function can also deteriorate, resulting in diabetes. Prolonged uncontrolled hyperglycaemia can result in deteriorating lung function and poor weight gain.
‣ CF-related liver disease. Blockages throughout the liver drainage architecture can result in hepatomegaly and portal hypertension. Some children require serial endoscopy and treatment of oesophageal varices.
‣ Infertility. The majority of males with CF will be infertile because CF is associated with an absent vas deferens. Females, while fertile, may also struggle to conceive or carry a pregnancy unless they are in good health.

Prognosis

CF was initially a post-mortem diagnosis. In the past 60 years, significant improvements have been made in diagnosis and treatment, resulting in a median survival age of 41 years. Childhood death is uncommon now. Death from CF is usually the result of respiratory failure.

Pertussis (Whooping Cough)

Whooping cough is caused by *Bordetella Pertussis*, and classically has an incubation period of 10-14 days. Children are infectious for approximately three weeks after onset of the classical symptoms. Pertussis is an example of an infectious disease controlled effectively by a successful vaccination programme. Most cases in the UK or other countries where vaccination uptake is good are in infants under 2 months or the unvaccinated child.

Clinical Features

The illness has a catarrhal phase (due to build-up of mucus) with fever that is followed by the paroxysmal cough, hence having the alternative name of "the 100 days cough". Imagine a child coughing in a persistent series, one after another until they have run out of air and then taking a large inhalation against an inflamed upper airway. The resulting sound can be described as a "whoop". This phase can be very prolonged and result in vomiting and apnoea in infants.

Investigations

‣ Postnasal swabs. These can be used to culture the bacteria or for direct immunofluorescence testing but are only useful in the first few weeks of the illness. After this period, serology for antibodies against pertussis may be utilised.
‣ Full blood count (FBC). This will demonstrate an elevated white cell count with a high lymphocytosis (up to 80% of total white count).

Imaging will be invariably normal and is not indicated, unless another alternative or concurrent diagnosis is suspected.

Prevention

Most western countries have vaccination programmes for pertussis.
‣ Mothers will be vaccinated antenatally.
‣ In the UK, pertussis immunisation occurs at 2, 3, and 4-months-old, followed by a preschool booster.

This will provide protection for 70% of patients and ameliorate illness in 30%. Children who have been vaccinated can still develop the illness. There has been a reduction in uptake of the pertussis vaccine in the UK and elsewhere, increasing the risk of the disease, both for the unvaccinated child and for the community.

Management

Most cases can be treated at home with good education and reassurance, particularly when explaining to parents that the cough can be present for a long time. There should be a low threshold for admitting children under six-months-old. Supportive oxygen therapy when a coughing paroxysm occurs may be required to avoid hypoxia.

Antibiotics

Antibiotic treatment with erythromycin can be used to reduce the infectiveness of the illness but is unlikely to alter the clinical course. It is recommended in cases that present within 21 days of onset of symptoms, otherwise it is unlikely to be effective.

Public Health

In many countries (including the UK), whooping cough is a notifiable disease; therefore, it is important to inform public health officials of the suspected diagnosis. Children with suspected or confirmed whooping cough should stay away from school or nursery for five days after starting antibiotics, or 21 days from the onset of the cough (whichever is sooner). Contact with young children should generally be avoided, particularly if they have not had their primary vaccination.

Prophylaxis

Children under one-year-old should be offered antibiotic prophylaxis if they are a close contact (generally people living in the same household) of someone diagnosed with pertussis.

Complications

In severe cases, the paroxysmal cough can result in sub-conjunctival haemorrhages, rib fractures, pneumothorax, hernia, post cough-fainting and even intra-ventricular haemorrhage or hypoxic brain injury.

Prognosis

Prognosis is excellent, although those under 6-months-old have a mortality rate one hundred times greater than that for adults.

Tuberculosis

Tuberculosis (TB) is one of the most common causes of infection-related deaths worldwide. The World Health Organisation (WHO) reports that there are more than nine million new cases per year, with a disproportionate amount in disadvantaged, malnourished and crowded areas. The highest rates are in South-East Asia, Africa and the Western Pacific. Rates are thought to have increased due to emigration and HIV epidemic. The most common cause is *Mycobacterium tuberculosis*, with rare infections by *M. bovis* and *M. africanum*. Mycobacteria are acid-fast bacilli, slow-growing and aerobic.

Key definitions to be aware of are:
> **Primary TB.** This is when TB infection first occurs.
> **Secondary TB.** This is from reactivation of latent TB. It may be precipitated by impaired immunity, e.g. due to HIV, malnutrition, or immunosuppressant therapy.
> **Miliary TB.** This occurs when primary infection is not adequately contained, and there is severe disease from haematogenous spread.
> **Active TB.** This is TB causing symptoms and contagious disease.
> **Latent TB.** This occurs when TB is present in the body, but is inactive, suppressed by the patient's immune system.

Most people infected with *M. tuberculosis* do not develop active disease (and therefore only have latent disease). Disease development is more likely in immunocompromised patients such as HIV-infected individuals.

Aetiology

Spread of TB is through droplet inhalation from patients with active disease. The droplets commonly settle in distal respiratory bronchioles or alveoli where they are phagocytosed by macrophages. These infected macrophages are unable to kill the bacilli, instead transporting them to the regional lymph nodes where they are able to spread to other organs via the lymphatic tract. The transition from TB infection to active TB occurs when the bacilli are able to overcome the immune defences. Primary active TB occurs when the mediastinal nodes enlarge causing cavitation and organism spread to the adjacent bronchi. Lymphohaematogenous dissemination can result in miliary TB or TB meningitis. Bacilli can also remain dormant in the apical posterior areas of the lung for several months or years with later progression of disease resulting in the development of secondary TB.

Clinical Features

Children with pneumonia, pleural effusion or a cavitating mass not responding to antibiotics should be considered for TB. A history of fever of unknown origin, faltered growth, a bloody cough, night sweats, weight loss, lethargy and unexplained lymphadenopathy are also common.

Investigations

> **Tuberculin skin test (TST).** This is an intradermal injection to the inner surface of forearm of tuberculin purified protein derivative. It results in a palpable raised hardened area (*Figure 9*). The size of the swelling needs to be measured in millimetres within 48-72 hours. The test is positive if it is greater than 5mm.
> **Chest X-ray.** This can show mediastinal enlargement, cavitating primary disease or lobar pneumonia.
> **Sputum culture.** This can be performed in older children relatively easily, but in those under 6-years-old,

early morning gastric aspirates may need to be used. Early morning gastric aspirates involve taking fluid samples from the stomach, which contains swallowed respiratory secretions from the night before. Alternatively, bronchial lavage may be required. Testing for acid fast bacilli using a Ziehl-Neelsen stain is the initial screening before culture results which can take up to eight weeks by conventional methods.

Rapid tuberculosis diagnostic tests are increasingly recognised as a gold standard for diagnosis of TB. They are based on nucleic acid amplification, and unlike sputum cultures, can give results within a few hours rather than potentially several weeks.

Management
Both latent and active TB should be treated. The ultimate goal of treatment is to achieve sterilisation of the TB lesion in the shortest time possible. Combination therapy is used to maximise clinical effect, and total

duration of treatment for active TB is usually at least six months. First-line treatment may include the following medications:
> **Rifampicin.** This works by inhibiting RNA polymerase in the bacteria, thus stopping RNA synthesis. Side effects include hepatitis.
> **Isoniazid.** This works by inhibiting the growth of the bacterial cell wall. Side effects include hepatitis, pancytopenia and peripheral neuropathy.
> **Pyrazinamide.** This inhibits bacterial growth. Side effects include joint pain and hepatitis.
> **Ethambutol.** This works by inhibiting the growth of the bacterial cell wall. Side effects include optic neuritis or hepatitis.
> **Streptomycin.** An aminoglycoside antibiotic. Side effects include neuropathy and nephropathy.

Multi-drug Resistant TB
Multi-drug resistant (MDR) TB is defined as TB resistant to at least Isoniazid and Rifampicin. It is an

increasing problem worldwide. Prophylactic treatment is also important. The BCG vaccination is offered to all babies born in areas with high TB rates or into a household with possible TB contacts. Recent contact with active TB should be treated despite a normal TST, particularly in those under 5-years-old or with HIV. Public health should also be notified as there is a risk of the disease spreading within the community.

Complications
Miliary TB and TB meningitis are the most deadly complications of primary TB. Respiratory complications include effusions, collapse, pneumothorax and bronchiectasis. Other systems may be affected too, including the small bowel, spleen, spine and the heart.

Prognosis
Full resolution is expected in non-MDR and non-immunocompromised individuals. Secondary TB can occur, but in high endemic areas, recurrent disease is more likely to be due to reinfection.

Primary Ciliary Dyskinesia
Once considered a milder form of CF, Primary Ciliary Dyskinesia (PCD) is the result of defective epithelial cilia that line the airways. Healthy cilia have a regular rhythmic pulse in unison allowing the airways to expel particulate matter. In PCD, cilia movement is either not in unison or static, resulting in mucous accumulation and poor airway clearance, which if untreated, can lead to recurrent infections, bronchiectasis and eventual respiratory failure.

Aetiology
Microscopic examination of a cilia cross-section reveals columns of proteins interlocked. This allows the cilia to move in uniform fashion. If the protein arrangement is disrupted or abnormal, the cilia movement is abnormal. This is what happens in PCD.

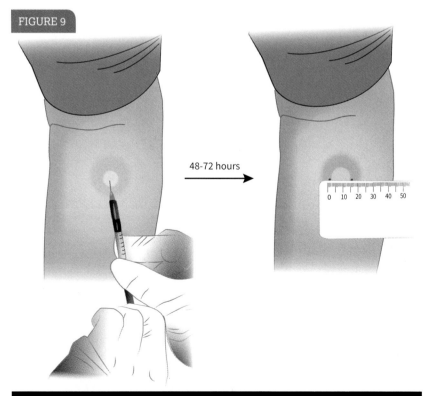

FIGURE 9

48-72 hours

Tuberculin Skin Test. The size of the bleb post injection is measured.

Clinical Features

- Recurrent chest infections. Similar to CF, the mucus build-up can allow bacteria to grow.
- Persistent wet cough. A constant build-up of mucus results in a moist-sounding cough.
- Unexplained neonatal respiratory distress. This is a common clinical feature with PCD in neonates.
- Conductive hearing defects. This is usually the result of a congested auditory canal. Grommet insertion can be devastating to these children as it can result in a constant foul smelling ear discharge as cilia clearance is affected here in the same way as in the chest.
- Sinusitis. Mucus build up can result in sinus pressure and pain.
- Dextrocardia. Cilia movement are not just vital for lung clearance. Embryologically, cilia beat patterns and directions dictate orientation of the developing organs. Abnormalities of heart orientation or abdominal organs can occur. Any child with dextrocardia should be investigated for PCD.

Investigations

Abnormal direction or static cilia is diagnostic of PCD. Nasal nitric oxide is also very sensitive as a detection tool, although the pathophysiology for this test is not fully understood. Research is ongoing as to a genetic cause for PCD. Several genes have been associated with cilia structure abnormalities.

Management

Similarly to CF, management is reliant on airway clearance techniques such as physiotherapy or inhaled therapies. There should be a low threshold for treating a suspected chest infection with antibiotics. PCD children also benefit from sinus rinse to treat the ENT symptoms which can be quite debilitating.

Prognosis

Mild cases can result in a normal life span. However, severe untreated disease will result in eventual respiratory failure.

Bronchiectasis

This term refers to an abnormal and fixed dilatation of the airways, which is usually the result of persistent and/or recurrent infections. Breakdown of the airway walls, due to persistent inflammation, reduces the ability to clear mucus and secretions and increases risk of infection.

Causes of bronchiectasis include:
- Chronic conditions, e.g. CF, PCD, immunodeficiency.
- Acute infections, e.g. measles.
- Obstruction, e.g. foreign body/tumour.

Clinical Features

Recurrent wet cough due to poor airway clearance along with episodes of haemoptysis and wheeze is characteristic. There is also a propensity to frequent infections. Patients often demonstrate clubbing of the finger nails.

Investigations

- Chest X-ray. This may show bronchial wall thickening.
- Chest CT scan. This is the gold standard test used for the diagnosis of bronchiectasis. It provides an indication of distribution, extent and severity (*Figure 10*).
- Sputum culture. While not needed for diagnosis, sputum culture can be useful for identifying persistent microbiology. For younger children unable to produce samples, sputum induction with nebulised hypertonic sodium chloride or a bronchoscopy may be of benefit.

Management

Similarly to other suppurative lung disease (CF or PCD), management is reliant on airway clearance techniques such as physiotherapy or inhaled therapies with a low threshold for treating a suspected chest infection with antibiotics. Lung function can be a poor indicator of an exacerbation. Sputum volume and colour is usually more telling.

Prognosis

A child with mild bronchiectasis can expect a normal life span. However, severe untreated disease will result in eventual respiratory failure.

FIGURE 10

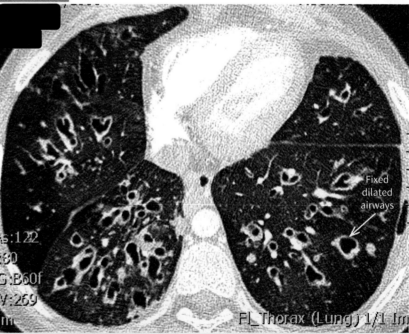

A slice from a CT scan of a child with cystic fibrosis. The image demonstrates bronchiectasis with fixed dilated airways, the result of scarring from recurrent infection.

Pneumothorax

A pneumothorax is defined as an air collection in the pleural space (*Figure 11*). This may be due to an underlying disease pathology (CF, asthma, severe infection) or traumatic causes. Most commonly, it is caused by a burst lung cyst. Tall, slim individuals appear to be more at risk. In these cases, consider whether the patient has an undiagnosed condition predisposing them, such as Marfan syndrome.

Clinical Features

A simple pneumothorax can be asymptomatic. Auscultation of the chest will reveal absent breath sounds and reduced air entry on the affected side and classically there will be a resonant percussion note. If tension is developing there will be signs of respiratory distress along with deviation of the trachea away from the affected side. This is an emergency situation, as hypoxia can develop.

Investigations

A chest X-ray will show a significant amount of air has accumulated in the pleural space. A tension pneumothorax is a clinical diagnosis, and should be treated immediately, as it is a medical emergency.

Management

- ▸ **Conservative.** Uncomplicated cases may resolve spontaneously, and require no active management. Oxygen therapy is helpful even in a non-hypoxic patient. This is because nitrogen (from the air in the pleural space) will diffuse into the lungs (filled with 100% oxygen) along its concentration gradient.
- ▸ **Needle aspiration.** This is necessary in tension cases and followed by a chest drain insertion. Aspirate from the second intercostal space in the mid-clavicular line.
- ▸ **Chest drain insertion.** This is used to prevent escaping air compromising the patient while the underlying defect repairs. The drain is usually inserted in the fifth intercostal space, in the mid-axillary line.
- ▸ **Surgical intervention.** Recurrent pneumothoraces or complicated cases may require surgical intervention such as pleurodesis where a substance is injected into the pleural space to encourage adhesion of the pleural layers.

Prognosis

In spontaneous isolated pneumothoraces, with early initiation of therapy, prognosis is excellent. However, there is a high incidence of recurrence, particularly in those with underlying lung disease.

IMPORTANT ADJUNCTS IN RESPIRATORY MANAGEMENT

Tracheostomies

A tracheostomy is an artificial opening in the trachea typically between the third and fourth tracheal rings. A tube is placed through the opening to bypass an airway obstruction, including congenital airway malformations or for long-term respiratory support. Most children with a tracheostomy depend upon

FIGURE 11

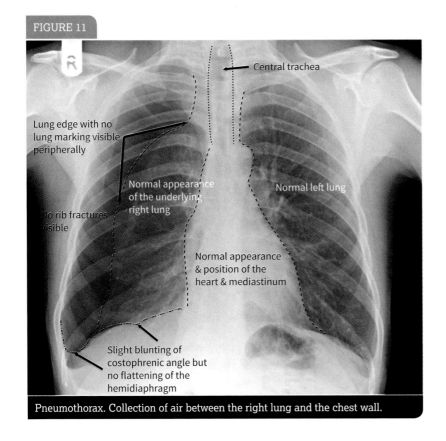

Central trachea

Lung edge with no lung marking visible peripherally

Normal appearance of the underlying right lung

Normal left lung

No rib fractures visible

Normal appearance & position of the heart & mediastinum

Slight blunting of costophrenic angle but no flattening of the hemidiaphragm

Pneumothorax. Collection of air between the right lung and the chest wall.

a patent tracheostomy tube to breathe. Secretions from the child's respiratory tract must be regularly suctioned to prevent blockages and respiratory difficulty. There are increasing numbers of patients with tracheostomies in the community.

Indications include:

> Subglottic stenosis.
> Tracheal stenosis.
> Laryngomalacia.
> Tracheomalacia.
> Bronchomalacia.
> Vocal cord paralysis.
> Craniofacial anomalies.
> Tumours (e.g. haemangioma).
> Trauma.
> Long-term mechanical ventilation.

Complications

All children with a tracheostomy must have a spare tube and emergency equipment with them at all times. They are at risk of a number of complications, including:

> Blockage.
> Decannulation/displacement of the tracheostomy tube.
> Infection- respiratory tract or around the insertion site.

Management

A common and life-threatening complication in patients with a tracheostomy is blockage of the tube. Therefore, if such a child has any suggestion of a compromised airway, it is important to suction the tracheostomy tube. If suction does not relieve the obstruction, the tube will need to be changed. Oxygen needs to be administered over the tracheostomy site as well as the mouth, since many tracheostomy patients still have a patent upper airway.

Oxygen Therapy

Indications

Oxygen is one of the most widely used treatments in medicine. Generally, any acutely unwell child should be given oxygen as it is easily accessible, simple to administer and has minimal side effects.

Common indications include:

> Low oxygen saturations, e.g. <92%.
> Low PaO_2, e.g. <65mmHg.
> Cardiorespiratory arrest.
> Severe respiratory distress.
> Seizures.
> Shock.

Methods of Delivery

Oxygen is either stored in transportable oxygen cylinders, or is available through an outflow circuit at the bedside. Adjusting the tap from either of these will vary the flow rate of

TABLE 5: Methods for administering oxygen therapy	
Method of Oxygen Delivery	Comments
Face mask	For delivery of high concentrations of oxygen. Not all children tolerate their use. For acute situations and short-term use. Must contain vents to allow CO_2 clearance.
Nasal cannulae	Deliver up to 2 L/min (24-30%). They can be used to provide a lower concentration of oxygen for a longer period. The child is able to speak and eat with the cannulae.
Nebuliser	Oxygen can be given via a nebuliser if medication to the airways needs to be given concurrently.
Headbox	A clear plastic box that surrounds a baby's head, and delivers humidified oxygen through it.
Wafting	A non-contact method of oxygen delivery, whereby a mask is held near the child. It may be utilised when conventional methods are not tolerated by the child.

oxygen, from 0-15 L/min. The oxygen tubing is then attached to a device (e.g. a face mask) and then oxygen is delivered the patient. When choosing the method of oxygen delivery, consider both the concentration of oxygen required and the age and co-operation of the child (*Table 5*).

Oxygen therapy can be placed into the following categories:

> **High concentration oxygen therapy.** This delivers a flow rate of >4 L/min (>30%) in acute situations.
> **Controlled oxygen therapy.** This delivers a specific concentration of oxygen to maintain saturations.
> **Long-term oxygen therapy (LTOT).** This is used to prevent chronic hypoxaemia, e.g. chronic lung disease, cystic fibrosis and pulmonary hypertension.

Note that humidified oxygen can be delivered via a facemask, head box or high flow nasal cannulae delivery systems. It is useful for long periods of high concentration oxygen therapy. Humidification prevents drying of mucous membranes and secretions.

Dangers of Oxygen Therapy

Oxygen is a very safe drug and should generally be administered with little hesitation. Certain groups are at high risk of oxygen toxicity:

> **Premature infants.** Oxygen therapy is associated with retinopathy of prematurity (p197).
> **Congenital heart disease.** High oxygen concentration closes the ductus arteriosus. The ductus arteriosus is needed to allow mixing of blood between the pulmonary and systemic circulations. Therefore, some patients with congenital heart disease may be given lower target oxygen concentrations.

REFERENCES AND FURTHER READING

Asthma
1 Asthma UK. www.asthma.org.uk
2 BTS/SIGN guidelines 101. British Guidelines on the Management of Asthma. 2014. https://www.brit-thoracic.org.uk/guidelines-and-quality-standards/asthma-guideline.

Bronchiolitis
1 Scottish Intercollegiate Guidelines Network (SIGN) 91. Bronchiolitis in Children. 2006. http://www.sign.ac.uk/pdf/sign91.pdf.

Pneumonia
1 BTS Guidelines; British Thoracic Society guidelines for the management of community acquired pneumonia in children. 2011. https://www.brit-thoracic.org.uk/document-library/clinical-information/pneumonia/paediatric-pneumonia/bts-guidelines-for-the-management-of-community-acquired-pneumonia-in-children-update-2011.

Cystic Fibrosis
1 CF Trust. www.cysticfibrosis.org.uk.
2 Newborn screening. www.newbornbloodspot.screening.nhs.uk/cf.
3 Royal Brompton and Harefield NHS Foundation Trust Clinical Guidelines: Care of Children with Cystic Fibrosis.2014. www.rbht.nhs.uk/childrencf.

Whooping Cough
1 NICE Guidelines. Whooping cough. 2015. http://cks.nice.org.uk/whooping-cough.

Tuberculosis
1 British Thoracic Society Guidelines. Tuberculosis. 2015. www.brit-thoracic.org.uk/guidelines-and-quality-standards.
2 World Health Organisation (WHO). Global tuberculosis control. 2010. http://www.who.int/tb/publications/en.

Pneumothorax
1 British Thoracic Society Guidelines. Pleural Disease Guideline.2010. www.brit-thoracic.org.uk/guidelines-and-quality-standards.

Tracheostomy
1 Great Ormond Street Hospital. Tracheostomy: care and management review. 2015. www.gosh.nhs.uk/health-professionals/clinical-guidelines/tracheostomy-care-and-management-review/#Other-care-needs.

Oxygen Therapy
1 Great Ormond Street Hospital. Oxygen therapy administration in a non-emergency situation. 2014. http://www.gosh.nhs.uk/health-professionals/clinical-guidelines/oxygen-therapy-administration-in-a-non-emergency-situation.

General
1 Wilmott, R, Boat, T, Bush A, Chernick V, Deterding R, Ratjen, F (2012). Kendig and Chernick's Disorders of the Respiratory Tract in Children. USA: Saunders.

RESPIRATORY MEDICINE

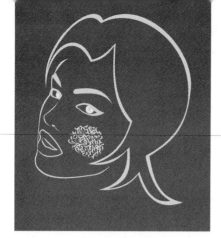

1.23
SKIN CONDITIONS
MAANASA POLUBOTHU

OVERVIEW OF THE SKIN

The skin is the largest organ in the body. Its key functions include:

> Barrier function. It prevents entry of water and electrolytes into the body through the surface.
> Immunosurveillance. Langerhans cells act as antigen-presenting cells. Macrophages and lymphocytes defend against microorganisms that breach its protective barrier.
> UV protection. Melanocytes contain the pigment melanin, which filters UV radiation from sunlight.
> Thermoregulation. This is orchestrated by sweat glands and blood vessels of the dermis, in addition to the insulating properties of the subcutaneous layer.
> Sensory function. Nerve endings detect touch, pain and temperature.
> Vitamin D synthesis. Vitamin D is converted into its active form in the basal and spinous layers of the epidermis under the influence of ultraviolet light from sunlight.
> Respiration. The skin accounts for up to 2% of respiration by absorbing oxygen and eliminating carbon dioxide.

There are three layers to the skin: the epidermis, dermis and the subcutaneous layer (*Figure 1*).

Epidermis

This is the thin, uppermost layer acting as a waterproof physical barrier. It is the first line of defence against the environment. The epidermis is immensely complex. It has four main layers: stratum basale, stratum spinosum, stratum granulosum and stratum corneum. Another layer, the stratum lucidum, is found on the palms and soles. The main cells of the epidermis are the keratinocytes. Other important cells are melanocytes (dendritic cells in the basal layer, containing melanin pigment) and Langerhans cells (dendritic antigen-presenting cells forming part of the immune surveillance system of the skin). The dermo-epidermal junction (DEJ) is the region that lies between the epidermis and the dermis holding it together. It is immunologically and genetically important; antibodies against various components of the DEJ are found in genetic and acquired skin conditions such as blistering diseases.

FIGURE 1

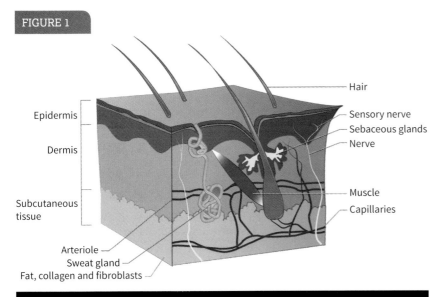

Hair
Sensory nerve
Sebaceous glands
Nerve
Muscle
Capillaries

Epidermis
Dermis
Subcutaneous tissue
Arteriole
Sweat gland
Fat, collagen and fibroblasts

Layers of the skin.

Dermis

The dermis lies below the dermo-epidermal junction. Important structures within the dermis include vasculature, cutaneous nerves, sweat glands (eccrine and apocrine glands) and the pilosebaceous unit which is composed of a hair bulb, sebaceous gland, arrector pili muscles and apocrine sweat glands. These structures lie in the dermal connective tissue which consists of collagen and elastin fibrils that give the skin its texture, structure and elasticity.

Subcutaneous Layer

This is the deepest layer of the skin and is made up of a network of adipocytes and collagen. It contains larger blood vessels and nerves and plays an important role in conserving energy and body heat.

SKIN DISORDERS

Atopic Eczema

Aetiology

Eczema refers to a group of conditions characterised by itchy, dry and inflamed skin. Atopic eczema is the most common type in children, affecting 20% of children in the UK. It results from impaired barrier function and usually starts in infancy. In those with atopic eczema, the risk of later developing asthma and hay fever is increased, the so-called "atopic march".

Clinical Features

Acute eczema presents with dry, erythematous, itchy skin. There is also increased skin temperature (vasodilatation), oedema, weeping (extravasation of serum from dilated vessels) and crusting (*Figure 2*). In severe cases, there are vesicles and occasionally bullae formation. There is an episodic pattern with periodic flares.

Two patterns of the condition are generally seen:
> Infantile eczema. This predominantly affects the face, neck, scalp (cradle cap) and extensor surfaces. The nappy area is mostly spared. The majority of cases clear within a few months but may progress.
> Childhood eczema. The distribution favours flexural surfaces, antecubital and popliteal fossae, the volar aspect of the wrists, neck and ankles. This is less weepy and wet than infantile eczema and there is marked lichenification.

Chronic eczema presents with lichenification, which describes thickening of the skin causing exaggeration of skin creases. Pigment changes and formation of papular eczema can be seen, especially in Asian or black skin.

Management

Atopic eczema can have a huge psychological impact, not only on the children who suffer from it but also their

FIGURE 2

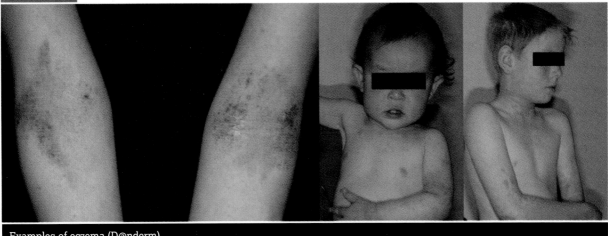

Examples of eczema (D@nderm).

331

families. Sleep disturbance and tiredness can occur, and school performance, growth, general well-being and happiness can be affected.

The general principles of management include the following:

- Establish the diagnosis, severity and extent of disease.
- Good education is vital. Give written and verbal advice to parents. Explain that atopic eczema is a chronic condition and the aim of treatment is adequate control. Explain about the recognition and management of flare ups.
- Determine and avoid exacerbating factors: stress, environmental allergens and irritants.
- Maintain skin hydration with generous and repeated applications of emollients.
- Stop soaps and shower gels and use soap substitutes.
- Use topical corticosteroids to minimise inflammation. Steroid phobia is a major issue causing under treatment of this condition in children. Explain that its benefits outweigh the risk when used correctly. Prescribe the lowest strength that is effective (*Table 1*).
- Treat pruritus using antihistamines.
- Initiate prompt and aggressive treatment of secondary infection with antibiotics or antivirals as appropriate.
- Second-line treatment includes topical calcineurin inhibitors (tacrolimus), bandages and stockinette garments.
- Third-line treatment includes phototherapy and systemic agents such as methotrexate, cyclosporine and azathioprine.

Complications

Short-term complications may include:

- Post-inflammatory hypo/hyperpigmentation.

TABLE 1: Examples of steroids at different potencies	
Potency	Example
Mild	1% hydrocortisone
Moderate	2.5% hydrocortisone
Strong	Betnovate/dermovate

- Secondary infections:
  - Bacterial. Bacterial infections are common. *Staphylococcus aureus* and *Streptococcus pyogenes* are commonly the culprit. These cause a golden crust and sometimes pustulation (impetiginized eczema). Mild localised infection can be treated with antiseptic washes and topical antibacterial ointments. Oral antibiotics are used alongside topical corticosteroids to treat widespread infections.
  - Viral. Chickenpox infection can be widespread and severe. Molluscum contagiosum is more common in children with eczema and can be spread by scratching. Eczema herpeticum is a serious complication caused by herpes simplex virus (*Figure 3*). It presents with monomorphic clusters of vesicles that erode and crust. Prompt diagnosis and treatment with systemic acyclovir is paramount. Same day dermatology referral is highly recommended. If there is eye involvement, an urgent ophthalmology referral is required as it can cause corneal scarring.
- Contact sensitivity.
- Photosensitivity.
- Erythroderma.

Prognosis

Most cases of eczema are mild. In 40% of cases, atopic eczema presenting in childhood will disappear in adulthood with no long-term complications.

Infantile Seborrhoeic Dermatitis

Aetiology

Infantile seborrhoeic dermatitis is a self-limiting eruption of non-inflammatory, erythematous, greasy plaques with yellow scales. It usually occurs in infants three–weeks-old to 12–months-old.

Clinical Features

Distribution favours the scalp, retroauricular areas, eyebrows and nasolabial folds; these are areas rich in sebaceous glands. It can also occur in the napkin area, around the umbilicus

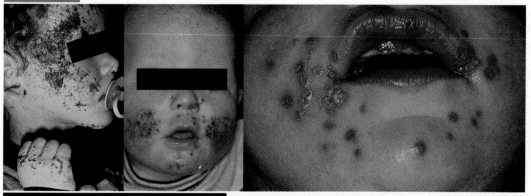

FIGURE 3

Examples of eczema herpeticum (D@nderm).

FIGURE 4

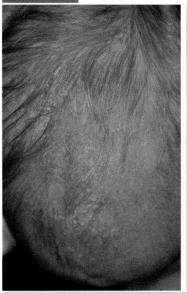
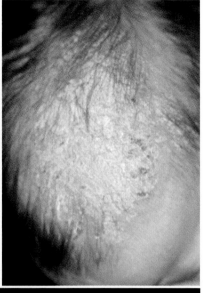

Seborrhoeic dermatitis (D@nderm).

the face. Guttate psoriasis is a form of psoriasis triggered by a throat or skin streptococcal infection. It presents suddenly, with widespread small plaques measuring up to 1 cm on the trunk and extremities.

Management

Management varies depending on disease severity and can include:

› Emollients.
› Vitamin D analogues.
› Tar preparations.
› Corticosteroids.
› Dithranol.

Second-line treatments include:

› Phototherapy.
› Systemic agents, such as retinoids, methotrexate or acitretin (in a minority of children).
› Biologic treatment with etanercept is now licensed for use in severe, refractory childhood psoriasis.

Complications

Associations include psoriatic arthritis in up to 48% of patients. This can affect the large or small joints but has a tendency to involve the distal small joints and may present with dactylitis. Additionally, nail changes such as pitting or onycholysis

and intertriginous areas. Lesions seen in the neck folds and axillae tend to be confluent, erythematous and greasy, but non-scaling. Seborrhoeic dermatitis may also manifest as "cradle cap", which favours the vertex and frontal areas of the scalp, in a "cap like" distribution (*Figure 4*). Pruritus, if experienced, tends to be mild. Infants generally thrive, with normal feeding and sleep.

Management

Parents should be offered reassurance and educated about simple skin care measures; the application of emollients, frequent shampooing and removal of scales with gentle brushing.

Prognosis

Most cases spontaneously resolve within a few weeks to months. Cases persisting for greater than 12 months may need further evaluation.

Psoriasis
Aetiology

Psoriasis is a common skin disorder affecting two percent of the population. The pathophysiology is not fully understood; an altered immune response and polygenic inheritance are thought to play vital roles. Although psoriasis can occur at any age, it is relatively

uncommon in children, with only 10% of cases presenting before 10-years-old.

Clinical Features

Psoriasis is characterised by intensely erythematous, well-demarcated, symmetrical plaques with adherent silvery scales. Common sites are the elbows, knees, lumbar region, ears, scalp and hairline (*Figure 5*). Psoriasis in children can present on

FIGURE 5

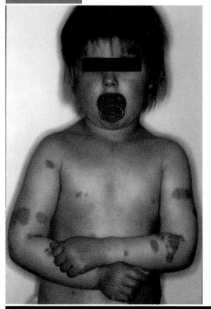
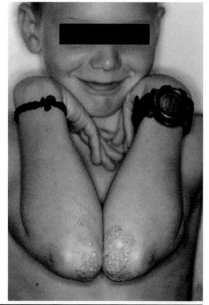

Psoriasitic plaques (D@nderm).

FIGURE 6

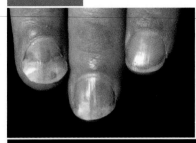
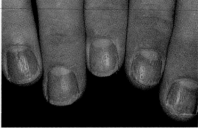

Nail changes in psoriasis: onycholysis (left), pitting (right) (D@nderm).

(separation of the nail from the nail bed) can be seen (*Figure 6*).

Prognosis

Psoriasis may completely resolve, particularly in mild cases that are reactive to an infection. However, the disease is often chronic, with a substantial psychosocial burden.

Acne Vulgaris

Aetiology

Acne is a common cutaneous condition affecting up to 90% of adolescents and young adults. It affects the pilosebaceous unit and is thought to be caused by a combination of the following factors:

> Sebaceous gland hypersensitivity to androgens.
> Increased sebum production, leading to duct blockage.

> Increased bacterial colonisation with the skin commensal flora *Propionibacterium acnes*.
> Inflammation.

Clinical Features

Acne presents in adolescence but can present as early as 8-years-old. The presentation varies and includes comedones (blackheads and whiteheads), papules, pustules, nodules, cysts and secondary scarring. It mainly affects areas with large hormone responsive sebaceous glands such as the face, back and chest, in a V-shape. It can extend to the lower back and waist (*Figure 7*).

Management

Treatment is important to prevent scarring. Response to treatment is slow and several agents may be tried in isolation or combination.

> Topical treatments. These are used in mild acne. They include antibiotics, benzoyl peroxide gels and topical retinoids.
> Oral antibiotics. In moderate acne, prolonged (at least three months) courses of oral antibiotics such as minocycline, doxycycline, lymecycline and erythromycin are added to the topical regimen. Tetracyclines should be avoided in children younger than 12-years-old to avoid permanent staining of the teeth.
> Oral retinoids. These are indicated in moderate, recalcitrant, nodular acne. Isotretinoin is teratogenic and effective contraception is imperative. In the UK, all females on retinoids are enrolled in the Pregnancy Prevention Programme, unless they choose to opt out. Although the most common side effect of isotretinoin is dryness of mucous membranes and skin, other side effects include hypercholesterolaemia, liver dysfunction, altered night vision, low mood, arthralgia and muscular pain. Isotretinoin is only prescribed by dermatologists in the UK and baseline bloods and a pregnancy test in females are required prior to initiating treatment.

Other possible treatments include hormone therapy in women (principally the oral contraceptive pill, but also potentially spironolactone). Rarely, intralesional injections of glucocorticosteroids may be used to treat a large, painful, nodulocystic lesion.

Prognosis

Eighty percent of acne cases resolve by the time a child reaches their 20s. However, it can have severe psychological implications and low mood and withdrawal are common.

Burns

Burns are the third leading cause of accidental death in high income countries.

FIGURE 7

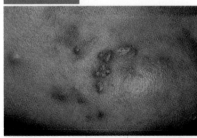
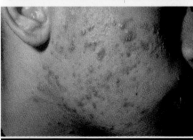
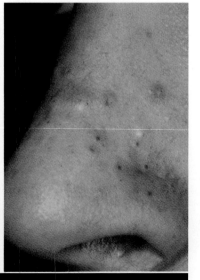

Acne. Note the presence of pustules (left image, top), secondary scarring (left image, bottom), and comedones (right image) (D@nderm).

TABLE 2: Classification of burns					
Type of Burn	1st Degree Burns (Superficial)	2nd Degree Burns (Partial Thickness)		3rd Degree Burns (Full Thickness)	4th Degree Burns
		Superficial Partial Thickness	Deep Partial Thickness		
Definition.	This involves only the epidermal layer of skin.	This involves the epidermis and portions of the dermis.	This extends into the dermis, damaging hair follicles and glandular tissue.	This destroys all of the epidermis and dermis and may extend to underlying subcutaneous tissue.	This involves full depth of skin plus underlying structures such as fascia, muscle and bone.
Presentation.	Painful, erythematous, dry lesion which blanches with pressure. It characteristically forms blisters within the first 24 hours between the epidermis and dermis.	Painful, erythematous, weeping lesion which blanches with pressure. It characteristically forms blisters within the first 24 hours between the epidermis and dermis.	Painful on pressure. It may be wet/dry, red/pale in appearance. Blanching may be sluggish or absent.	Painless lesion. The colour ranges from white to grey to black. Non-blanching. The non-viable dermis appears as an eschar which eventually separates.	As per third degree burns, with underlying muscle/bone potentially visible.
Prognosis.	Heals within 7 days without scarring.	Heals within 7 to 21 days; may cause pigment change but rarely scar.	If no secondary complications, this will heal within 3 to 9 weeks. Hypertrophic scarring is common.	This may not always spontaneously heal and typically results in severe scarring and contractures. Surgery may be indicated.	Always requires hospitalisation.

Aetiology

Scalds account for 60-80% of burns in children. Other causes of burns in children include fire-related burns, chemical burns and electrical burns. Deeper burns are more common in young children due to a relatively thin dermis and epidermis. It is important to remember that burns may be the presenting feature of child abuse. Patterns of burns that may raise suspicion include deep symmetrical burns of the extremities in a "glove-and-stocking" distribution which suggests a submersion injury, cigarette burns or burns in distinct shapes that suggest branding with an implement.

Clinical Features

A common classification system for burns is shown in *Table 2*.

Burn Surface Area

In children, surface area of burns is often calculated using the Lund-Browder chart. It attributes percentages to each body part and allows for a rapid assessment of the extent of skin involvement (*Figure 8*). Morbidity and mortality increase with higher surface area. Burns greater than 10% in a child are very serious and will require hospitalisation.

Management

Burns are potentially life-threatening injuries, especially in children. Improved survival is associated with early identification of associated injuries, adequate fluid resuscitation and prompt referral to a burns unit for specialist care. Mortality from burns increases as body surface area of thermal injury increases and in the presence of inhalation injury. The pattern of burns should be fully documented at presentation.

Clinicians should adopt an initial ABC approach, with special consideration to:

Airway and Breathing

- Examine the oropharynx for evidence of inhalation injury. If suspected consider early intubation to avoid acute airway obstruction due to laryngeal oedema.
- Provide high flow supplemental oxygen therapy to all fire-related burns patients to treat possible carbon monoxide poisoning.
- Consider carbon monoxide poisoning and monitor carboxyhaemoglobin levels from arterial blood. Especially in cases of reduced mental status or metabolic acidosis (N.B. pulse oximetry and arterial oxygen levels are frequently normal in carbon monoxide poisoning).
- Circumferential burns of the chest wall may compromise respiration by reducing chest wall compliance: this may require immediate surgery (escharotomy) to release the constriction caused by eschar (tough, inelastic mass of burnt tissue).

Circulation

- Monitor closely for signs of hypovolaemic shock.
- Aggressive fluid resuscitation may be necessary.
  - Establish adequate vascular access early.
  - Consider bladder catheterisation to monitor urine output.
- Metabolic acidosis may indicate inadequate tissue perfusion or carbon monoxide poisoning.
- An ECG should be immediately sought in suspected cases of carbon monoxide poisoning to assess for myocardial ischaemia.
- The Parkland formula is frequently used to calculate the fluid deficit which needs to be replaced. Typically, half is replaced in the first 8 hours,

FIGURE 8A

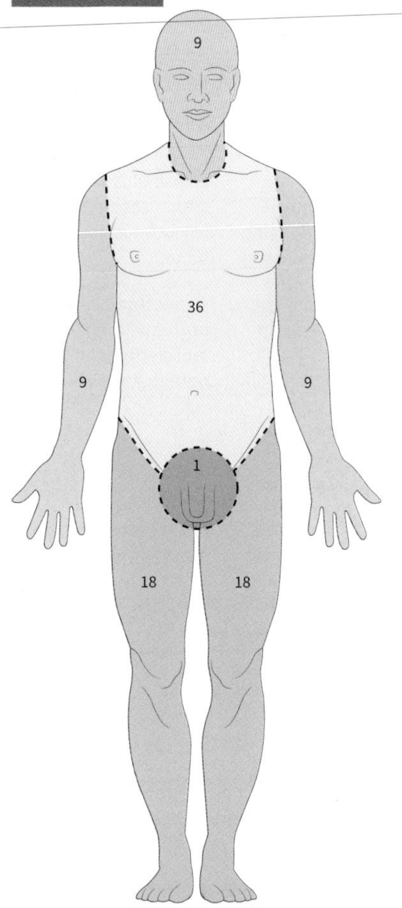

FIGURE 8B

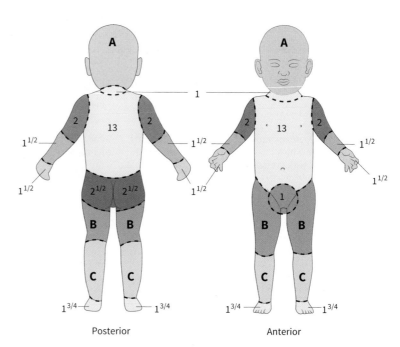

Lund and Browder chart in adults: percentage of body covered by burns (except genitalia, numbers refer to front and back combined).

Posterior   Anterior

Body part		Age (years)				
		0	1	5	10	15
A.	½ of head.	9.5	8.5	6.5	5.5	3.5
B.	½ of 1 thigh.	2.75	3.25	4	4.25	4.75
C.	½ of 1 lower leg.	2.5	2.5	2.75	3	3.5

Lund and Browder chart in children: percentage of body covered by burns.

and the other half over the next 16 hours. The deficit is calculated as:

Volume (ml) = 4 x body weight (kg) x % of total skin surface burned

e.g. if 20kg, with 10% burns:
Volume = 4 x 20 x 10 = 800 ml

Disability

- Hypoglycaemia or hyperglycaemia may occur. Monitor blood glucose levels carefully and consider adding 5% dextrose or insulin to parenteral fluids as indicated.
- Altered consciousness levels may indicate carbon monoxide poisoning.

Exposure

- Ensure the entire body is exposed, to identify and treat all burns and associated injuries.

Initial management additionally comprises:

- Debriding any bullae and removing any necrotic tissue. Look at the base of the bullae to identify the depth of a burn. Necrotic tissue may become infected if not removed.
- Cleansing the burn with chlorhexidine solution or equivalent and applying a suitable dressing.
- Topical and parenteral antimicrobials should be considered to prevent/treat secondary bacterial infections.
- Adequate analgesia is important and often morphine is indicated.
- Adequate nutrition in the acute phase is important to support the metabolic demands of catabolism of trauma, heat loss, and the demand of tissue regeneration. This may require the

insertion of a nasogastric tube.
- Monitor closely for signs of compartment syndrome, infection and cellulitis around the burn.
- Consider tetanus prophylaxis in any child that is not immunised.

Children with significant burns should be transferred to a burns centre when clinically stable for specialist management by surgeons and tissue viability specialists. Surgery, including debridement and skin grafting, may be indicated in severe cases.

Complications

Morbidity following a burn may result from:

- **Local injury.** Burns cause tissue destruction and decreased perfusion.

- **Fluid loss.** Following a burn there is an inflammatory response leading to release of vasoactive mediators and increased capillary permeability, resulting in accumulation of fluid in the interstitial space. Fluid loss contributes considerably to morbidity. Children need to be monitored closely for signs of hypovolaemic shock.
- **Metabolic response.** Due to a stress response, children with severe burns develop a hypermetabolic response post resuscitation. There is an increased release of catecholamines, glucagon and cortisol; a dramatic increase in energy expenditure and protein metabolism; and a hyperdynamic circulation.
- **Secondary bacterial infection.** Breach of the skin's protective barrier and the presence of necrotic debris predispose to bacterial infection. Intravenous and topical antibiotics should be considered at an early stage.
- **Toxic shock syndrome.** Causative organisms which may thrive at a burn site include *Staphylococcus aureus* and *Streptococcus pyogenes*. Toxic shock syndrome is not caused by the bacterial infection itself, but rather by bacterial toxins. These cause a systemic reaction, resulting in pyrexia, hypotension, malaise, confusion, diffuse macular erythroderma and multiorgan dysfunction. The rash desquamates after one to two weeks. Treatment involves supportive therapy and broad spectrum antibiotics.
- **Compartment syndrome.** Eschar is burnt, denatured skin, which is tough and inelastic and overlies deep burns. If circumferential, it may lead to compartment syndrome that requires prompt treatment.

Prognosis
Outcomes depend on the degree and severity of the burns. Children are at a particular risk of developing contractures around scars. This is because the scars cannot expand to keep pace with overall growth of the child; this will potentially require surgical release.

Cellulitis
Aetiology
Cellulitis is an infection of soft tissue caused by bacteria breaching the skin's physical barrier. It is normally caused by pathogens that colonise skin, such as *Staphylococcus aureus* and β haemolytic streptococcal infections. Predisposing factors include trauma, insect bites and underlying medical conditions such as diabetes mellitus, immune deficiencies and chronic venous insufficiency.

Clinical Features
Clinically, cellulitis presents with erythema, oedema, tenderness and increased temperature of the skin. There may also be evidence of an entry wound. It can be superficial, affecting the upper dermis only, or may be deeper, extending to the deeper dermis and subcutaneous fat. Skin abscesses may develop, identified by swelling and purulent discharge and should be evaluated promptly as they may need surgical drainage.

Management
Treatment involves simple measures such as elevation and appropriate antibiotic cover.

Mild cellulitis can be treated with oral antibiotics but intravenous antibiotics should be instituted promptly if cellulitis is rapidly progressive and the child is systemically unwell. Intravenous antibiotics should also be considered in neonates with cellulitis in whom absorption of oral antibiotics can be poor. Marking the area before starting therapy is useful as a guide to whether the infection is improving or spreading.

Special consideration should be given to children with periorbital cellulitis as these infections can progress rapidly and threaten vision. Evaluation by an ophthalmologist is crucial. If proptosis or involvement of the orbit is suspected, immediate imaging is indicated p55.

Impetigo
Aetiology
Impetigo is a highly contagious superficial bacterial skin infection, commonly caused by *Staphylococcus aureus* or *Streptococcus pyogenes*. It can affect people of any age but is most frequently seen in children 2 to 5-years-old.

Clinical Features
Lesions favour the face and extremities. They initially appear as papules which progress to pustules that rupture producing a gold adherent crust with surrounding erythema (*Figure 9*). It may occasionally present as clear fluid filled blisters (bullous impetigo).

Management
Treatment depends on the severity of the infection. Topical antiseptic washes and topical antibiotic preparations (e.g. fusidic acid) are sufficient in mild cases. The addition of oral antibiotics (e.g. flucloxacillin) is recommended if the infection is extensive or not responding to topical preparations. If the infection is recurrent or is slow responding, swabbing and treating carrier sites, such as the nose, is important. Identifying and treating infected contacts or using prolonged oral antibiotic courses along with topical antibacterials may be necessary for eradication.

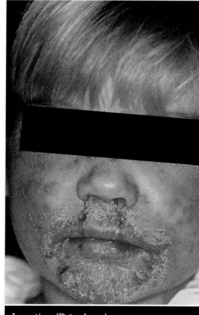

FIGURE 9

Impetigo (D@nderm).

Viral Warts

Aetiology

Cutaneous warts occur commonly in children and are caused by the human papillomavirus family (HPV), of which there are over 150 identified types. Infections occur by skin-to-skin contact, particularly if there is a breach in the skin barrier. These viruses affect the skin and mucous membranes and typically cause hyperproliferative lesions after a two to six month incubation period.

Clinical Features

Several types of wart are seen:

› Common warts (verruca vulgaris) represent approximately 70% of all cutaneous warts and occur in up to 10% of all school-age children. They commonly present as firm papules measuring 1-10 mm or larger. They are hyperkeratotic and sometimes have vegetations. They occur at sites of trauma such as the hands, fingers and knees.

› Palmar lesions are also common, disrupting the fingerprint. Return to normal fingerprints is a sign of resolution. When similar warts occur on the plantar surface of the feet, they are termed plantar warts (verruca plantaris).

› Flat warts (verruca plana) are sharply defined, round or oval papules measuring 1-5 mm with flat surfaces. They commonly occur on the face, dorsa of the hands, and shins.

Management

Spontaneous regression occurs in most cases within two years. Therefore, aggressive therapy that may cause scarring should be avoided. Treatment, if necessary, most frequently involves salicylic acid in different strengths, ranging between 10-40%, depending on the size of the wart. Cryotherapy is also an option if tolerated by children. However, it is generally avoided on the feet as it can be exquisitely painful and affect mobility.

Molluscum Contagiosum

Aetiology

Molluscum contagiosum is a self-limiting epidermal viral infection caused by the molluscum contagiosum virus (MCV). Infection is spread by skin-to-skin contact and the incubation period is between two and six weeks. It colonises the epidermis and infundibulum of the hair follicles causing a chronic localised infection of the skin. It is more common in those with immunodeficiencies.

Clinical Features

Lesions appear as flesh-coloured, dome-shaped papules (*Figure 10*). They are 2-5 mm in diameter and have a central indentation. Lesions can occur anywhere on the body, favouring the trunk, axillae and antecubital/popliteal fossae.

Management

Children should be advised to cover exposed lesions and avoid sharing towels. Molluscum is a self-limiting infection and usually clears within 6 to 12 months. Treatment is considered to reduce spread of infection or to reduce psychological distress. Rapid resolution can be achieved by cryotherapy, curettage and electrodessication (using an electric current to remove

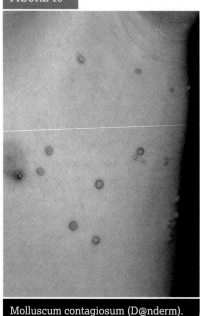

Molluscum contagiosum (D@nderm).

the lesion). Imiquimod (an immune response modifier) 5% cream may also be effective.

Hand-Foot-and-Mouth Disease

Aetiology

Hand-foot-and-mouth disease describes a highly contagious viral infection that is common in infants and children. It can be caused by a number of enterovirus serotypes, commonly coxsackievirus A16 and enterovirus 71. The incubation period is between three to five days and transmission is via the faeco-oral route or contact with vesicle fluid.

Clinical Features

The clinical syndrome is characterised by oral lesions, vesicular exanthum on the distal extremities and mild constitutional symptoms, namely fever. The oral lesions start as macules on the hard palate, tongue and buccal mucosa. They initially turn into greyish vesicles and eventually become painful punched out ulcers measuring between 5 and 10 mm. Cutaneous lesions appear with, or shortly after, the oral lesions. The lesions erupt as erythematous macules and papules and then turn into vesicles (*Figure 11*). They characteristically occur on the palms, soles, sides of the fingers, and the buttocks, but can occur anywhere. They can be linear in shape, can crust or erode and generally heal without scarring.

Management

The diagnosis is based on the history and clinical findings. The illness is self-limiting and resolves within seven days.

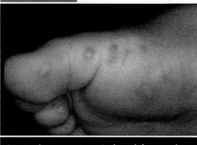

FIGURE 11

Vesicular eruptions in hand-foot-and-mouth disease (D@nderm).

Tinea or Dermatophyte Infections (Ringworm)

Aetiology

"Tinea" refers to a cutaneous infection with dermatophyte fungus (ringworm) (*Figure 12*). Common non-dermatophyte fungal infections include infections with *Candida* species and moulds.

Clinical Features

Depending on which part of the body it affects, tinea is given a specific designation: tinea capitis (head), tinea faciei (face), tinea corporis (body), tinea manuum (hand), tinea pedis (foot), tinea unguium (nail) and tinea cruris (groin). Tinea capitis is common in children and usually presents as a bald, scaly, erythematous patch. Pustules or black spots may be present. Kerion refers to abscess formation with a tinea infection and the most common anatomical location is the scalp.

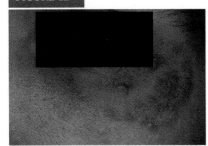
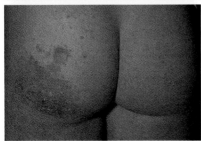
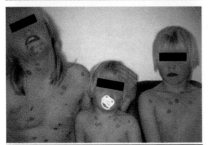

FIGURE 12

Examples of fungal infections. Note that these are contagious, and the third example shows three siblings acquiring the same infection (D@nderm).

Management

The diagnosis is made with mycological identification of the fungus by skin scrapings, nail clippings or hair plucking. The licensed treatment is oral griseofulvin (10-20 mg/kg). The duration of the treatment depends on the location of the infection. Tinea capitis requires a six week course of treatment.

Scabies

Aetiology

Scabies is an extremely contagious superficial epidermal infestation caused by the mite *Sarcoptes scabiei* var. *hominis*. It is spread by skin-to-skin contact and has an incubation period of three to six weeks. Mites burrow into the superficial layers of the skin and deposit faeces in tunnels.

Burrows have predilection to the following sites: web spaces of the hands and toes, wrists, lateral aspects of the palms, extensor surfaces of the elbows and knees, axillary folds and the periumbilical and genital areas. Immediate and delayed hypersensitivity reactions to the mite, its faeces or eggs may occur, causing eczematous rashes and occasionally scabietic nodules. Hyperinfestations with >10^6 mites were previously referred to as Norwegian scabies. Norwegian scabies is more likely to occur in immunocompromised individuals or in those with neurological disorders. Complications include lymphadenopathy and secondary bacterial infections, which can be suggested by tenderness of the lesions.

Clinical Features

The diagnosis is based on the clinical findings of burrows, papules and nodules, plus a history of affected contacts. If possible, microscopic visualisation of the mite, ova or mite faeces extracted from a scabietic burrow is diagnostic. The diagnosis can be easily missed and should be considered in any patient of any age with persistent severe pruritus, especially if there is a family history of similar symptoms.

Management

Treating the affected individual and all physical contacts, whether symptomatic or not, at the same time is very important. The recommended treatment is with two applications of 5% permethrin cream, one week apart. The cream should be applied to all areas of the body excluding the head, left overnight and washed off in the morning. A single dose of oral ivermectin is also effective. However, this should not be used in infants or young children. All bedding and clothing should be washed in a hot cycle for eradication. It is important to remember that eczematous rashes can persist post-treatment. Short courses of topical or oral steroids may be necessary.

Pediculosis Capitis (Head lice)

Aetiology

Head lice are also known as the insect *Pediculus humanus capitis*. It attaches to and feeds from the scalp of the host. Head lice are translucent mobile insects measuring 3-4 mm in length. The life span of the head louse is one month; adult lice can survive up to 48 hours without a host. It is a common infestation worldwide; the prevalence in schoolchildren ranges from 10-40%. Transmission is by head-to-head contact. Adolescents and adults tend to be less affected than children.

Clinical Features

The main symptom of head lice infestation is pruritus. The degree of itching is variable and can be absent. It is thought to be due to an allergic reaction to the louse saliva. Persistent scratching can cause excoriations to the scalp and neck, secondary bacterial infections and posterior cervical lymphadenopathy.

The diagnosis is based on the presence of lice or their ova (nits), which are cemented to the hair shafts. The occipital and postauricular scalp regions are areas of predilection.

Management

Topical pediculicides, such as permethrin, phenothrin and malathion, have been the standard treatment for head lice. The use of the oral anthelmintic agent ivermectin is rarely justified. Due to worldwide observation of resistance to topical treatments, lack of commercial availability or simply poverty, alternative methods such as removal of lice by hands (nit-picking), wet combing with a fine-toothed net comb and application of topical asphyxiation agents, such as petrolatum and dimethicone, are widely used.

Urticaria
Aetiology

Urticaria occurs due to plasma leakage from permeable blood vessels. These reactions are due to allergic or non-allergic mast cell stimulation, resulting in histamine release along with other cytokines. It is defined as acute if the duration is less than six weeks and chronic if more than six weeks. In 85% of cases, the episodes are isolated.

▸ Acute urticaria is commonly associated with trigger factors, such as bacterial and viral infections, drugs (aspirin, non-steroidal anti-inflammatory drugs [NSAIDS], codeine and antibiotics), food, pollen, bites and stings.

▸ Chronic urticaria is also termed idiopathic or "ordinary" urticaria. A circulating autoantibody has been identified in a proportion of these patients. In these patients, triggering factors, such as viral infections or certain medications, may exacerbate the condition.

Clinical Features

Urticaria, or hives, presents as common itchy, raised, blotchy, red rashes that occur without surface change or scaling (*Figure 13*). Urticaria can be associated with underlying swelling of the skin, known as angioedema, causing swelling of the mucous membranes. Urticaria can also be an early sign of anaphylaxis, a life-threatening allergic reaction which requires urgent treatment with adrenaline, antihistamines and corticosteroids (p144).

Management

Urticaria is a self-limiting condition and an important part of management is educating patients on its time course. Excluding precipitating factors and avoiding possible triggers is essential. Cooling anti-pruritics, such as menthol in aqueous cream preparations, can be useful. First-line treatment includes non-sedating antihistamines, followed by sedating antihistamines. Short courses of oral prednisolone can be used in severe episodes but should be avoided in chronic urticaria. Second line treatment includes montelukast and mast cell stabilising agents. Cyclosporine is licensed for use in severe urticaria.

Erythema Nodosum
Aetiology

Erythema nodosum is the most common type of panniculitis in both adults and children. Although it has a female predilection in adults, the incidence is equal in both genders in children. Around 70% of erythema nodosum cases in children are related to infectious aetiology; β-haemolytic streptococcal infection is the most common cause. Non-infectious aetiologies include inflammatory bowel disease and sarcoidosis. Drug-related cases are much less common in this age group.

Clinical Features

Clinically, this condition presents with sudden onset of tender, erythematous nodules and plaques. These are symmetrically distributed on the anterior shins, ankles and occasionally knees (*Figure 14*). They eventually evolve to bruise-like plaques and heal without scarring.

Management

The diagnosis is made clinically; however, a biopsy is diagnostic as it shows the classic septal panniculitis without vasculitis picture. The treatment includes addressing the underlying cause, such as treating any infection or controlling inflammatory bowel disease. Mild cases are treated with bed rest and non-steroidal anti-inflammatory medication to improve pain and inflammation. Short courses of oral steroids can be used once any underlying infection is completely treated.

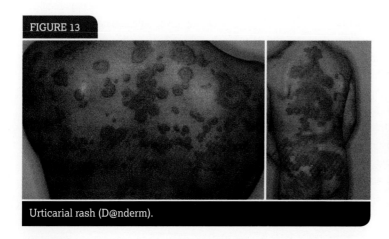

FIGURE 13

Urticarial rash (D@nderm).

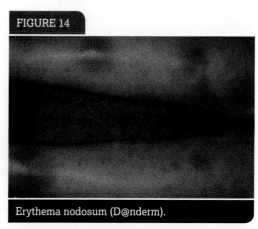

FIGURE 14

Erythema nodosum (D@nderm).

REFERENCES AND FURTHER READING

Eczema

1   NICE CG57. Atopic eczema in children. 2013. https://www.nice.org.uk/guidance/cg57.

Burns

1   Jeschke MG, Herndon DN. Burns in children: standard and new treatments. Lancet. 2014; 383:1168-78.

Miscellaneous

1   Jones SL. Oxford Specialist Handbooks in Paediatrics: Paediatric Dermatology. Oxford: Oxford University Press; 2010.

2   Irvine PH, Yan A. Harper's Textbook of Pediatric Dermatology. Third Edition. Hoboken: Wiley Blackwell; 2011.

341

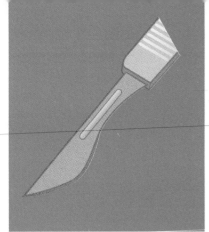

1.24
SURGERY

MAY BISHARAT

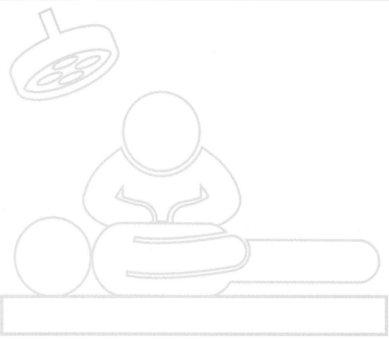

CONTENTS

GENERAL SURGERY

Infantile Pyloric Stenosis

Infantile pyloric stenosis (IPS) is characterised by gradual thickening of the pyloric muscle, which eventually results in complete gastric outlet obstruction.

Aetiology

The aetiology of IPS remains unclear but some evidence suggests a neurogenic cause. The neuronal nitric oxide synthase gene has been linked to the condition. The incidence of IPS is one to three per 1000 live births. The condition is more prevalent in:

›   Males (four times more common).
›   Firstborns.
›   Those with a strong family history.

Clinical Features

Typically, infants with pyloric stenosis present with non-bilious vomiting that commences between three to four weeks of age. The vomiting is usually described as projectile, and can be associated with haematemesis secondary to oesophagitis. Prolonged vomiting typically leads to:

›   Lethargy.
›   Weight loss (or failure to gain weight) despite being a hungry baby.
›   Constipation.

On examination, infants appear thin, but hungry, and may display signs of dehydration. Occasionally, visible gastric peristalsis can be seen. A palpable pyloric tumour (olive-shaped mass) in the epigastrium or right upper quadrant is diagnostic of the condition but is often difficult to feel and can often only be detected by an experienced clinician. If unsure, a "test feed" should be performed by offering the infant dextrose water. This relaxes the abdominal muscles, allowing deep palpation, and stimulating the pylorus to contract. The examining hand needs to be placed in the right upper quadrant to appreciate the thickened pylorus.

Investigations

›   Blood tests. A blood gas will show a hypochloraemic, hypokalaemic, metabolic alkalosis. This is caused by excessive vomiting and loss of gastric fluid (mainly hydrogen and chloride). As dehydration worsens, the patients also develop a paradoxical aciduria. With worsening dehydration, sodium conservation becomes the kidneys' priority. The renal tubules reabsorb sodium in exchange for potassium and hydrogen, resulting in acidic urine. Electrolytes will need to be regularly monitored.
›   Ultrasound of the abdomen. If the test feed is positive (the pylorus was palpable), no further investigations are needed. If, however, the test feed is inconclusive, an ultrasound scan

is recommended. The following three criteria need to be met to confirm IPS on ultrasound (*Figure 1*):

›   Pyloric muscle thickness > 4 mm.
›   Pyloric muscle length > 18 mm.
›   Failure of fluid passage beyond the pylorus despite vigorous gastric peristalsis.

›   Contrast studies. This is usually reserved for cases where ultrasonography is inconclusive. The "string sign" is the diagnostic term given to the delayed passage of a small amount of contrast through a thin, long pyloric canal. One advantage of contrast studies is the ability to detect other conditions, such as malrotation.

Differential Diagnosis

The main differential diagnoses are:

›   Gastroesophageal reflux disease (GORD).
›   Malrotation.
›   Sepsis.

In these cases, vomiting is usually non-projectile, and in malrotation is bile stained.

Management

›   Medical. Preoperative rehydration and correction of electrolyte imbalances is of paramount importance: surgery is deferred until this has happened. A nasogastric (NG) tube allows (i) the stomach to be decompressed (ii) losses to be measured, and (iii) losses to be replaced accurately. Oral feeds are stopped. There are three aspects to fluid management:
    ›   Fluid boluses. Given for initial dehydration. Boluses of 0.9% sodium chloride are given.
    ›   Maintenance fluids. Given since the patient is kept nil by mouth e.g. 100ml/kg of 5% dextrose/0.9% sodium chloride. Potassium is added as per serum levels, and sodium may need to be adjusted.

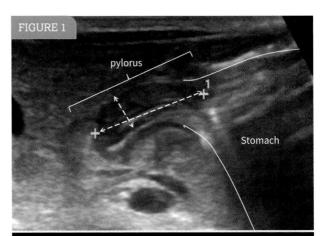

FIGURE 1

Ultrasound of the pylorus demonstrating pyloric stenosis. The pyloric muscle is thickened and elongated (21cm x 5.5cm). The numbers and appearance are diagnostic of pyloric stenosis.

> › Replacement fluids. Given to replace NG tube losses, e.g. 0.9% sodium chloride with 10% potassium chloride. Replacement fluids have to be potassium rich due to the high potassium content of gastric fluid. The rate of infusion is adjusted according the rate of gastric losses, and therefore higher concentrations of potassium are not recommended due to the risk of hyperkalaemia.

› Surgical. Definitive treatment for the condition is Ramstedt's pyloromyotomy. This can be performed via a right upper quadrant or a supraumbilical incision. Recently, a laparoscopic approach has been advocated, but this is not yet widely practiced. In all approaches, an incision is made along the length of the pyloric swelling, down to the mucosa.

Complications

The main presurgical issues are electrolyte imbalance and dehydration. Complications of Ramstedt's pyloromyotomy include bleeding, perforation and wound infection.

Prognosis

Recovery is usually uneventful. Infants are discharged 24-48 hours following the procedure once feeding has been re-established. Patients usually suffer no long-term complications.

Acute Appendicitis

Acute appendicitis is an acute inflammation of the appendix, commonly caused by obstruction of the lumen by mucosal swelling or a faecolith. Appendicitis can occur at any age, but is uncommon in children under 4–years-old and is therefore more difficult to diagnose. The condition can be associated with the presence of serous (reactive) free fluid in the peritoneal cavity.

A perforated appendicitis is an extensive inflammation of the appendix that has resulted in microscopic or macroscopic perforations. The condition is associated with the presence of free pus in the peritoneal cavity. This can either be contained by omentum or spread all over the peritoneal cavity (peritonitis).

An appendix mass is appendicitis (usually perforated) that has been walled and sealed off from the rest of the peritoneal cavity by omentum and loops of small bowel. The mass is usually palpable on clinical examination.

Aetiology

Risk factors for acute appendicitis are poorly understood. Some patients suffer from a pre-existing viral illness. Others may have a history of a "grumbling appendix" with previous intermittent symptoms of appendicitis and spontaneous recovery.

Clinical Features

› Pain. Periumbilical colicky pain that shifts to the right iliac fossa and becomes constant and severe. The main aggravating factor is movement. On palpation, there is typically tenderness and localised guarding. In some cases of perforated appendicitis the children have generalised guarding and peritonitis.

› Gastrointestinal upset. The child is frequently nauseous, off their food and occasionally has vomited.

› Fever. A temperature >39°C makes perforated appendicitis likely. Perforation is also accompanied by tachycardia and moderate dehydration.

If in doubt, the "jump test" is extremely useful. Only a child with no significant intra-abdominal pathology is able to jump up and down a few times without significant pain.

Investigations

The diagnosis of appendicitis is made clinically. The decision to remove an inflamed appendix does not depend on blood test results. Tests are performed to support the diagnosis, as a baseline for future developments and to ensure a safe anaesthetic approach.

› Inflammatory markers. The white cell count is usually elevated, as is the C-reactive protein (CRP). However, CRP may lag behind the clinical picture, so if the child presents early in the course of his illness, this test can potentially be normal.

› Renal function/electrolytes. If the patient is very unwell, especially if they are very young, dehydration and electrolyte imbalances can be dangerous, requiring preoperative correction.

› Urinalysis. May have a urinary tract infection (UTI). Frequently, patients with acute appendicitis have some white blood cells in the urine, but no nitrites. This is due to mechanical irritation of the bladder by a pelvic appendix.

› Pregnancy test. Mandatory in any girl over 12-years-old presenting with abdominal pain.

› Ultrasonography. Ultrasound can identify features consistent with appendicitis. It is especially useful in patients where other potential causes for the pain are being sought (e.g. ruptured ovarian cyst, intussusception). The test carries a significant false negative result risk (low sensitivity).

Differential Diagnosis

If symptoms and signs are typical, diagnosis may be clear. However, other conditions to consider include:

› Nonspecific abdominal pain of childhood. This is very common and usually resolves spontaneously.
› UTI.
› Ectopic pregnancy.
› Meckel's diverticular disease (inflammation or perforation).
› Ovarian pathology.
› Constipation.

Management

› Surgical. For acute appendicitis, the appendix is removed either via an open or laparoscopic approach. The peritoneal cavity is entered, the appendix is identified and the diagnosis is confirmed. The appendix is then removed, peritoneal swabs are taken and the wound/wounds are closed.

› Antibiotics are given for 24 hours if there is mild inflammation and for several days if the inflammation is significant.

› If the appendix is perforated, a thorough washout with copious amounts of washout fluid is performed to decrease the risk of abscess formation. Antibiotics are given for a further 5-10 days afterwards, ensuring anaerobe and gram negative cover, for example giving co-amoxiclav and gentamicin.

› Medical. Tremendous debate surrounds the treatment of an appendix mass. Most units manage the patient conservatively, by commencing IV antibiotics followed by oral therapy on improvement. The resolution of the mass is monitored clinically and by ultrasound. An interval appendectomy (elective removal of the now non-inflamed appendix) is offered after a period of six to eight weeks.

› Conservative. In cases with significant abdominal pain, but an unclear diagnosis, the patients should be actively managed by admitting, and regularly re-examining to see whether the pain progresses/localises, or if it settles.

Complications

Complications are more common in children who present with perforated appendicitis. These include:

› Wound infection/breakdown.
› Electrolyte derangement/dehydration.
› Pelvic collection.
› Bowel obstruction due to adhesions.

Prognosis

Recovery is complete in most patients, particularly those who present early.

Intussusception

Intussusception is invagination of a proximal segment of bowel into another more distal part (*Figure 2*). It occurs most commonly in infants aged between two months and two years, with the majority of cases occurring before the first birthday. Male infants have a slightly higher risk of developing the condition (M:F, 3:2). The incidence ranges between one and four cases per 1000 live births.

Aetiology

Most cases of intussusception are idiopathic. However, the condition is more common in winter and spring, suggesting a link to viral infections (gastroenteritis, respiratory infections). Viral infection is believed to cause swelling of the Peyer's patches, aggregates of lymphoid tissue in the distal ileum, which in turn encourages intussusception.

In up to 10% of cases, a pathological lead point can be found. These can include Meckel diverticulae, Peutz-Jeghers polyps and small bowel lymphoma.

Intussusception can arise anywhere in the small or large bowel. Different types include:

› Small bowel into small bowel.
› Small bowel into large bowel.
› Large bowel into large bowel.
› Large bowel into rectum.

The most common type of intussusception occurs in the terminal ileum and passes through the ileocaecal valve. This usually draws the mesentery of the small bowl into the intussusception, and venous congestion ensues. Soon after, arterial occlusion occurs, leading to ischaemia, necrosis and perforation.

Clinical Features

Children with intussusception usually present with:

› Abdominal pain. Sudden colicky abdominal pain. Parents typically describe bouts of severe pain that occur every 10–20 minutes. The pain is usually associated with drawing up of legs, and screaming. Children are typically well and asymptomatic between bouts of colic.

› Pale episodes. Particularly in association with pain.

› Vomiting. Some children vomit with the pain. This can be a reflex to pain or intestinal obstruction due to the intussusception.

› "Redcurrant jelly" stool. A mixture of blood and mucus.

On clinical examination, children may appear weak and dehydrated, tachycardic or even lethargic. If the abdomen is

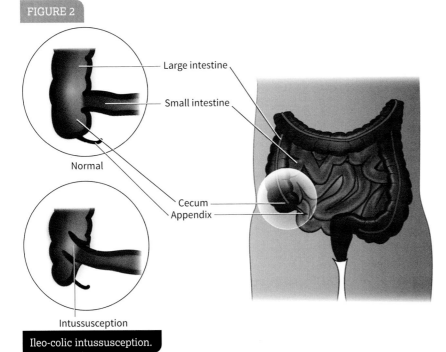

FIGURE 2

Large intestine

Small intestine

Normal

Cecum
Appendix

Intussusception

Ileo-colic intussusception.

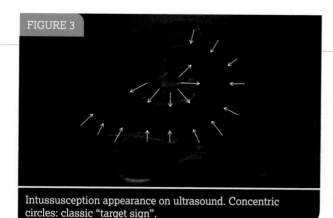

FIGURE 3

Intussusception appearance on ultrasound. Concentric circles: classic "target sign".

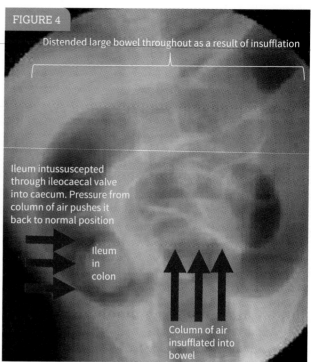

FIGURE 4

Distended large bowel throughout as a result of insufflation

Ileum intussuscepted through ileocaecal valve into caecum. Pressure from column of air pushes it back to normal position

Ileum in colon

Column of air insufflated into bowel

Abdominal X-ray taken during an air reduction enema. Air is insufflated via a catheter into the rectum. The column of air gradually reduces the intussuscepted ileum out of the colon.

examined between bouts of pain, a sausage-shaped mass can frequently be felt in the right upper quadrant. Occasionally children have an extremely distended abdomen or can have frank peritonitis (rigid abdomen) and sepsis.

Investigations

Blood tests may point towards inflammation, electrolyte derangement, dehydration and significant bleeding. However, the gold standard investigation is an ultrasound scan of the abdomen. The classic sign is the "target sign" (or doughnut sign) on transverse section, which represents the two concentric lumina of bowel (*Figure 3*). An abdominal X-ray may reveal features of small bowel obstruction.

Management

Non-Operative Management

Appropriate fluid resuscitation should occur prior to any intervention as children with intussusception will have suffered huge third space losses of fluid. IV antibiotics (broad spectrum, like co-amoxiclav) should be administered promptly.

Following adequate resuscitation, a pneumatic reduction enema is performed:

>   A catheter is inserted into the rectum of the child in the radiology department and air is insufflated under fluoroscopic screening.
>   The pressure generated by the air, in 75-80% of cases, is sufficient to achieve a complete reduction (*Figure 4*).

Patients who fail air enema, have a highly distended abdomen, or who are peritonitic will require an urgent laparotomy.

Operative Management

A right transverse incision is made and the intussusception is identified. In 50-60% of cases, a simple manual reduction is possible. In the remainder of cases, the bowel is either too oedematous to allow a successful reduction or has become non-viable. In such cases, a resection of the affected bowel with end-to-end anastomosis is performed.

Following a successful air reduction enema, fluids can be reintroduced after 12–24 hours and patients are discharged

48 hours later. Patients who undergo an open manual reduction have a similar post-operative course, whereas children who undergo bowel resection have a slightly longer recovery period.

Complications

If left untreated, intussusception can lead to:

>   Ischaemia.
>   Necrosis.
>   Haemorrhage.
>   Perforation.
>   Infection/peritonitis.

Complications can also be iatrogenic, with one percent of air reduction enemas leading to perforation.

Prognosis

Mortality is approximately one percent and is mainly related to inadequate fluid resuscitation or diagnostic delay. Recurrence occurs in 10% of cases. Approximately 30% occur in the first 24 hours post reduction and 70% present within six months. In children with more than one recurrence, investigations for a pathological lead point need to be performed.

Inguinal Hernia

An inguinal hernia is the protrusion of peritoneal cavity contents through the inguinal canal. The incidence of inguinal hernias is approximately one to two percent, but is much higher in pre-term infants (up to 20%). The male to female ratio is four to one. The condition is more common on the right, although 10% of cases are bilateral.

Aetiology

Inguinal hernias are typically "indirect" inguinal hernias in children, i.e. the abdominal contents do not herniate through a weakness in the abdominal wall (direct); rather, they follow through a patent processus vaginalis (PPV). Ninety-five percent are present in the groin only; the rest are inguino-scrotal (*Figure 5*). Direct hernias are very rare in children.

The processus vaginalis (PV) is a peritoneal elongation that passes through the inguinal canal. Gender determines contents:

➤ In boys, the testis descends into the scrotum through this channel.
➤ In girls, the round ligament is present in the canal.

The PV is patent at birth in most babies, but closes soon after birth. If the channel remains open, a patent processus vaginalis (or PPV) is the outcome.

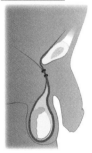

Nomal · Hydrocoele

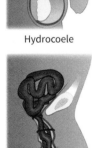

Inguinal hernia · Inguinoscrotal hernia

Patent processus vaginalis. In the hydrocoele, only fluid connects with the scrotum. In a hernia, loops of bowel pass through, either into the inguinal canal (inguinal hernia) or into the inguinal canal and scrotum (inguinoscrotal hernia).

Clinical Features

➤ Reducible lump. A hernia usually manifests as a reducible lump in the groin that occasionally extends into the scrotum or labium. This may be present from birth.
➤ Intermittent lump. Older children may report the intermittent appearance of a lump on laughing, coughing or straining. It may only appear after standing for a long period. The lesion is frequently not present on examination, and in children, manoeuvres to increase the intra-abdominal pressure (e.g. laughing, coughing, straining) should be used.
➤ Discomfort. Unobstructed hernias are usually painless, but there may still be discomfort or heaviness at the site.

Some children can present with a strangulated or "stuck" inguinal hernia, where the blood supply has become compromised. The skin overlying the hernia may be oedematous, erythematous or discoloured. It is also associated with nausea, vomiting, severe pain and tachycardia. The child may have inconsolable crying and be off food. Incarcerated hernias are a surgical emergency.

It is important to note:

➤ The classic "adult" teaching of "hydrocoeles transilluminate and hernias do not" does not apply to young infants, as hernias can brightly transilluminate as well. The bowel wall in young infants tends to be paper thin and light can easily shine through. Additionally, feeds for babies are more liquid in consistency anyway, making them naturally transilluminate.
➤ The "adult" examination mantra of "it's a hernia if you can't go above it and a hydrocoele if you can" does not apply to young infants. You cannot go above either in children.

Investigations

The diagnosis is usually evident from the clinical history and examination. In some cases however, confirmation of the diagnosis is required, or the exclusion of a contralateral hernia is needed. In those cases ultrasonography can be useful.

Differential Diagnosis

Hydrocoeles and inguinal lymphadenopathy are both common groin conditions that need differentiating from inguinal hernias. Ascertaining the position of the testes is important in male patients. If the gonads have not descended into the scrotum, the lump in the groin could represent an undescended testis.

Management

The approach to management depends on the age and mode of presentation. Unlike with adults, all children with hernias need to be operated on.

➤ In young babies (under six months of age), the hernia should be operated on within two weeks of presentation, as there is a high risk (50%) of strangulation.
➤ In older children, the risk of strangulation is markedly less. The hernia can therefore be dealt with electively. An irreducible inguinal hernia is a surgical emergency as both the hernia contents and the testis are at high risk of ischaemia.

If a child presents with an irreducible hernia, all attempts should be made at non-surgical reduction of the hernia prior to surgery. The likelihood of success is increased by:

➤ Relaxing the patient.
➤ Putting them in the head down position.
➤ Giving adequate analgesia (morphine).

The tissue oedema associated with incarceration makes surgery more technically demanding, therefore the risk of damage to the vas deferens and vessels increases, and the risk of testicular atrophy increases as well. If reduction is successful, surgery should be postponed for 48 hours – this allows for a reduction of tissue oedema. If closed reduction fails, an emergency (open) procedure is needed.

Surgery involves herniotomy, which may be laparoscopic or open. This aims to identify the hernia sac, separate it from the vas deferens and blood vessels, and close the muscle, fat and skin layers.

Complications

An untreated inguinal hernia may become strangulated, leading to bowel ischaemia. It may also lead to bowel obstruction, or perforation. Surgery is a relatively low risk procedure, particularly if done electively.

Complications include:

> Infection.
> Bleeding.
> Testicular atrophy.
> Damage to spermatic cord structures (vas deferens, blood vessels, nerves).

Prognosis

Most children that undergo an elective herniotomy can go home the same day. The success rate is generally very high with a low rate of recurrence. Premature babies that undergo the procedure must remain in hospital for a period of 24–48 hours to observe for respiratory apnoeas.

Hydrocoele

A hydrocoele (meaning a collection of water) occurs if a narrow or microscopic PPV persists. In females, the fluid collection is termed "a hydrocoele of the canal of Nuck". In males, most present as a swelling in the scrotum (fluid in the tunica vaginalis). Some present as an isolated swelling in the cord termed "hydrocoele of the cord".

Clinical Features

Typically parents present after noticing a swelling in the child's groin. The child is usually asymptomatic, but may present with pain. Aetiology is similar to that of inguinal hernias. Some hydrocoeles appear after a viral illness or commencement of peritoneal dialysis. Spontaneous resolution occurs in 90% of cases before the child's second birthday. No evidence exists to suggest a hydrocoele has a negative impact on fertility.

Management

Surgery is only indicated if the hydrocoele persists beyond the child's second birthday, as spontaneous resolution is likely before then. This is done mainly for cosmetic reasons and pain relief. The procedure is termed "ligation of PPV" and is similar to that of an inguinal herniotomy. The sac needs to be identified, separated from vas deferens and vessels and then ligated. The hydrocoele is drained prior to closure. Recurrence is rare.

Umbilical Hernia

An umbilical hernia is a congenital defect in the umbilicus that leads to protrusion of omentum and occasionally gut through the defect. This is the most common hernia in children. The hernia is covered by a sac and skin. Most are asymptomatic and present because of aesthetic concerns the parents have. Spontaneous resolution of the umbilical hernia occurs in 90% of patients before their first birthday. A further 5% resolve before five-years-old.

Surgery is only indicated if the child is symptomatic or the child is more than three-years-old. It is performed as an elective day case. The incision is infra-umbilical, the sac is excised, and the defect is closed followed by skin closure. A pressure dressing is applied for 48 hours to prevent haematoma formation.

Divarication of Recti

This large bulge appears between the two recti of the rectus abdominis on contracting the muscle. This is a very frequent finding in infants and may alarm parents. No surgical intervention is needed for this condition, and it resolves naturally as the child ages.

UROLOGY

Undescended Testes

Undescended testes (UDT) refers to the absence of one or both testes in the scrotum. The incidence of UDT in term male infants at birth is three to five percent, making it the most common congenital abnormality of male genitalia. The incidence is higher (21-33%) in premature babies. This decreases to 1.5% at 3-months-old, and remains at this level in older children. The condition more commonly affects the right testicle, although bilateral UDTs are present in 10-20% of cases.

Undescended testicles should be classified as:

> Palpable (80%) or impalpable (20%) (*Table 1*). The condition of having impalpable testes is called cryptorchidism.
> Retractile or non-retractile. Retractile testes are testes that are present in the inguinal canal but can be manoeuvred into the base of the scrotum. Retractile testes remain in the scrotum for a few seconds before returning to their original position.

TABLE 1: The classification of undescended testes		
Palpable.	Imperfectly descended.	External inguinal ring. Superficial inguinal pouch. Gliding testis.
	Ectopic.	Lateral abdominal wall. Femoral. Base of penis. Perineal. Crossed ectopia.
Impalpable.	Absent.	Primary failure. Vascular injury.
	High location.	Intra-abdominal. High intra-canalicular.

Note here that this section refers to undescended testes in a baby that has otherwise normal male genitalia. Ambiguous genitalia is covered on p78.

Aetiology
There are two stages for testicular descent:

1 The "trans-abdominal phase" occurs in the first trimester of foetal development and is dependent on the Müllerian-inhibiting substance (MIS) and insulin related growth factor (IRGF). Descent occurs from around the kidneys down to the internal inguinal ring.
2 The "inguino-scrotal stage" occurs in the third trimester and depends on testosterone. This in turn depends on a functioning hypothalamic-pituitary axis. Descent occurs through the inguinal canal, down to the bottom of the scrotum.

What causes testicular maldescent is unclear, but it is believed to arise due to a fault in the testis itself or to hormonal/mechanical factors, or a combination of factors. UDTs are also associated with other conditions such as:

> Genetic conditions. Prader-Willi syndrome, Kallmann syndrome.
> Endocrine conditions. Congenital adrenal hyperplasia.
> Abdominal wall abnormalities. Exomphalos, gastroschisis.

Investigations
The diagnosis of undescended testes is clinical, but laparoscopy may be required to identify the location of the testis if it is not palpable. Ultrasonography scans (USS) and magnetic resonance imaging (MRI) are not needed to establish the diagnosis, as laparoscopy is both diagnostic and therapeutic.

Management
Treatment is surgical, but the exact approach depends on three factors:

> Patient age.
> Unilateral versus bilateral.
> Palpable versus impalpable.

Palpable Testes
All palpable UDT testicles (regardless of whether they are unilateral or bilateral) should be treated with an elective inguinal orchidopexy. This is done as follows:

> The vas deferens and testicular vessels are separated from the processus vaginalis (this increases the length of the cord structures).
> The testis is brought down to the scrotum.

The procedure is usually delayed until after the infant is 3-months-old, to give the testes a chance to descend independently. In bilateral cases, most surgeons prefer to perform the procedures three to six months apart, as this minimises the risk of complications.

Impalpable Testes
All impalpable undescended testicles require laparoscopy. The surgical procedure depends on what is identified:

> The testicle is visualised in the abdomen. The testicle is brought into the scrotum. If the cord is short, this may need to be a two-stage procedure.
> The vas and vessels are blind ending, or are attached to a small testicular remnant. This implies intrauterine torsion has occurred. The remnant requires removal.
> The vas and vessels are seen entering the inguinal canal. A groin exploration is necessary. On the occasion a small testis can be identified, this can be brought into the scrotum. On most occasions, however, the testicular remnant is tiny, with no residual normal function (so called nubbins). This requires excision due to the possibility of malignant transformation.

Bilateral impalpable testes require joint endocrine and paediatric surgical management. Karyotyping and hormonal work up are necessary first, to confirm testicular tissue is likely to be present. If so, laparoscopic exploration should occur as above.

Complications
> Fertility. Fertility potential for a normal man with bilateral descended testes is approximately 90%. This drops to 80-85% for a man with a treated unilateral UDT, and to 10-40% for a man with treated bilateral UDTs. Patients with intra-abdominal testes have significantly lower sperm count than those with palpable gonads. It is thought that the high temperature in the abdominal cavity or inguinal canal (in comparison to the cooler scrotal temperature) causes a reduction in the number of germ cells in the testicles. However, early surgery (ideally at around nine-months-old) prevents loss of significant numbers of germ cells and improves fertility.
> Malignancy. The risk of testicular cancer (seminoma) is approximately 30 times higher in those with UDT than those with bilaterally descended testicles. Malignant transformation may be due to intra-abdominal temperatures. However, early surgery reduces this risk.
> Cosmetic/psychological. Without treatment, this is can be a significant issue, particularly as the child gets older.

Prognosis
Prognosis depends on age of treatment, and specific pathology, but early intervention can reduce the risk of malignancy and improve fertility.

Phimosis
Phimosis is a narrowing of the opening of the foreskin, preventing its full retraction.

Normal foreskin retraction, phimosis and paraphimosis are all shown in *Figure 6*.

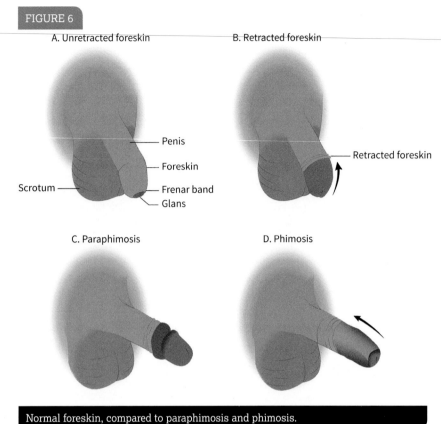

A. Unretracted foreskin

Penis
Foreskin
Scrotum
Frenar band
Glans

B. Retracted foreskin

Retracted foreskin

C. Paraphimosis

D. Phimosis

Normal foreskin, compared to paraphimosis and phimosis.

Aetiology

Phimosis can be physiological or pathological. Almost all male infants are born with prepucial adhesions. These are present between the glans penis and the foreskin, resulting in a non-retractile foreskin at birth. The incidence of prepucial adhesions declines with age. At their first birthday, only 20-30% of boys have a fully retractable foreskin. By school entry, almost 90% of boys are able to fully retract their foreskin.

Clinical Features

Occasionally, the child suffers with recurrent infections of the foreskin and glans (balanoposthitis). Frequently, parents complain that the child has "ballooning" of the foreskin on micturition. This is normal. It simply means some urine is getting trapped between the glans and the foreskin.

Management

For children with symptomatic phimosis, a topical corticosteroid cream is prescribed. The corticosteroid cream is used to thin the skin for a period of four weeks, and parents are advised to continue gently retracting the foreskin in the bath. This combination of corticosteroid cream and gentle retraction is frequently sufficient to achieve full symptom relief.

There are two surgical options:

> Foreskin-preserving surgery may be trialled. This involves prepucial adhesiolysis or dividing the prepucial adhesions, although there is a high recurrence risk.
> Definitive surgical management is circumcision. Excision of the foreskin is either "free hand" or by use of a device like the PlastiBell.

Complications

Fifteen percent of circumcisions have complications. These include:
> Bleeding. This is the leading cause of morbidity and mortality.
> Inclusion cysts. This is caused if keratinised skin is inverted in the repair.
> Damage to the glans and urethra. This can lead to fistula formation or meatal stenosis.
> Infection.

Other indications for circumcision include Balanitis Xerotica Obliterans, as an absolute indication. However, recurrent infection, or those with high grade vesicoureteric reflux (at risk of severe UTIs) are a relative indication.

Paraphimosis

Paraphimosis is a circumferential tightening along the corona of the glans, resulting from a retracted foreskin. This is associated with restricted perfusion of the glans penis, leading to swelling, pain and difficult micturition.

Urgent reduction is necessary to prevent continued blood flow compromise to the glans. This can be achieved with compression of the glans to reduce its swelling, along with cold compresses. Occasionally, a surgical split in the foreskin is necessary to achieve reduction. Formal circumcision is not necessary after reduction.

Balanitis Xerotica Obliterans

Balanitis Xerotica Obliterans (BXO) is a progressive inflammatory condition of the foreskin and glans, and can be caused by recurrent infections. Affected areas are inflamed and progressively become scarred. The main danger of the condition in children is that the progressive scarring affects the anterior urethral meatus, leading to urethral stenosis. Children with BXO frequently complain of painful micturition, difficulty in initiating micturition, itchiness and burning. Performing a circumcision can halt the disease progress, and is therefore the gold standard management.

Hypospadias

Hypospadias (*Figure 7*) is a congenital disorder of the penis that has three components:
> Chordee. This is a ventral curvature in the shaft of the penis. This is due to the incomplete development

FIGURE 7

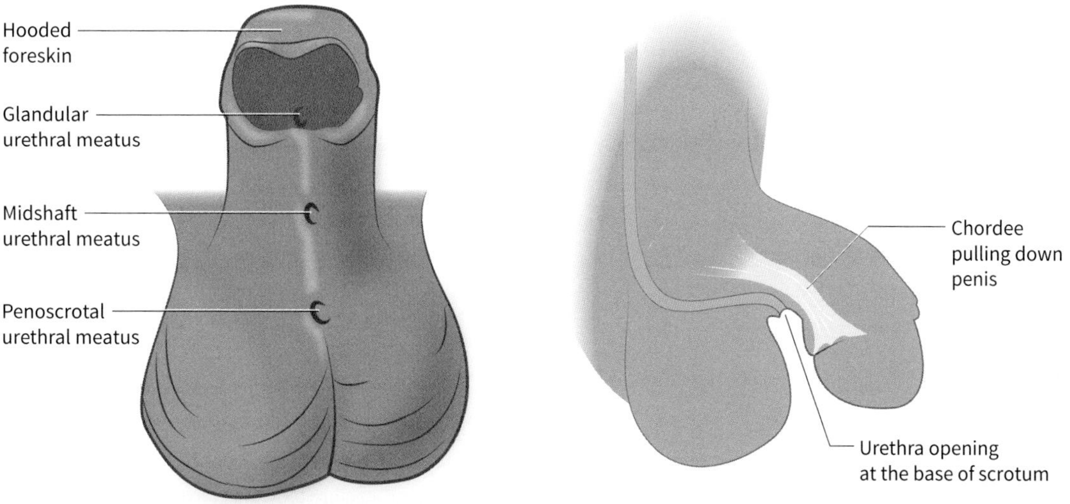

Hooded foreskin

Glandular urethral meatus

Midshaft urethral meatus

Penoscrotal urethral meatus

Chordee pulling down penis

Urethra opening at the base of scrotum

The three features of hypospadia: hooded foreskin, locations of the meatus (distal 50%, shaft 30%, penoscrotal 20%), and chordee.

of the corpora spongiosa and the distal urethra.

- Hooded foreskin. This a foreskin that is deficient ventrally. Therefore, there is excess skin dorsally, giving the foreskin a hooded appearance.
- Abnormal site of anterior urethral meatus.

Aetiology

The exact aetiology is unclear. The incidence of hypospadias is one in 300 live male births. Children with hypospadias have a higher than average incidence of other urogenital anomalies, such as undescended testes and kidney and bladder anomalies.

The incidence of hypospadias is higher in:

- Children affected by the VACTERL association (vertebral anomalies, anorectal malformation, cardiac defects, trachea-oesophageal fistula, renal anomalies, limb defects).
- Siblings and offspring of affected individuals.

Clinical Features

Babies with the condition are asymptomatic, and the diagnosis is usually picked up on routine baby checks. A child with bilateral undescended testes and a severe

(penoscrotal) hypospadias has to be referred for urgent karyotyping and hormonal analysis. The danger is missing a female infant (with congenital adrenal hyperplasia) that has developed clitoromegaly due to the virilising effects of testosterone.

Management

Management is surgical. Timing of surgery can vary; it is frequently dependent on the severity of the condition and surgeon's preference. It is very important that the parents are made aware not to circumcise their child, as the foreskin may be needed during surgery.

Generally, repair should be complete before the boy undergoes toilet training (around the second birthday). The argument against very early surgery is that the structures are very small and the risk of developing complications is higher. Mild (distal) hypospadias is usually managed as a one-step procedure (typically around the first birthday). If the child has a severe (proximal) hypospadias, a two-stage repair is frequently necessary.

The principles of surgery are:

- Correction of penile curvature (chordee).
- Reconstruction of a urethra (urethroplasty): if the urethral plate is well-developed, it can be tabularised

around a catheter. If the plate is narrow, either an incision into the urethral plate or incision and skin grafting is needed. The most common sites for skin grafting are the preserved foreskin, the buccal mucosa and skin from behind the ear.

- Reconstruction or removal of the foreskin at the end of the procedure.

Complications

Depending on the severity of the condition and the skill of the surgeon, complications happen in two to forty percent of cases. These include:

- Fistula. This complication commonly occurs at the site of the original urethral opening. It can happen secondary to infection or a stricture, as the urine flow will follow the path of least resistance.
- Urethral stricture. This will require dilatation or reconstruction.
- Breakdown of the repair. This requires a second procedure.

Prognosis

Prognosis is generally good, particularly with newer surgical techniques. Although patients have decreased satisfaction with their genital appearance, they are generally able to have a normal sex life in adulthood.

Pelvi-Ureteric Junction (PUJ) Obstruction

Aetiology

PUJ obstruction can occur due to intrinsic, mural and extrinsic causes.

> Intrinsic. Narrowed segment of ureter.
> Mural. Abnormal ureteric folds.
> Extrinsic. Crossing vessels (compressing the ureter).

This is the most common obstructive uropathy. Most frequently, PUJ obstruction is picked up antenatally, during routine antenatal scans. In older children, it can present with loin pain or UTIs, but may also be an incidental finding on a scan looking for other pathology.

Investigations

Ultrasonography is used both antenatally and postnatally to detect PUJ. The antero-posterior diameter (AP diameter) of the renal pelvis is an excellent indicator of the severity of obstruction:

> If the AP diameter is >40mm, it is most likely that the child will require surgery.
> If the AP diameter is <20mm, almost all patients will improve and not require intervention.

In those with an antenatal diagnosis, the scan should be repeated postnatally on day 6, and week 6. If there is very significant PUJ obstruction, or it is bilateral, USS should be performed earlier.

In a neonate with bilateral hydronephrosis, the main differentials that need to be excluded at birth are high grade VUR and posterior urethral valves. Posterior urethral valves are more common if there is bilateral hydronephrosis and poor urinary stream. These can both be excluded using MCUG (micturating cystourethrography). In MCUG, contrast is injected into the bladder and images are taken during micturition (bladder contraction).

MAG3 renography (^{99}TC-Mercaptoacetyltriglycerine) is performed at three months of age, and is useful for determining renal function.

Management

In the immediate newborn period, it is important that any baby with antenatally diagnosed PUJ obstruction passes a good stream of urine. Prophylactic trimethoprim should be commenced to prevent UTIs.

Dilatation of the renal pelvis should be monitored via serial USS.

> If the dilatation is stable, scans should be repeated every three months.
> If the dilatation improves, the patient is discharged.
> If dilatation increases or the patient deteriorates, surgery is performed. The standard operation for a PUJ obstruction is called a pyeloplasty. The obstructing part of the proximal ureter is excised and the two remaining ends are anastomosed over a stent (removed later).

Complications

Complications of the procedure include:

> Anastomotic leak.
> Narrowing at the site of anastomosis.
> Continued deterioration of renal function.

Prognosis

Generally, the prognosis is good. Renal function becomes static, and occasionally may improve post procedure.

Vesico-Ureteric Junction (VUJ) Obstruction

Aetiology

An obstruction at the VUJ can be due to a narrowing, stricture or stenosis of the lower ureter. It could also be secondary to a neuropathic bladder. The condition leads to pathological dilatation of kidney and ureter (hydroureteronephrosis). Most cases are antenatally diagnosed. If children present later in life, they usually present with severe sepsis due to the obstruction. Investigations are identical to that for PUJ.

Management

Treatment involves re-implantation of the ureter or stenting. If the condition has only caused mild to moderate impairment in renal function, stenting is advisable. The stent is left in situ for a period of six months, after which it is removed and tests are repeated. Half of all cases will have resolved by then, but the remaining half will require a re-implantation of the ureter.

If the condition has caused severe damage to the kidney, both the kidney and ureter will require removal to prevent recurrent bouts of sepsis.

Vesico-Ureteric Reflux

Vesico-ureteric reflux (VUR) involves the backwards movement of urine from the bladder into the ureter. The incidence is 1 in 100, but increases to 30 in 100 in children with UTIs. The incidence is much higher amongst siblings (30%) and offspring (50%) of affected patients.

Aetiology

The normal ureter enters the bladder diagonally. It runs in a submucosal tunnel towards its opening (ureteric orifice) in the bladder trigone. This layout provides a flap-valve mechanism that prevents reflux of urine from the bladder into the ureter.

If the natural anti-reflux mechanism fails, "primary" reflux occurs. Other causes are labelled "secondary" reflux. These are both summarised in *Table 6*.

The occurrence of renal damage and scarring secondary to VUR requires a combination of two things (damage does not occur unless both factors are present):

> Reflux. Urine refluxes into the kidney.
> Infection. The first infection is believed to cause the highest degree of damage.

FIGURE 8

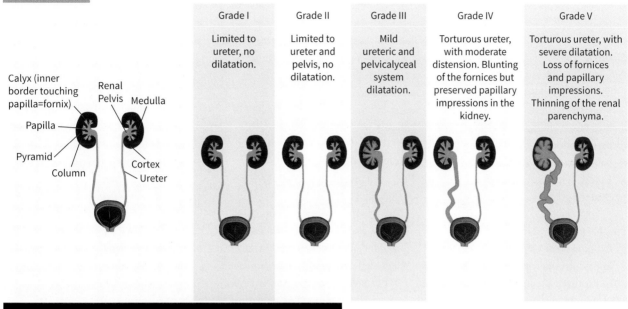

Grade I	Grade II	Grade III	Grade IV	Grade V
Limited to ureter, no dilatation.	Limited to ureter and pelvis, no dilatation.	Mild ureteric and pelvicalyceal system dilatation.	Torturous ureter, with moderate distension. Blunting of the fornices but preserved papillary impressions in the kidney.	Torturous ureter, with severe dilatation. Loss of fornices and papillary impressions. Thinning of the renal parenchyma.

Grading of VUR by the International Reflux Study Committee (1981).

TABLE 6: Aetiology of vesico-ureteric reflux

Primary VUR	Abnormally situated ureteric orifice.
	Larger than normal orifice.
	Short submucosal tunnel.
Secondary VUR	Obstructive: posterior urethral valves, meatal stenosis.
	Neuropathic bladder: spina bifida, spinal injury.
	Dysfunctional bladder.

Progressive renal scarring leads to loss of function. This, in turn, leads to renal failure and hypertension. Up to 15% of all cases of VUR develop end-stage renal failure.

The grades of VUR reflux are summarised in *Figure 8*. Grade I and II resolve relatively quickly, but the higher the grade, the greater the chance of renal scarring.

Clinical Features
VUR can be picked up:
› Most commonly, during the investigations arising after a UTI (p304).
› As part of the work up for antenatal hydronephrosis.
› Incidental findings (e.g. the finding of a scarred atrophic kidney on ultrasound for other reasons).
› Patients present with hypertension and/or end stage renal disease (rarely).

Investigations
MCUG is the gold standard for diagnosing reflux. Contrast is injected into the bladder, and images are taken during micturition (bladder contraction). Any reflux can subsequently

be seen. DMSA (dimercaptosuccinic acid) scanning is a nuclear medicine imaging modality that is very useful for the detection of any renal scarring. Hydronephrosis (distension and dilatation of the renal pelvis and calyces) can be seen on ultrasound (*Figure 9*).

Management
Medical
The aim is to treat ongoing UTIs and prevent any further episodes. Medical treatment options for VUR include:
› Prophylactic antibiotics.
› Laxatives (to treat any associated constipation).

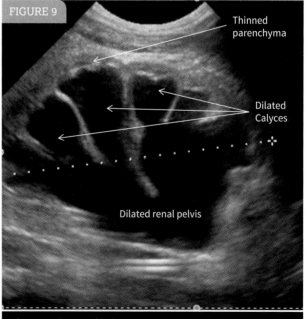

Ultrasound scan of kidney, showing hydronephrosis. There is dilatation of the pelvicalyceal system, and thinning of the renal parenchyma.

- Anticholinergics (bladder relaxant to control overactivity) and bladder training.

Surgical

Surgery is considered if:

- The patient (whilst on adequate prophylaxis) develops breakthrough infections or suffers from deterioration in renal function.
- New renal scars.
- Failure of medical treatment.
- Bilateral grade IV-V disease.

Possible procedures include:

- Circumcision. Circumcision can be offered to boys with VUR. Studies have proven a reduced incidence of UTI in this group.
- STING procedure. This is a very simple procedure that involves cystoscopy, identification of the refluxing ureteric orifice (UO) and injecting a bulking agent submucosally around the urethral orifice to prevent reflux. This procedure is performed as a day case and has a 75% success rate.
- Re-implantation of ureters. This aims to increase the length of the submucosal tunnel through which the ureter enters the bladder.
- Nephrectomy. Occasionally, if the kidney is poorly functioning, a nephrectomy is offered to prevent recurrent infections and hypertension.

Complications

The most significant complications relate to recurrent UTIs and renal dysfunction.

Prognosis

The majority of grade I cases, and about half of grade II and III cases, resolve spontaneously after a few years. Surgical procedures, when required, have a high success rate, but there may still be significant residual renal damage.

Posterior Urethral Valves

Posterior urethral valves (PUV) are membranes or leaflets present in the posterior urethra in males.

Aetiology

The vast majority of PUVs obstruct the outflow of urine from the bladder. As these valves develop in early intrauterine life, the effect of the back-pressure on the bladder and kidneys is severe and destructive. PUVs remain the most common cause of renal failure in children.

Clinical Features

PUVs can present antenatally (2/3) or postnatally (1/3):

- Antenatally. Present on routine ultrasound scan with distended bladder and posterior urethra (key hole sign), along with severe unilateral or bilateral hydronephrosis. In severe cases, there is also reduction in the amount of amniotic fluid surrounding the foetus. This is a bad prognostic sign, as it means that the foetus cannot bypass the bladder obstruction.
- Postnatally. This may present in a variety of different ways, including:
  - Difficulty in passing urine (at any stage after birth).
  - UTIs, usually severe requiring hospitalisation and IV antibiotics.
  - Renal failure.

Investigations

- Ultrasound. If the child was diagnosed antenatally, an ultrasound is obtained within the first 24-48 hours of life. This will confirm the presence of hydronephrosis, a large thickened bladder and possibly a distended posterior urethra.
- MCUG (micturating cystourethrogram). This is the gold standard. It will confirm bladder and urethral abnormalities, as well as demonstrate reflux into one or both ureters. Occasionally, the valves themselves are visible.

Management

- Drainage of the bladder. Immediately after birth, post any immediate resuscitation, the bladder must be drained via a urinary catheter. If this is difficult to pass, a suprapubic catheter may be required.
- Antibiotics. Empirical prophylactic antibiotics are started because of the risk of urinary stasis and reflux, which predispose to infection.
- Stabilisation of kidney function. Kidney function has to be checked frequently and electrolyte abnormalities need to be corrected.
- Valve ablation. This procedure is done with cystoscopy: the valves are identified and divided with a cold knife, diathermy or laser. If ablation is not possible (e.g. unavailable equipment, too small a baby), a definitive drainage procedure is needed. This is a vesicostomy, where the bladder is brought out as a stoma to the anterior abdominal wall, and is allowed to drain into a nappy.

Complications

- Renal failure. Thirty percent of children with PUVs will develop renal failure and require dialysis and transplant.
- Dysfunctional abnormal bladder. This may occur even after successful valve ablation. A dysfunctional bladder increases the risk of UTIs, vesicoureteric reflux disease, incontinence and renal failure.
- Infertility. Abnormal ejaculation and abnormal semen content.

Prognosis

Infants with posterior urethral valves require long-term follow up due to the risk of complications, as described above. These may still occur, even with treatment.

NEONATAL SURGERY

Necrotising Enterocolitis

Necrotising enterocolitis (NEC) is an inflammatory condition that affects the intestines of newborn infants upon introduction of feedings. The condition is most common in premature infants, occurring in three out of 10, 000 live births.

Aetiology

NEC can affect the gastrointestinal system at any site from the stomach to the rectum, but the most commonly affected segments are the terminal ileum and ascending colon.

The aetiology of NEC is still poorly understood but is believed to be multifactorial:

- Toxins and bacteria. The neonatal gut is sterile until feeding starts. The flora that colonises the neonatal gut differs between premature and term babies, as well as between breastfed and formula fed ones. It also varies with the type of formula, the neonatal unit where the baby is situated and the maternal flora. Bacteria produce toxins and, when combined with other factors, the bacteria can translocate into the bloodstream and cause sepsis.
- Mucosal intestinal barrier. The premature mucosal barrier is not as tight and strong as that of a term baby. This weak barrier is thought to allow translocation of gut organisms.
- Milk/ formula. Evidence suggests that formula fed infants have a six times higher risk of developing NEC, when compared to their breastfed counterparts. Casein (from cow's milk based formulas) is thought to damage the immature mucosa.
- Intestinal blood flow. Decreased intestinal blood flow can contribute to the development of NEC. In babies with other comorbidities, such as cardiac issues and sepsis, blood is shunted away from the gut. This hypoperfusion weakens the mucosal barrier even further leading to translocation of microorganisms.

Clinical Features

The classic history of NEC is its appearance in a previously stable premature baby upon starting feeds. The baby suddenly stops tolerating feeds, develops abdominal distension/ tenderness, presents with blood in the stools and becomes haemodynamically unstable.

NEC symptoms occur across a spectrum ranging from "possible" NEC to fulminant disease. The best known severity classification is the Bell classification, which subdivides NEC into three stages (*Table 7*).

Investigations
Blood Tests

It is important to take bloods for full blood counts (FBC), clotting, biochemistry profile including C-reactive protein

(CRP), coagulation screens and blood cultures. Stool cultures can also be sent for microscopy, culture & sensitivity (MC&S) analysis and virology. Blood gases should also be measured, looking specifically for metabolic acidosis and elevated lactate.

Imaging

The investigation of choice is an abdominal X-ray (*Table 7*). Occasionally, a lateral shoot-through film is useful for demonstrating free air. Abdominal X-rays are often repeated to measure the progression of the disease. X-ray signs include:

- Small bowel dilatation, which is the earliest and most common sign.
- Pneumatosis intestinalis (mottled appearance from gas in the bowel wall), which is diagnostic for NEC (*Figure 10*).
- A fixed dilated loop of bowel, across several X-rays, which is also a worrying feature.

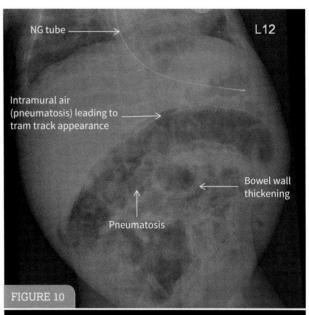

FIGURE 10

Abdominal X-ray of a neonate with NEC: note the evidence of pneumatosis (air bubbles) in the bowel wall.

Stage	Systemic signs	Abdominal signs	Radiographic signs	Treatment
Stage I (suspected).	Temperature instability, apnoea, bradycardia, lethargy.	Large NG aspirates, vomiting, abdominal distension, blood in stool.	Normal or intestinal dilation.	Nil by mouth (NBM), antibiotics (at least three to five days)
Stage II (moderately ill).	Same as above, plus mild metabolic acidosis and thrombocytopenia.	Same as above, plus absent bowel sounds, abdominal tenderness, abdominal cellulitis, right lower quadrant mass.	Intestinal dilation, ileus, pneumatosis intestinalis (gas in bowel wall).	NBM, antibiotics (14 days).
Stage III (advanced, severely ill, intact or perforated bowel – surgical NEC).	Same as above, plus hypotension, combined respiratory and metabolic acidosis, disseminated intravascular coagulation, and neutropenia.	Same as above, plus signs of peritonitis, marked tenderness, and more marked abdominal distension.	As above plus ascites or pneumoperitoneum (free gas in peritoneal cavity on X-ray).	NBM, antibiotics (14 days), fluid resuscitation, inotropic support, ventilator therapy, surgery.

TABLE 7: Simplified Bell classifcation for severity of NEC

Differential Diagnosis

The main differentials for NEC are intestinal obstruction and sepsis. However, the differential diagnosis is broad for a severely compromised neonate.

Management

Medical Management

Initial medical management for NEC is:

▸ Making the patient nil by mouth (NBM) and commencing intravenous fluids/total parenteral nutrition (TPN). The patient is likely to be NBM for 7 to 14 days, and TPN provides nutrition.

▸ Inserting a large bore nasogastric (NG) tube on free drainage.

▸ Administering broad spectrum intravenous antibiotics (e.g. amoxicillin, gentamicin and metronidazole).

After this period, feeds are gradually introduced and increased with great caution, as the mucosa of the small bowel has lost significant absorptive area.

Management Specific to Bell Stage

▸ Stage I. Babies with stage I disease are usually stable.

▸ Stage II. Babies with stage II disease may require support with inotropes, morphine infusions and intubation/ventilation. These patients need frequent assessment to ensure they are not displaying signs of imminent perforation or peritonitis (stage III). This involves regular clinical assessment of the abdomen, bloods and serial abdominal X-rays.

▸ Stage III. Stage III patients require consideration for urgent surgical intervention. Intraoperative findings vary from a small blowout hole (usually in the terminal ileum) to fulminant NEC, leading to necrosis of the entire GI tract. If the child has a small patch, a limited resection and anastomosis may be performed. A safer option is usually to divert the intestinal contents away from the affected bowel. This is done by diverting the proximal bowel to the skin (into a stoma) so that it bypasses the diseased segment. If NEC totalis (involving the entire GIT) is present, the bowel is left unresected and simply reduced into the peritoneal cavity. This option has a bleak prognosis.

Once a stoma is fashioned, the patient should continue their IV antibiotic treatment and TPN and remain NBM for at least 14 days.

Stomas are reversed at about three months from the laparotomy, after contrast studies have excluded the presence of a stricture in the distal bowel.

Complications

Surgical complications include:

▸ **Wound breakdown.** A NEC laparotomy wound is especially prone to breakdown.

▸ **Stoma site necrosis.** The stoma can become necrotic as part of the disease process.

▸ **Stricture.** A stricture may occur at the site of anastomosis/from the disease process. This often requires surgical intervention.

▸ **Short gut/TPN dependence.** Short gut is the main long-term complication of NEC. Frequently, children with short gut are TPN dependent. This, in turn, can have a negative effect on the liver (TPN-related liver cirrhosis). If the patients continue to deteriorate, they soon become candidates for small bowel / liver transplants.

Prognosis

Mortality varies depending on severity, but it can be as high as 50% for critically ill patients.

Congenital Diaphragmatic Hernia

Congenital Diaphragmatic Hernia (CDH) frequently results in segments of bowel (or even the liver and other abdominal organs) herniating into the thoracic cavity. This is associated with lung hypoplasia (due to pressure of the gut on the lungs), which is the main cause of morbidity and mortality in CDH patients.

Aetiology

Development of the diaphragm in the embryo occurs around the eighth week of gestation and is a complex process. Failure of fusion of various segments can lead to a defect in the diaphragm. The incidence of CDH is approximately one in 3000 births in the UK; 80% are left sided.

Clinical Features

CDH neonates often develop respiratory distress in the first few minutes of life. Examination frequently shows a mediastinal shift with a scaphoid abdomen. Occasionally, chest auscultation will reveal bowel sounds. Associations can emerge between CDH and other anomalies, such as cardiac defects and trisomy 13 and 18.

Differential Diagnosis

Respiratory distress in the immediate newborn period has a wide differential diagnosis, including:

▸ Sepsis.
▸ Pneumonia.
▸ Respiratory Distress Syndrome.
▸ Meconium aspiration.
▸ Pneumothorax.
▸ Cardiac disease.

Investigations

Approximately 50% of cases of CDH are diagnosed by antenatal sonography. In most cases, the CDH is an isolated finding; however, some cases can show an associated anomaly.

Postnatally the diagnosis is confirmed with a chest X-ray (*Figure 11*). This typically reveals:

▸ Loops of bowel in the chest cavity.
▸ Paucity of bowel loops in the abdomen.
▸ An absent diaphragmatic outline.
▸ Occasionally, the tip of the NG tube is in the thorax (signifying an intra-thoracic stomach).

If the diagnosis remains unclear an ultrasound scan can help, by demonstrating the defect in the diaphragmatic muscle. Dubious cases can also benefit from GI contrast studies, as the contrast can reveal the presence of bowel in the thoracic cavity.

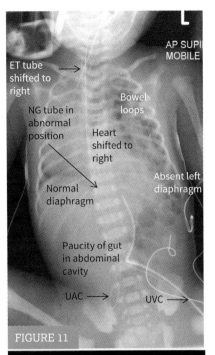

FIGURE 11

Chest and abdominal X-ray demonstrating a congenital diaphragmatic hernia. Loops of bowel are scant in the abdomen and extend into the left chest cavity. The mediastinum is shifted to the right, as demonstrated by the ET tube and the heart being on the right hand side. The NG tube may be insufficiently advanced as it is only just extending below the right diaphragm. The left diaphragm cannot be seen because of the degree of herniation.

Management

If the condition was diagnosed on antenatal scans, delivery should be planned at a centre that provides neonatal intensive care and paediatric surgery. Neonatal resuscitation involves insertion of a NG tube (to prevent distension of the stomach) and intubation/ventilation.

Surgical repair of the diaphragmatic defect is only performed once the infant is in a stable condition. The procedure begins with a subcostal incision and the defect is then repaired using remnants of muscle (primary repair) or prosthetic material (patch repair). Both laparoscopic and thoracoscopic CDH repairs are now performed.

In recent years, foetal surgery has undergone some trials but it is not yet widely adopted. Inserting a balloon into the foetal trachea to promote lung expansion is currently reserved for cases with poor outcome indicators.

Complications

Patients who are well enough to undergo CDH repair show some long-term sequelae:

➤ Respiratory insufficiency secondary to the pulmonary hypoplasia.
➤ Neurological and developmental issues secondary to hypoxia in the newborn period.
➤ Gastro-oesophageal reflux disease. This might be so severe that medical anti-reflux treatment is insufficient and a fundoplication is required.
➤ Chest wall and spine deformity. Some require surgical correction.
➤ Recurrence of the diaphragmatic hernia. This is more common following use of a synthetic patch.

Prognosis

Despite advances in antenatal and neonatal care, the mortality of the condition remains approximately 60%. The major determinant of survival is pulmonary hypoplasia, while presence of associated cardiac defects increases mortality to over 90%. Antenatal diagnosis gives a worse prognosis, as it is associated with a significantly greater lung hypoplasia.

Tracheo-Oesophageal Fistula/Oesophageal Atresia (TOF/OA)

In most instances, oesophageal atresia and tracheo-oesophageal fistulae occur together. The incidence of this condition is around one in 4000 live births.

In oesophageal atresia (OA), a portion of the mid-oesophagus is missing. The gap between the two remaining ends can be short (more common) or long (less frequent).

A tracheo-oesophageal fistula (TOF), by contrast, is a communication between the oesophagus and the trachea. This can occur as an isolated defect (an H-type fistula), but is very rare. The most common variant is a blind ending upper pouch of oesophagus, with the lower oesophagus connecting to the trachea; this is called a "distal" pouch fistula. This variant accounts for more than 85% of TOF/OA cases (*Figure 12*).

FIGURE 12

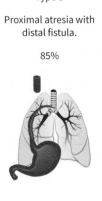
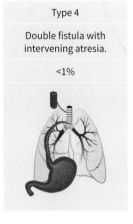

Type 1	Type 2	Type 3	Type 4	Type 5
Isolated oesophageal atresia.	Proximal fistula with distal atresia.	Proximal atresia with distal fistula.	Double fistula with intervening atresia.	Isolated fistula (H-type).
8%	2%	85%	<1%	4%

Classification of TOF/OA.

Aetiology

Approximately half of all cases of TOF/OA have one or more associated abnormalities. The most common ones are part of the VACTERL association [V: vertebral anomalies, A: anorectal malformations, C: cardiac anomalies, T: tracheo-oesophageal anomalies, R: renal tract anomalies, L: limb anomalies (typically radial aplasia)].

Clinical Features

Some cases of TOF/OA are diagnosed antenatally, based on evidence of polyhydramnios (baby cannot swallow amniotic fluid) and/or a small stomach (lack of swallowed fluid in stomach). After birth, the baby might produce lots of mucus, drool or aspirate either secretions or a feed (becoming cyanotic).

Investigations

Classically, a nasogastric tube is passed, but it cannot pass beyond a certain point. Frequently, it curls up in the upper pouch of the oesophagus (*Figure 13*). A chest X-ray will demonstrate a curled tube in the upper pouch and gas in the remainder of the intestines.

Any child with TOF/OA should have an echocardiogram and an ultrasound of the renal tract to rule out associated abnormalities.

Management

A special tube (Replogle tube) is passed into the upper pouch and put on continuous suction to drain pooling saliva and prevent aspiration.

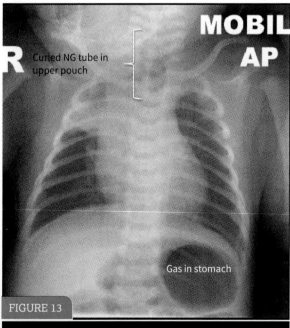

Curled NG tube in upper pouch

R

Gas in stomach

FIGURE 13

Tracheo-oesophageal fistula (TOF) with oesophageal atresia (OA). Oesophageal atresia is confirmed by the coiled NG tube. With an atresia, the only way air can enter the stomach is via a fistula; therefore, a tracheo-oesophageal fistula must be present.

Surgery is the definitive treatment. It involves:

▸ Approaching via a right-sided thoracotomy.
▸ Identifying and dividing the fistula between the lower oesophagus and the trachea.
▸ Joining the two parts of the oesophagus.
▸ A feeding tube is placed, crossing the anastomosis, which can be used to commence early feeding.

Occasionally, the patient has no TOF, and the condition is an isolated OA. Frequently, the gap between the two parts of the oesophagus is too great to allow primary anastomosis. In such situations, a feeding gastrostomy is fashioned (to allow enteral feeds) and the child is scheduled for a gastric pull up a few months later (to join up the stomach and the upper oesophagus within the chest).

Complications

Complications prior to treatment relate to aspiration. Problems encountered post-surgery may include:

▸ Stricture of the oesophagus. This is a common problem. Children may require frequent dilatations to stretch the scar tissue.
▸ Oesophageal dysmotility. This can cause difficulty in swallowing and is a common long-term problem in these children.
▸ Anastomotic leak.

Prognosis

Patients with isolated TOFs, diagnosed antenatally, have a very good prognosis. However, those with comorbidities, or who are too unwell for early repair, face a more unpredictable outcome.

Anorectal Malformation

An anorectal malformation (ARM) is an abnormally situated or absent anus (*Figure 14-5*). The incidence is approximately one in 4000 live births, with a higher incidence in males.

Abnormalities vary and may include:

▸ Persistence of a cloaca. This is a single opening for the urinary, intestinal and reproductive tract.
▸ Rectum ending in a blind pouch (atresia) with no distal anus.
▸ Diversion of faeces through a fistula, and no anus. This may be from the rectum to:
  › The urethra (recto-urethral fistula).
  › The bladder (recto-vesical fistula).
  › The vestibule of the vagina (recto-vestibular fistula).
  › The skin (recto-perineal fistula).

Associated Abnormalities

As with TOF/OA, the cause of ARM is not known. More than 50% of all cases are associated with other congenital anomalies, with urogenital ones being most common. ARM is commonly associated with the VACTERL association (V: vertebral

Missing/closed off anal opening

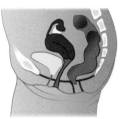

Opening in wrong place and too small

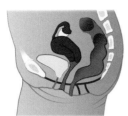

Rectum connects to vagina

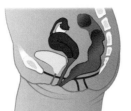

Cloaca: bladder, uterus and anus all form a single opening

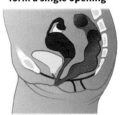

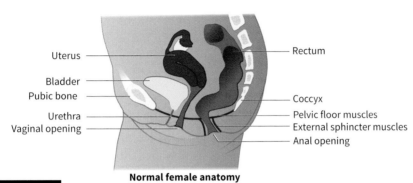

Uterus — — Rectum

Bladder
Pubic bone — — Coccyx

Urethra — — Pelvic floor muscles
Vaginal opening — — External sphincter muscles
— Anal opening

Normal female anatomy

FIGURE 14

Anorectal abnormalities in females.

Missing/closed off anal opening

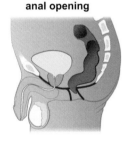

Opening in wrong place and too small

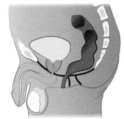

Rectum connects to urethra or bladder

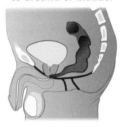

High rectum connects to bladder

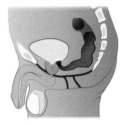

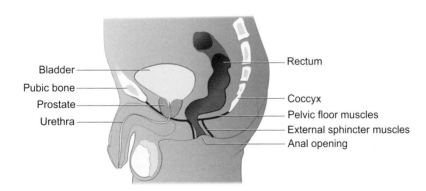

Bladder — — Rectum
Pubic bone
Prostate — — Coccyx
Urethra — Pelvic floor muscles
— External sphincter muscles
— Anal opening

Normal male anatomy

FIGURE 15

Anorectal abnormalities in males.

anomalies, A: anorectal malformations, C: cardiac anomalies, T: tracheo-oesophageal anomalies, R: renal tract anomalies, L: limb anomalies (typically radial aplasia)).

Clinical Features

The condition is usually diagnosed during the routine baby check, when the absence/abnormal position of the anus is noted. It may also be picked up after delayed passage of meconium. If an obstructive defect is present, babies tend to remain well for 24-48 hours before symptoms of large bowel obstruction occur.

359

Further Assessment

Anorectal anomalies can have a high or low position, determined by whether the rectum ends above (high) or below (low) the puborectalis muscle. Children with low lesions have a higher chance of achieving continence later in life.

A high lesion is more likely if the perineum is not well formed, i.e. there is no deep perineal cleft between the buttocks. Conversely, a low lesion is present if the child passes faeces from the vagina or perineum (as this implies a recto-vaginal or recto-perineal fistula). Faeces coming out of the urethra could mean a high lesion (fistula to the bladder above the puborectalis sling), or a low lesion (fistula to the urethra below the puborectalis sling), and so the presence of faeces is non-discriminatory.

Fistulas can be identified by several methods:

1   By physically identifying a fistula (in the perineum or vagina).
2   By seeing meconium in the nappy, despite an absent anus.
3   By analysing the urine for meconium– its presence will confirm a recto-urethral or recto-vesicular fistula.

Identifying any co-existing anomalies (renal, cardiac, spine) is important prior to planning definitive treatment. Examine the baby to ensure that the infant has passed urine, has no murmurs, and has a normal sacrum on examination.

Imaging

Obtain an abdominal X-ray. This may show large bowel obstruction, although it should be taken after 24 hours of life, as swallowed air takes at least one day to get to the most distal end of the bowel. A renal ultrasound should be performed in all cases, as well as an echocardiogram if there is any suspicion of a cardiac lesion.

Management

Once an anorectal malformation is identified, it is important to keep the baby's GI tract decompressed by passing an NG tube and keeping them NBM. Definitive management is surgical.

Low Lesion

The procedure to treat an ARM is a posterior sagittal anorectoplasty (PSARP). The aim of this procedure is to create a new anus for the baby and bring the rectal tube through to the anal sphincter muscle complex. If the anomaly has a low position, then this can be performed within the first three days of life.

High Lesion

For lesions with high positions, a defunctioning colostomy is formed first, to allow the distended bowel to return to its normal size. Contrast is then placed in the distal lumen of the stoma (the part that connects the stoma to the abnormal anorectum). This test is called a distal colostogram, and can identify any fistula. PSARP and colostomy closure are then performed at a later stage.

Complications

Complications following PSARP include:

>   Breakdown of the repair. Usually secondary to infection. This will require re-operation.
>   Anal stenosis. This complication is very common. It is therefore mandatory to teach parents to perform regular dilatations to the new anus to prevent this complication from developing.
>   Infections of the urinary tract. This can be due to the fistula or due to associated urogenital anomalies. It is important to remember that all patients with ARM have to be placed on prophylactic antibiotics.

Those requiring a colostomy may develop prolapse at the colostomy site, or a stricture.

Prognosis

The main prognostic factor for children with ARM is continence. This is a complex issue that involves chronic constipation, inability to control flatus, and faecal soiling. Better continence outcomes are usually obtained with patients with low (rather than high) anomalies. Children who have an associated sacral anomaly (and subsequent abnormal innervation to the sphincter muscles) have the worst continence outcomes.

Gastroschisis

Gastroschisis is an open defect in the anterior abdominal wall that results in protrusion of abdominal contents (mainly bowel) (*Figure 16*). The incidence of gastroschisis is one in 5000 live births. The condition is more common in infants of mothers who are:

>   Very young.
>   Smokers.
>   Substance abusers.

Aetiology

The defect is relatively small (<4cm), and loops of small and large bowel may protrude. The defect is mostly present on the right of the midline. Occasionally the stomach, bladder, ovaries or even testes can also protrude. The herniating organs are NOT covered with peritoneum. This is important for differentiation of this condition from exomphalos.

The presence of associated anomalies is rare in gastroschisis. However, the loops of bowel failed to undergo the normal rotation process; therefore, a malrotation or non-rotation anomaly is associated with the condition. Compromise of the blood supply to the protruding extra-abdominal loops of bowel can result in an atresia. This occurs in 5–10% of cases.

Clinical Features

After delivery, the diagnosis can easily be confirmed by inspection of the newborn. The protruding loops of bowel can appear entirely normal, can be thickened and dilated, or may be matted together. The baby can be dehydrated secondary to the third space losses.

Investigations

The condition can be picked up on the foetal anomaly scan. After 32 weeks gestation, the antenatal scan frequency for babies with gastroschisis increases to

FIGURE 16

Gastroschisis.

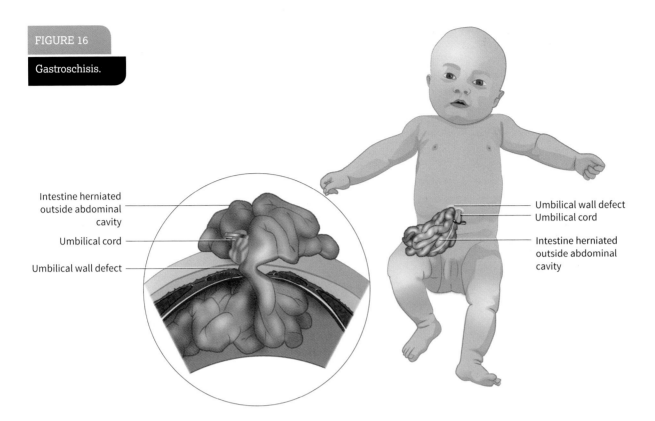

FIGURE 16

Gastroschisis.

Intestine herniated outside abdominal cavity

Umbilical cord

Umbilical wall defect

Umbilical wall defect
Umbilical cord

Intestine herniated outside abdominal cavity

once per week to pick up very dilated or thickened loops of gut. If any such findings appear, an early delivery is considered, as the risk of intrauterine death is high. Vaginal delivery does not increase the risk of infection or damage to the gut, and is the preferred mode of delivery.

Management

Neonatal resuscitation includes establishing venous access and rehydration. The infant also requires:

▸ An NG tube, to drain the stomach and increase the available space in the abdominal cavity.

▸ Broad spectrum antibiotics.

▸ Maintenance and replacement fluids, as necessary.

To close the defect, two options are available.

▸ Primary closure. The gut is reduced into the abdominal cavity and the defect is closed.

▸ Preformed silo. Loops of bowel are inserted into a pre manufactured plastic bag and suspended from the roof of the incubator (*Figure 17*). Gravity gradually allows the gut to descend into the abdomen. The process is helped along twice a day by gently pushing the loops into the abdomen. After all the bowel is reduced, formal closure can be performed (with or without sutures).

Complications

Acutely, an elevated intra-abdominal pressure may exist after reduction of the gut. This can lead to compression of the thoracic cavity and breathing difficulty. Ventilator support is frequently indicated for these babies for a few days after closure.

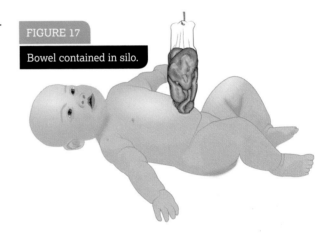

FIGURE 17

Bowel contained in silo.

In the long-term, the gut will commonly malfunction for a significant number of months prior to improvement. This is due to the gut having developed in an abnormal environment (surrounded by amniotic fluid). Feeds must be commenced at a very slow pace, with very small increments in volume. In the interim, the patient requires TPN.

Prognosis

Survival of this condition is 90% in high income countries. The mortality in countries with no access to TPN is 100%. Long-term morbidity is due to gut dysmotility. Mortality is mainly related to TPN, both from associated liver cirrhosis and line sepsis.

Exomphalos

Exomphalos is an umbilical herniation. In contrast to gastroschisis, the exomphalos defect is covered by a membrane (*Figure 18*). The inner lining is peritoneum, the outer is amnion.

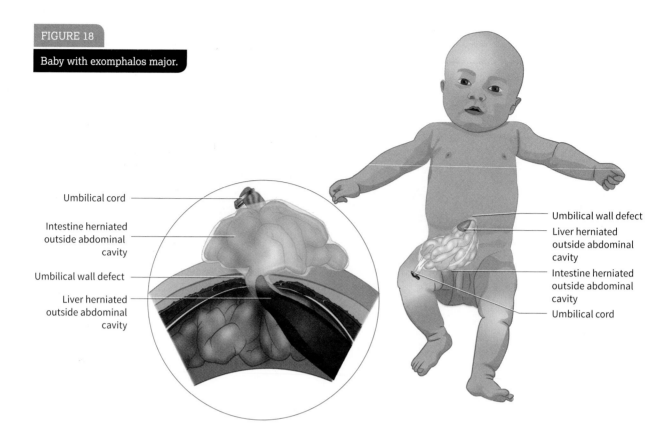

Baby with exomphalos major.

Umbilical cord

Intestine herniated outside abdominal cavity

Umbilical wall defect

Liver herniated outside abdominal cavity

Umbilical wall defect

Liver herniated outside abdominal cavity

Intestine herniated outside abdominal cavity

Umbilical cord

Aetiology

There are two types of exomphalos. The incidence of each condition is one in 7000 live births.

> Exomphalos minor. This is also known as hernia of the umbilical cord. Classically, the defect is small (<4cm) and contains only loops of bowel.
> Exomphalos major. This is a midline defect of the anterior abdominal wall. The defect is large (5–20cm in diameter) and contains the small and large bowel, liver and occasionally the stomach and spleen.

Exomphalos minor is frequently an isolated finding; however, exomphalos major is associated with other congenital anomalies in 50% of cases (particularly cardiac conditions). A high proportion of cases can have potentially fatal chromosomal anomalies.

Clinical Features

Exomphalus is usually antenatally diagnosed and managed from birth. In a proportion of cases, the covering membrane ruptures either during delivery or in utero. A large exomphalos may be associated with significant respiratory compromise.

Investigations

Investigations are directed towards uncovering associated anomalies (cardiac echo, renal scans, karyotyping).

Management

Exomphalos minor can be operated on soon after birth. The procedure involves excision of the membrane, reduction of the organs into the abdomen, and closure of the midline defect. The baby can usually be discharged within 48 hours.

In exomphalos major, surgery is avoided in the early period as the defect is too large for closure. The sac is covered with dressings and is allowed to keratinise over time. The defect is closed at a later stage (can be several years, depending on the size of the defect and associated anomalies the child may have).

Complications

The immediate post-operative period for exomphalos major patients can be difficult, as the intra-abdominal pressure is hugely increased, frequently necessitating ventilator support and gut rest with TPN.

Prognosis

Prognosis depends on associated conditions. If the child has no serious comorbidities, prognosis is usually excellent.

Table 8 provides a comparison of umbilical hernia, gastroschisis and exomphalos.

Duodenal Obstruction

Duodenal obstruction occurs in one in 5000 live births. It is a congenital obstruction of the duodenum that can either be due to stenosis or atresia.

Aetiology

Duodenal obstruction is believed to result from failure of canalisation of the duodenum in the early gestational period. Fifty percent of the cases are associated with other congenital anomalies. Twenty percent of patients have congenital heart disease and 30% have Down syndrome. Eight percent of

TABLE 8: Comparison of umbilical hernia, gastroschisis and exomphalos

	Umbilical Hernia	Exomphalos	Gastroschisis
Frequency.	One in 5.	One in 7000 (incidence for minor and major).	One in 5000.
Genetics.	Sporadic.	Familial occurrence. Associated with syndromes, e.g. Beckwith-Wiedemann syndrome, Down syndrome.	Sporadic.
Location of abnormality.	Over umbilicus.	Over umbilicus.	Usually to the right of the umbilicus.
Size of defect.	Small.	Can be very large (e.g. 15cm).	Small-medium (Usually<5 cm).
Organ herniation.	Small bowel.	Small bowel, but also potentially liver, spleen, stomach, gonad or gall bladder.	Small bowel.
Appearance of skin over abnormality.	Normal.	Defect in skin: membrane covering exomphalos (comprised of peritoneum and amniotic layers).	Defect in skin: no skin or membrane covering the defect.
Associated abnormalities	Rare.	Common, particularly cardiac and renal defects.	Less common, but may be associated with bowel atresia.
Bowel complications.	Rare.	Rare: bowel function typically normal.	Bowel may be inflamed. Risk of obstruction, gut dysmotility, gastro-oesophageal reflux disease (GORD).
Management.	Conservative.	Small defects can be operated on soon after birth. Large defects are left open to keratinise over, and surgically repaired later.	Most cases are managed with a "silo" suspended from the roof of the incubator, with gravity assisting gut descent into the abdomen. If there is ischaemia of the bowel/atresia, surgery is performed earlier.

all patients with Down syndrome have duodenal atresia.

Clinical Features

Fifty percent of patients with duodenal atresia have polyhydramnios on antenatal scans. Frequently, a large distended stomach and collapsed distal bowel are also identified. Classically, a baby born with the condition develops either clear or bilious vomiting hours after birth. The obstruction is usually distal to the ampulla, thereby giving rise to bilious vomiting. Inspection frequently reveals a marked distension in the left upper quadrant.

Investigations

The classic "double bubble" sign can be seen on a plain abdominal X-ray (*Figure 19*). The distal bowel is usually devoid of air. If some air is present in the distal segments of the bowel, an upper GI contrast study might be beneficial, as this will clarify the level of any obstruction.

Differential Diagnosis

Duodenal obstruction can be caused by duodenal atresia or stenosis.

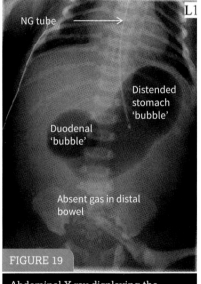

NG tube

L1

Distended stomach 'bubble'

Duodenal 'bubble'

Absent gas in distal bowel

FIGURE 19

Abdominal X-ray displaying the double bubble sign.

Intrinsic obstruction can be due to a duodenal web leading to the "wind sock deformity" (a classic sign on a contrast study, showing a contrast filled sac in the duodenum, with a lucent line distal to it, representing the web). If the duodenal web perforates, presentation can be delayed. Other differential diagnoses include annular pancreas (ring of pancreatic tissue surrounding the duodenum) and malrotation.

Management

An NG tube allows decompression of the stomach and decreases the risk of aspiration. Definitive management is surgical. A preoperative echocardiogram is essential to identify any associated congenital heart disease.

On laparotomy, the obstruction is bypassed by performing a duodeno-duodenostomy. An NG tube is left in situ (for drainage of the distended stomach) and frequently the anastomosis is bridged with a trans-anastomotic tube that can be utilised for feeding.

Prognosis

This depends on comorbidities, but generally infants can tolerate normal feeds within a few weeks and have no long-term morbidities.

Ileal and Jejunal Atresias

Ileal and jejunal atresias are obstructions in the small bowel that occur secondary to a vascular occlusion in utero. They are classified as Grade I-IV (*Table 9*).

TABLE 9: Classification of intestinal atresias	
Type of atresia	
I.	Mucosal web with intact bowel.
II.	The blind ends are separated by a fibrous band.
IIIa.	The blind ends are disconnected.
IIIb.	Large defect in the mesentery, with a significant loss of gut length.
IV.	Multiple atresias that look like a "string of sausages"; significant loss of gut length.

Clinical Features

Cases present with bilious vomiting and abdominal distension. Vomiting is a more prominent feature in more proximal obstructions. The infant may also fail to pass meconium. Abdominal radiographs are suggestive of the diagnosis. A lower GI contrast study can be diagnostic.

Management

Definitive management is surgical. Laparotomy identifies the type of atresia. Where possible, an end-to-end anastomosis is formed. Long-term outcome depends on the length of remaining gut.

Meconium Ileus

Aetiology

Meconium ileus is an obstruction of the distal ileum by abnormally thick meconium. It occurs in 5-10% of neonates with cystic fibrosis.

Clinical Features

The classic presentation is a baby who does not open their bowels in the first 48 hours of life. Normal meconium is passed within this time frame, but if it is abnormally thick, it can cause an obstruction. Other features that then ensue are those associated with obstruction, including abdominal distension and vomiting.

Differential Diagnosis

Passage of meconium can be delayed for a variety of causes, including:

› Meconium ileus.
› Ano-rectal malformation.
› Hirschsprung disease.

Investigations

Abdominal X-rays show features of small bowel obstruction, with thickened and dilated loops of bowel. A gastrografin enema can be diagnostic for the obstruction, as well as therapeutic (by breaking up the obstructing material). Investigation for cystic fibrosis is mandatory due to the association with meconium ileus.

Management

If the enema fails, a laparotomy with formation of temporary ileostomy is necessary. Rectal washouts (using small amounts of 0.9% sodium chloride) can be helpful to remove stool.

Malrotation with Midgut Volvulus

Aetiology

The ability to differentiate normal rotation, malrotation and volvulus is important (*Figure 20*):

› Normal rotation. The gut develops and matures outside the abdominal cavity in the foetus. The intestines rotate 270 degrees counter clockwise whilst returning into the abdominal cavity during the 11th week of gestation.

› Malrotation. An aberration of the normal rotation process. This can happen to various degrees, but classically the

Normal

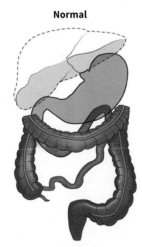

Malrotation

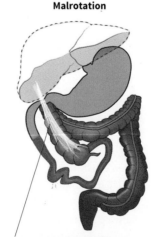

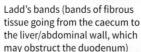
Ladd's bands (bands of fibrous tissue going from the caecum to the liver/abdominal wall, which may obstruct the duodenum)

Midgut volvulus

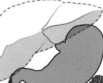

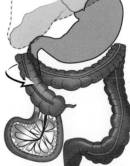

FIGURE 20

Normal rotation, with the DJ flexure left of the midline (left). Malrotation, with the DJ flexure right of the midline (middle). Midgut volvulus, twisting around the mesentery (right).

duodenal-jejunal (DJ) flexure comes to lie on the right of the midline instead of the left.

> Midgut volvulus. In patients with malrotation, the gut mesentery has a narrow base and can twist on its own axis, resulting in a midgut volvulus. The mesentery contains the superior mesenteric blood vessels. This leads to compromise of the blood flow and a mechanical obstruction. The consequences of this condition are catastrophic.

The true incidence of malrotation in the general population is unknown, as a proportion will remain asymptomatic throughout life. The incidence of symptomatic malrotation is one in 5000 live births. Congenital anomalies occur in approximately 70% of children with malrotation.

Clinical Features

Thirty percent of cases present in the first week of life and 75% will present within the first month. The classic presentation is a previously well infant that develops bilious vomiting.

During early presentation, the abdomen examines normally; however, as the condition progresses, the abdomen becomes distended, tender and occasionally peritonitic. Blood per rectum is typically a late feature of the condition and signifies gut ischaemia. At this stage, the child is extremely ill and shows hypotension, respiratory distress, severe metabolic acidosis and sepsis.

Investigations

Ultrasonography in experienced hands can be useful for screening for malrotation. However, when the condition is suspected, an urgent upper GI contrast study is the gold standard diagnostic tool. The normal position of the DJ flexure is on the left of the midline, above the level of the pylorus. If the position of the DJ flexure is displaced to the right of the midline, with complete or incomplete obstruction of the duodenum (corkscrew sign- *Figure 21*), the diagnosis of malrotation with midgut volvulus is confirmed and intervention is urgently needed.

Differential Diagnosis

Other conditions presenting with bilious vomiting include:
> Duodenal/intestinal atresia.
> Hirschsprung disease.
> Anorectal malformation.

Management

Malrotation with a midgut volvulus is a paediatric surgical emergency. Dead gut can lead to death of the patient in a few hours. Initial resuscitation involves aggressive fluid management, NG drainage and IV broad spectrum antibiotics. An emergency laparotomy should be undertaken as soon as possible:
> A transverse incision is made, and the twisted gut is untwisted and observed.

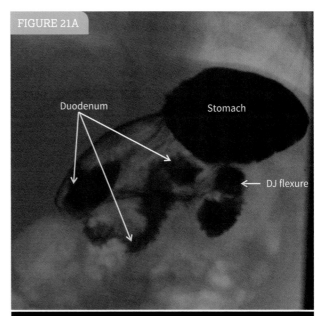

FIGURE 21A

Abdominal X-ray showing normal bowel. The duodeno-jejunal (DJ) flexure is to the left of the midline.

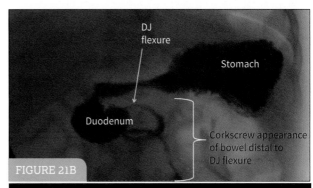

FIGURE 21B

Abdominal X-ray demonstrating malrotation. The duodeno-jejunal (DJ) flexure is on the right of the midline and the small bowel has twisted on itself, giving a corkscrew appearance.

> If the gut is viable, Ladd bands (peritoneal bands between the caecum and abdominal wall/liver) are divided, an appendicectomy is performed and the gut is reduced into the peritoneal cavity.
> If necrotic gut is present, it can be excised and stomas formed. If, however, the entire midgut is necrotic, many surgeons would simply reduce the gut back into the peritoneal cavity and commence palliative care for the child.

Prognosis

Mortality is approximately 5% for patients without significant loss of gut. It is higher for patients who lose significant lengths of gut (short gut). Complications of short gut syndrome include liver failure secondary to TPN, and sepsis (especially from central venous catheters).

Hirschsprung Disease

Hirschsprung disease (HD) is a congenital absence of ganglion cells in nerve plexuses that innervate the GI tract. This aganglionosis begins at the internal anal sphincter and extends proximally for a variable distance (*Table 10*). It affects one in 5000 births, with a male preponderance of four to one for short segment disease (recto-sigmoid aganglionosis) and two to one for long segment disease (ascending or transverse colon aganglionosis). Approximately 10-20% of all cases are familial. Approximately 15% of children with HD have trisomy 21.

Aetiology

The main pathological feature of HD is the absence of ganglion cells in the submucosal and intermyenteric plexuses of the GI tract. Different segments are affected differently:

- The distal segment appears aganglionic on histological examination.
- The transition zone is hypoganglionic.
- The proximal segment will appear normally ganglionated.

Macroscopically, the distal segment of bowel appears contracted and aperistaltic. The transition zone can be of variable length and usually is cone shaped. The proximal segment is hypertrophied and dilated.

The colonic mucosal barrier and the immune function of the gut in patients with HD is also suboptimal, predisposing patients to enterocolitis (a serious

infection of the bowel that can lead to death).

Clinical Features
Neonatal Presentation

Approximately 90% of children with HD present in the neonatal period with failure to pass meconium in the first 48 hours of life. This can be associated with progressive abdominal distension and bilious vomiting. A digital rectal exam classically causes an explosive expulsion of air and faeces, with marked decompression of the distended abdomen. Occasionally, a mucus plug can be passed.

Late Presentation

In a minority of children, the condition goes undiagnosed in early infancy, and they present later in life with severe constipation and faltering growth. Late presentation is more likely in short segment Hirschsprung disease.

Investigations

The gold standard diagnostic test is rectal biopsy. In infants, a suction rectal biopsy can be performed at the bedside. Older children will require a general anaesthetic for the procedure. Often, for this reason, anorectal manometry is used in older children. The reflex relaxation of the internal anal sphincter is absent in patients with HD, and this can be measured.

Other studies that might be helpful are plain abdominal X-rays and lower GI contrast studies. A plain abdominal X-ray in the symptomatic neonate frequently reveals distended thickened loops of bowel with a striking paucity of air in the rectum. A lower GI contrast study reveals a normal calibre rectum, a cone shaped transition zone and a very distended segment of proximal bowel (*Figure 22*). The large bowel can appear normal in patients with total colonic aganglionosis.

Differential Diagnosis

Delayed passage of meconium may also be due to:

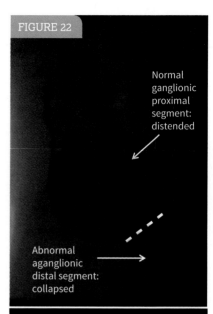

FIGURE 22

Normal ganglionic proximal segment: distended

Abnormal aganglionic distal segment: collapsed

Hirschsprung disease. Lower GI contrast study. The transition zone between a non-relaxing distal aganglionic segment and a very distended upper ganglionic segment is evident.

- Meconium ileus secondary to cystic fibrosis.
- Meconium plug syndrome.
- Premature gut.

Management

After the diagnosis of HD is confirmed, the bowel needs to be adequately decompressed. This can be achieved using regular rectal washouts or, if needed, by formation of a colostomy or ileostomy. The next step is surgery. The basic principle is to remove the aganglionic segment and join the normal ganglionic bowel to the internal anal sphincter. Several procedures have been described; these include the Duhamel, Swenson and Soave procedures.

Complications

Even after surgery, the following complications should be kept in mind:

- **Enterocolitis.** Enterocolitis is a potentially fatal condition that can affect children with HD pre and post operatively (despite adequate resection of the aganglionic segment). The condition presents with abdominal distension and tenderness, explosive

TABLE 10: Extent of gut involvement in Hirschsprung's disease	
Extent of gut involvement	**% of patients affected**
Recto sigmoid	75%
Ascending or transverse colon	17%
Total colonic aganglionosis	8%
Total intestinal aganglionosis	< 1%

- foul smelling motions, blood in the stools, signs of systemic sepsis and severe dehydration.
- › Faecal soiling. This may be a result of chronic constipation and overflow, or might be due to damage to the sphincter complex due to surgery.
- › Chronic constipation. This requires long-term laxative use.

Prognosis
Prognosis is generally good, particularly for short segment Hirschsprung disease. The majority of children will have relatively normal lives.

Biliary Atresia
Aetiology
Biliary atresia is an inflammatory process of extra hepatic bile ducts. If left to run its natural course, it leads to cholestasis, liver cirrhosis, liver failure and death. It is the most common surgical cause

of conjugated hyperbilirubinaemia in the neonate. The condition affects one in 15,000 live births. The cause is unknown, but in utero viral infections, autoimmune disorders and genetic theories have been postulated. Three subtypes are recognised (*Figure 23*). Note: this atresia only affects the extra-hepatic, not the intrahepatic ducts.

Clinical Features
Babies born with biliary atresia are usually term, with normal birth weights. Soon after birth, jaundice develops and worsens (*Figure 24*). Subsequently, the classic dark urine and pale stools develop, implying that only limited bile is getting into the gut. It is extremely important to investigate every baby with obstructive jaundice that fails to improve/resolve within the first two-three weeks of life.

Investigations
Blood Tests
› Serum bilirubin (SBR). The key feature here is conjugated hyperbilirubinaemia, with an elevated conjugated fraction of the total bilirubin (greater than 20–25%). Note that conjugated hyperbilirubinemia has a wide differential diagnosis,

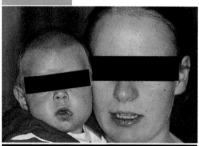
FIGURE 24
Jaundice secondary to biliary atresia (D@nderm).

Type I
Atresia of the common bile duct.

Type II
Atresia of the common hepatic duct and the common bile duct.

Type III
(>90% of patients). Atresia of the right and left hepatic ducts to the level of the porta hepatis.

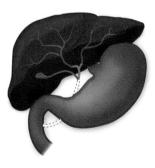
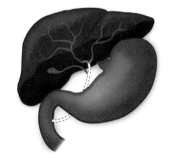
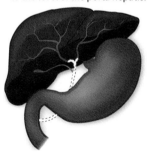

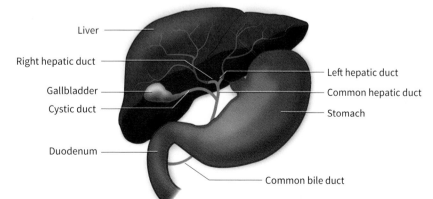

Liver — Right hepatic duct — Gallbladder — Cystic duct — Duodenum — Left hepatic duct — Common hepatic duct — Stomach — Common bile duct

Normal

FIGURE 23
Classification of biliary atresia.

and patients will be screened for a wide range of possible pathologies at this stage.

Imaging

- Ultrasound. Several changes are possible, including the absence of dilated intrahepatic ducts.
- HIDA (hepatobiliary iminodiacetic acid) scan. A radionuclide scan can be useful in establishing the diagnosis, as the conjugated bilirubin is taken up by the liver but not excreted.
- MRCP (magnetic resonance cholangiopancreatography). This may prove very effective in the future, but is not routinely used as it is very costly.

A liver biopsy gives the definitive diagnosis.

Differential Diagnosis

Biliary atresia is usually picked up because of prolonged jaundice. Key other causes of prolonged jaundice include:

- UTIs.
- Hypothyroidism.
- G6PD deficiency.
- Haemolytic anaemia.
- Physiological/breast milk jaundice.

Management

Definitive management is surgical. Dissection of abnormal tissue of the atretic bile ducts close to the porta hepatis results in biliary drainage. The draining component is anastomosed to a loop of jejunum (a Roux loop). The procedure is hence called Kasai porto-enterostomy.

Post operatively children require antibiotics (to prevent cholangitis e.g. cephalexin), medium chain triglyceride rich formula, and Vitamin A, D, E, K supplementation.

Complications

Liver fibrosis and cirrhosis can develop, even with surgical treatment. Sepsis is a particular concern, secondary to gut organisms ascending into the biliary system (cholangitis).

Prognosis

Even following a Kasai procedure, 80% of children still require a liver transplant.

Choledochal Cysts

Congenital biliary tract dilatations are known as choledochal cysts.

Clinical Features

The classic triad for presentation is jaundice, abdominal pain and an abdominal mass, but this only occurs in 15% of patients.

Investigations

Ultrasonography can visualise the extrahepatic bile ducts, but MRCP and endoscopic retrograde cholangiopancreatography (ERCP) can detail the anatomy further. Some cases are diagnosed in utero via antenatal ultrasound.

Complications

If untreated, complications may include:

- Cyst rupture and bile peritonitis.
- Malignant transformation: choledochocarcinoma.
- Cholangitis.
- Pancreatitis.
- Liver cirrhosis and portal hypertension.
- Choledocholithiasis.

Management

Management requires surgery. Cyst excision, cholecystectomy and hepatico-enterostomy (forming a communication between the hepatic duct and the gut) are the procedures of choice.

REFERENCES AND FURTHER READING

Pyloric Stenosis

1. Burkitt HG, Quick CR. (Eds). The acute abdomen in children. In: Essential Surgery : Problems, Diagnosis and Management. Third Edition. Harcourt Publishers Limited. London; 2002. 596.
2. Tam PK, Wong KK . Infantile Hypertrophic Pyloric Stenosis. In : Burge DM, Griffiths DM, Steinbrecher HA, et al. (Eds). Paediatric Surgery. Second Edition. London: Edward Arnold Publishers Ltd; 2005. 191-6.

Acute Appendicitis

1. Burkitt HG, Quick CR. (Eds). The acute abdomen in children. In : Essential Surgery : Problems, Diagnosis and Management. Third Edition. London: Harcourt Publishers Ltd; 2002. 599.
2. Peter SD. Appendicitis. In: Holcomb GB III, Murphy JP (Eds). Ashcraft's Pediatric Surgery. Fifth Edition. Philadelphia: Elsevier Inc; 2010. 549-56.
3. Puri P, Mortell A. Appendicitis. In: Stringer MD, Oldham KT, Mouriquand PD (Eds). Pediatric Surgery and Urology Long –Term Outcomes. Second Edition. New York: Cambridge University Press; 2006. 374-83.
4. Surana R. Abdominal pain . In: Burge DM, Griffiths DM, Steinbrecher HA, et al. (Eds). Paediatric Surgery. Second Edition. London: Edward Arnold Publishers Ltd; 2005. 231-5.

Intussusception

1. Burkitt HG, Quick CR. (Eds). The acute abdomen in children. In: Essential Surgery: Problems, Diagnosis and

Management. Third Edition. London: Harcourt Publishers Ltd; 2002. 576-8.

2   Cusick E, Woodward MN. Intussusception. In: Burge DM, Griffiths DM, Steinbrecher HA, et al. (Eds). Paediatric Surgery. Second Edition. London: Edward Arnold Publishers Ltd; 2005. 197-9.

3   Ignacio RC and Fallat ME. In: Holcomb GB III, Murphy JP (Eds). Ashcraft's Pediatric Surgery. Fifth Edition. Philadelphia. Elsevier Inc; 2010. 508-16.

Inguinal Hernia

1   MacKinnon AE. Hereniae and Hydroceles. In: Burge DM, Griffiths DM, Steinbrecher HA, et al. (Eds). Paediatric Surgery. Second Edition. London: Edward Arnold Publishers Ltd; 2005. 301-9.

Hydrocoele

1   Burkitt HG, Quick CR. (Eds). The non- acute abdominal problems in Children. In : Essential Surgery: Problems, Diagnosis and Management. Third Edition. London:Harcourt Publishers Ltd; 2002. 600-1.

2   MacKinnon AE. Hereniae and Hydroceles. In: Burge DM, Griffiths DM, Steinbrecher HA, et al. (Eds). Paediatric Surgery. Second Edition. London: Edward Arnold Publishers Ltd; 2005. 301-6.

Umbilical Hernia

1   Burkitt HG, Quick CR. (Eds). The non- acute abdominal problems in children. In:Essential Surgery: Problems, Diagnosis and Management. Third Edition. London: Harcourt Publishers Ltd; 2002. 601.

2   Grosfeld JL, O'Neill JA Jr, Coran AG, et al. (Eds). Pediatric Surgery. Volume 2. Sixth Edition. Philadelphia: Mosby Inc; 2006.

Divarication of Recti

1   Burkitt HG, Quick CR. (Eds). The non- acute abdominal problems in Children. In:Essential Surgery: Problems, Diagnosis and Management. Third Edition. London: Harcourt Publishers Ltd; 2002. 601.

2   MacKinnon AE. Hereniae and Hydroceles. In: Burge DM, Griffiths DM, Steinbrecher HA, et al. (Eds). Paediatric Surgery. Second Edition. London: Edward Arnold Publishers Ltd; 2005. 301-6.

Undescended Testes

1   Bisharat M. The Ideal Age for Orchidopexy in Children with Undescended Testes : Impact of Fertility and Malignancy. MSc Thesis. University of Cardiff; 2011.

2   Hutson JM. Undescended testes. Stringer MD, Oldham KT, Mouriquand PD (Eds). Pediatric Surgery and Urology Long –Term Outcomes. Second Edition. New York: Cambridge University Press; 2006. 652-62.

3   Madden NP. Testis, hydrocoele and varicoele. In: Thomas DF, Duffy PG, Rickwood AM (Eds). Essentials of Paediatric Urology. Second Edition. London: Informa Healthcare; 2008. 247-57.

Phimosis

1   Burkitt HG, Quick CR. (Eds). The non- acute abdominal problems in Children. In : Essential Surgery : Problems, Diagnosis and Management. Third Edition. London: Harcourt Publishers Ltd.; 2002. 603.

2   Huttun KA. The prepuce. In: Thomas DF, Duffy PG, Rickwood AM (Eds). Essentials of Paediatric Urology. Second Edition. London: Informa Healthcare; 2008. 234-45.

3   Verleyen P and Bogaert G. The prepuce, hypospadias and other congenital anomalies of the penis. In : Burge DM, Griffiths DM, Steinbrecher HA, et al. (Eds). Paediatric Surgery. Second Edition. London: Edward Arnold Publishers Ltd.; 2005. 533-35.

Paraphimosis

1   Burkitt HG, Quick CR. (Eds). The non- acute abdominal problems in Children. In : Essential Surgery : Problems, Diagnosis and Management. Third Edition. London: Harcourt Publishers Ltd.; 2002. 603.

2   Huttun KA. The prepuce. In: Thomas DF, Duffy PG, Rickwood AM (Eds). Essentials of Paediatric Urology. Second Edition. London: Informa Healthcare; 2008. 234-45.

3   Verleyen P and Bogaert G. The prepuce, hypospadias and other congenital anomalies of the penis. Burge DM, Griffiths DM, Steinbrecher HA, et al. (Eds). Paediatric Surgery. Second Edition. London: Edward Arnold Publishers Ltd.; 2005.

Balanitis Xerotica Obliterans

1   Burkitt HG, Quick CR. (Eds). The non- acute abdominal problems in Children. In : Essential Surgery : Problems, Diagnosis and Management. Third Edition. London: Harcourt Publishers Ltd.; 2002. 603.

2   Huttun KA. The prepuce. In: Thomas DF, Duffy PG, Rickwood AM (Eds). Essentials of Paediatric Urology. Second Edition. London: Informa Healthcare; 2008. 234-45.

3   Verleyen P and Bogaert G. The prepuce, hypospadias and other congenital anomalies of the penis. Burge DM, Griffiths DM, Steinbrecher HA, et al. (Eds). Paediatric Surgery. Second Edition. London: Edward Arnold Publishers Ltd.; 2005. 533-5.

4   British Medical Association. Symposium on circumcision: The law and ethics of circumcision: guidance for doctors. J Med Ethics 2004;30:259-63 doi:10.1136/jme.2004.008540

Hypospadias

1. Stringer MD, Oldham KT, Mouriquand PD (Eds). Pediatric Surgery and Urology Long-Term Outcomes. Second Edition. New York: Cambridge University Press; 2006.
2. Wilcox DT and Mouriquand PD. Hypospadias. In: Thomas DF, Duffy PG, Rickwood AM (Eds). Essentials of Paediatric Urology. Second Edition. London: Informa Healthcare; 2008. 213-31.

Vesico-Ureteric Junction Obstruction

1. Thomas DF. Upper tract obstruction. In: Thomas DF, Duffy PG, Rickwood AM (Eds). Essentials of Paediatric Urology. Second Edition. London: Informa Healthcare; 2008. 87-92.

Vesico-Ureteric Reflux

1. Minevich E and Sheldon CA. Urinary tract infection and vesicoureteral reflux. In: Holcomb GB III, Murphy JP (Eds). Ashcraft's Pediatric Surgery. Fifth Edition. Philadelphia: Elsevier Inc.; 2010. 721-30.
2. Thomas DFM, Subramaniam R. Vesicoureteric reflux. In: Thomas DF, Duffy PG, Rickwood AM (Eds). Essentials of Paediatric Urology. Second Edition. London: Informa Healthcare; 2008. 57-72.

Posterior Urethral Valves

1. SN Cenk Buyukunal. Lower urinary tract obstruction. In: Burge DM, Griffiths DM, Steinbrecher HA, et al. (Eds). Paediatric Surgery. Second Edition. London: Edward Arnold Publishers Ltd.; 2005. 483-7.
2. Thomas DF, Duffy PG, Rickwood AM (Eds). Essentials of Paediatric Urology. Second Edition. London: Informa Healthcare; 2008.

Necrotising Enterocolitis

1. Boston V. Necrotising Enterocolitis. In: Burge DM, Griffiths DM, Steinbrecher HA, et al. (Eds). Paediatric Surgery. Second Edition. London: Edward Arnold Publishers Ltd.; 2005. P 167-72.
2. Henry MC, Moss RL. Necrotizing enterocolitis. In: Stringer MD, Oldham KT, Mouriquand PD (Eds). Pediatric Surgery and Urology Long –Term Outcomes. Second Edition. New York: Cambridge University Press; 2006. 329-49.
3. Henry MC, Moss RL. Necrotising enterocolitis. In: Holcomb GB III, Murphy JP (Eds). Ashcraft's Pediatric Surgery. Fifth Edition. Philadelphia: Elsevier Inc.; 2010. 439-55.

Congenital Diaphragmatic Hernia

1. Stolar CJ, Dillon PW. Congenital diaphragmatic hernia and eventration. In: Grosfeld JL, O'Neill JA Jr, Coran AG, et al. (Eds). Pediatric Surgery. Volume 1. Sixth Edition. Philadelphia: Mosby Inc.; 2006. 931-50.
2. Tsao K, Lally KP. Congenital diaphragmatic hernia and eventration. In: Holcomb GB III, Murphy JP (Eds). Ashcraft's Pediatric Surgery. Fifth Edition. Philadelphia: Elsevier Inc.; 2010. 304-21.

Oesophageal Atresia/ Tracheo-Oesophageal Fistula

1. Harmon CM, Coran AG. Congenital anomalies of the esophagus. In: Grosfeld JL, O'Neill JA Jr, Coran AG, et al. (Eds). Pediatric Surgery. Volume 1. Sixth Edition. Philadelphia: Mosby Inc.; 2006. 1051-80.
2. Klaas B . Esophageal atresia and tracheoesophageal malformations. In: Holcomb GB III, Murphy JP (Eds). Ashcraft's Pediatric Surgery. Fifth Edition. Philadelphia: Elsevier Inc.; 2010. 345-61.

Anorectal Malformation

1. Levitt MA, Pena A. Imperforate anus and cloacal malformations. In: Holcomb GB III, Murphy JP (Eds). Ashcraft's Pediatric Surgery. Fifth Edition. Philadelphia: Elsevier Inc.; 2010. 468-90.

Gastroschisis/ Exomphalos

1. Burkitt HG, Quick CR. (Eds). The acute abdomen in Children. In: Essential Surgery : Problems, Diagnosis and Management. Third Edition. London: Harcourt Publishers Ltd.; 2002. 594.
2. Kelleher C, Langer JC. Congenital abdominal wall defects. In: Holcomb GB III, Murphy JP (Eds). Ashcraft's Pediatric surgery. Fifth Edition. Philadelphia: Elsevier Inc.; 2010. 625-32.
3. Nielsen OH. Abdominal Wall Defects. In: Burge DM, Griffiths DM, Steinbrecher HA, et al. (Eds). Paediatric Surgery. Second Edition. London: Edward Arnold Publishers Ltd.; 2005. 188-90.

Duodenal Obstruction, Ileal/Jejunal Atresia

1. Aguayo P, Ostlie DJ. Dudenal and intestinal atresia and stenosis. Holcomb GB III, Murphy JP (Eds). Ashcraft's Pediatric Surgery. Fifth Edition. Philadelphia: Elsevier Inc.; 2010. 400-5.

Meconium Ileus

1. Caty MG, Escobar MA. Meconium disease. In: Holcomb GB III, Murphy JP (Eds). Ashcraft's Pediatric Surgery. Fifth Edition. Philadelphia: Elsevier Inc.; 2010. 425-36.
2. Ziegler MM. Meconium ileus. In: Grosfeld JL, O'Neill JA Jr, Coran AG, et al. (Eds). Pediatric Surgery. Volume 2. Sixth Edition. Philadelphia: Mosby Inc.; 2006. 1289-303.

Malrotation

1. Little DC, Smith SD. Malrotation. In: Holcomb GB III, Murphy JP (Eds). Ashcraft's Pediatric Surgery. Fifth Edition. Philadelphia: Elsevier Inc.; 2010. 416-24.

Hirschsprung's Disease

1   Burkitt HG, Quick CR. (Eds). The acute abdomen in children. In: Essential Surgery : Problems, Diagnosis and Management. Third Edition. London: Harcourt Publishers Ltd.; 2002. 592-3.

2   Georgeson KE. Hirschsprung's disease. In: Holcomb GB III, Murphy JP (Eds). Ashcraft's Pediatric Surgery. Fifth Edition. Philadelphia: Elsevier Inc.; 2010. 456-67

3   Whan EB. Hirschsprung's Disease. In: Burge DM, Griffiths DM, Steinbrecher HA, et al. (Eds). Paediatric Surgery. Second Edition. London: Edward Arnold Publishers Ltd.; 2005. 147-53.

Biliary Atresia/ Choledochal Cysts

1   Yamataka A, Kato Y, Miyano T. Biliary tract disorders and portal hypertension. In: Holcomb GB III, Murphy JP (Eds). Ashcraft's Pediatric Surgery. Fifth Edition. Philadelphia: Elsevier Inc.; 2010. 557-66.

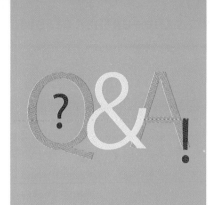

CONTENTS

CONTENTS

CASE 1
A 14-year-old girl presenting with self-harm

Jennifer, a 14-year-old girl, is brought in by her mum after having self-harmed by cutting her arm with a razor. On assessment, the cuts are shallow and horizontal, with no active bleeding. The girl is quiet and withdrawn, but appears otherwise well. This is her first episode of self-harm. When asked whether she wanted to kill herself, she shrugs. Observations are within normal limits. After being reassured that her cuts do not require further treatment, both Jennifer and her mother are keen to go home.

Questions

Q1 Which of the following would be the best way to manage Jennifer?
A Jennifer should be sectioned because she is suicidal
B She should be discharged home in her mother's care, because she is a child
C She should be assessed before discharge by the child and adolescent mental health team, either in the ED or as an inpatient
D She should be discharged on her own because she has been assessed as Gillick competent

Q2 When you speak to Jennifer alone, she tells you she has a 16-year-old boyfriend that her mother doesn't know about. On questioning, she admits that they are having sex but that "he doesn't like condoms". Which of the following is/are correct? Select all that apply.
A You have a duty to inform the police because she is having underage sex

B You should encourage her to talk to her mother about her boyfriend
C You have a duty to tell her mother that she is having sex because she is under 16, but you don't need to tell Jennifer before you do this
D If Jennifer has been assessed as Gillick competent, you do not need to do anything about this
E If she requests it, Jennifer can be prescribed the pill without telling her mother

Q3 You want to give Jennifer further advice regarding sexual health. Which of the following is/are correct? Select all that apply.
A Jennifer should go on the pill so that she doesn't need to use condoms
B She should not be given any contraception, as this is encouraging her to have sex underage
C A coil is the best choice for her because she is young and hasn't had children yet
D She can go on her own for a sexual health screen
E Telling her about all the different methods of contraception will be confusing for her

For answers see page 390

CASE 2
A 3-year-old boy presenting with stridor

A 3-year-old boy is brought in by ambulance to ED, as his parents were concerned about his breathing. Yesterday, he had a hoarse voice, runny nose and temperature, but awoke this morning very distressed, with a barking cough and high-pitched noise on inspiration. His parents reported he seemed unable to catch his breath. Now that he has stopped crying, his breathing is less noisy.

Observations are within normal limits, apart from a mild tachycardia (HR 150 bpm), and a temperature of 37.9°C. His cough has a barking quality, and at rest, you can just hear a soft, high-pitched noise on inspiration. He has tracheal tug, mild intercostal recession and mild reduced air entry. He is interacting well with you during your examination and is not drooling.

Questions

Q1   What is the most likely diagnosis?
   A   Epiglottitis
   B   Bacterial tracheitis
   C   Anaphylaxis
   D   Inhaled foreign body
   E   Croup

Q2   What first-line treatment should this patient receive?
   A   Oral dexamethasone
   B   Intramuscular adrenaline
   C   Nebulised budesonide
   D   Oral antibiotics

Q3   Which symptom(s) would make you worry about a diagnosis of acute epiglottitis? Select all that apply.
   A   Sore throat
   B   Drooling
   C   Constant barking cough
   D   High fever >38.5°C
   E   Onset over days not hours

For answers see page 391

CASE 3
A 14-year-old boy presenting with a limp

Jonah is a 14-year-old boy who presents to the ED with a two week history of a limp and left knee pain that has been increasing in severity and now prevents him from doing exercise. His mother is worried as it has not been getting better. He is overweight and does not enjoy sports at school. There is no clear history of trauma. Observations are within normal limits, and he feels otherwise well.

On examination, there is an antalgic gait. On palpation, there is no hip/knee effusion, or any localised skin changes. Hip rotation is restricted on active movement and painful on passive movement. There is no pain or restriction of movement in the knee.

Questions

Q1   What is the most useful next step?
   A   AP and lateral knee X-ray
   B   FBC, CRP and ESR
   C   MRI knee

   D   AP and frog-leg lateral hip X-ray
   E   MRI hip
   F   Thyroid function tests

Q2   Given the above information what is the most likely diagnosis?
   A   Perthes' disease
   B   Blount's disease
   C   Knee septic arthritis
   D   Slipped upper femoral epiphysis
   E   Osgood-Schlatter disease

Q3   How should this child be treated?
   A   Rest, ice and elevation of knee
   B   Intravenous antibiotics
   C   Bed rest and traction
   D   Fixation of the femoral epiphysis with threaded pins/screws
   E   Conservative management, with observation only

For answers see page 392

CASE 4
A 10-month-old presenting with fever

A 10-month-old boy presents to ED with a three week history of fever. His parents tell you they have been unable to control his temperature with paracetamol and that it was 39°C when measured at home. The fever seemed to subside for a few days last week before coming back again. The parents also tell you that they have both had a tummy bug, with diarrhoea and vomiting, starting two days ago. You see the infant is flushed, but he has no coryzal symptoms. At present, he is afebrile and is tolerating oral fluids but not any other feeds. He has vomited once this morning, and is also having several episodes of diarrhoea a day. He is normally fit and well, with no previous hospital admissions.

On general inspection, the infant appears well and is active, though slightly irritable. Examination shows that he has normal heart sounds, a clear chest, a soft non-tender abdomen, no rashes and a normal ENT examination. Mucous membranes are slightly dry. He is passing urine normally, but his stools are more liquid than normal. His observations are within normal limits. A urine culture collected two days ago at the GP surgery via a bag sample showed a "mixed growth", with a 1+ white blood cell count.

Questions

Q1   Mark the following statements true or false.
   A   A lumbar puncture should be performed on this child
   B   A fever of 39°C suggests it is more likely to be a bacterial infection
   C   This boy has a prolonged fever
   D   Body temperature can be reliably measured using an axillary digital thermometer
   E   This boy has very worrying symptoms/signs for a child with fever

Q2   What is the most likely diagnosis?
   A   Gastroenteritis
   B   Urinary tract infection
   C   Viral tonsillitis
   D   Upper respiratory tract infection
   E   Sepsis

Q3   What is the best management option?
   A   Discharge home with written and verbal advice
   B   Start IV antibiotics and take blood cultures
   C   Start IV fluids
   D   Keep him nil by mouth in case he has an acute abdomen
   E   Admit him into a bay on the paediatric ward

For answers see page 394

CASE 5
A 20-day-old boy presenting with fever, vomiting, and lethargy

A 20-day-old boy is brought into ED by his parents, who are concerned that he has been sleepier than usual and hasn't been waking for feeds. They have also noticed he has been hot for the last 12 hours and has vomited milky fluid twice during this time. He was born by spontaneous vaginal delivery and has an uncomplicated antenatal history. There were no problems at birth.

On examination, his respiratory rate was 80 breaths/min (tachypnoeic) with SpO_2 95% in air, pulse 180 bpm (tachycardic), a normal BP and temperature of 39°C. He is mottled, with cold hands and feet and a capillary refill time of 4 seconds. He is sleepy, but he opens his eyes spontaneously when roused and cries weakly. Blood glucose is 3.5 mmol/L. He moves all his limbs but is floppy. He has no rash and his fontanelle is not bulging. His heart sounds are normal, his chest is clear with no recession, and his abdomen is soft and not distended, with bowel sounds audible.

Questions
Q1   What is the first priority in managing this child?
   A   Get IV access, give a fluid bolus and give broad spectrum IV antibiotics
   B   Give oral antibiotics
   C   Get a urine sample
   D   Give paracetamol
   E   Give oral rehydration salts

Q2   A full septic screen is performed. A lumbar puncture and blood cultures are taken and the child had a chest X-ray. Which investigation is required to complete the septic screen?
   A   Throat swab
   B   Urine microscopy, culture and sensitivity
   C   CT head
   D   Abdominal ultrasound
   E   Nasopharyngeal aspirate

Q3   You get a phone call from the microbiology lab saying that the blood culture grows gram-negative diplococci. Which of the following bacteria would fit this picture?
   A   Group A streptococcus
   B   Group B streptococcus
   C   *Staphylococcus aureus*
   D   *Escherichia coli*
   E   Group B *Neisseria meningitidis*

For answers see page 395

CASE 6
An 11-year-old boy presenting with chronic abdominal pain

Matt is an 11-year-old boy who presents via the outpatient clinic, unwell with abdominal pain for three months, significant weight loss and bloody diarrhoea. His symptoms make you suspect inflammatory bowel disease. He gets admitted for further tests to the ward, including blood tests and colonoscopy to confirm the diagnosis. Observations are within normal limits. He is very nervous and refuses to have blood tests or consider having any procedures. His mother is with him, and his parents are keen that he is investigated, as he requires a diagnosis to allow appropriate treatment to be commenced.

Questions
Q1   Regarding consent, mark the following statements true or false.
   A   Matt definitely does not have capacity
   B   Matt's mother can consent on behalf of her child
   C   The doctors should bypass asking for consent, as this is a potentially serious condition

Q2   What should happen next?
   A   The decision to perform the investigations should be delayed until Matt has the ability to consent
   B   Ideally, consent should be sought from the mother, but if she does not agree with treatment, then treatment should proceed either through a court order or immediately if the case is life threatening
   C   A compromise should be made whereby treatment is started empirically so that Matt can avoid blood tests and a colonoscopy

For answers see page 397

CASE 7
An 8-year-old child presenting with persistent chest infections

A primary care physician has referred an 8-year-old boy to the paediatric clinic due to recurrent chest infections. He appears to be requiring a course of antibiotics every month and has a persistently wet-sounding cough. He is on the 50th centile for height and the 0.4th centile for weight. Mum tells the paediatrician that her son had poor weight gain in infancy. He has been treated for constipation and "difficult to control" asthma, although she expresses some confusion regarding inhaler use. Observations are within normal limits.

You perform a sweat test that yields a chloride result diagnostic of cystic fibrosis. He is admitted to the paediatric unit for education, counselling and treatment in the form of intravenous antibiotics and intensive physiotherapy. After ten days of treatment, his lung function has not improved from admission. He feels short of breath and tight chested. His blood results show an elevated IgE of 1300 IU/mL (ref 0-63 IU/mL).

Questions

Q1 What is the most likely reason for the child's faltering growth?

    A He likely has pancreatic insufficiency

    B He has been frequently unwell

    C He has undiagnosed coeliac disease

    D His faltering growth is secondary to asthma medication

Q2 On which chromosome is the gene defect located in CF?

    A Chromosome 21

    B Chromosome 13

    C Chromosome 7

    D Chromosome 2

Q3 What is the next most important test to be performed following a positive diagnosis on the sweat test?

    A Stool sample analysis for faecal elastase

    B Extended genetic testing

    C Coeliac screen

    D Random blood glucose

Q4 What diagnosis is most likely to account for the failure in treatment to improve the child's symptoms and an elevated total IgE?

    A Meconium ileus

    B Distal intestinal obstructive syndrome

    C Allergic bronchopulmonary aspergillosis

    D CF-related diabetes

For answers see page 398

CASE 8
A 5-year-old boy with unstable asthma

A 5-year-old boy attends the paediatric outpatient clinic. He has a diagnosis of asthma and is on beclomethasone 100 micrograms MDI 2 puffs BD, and salbutamol 100 micrograms MDI 2-10 puffs PRN. Observations are within normal limits.

Lately, he has been using more of his salbutamol inhaler during the day on minimal exercise and even when at rest. He is also waking in the night coughing and short of breath, which is relieved with five puffs of salbutamol. You are asked to review his asthma therapy.

Questions

Q1 What would be the next treatment step?

    A Increase his inhaled corticosteroid

    B Add in a leukotriene receptor antagonist

    C Add in a long acting $\beta 2$ agonist

    D Add oral corticosteroids

Q2 Which method of drug delivery would be the most appropriate for a 5-year-old?

    A Metered dose inhaler on its own

    B Metered dose inhaler with a spacer device and a mouth piece

    C Metered dose inhaler with a spacer device and a facemask

    D A breath-activated inhaler

Q3 What is a common side effect with the use of leukotriene receptor antagonists such as Montelukast?

    A Dry mouth

    B Oral candidiasis

    C Disturbed sleep

For answers see page 399

CASE 9
A 6-year-old girl presenting with wheeze and breathlessness

A 6-year-old girl attended ED with a 24 hour history of worsening cough and a runny nose. In the last four hours, her parents had noticed that she was very quiet and her breathing had become rapid and wheezy. She has a history of viral-induced wheeze, which has been managed in the community with inhaled salbutamol. Between these episodes, she has often woken up coughing at night. Her father, who has brought her in, states that the family has moved into a new house two days ago.

On examination, her respiratory rate is 60 breaths/min (tachypnoeic), SpO_2 is 91% on room air, pulse is 150 bpm (tachycardic) and temperature is 37.2°C. She is sitting upright and refuses to lie down. She can only talk in short sentences. She has subcostal and intercostal recession, as well as tracheal tug. Auscultation reveals decreased air entry and expiratory wheeze throughout her chest. Her heart sounds are normal and her abdomen is soft, with normal bowel sounds. She is not coryzal and her throat and ears are not erythematous. Her GCS is 15/15.

Questions

Q1 What is the most likely diagnosis?

    A Bronchiolitis

    B Acute exacerbation of asthma

    C Pneumonia

    D Foreign body inhalation

    E Viral-induced wheeze

Q2 A nurse starts high-flow oxygen via a non-rebreather mask and asks you what to do next. Which step would be the most appropriate?

 A Inhaled ipratropium bromide from a metered dose inhaler via a spacer

 B Inhaled salbutamol from a metered dose inhaler via a spacer

 C Start oral amoxicillin

 D Nebulised ipratropium bromide driven with oxygen

 E Nebulised salbutamol driven with oxygen

Q3 Which of the following would be required on discharge? Select all that apply.

 A Review of inhaler technique

 B Epipen

 C Sweat test

 D Prophylactic antibiotics

For answers see page 400

CASE 10
A 7-year-old boy presenting with fever and a cough

A 7-year-old boy presents to the ED. He has been coughing for the past six days, which keeps him awake at night, with temperatures of up to 38.5°C. He has a reduced appetite but is drinking adequately. He is a previously well child, on no regular medication and is fully vaccinated.

You auscultate his chest and hear crackles on the right apex and no breath sounds below this point, with a dull percussion note throughout the right lung field. He has a respiratory rate of 40 breaths/min (tachypnoeic) and requires 2L of oxygen delivered via a nasal cannula to maintain saturations above 92%. HR is 140 bpm (tachycardic). A chest X-ray shows consolidation of the right lung, with a large associated effusion.

Questions

Q1 What is the most likely organism to cause community acquired pneumonia in this age group?

 A Group A streptococcus

 B *Streptococcus pneumoniae*

 C Mycoplasma

 D *Staphylococcus aureus*

Q2 What would be the most appropriate treatment course for this child?

 A Discharge with oral broad spectrum antibiotics and follow up arrangements

 B Back-to-back salbutamol nebulisers and oral corticosteroids

 C Admit to hospital and start on broad spectrum antibiotics

 D Intubation, ventilation and transfer to the nearest paediatric intensive care unit

Q3 Once treatment and management has been established, which of the following would be the most useful next step investigations for management of the effusion?

 A Chest CT

 B Chest ultrasound scan

 C Needle aspiration

 D Lung biopsy

For answers see page 402

CASE 11
An 8-month-old baby presenting with respiratory distress and poor feeding

An 8-month-old baby girl is brought into ED by her parents. She has been coughing and unsettled for the past two days with coryzal symptoms and a temperature of 37.9°C. She is feeding less than she would usually, taking approximately one-third of her usual volume of milk and not tolerating solid food. She is also producing fewer wet nappies.

Examination reveals a respiratory rate of 50-60 breaths/min (tachypnoeic), with nasal flaring and head bobbing. Her saturations in room air are 95%. HR is 165 bpm (tachycardic). When auscultating her chest, wheeze and crackles are heard bilaterally.

Questions

Q1 What is the most likely diagnosis?

 A Pneumonia

 B Croup

 C Viral induced wheeze

 D Bronchiolitis

Q2 What would be the most appropriate course of action?

 A Discharge and advise the use of nasal sodium chloride drops

 B Admit for observation and feeding support

 C Perform a chest X-ray

 D Start a course of antibiotics

Q3 Which of the following is the most appropriate initial care? Select all that apply.

 A Oral corticosteroids

 B Nebulised salbutamol

 C Nebulised hypertonic sodium chloride

 D Nebulised adrenaline

 E Supportive management

For answers see page 403

CASE 12
A 6-year-old girl presenting with a possible allergic reaction

A 6-year-old girl is brought in to paediatric ED by ambulance. She had eaten prawns at dinner and 30 minutes later, she complained of tingling of her tongue and difficulty breathing. She then vomited twice. Her parents called an ambulance after noticing that her breathing was fast and noisy and her lips and face appeared swollen. She has a history of eczema, which is controlled with 1% hydrocortisone cream and emollients. On examination, RR is 40 breaths/min (tachypnoeic), with SpO_2 90% in air, HR is 150 bpm (tachycardic), BP is 75/40 mmHg (hypotensive) and temperature is 37°C. She has widespread facial swelling involving her lips, and an urticarial rash on her chest. She has quiet stridor, with tracheal tug and intercostal recession. On auscultation, she has decreased air entry bilaterally, with expiratory wheeze throughout her chest. Her capillary refill centrally is three seconds and she has cold hands.

Q1   What medication should be given to this patient immediately?
   A   IM adrenaline (1:10 000)
   B   IM adrenaline (1:1 000)
   C   IV adrenaline (1:10 000)
   D   IV adrenaline (1:1 000)
   E   Nebulised adrenaline (1:1 000)

Q2   Which of the following is the most worrying symptom in this patient?
   A   Wheeze
   B   Hypotension
   C   Vomiting
   D   Stridor
   E   Tachycardia

Q3   What type of hypersensitivity reaction is this girl likely to be experiencing?
   A   Type I
   B   Type II
   C   Type III
   D   Type IV
   E   Type V

For answers see page 404

CASE 13
A 5-year-old girl presenting with burns

A 5-year-old girl is brought to ED by ambulance after being retrieved from a house fire. On arrival, she looks well. Her RR is 35 breaths/min (tachypnoeic) with saturations of 98% in air, HR is 150 bpm (tachycardic) and temperature is 37°C.

She appears to have no obvious injury but seems tired and keen to sleep. There is soot around her mouth and she has a hoarse cry. Her mucous membranes appear dry and she has reduced skin turgor and reduced urine output. She had been well throughout the day, eating and drinking normally.

Q1   Which of the following features would be concerning in this patient? Select all that apply.

   A   Poor urine output
   B   Decreased mental status
   C   Soot-tinged sputum
   D   Hoarse cry

Q2   What is the most important priority in her management?
   A   Insertion of at least two wide bore cannulas to institute aggressive fluid resuscitation
   B   Chest X-ray
   C   Administration of high flow oxygen
   D   Transfer to a burns centre for specialist management

Q3   What feature would be most suggestive of carbon monoxide poisoning?
   A   Elevated arterial $PaCO_2$ on blood gas
   B   Low oxygen saturations on pulse oximetry
   C   Elevated carboxyhaemoglobin level
   D   Metabolic alkalosis on a blood gas
   E   A respiratory rate of 28 breaths/min

For answers see page 405

CASE 14
A 1-hour-old baby presenting with suspected sepsis

Baby Smith was born today (01.01.15, Hospital Number: 334335X) at 39 weeks gestation, weighing 4 kg. Mum had a fever during labour on a background of Group B streptococcus colonisation. The baby has developed significant respiratory distress and is unable to tolerate oral feeds. The midwife at delivery was concerned about "foul smelling" liquor and suspected chorioamnionitis. Observations are within normal limits.

Question
Your registrar has admitted the baby to NICU (under Dr Daniels). You are asked to prescribe cefotaxime (50 mg/kg BD) and maintenance intravenous fluids (at 60 mL/kg/day), as the baby is nil by mouth (NBM). Use this information to fill out the prescription chart (Chart 1a). Note that many units have dedicated gentamicin charts, but for the purpose of this exercise, a generic chart will be used.

For answers see page 406

CASE 15
A 6-year-old boy presenting with an infective asthma exacerbation

David Hodgkins (DOB 15/02/2008, hospital number: SM506901) is a 6-year-old boy with known asthma who has presented with difficulty in breathing and wheeze. He weighs 20 kg and had an anaphylactic reaction to penicillin at 3-years-old.

CHART 1A: BLANK PRESCRIPTION CHART FOR CLINICAL CASE 14

Name				Weight				Known allergies			
Date of birth				Gestation							
Hospital number				Consultant							
Admission date				Ward				Signature:		Date:	

REGULAR MEDICATIONS

			Date Time								
Drug			02								
Dose	Freq	Route	06								
			10								
Start	Stop/review		14								
Signature			18								
Indication			22								
Drug			02								
Dose	Freq	Route	06								
			10								
Start	Stop/review		14								
Signature			18								
Indication			22								

FLUID PRESCRIPTIONS

Date	Fluid	Additive	Volume	Route	Rate	Signature	Given	Batch

He is febrile, with focal crepitations on his chest. You suspect a lower respiratory tract infection. He has not been eating or drinking. He is to be admitted to Puffin ward under Dr Ross.

Question

Please write up a drug chart (Chart 2a) for him to include:

> Ten puffs of salbutamol inhaler every four hours
> An appropriate choice of oral antibiotics
> 2/3 maintenance fluids
> 30mg oral prednisolone once per day

For answers see page 407

CASE 16
A 12-year-old girl presenting with abdominal pain

A 12-year-old girl presents with a 36-hour history of vague central abdominal pain that has shifted to the right iliac fossa.

She is otherwise well. Her periods started four months ago but have been irregular: her last one was one week ago. She has vomited twice since the onset of pain, and complains of dysuria. Whilst waiting to be seen, the child had a bout of watery diarrhoea.

On examination, her HR is 120 bpm (tachycardic) and her temperature is 37.8°C, but all other observations are within normal limits. She is coryzal. She is tender over both sides of her abdomen.

Questions

Q1 Which of the following conditions is on your list of differential diagnoses? Select all that apply.

A Urinary tract infection
B Acute appendicitis
C Ovarian pathology
D Nonspecific abdominal pain
E Gastroenteritis

CHART 2A: BLANK PRESCRIPTION CHART FOR CLINICAL CASE 15

Name	Weight	Known allergies		
Date of birth	Age			
Hospital number	Consultant			
Admission date	Ward	Signature: Date:		

REGULAR MEDICATIONS

		Date / Time									
Drug		02									
Dose	Freq	Route	06									
			10									
Start	Stop/review	14									
Signature		18									
Indication		22									
Drug		02									
Dose	Freq	Route	06									
			10									
Start	Stop/review	14									
Signature		18									
Indication		22									

FLUID PRESCRIPTIONS

Date	Fluid	Additive	Volume	Route	Rate	Signature	Given	Batch

Q2   Please match the following condition to the most important diagnostic modality.

Match:

    A   Acute pancreatitis
    B   Acute appendicitis
    C   Gastroenteritis
    D   Urinary tract infection
    E   Ruptured ovarian cyst
    F   Mesenteric adenitis
    G   Meckel's diverticulitis

To:

    i.   Ultrasound scan
    ii.   Urine microscopy, culture and sensitivity
    iii.   Clinical assessment, FBC, CRP and observation
    iv.   Amylase
    v.   Stool cultures

Initial investigations come back. Urinalysis is negative, full blood count shows a mild leucocytosis, with a CRP <1. Stool cultures are pending. She is reviewed by the surgeons, and pain appears to be settling. After some oral fluids and a period of observation, she feels better. The diagnosis of gastroenteritis is made and she is discharged. However, she re-presents after five days, with a high temperature (39.8°C) and a palpable mass in the right iliac fossa.

Q3   What is the most likely diagnosis?
    A   Acute appendicitis
    B   Appendix mass
    C   Ovarian tumour
    D   Concealed pregnancy

For answers see page 409

CASE 17
A 1-minute-old baby requiring resuscitation

A term baby is born in poor condition, and you are asked to review them urgently. There were no concerns during pregnancy, but labour was prolonged and forceps were used to deliver the baby. The baby is now on the neonatal resuscitaire. On initial assessment, the baby is blue, floppy and breathing irregularly, with a slow HR. He is showing no other activity when stimulated.

Questions

Q1 What would be your first step in managing this baby?
   A Dry the baby, and put them under a radiant heater
   B Give inflation breaths
   C Intubate the baby
   D Start CPR
   E Give ventilation breaths

Q2 What is the baby's initial APGAR score?
   A 4
   B 2
   C 7
   D 5
   E 3

Q3 Which of the following symptoms and signs are indicative of hypoxic ischaemic encephalopathy? Select all that apply.
   A Poor cord blood gases
   B Irritability
   C Absent suck reflex
   D Seizures

For answers see page 410

CASE 18
An 18-hour-old baby presenting with jaundice

Baby Smith is 18-hours-old and is now jaundiced. The baby's mother is blood group AB –ve and this is her second baby. The pregnancy was unremarkable and regarded as low risk. The baby was born by normal vaginal delivery and has been feeding well on the breast. Observations are within normal limits. There are no other concerns noted.

Questions

Q1 Which two of the following diagnoses would you consider most likely in a baby presenting with jaundice in the first 24 hours of life?
   A Infection
   B Haemolytic disease of the newborn
   C Biliary atresia
   D Hypothyroidism
   E Breast milk jaundice

Q2 The baby's blood group is checked. Given that mum is AB –ve, which of the following blood groups for the baby would make you concerned about a possible haemolytic anaemia?
   A A –ve
   B B –ve
   C AB –ve
   D O –ve
   E A +ve
   F B +ve

Q3 The bilirubin levels are high, and a decision is made to start phototherapy. What is the most important complication of hyperbilirubinaemia that treatment aims to prevent?
   A Liver failure
   B Renal failure
   C Anaemia
   D Kernicterus
   E Weight loss

For answers see page 411

CASE 19
A 6-hour-old baby presenting with difficulty in breathing

Baby Fahad was born at 35+5 weeks gestation by normal vaginal delivery. The mother gave a urine sample during her pregnancy that grew group B streptococcus. At six hours of life, the baby started grunting and became tachypnoeic, with a respiratory rate of 90 breaths/min (tachypnoeic). Saturations were 100% in air, HR was 170 bpm (tachycardic), and temperature was 37°C. The baby was transferred to the neonatal unit, where a chest X-ray showed a right lower lobe pneumonia.

Questions

Q1 Which of the following might commonly cause respiratory distress in a newborn baby? Select all that apply.
   A Infection
   B Jaundice
   C Atrial septal defect
   D Transient tachypnoea of the newborn
   E Respiratory distress syndrome

Q2 Which of the following are risk factors for infection in a baby? Select all that apply.
   A Maternal fever during labour
   B Prolonged rupture of membranes
   C Meconium staining at delivery
   D A low APGAR score at one minute
   E Prematurity

Q3 What bacteria are commonly implicated in early onset neonatal infection? Select all that apply.
   A *E. coli*

B   Group B *Streptococcus*
C   Coagulase negative *Staphylococcus*
D   *Klebsiella*
E   *Streptococcus pneumoniae*

For answers see page 413

CASE 20
A 1-day-old baby with an abnormal newborn baby examination

A baby is now 24-hours-old and is awaiting discharge. A baby check is required. The baby was born by forceps-assisted delivery and the mother is concerned about a swelling on the top of the head.

Questions

Q1   You start by examining the eyes, but are unable to elicit the red reflex. Which two of the following pathologies would you be particularly concerned about?
   A   Cataracts
   B   Retinoblastoma
   C   Glioblastoma
   D   Cerebral palsy
   E   Kernicterus

Q2   Which of the following may be considered normal in a newborn baby? Select all that apply.
   A   Soft symmetrical breast tissue
   B   Small amounts of vaginal bleeding
   C   A single, painless, round, blue, discoloured skin lesion
   D   A widespread erythematous rash, blanching, which looks urticarial in nature
   E   A left sided inguinal hernia

Q3   The baby is felt to have a cephalohaematoma secondary to birth trauma. Which of the following are possible complications of cephalohaematoma? Select all that apply.
   A   Jaundice
   B   Anaemia
   C   Kernicterus
   D   Raised intracranial pressure
   E   Infection

Q4   On examining the baby's hips, on the right side, the Barlow and Ortolani tests show the hip is dislocatable and relocatable. Which investigation is best suited to assessing for congenital dislocation of the hip?
   A   MRI hip
   B   X-Ray hip
   C   Ultrasound of the hip
   D   CT Hip
   E   Laparoscopic exploration of hip

For answers see page 414

CASE 21
A 24-month-old presenting with developmental delay

Kayden, a 24-month-old boy, was referred to the Community Paediatrician as he has not said any words yet. When watching him play, you notice there is no eye contact and no obvious symbolic or imitative play. He is lining bricks in colour order. On developmental assessment, you note he can walk and run quite steadily and is able to jump but not hop or stand on one leg. He can hold a pen with a palmar grasp and is able to scribble back and forth and circularly. He can pick up a raisin from the floor with no trouble, demonstrating a good pincer grasp, and is able to build a tower of 6 bricks. He is not pointing. He rarely makes vocal noises but recently starting babbling/trying to imitate sounds of others. He has been known to smile—they think from about 2 months old—but he is not yet waving. He has stranger anxiety.

Questions

Q1   What best describes Kayden?
   A   Fine motor delay
   B   Fine motor and speech and language delay
   C   Social and fine motor delay
   D   Delayed social development
   E   Social and speech and language delay

Q2   What is the most important initial investigation?
   A   Genetic blood tests
   B   Thyroid function tests
   C   Hearing test
   D   TORCH screen
   E   Visual acuity test

Q3   In relation to autistic spectrum disorder, mark the following statements true or false.
   A   It is linked to the MMR vaccine
   B   It can be seen with an underlying diagnosis of tuberous sclerosis
   C   Early diagnosis and intervention is proven to improve outcome and level of functioning
   D   It can be associated with neurofibromatosis
   E   Drugs can significantly alter outcome

Q4   Which of the following conditions may be associated with autistic spectrum disorder? Select all that apply.
   A   ADHD
   B   Tourette's syndrome
   C   Depression
   D   High IQ
   E   Resistance to change or new experiences

For answers see page 415

CASE 22
An 8-year-old boy presenting with behavioural problems

An 8-year-old boy, Sam, was referred to the Community Paediatrician for concerns over his concentration ability. He cannot sit still for more than five minutes at home and is not completing his homework. He is constantly restless, and can be aggressive and rude to his parents at home. At school, his teachers report that he can be fidgety and restless, but with encouragement he concentrates well and completes his work. He can be aggressive to other children but responds to authority figures disciplining him. On further questioning, Sam's mother has suffered from depression for a long time and there have been periods of severe episodes, during which concerns were raised about neglect and there was social services involvement. She has been struggling to manage his behaviour for a while. He does not have a set bedtime or a set pattern to meals. His meals generally consist of fast food. His father has not been around for the past few years.

Sam is suspected to have ADHD.

Questions
Q1 In relation to Sam and attention deficit hyperactivity disorder (ADHD), mark the following statements true or false.
A Symptoms of ADHD must be pervasive in various areas of life for a diagnosis
B ADHD can be screened for using the Conner's questionnaire
C Hyperactivity, inattention and rigidity in behaviour are the three themes used in diagnosis
D Incidence is increased in VLBW (very low birth weight) babies
E Neglect and lack of emotional warmth can lead to behaviours similar to that seen in ADHD
F Lack of structure and routine can lead to difficult and defiant behaviour, poor concentration and hyperactivity
G Mental health disorders in parents can have significant impacts on a child's behaviour
H Sam's diet may be contributing to his behaviour

For answers see page 417

CASE 23
An 8-month-old presenting with a fall

Charlie, an 8-month-old girl, has been brought to ED because, about a day ago, her mother reported that she was crawling on a wooden floor and seemed to fall forward over her right arm. She has not been moving this as much or using it since the incident. An X-ray shows a spiral fracture of the humerus. At the time of the incident, the mother did not feel Charlie needed to come to hospital but attended now as Charlie had continued not to move or use it as much.

On assessment, Charlie seems developmentally normal and is otherwise well. HR is 170 bpm (tachycardic), but all other observations are within normal limits. She has had no previous fractures. However, Charlie's 4-year-old brother has presented to the ED six times in the last year with various complaints.

Charlie's parents have recently divorced, and her mother is currently unemployed. The mother denies any social services involvement.

Non-accidental injury (NAI) is suspected.

Q1 Which of the following factors increase the possibility of non-accidental injury (NAI)? Select all that apply.
A The father is not in ED with them
B The mechanism of injury
C The delay in presentation
D Charlie has had no previous fractures

Q2 Social services are contacted and do not know the family. Which answer represents the best next course of action?
A Explain to the mother we think she is lying and that we are likely to remove her child from her care
B Put the arm in a sling and discharge home with fracture clinic follow up as per orthopaedic advice
C Explain to the mother that, given Charlie's age and concerns, the mechanism given does not entirely explain the injury sustained; therefore, we have a legal duty of care to Charlie to investigate this further, including investigations for Charlie, and discussions with police and social services. The fracture will also be managed by being put in a sling, but Charlie will need to remain in hospital pending a safeguarding plan
D Call the police to come to ED

For answers see page 418

CASE 24
An 18-month-old presenting with a seizure

Chris is an 18-month-old boy brought by ambulance to ED after having an "abnormal episode" an hour previously. It happened whilst his mother was changing the nappy, and he began to breathe irregularly whilst his eyes rolled back. He lost consciousness and his mother caught him in her arms. She then noticed that he started to jerk all four limbs rhythmically. He was slightly blue around the lips but did not stop breathing. His father immediately called an ambulance, as the episode was very frightening and they were not sure what was happening. The episode lasted no longer than 5 minutes and had stopped by the time the ambulance arrived. Chris was initially drowsy, but is better now and has taken some milk in the waiting room. The parents inform you that he has had a bit of a cold in the last day or so, but he has been well with it, and during the episode he "felt hot to touch". Chris was born at term with no complications, has no significant past medical history and is up to date with his immunisations. Of note, his father tells you that he himself had "fits with fever" as a child.

On initial examination, RR is 38 breaths/min (tachypnoeic) with saturations of 98% in air, HR is 150 bpm (tachycardic), with a normal BP. He is febrile, at 38.9°C. He looks unsettled. Both neurological and systemic examinations are normal. Chris is moving his head around and he has his eyes open without evident discomfort. He does not have a rash. His tonsils look red and inflamed and he has a runny nose. Chris is given some paracetamol and appears brighter, alert and settled. His HR and respiratory rate stabilise and his temperature settles. The parents are very concerned and ask you what has happened.

Questions

Q1 What is the most likely diagnosis?
- A Epilepsy
- B Simple febrile seizure
- C Complex febrile seizure
- D Status epilepticus
- E Meningitis

Q2 Which investigations are indicated? Select all that apply.
- A Blood culture
- B Urine dipstick/culture
- C Lumbar puncture
- D Blood glucose
- E CT or MRI

Q3 What is the most appropriate management plan? Select all that apply.
- A Start antibiotics
- B Administer antiepileptic medication
- C Provide anti-pyretic medications
- D Recommend prophylactic anti-epileptics
- E Educate parents

Q4 What is/are the complication(s) associated with the diagnosis? Select all that apply.
- A Brain damage
- B Epilepsy
- C Increased mortality
- D Poorer cognition and performance at school
- E Recurrence of febrile seizure

For answers see page 419

CASE 25
A 7-year-old presenting with fever

Holly is a 7-year-old girl who is brought to ED by her parents because of a persisting temperature, lethargy and headache. She was seen by her primary care physician three days previously for fever and a widespread non-specific rash. She was diagnosed as having a viral illness. On further questioning,

you discover she has been closing her eyes to light, become drowsier and is "not herself". She has started vomiting since this morning. She has no other significant past medical history, is up to date with her immunisations and is not on any regular medication. You ask the parents about any illnesses in the family and her mother reveals that she has had recurrent cold sores, including one last week.

On examination, she is lethargic and intermittently awake. A maculopapular rash on her arms and legs blanches to pressure. She complains of tenderness during examination of her arms and legs. Her neck is very stiff. Observations reveal RR of 35 breaths/min (tachypnoeic) with saturations of 93% in air; HR is 130 bpm (tachycardic), BP is 100/55 mmHg (borderline hypotensive), capillary refill is 2-3 seconds, and temperature is 38 °C. She appears confused and tells her mum about seeing "teddies on the wall".

Systemic examinations are normal. Her lung fields are clear and heart sounds are normal. Pupils are equal and responsive to light. Neurological exam shows neck stiffness and generalised weakness. Kernig's sign is positive, and there is obvious photophobia.

Q1 What is the most likely diagnosis?
- A Febrile seizure
- B Meningoencephalitis
- C Vasculitis
- D Space occupying lesion
- E Cerebrovascular accident

Q2 What is the immediate management? Select all that apply.
- A Fluid resuscitation
- B Lumbar puncture
- C IV antibiotics
- D CT head
- E IV aciclovir

Q3 Which is/are recognised complication(s) of this condition? Select all that apply.
- A Hearing loss
- B Hydrocephalus
- C Seizures
- D Neurodevelopmental delay
- E Subdural effusion

For answers see page 420

CASE 26
A 15-year-old presenting with recurrent headaches

Sarah is a 15-year-old girl who has had a two year history of recurrent headaches. The headaches are scored 7/10 in severity, frontal, mainly on the left side and throbbing in nature. The pain is consistent throughout the day. The pain is associated with nausea. There are no associated visual symptoms. The pain lasts for several hours and resolves after resting with the lights turned off. There is no aggravation on leaning forward. The headache does not occur on waking. She occasionally takes paracetamol, which marginally helps. The headaches also tend to worsen when she has her period. In between, she is well in herself and competes at a national level for her school swimming team. She has no other significant past medical history and is not on any regular medication. Her mother and sister have migraines.

On examination, she is a tall girl of athletic build, plotting on the 75th centile for height and the 50th centile for weight. Observations are within normal limits. Her neurological examination, including cranial nerves, peripheral nerves and fundoscopy, is normal. Cardiovascular, respiratory and abdominal examinations are normal.

Q1 What is the most likely diagnosis?
  A Tension headache
  B Migraine
  C Brain tumour
  D Subarachnoid haemorrhage

Q2 What is/are the risk factor(s) for this condition? Select all that apply.
  A Family history
  B Stress
  C Head trauma
  D Meningitis

Q3 Which treatment is particularly good for prevention of severe, recurrent headaches caused by this disorder?
  A NSAIDs
  B Sumatriptan
  C Paracetamol
  D Propranolol

For answers see page 422

CASE 27
A 9-month-old girl presenting with poor weight gain and lethargy

A 9-month-old girl presents with poor weight gain since she started solid foods three months ago. She has been bottle fed from birth and her mother has been trying to feed her some rusks and toast for breakfast. Mum has also noticed that her daughter seems more lethargic than normal. On examination, she has mouth ulcers and looks pale. Observations are within normal limits. A full blood count shows a haemoglobin level of 90 g/L. Mum was diagnosed with type 1 diabetes mellitus at age six. Coeliac disease is suspected.

Questions
Q1 Which of the following are implicated in the aetiology of coeliac disease? Select all that apply.

  A HLA-DR3
  B Smoking
  C HLA-DQ8
  D High alcohol consumption
  E Fat-rich diet

Q2 Which patient is most likely to test positive for coeliac disease?
  A A 10-year-old boy with weight loss, heat intolerance and increased appetite
  B A 12-year-old girl with type 1 diabetes mellitus
  C A 12-year-old girl who eats a gluten-free diet
  D An 8-year-old boy with sudden onset diarrhoea
  E A 16-year-old girl with weight loss and chronic diarrhoea

Q3 The best initial investigation for coeliac disease is:
  A IgA serology
  B Endomysial antibodies and tissue transglutaminase antibody serology
  C Tissue transglutaminase antibody serology only
  D Food and symptom diary
  E Endoscopy and biopsy

Q4 Which condition has an association with coeliac disease?
  A Type 1 diabetes mellitus
  B Bacterial gastroenteritis
  C Cystic fibrosis
  D Irritable bowel syndrome
  E Cow's milk protein intolerance

For answers see page 423

CASE 28
A 2-month-old boy presenting with vomiting and diarrhoea

A 2-month-old boy is admitted with a one day history of vomiting and diarrhoea. On examination, he appears unwell but is sleeping. There is no sign of respiratory distress. Observations show a respiratory rate of 62 breaths/min (tachypnoeic), a HR of 170 bpm (tachycardic), BP of 60/40 mmHg (hypotensive), capillary refill of 4 seconds, and a temperature of 38.7°C. Mucous membranes are dry. He is not tolerating oral fluids.

Blood samples are taken for blood cultures, a full blood count, CRP, and urea and electrolytes. The results show an elevated neutrophil count of 17.1×10^9/L and sodium of 136 mmol/L. CRP is normal, at 1 mg/L. Other blood parameters are normal. A stool sample and a urine sample are also taken for microscopy. A 20ml/kg 0.9% sodium chloride bolus is given, and IV fluids are commenced. Broad spectrum IV antibiotics are started for possible sepsis. A lumbar puncture is performed once stable. Blood, urine and CSF cultures are negative after 48 hours, but the cultured stool sample has grown *Campylobacter jejuni*.

Questions

Q1 What is the most important differential diagnosis to exclude acutely in this case?

  A Meningitis

  B Pneumonia

  C Crohn's disease

  D Cow's milk protein intolerance

  E Toddler's diarrhoea

Q2 Which group of children are most at risk of a severe gastrointestinal infection?

  A Over 1-year-old

  B Under 6-months-old

  C Those that have had recent contact with a relative who has food poisoning

  D Those that have been previously treated for leukaemia

Q3 Which of the symptoms or signs below are red flags for dehydration? Select all that apply.

  A Altered consciousness

  B Dry mucous membranes

  C Tachycardia

  D Tachypnoea

For answers see page 425

CASE 29
A 6-week-old girl presenting with vomiting and distress after feeds

A 6-week-old girl is admitted with a history of non-projectile vomiting and crying after every feed over the past two weeks. The pregnancy and delivery were uneventful. She has been bottle fed from birth. She appears well and has been gaining weight as expected, along the 50th centile. The parents also mention that she always seems hungry, despite being bottle fed four ounces every three hours. She is passing urine and faeces normally. On examination, observations are within normal limits, but she is uncomfortable and cries when lying supine, particularly after feeds, arching her back at the same time.

Questions

Q1 What is the most likely diagnosis in this case?

  A Gastroenteritis

  B Gastro-oesophageal reflux disease

  C Pyloric stenosis

  D Cow's milk protein intolerance

  E Infantile colic

Q2 Regarding the likely diagnosis, mark the following statements true or false.

  A The parents can be reassured that it is likely to self-resolve with age

  B Investigations should always be carried out to rule out a more serious disorder

  C Thickening feeds may be useful

  D It is a lifelong condition with multiple complications

  E Surgery is never required

Q3 What is the most appropriate investigation in a mild case of this disease?

  A Oesophageal pH monitoring

  B Barium meal

  C Upper gastrointestinal endoscopy

  D Full blood count

  E None of the above; diagnosis is based on clinical history and examination

For answers see page 426

CASE 30
A 12-year-old boy presenting with weight loss and abdominal pain

A 12-year-old boy presents with weight loss, lethargy, poor appetite and abdominal pain over the past four months. On further questioning, he has also had loose stools. HR is 120 bpm (tachycardic), but all other observations are within normal limits. On examination, he looks pale and displays tenderness in the right iliac fossa. Blood tests show haemoglobin of 97 g/L, CRP 63 mg/L and albumin 20 g/L. A stool sample is taken for microscopy and culture.

The patient is admitted to hospital for further investigations and treatment.

Questions

Q1 What is the most likely diagnosis?

  A Gastroenteritis

  B Appendicitis

  C Mesenteric adenitis

  D Inflammatory bowel disease

  E Coeliac disease

Q2 What one further investigation is most important to confirm the likely diagnosis?

  A Flexible sigmoidoscopy

  B Colonoscopy

  C Antibody testing

  D Urea and electrolytes

  E Faecal calprotectin

For answers see page 427

CASE 31

A pregnant lady with concerns about Down syndrome

A 46-year-old married woman who is 12 weeks pregnant presents to the antenatal clinic with concerns about Down syndrome, as she is aware of a screening programme offered to pregnant women. She already has one child with autistic spectrum disorder. She smoked in her youth but quit five years ago. She is offered screening and is aware of the risks of further testing.

Questions

Q1   In the UK, what are the components of the screening test that this pregnant woman is offered?

   A   Nuchal translucency scan, β-hCG, PAPP-A

   B   β-hCG, uE3, AFP, Inhibin-A

   C   Nuchal translucency scan, β-hCG

   D   Chorionic villus sampling

   E   Amniocentesis

Q2   In this case, what is her biggest risk factor for Down syndrome?

   A   Full-term pregnancy

   B   Older maternal age

   C   Multiparity

   D   Previous child with autistic spectrum disorder

   E   Previous smoking history

After screening, she discovers that she has a high risk of having a child with Down syndrome. She declines further diagnostic testing. Her daughter is born at full term and the doctors have a strong clinical suspicion of Down syndrome, which is confirmed on chromosomal testing. They also notice that she has a heart murmur, so she is sent for an echocardiogram, which demonstrates an atrial septal defect.

Q3   What services should be involved in the care of patients with Down syndrome? Select all that apply.

   A   Speech and language therapy

   B   Physiotherapy

   C   Paediatrician follow-up

   D   Social services

   E   Dieticians

For answers see page 428

CASE 32

A 9-year-old boy with acute onset testicular pain

A 9-year-old boy is brought to the ED with acute right-sided groin and scrotal pain. He is also complaining of suprapubic pain and has vomited twice since the onset of pain two hours ago. However, he has subsequently had a large meal, which he has kept down. He states that he was playing football the day before and that one of the other boys kicked him in the groin. HR is 130 bpm (tachycardic), but all other observations are within normal limits. On examination, his right testis is found to be higher than the left one. It is extremely tender, and the skin of his scrotum is swollen and red.

Questions

Q1   What is the next step in the management of this child?

   A   An USS of his scrotum to visualise testicular blood flow

   B   Commence IV antibiotics to treat possible epididymo-orchitis

   C   Contact the anaesthetic team after the child has been appropriately fasted

   D   Refer to the surgical team (paediatric if available) to organise an urgent scrotal exploration, despite inadequate fasting

   E   Prescribe analgesia, anti-emetics and scrotal support and ask the family to come to the next available clinic appointment

Q2   Mark the following statements true or false.

   A   Testicular torsion is not related to trauma

   B   Doppler USS is 100% sensitive and 100% specific in the diagnosis of testicular torsion

   C   At six hours post-torsion, approximately 85% of testes will survive

   D   Following operative detorsion of a twisted testis, the contralateral testis should undergo fixation

   E   If a paediatric orchidectomy is necessary, implantation of a suitable prosthesis should be carried out during the same operation

For answers see page 430

CASE 33

A 2-month-old presenting with irritability and shortness of breath

You are called to assess a 2-month-old baby presenting with a six hour history of decreased feeding, irritability and shortness of breath. The initial observations are RR 60 breaths/minute (tachypnoeic), oxygen saturation of 95% on room air, HR 280 bpm (tachycardic- confirmed on HR monitor), BP 90/55 mmHg (normal), capillary refill time 3-4 seconds and temperature 37.5°C. The baby is alert on the "alert, voice, pain, unresponsive" (AVPU) scale.

The child is irritable and crying, with good tone throughout and a soft non-bulging anterior fontanelle. He has moist mucous membranes. He has warm peripheries and palpable, symmetrical femoral pulses. Respiratory examination reveals a few scattered crepitations throughout the lung field but good air entry bilaterally. He has a soft abdomen, with no palpable

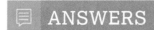

ANSWER TO CASE 1
A 14-year-old girl presenting with self-harm

Q1 Which of the following would be the best way to manage Jennifer?

The correct answer is C. She should be assessed before discharge by the child and adolescent mental health team, either in the ED or as an inpatient.

When dealing with a child that has presented with self-harm, it is important to get an accurate assessment of their risk of further self-harm or completed suicide. A formal assessment is required by the child and adolescent mental health team before discharge. Their role is to make a discharge plan to keep the child or young person safe.

A Jennifer should be sectioned because she is suicidal – Incorrect. Although this is a possibility, it would be very rare to need to section a patient following self-harm. This patient appears to be cooperative and not an immediate risk to her own safety, so there are other options that are more appropriate.

B She should be discharged home in her mother's care because she is a child – Incorrect. Children and young people should generally be admitted following a significant episode of self-harm. This could be admission to a paediatric or adolescent ward, if available. In some circumstances, review by the mental health team may occur in the ED, and if a plan is put in place for a safe discharge, this can be followed, but it is not the norm.

C She should be assessed before discharge by the child and adolescent mental health team, either in the ED or as an inpatient – Correct. Usually patients are only discharged from the ward after being formally assessed by child and adolescent mental health services. This may happen in the ED, depending on when the young person attends. If an assessment is not available on the same day, she should be admitted until she is assessed. It is also important to consider child protection concerns, and it may be appropriate to inform social care.

D She should be discharged on her own because she has been assessed as Gillick competent – Incorrect. As above, she should be admitted. Irrespective of her Gillick competence, she cannot refuse treatment that is deemed in her best interests.

Key Point

Ensure all children presenting to hospital with self-harm have a formal specialist assessment of their risk of suicide before discharge.

Q2 When you speak to Jennifer alone, she tells you she has a 16-year-old boyfriend that her mother doesn't know about. On questioning, she admits that they are having sex but that "he doesn't like condoms." Which of the following is/are correct?

The correct answers are B. You should encourage her to talk to her mother about her boyfriend and E. If she requests it, Jennifer can be prescribed the pill without telling her mother.

When reviewing a child or young person, it is important to be aware of any possibility of abuse or exploitation. However, it doesn't necessarily follow that a relationship such as this is harmful. Sharing such information has to be balanced against the autonomy and confidentiality of the patient. Although Jennifer should be encouraged to openly discuss important issues with her parents, if there are no specific concerns about this relationship beyond age, it would be an unnecessary breach of confidentiality for the parents to be informed without explicit consent.

A You have a duty to inform the police because she is having underage sex – Incorrect. Although she is under 16, if she is having consensual sex with someone close to her age, the police do not need to be informed. However, if abuse or exploitation is suspected, social services need to be informed. If she was under 13, this would always be reported, regardless of the nature of the relationship.

B You should encourage her to talk to her mother about her boyfriend – Correct. It is good practice to encourage young people to confide in their parents, even if they are reluctant. However, this cannot be forced. Be aware that, within some cultures, this may be particularly difficult for the young person or, in extreme cases, it may put the young person in harm's way.

C You have a duty to tell her mother that she is having sex because she is under 16, but you don't need to tell Jennifer before you do this. – Incorrect. This should only be done if there are concerns about the child's safety. If this was the case, it is good practice to inform a young person before breaking confidentiality.

D If Jennifer has been assessed as Gillick competent, you do not need to do anything about this – Incorrect. Although she may be Gillick competent relative to this decision, it is an important opportunity to give advice and any treatment required.

E If she requests it, Jennifer can be prescribed the pill without telling her mother. – Correct. If she is Gillick competent, she can have this medical treatment confidentially.

🔑 Key Point

Although safeguarding concerns are important, do not forget about the right to confidentiality of a child or young person. It should only be broken if doing so may prevent a clear, significant harm.

Q3 You want to give Jennifer further advice regarding sexual health. Which of the following is/are correct?

The correct answer is D. She can go on her own for a sexual health screen.

Seeing a young person in the Emergency Department provides a good opportunity for further health promotion. Jennifer should be fully informed about her options with regard to contraception, including how to access contraceptive services. Barrier methods are important if there is any risk of sexually transmitted infections.

A Jennifer should go on the pill so that she doesn't need to use condoms – Incorrect. She may choose to start taking the pill, but condoms are recommended in addition, to reduce the risk of sexually transmitted diseases.
B She should not be given any contraception as this is encouraging her to have sex underage – Incorrect. There is no evidence to back up this statement, and it is important to promote "safe sex".
C A coil is the best choice for her because she is young and hasn't had children yet – Incorrect. Although coils are a very effective form of long-acting reversible contraception, it may be slightly more difficult to insert a coil in younger patients. As such, contraceptive implant use is preferable.
D She can go on her own for a sexual health screen – Correct. This makes sexual health services much more accessible to adolescents.
E Telling her about all the different methods of contraception will be confusing for her – Incorrect. Giving Jennifer all of the information about available forms of contraception will enable her to make the most appropriate choice for her. This gives her autonomy over her own care and increases the chances that she will use contraception effectively.

🔑 Key Point

Just as with an adult patient, with adolescents, the duty of a doctor involves ensuring patients have the full information required to make informed decisions.

ⓘ IMPORTANT LEARNING POINTS

- When dealing with self-harm, it is important to assess the risk of further self-harm or suicide. This should be followed by referring or sign-posting other services that are available to support the young person. These can be general (for example, community mental health teams) or specific to an individual problem (for example, drug addiction).
- Sexually active adolescents have a right to access contraceptive services. They should be fully informed of their options, including how to access care.
- Encourage sexually active adolescents to have a sexually transmitted disease screening, if they haven't done so already.
- It is important to be very aware of the possibility of abuse or exploitation in any relationship. If this is suspected, then it is appropriate to break confidentiality in the best interest of the patient.

ANSWER TO CASE 2
A 3-year-old boy presenting with stridor

Q1 What is the most likely diagnosis?

The correct answer is E. Croup.

The five options given are the five commonest causes of stridor, which should be considered in the differential diagnosis of any case with stridor.

A Epiglottitis – Incorrect. Stridor is present, but children with epiglottitis appear unwell, with high fevers and drooling.
B Bacterial tracheitis – Incorrect. Unlike children with croup, these children are toxic, with rapidly progressive airway obstruction. Onset is not as rapid as with epiglottitis. Bacterial tracheitis is rare but very serious. It can be difficult to differentiate clinically from epiglottitis, but the treatment is the same.
C Anaphylaxis – Incorrect. Anaphylaxis is associated with an urticarial rash, wheeze, shock, and often vomiting and diarrhoea. This patient has no clear precipitant for anaphylaxis and none of the other features.
D Inhaled foreign body – Incorrect. A barking cough and infective symptoms make this unlikely. However, sudden-onset respiratory distress can be a sign of foreign body inhalation, particularly in a young child. It is important to ask about the possibility of foreign body inhalation specifically in the history.
E Croup – Correct. The progressive nature of the symptoms and worsening overnight are classical of croup. The patient is interacting well, with only a low-grade fever, and is not tachycardic. All these features suggest that, despite presence

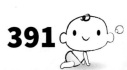

of stridor, this patient has croup rather than epiglottitis or bacterial tracheitis.

⚲ Key Point

Croup is a common presenting complaint in emergency paediatrics. It is suggested by a hoarse voice, barking cough and stridor, and a history over days rather than hours.

Q2 What first-line treatment should this patient receive?

The correct answer is A. Oral dexamethasone.

Treatment of croup depends on its severity. This case would be considered moderate, owing to i) inspiratory stridor at rest, ii) mild intercostal recession with tracheal tug and iii) decreased air entry. This suggests a need for oral corticosteroid treatment.

A   Oral dexamethasone – Correct. This rapidly decreases laryngeal mucosal inflammation, reducing stridor and the work of breathing.

B   Intramuscular adrenaline – Incorrect. This would only allow short-term improvement of symptoms and can cause upsetting side effects. However, nebulised adrenaline may be used in severe cases.

C   Nebulised budesonide – Incorrect. This is not routinely used in the management of croup, as oral steroids are usually sufficient.

D   Oral antibiotics – Incorrect. This is not used in the management of croup, which is a viral infection. Intravenous antibiotics are given in epiglottitis as it is secondary to a bacterial infection.

⚲ Key Point

The key goal in treating croup is to reduce laryngeal mucosal inflammation. This is done using oral corticosteroids, although this may not be necessary in mild cases.

Q3 Which symptom(s) would make you worry about a diagnosis of acute epiglottitis?

The correct answers are B. Drooling, and D. High fever >38.5°C.

Croup and epiglottitis are often confused. Croup is a viral infection, associated with a barking cough and milder onset of symptoms. Children with croup are usually well, although severe cases can occur with airway obstruction requiring intubation and ventilation. Epiglottitis, on the other hand, is a more rapid onset,

severe illness. The throat is often so sore that the patient cannot swallow their own saliva and presents with drooling.

A   Sore throat – Incorrect. Sore throat is a common symptom of both croup and epiglottitis; therefore, it does not differentiate the two conditions.

B   Drooling – Correct. Children with epiglottitis have an extremely sore throat which inhibits swallowing, so they drool saliva. Children with croup will have a milder sore throat and will still swallow.

C   Constant barking cough – Incorrect. Constant barking cough is highly suggestive of croup. The bark is produced by air being forced through a swollen, constricted larynx.

D   High fever >38.5°C – Correct. Croup is a viral infection, whereas epiglottitis is a bacterial infection caused by *Haemophilus influenzae* or *Staphylococcus aureus*. Therefore a high fever is more often seen with epiglottitis, whereas a low grade fever is more often seen with croup.

E   Onset over days not hours – Incorrect. Epiglottitis usually has a very fast onset, with symptoms developing over hours rather than days. Croup will usually have preceding coryzal symptoms or hoarseness for at least 24 hours before the onset of stridor.

⚲ Key Point

Drooling and high fever associated with stridor should prompt concerns of epiglottitis.

ⓘ   IMPORTANT LEARNING POINTS

- Epiglottitis is now a rare diagnosis in emergency paediatrics due to widespread uptake of the *Haemophilus influenzae* type B vaccine. Cases can occur due to other bacteria such as *S. aureus*.

- The presence of a hoarse voice and barking cough, accompanied by a soft stridor, is classical of croup.

- Systemic corticosteroids are widely used in the treatment of moderate croup, often in the form of oral dexamethasone.

ANSWER TO CASE 3
A 14-year-old boy presenting with a limp

Q1 What is the most useful next step?

The correct answer is D. AP and frog-leg lateral hip X-ray.

Establishing the location of orthopaedic pathology is key to making an accurate diagnosis, and orthopaedic principles dictate that the joints above and below the area of concern should be examined. Knee pain can radiate from the hip without any knee pathology. SUFE is best diagnosed using measurements ascertained from AP pelvis and frog-leg lateral views of the affected hip. MRI hip is the modality of choice if there is clinical suspicion but lack of radiological findings on X-ray.

A AP and lateral knee X-ray – Incorrect. Two views of the knee will allow a thorough radiological evaluation of the pain. While a knee X-ray may exclude any fractures, it will not identify soft tissue injuries. As seen in this case, radiographs are best requested after identifying an area of concern with a full history and clinical examination, to eliminate unnecessary radiation exposure. This appears to be a case of referred pain from the hip to the knee, rather than a primary knee problem.

B FBC, CRP and ESR – Incorrect. Blood tests should be considered if the X-rays are normal. If SUFE is proven on X-ray, then bloods are unnecessary. Inflammatory markers may be elevated in cases of septic arthritis and can be a useful adjuvant to help confirm a diagnosis. As the child is afebrile and otherwise well, septic arthritis is unlikely. Bloods can also demonstrate presence of haematological malignancies.

C MRI knee – Incorrect. MRI knee would only be indicated if soft-tissue knee pathology was likely, following history and examination.

D AP and frog-leg lateral hip X-ray – Correct. AP and, more helpfully, frog-leg lateral X-rays allow measurements to be made that can help identify subtle slips. From an AP pelvis, Klein's line can be drawn along the superior border of the femoral neck and should intersect the growth plate. From the frog-leg lateral, the Southwick angle can be measured. This calculates the angulations of the femoral head relative to the femoral shaft.

E MRI hip – Incorrect. Although not an initial imaging modality, MRI of the affected hip can help to highlight so-called "pre-slip" condition, such as growth plate widening and increased signal in the femoral metaphysis. This is usually indicated if initial hip radiographs are inconclusive.

F Thyroid function tests – Incorrect. In a child presenting with the above features in the normal age range for SUFE, endocrine tests such as thyroid function tests are not routinely indicated unless the patient has co-existing features of endocrine disorders. If the child was found to have a SUFE and was either under 10-years-old or below the 50th percentile for their weight, an endocrine cause is more likely.

♀ Key Point

Consider imaging in a logical manner: What is most readily available? What limits radiation exposure? What modality is most feasible for children? AP pelvis and frog-leg lateral X-rays allow precise measurements that can help to identify subtle slips. In the case of an inconclusive hip radiograph with a good history and examination of a potential SUFE, an MRI should be sought to highlight subtle slips and "pre-slip" conditions.

Q2 *Given the above information what is the most likely diagnosis?*

The correct answer is D. Slipped upper femoral epiphysis.

SUFE should be considered in any overweight 11 to 15-year-old child presenting with a limp and hip or knee pain. The opposite side should be examined, as bilateral SUFE occurs in around 30% of cases.

A Perthes' disease – Incorrect. While Perthes' disease can present with referred hip pain and a limp, the age of presentation tends to be in a younger paediatric age group (median age 6-years-old). Perthes' disease in patients over 14-years-old is rare and tends to be from an earlier missed diagnosis that results in avascular necrosis.

B Blount's disease – Incorrect. Blount's disease is a growth disorder of the tibia resulting in progressive varus angulation of the tibia. It is only seen in younger children/toddlers. While the main risk factor is obesity affecting the proximal tibial growth plate, there is no evidence of bowing of the lower leg in the above case.

C Knee septic arthritis – Incorrect. A two week history in an afebrile and well child without an effusion makes a diagnosis of a septic joint less likely.

D Slipped upper femoral epiphysis – Correct. Risk factors for SUFE include childhood obesity and being of African or Pacific Island descent. SUFE is a Salter-Harris type I injury due to forces on the proximal femoral growth plate. Typical presentation is with hip or referred knee pain and a limp, with the opposite hip often also affected.

E Osgood-Schlatter Disease – Incorrect. Osgood-Schlatter disease is due to inflammation of the patella ligament at its insertion onto the tibial tuberosity at the knee. A painful, palpable bump often occurs over the tibial tubercle. It predominantly affects sporty male children between 9 and 16-years-old, though inactive children can also have this condition.

⚷ Key Point

SUFE should be considered in the overweight child in their early teenage years presenting with unilateral or bilateral hip or knee pain. A missed diagnosis can result in femoral growth disturbance and permanent loss of function and has medico-legal implications.

Q3 How should this child be treated?

The correct answer is D. Fixation of the femoral epiphysis with threaded pins/screws.

Both stable and unstable SUFEs should be fixed to prevent further slip and allow the growth plates to fuse.

A   Rest, ice and elevation of knee – Incorrect. In a patient with a SUFE, the parents and child should be advised that the knee pain is in fact referred from the hip and should resolve upon treatment of the hip pain.

B   Intravenous antibiotics – Incorrect. There is no evidence of infection.

C   Bed rest and traction – Incorrect. Although the child with a confirmed SUFE should be treated with bed rest to prevent further slip, this is not a definitive treatment and should only be used while awaiting definitive fixation. There is no place for traction in SUFE.

D   Fixation of the femoral epiphysis with threaded pins/screws – Correct. This is the appropriate management of SUFE with minor displacement of the femoral head and prevents further slip while the growth plate fuses. Often, the surgeon will fix the opposite side at the same time.

E   Conservative management with observation only – Incorrect. The underlying pathology needs to be actively corrected.

⚷ Key Point

Any patient with a SUFE diagnosed on imaging should be treated with percutaneous pinning of the femoral epiphysis. This prevents further slip of the growth plate and allows the growth plate to fuse with age, as per the normal time course.

ⓘ **IMPORTANT LEARNING POINTS**

- A child presenting with knee pain must have their hip examined to exclude referred pain.
- Any overweight child 11 to 15-years-old presenting with hip or knee pain should be investigated for SUFE.
- AP and lateral frog-leg views of both hips should be sought and can be used to ascertain Klein's line (AP view) and the Southwick angle (frog-leg view) to objectively highlight subtle slips.
- Percutaneous pinning remains the treatment of choice to prevent further slip.

ANSWER TO CASE 4
A 10-month-old presenting with fever

Q1 Mark the following statements true or false.

A   A lumbar puncture should be performed on this child – False. A lumbar puncture is not indicated, as there are no signs or symptoms of meningitis or encephalitis. It is important to check for neck stiffness and a bulging fontanelle (the anterior fontanelle is difficult to feel after 1–year-old, but it can be open until 19–months-old), to assess the level of consciousness and to examine for any focal neurological signs.

B   A fever of 39°C suggests it is more likely to be a bacterial infection – False. The height or duration of fever does not reliably distinguish between bacterial and viral infection, nor does it reflect the severity of the illness. Regardless, fever algorithms suggest that children with temperatures of unknown origin should be investigated.

C   This boy has a prolonged fever – False. This child does not have a prolonged fever, as the parents reported the child's fever got better in the last week, for a few days. It is important to take a detailed history of the fever in any child presenting with a temperature.

D   Body temperature can be reliably measured with an axillary digital thermometer – True. Body temperature can be reliably measured with an electronic/chemical dot thermometer in the axilla or infrared tympanic thermometer in children more than 1-month-old.

E   This boy has very worrying symptoms/signs for a child with fever – False. This boy is over 3-months-old and is otherwise well. Red flag features are listed on p153.

⚷ Key Point

This child has a fever, but fever in and of itself does not mean the child must be sick. There are no red flag features, and the child is clinically well.

Q2 What is the most likely diagnosis?

The correct answer is A. Gastroenteritis.

This child is likely to have an infection. The debate here is whether it is a urinary tract infection (UTI), gastroenteritis, or both. The evidence for gastroenteritis is strong, with the child having sick contacts, as well as symptoms himself. The result of the urine test is likely to be a contaminant.

A   Gastroenteritis – Correct. The history that the parents provided suggested a possible diagnosis of norovirus-induced gastroenteritis. Norovirus, commonly known as the winter vomiting bug, is the most common cause of gastroenteritis in the UK. Since the widespread administration of the rotavirus vaccine, norovirus has overtaken rotavirus as the main cause of gastroenteritis in children.

B Urinary tract infection – Incorrect. A bag urine sample showing a "mixed growth" can be a contamination from the perineum rather than a true UTI, particularly if there is no significant white cell response.

C Viral tonsillitis – Incorrect. Tonsillitis is less common in infants. In this case, there is adequate oral intake and no localising signs of tonsillitis.

D Upper respiratory tract infection – Incorrect. There was no cough or coryzal symptoms, which would make this diagnosis less likely.

E Sepsis – Incorrect. Measuring vital signs would be necessary to be completely sure, but the child appears too well to be septic.

🔑 Key Point

Often the clinical history points to two possible focuses of infection. In this type of scenario, use investigations to narrow down the differential diagnosis. It is possible, but less likely, that there are two sources of infection.

Q3 What is the best management option?

The correct answer is A. Discharge home with written and verbal advice.

Gastroenteritis is best managed at home if the child is a) tolerating oral fluids, b) haemodynamically stable, and c) otherwise well. It is particularly important to try and keep such patients out of hospital because of the risk of passing the infection to other vulnerable children on the ward.

A Discharge home with written and verbal advice – Correct. This is a well patient, with likely gastroenteritis. If they are tolerating oral fluids, they should be managed at home. This scenario involves dealing with ambiguous results from a test that wasn't needed. If any ambiguity existed, or if the child had urinary symptoms, it would be worth retesting a new urine sample.

B Start IV antibiotics and take blood cultures – Incorrect. There is no evidence of a systemic infection.

C Start IV fluids – Incorrect. This infant can tolerate oral fluids and is not dehydrated.

D Keep him nil by mouth in case he has an acute abdomen – Incorrect. The child has not presented with signs of an acute abdomen, so this approach is unnecessarily cautious.

E Admit him into a bay on the paediatric ward – Incorrect. No specific inpatient treatment is needed. However, if he were admitted to the ward, it would have to be to a cubicle due to the risk of infecting other patients.

🔑 Key Point

Management depends on i) the most likely diagnosis and ii) whether the child is septic/unwell. In a child with likely gastroenteritis who is tolerating oral fluids, management is best delivered at home.

> ℹ️ **IMPORTANT LEARNING POINTS**
>
> - It is imperative to recognise the sick child by looking for the red flags associated with fever, p153. The next step is identifying a possible focus for infection and then determining a management plan.
> - A useful checklist when assessing a child with fever is to rule out the "big five" illnesses: sepsis, meningitis, pneumonia, UTI and osteomyelitis.
> - More than one infection may be causing the fever, but it is more likely that there is a single culprit.
> - Initial treatment for a UTI is usually initiated based on clinical symptoms, but in the well child, it is possible to wait for test results before starting any antibiotics (like a repeat urine sample, in this case).

ANSWER TO CASE 5
A 20-day-old boy presenting with fever, vomiting, and lethargy

Q1 What is the first priority in managing this child?

The correct answer is A. Get IV access, give a fluid bolus and give broad spectrum IV antibiotics.

This child is severely unwell, in septic shock. He requires urgent resuscitation using an ABCDE approach. Vital to this is giving fluid boluses – up to 60 mL/kg may be given in the first 30 minutes, in 20 mL/kg aliquots, reassessing each time, and broad spectrum antibiotics.

A Get IV access, give a fluid bolus and give broad spectrum IV antibiotics – Correct. This infant presents with signs of shock: tachycardia, tachypnoea, cold peripheries, mottling and decreased conscious level. Shock needs to be treated immediately with fluid boluses of 20 mL/kg and broad spectrum antibiotics need to be given urgently. If IV access cannot be obtained immediately, intraosseous access should be sought. If possible, a blood culture should be obtained prior to giving antibiotics. Broad spectrum antibiotics (Benzylpenicillin and Gentamicin, or Ceftriaxone) should be given until culture results are available.

B Give oral antibiotics – Incorrect. This child is in septic shock and therefore requires IV, not oral, antibiotics.

C Get a urine sample – Incorrect. A positive urine culture could provide a source of infection in a child presenting with sepsis. It is likely the child will be catheterised, and a urine sample will be obtained this way. However, treating shock and giving antibiotics is more urgent in this infant. If delay is minimised, the urine sample should ideally be obtained before the antibiotics are given.

D Give paracetamol – Incorrect. Fever can be treated if the infant is febrile, but intravenous fluids are more urgent.

E   Give oral rehydration salts – Incorrect. Oral rehydration salt solutions are life-saving where IV fluids are not indicated, or not available. It would be appropriate to use an oral rehydration salt solution if dehydration was mild or moderate, but much larger volumes of fluids can be given faster via the IV route.

♀ Key Point

Fluid resuscitation and broad spectrum antibiotics should be given as soon as possible once the diagnosis of septic shock is made. Rapid reassessment should occur afterwards, as several boluses may be required.

Q2 A full septic screen is performed. A lumbar puncture and blood cultures are taken and the child had a chest X-ray. Which investigation is required to complete the septic screen?

The correct answer is B. Urine microscopy, culture and sensitivity.

Although this patient is in septic shock, there is no clear focus of infection. A full septic screen should be taken so that antibiotic therapy can be targeted to any identified organism. Note that shock is a contraindication for a lumbar puncture.

A   Throat swab – Incorrect. A throat swab is not a routine part of a septic screen. However, it provides useful information regarding nasopharyngeal carriage of meningococci, Group A streptococci and other organisms.

B   Urine microscopy, culture and sensitivity – Correct. A clean catch sample will reduce the likelihood of contamination from organisms colonising the perineum. If an urgent urine result is needed, a suprapubic aspiration or catheter urine sample can be obtained. However, if the child has already had antibiotics, the result may be falsely negative.

C   CT head – Incorrect. A CT head is performed in a child presenting with focal neurological signs to rule out a space-occupying lesion. There are no concerns about a space-occupying lesion here.

D   Abdominal ultrasound – Incorrect. Abdominal ultrasound is a useful investigation if the child had a distended abdomen or signs of intraabdominal pathology.

E   Nasopharyngeal aspirate – Incorrect. Nasopharyngeal aspirate can be sent to check for viruses and bacteria. Influenza with or without bacterial co-infection can present with sepsis. It is only done when there are respiratory symptoms.

♀ Key Point

A septic screen for infants under one month includes:
> Full blood count and C-reactive protein
> Arterial blood gas
> Blood culture

> Urine MC&S
> Chest X-ray (if respiratory signs are present)
> Stool culture (if diarrhoea is present)
> Lumbar puncture

Q3 You get a phone call from the microbiology lab saying that the blood culture grows gram-negative diplococci. Which of the following bacteria would fit this picture?

The correct answer is E. Group B Neisseria meningitidis.

Gram stain is a technique that identifies the type of cell wall of the bacteria. Gram stain can be positive (red) or negative (blue). Cocci describes their circular shape under the microscope. Bacilli describes rod-shape bacteria.

A   Group A streptococcus – Incorrect. Group A streptococci are gram-positive cocci in chains. Group A streptococci commonly cause pharyngitis but can also cause severe disease, including sepsis and multi-organ failure.

B   Group B streptococcus – Incorrect. Group B streptococci are gram-positive cocci in chains. Group B Streptococci colonise 15-40% of pregnant women's vaginal tracts and can cause sepsis and meningitis in newborn infants.

C   *Staphylococcus aureus* – Incorrect. *Staphylococcus aureus* are gram-positive cocci in clusters. It colonises skin and can cause skin, bone and heart infections, as well as more severe disease including sepsis and multi-organ failure.

D   *Escherichia coli* – Incorrect. *Escherichia coli* (*E. coli*) is a gram-negative bacillus. It is a frequent cause of sepsis in infants less than 3-months-old.

E   Group B Neisseria meningitidis – Correct. Neisseria meningitidis is a gram-negative diplococci (a couple of cocci). Group B is the most common serogroup in Europe. Other groups include A, C, Y and W135. It can cause sepsis (25% of cases), meningitis (15% of cases), or both (60% of cases).

♀ Key Point

Basic microbiology will help the interpretation of initial blood culture results before a specific organism is identified. This may help deciding on empirical therapy.

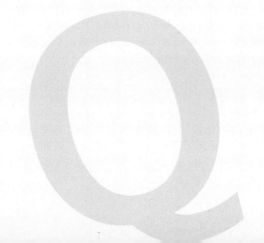

- When assessing a child with sepsis, remember to take a systematic ABCDE approach.
- Do not delay antibiotics or fluid resuscitation. Up to three 20 mL/kg boluses may be given in the first 30 minutes after presentation, regardless of the pathogen.
- Meningococcal sepsis can present without the typical non-blanching rash, as may be the case in the scenario here. Blood culture is the gold standard investigation; however, sensitivity is greater with PCR testing to confirm meningococcal disease.

ANSWER TO CASE 6
An 11-year-old boy presenting with chronic abdominal pain

Q1 Regarding consent, mark the following statements true or false.

A Matt definitely does not have capacity – False. As a minor, Matt is unlikely to have capacity. However, the test of capacity depends on what the task is. Matt is likely to have capacity to refuse the procedure of a blood test, if he shows understanding of what the procedure involves. However, he is unlikely to have capacity to understand the consequences of refusing the tests and the longer term consequences. In children and young people (CYP) under 16-years-old, the ability to have capacity to consent for themselves is termed "Gillick" or "Fraser" competency. A CYP under 16-years-old cannot refuse treatment, and consent should be taken from someone with parental responsibility (as long as they also have capacity).

B Matt's mother can consent on behalf of her child – True. As the biological mother, Matt's mother has parental responsibility, giving her the right to consent on behalf of her child to treatment.

C The doctors should bypass asking for consent, as this is a potentially serious condition – False. Although, in emergency situations, doctors can potentially proceed without explicit consent, it should always be sought. Written consent is preferable where appropriate.

♀ Key Point

All children less than 16-years-old are assumed not to have capacity, unless they meet the criteria for competence. However, in England and Wales, they cannot refuse treatment. Over 16-years-old, capacity is presumed to consent for and to refuse treatment.

Q2 What should happen next?

The correct answer is B. Ideally, consent should be sought from the mother, but if she does not agree with treatment,

then treatment should proceed either through a court order, or immediately if the case is life threatening.

Matt is unwell and requires a diagnosis before treatment is initiated. In this case, there would be time to seek consent legally.

A The decision to perform the investigations should be delayed until Matt has the ability to consent – Incorrect. It may take time for Matt to understand the consequences of his refusal and although it is better that he is involved in the decision, it would be difficult to wait, as it is not clear how long he would take to understand.

B Ideally, consent should be sought from the mother, but if she does not agree with treatment, then treatment should proceed either through a court order, or immediately if the case is life threatening – Correct. If possible, consent should always be sought. The risks, benefits of and alternatives to the treatment plan should be discussed with the mother. In the majority of cases, consent will usually be provided by a mother following a reasoned discussion, after which she should be asked to sign a consent form. If the mother refuses investigations and treatment, then legal advice should be sought, social services involved, and it may be necessary to obtain a court order to proceed.

C A compromise should be made whereby treatment is started empirically so that Matt can avoid blood tests and a colonoscopy – Incorrect. The diagnosis is not yet clear, and there is a potential for harm from delaying a diagnosis or instigating the wrong treatment. Therefore, it would not be in Matt's best interest to wait.

♀ Key Point

It is important to involve and inform parents of their child's treatment. Children are treated without parental consent only in exceptional circumstances.

- Consent for a medical procedure on a child can be obtained from the child (if they have capacity), from someone with parental responsibility or from a court.
- Parental responsibility is generally possessed by the biological mother, the biological father and those that have legally acquired parental responsibility since the child's birth.
- The child's best interests are paramount when making a decision regarding their healthcare. Involve the child and family fully in discussions about their care.
- Where there is refusal to accept treatment believed to be in the best interests of the child, recourse to the courts may be necessary.

ANSWER TO CASE 7
An 8-year-old child presenting with persistent chest infections

Q1 What is the most likely reason for the child's faltering growth?

The correct answer is A. He likely has pancreatic insufficiency.

Faltering growth has a diverse range of causes, and it is important to check for non-organic causes, such as inappropriate diet or neglect, in all cases. Chronic disease can affect growth through multiple mechanisms. Many chronic diseases are associated with a higher baseline metabolic requirement. IBD is associated with poor nutrient absorption from the gut. CF is associated with recurrent infections and poor pancreatic function.

A He likely has pancreatic insufficiency — Correct. Many CF gene mutations are associated with insufficient pancreatic function. In countries without a newborn screening programme, the commonest method of detecting CF is faltering growth (before the onset of frequent chest symptoms).

B He has been frequently unwell — Incorrect. Although frequent infections do increase the risk of faltering growth, it depends on the nature of the infections. Difficult to control asthma may be associated with frequent and prolonged infections, although this may not necessarily be the case, particularly if compliance is an issue.

C He has undiagnosed coeliac disease — Incorrect. While the two diagnoses can coexist, this is not the most likely explanation. Poor weight gain in infancy may be related to weaning and introduction of gluten. Further investigation may be necessary.

D His faltering growth is secondary to asthma medication — Incorrect. Long-term steroid use is associated with a potential reduction in final height, but it is a minimal change, and it certainly isn't associated with being tall and thin.

⚲ Key Point

It is vital to establish pancreatic function in a child with newly diagnosed CF. The demands of the disease on growth and nutrition can be worse than the respiratory consequences.

Q2 On which chromosome is the gene defect located in CF?

The correct answer is C. Chromosome 7.

Chromosome 7 is the location of the gene defect coding for CFTR, the protein that controls chloride movement across the cell membrane. In the UK, approximately 85% of CF patients have at least one of the p.phe508del (formally known as delta F508)

defects. Defects can be categorised into classes that reflect the underlying changes to the CFTR receptor protein.

⚲ Key Point

All gene mutations for CF are localised to Chromosome 7.

Q3 What is the next most important test to be performed following a positive diagnosis on the sweat test?

The correct answer is A. Stool sample analysis for faecal elastase.

Although a positive sweat test confirms the diagnosis of CF, further testing is required to establish possible complications of the disease (particularly pancreatic dysfunction/diabetes) and any possible genetic abnormalities, some of which may be treatable.

A Stool sample analysis for faecal elastase – Correct. The absence of elastase in the faecal matter would suggest pancreatic insufficiency as explaining the poor weight. Undernourished children will struggle to fight infections. Enzyme therapy would be needed.

B Extended genetic testing – Incorrect. A positive sweat test may occur without a genetic defect being identified. The specific genotype is needed, however, as there is now a drug available for patients with the p.Arg117His (formally known as G551D) gene defect.

C Coeliac screen – Incorrect. Both pathologies may co-exist, but they are not usually associated.

D Random blood glucose – Incorrect. This should be undertaken regularly to monitor for CF-related diabetes but is not an immediate priority. Insulin function analysis, such as a glucose tolerance test or continuous glucose monitoring, should be undertaken annually as well.

⚲ Key Point

A low faecal elastase level is diagnostic of pancreatic insufficiency in CF.

Q4 What diagnosis is most likely to account for the failure in treatment to improve the child's symptoms and an elevated total IgE?

The correct answer is C. Allergic bronchopulmonary aspergillosis.

Allergic bronchopulmonary aspergillosis (ABPA) is an allergic reaction to the fungus Aspergillus, *which can grow in cavities in the chest. A diagnosis of ABPA usually needs symptoms of wheeze, chest X-ray findings demonstrating cavitation, elevated IgE and elevated blood titres to* Aspergillus. *The treatment includes antifungal medication and high dose corticosteroids.*

A Meconium ileus – Incorrect. This diagnosis is made in neonates with a congenital bowel obstruction due to dehydrated mucus. Any affected child requires an urgent sweat test after treatment of the obstruction. This condition is not seen outside the neonatal period.

B Distal intestinal obstructive syndrome – Incorrect. There is a bowel obstruction risk in CF children due to dehydration of their faecal matter. Severe obstruction may impact diaphragm movement and therefore respiratory effort. However, it does not account for the elevated total IgE.

C Allergic bronchopulmonary aspergillosis – Correct. With an elevated IgE and symptoms of treatment-resistant respiratory distress, one should consider ABPA.

D CF-related diabetes – Incorrect. Hyperglycaemia may impact respiratory function, but it is not associated with IgE level changes.

♀ Key Point

Complications of CF should be considered in the management of children with CF when symptoms do not improve.

ⓘ IMPORTANT LEARNING POINTS

- In the absence of a newborn screening programme, CF usually presents as faltering growth and recurrent chest infections.
- A sweat test is required for diagnosis, following which pancreatic function must be established. This is done via a faecal elastase test.
- If a child is being treated for a chest exacerbation with antibiotics and is not responding, other chest pathologies should be considered, such as ABPA.

ANSWER TO CASE 8
A 5-year-old boy with unstable asthma

Q1 What would be the next treatment step?

Correct answer is C. Add in a long acting β2 agonist.

This young man is currently on inhaled corticosteroids (preventer) and inhaled short acting β2 agonists (reliever). To improve control of his asthma, treatment escalation is required, and may involve either a leukotriene receptor antagonist or a long acting β2 agonist (LABA). The latter is preferred in children more than 5-years-old. It is also important to review inhaler technique and compliance, as non-adherence is the commonest reason for treatment failure.

A Increase his inhaled corticosteroid — Incorrect. He is already receiving a total of 400 micrograms of corticosteroid daily. This is a moderate dose and alternative therapies should be investigated before increasing the dose.

B Add in a leukotriene receptor antagonist — Incorrect. This would be an option, but as he is over 5-years-old, the LABA would be more suitable.

C Add in a long acting β2 agonist — Correct. This will hopefully give more sustained control of his symptoms throughout the day and night.

D Oral corticosteroids — Incorrect. Oral corticosteroids have significantly more side effects than inhaled agents. They are therefore reserved for the most severe cases, when other treatment options have been exhausted.

♀ Key Point

Chronic asthma management should escalate in a stepwise fashion, assessing medication effectiveness and adherence at each step before increasing dosages or adding new therapies (p315).

Q2 Which method of drug delivery would be the most appropriate for a 5-year-old?

Correct answer is B. Metered-dose inhaler with a spacer device and a mouth piece.

One of commonest mistakes amongst health professionals is prescribing the wrong spacer device. Take time to review available devices, and the patient group each device is designed for. The spacer should be prescribed just like the inhaler.

A Metered-dose inhaler on its own — Incorrect. Most of the medication will be hitting the back of the throat. Therefore, it is always recommended that a spacer is used with an MDI.

B Metered-dose inhaler with a spacer device and a mouth piece — Correct. He is old enough to form a seal around a mouthpiece, insuring all the dose is in his airway and not hitting his face.

C Metered-dose inhaler with a spacer device and a facemask — Incorrect. Facemasks are unnecessary in children over 5-years-old, as they are usually able to form a seal around the mouthpiece with their mouths. Exceptions may include those with developmental delay.

D A breath-activated inhaler — Incorrect. Breath-activated inhalers are usually only appropriate for those over 6-years-old, as they require more technical skill to use correctly. The technique can be tested using a dummy device that whistles when used appropriately. Older children may prefer them to using a spacer.

♀ Key Point

Metered dose inhalers should always be prescribed with a spacer. If the child cannot form a seal around a mouthpiece, an additional facemask is required.

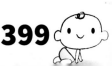

Q3 What is a common side effect with the use of leukotriene receptor antagonists, such as Montelukast?

The correct answer is C. Disturbed sleep.

Leukotriene receptor antagonists are non-steroidal anti-inflammatory medications. They come in oral tablet form and are an effective way to manage moderate asthma. Side effects include nausea, headache, abdominal pain, rashes and diarrhoea. Nightmares can potentially be a very troublesome side effect.

A Dry mouth — Incorrect. This can be a side effect of using an MDI directly into the mouth or any oral powder drug inhalation. However, leukotriene receptor antagonists are given as tablets.

B Oral candidiasis — Incorrect. This is a side effect of inhaler corticosteroids, not leukotriene receptor antagonists.

C Disturbed sleep — Correct. Leukotriene receptor antagonists can result in nightmares. If this occurs, the medication should be discontinued and alternative treatments explored.

⚲ Key Point

Any change in treatment should be followed up. This involves assessing whether asthma control is improved, but also involves exploring potential side effects. Be aware that parents may not realise that disturbed sleep might be caused by a new medication.

ⓘ IMPORTANT LEARNING POINTS

- The treatment of chronic asthma requires a stepwise approach of increasing and decreasing treatment depending on symptoms (p315).
- Consider the medication a child can take, depending on age, the side effects of those drugs and how they are administered. Benefits need to be weighed against side effects.
- Ensure both the right treatment and the right delivery method are prescribed. Check the inhaler technique at every asthma review, and ensure that local asthma services are being utilised (e.g. dedicated asthma nurses).
- Ensure all children have an asthma plan with their regular treatment and know what to do if they have an acute exacerbation. Always give written advice where possible.

ANSWER TO CASE 9

A 6-year-old girl presenting with wheeze and breathlessness

Q1 What is the most likely diagnosis?

The correct answer is B. Acute exacerbation of asthma.

Respiratory distress is a very common presenting complaint for children in ED. Asthma, pneumonia, anaphylaxis, bronchiolitis and viral-induced wheeze are important differentials to consider depending on the age of the child. Foreign body inhalation is a rare, but potentially catastrophic, event.

A Bronchiolitis – Incorrect. Bronchiolitis occurs in children up to 2-years-old and is less common in those over 1-year-old. Infants with bronchiolitis usually have fever, coryzal symptoms, cough and wheeze. Fine end-inspiratory crackles are also heard.

B Acute exacerbation of asthma – Correct. Although this patient does not yet have a formal diagnosis of asthma, she has had repeated admissions with viral-induced wheeze, suggesting she has hyper-reactive airways. She also has interval symptoms of coughing at night. It is possible that moving house may have precipitated the asthma exacerbation.

C Pneumonia – Incorrect. This is an important differential to consider, but there is no history of fever and no coarse inspiratory crackles on auscultation. Wheeze is also rare with pneumonia, although it can sometimes be heard due to air being forced through bronchioles congested by consolidation and mucus.

D Foreign body inhalation – Incorrect. This is an important diagnosis not to miss. It presents with sudden onset breathlessness after a choking event. The wheeze is focal and monophonic. It is an emergency, requiring urgent removal of the foreign body under bronchoscopic guidance.

E Viral-induced wheeze – Incorrect. This is unlikely, given the interval symptoms of nocturnal cough, the history of wheezy episodes and the episodes persisting over the age of 5-years-old.

⚲ Key Point

A wheezy child presenting with a previous history of wheeze and interval symptoms is suggestive of asthma. Reversibility tests could be performed to support the diagnosis.

Q2 A nurse starts high flow oxygen via a non-rebreather mask and asks you what to do next. Which step would be the most appropriate?

The correct answer is E. Nebulised salbutamol driven with oxygen.

The patient's SpO₂ is <92%, she can't speak in full sentences and her pulse is >140 bpm with a respiratory rate of 60 breaths/min, indicating she has a severe acute exacerbation of asthma. In this scenario, both oxygen and bronchodilator therapy are required. The only way to deliver them simultaneously is via an oxygen-driven nebuliser. Other treatments to consider after this are ipratropium bromide via an oxygen-driven nebuliser, further repeat nebulisers and then intravenous magnesium sulphate, salbutamol or aminophylline.

A   Inhaled ipratropium bromide from a metered dose inhaler via a spacer – Incorrect . This patient is hypoxic and requires oxygen; therefore, all inhaled medications must be delivered via an oxygen driven nebuliser rather than a spacer. Salbutamol is the first-line medication in exacerbations of asthma, not ipratropium bromide.

B   Inhaled salbutamol from a metered dose inhaler via a spacer – Incorrect. This patient has a severe exacerbation of her asthma and is hypoxic; therefore, she requires oxygen and should receive bronchodilators via an oxygen-driven nebuliser.

C   Start oral amoxicillin – Incorrect. Antibiotics are not routinely used in treating exacerbations of asthma. They are, however, required if the asthma exacerbation is secondary to a bacterial pneumonia. This may be suggested by fever, localised crepitation and/or a heterogeneous opacity on chest X-ray. Asthmatic patients, if not well controlled, can be prone to developing chest infections, as mucus gets trapped in the lungs and acts as a breeding ground for bacteria.

D   Nebulised ipratropium bromide driven with oxygen – Incorrect. The delivery method is correct but this is not the first-line drug and is only used in conjunction with salbutamol.

E   Nebulised salbutamol driven with oxygen – Correct. This is the correct drug and the correct delivery method.

⚷ Key Point

Hypoxic asthmatic patients need to be given bronchodilators via oxygen-driven nebulisers; otherwise, they may become more hypoxic.

Q3 Which of the following would be required on discharge?

The correct answer is A. Review of inhaler technique.

This patient has a new diagnosis of asthma. As this is a chronic illness, it is important to maximise patient education whilst in hospital: often an asthma specialist nurse will be able to see the patient on the wards. Education should cover knowing how and when to administer medication, how to prevent exacerbations and when to present to hospital.

A   Review of inhaler technique — Correct. Although the child has had previous viral induced wheeze, she is now going home with a new diagnosis of a chronic condition. Once stabilised, she is likely to be sent home on a salbutamol-reducing regime as her treatment is gradually reduced in the community. It is vital to know that the inhaler and spacer are being used correctly. More generally, "asthma action plans" are initiated. These ensure families know how to manage the asthma, what services are available to them in the community and when to re-present to hospital.

B   Epipen — Incorrect. Whilst the child may be atopic, there is no evidence that she has allergies which could put her at risk of anaphylaxis.

C   Sweat test — Incorrect. There is no evidence of cystic fibrosis. This presents with recurrent chest infections and faltering growth, not wheezy episodes.

D   Prophylactic antibiotics — Incorrect. Prophylactic antibiotics do not have a role in prevention of asthma exacerbation unless the child has a very severe case; these are prescribed only by asthma specialists.

⚷ Key Point

Discharge from hospital is a vital opportunity to share knowledge on the community management of chronic conditions, particularly in a new diagnosis. Severe asthma exacerbation can be prevented by appropriate treatment and utilisation of emergency care facilities. This needs to be communicated to the family.

ⓘ IMPORTANT LEARNING POINTS

- Asthma is a common cause of morbidity. It is more likely in those with a personal history or family history of atopy, eczema or asthma.

- Severe exacerbation of asthma requires prompt identification and treatment. Bronchodilator therapy and corticosteroid therapy should be delivered promptly.

- If the patient is hypoxic, bronchodilators should be delivered via oxygen-driven nebulisers. Otherwise, in a non-hypoxic patient, using a MDI with a spacer is equally effective.

- On discharge, it is important to ensure the child and family are comfortable using an inhaler correctly. Patients and parents should be educated on the signs of deterioration, recognising when exacerbations can be managed at home, how much medication is safe to administer at home and when they should seek help.

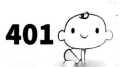

ANSWER TO CASE 10
A 7-year-old boy presenting with fever and a cough.

Q1 What is the most likely organism to cause community acquired pneumonia in this age group?

The correct answer is B. *Streptococcus pneumoniae.*

The history, examination findings and chest X-ray findings are all consistent with a right-sided pneumonia. It is likely to be a typical community-acquired pneumonia since i) the patient has not been in hospital recently, and ii) there is no recent travel or immune deficiency. Certain bacteria are more common in different age groups. Streptococcus pneumoniae *is the commonest pathogen for a child of his age.*

A Group A streptococcus – Incorrect. Children with Group A streptococcus can be very unwell and require significant amounts of resuscitation. It is usually treated with a penicillin, but significant amounts of fluid may be required to treat associated septic shock.

B *Streptococcus pneumoniae* – Correct. Although the UK vaccination schedule includes a vaccination against the most common *Streptococcus pneumoniae* serotypes, it is still the most common cause of community acquired pneumonia. A rise in infection with non-vaccinated serotypes of the bacteria has been observed. It is usually treated with a penicillin.

C Mycoplasma – Incorrect. This is more common in older children, and once diagnosed, requires macrolide antibiotic treatment. Classically, there is bilateral consolidation on the chest X-ray, predominantly affecting the hilar regions.

D *Staphylococcus aureus* – Incorrect. This is more common in the infant age group and in those with indwelling lines or where there is immune deficiency. Abscess formation may be seen on chest X-ray. Flucloxacillin is a good initial therapy.

⚲ Key Point

For community-acquired pneumonia, use a broad spectrum antibiotic until a specific organism is isolated. If there is a strong suspicion of a particular infection (e.g. mycoplasma in bilateral hilar consolidation), ensure this organism is also covered by the initial therapy choice.

Q2 What would be the most appropriate treatment course for this child?

The correct answer is C. Admit to hospital, and start on broad spectrum antibiotics.

The pneumonia is compromising this child's ability to breath and he needs support in the form of oxygen. He needs to be admitted and observed while treatment is administered, because of the risk of deterioration. Whilst antibiotic therapy is necessary, this scenario would only merit oral therapy. However, practice varies between clinicians and indications for intravenous antibiotics are hotly debated.

A Discharge with oral broad spectrum antibiotics and follow up arrangements – Incorrect. This patient needs admission and monitoring to ensure he doesn't deteriorate any further, as well as continuing oxygen to maintain his saturations. He also has signs consistent with a pleural effusion that possibly needs drainage.

B Back-to-back salbutamol nebulisers and oral corticosteroids – Incorrect. This patient has no wheeze or symptoms suggestive of bronchoconstriction.

C Admit to hospital, and start on broad spectrum antibiotics – Correct. Broad spectrum treatment may include a penicillin and a macrolide. He may also require intravenous fluids if oral fluids are not tolerated.

D Intubation, ventilation and transfer to the nearest paediatric intensive care unit – Incorrect. At the moment, his needs can be met on a general paediatric ward, however, if he were to deteriorate he may need the expertise of paediatric intensive care. Indications would be i) failed oxygenation, ii) circulatory shock resistant to fluid boluses, or iii) impending respiratory failure suspected if showing signs of tiring/deterioration. If a chest drain is needed, this may not be manageable locally.

⚲ Key Point

A child showing signs of distress needs careful monitoring to ensure they don't deteriorate. In general, and unlike adults, children tend to compensate with illness until a point at which they can deteriorate very quickly.

Q3 Once treatment and management has been established, which of the following would be the most useful next step investigations for management of the effusion?

The correct answer is B. Chest ultrasound scan.

With a large consolidation of the lung, there is often also a fluid collection (a parapneumonic effusion), as in this case. This not only can compromise ventilation but fluid may be loculated by fibrin sheaths making it difficult for antibiotics to reach, should it also be infected. Ultrasound can sufficiently identify the size and location of the effusion, as well as the best location site to aspirate/drain it.

A Chest CT – Incorrect. CT is one of the best modalities to assess the lung parenchyma and pleural space. If an effusion is present, it will be demonstrated on CT, but an ultrasound is adequate to demonstrate this without the radiation exposure.

B Chest ultrasound scan – Correct. This is done to clarify the size and location of the suspected effusion, which may need to be drained to allow the chest to recover.

C Needle aspiration – Incorrect. Needle aspiration should not occur until the location and presence of an effusion is confirmed. Aspirated fluid may be useful to identify any infectious pathogen.

D Lung biopsy – Incorrect. There is no indication for lung biopsy in this case. Lung biopsy is rarely done in paediatrics. It is used predominantly i) in suspected malignancy, ii) in investigating interstitial lung disease and iii) as part of the post lung transplant monitoring process. All these indications are uncommon in general paediatrics.

⚲ Key Point

In the case of a complete consolidation, it is important to rule out a concurrent pleural effusion. As a benchmark, fluid collection greater than 2 cm from skin to lung may need drainage. Advice should be sought from a respiratory physician.

ⓘ IMPORTANT LEARNING POINTS

- Community-acquired pneumonia is common and usually treated with oral antibiotics at home. When considering antibiotic treatment, consider the most likely causative organism.
- If a child shows signs of significant respiratory distress, admission and more invasive treatment may be required. However, there has been a move towards using oral antibiotics rather than intravenous antibiotics, unless the patient i) is nil by mouth, ii) has malabsorption, iii) has signs of septicaemia, or iv) has developed severe complications, such as a lung abscess.

ANSWER TO CASE 11
An 8-month-old baby presenting with respiratory distress and poor feeding

Q1 What is the most likely diagnosis?

The correct answer is D. Bronchiolitis.

Given the child's age and symptoms, this is the most likely diagnosis, particularly in the winter months. It is commonly caused by respiratory syncytial virus. Children are classically unwell for three to five days, with deteriorating symptoms before they start to improve.

A Pneumonia – Incorrect. The presence of wheeze and the bilateral nature of the chest signs is more suggestive of bronchiolitis than pneumonia. Pneumonia in this age will usually have higher temperatures and no wheeze.

B Croup – Incorrect. This would present with an inspiratory stridor and barking cough. Additionally, croup usually has a quicker onset. Croup is a viral infection of the upper airways, whereas bronchiolitis is a viral infection of the lower airways.

C Viral-induced wheeze – Incorrect. Viral-induced wheeze is a phenomenon seen in young children, and on auscultation, crackles are usually not present.

D Bronchiolitis – Correct. The age and clinical presentation is very suggestive of bronchiolitis.

⚲ Key Point

An unwell infant with respiratory distress, crackles, wheeze and an intercurrent upper respiratory tract infection is likely to be diagnosed with bronchiolitis, particularly in the winter months.

Q2 What would be the most appropriate course of action?

The correct answer is B. Admit for observation and feeding support.

Two key factors in this case necessitate admission. First, whilst she is maintaining her saturations, it is leading to significant respiratory distress. When she is asleep and not putting in as much effort, it is highly likely that her saturations will drop and she will require oxygen support. Secondly, regarding feeding, she is taking in less than half her usual amount of fluid. This is likely due to exhaustion from the additional respiratory effort. Smaller and more frequent feeds could be tried initially, but it may be the case that nasogastric feeding or intravenous fluids are required to maintain hydration.

A Discharge and advise the use of nasal sodium chloride drops – Incorrect. In milder cases, this may alleviate some of the respiratory distress caused by the blocked nasal passages, but this child is too unwell and needs additional monitoring.

B Admit for observation and feeding support – Correct. She needs feeding support, and this may entail nasogastric feeds. Oxygen may be required during the course of the hospital stay.

C Perform a chest X-ray – Incorrect. Chest X-rays have no clinical value in bronchiolitis, unless i) another diagnosis is suspected, ii) a complication such a pneumothorax may have developed, or iii) the patient has been intubated, and the position of the endotracheal tube needs to be checked.

D Start a course of antibiotics – Incorrect. Bronchiolitis is due to a viral infection; therefore, antibiotics have no place in its management.

Key Point

A child with respiratory distress and poor feeding will require observation initially to ensure they remain stable. If they are going to deteriorate and need further interventions, the best place for them would be in hospital, even if they are not receiving active treatment.

403

Q3 Which of the following is the most appropriate initial care?

The correct answer is E. Supportive management.

Despite many studies on the best forms of treatment, nothing has been shown to make a significant improvement in the management of bronchiolitis. Anecdotally, many clinicians may feel that certain treatments are helpful, such as hypertonic saline, salbutamol or ipratropium bromide, but no clear evidence supports this. Supportive measures remain the mainstay management.

A   Oral corticosteroids – Incorrect. Although this is often incorrectly prescribed, it exacerbates rather than improves bronchiolitis.

B   Nebulised salbutamol – Incorrect. There is no evidence that this works, particularly in those under six-months-old that have not developed β2 receptors. Some clinicians favour a trial of salbutamol, particularly in older infants with an atopic history.

C   Nebulised hypertonic sodium chloride – Incorrect. Although previous evidence showed a benefit, the most recent data have not indicated any benefit to nebulised hypertonic sodium chloride on either length of hospital stay or outcome.

D   Nebulised adrenaline – Incorrect. There is no evidence of effectiveness for this treatment.

E   Supportive management – Correct. Management involves supportive care only.

⚷ Key Point

The management of bronchiolitis is entirely supportive. This involves respiratory support (with oxygen and with ventilatory support, if required, including high flow nasal cannulae oxygen, CPAP and intubation) and feeding support (with feeding plans and consideration of either nasogastric feeds or intravenous fluids, if required).

ⓘ IMPORTANT LEARNING POINTS

- Bronchiolitis is extremely common in infancy, particularly in the winter months. Most children will have a short disease course and can be managed at home safely.
- If a child is working hard to maintain adequate oxygenation when awake, they will likely require respiratory support when sleeping.
- Often, a child's ability to feed and remain adequately hydrated is the deciding factor on whether they should be admitted.
- No treatment interventions have been shown to improve outcomes in the management of bronchiolitis, although they are often attempted to see if they have any effect.

ANSWER TO CASE 12
A 6-year-old girl presenting with a possible allergic reaction

Q1 What medication should be given to this patient immediately?

The correct answer is B. IM adrenaline (1:1000).

If any life-threatening symptoms of anaphylaxis are present, IM adrenaline concentration 1:1000 should be administered as soon as possible. Concentration 1:1000 = 1 g adrenaline in 1000 mL = 1 mg/mL. The dose of adrenaline required is 10 microgram/kg = 0.01 mL/kg.

Q2 Which of the following is the most worrying symptom in this patient?

The correct answer is D. Stridor.

Solve airway problems before moving on to breathing, and solve breathing problems before moving on to circulation, as airway obstruction will cause cardiorespiratory arrest first.

A   Wheeze – Incorrect. Wheeze occurs because of bronchospasm and swelling of the bronchiolar mucosa. It should be treated with nebulised salbutamol, after any airway problems are addressed.

B   Hypotension – Incorrect. Hypotension is due to vasodilatation and increased capillary leak from release of vasoactive substances. It requires treatment with an IV fluid challenge of 20 mL/kg of crystalloid, but it needs to be addressed after airway and breathing issues.

C   Vomiting – Incorrect. This is unlikely to immediately compromise the patient. Treating the anaphylaxis appropriately with IM adrenaline and addressing ABC in turn is the first concern.

D   Stridor – Correct. Stridor indicates laryngeal oedema and imminent upper airway obstruction, and should be treated first with IM adrenaline.

E   Tachycardia – Incorrect. Tachycardia occurs in anaphylaxis to maintain or increase cardiac output in the face of hypotension (falling stroke volume) and increased tissue demands for oxygen. Together with hypotension, it indicates circulatory compromise, which requires treatment. However, circulatory compromise should be addressed after airway and breathing issues.

⚷ Key Point

Regardless of other factors, a patient is more likely to die from an airway issue than breathing or circulation problems. As such, this should be prioritised. The reality in anaphylaxis is that adrenaline treats airway, breathing and circulation problems simultaneously, but the above principle is still important to remember.

Q3 What type of hypersensitivity reaction is this girl likely to be experiencing?

The correct answer is A. Type I.

A Type I – Correct. Anaphylaxis is a Type I hypersensitivity reaction mediated by antigens crosslinking IgE antibodies attached to mast cells and basophils, causing release of histamine and production of other chemicals causing vasodilatation and oedema.

B Type II – Incorrect. Type II hypersensitivity reactions are mediated by IgM or IgG binding to antigens on specific cells in the human body, erroneously leading to activation of complement and formation of membrane attack complexes. Membrane attack complex formation results in destruction of the cell, e.g. autoimmune haemolytic anaemia.

C Type III – Incorrect. Type III hypersensitivity reactions are mediated by IgG erroneously binding to antigens on cells in the human body (opsonisation). Opsonised cells are destroyed by phagocytosis by neutrophils, e.g. systemic lupus erythematosus.

D Type IV – Incorrect. Type IV hypersensitivity reactions (also known as delayed-type hypersensitivity reactions) are mediated by T cells, which recognise an antigen that is not usually considered a pathogen and recognise macrophages rather than antibodies. Contact dermatitis is a delayed-type hypersensitivity reaction.

E Type V – Incorrect. Type V is sometimes considered as a subcategory of type II. Type V reactions cause autoimmune diseases like Graves' disease, where an antibody (IgG or IgM) produced by the body attaches to receptors they are not designed for. Either this falsely activates the receptor or it prevents the receptor's usual substrate from activating it.

Key Point

The key features of anaphylaxis are respiratory (stridor/wheeze), cardiac (hypotension, tachycardia, shock), skin (urticaria, angioedema) and gastrointestinal (abdominal cramping, nausea, vomiting, diarrhoea).

IMPORTANT LEARNING POINTS

- Anaphylaxis is a serious and life-threatening allergic reaction. Prompt diagnosis and treatment is critical to prognosis.
- Recognition is not always easy, as the symptoms may mimic other disorders. If reasonable suspicion exists, treatment should not be delayed.
- Adrenaline is lifesaving in anaphylaxis. Knowledge of doses, routes and delivery is essential. This information for all age groups is available from the resuscitation council and will be readily available in all EDs.
- Patient education is critical to the future management of anaphylaxis. All patients require an anaphylaxis plan on discharge and adrenaline to take home in an auto-injectable device.

ANSWER TO CASE 13
A 5-year-old girl presenting with burns

Q1 Which of the following features would be concerning in this patient?

The correct answers are A. Poor urine output. B. Decreased mental status, C. Soot-tinged sputum and D. Hoarse cry.

This patient is at risk of having suffered smoke inhalation and thermal injury. Also note that they may have had an underlying illness that either led to the fire being caused, or made it difficult for them to escape it.

A Poor urine output – Correct. Poor urine output is always worrying (hypovolaemia, acute kidney injury) although it may be seen due to significantly reduced oral intake. It would be particularly concerning if there was a significant thermal injury or evidence of underlying illness.

B Decreased mental status – Correct. Decreased mental status is a sign of severe carbon monoxide poisoning and hypoxia.

C Soot-tinged sputum – Correct. Soot tinged sputum suggests an inhalation injury, which may rapidly progress to pulmonary oedema or upper airway obstruction.

D Hoarse cry – Correct. A hoarse cry suggests an inhalation injury and is worrying, as it may suggest laryngeal oedema and impending airway obstruction.

Key Point

Smoke inhalation is particularly concerning because of potential damage to the airways. Soot-tinged sputum, soot around the mouth and a hoarse cry are all suggestive of inhalation injury.

Q2 What is the most important priority in her management?

The correct answer is C. Administration of high flow oxygen.

Although all patients should be assessed using an ABCDE approach, in this patient, there is a strong suspicion of smoke inhalation. This may mean both carbon monoxide poisoning and burns to the airway. High-flow oxygen is vital to the treatment of carbon monoxide poisoning.

A Insertion of at least two wide bore cannulas to institute aggressive fluid resuscitation – Incorrect. Aggressive fluid resuscitation is lifesaving in the case of a sustained thermal burn but in the case described above, a child with a potential inhalation injury, aggressive use of fluid can worsen pulmonary oedema. There is no indication of clinical dehydration; therefore, fluids are not warranted at this stage.

B Chest X-ray – Incorrect. A chest X-ray can be useful in those with suspected inhalation injury, even in those with no respiratory compromise, to serve as a baseline for pulmonary oedema which may develop. However, it is not a priority and should not delay treatment.

C Administration of high flow oxygen – Correct. In all fire-related presentations, high flow oxygen should be administered even if oxygen saturations are normal. It speeds up the formation of oxyhaemoglobin to replace carboxyhaemoglobin.

D Transfer to a burns centre for specialist management – Incorrect. Transfer to a specialist burns unit is indicated for all cases of inhalation injuries and moderate/severe thermal burns. However, it is not initial management. Patients should all be stabilised prior to transfer.

♀ Key Point

Fires can result in multiple pathologies including thermal burns to the skin/airway, and smoke/carbon monoxide inhalation.

Q3 What feature would be most suggestive of carbon monoxide poisoning?

The correct answer is C. Elevated carboxyhaemoglobin level.

Carbon monoxide poisoning can be difficult to diagnose, since oxygen saturation can be falsely reassuring. The key investigation required is an arterial blood gas.

A Elevated arterial $PaCO_2$ on blood gas – Incorrect. Arterial carbon dioxide concentration is often normal.

B Low oxygen saturations on pulse oximetry – Incorrect. Oxygen saturation in carbon monoxide poisoning is often normal using standard pulse oximetry, as oxyhaemoglobin and carboxyhaemoglobin absorb light at similar wavelengths.

C Elevated carboxyhaemoglobin level – Correct. Carbon monoxide poisoning leads to the formation of carboxyhaemoglobin; therefore, this is elevated. This can be measured on a blood gas or a specific carboxyhaemoglobin pulse oximeter.

D Metabolic alkalosis on a blood gas – Incorrect. A picture of metabolic acidosis is seen in carbon monoxide poisoning.

E A respiratory rate of 28 breaths/min – Incorrect. A respiratory rate of 28 breaths/min is in the normal range (20-30 breaths/min) at 5-years-old. Tachypnoea can be a symptom of carbon monoxide poisoning, but it is nonspecific and respiratory rate can be normal even with significant inhalation.

♀ Key Point

Do not be misled by normal oxygen saturations, or a normal $PaCO_2$ on a blood gas. Look at the carboxyhaemoglobin on the blood gas and assess whether metabolic acidosis is present.

ⓘ IMPORTANT LEARNING POINTS

- Burns are a major source of morbidity and mortality in children. Early identification of associated injuries, fluid resuscitation, analgesia and early referral to a specialist burns centre improve survival.
- Initial assessment and management of burn injuries should follow an ABC structure.
- In cases of moderate to severe thermal injury, fluid loss can be life-threatening and requires aggressive fluid management.
- All cases of fire-related injury require prompt assessment for evidence of inhalational injuries and carbon monoxide poisoning, as both can be life-threatening.
- All moderate to severe burns should be discussed with a specialist burns centre and may require transfer for further management once the patient is stabilised.

ANSWER TO CASE 14
A 1-hour-old baby presenting with suspected sepsis

This is a very common neonatal scenario. Note the chart is filled out in black ink in legible capital letters. It is good practice to write the dose in mg/kg, as well as mg, so that the calculation can be checked by the nurses. Include your contact details with every prescription. Gentamicin levels are often performed before the third dose of gentamicin, and this should be written on the drug chart.

Remember that neonatal fluids start at 60 mL/kg/day of 10% glucose, so 60 mL x 4 kg = 240 mL/day = 10 mL/hour, as prescribed in *Chart 1b* below.

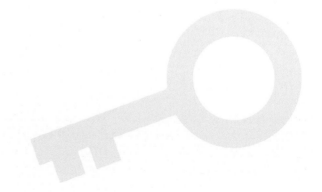

CHART 1B: PRESCRIPTION CHART FOR CLINICAL CASE 14

Name	BABY SMITH	Weight	4kg	Known allergies

NO KNOWN DRUG ALLERGIES

Date of birth	01/01/2015	Gestation	39 WEEKS

Hospital number	334335X	Consultant	DR DANIELS

Signature: A.Jones JONES Blp 1234   Date: 1/1/15

Admission date	01/01/2015	Ward	NICU

REGULAR MEDICATIONS

	Date / Time	1/1	2/1	3/1	4/1	5/1	6/1	7/1	8/1	9/1
Drug CEFOTAXIME 50mg/kg	02									
Dose 200mg Freq BD Route IV	06									
	(10)									
Start 1/1/15 Stop/review 3/1/15	14									
Signature A.Jones JONES 1234	18									
Indication Suspected sepsis review with blood culture results	(22)									

FLUID PRESCRIPTIONS

Date	Fluid	Additive	Volume	Route	Rate	Signature	Given	Batch
1/1/15	10% GLUCOSE (60ml/kg/day)	–	500ml	IV	10ml/hour	A.Jones JONES 1234		

ANSWER TO CASE 15
A 6-year-old boy presenting with an infective asthma exacerbation

The allergy status should include the allergen and the reaction seen. Normal first-line antibiotics for a lower respiratory tract infection would be amoxicillin, but this cannot be used in this case. A macrolide is a suitable alternative. The fluid prescription is calculated as below:

(10 x 100 mL/day) + (10 x 50 mL/day) = 1500 mL/day full maintenance

= 62.5 mL/hour full maintenance
= 41.6 mL/hour at 2/3 maintenance (rounded to 42 mL /hour)

The full prescription is shown in **Chart 2b.**

CHART 2B: COMPLETE PRESCRIPTION CHART FOR CLINICAL CASE 15

Name				Weight		Known allergies	
DAVID HODGKINS				20kg		PENICILLIN (ANAPHYLAXIS)	

Date of birth	Age	
15/02/2008	6 YEARS	

Hospital number	Consultant	
SM506901	Dr. ROSS	

Admission date	Ward	Signature: A.Jones Jones Blp 1234	Date: 1/1/15
01/01/2015	PUFFIN		

REGULAR MEDICATIONS

			Date / Time	1/1	2/1	3/1	4/1	5/1	6/1	7/1	8/1	9/1
Drug SALBUTAMOL			(02)									
Dose 10 PUFFS	**Freq** 4 hrly	**Route** INH (spacer)	(06)									
			(10)									
Start 1/1/15	**Stop/review** 3/1/15		(14)									
Signature A.Jones JONES 1234			(18)									
Indication Asthma			(22)									
Drug CLARITHROMYCIN			02									
Dose 187.5mg	**Freq** BD	**Route** ORAL	06									
			(10)									
Start 1/1/15	**Stop/review** 6/1/15		14									
Signature A.Jones JONES 1234			18									
Indication Pneumonia			(22)									
Drug PREDNISOLONE			02									
Dose 30mg	**Freq** OD	**Route** ORAL	06									
			(10)									
Start 1/1/15	**Stop/review** 4/1/15		14									
Signature A.Jones JONES 1234			18									
Indication Asthma exacerbation.			22									

FLUID PRESCRIPTIONS

Date	Fluid	Additive	Volume	Route	Rate	Signature	Given	Batch
1/1/15	0.9% SODIUM CHLORIDE + 5% GLUCOSE (2/3 maintenance)	–	500ml	IV	42ml/hour	A.Jones Jones 1234		

ANSWER TO CASE 16
A 12-year-old girl presenting with abdominal pain

Q1 Which of the following conditions is on your list of differential diagnoses?

The correct answers are A. Urinary tract infection, B. Acute appendicitis, C. Ovarian pathology and E. Gastroenteritis.

In any child presenting with abdominal pain, all of the following need to be considered. Additionally, in women of childbearing age, a urine pregnancy test should always be performed.

A Urinary tract infection – Correct. This child has a key symptom: dysuria. UTI should always be suspected in a pyrexic child with abdominal pain, and it is important to obtain a urinalysis to confirm or exclude the diagnosis. Note that it is common for children with appendicitis to have leucocytes in the urine. A pelvic appendix can irritate the bladder, resulting in urinary leucocytes and dysuria. This will not result in nitrites on urinalysis, as there is urinary inflammation, not infection.

B Acute appendicitis – Correct. A history of colicky, vague, periumbilical pain that shifts to the right iliac fossa and becomes constant and severe with a low grade pyrexia is classic of appendicitis, and this child requires a surgical review.

C Ovarian pathology – Correct. Ruptured ovarian cysts or a twisted ovary (similar in pain to testicular torsion) have to be considered in peripubertal girls with lower abdominal pain. The presence of a low grade temperature does not exclude the condition, as any peritoneal irritation and inflammation can lead to a rise in temperature and pulse rate.

D Nonspecific abdominal pain – Incorrect. This is a common diagnosis in any child presenting with abdominal pain after pathology has been excluded. However, the presence of diarrhoea and vomiting, as well as right iliac fossa pain, make the diagnosis less likely.

E Gastroenteritis – Correct. The presence of vomiting and diarrhoea support the diagnosis. However, it is important to remember that an inflamed appendix can irritate the rectum (similar to bladder irritation) and cause frequent loose motions.

♀ Key Point

Appendicitis can cause symptoms and signs which mimic gastroenteritis or a UTI. If in doubt, surgical review, further observations and investigation with an ultrasound may be helpful.

Q2 Please match the following condition to the most important diagnostic modality

A Acute pancreatitis   iv. Amylase

Acute pancreatitis is rare in children, but should be suspected in children with predisposing factors such as gallstones, choledochal cysts or congenital bile duct malformations, and in children who have sustained trauma to the upper abdomen (e.g. handle bar injury after falling off a bike). Amylase is not a routine test that is required for children with lower abdominal pain.

B Acute appendicitis   iii. Clinical assessment, FBC, CRP and observation

The history and the abdominal examination are the most important discriminators for acute appendicitis. Inflammatory markers may also help, and sometimes an abdominal ultrasound is used to assess the appendix. However, blood test results are non-specific and ultrasound is often normal even in appendicitis. The best approach to take with children with possible early appendicitis is a period of observation in hospital, with analgesia and intravenous fluids if necessary. The child is reassessed every 3-6 hours until the clinical picture becomes clearer. If a child has a significant intra-abdominal pathology, the signs of localised peritonitis will gradually worsen. The child will develop guarding, percussion and rebound tenderness. If the child improves, the diagnosis of nonspecific abdominal pain can be made.

C Gastroenteritis   iii. Clinical assessment, FBC, CRP and observation

Occasionally, children with gastroenteritis present with severe abdominal pain. This is rare, but children with this condition can become very unwell and require surgical attention. Usually, gastroenteritis is a clinical diagnosis, requiring no investigations. Stool cultures are only necessary in unusual cases, e.g. specific food poisoning, prolonged diarrhoea, rectal bleeding and recent travel abroad.

D Urinary tract infection   ii. Urine microscopy, culture and sensitivity

The diagnosis of a true UTI is based on a significant growth of the organism on culture, ideally from a clean catch urine sample, and associated with a white cell response in the urine.

E Ruptured ovarian cyst   i. Ultrasound scan

This diagnosis needs to be considered, particularly in peripubertal girls who present with acute onset of severe pain.

F Mesenteric adenitis   iii. Clinical assessment, FBC, CRP and observation

It can be very difficult to differentiate this condition from acute appendicitis. In the history, some children with mesenteric adenitis have experienced a recent febrile illness with neck

lymphadenopathy and a respiratory tract infection. The natural history of the condition is that it improves after 24-48 hours.

G   Meckel's diverticulitis   iii. Clinical assessment, FBC, CRP and observation

This condition cannot be differentiated easily from acute appendicitis. Rectal bleeding may be one identifying factor (sometimes painless). The child can also present with acute catastrophic bleeding per rectum. Often such patients are booked for an appendicectomy. When the appendix is found to be normal, the surgeon must search for other causes. The diagnosis is then made on inspection of the small bowel. The Meckel's diverticulum is then excised and a small bowel anastomosis is fashioned. Where there is suspicion of Meckel's diverticulitis, the child should be referred for a surgical opinion and further investigation, e.g. Meckel's scan.

⚲ Key Point

Whilst a specific test can confirm one or more of the possible diagnoses, frequently a period of observation is needed for the condition to declare itself. A surgical opinion can be helpful.

Q3 What is the most likely diagnosis?

The correct answer is B. Appendix mass.

A   Acute appendicitis – Incorrect. The history is too long for the diagnosis of "simple" acute appendicitis. It is more likely that this was the diagnosis at the child's first attendance to hospital, and the mass represents a complication.

B   Appendix mass – Correct. The diagnosis on the child's first attendance was acute appendicitis not gastroenteritis. The omentum has sealed off the inflamed/perforated appendix. This means that the perforation is contained to the right iliac fossa. This explains the improvement of the general symptoms. The diagnosis is confirmed on ultrasound. Management of appendix mass includes a prolonged period of antibiotics, followed by an interval appendicectomy.

C   Ovarian tumour – Incorrect. The rapid growth of this mass, along with the septic picture, make this diagnosis unlikely.

D   Concealed pregnancy – Incorrect. The infective symptoms make this unlikely. Nonetheless, it is important to perform a pregnancy test on all females aged 12 and over who present with abdominal pain.

An appendix mass can be the aftermath of "missed" appendicitis.

ⓘ IMPORTANT LEARNING POINTS

- Nonspecific abdominal pain is responsible for over 60% of presentations with abdominal pain.
- If the diagnosis is unclear at the time of presentation, a period of observation is recommended.
- Analgesia will never "mask" peritonitis and should always be offered.
- An appendiceal mass can be treated conservatively with antibiotics, followed by an elective interval appendicectomy a few weeks after resolution.

ANSWER TO CASE 17
A 1-minute-old baby requiring resuscitation

Q1 What would be your first step in managing this baby?

The correct answer is A. Dry the baby, and put them under a radiant heater.

The most important step following the delivery of a baby is to dry and wrap them to keep it warm. A cold baby will deteriorate quickly and respond less well to resuscitation if required. If it is not breathing despite being warm and dry, inflation breaths are needed to help with the baby's first breaths as the lungs will have never opened before.

A   Dry the baby, and put them under a radiant heater – Correct. The first step is warming and drying the baby. This should be done with all babies regardless of how well it looks after being delivered. Extremely premature babies should be placed in a plastic bag and placed under a radiant heater, as they lose heat rapidly.

B   Give inflation breaths – Incorrect. Inflation breaths are sustained pressure breaths given to the baby to help open the lungs for the first time. They are required if the baby is still not breathing after being warmed and dried. Resuscitation is less effective if the infant is cold.

C   Intubate the baby – Incorrect. Intubation is rarely required in neonatal resuscitation. The majority of babies respond to the stimulation of drying and wrapping. Occasionally inflation breaths or ventilation breaths are required. Intubation is required if the airway cannot be opened despite manoeuvres.

D   Start CPR – Incorrect. This should only be started if there is a poor HR despite effective inflation and ventilation breaths.

E   Give ventilation breaths – Incorrect. Ventilation breaths are designed to support breathing once the lungs have already been opened with the more sustained inflation breaths.

⚕ Key Point

The majority of newborn babies are born without requiring any form of resuscitation. It is rare for inflation breaths to be needed, and even rarer for CPR or drugs to be needed.

Q2 What is the baby's initial APGAR score?

The correct answer is E. 3.

*APGAR scores are simple to calculate, and give an indication of degree of compromise. The APGAR is calculated at 1, 5, and 10 minutes of age (**Figure 1**).*

Feature	0	1	2
Appearance.	White / Pale.	Blue.	Pink.
Pulse.	Absent.	<100 bpm.	>100 bpm.
Grimace (reflex irritability).	Unresponsive.	Grimace/ feeble cry when stimulated.	Pulls away/cries when stimulated.
Activity (tone).	None.	Some flexion.	Flexed arms and legs that resist extension.
Respiration.	Absent.	Weak and irregular.	Strong cry.

FIGURE 1

Calculating APGARs

Q3 Which of the following symptoms and signs are indicative of hypoxic ischaemic encephalopathy? Select all that apply.

The correct answers are A. Poor cord blood gases, B. Irritability, C. Absent suck reflex, and D. Seizures.

Acute intrapartum events are still a significant cause of neonatal mortality. Hypoxic ischaemic encephalopathy results from oxygen deprivation to the newborn infant. Primary brain damage cannot be prevented. Therapeutic cooling has been shown to reduce secondary brain damage, which is why it is important to diagnose hypoxic ischaemic encephalopathy early. Defining whether a baby has suffered significant birth asphyxia hinges on establishing whether a significant insult has occurred at birth and if there is a significant neurological insult (i.e. is encephalopathy present?).

A Poor cord blood gases – Correct. This indicates a significant perinatal insult to baby. However, a baby may have a significant perinatal insult, but still be born in good condition, and have no neurological signs.

B Irritability – Correct. This may indicate an encephalopathy, but is also associated with sepsis.

C Absent suck reflex – Correct. This indicates a neurological deficit.

D Seizures – Correct. This is secondary to ischaemia and hypoxia. Seizures can be difficult to control and often require treatment.

⚕ Key Point

A significant insult in a baby is suggested by poor APGAR scores, continued need for resuscitation and poor cord blood gas results. Features of encephalopathy in a baby include altered state of consciousness, abnormal tone, abnormal reflexes, abnormal posture and seizures.

ⓘ IMPORTANT LEARNING POINTS

- Neonatal resuscitation is rarely required. Warming and drying of the baby is needed at all deliveries. Without this step, all other attempts at resuscitation are likely to be futile.
- When giving inflation or ventilation breaths, observe for chest wall movements. This will help decide whether the breaths are effective.
- Remember that APGAR scoring is not done just once; it is done at least three times: at 1 minute, 5 minutes and 10 minutes.
- Calculating APGAR scores can provide a tool for assessing how unwell a baby is at birth. When combined with cord blood gases and clinical examination, an informed decision regarding cooling can be made.

ANSWER TO CASE 18
An 18-hour-old baby presenting with jaundice

Q1 Which two of the following diagnoses would you consider most likely in a baby presenting with jaundice in the first 24 hours of life?

The correct answers are A. Infection and B. Haemolytic disease of the newborn.

If jaundice occurs within the first 24 hours of life, it is more likely that the baby will require an exchange transfusion to prevent kernicterus. Treatment should be started without delay. Jaundice presenting after the first 24 hours has other causes and unless very high, it often responds to good fluid intake and phototherapy. Prolonged jaundice (of greater than two weeks) can be caused by breastfeeding, but it is important to consider other more serious causes such as hypothyroidism and biliary atresia. Late detection of these conditions can be life limiting or lead to lifelong consequences.

411

A Infection – Correct. Infection is an important cause of jaundice in the first day of life. It is important to remember that infection markers alone are inaccurate at identifying infection in neonates, especially in the early stages.

B Haemolytic disease of the newborn – Correct. This is due to blood group incompatibility between the mother and baby. A direct Coombs test (direct antiglobulin test) is able to establish the likelihood of haemolysis. A blood film can also provide evidence of haemolysis. It is important to establish the blood group of both the baby and the mother to see if a setup for blood group incompatibility exists.

C Biliary atresia – Incorrect. Biliary atresia is a cause of prolonged jaundice. It is associated with a conjugated hyperbilirubinaemia, pale stools and a need for urgent surgical intervention.

D Hypothyroidism – Incorrect. Hypothyroidism is a cause of prolonged jaundice. Treatment with thyroxine in the neonatal period can prevent the developmental delay and abnormal facies that are a hallmark of this condition when left untreated.

E Breast milk jaundice – Incorrect. Breast milk jaundice is a cause of prolonged jaundice that is a diagnosis of exclusion. No treatment is required and mothers should be encouraged to continue breastfeeding.

♀ Key Point

All babies have hyperbilirubinaemia when compared to expected adult levels. The human eye is highly inaccurate at predicting bilirubin levels. Clinical jaundice is indicative of higher bilirubin levels that may require treatment. It is important to investigate and initiate treatment early in babies who have jaundice in the first 24 hours.

Q2 The baby's blood group is checked. Given that mum is AB -ve, which of the following blood groups for the baby would make you concerned about a possible haemolytic anaemia?

The correct answers are E. A+ve, and F. B+ve.

Blood group and Rhesus incompatibility are important causes of jaundice that presents in the first day of life. These causes are more likely to lead to kernicterus if not treated. Phototherapy and an exchange transfusion can be used to reduce the hyperbilirubinaemia and prevent kernicterus. Kernicterus is caused when bilirubin passes through the blood-brain barrier and binds irreversibly to neuroreceptors in the basal ganglia of the brain. It has lifelong complications. Table 1–2 highlights those at risk of rapid haemolysis.

♀ Key Point

Identifying and treating jaundice in the first day of life is vital in preventing kernicterus.

Q3 The bilirubin levels are high, and a decision is made to start phototherapy. What is the most important complication of jaundice that treatment aims to prevent?

The correct answer is D. Kernicterus.

At high levels, bilirubin passes the blood brain barrier and binds irreversibly with the neuroreceptors in the basal ganglia of the brain. The likely consequences include cerebral palsy and a Parkinsonian disorder.

A Liver failure – Incorrect. Liver failure is a potential cause of jaundice, rather than a consequence of it.

B Renal failure – Incorrect. Renal failure is not a cause of jaundice, although dehydration may lead to both renal failure and hyperbilirubinaemia.

C Anaemia – Incorrect. Anaemia itself is not caused by jaundice; however, anaemia in the presence of early jaundice may suggest rapid haemolysis.

D Kernicterus – Correct. Kernicterus is due to deposition of bilirubin in the basal ganglia. It can cause irreversible brain damage.

E Weight loss – Incorrect. Weight loss is not a complication of jaundice, though poor feeding and weight loss may be associated with worsening jaundice.

♀ Key Point

Kernicterus is highly preventable but has lifelong consequences. Severe hyperbilirubinaemia may be treated with phototherapy, immunoglobulins and exchange transfusion.

TABLE 1: Possible combinations of Rhesus antigens between mother and baby

Mum.	Rhesus Positive	Rhesus Positive	Rhesus Negative	Rhesus Negative
Baby.	Rhesus Positive	Rhesus Negative	Rhesus Positive	Rhesus Negative
High risk of haemolysis.	NO	NO	YES	NO

TABLE 2: Possible combinations of ABO antigens between mother and baby

Mum.	A	A	A	A	B	B	B	B	AB	AB	AB	AB	O	O	O	O
Baby.	A	B	AB	O	A	B	AB	O	A	B	AB	O	A	B	AB	O
High risk of haemolysis.	NO	YES	YES	NO	YES	NO	YES	NO	NO	NO	NO	NO	YES	YES	YES	NO

> **IMPORTANT LEARNING POINTS**
>
> - All babies that are jaundiced should have their bilirubin measured.
> - The causes of jaundice can be categorised into those that present before 24 hours, after 24 hours and prolonged jaundice. The most worrying causes tend to present in the first 24 hours (due to blood group incompatibility and infection).
> - Once bilirubin levels are measured, treatment (if indicated) should be started as soon as possible. Adequate fluid intake should be ensured and the bilirubin level monitored regularly to ensure adequate response to treatment.

ANSWER TO CASE 19
A 6-hour-old baby presenting with difficulty in breathing

Q1 Which of the following might commonly cause respiratory distress in a newborn baby? Select all that apply.

The correct answers are A. Infection, D. Transient tachypnoea of the newborn and E. Respiratory Distress Syndrome.

There are many causes of respiratory distress in the newborn. A worrying cause is infection. It is important to consider antibiotic treatment for babies with respiratory distress, as inflammatory markers in this age group may be inaccurate, particularly in the early stages of sepsis.

A Infection – Correct. This is a common cause of respiratory distress, particularly in babies with antenatal risk factors for infection such as maternal Group B streptococcal colonisation. The respiratory distress may be a result of a congenital pneumonia, or it may be a non-specific sign of infection elsewhere.

B Jaundice – Incorrect. Jaundice is a clinical sign of hyperbilirubinaemia and not a cause of respiratory distress.

C Atrial septal defect – Incorrect. There may be a patent foramen ovale or atrial septal defect in newborn babies, but this is usually asymptomatic. Complex congenital cardiac abnormalities may cause tachypnoea, which is classically seen in the absence of other signs of respiratory distress in the newborn baby.

D Transient tachypnoea of the newborn – Correct. This is respiratory distress due to slow lung adaptation to extra-uterine life. It is more common in babies born by Caesarean section. It is self-limiting and usually resolves by 4-hours-old. It is commonly present from birth and does not require treatment.

E Respiratory distress syndrome – Correct. Respiratory distress syndrome is caused by surfactant deficiency and resultant poor lung compliance. It is more common in preterm infants but can present in infants of diabetic mothers or severe sepsis at any gestation.

Key Point

Always consider treating for infection in any tachypnoeic baby, particularly if it persists beyond four hours of life.

Q2 Which of the following are risk factors for infection in a baby?

The correct answers are A. Maternal fever during labour, B. Prolonged rupture of membranes, and E. Prematurity.

Sepsis remains a leading cause of neonatal mortality globally. Looking for risk factors of infection are important in guiding early treatment of neonates given the inaccuracies of using inflammatory markers in predicting sepsis in this age group. Risk factors for sepsis also include invasive group B streptococcal infection affecting a previous baby, suspected or confirmed maternal septicaemia and suspected or confirmed infection in another baby of a multiple pregnancy (e.g. twins).

A Maternal fever during labour – Correct. This is an important risk factor, and may be a sign of maternal infection or chorioamnionitis.

B Prolonged rupture of membranes – Correct. This increases the risk of ascending infection through the vagina, because there is no longer an intact membrane separating the foetus from the external environment. Antibiotics can be given to the mother to reduce the risk of ascending infection.

C Meconium staining at delivery – Incorrect. This is a non-specific sign of foetal distress, and does not represent a significantly increased risk of infection.

D A low APGAR score at one minute – Incorrect. Low APGAR score at one minute bears little correlation with infection.

E Prematurity – Correct. Premature babies are at increased risk of infection. An infection may trigger the onset of premature labour. Prematurity is also associated with a comparatively weaker immune system.

413

⚥ Key Point

It is important to be aware of risk factors for infection in neonates. Babies can present non-specifically and become rapidly unwell. Infection is a leading cause of morbidity and mortality in the neonatal population, but early treatment improves outcomes.

Q3 What bacteria are commonly implicated in early onset neonatal infection?

The correct answers are A. *E. coli*, and B. Group B *Streptococcus*.

Knowing which bacteria are more likely to be present in different settings helps to guide antibiotic therapy. Blood cultures can take days to give a positive result and can remain negative even in the presence of overwhelming sepsis. Early onset infections are normally transmitted from the birth canal.

A   *E. coli* – Correct. This is a common early onset infection.

B   Group B *Streptococcus* – Correct. Group B *Streptococcus* sepsis is a leading cause of neonatal death globally. The bacteria rarely causes any maternal symptoms and can be detected in urine samples, high vaginal swabs or placental swabs. A previous baby with invasive Group B streptococcal infection is a major risk factor for infection in the current baby.

C   Coagulase negative *Staphylococcus* – Incorrect. This pathogen should be considered in babies with long term indwelling lines, but it is not a cause of early onset sepsis. It is commonly isolated in blood cultures, as it is part of the normal skin flora. In the absence of long-term indwelling lines, it can be considered a likely contaminant.

D   *Klebsiella* – Incorrect. This is not a common cause of early sepsis in babies in the UK. *Klebsiella* is more prevalent in the developing world. It is a cause of late-onset sepsis globally.

E   *Streptococcus pneumoniae* – Incorrect. This is not common in the neonatal period.

⚥ Key Point

Although a broad spectrum approach to antibiotics in neonates is required, knowing the prevalence of bacterial flora allows for at least some rationalisation of antibiotic therapy. This prevents resistance to the most potent antibiotics and is the reason why early-onset and late-onset neonatal sepsis are usually treated with different antibiotics.

ANSWER TO CASE 20
A 1-day-old baby with an abnormal newborn baby examination

Q1 You start by examining the eyes, but are unable to elicit the red reflex. Which two of the following pathologies would you be particularly concerned about?

The correct answers are A. Cataracts, and B. Retinoblastoma.

A   Cataracts – Correct. This is the commonest cause of an absent red reflex and can be corrected with a simple operation. Late diagnosis can result in failure of development of the occipital region of the brain and long-term disability.

B   Retinoblastoma – Correct. This is the most worrying cause of an absent red reflex. Often there will be a white reflex rather than a red reflex. There may be a family history of retinoblastoma, since this is an autosomal dominant condition.

C   Glioblastoma – Incorrect. This is very uncommon in newborn babies and would not present with an absent red reflex. It may be noted on an antenatal ultrasound scan.

D   Cerebral palsy – Incorrect. This is an acquired motor defect not diagnosed at the newborn examination.

E   Kernicterus – Incorrect. This is a result of severe jaundice affecting the basal ganglia. It would not present with an absent red reflex.

⚥ Key Point

A red reflex examination is part of the routine baby check at birth and at 6 weeks of age. If it is not possible to elicit a red reflex, urgent ophthalmological review is required.

Q2 Which of the following may be considered normal in a newborn baby?

The correct answers are A. Soft symmetrical breast tissue, B. Small amounts of vaginal bleeding, C. A single, painless, round, blue, discoloured skin lesion, D. A widespread erythematous rash, blanching, which looks urticarial in nature.

A Soft symmetrical breast tissue – Correct. This is normal and can result from the effects of maternal oestrogen. Small amounts of milky discharge may also be present.

B Small amounts of vaginal bleeding – Correct. Babies can have "withdrawal bleeds". This is a result of the withdrawal of maternal oestrogen. It causes the endometrium to build up in the foetal uterus, and then break down after withdrawal of maternal hormones after birth.

C A single, painless, round, blue, discoloured skin lesion – Correct. This is a Mongolian blue spot and is entirely benign. It is more common in Afro-Caribbean babies and may persist into adulthood. Mongolian blue spots should be documented at birth as they can be difficult to differentiate from bruises. This can avoid unnecessary concern about child protection if the child presents to healthcare professionals later in life.

D A widespread erythematous rash, blanching, which looks urticarial in nature – Correct. This is erythema neonatorum (or erythema toxicum). It is normal and resolves with time. This is the most common rash seen in neonates.

E A left sided inguinal hernia – Incorrect. This should always be referred to paediatric surgeons, as it requires surgical intervention.

Key Point

There is a wide range of normal variations in babies. Rashes and skin lesions, such as Mongolian blue spots and erythema neonatorum, are the most common normal findings that cause parents concern.

Q3 The baby is felt to have a cephalohaematoma secondary to birth trauma. Which of the following are possible complications of cephalohaematoma?

The correct answers are A. Jaundice, and B. Anaemia.

A Jaundice – Correct. The breakdown of the red cells in a haematoma can result in hyperbilirubinaemia and subsequent jaundice. Therefore, parents should be asked to monitor for this.

B Anaemia – Correct. A large bleed can result in anaemia.

C Kernicterus – Incorrect. Although broken red cells in a haematoma will release bilirubin, it is unlikely they will lead to levels that cause kernicterus. This is especially true if jaundice can be monitored and treatment started early if needed.

D Raised intracranial pressure – Incorrect. Cephalohaematomas are outside of the skull, therefore, they do not increase the intracranial pressure.

E Infection – Incorrect. A cephalohaematoma does not increase the risk of infection to the neonate.

Key Point

Cephalohaematomas are common and usually self-limiting. They may occasionally result in jaundice as the haematoma breaks down, and also have the potential to cause anaemia if they are large enough.

Q4 On examining the baby's hips, on the right side, the Barlow and Ortolani tests show the hip is dislocatable and relocatable. Which investigation is best suited for assessing for congenital dislocation of the hip?

The correct answer is C. Ultrasound of the hip.

Infants with possible congenital dislocation of the hip should initially be investigated by ultrasound. This is a simple investigation, with a very high sensitivity. The other investigations are either unnecessarily invasive, expensive, or give unwarranted radiation.

Key Point

All babies with suspected congenital dislocation of the hip should be referred for an ultrasound scan of the hip.

(i) IMPORTANT LEARNING POINTS

- Babies with absent red reflexes should be referred to ophthalmologists, as this can be a sign of cataracts or a retinoblastoma.
- Suspected hip dislocations require an ultrasound of the hip and possible referral to an orthopaedic surgeon.
- It is important to give parents adequate discharge advice and answer any questions they may have before going home. This prevents unnecessary anxiety and ensures that parents know what to look for that may prompt seeking of medical advice. In the case of cephalohaematoma, they should be aware of the possibility of the child becoming jaundiced.

ANSWER TO CASE 21
A 24-month-old presenting with developmental delay

Q1 What best describes Kayden?

The correct answer is E. Social and speech and language delay.

Kayden's developmental assessment is summarised in the table below. His fine motor skills are age appropriate. He is not pointing, but all other fine motor milestones are normal. This is likely to represent a delay in social communication. Social

development is less than a year: there is no pointing or waving, play skills are underdeveloped, and the quality of the social communication is poor.

He is presenting with signs of autistic spectrum disorder (**Table 3**).

TABLE 3: Developmental assessment for Kayden.		
Domains	**Skills**	**Developmental Age**
Fine Motor.	Fine pincer grasp. Circular scribble. Able to build a tower of 6 bricks.	2 years.
Gross Motor.	Runs and jumps.	2 years.
Speech and Language.	Minimal vocalisations. Babbles/imitates others.	8-9 months.
Social.	Smiles. Stranger anxiety. Not waving or pointing. No symbolic/imitative play.	9 months.

⚷ Key Point

The combination of social and speech and language delay is highly suggestive of autistic spectrum disorder.

Q2 What is the most important initial investigation?

The correct answer is C. Hearing test.

It is important to identify potentially treatable causes of developmental delay, and in the case of speech delay, hearing impairment is a clear potential cause that needs to be ruled out. Newborn screening is not 100% sensitive for detecting congenital hearing loss, and hearing loss may be acquired (e.g. secondary to persistent ear infections).

A Genetic blood tests – Incorrect. Although genetic tests may be indicated at some stage, there is no specific concern for an underlying genetic disorder at present.
B Thyroid function tests – Incorrect. There is no current clinical concern for hypothyroidism given the history.
C Hearing test – Correct. This is vital in anyone presenting with language delay. There may be a treatable problem that, if identified, could prevent further delay.
D TORCH screen – Incorrect. A TORCH screen looks for infection (toxoplasmosis, other, rubella, cytomegalovirus, herpes simplex). It would only be done if there was a specific concern.
E Visual acuity test – Incorrect. There are no current concerns about vision.

⚷ Key Point

Hearing impairment can commonly present with speech and language delay. It is important that this is picked up early because the earlier it is detected, the better the prognosis.

Q3 In relation to autistic spectrum disorder, mark the following statements true or false.

Treatment of autistic spectrum disorder involves a multidisciplinary team approach. Speech and language therapy form the mainstay of treatment, but there are also psychosocial and behavioural interventions that can be helpful. Pharmacotherapy is very rarely used. Antipsychotics may be considered in the rare circumstance where behaviour remains extremely challenging despite other interventions. Melatonin might also be considered for sleep problems.

A It is linked to the MMR vaccine – False. Although the specific inheritance pattern is not completely understood, genetics evidently plays a significant role. MMR is not implicated in causation. However after the release of Wakefield's report, falsely claiming a link between MMR and autism, the significant decline in the uptake of the MMR vaccine has led to an increase in measles and its complications.
B It can be seen with an underlying diagnosis of tuberous sclerosis – True. About 10-15% of children with autism have a diagnosable underlying cause including tuberous sclerosis, fragile X syndrome, and phenylketonuria.
C Early diagnosis and intervention is proven to improve outcome and level of functioning – True. Early detection and intensive behavioural intervention before the age of 2 have been shown to alter outcome.
D It can be associated with neurofibromatosis – False. It is not associated with neurofibromatosis. ADHD is associated with neurofibromatosis.
E Drugs can significantly alter outcome – False. Medication does not significantly alter outcome, and is very rarely given for ASD. Usually, it is in the context of comorbidities, e.g. epilepsy, although, very rarely, anti-psychotics may be used.

⚷ Key Point

There is no proven link between autism and the MMR vaccination.

Q4 Which of the following conditions may be associated with autistic spectrum disorder? Select all that apply.

The correct answers are A. ADHD, B. Tourette's Syndrome, C. Depression, D. High IQ, and E. Resistance to change or new experiences.

Autistic spectrum disorder classically presents with symptoms in three key domains: social interaction, social communication, and rigidity of thought/behaviour.

A ADHD – Correct. These two conditions often overlap.
B Tourette's Syndrome – Correct. This is a known association.
C Depression – Correct. There is an increased incidence of depression.

D High IQ – Correct. However, it is more commonly associated with a low IQ and learning difficulties. Children diagnosed with high functioning autism, previously known as Asperger's syndrome, may have a higher than average IQ. Those with exceptionally high abilities are known as having "savant autism", but this is rare.

E Resistance to change or new experiences – Correct. This is a marker of rigidity of thinking and imagination.

♀ Key Point

Autistic spectrum disorder is associated with multiple comorbidities, such as ADHD, Tourette's and epilepsy. In addition, it may be linked to an underlying diagnosis, such as tuberous sclerosis, fragile X syndrome or phenylketonuria.

ⓘ IMPORTANT LEARNING POINTS

- Autistic spectrum disorder is a developmental disorder characterised by symptoms in three domains: social interaction, social communication, and rigidity of thought/behaviour.
- It is associated with many co-morbidities, and in a small proportion, underlying conditions such as Fragile X syndrome.
- Children vary dramatically in the severity of the condition: many will function with relatively little support, whilst others never develop any speech, remain un-toilet trained, and have severe learning difficulties.
- Management is complex but largely supportive. It includes speech and language therapy, behavioural support, and education for parents and siblings. There are many schools designed specifically to support children with autistic spectrum disorder.

ANSWER TO CASE 22
An 8-year-old boy presenting with behavioural problems

Q1 In relation to Sam and ADHD, mark the following statements true or false.

A Symptoms of ADHD must be pervasive in various areas of life for a diagnosis – True. The symptoms need to be present at home, school and in other interactions, e.g. with other family members.

B ADHD can be screened for using the Conner's questionnaire – True. With the limited information available about the exact situation at school, and the features mentioned being suggestive of ADHD, it would be important to look at this further. One method would be using a Conner's questionnaire. This is a long series of questions that parents and school staff will fill in. From this, a score will be generated which strongly supports, but does not make, the diagnosis. Diagnosis is done clinically by specialists.

C Hyperactivity, inattention and rigidity in behaviour are the three themes used in diagnosis – False. The three themes required for diagnosis are hyperactivity, inattention and impulsiveness. Rigidity in behaviour and thinking is a feature of autistic spectrum disorder.

D Incidence is increased in VLBW babies – True. There is an association with features of ADHD and premature and VLBW babies.

E Neglect and lack of emotional warmth can lead to behaviours similar to that seen in ADHD – True. Neglect and lack of emotional warmth are recognised as a cause of similar behavioural traits. Often when children are taken into care for reasons such as chronic neglect, ADHD-like behaviour disappears.

F Lack of structure and routine can lead to difficult and defiant behaviour, poor concentration and hyperactivity – True. Children respond well to clear rules, routine, discipline, positive encouragement, and emotional warmth. In cases where this is not the case, parenting courses and a change in parenting behaviour can positively alter the behaviour of the child.

G Mental health disorders in parents can have significant impacts on a child's behaviour – True. Mental health problems can potentially affect the interaction of parents with their children, leading to less consistent responses, lack of emotional warmth, and poor insight into the emotional needs of the child. This can have a significant impact on a child's behaviour and can cause attachment disorders.

H Sam's diet may be contributing to his behaviour – True. It is generally accepted that additives (including food colourings, preservatives and flavourings) and salicylates (found in most fruits, tea and coffee) can cause hyperactivity, fidgeting and poor concentration, although it is also clear that susceptibility plays a part. The definitive evidence from randomised controlled trials is less clear on sugar.

ⓘ IMPORTANT LEARNING POINTS

- ADHD is a condition characterised by three themes: i) hyperactivity, ii) inattention, and iii) impulsiveness.
- The condition usually has an early onset, is chronic, and is associated with moderate impairment to emotional, educational, and social functioning.
- For a diagnosis of ADHD, symptoms must be chronic and pervasive across various areas of life.
- It is important to remember that many different environmental factors can lead to behavioural traits similar to those of ADHD, and these must be considered before making a diagnosis.
- Management involves an MDT approach with education, behavioural intervention, medication and ensuring a healthy, nutritionally balanced diet. First-line medication is usually methylphenidate, if required.

ANSWER TO CASE 23
An 8-month-old presenting with a fall

Q1 Which of the following factors increase the possibility of NAI?

The correct answers are B. The mechanism of injury, and C. The delay in presentation.

Assessment of possible NAI involves looking at the clinical history as well as the specific injury sustained and the developmental stage of the child. There should be a strong suspicion of NAI in spiral, oblique or metaphyseal fractures. Be wary of NAI if the clinical history suggests a possible attempt to cover up the injury (for example, a delayed presentation).

A The father is not in the ED with them – Incorrect. There may be many reasons why he is not there, and it is usual for children to present with just one parent.

B The mechanism of injury – Correct. A non-mobile (i.e. not walking or cruising) child is very unlikely to sustain a fracture unless there is a significant mechanism of injury. This particular mechanism is very unlikely to have had enough force to cause a fracture in Charlie. Of course, this could represent underlying bone fragility, and signs of osteogenesis imperfecta should be looked for. Vitamin D deficiency should be considered in breastfed babies or if there are any suggestive features on the X-rays.

C The delay in presentation – Correct. Delay in presentation increases the suspicion of, but does not confirm, NAI.

D Charlie has had no previous fractures – Incorrect. This should not affect the suspicion of NAI, although questions might be asked if there were an unusual number of fractures in the history.

⚲ Key Point

It is vital that the mechanism given for any injury is considered in regard to its plausibility and in the context of the developmental stage and age of the patient.

Q2 Social services are contacted and do not know the family. Which answer represents the best next course of action?

The correct answer is C. Explain to the mother that, given Charlie's age and concerns, the mechanism given does not entirely explain the injury sustained; therefore, we have a legal duty of care to Charlie to investigate this further, including investigations for Charlie, and discussions with police and social services. The fracture will also be managed by being put in a sling, but Charlie will need to remain in hospital pending a safeguarding plan

At the point of identifying possible NAI, it is the responsibility of whoever is involved to ensure that management proceedings are

initiated. This does not necessarily mean being confrontational with the parents. Indeed, parents are usually compliant with proceedings when it is emphasised that the best interests of the child are being put first, and that currently there is no clear medical explanation for the injuries. Rare diagnoses like osteogenesis imperfecta are sometimes picked up during investigations done in the context of suspected NAI.

A Explain to the mother we think she is lying and that we are likely to remove her child from her care – Incorrect. This is the wrong way to approach a conversation with the mother. It is important to be honest and open about the reasons for concern but the way in which this is communicated is vital. The decision to remove a child is made by social services after a complete investigation.

B Put the arm in a sling and discharge home with fracture clinic follow up as per orthopaedic advice – Incorrect. This case cannot be managed without considering safeguarding concerns and it may be that the home is not considered a place of safety.

C Explain to the mother that, given Charlie's age and concerns, the mechanism given does not entirely explain the injury sustained; therefore, we have a legal duty of care to Charlie to investigate this further, including investigations for Charlie, and discussions with police and social services. The fracture will also be managed by being put in a sling, but Charlie will need to remain in hospital pending a safeguarding plan – Correct. This explanation fully explains to the mother what the concerns are and what will be happening, without being confrontational and accusatory.

D Call the police to come to ED – Incorrect. This is not the role of the medical professionals. Social services should be contacted and they can contact the police. There are exceptions to this; for example, the police may be contacted if the mother absconded with the child and it was felt the risk was high enough that the mother and child needed to be brought back in.

⚲ Key Point

Management of safeguarding concerns can be challenging and anxiety inducing to professionals, but having an open and honest dialogue with parents is paramount. Good inter-agency communication is also vital in helping prevent future maltreatment.

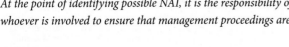

- Child abuse can be physical abuse, emotional abuse, sexual abuse or neglect.
- NAI may present through a child attending ED with injuries that do not fit the explanation offered by the parents. However, be aware that abuse can present in a wide range of manners, including inappropriate behaviour around parents/strangers, evidence of inadequate care, such as poor hygiene or persistent nappy rash, developmental delay and poor educational achievements.
- Investigations likely to be performed in suspected NAI are: skeletal survey, CT head and ophthalmology assessment (for retinal haemorrhage).
- Social services should be involved early. A child should never be sent home if there is strong suspicion of physical or other abuse by the caregiver.

ANSWER TO CASE 24
An 18-month-old presenting with a seizure

Q1 What is the most likely diagnosis?

The correct answer is B. Simple febrile seizure.

Febrile seizures (or febrile convulsions) are the most common cause of seizures in children aged between 6-months-old and 6-years-old. Children are diagnosed clinically and temperatures of at least 38°C are required for a diagnosis. An episode lasting less than 15 minutes is classified as simple, greater than 15 minutes as complex and over 30 minutes as status. The diagnosis is based on a clinical history and assessment, in the absence of infection of the central nervous system, metabolic imbalance or history of afebrile seizures.

A Epilepsy – Incorrect. The clinical diagnosis of epilepsy requires two unprovoked seizures more than 24 hours apart, or one seizure with clinical evidence of a probability of further seizures.

B Simple febrile seizure – Correct. The episode described by the parents is consistent with a seizure, including loss of consciousness, limb jerking, irregular breathing and post-ictal drowsiness, which has improved by an hour. Since the seizure lasted for less than 15 minutes, it is classified as simple. The child is in the correct age range (6-months-old to 6-years-old) to be diagnosed for this condition and there seems to be an URTI focus. Symptoms such as pallor and incontinence are not diagnostic of a seizure by themselves, as they can be seen in other situations such as syncope.

C Complex febrile seizure – Incorrect. Complex febrile seizures are, by definition, seizures that include any of the following: last longer than 15 minutes, have a focal element, the seizure recurred in the same febrile illness or within 24 hours, or incomplete recovery in one hour.

D Status epilepticus – Incorrect. Status epilepticus is, by definition, seizures which last longer than 30 minutes.

E Meningitis – Incorrect. Although meningitis may cause seizures, it is unlikely, as the child has fully recovered, with no signs of meningism. Classical signs of meningitis are neck stiffness, photophobia, vomiting and headache. In younger children, the absence of neck stiffness and photophobia do not exclude meningitis, and other signs such as irritability may be more significant.

⚷ Key Point

Simple febrile seizures are primary, generalised, tonic-clonic seizures which last for a maximum of 15 minutes and do not recur in 24 hours or in the same illness. They occur in the 6-months-old to 6-years-old age group.

Q2 Which investigations are indicated? Select all that apply.

The correct answers are B. Urine dipstick/culture and D. Blood glucose.

Although the diagnosis of febrile convulsion is made clinically, a source of infection should be sought. Here, the likely diagnosis is an URTI, but a urine dipstick is also justifiable. It is easy to perform and can rule out a common source of infection. Any funny turn or seizure should be accompanied by investigating blood glucose to rule out hypoglycaemia as a cause. If no focus of infection is obvious, the child should be referred to a paediatrician and admitted to hospital, pending further assessments and investigations.

A Blood culture – Incorrect. This is not indicated in a simple febrile seizure. However, persistent symptoms and signs, such as fever, irritability, or tachycardia in the presence of a normal temperature and no other cause (e.g. pain) may indicate bacterial sepsis.

B Urine dipstick/culture – Correct. This is often done routinely in cases of febrile seizures, as it is a simple diagnostic test.

C Lumbar puncture – Incorrect. Lumbar punctures are not indicated unless meningitis is suspected.

D Blood glucose – Correct. Hypoglycaemia is a common cause for seizures and should always be ruled out in a first seizure.

E CT or MRI – Incorrect. This is not indicated in a simple febrile seizure unless the clinical presentation is consistent with meningitis or a cerebral abscess (e.g. focal neurological signs).

⚷ Key Point

The diagnosis of febrile convulsion is a clinical one, requiring a typical seizure, plus a clear focus of infection. UTIs, chest infections and hypoglycaemia need to be considered.

Q3 What is the most appropriate management plan? Select all that apply.

The correct answer is C. Provide anti-pyretic medications, and E. Educate parents.

Anti-pyretic medications reduce discomfort associated with fever, but are now not thought to prevent further convulsions. Recognition of a developing fever and removal of clothing may also help. Benzodiazepines can be given by the ambulance crew or ED if the seizure has failed to terminate after five minutes. Parents should be reassured and educated about the risks of recurrence and how to recognise and manage fever and febrile seizures (i.e. recovery position and keeping them safe). They should be advised to return to hospital if there are prolonged symptoms or a clinical deterioration. After a first febrile convulsion, children should be observed until they have had a complete recovery. There should be a low threshold for admission, especially if the child is less than 1-year-old.

A   Start antibiotics – Incorrect. The likely diagnosis is a viral URTI, requiring supportive management only. If a bacterial cause, such as a UTI or pneumonia, is suspected, then antibiotics are indicated.

B   Administer antiepileptic medication – Incorrect. The seizure has self-resolved. Rectal or oral diazepam/lorazepam or buccal midazolam can be effective treatments if episodes are prolonged or repeated.

C   Provide anti-pyretic medications – Correct. Anti-pyretic medications are effective in reducing discomfort.

D   Recommend prophylactic anti-epileptics – Incorrect. Prophylactic anti-epileptics are not recommended. Even though there is a slight increase in risk of developing epilepsy compared to the background population, it is still very small.

E   Educate parents – Correct. Parents should be educated about the risks of recurrence (1 in 6 children who have had febrile convulsions have further febrile convulsions) and how to manage future febrile seizures. In children with recurrent febrile convulsions or a complex history, it may be appropriate to advise the use of benzodiazepines if seizures fail to terminate in five minutes. Parents will require education and training in this situation, including basic life support training.

Key Point

Education and reassurance is an important part of management of future events and in explaining to the parents what has happened.

Q4 What is/are the complication(s) associated with the diagnosis? Select all that apply.

The correct answers are B. Epilepsy and E. Recurrence of febrile seizure.

Simple febrile seizures are not associated with brain damage or increased mortality. The overall risk of recurrence is 1 in 6, and the risk of developing epilepsy is slightly increased, although still small. This risk is increased in those with recurrent complex febrile seizures.

A   Brain damage – Incorrect. There is no evidence to suggest that any form of brain damage occurs.

B   Epilepsy – Correct. There is a slightly increased risk of developing epilepsy compared to the general population, but this is still very small.

C   Increased mortality – Incorrect. There is no increased mortality associated with simple febrile seizures.

D   Poorer cognition and performance at school – Incorrect. There is no evidence that children with simple febrile seizures have poorer cognition or performance at school.

E   Recurrence of febrile seizure – Correct. One in 6 febrile seizure patients have recurrence of simple febrile seizures.

Key Point

The main complication of simple febrile seizures is recurrence, which occurs in 1 in 6 cases. The risk of developing epilepsy for children with simple febrile seizures is 1 in 50, but this increases to 1 in 20 for those with complex febrile seizures.

IMPORTANT LEARNING POINTS

- Simple febrile seizures are common and are very frightening for parents when they occur. Management is supportive, as the seizures invariably self-terminate very quickly.
- It is important to consider hypoglycaemia, UTI, chest infection and tonsillitis as possible triggers, although viral infections are the most common association.
- There is a small absolute increase in the risk of epilepsy, but the main point to inform parents of is that febrile seizures may recur in future illnesses and advise them accordingly.

ANSWER TO CASE 25
A 7-year-old presenting with fever

Q1 What is the most likely diagnosis?

The correct answer is B. Meningoencephalitis.

The temperature suggests an infective process, while the headache, vomiting, drowsiness, photophobia and confusion all point to a cerebral cause. Photophobia, vomiting and neck stiffness are suggestive of meningeal irritation. Confusion, although non-specific, may be related to encephalopathy. The previous cold sores indicate herpes simplex infection, which could be the culprit virus. Note that children with meningitis, particularly in the early stages, may present with non-specific signs and symptoms, such as irritability and poor feeding, especially in the neonatal or toddler age group. Older children have more classical signs. These patients commonly may have initial symptoms and signs that are attributed to a non-specific viral illness. They may not be "diagnosed", as they may not seek medical advice.

A Febrile seizure – Incorrect. There has been no seizure, so by definition this is wrong.

B Meningoencephalitis – Correct. The symptoms and signs are suggestive of meningoencephalitis, as described above. This necessitates urgent treatment.

C Vasculitis – Incorrect. Connective tissue diseases, such as Kawasaki disease and SLE, may present with a rash, irritability, fever and photophobia. However, this is not the most likely diagnosis. The history is too short, the rash is atypical and there are no joint symptoms.

D Space occupying lesion – Incorrect. Malignancies can present with neurological symptoms, either through primary CNS tumours, brain metastasis or a paraneoplastic syndrome. However, there are usually other clues to the diagnosis, and the onset of symptoms is much slower. Fever is more unusual with malignancy, although it can happen.

E Cerebrovascular accident – Incorrect. Strokes are rare in this age group and are usually accompanied by a focal neurological deficit. Groups such as those with sickle cell disease are at a high risk.

Key Point

A child with irritability, photophobia, fever and neck stiffness, with or without confusion, should be suspected to have meningoencephalitis until proven otherwise.

Q2 What is the immediate management? Select all that apply.

The correct answers are A. Fluid resuscitation, C. IV Antibiotics, and E. IV Aciclovir.

Meningoencephalitis is a medical emergency which results in significant morbidity and mortality. Intravenous access should be gained and blood cultures/viral PCR taken. Ideally, a LP should be performed before treatment, but this patient is too haemodynamically unstable for this and has signs that may suggest raised ICP. As such, immediate treatment with antibiotics and fluids should not be delayed. Other contraindications are shown on p640.

In children with signs of shock, an immediate IV or IO fluid bolus of 20 mL/kg 0.9% sodium chloride should be given over 10 minutes. Caution should be exercised, however, since the confusion in this patient may be a sign of cerebral oedema, which can be worsened by fluid boluses. A broad spectrum

antibiotic with good blood-brain barrier penetration, such as IV ceftriaxone, is required, along with IV aciclovir.

A Fluid resuscitation – Correct. This patient is in septic shock and requires restoration of fluid volume in order to maintain adequate tissue perfusion. Care must be taken if raised ICP is suspected.

B Lumbar puncture – Incorrect. This should not be done in any patient who is haemodynamically unstable. It must be performed after the child has been stabilised, has no signs of raised ICP and is not thought to be at risk of coning. If the child is stable, then ideally it should be done before antibiotic administration, since partial treatment of the meningitis may prevent the growth of organisms on CSF culture.

C IV antibiotics – Correct. IV ceftriaxone should be administered as soon as possible in patients with suspected meningoencephalitis, immediately after the blood cultures are taken. IV aciclovir is also recommended and the CSF should be sent for herpes PCR.

D CT head – Incorrect. Whilst it will be important to scan the child's head, the immediate priority is to stabilise the child. There is a risk of further deterioration during the scan without any initial management; therefore, it is not indicated as immediate management. The patient may have developed a cerebral abscess or cerebral oedema which the CT would help identify. There may also be a completely different and as yet unrecognised pathology, such as an intracranial bleed or a tumour.

E IV aciclovir – Correct. This is likely to be viral meningitis, particularly given the confusion and the recent cold sore. Therefore, IV aciclovir should be administered.

Key Point

Meningoencephalitis is initially diagnosed clinically, with treatment starting pre CSF or blood culture results. Give fluid boluses as necessary, broad spectrum antibiotics and antivirals.

Q3 Which is/are recognised complication(s) of this condition? Select all that apply.

The correct answers are A. Hearing loss, B. Hydrocephalus, C. Seizures, D. Neurodevelopmental delay and E. Subdural effusion.

The most common complications of bacterial meningitis are hearing loss, seizures, subdural effusions, neurological deficits, psychosocial disturbance, behavioural disturbance and renal disease. Viral meningitis is usually self-limiting, with no long term sequelae, and is classically caused by enteroviruses. HSV meningoencephalitis, unlike the other causes of viral meningitis, is associated with significant morbidity and mortality, particularly in neonates.

421

A Hearing loss – Correct. Sensorineural hearing loss is the most common complication of bacterial meningitis. It is caused by cochlear infection and occurs in 5-30% of children with meningitis. Children should undergo hearing assessment after discharge from hospital.

B Hydrocephalus – Correct. Hydrocephalus is a recognised complication of meningoencephalitis.

C Seizures – Correct. Seizures can occur acutely due to raised ICP and cerebral irritation.

D Neurodevelopmental delay – Correct. It can affect all domains of development.

E Subdural effusion – Correct. Subdural effusions affect 10-30% of children with meningitis and often develop within days. They occur most commonly in infants. Although most cases of subdural effusions will be asymptomatic, presentation is usually with a bulging fontanelle, enlarged head size (monitor head circumference daily) and seizures.

Key Point

Most children recover fully from viral meningitis. However, HSV meningoencephalitis and bacterial meningitis have a significant morbidity and mortality.

IMPORTANT LEARNING POINTS

- Meningoencephalitis can present very non-specifically in children. Neonates present with non-specific symptoms and signs and babies with a temperature above 38°C will often have a lumbar puncture as part of a septic screen.
- Once meningoencephalitis is suspected, the priority is fluid resuscitation and rapid administration of antibiotics (and antivirals, if indicated).
- Bacterial meningitis has a much worse prognosis than viral meningitis. Since the two are difficult to differentiate clinically, antibiotics are usually given. Antiviral cover is given if there is suspicion of encephalopathy, especially if there is confusion or seizures.

ANSWER TO CASE 26
A 15-year-old presenting with recurrent headaches

Q1 What is the most likely diagnosis?

The correct answer is B. Migraine.

Headaches are common in children (40% of children annually by 7-years-old and 75% of children by 15-years-old), with frequency increasing with age. The history above is suggestive of migraine, due to the nature and pattern of the pain, with pain-free intervals. These headaches are often unilateral, throbbing and associated with nausea and vomiting. These children may experience auras as part of a classical migraine. These can include small areas of visual field loss (scotomas) and white zigzag lines (fortification spectra). There may be neurological signs or symptoms (e.g. visual disturbance, paraesthesia, weakness) before, during or after the attack, although these should self-resolve. Neurological symptoms should prompt referral to a neurologist. There may be an association with autonomic features, abdominal pain and nausea.

A Tension headache – Incorrect. The history is not typical of tension headaches. These tend to be symmetrical, of gradual onset, non-throbbing, feeling like a band of pressure or tightness across the head and not affected by physical activity.

B Migraine – Correct. There is a clear history of episodes with symptom-free periods. The history is classic of a migrainous headache.

C Brain tumour – Incorrect. This is unlikely, given the lack of other features, such as the headache being worse in the morning, vomiting and focal neurology.

D Subarachnoid haemorrhage – Incorrect. Children are more likely to present acutely with neurocognitive and/or neurological deficits.

Key Point

Migraines are a common cause of chronic headaches in school-aged children. They are characterised by unilateral throbbing pain and may be associated with aura, nausea and/or vomiting.

Q2 What is/are the risk factor(s) for this condition? Select all that apply.

The correct answers are A. Family history, and B. Stress.

Recognised risk factors for migraine include family history, triggers (such as sleep pattern, stress and menstruation) and frequent analgesia use.

A Family history – Correct. Migraines are familial and 90% of children have a first or second-degree family member with recurrent headaches.

B Stress – Correct. Triggers include stress, menstruation, not eating food at regular intervals, irregular or inadequate sleep, dehydration and weather changes.

C Head trauma – Incorrect. Migraines are not typically associated with head trauma. Any lasting headache that occurs after trauma to the head should be investigated further.

D Meningitis – Incorrect. There are no associations between migraines and an infective process.

♀ Key Point

Migraines are associated with triggers. These vary from individual to individual and may include: menstruation, sleep deprivation, stress and certain foods/drink (e.g. red wine, cheese or chocolate).

Q3 Which treatment is particularly good for prevention of severe, recurrent headaches caused by this disorder?

The correct answer is D. Propranolol.

For those with migraines, drinking adequate fluids, having a good sleep regime and avoiding identifiable triggers should be discussed. Simple analgesia alone may be effective. For 12 to 17-years-olds, nasal triptan may be preferred to oral triptan and is used at the onset of a migraine. Anti-emetics can be given to relieve nausea and vomiting. If migraines are truly problematic and not responding to these treatments, prophylactic propranolol, pizotifen or topiramate may be considered. Topiramate has an unclear mechanism of action, but it may relate to its effect on sodium channels in the brain. These medications have side effects and therefore should be used only if necessary and under specialist advice.

A NSAIDs – Incorrect. NSAIDs are commonly used analgesics for acute migraine and non-specific headaches.

B Sumatriptan – Incorrect. Sumatriptan is commonly used to treat acute migraine by acting via serotonin receptors.

C Paracetamol – Incorrect. Paracetamol is an effective analgesic but is not the typical first line medication recommended.

D Propranolol – Correct. Propranolol may be effective in recurrent migraines as prophylaxis, as this patient has been suffering for two years. An alternative is pizotifen, which is usually taken at night but is not popular with young girls as it leads to an increase in appetite and potential weight gain. Topiramate is another option.

♀ Key Point

The mainstay of management for migraines is lifestyle modification and avoidance of triggers. Simple analgesia, rest and avoidance of light are usually all that is needed. If prophylactic medication is required, propranolol, pizotifen or topiramate should be considered.

ⓘ IMPORTANT LEARNING POINTS

• Headaches are very common in children, and it is important to be able to differentiate those that require further investigations and those that do not.

• Red flag symptoms for headaches include focal neurological features, waking at night with the pain, headaches that are worse in the morning, headaches that are worse on coughing or stooping, increasing frequency or severity, confusion, change in personality, abnormal gait, growth failure, diplopia or facial nerve palsy, visual field effects or development of seizures. Such features indicate a need for further investigation to exclude a more sinister cause, such as a brain tumour.

• Migraines can be managed conservatively, but in severe cases, sumatriptan is given acutely, and propranolol, pizotifen, or topiramate for prophylaxis.

ANSWER TO CASE 27
A 9-month-old girl presenting with poor weight gain and lethargy

Q1 Which of the following are implicated in the aetiology of coeliac disease?

The correct answer is C. HLA-DQ8.

Coeliac disease is an immune reaction to the gliadin peptide of gluten found in particular foods. However, the autoimmune process also requires a genetically susceptible person to be exposed to environmental factors. Smoking, alcohol consumption and fatty diets are not factors that influence the development of coeliac disease. HLA-DQ2 and HLA-DQ8 have been linked to the development of coeliac disease. The main management requires the removal of gluten from the diet to prevent the immune response.

♀ Key Point

Coeliac disease only occurs in genetically and immunologically susceptible individuals who have been exposed to necessary environmental factors.

Q2 Which patient is most likely to test positive for coeliac disease?

The correct answer is E. A 16-year-old girl with weight loss and chronic diarrhoea.

Coeliac disease is a disease characterised by an immune reaction to gliadin peptides in gluten. It is often asymptomatic and should be screened for in patients with associated conditions.

423

A A 10-year-old boy with weight loss, heat intolerance and increased appetite – Incorrect. This boy may have hyperthyroidism, which warrants investigation, but heat intolerance and increased appetite are not symptoms associated with gluten intolerance.

B A 12-year-old girl with type 1 diabetes mellitus – Incorrect. This girl is likely to be screened for coeliac disease, as type 1 diabetes mellitus has an association with coeliac disease, but she has no active features of disease.

C A 12-year-old girl who eats a gluten-free diet – Incorrect. This girl has already removed the gluten from her diet; therefore, even if she had coeliac disease before the diet change, any investigations would be negative as the immune response would not take place. If she starts eating gluten again and has symptoms, then investigation is warranted.

D An 8-year-old boy with sudden onset diarrhoea – Incorrect. This boy is more likely to have gastroenteritis, as the history is very acute.

E A 16-year-old girl with weight loss and chronic diarrhoea – Correct. This girl may have coeliac disease and warrants investigation.

Key Point

Coeliac disease tends to present with chronic non-specific symptoms, including weight loss, abdominal pain, diarrhoea, vomiting and faltering growth in children. Toddlers may present with buttock wasting due to weight loss and a protuberant abdomen, as well as irritability.

Q3 The best initial investigation for coeliac disease is:

The correct answer is B. Endomysial antibodies and tissue transglutaminase antibody serology.

Coeliac disease shares many common symptoms with other pathologies and usually requires endoscopy for definitive diagnosis. However, initial less invasive testing is required first, as simple blood tests can be effective in ruling out the disease.

A IgA serology – Incorrect. IgA antibodies alone will not diagnose coeliac disease. However, IgA deficiency may give falsely negative endomysial/tissue transglutaminase antibody results. Therefore if a strong clinical suspicion remains despite negative antibody testing, IgG antibodies should be checked.

B Endomysial antibodies and tissue transglutaminase antibody serology– Correct. Endomysial antibodies and tissue transglutaminase antibodies are produced by B-lymphocytes in the immune response to gliadin; therefore, these antibodies are the most specific markers of coeliac disease.

C Tissue transglutaminase antibody serology only – Incorrect. Although this is useful, when done in combination with endomysial antibodies, the sensitivity is higher.

D Food and symptom diary – Incorrect. A food and symptom diary, although helpful when the symptom history is unclear, will not show the immunological responses occurring in the disease and is therefore inadequate for diagnosis. Symptoms may not always correlate to the food being eaten as the immune response is a chronic process.

E Endoscopy and biopsy – Incorrect. Endoscopy and biopsy are highly invasive procedures that should not be carried out on everyone with the non-specific symptoms found in coeliac disease. Endoscopy should be used after blood tests to give a definitive diagnosis.

Key Point

Coeliac disease is an immune process in which a blood test looking for specific antibodies is the most appropriate initial investigation which can then be followed up by tissue biopsy on endoscopy.

Q4 Which condition has an association with coeliac disease?

The correct answer is A. Type 1 diabetes mellitus.

Coeliac disease is associated with many other conditions, particularly autoimmune disorders. Many of these, like Type 1 diabetes, have such a strong association that it merits routine screening for them in a new diagnosis of coeliac disease.

A Type 1 diabetes mellitus – Correct. Type 1 diabetes mellitus is another autoimmune condition that is linked to coeliac disease.

B Bacterial gastroenteritis – Incorrect. Bacterial gastroenteritis is an acute infection of the gut that has no association with the development of coeliac disease. However, rotavirus infection in children may increase the risk of developing coeliac disease.

C Cystic fibrosis – Incorrect. Cystic fibrosis is an inherited condition that has no association with coeliac disease.

D Irritable bowel syndrome – Incorrect. Irritable bowel syndrome is a diagnosis given to many patients when no cause can be found for their gastrointestinal symptoms. However it does not have any association with coeliac disease.

E Cow's milk protein intolerance – Incorrect. Cow's milk protein intolerance is common in infants but does not have any association with coeliac disease.

Key Point

Coeliac disease is associated with a number of autoimmune diseases due to both the genetic susceptibility required in autoimmune diseases and the link between HLA and autoimmune diseases.

424

IMPORTANT LEARNING POINTS

(i) IMPORTANT LEARNING POINTS

- Coeliac disease is an autoimmune condition characterised by an immune response to gliadin, found in wheat, barley and rye.
- It can be asymptomatic or it can present with non-specific symptoms, including weight loss, chronic diarrhoea, vomiting and abdominal pain.
- Blood tests for IgA endomysial antibodies and IgA tissue transglutaminase antibodies can be useful in detecting the disease and identifying individuals who require further testing.
- The majority of cases can be resolved by changing to a gluten-free diet. However, in some patients, a more severe, refractory coeliac disease can occur, which needs specialist input.
- The most important complications in children relate to malabsorption and associated failure to thrive. Long-term complications include nutritional deficiency, stunted growth and delayed milestones.

ANSWER TO CASE 28
A 2-month-old boy presenting with vomiting and diarrhoea

Q1 What is the most important differential diagnosis to exclude acutely in this case?

The correct answer is A. Meningitis.

The symptoms presented could represent any infection in a child less than 1-year-old. It is important to rule out serious infections and treat empirically if there is any suspicion of meningitis or septicaemia.

A Meningitis – Correct. Meningitis can present very non-specifically in children, particularly those under three-months-old. Therefore, when children under three-months-old present with a fever, they invariably undergo a lumbar puncture and are treated with broad spectrum antibiotics that have good CNS penetration.

B Pneumonia – Incorrect. This is a serious infection in young children that can be investigated using a chest X-ray. However there is no respiratory distress in this case.

C Crohn's disease – Incorrect. Crohn's disease tends to present in older children, with more chronic symptoms.

D Cow's milk protein intolerance – Incorrect. Cow's milk protein intolerance is not associated with a fever and is more likely to present with symptoms for a longer period.

E Toddler's diarrhoea – Incorrect. Toddler's diarrhoea occurs in well children and is not associated with vomiting or fever. It also occurs in an older age group than seen in this case.

♀ Key Point

In any child under 3-months-old with a temperature above 38°C, meningitis should be strongly suspected. A lumbar puncture is invariably performed if they are unwell, and broad spectrum antibiotics should be commenced.

Q2 Which group of children are most at risk of a severe gastrointestinal infection?

The correct answer is B. Under 6-months-old.

It is important to recognise children who are most at risk of developing severe infections, as they are likely to require hospital admission, IV fluids and antibiotics if their illness progresses.

A Over 1-year-old – Incorrect. Children under 5-years-old are more likely to get an infection. However, the risk of a severe infection decreases as the child gets older, even within the under-five age group.

B Under 6-months-old – Correct. Children under 6-months-old are more likely to get severe infections, as their immune systems are less developed and they have been exposed (i.e. developed immunity) to fewer pathogens. In this age group, identifying the source of the infection may also be difficult as the presentation is often non-specific.

C Those that have had recent contact with a relative who has food poisoning – Incorrect. Gastroenteritis caused by food poisoning is likely to have been transmitted from the food eaten by the relative, and as long as the child is not exposed to the same source, the risk of developing food poisoning is low.

D Those that have been previously treated for leukaemia – Incorrect. Whilst the child was being treated for leukaemia, they would have been immunosuppressed and at an increased risk of infection. However, once in remission, the risk would return to the same level as their peers.

♀ Key Point

Gastroenteritis tends to be a self-limiting condition. However, in children under 6-months-old and in children who are immunosuppressed, this simple infection can become serious and require hospital admission.

Q3 Which of the symptoms or signs below are red flags for dehydration?

The correct answers are A. Altered consciousness, C. Tachycardia, and D. Tachypnoea.

Assessing dehydration in gastroenteritis is very important in deciding whether the child can be treated at home or needs hospital admission. Dehydration also requires treatment with fluids either with ORS or with IV fluids.

A Altered consciousness – Correct. Altered consciousness can be assessed both on clinical history and examination. The parents may express that the child seems more lethargic or irritable than normal, and on examination the child may be difficult to rouse.

B Dry mucous membranes – Incorrect. Dry mucous membranes are a sign of dehydration. However, in children who tend to breathe through their mouths, mucous membranes can be dry without dehydration being the cause.

C Tachycardia – Correct. Tachycardia is a "red flag" sign that should be recorded in the examination of the patient.

D Tachypnoea – Correct. Tachypnoea is a "red flag" sign that is present in dehydration as well as other conditions.

⚥ Key Point

Red flag symptoms are important in measuring the severity of dehydration from gastroenteritis. However, be aware that many red flags are non-specific, with many overlapping with sepsis. Therefore, the very unwell child with dehydration should be carefully assessed for signs of shock and its possible causes.

ⓘ IMPORTANT LEARNING POINTS

- Gastroenteritis is usually a mild, self-resolving condition that can be managed at home.
- It is important to consider meningitis in any pyrexial patient if they are under three-months-old and if there is no clear focus.
- The main symptoms of gastroenteritis are diarrhoea and vomiting. Other symptoms include abdominal pain and poor feeding.
- Gastroenteritis is most likely to be caused by a virus. However, bacterial and protozoal infections can also occur.
- In patients who are dehydrated but tolerating fluids, ORS should be used to rehydrate the patient. If the patient stops tolerating fluids, NG or IV fluids may have to be initiated.

ANSWER TO CASE 29
A 6-week-old girl presenting with vomiting and distress after feeds

Q1 What is the most likely diagnosis in this case?

The correct answer is B. Gastro-oesophageal reflux disease.

The symptoms presented of vomiting and distress after feeds, with the background of normal weight gain, make gastro-oesophageal reflux disease (GORD) the most likely diagnosis. It is important in such a young child to consider infection as the cause of vomiting and to ensure that there is no evidence of intestinal obstruction.

A Gastroenteritis – Incorrect. This infective cause of vomiting would have an acute presentation. It is important to check for fever and a history of diarrhoea.

B Gastro-oesophageal reflux disease – Correct. Chronic vomiting after feeds, accompanied with crying, makes this the most likely diagnosis. Good weight gain shows that some digestion is occurring, and in this case, the parents may be overfeeding as well. Back arching is associated with oesophagitis secondary to reflux.

C Pyloric stenosis – Incorrect. Pyloric stenosis presents with projectile vomiting after feeds, and although she is in the correct age range, the vomiting in this case was not forceful. The child with pyloric stenosis is also more likely to be clinically unwell.

D Cow's milk protein intolerance – Incorrect. This may present with vomiting and discomfort. However, back arching isn't expected. Cow's milk protein intolerance can also present with lower GI symptoms or colic. As the baby has been bottle fed from birth and symptoms started only two weeks ago, cow's milk protein intolerance is less likely.

E Infantile colic – Incorrect. Infantile colic presents with inconsolable crying, whereas, in this case, the main complaint is vomiting.

⚥ Key Point

Gastro-oesophageal reflux disease is common in young children and classically presents with non-forceful vomiting and distress after feeds.

Q2 Regarding the likely diagnosis, mark the following statements true or false.

The assessment and management of an infant with GORD should be focused on providing the correct advice for parents and trying to manage the condition non-pharmacologically at first. If this fails, then pharmacological and eventually surgical management can be considered.

A The parents can be reassured that it is likely to self-resolve with age – True. GORD is a common condition in infants that normally resolves as the diet becomes more solid, as the child spends more time in an upright position and as the oesophageal sphincter tone matures.

B Investigations should always be carried out to rule out a more serious disorder – False. Investigations are rarely required in GORD and should only be performed if the symptoms are severe; e.g. weight loss, failure to gain weight or after unsuccessful pharmacological treatment.

C Thickening feeds may be useful – True. One pharmacological solution for GORD is to add a thickener to the feeds so reflux is less likely.

D It is a lifelong condition with multiple complications – False. While GORD can last into adolescence and adulthood, most cases resolve by 2-years-old.

E Surgery is never required – False. In severe GORD, where pharmacological interventions have failed, fundoplication may be considered as a treatment. However, fundoplication has a high failure rate and a high level of morbidity.

Key Point

GORD is common in infancy and parents should be advised that their child is likely to grow out of it. However, in some severe cases, medications and surgery may be required.

Q3 What is the most appropriate investigation in a mild case of this disease?

The correct answer is E. None of the above; diagnosis is based on clinical history and examination.

In GORD, investigations are rarely required as the diagnosis should be made from clinical history and examination. Investigations should be used to exclude differential diagnoses in situations where the diagnosis is unclear or pharmacological treatments have failed.

A Oesophageal pH monitoring – Incorrect. Whilst pH monitoring can confirm this diagnosis, this invasive test is unnecessary in mild cases where there is already clinical suspicion of GORD.

B Barium meal – Incorrect. This test used to be one of the main investigations but is less commonly performed now. It is helpful to exclude other causes of vomiting, such as malrotation.

C Upper gastrointestinal endoscopy – Incorrect. This test would be used if biopsies were needed to rule out oesophagitis or if any anatomical abnormality was suspected.

D Full blood count – Incorrect. A full blood count can be used in GORD to assess anaemia from malabsorption of iron, vitamin B_{12} or folate.

E None of the above; diagnosis is based on clinical history and examination – Correct. A diagnosis of mild gastro-oesophageal reflux disease should be made on the basis of clinical history and examination, and the appropriate advice should then be given to the parents.

Key Point

Gastro-oesophageal reflux disease can usually be diagnosed on the basis of clinical history and examination alone.

> ⓘ **IMPORTANT LEARNING POINTS**
>
> - Gastro-oesophageal reflux disease usually resolves as the child develops and grows older, due to changes in diet and activity, and improvement in sphincter tone.
> - The main symptoms are vomiting and distress after feeds, which may be accompanied by behavioural signs of abdominal pain, including drawing up of the knees and back arching.
> - It can usually be diagnosed on the basis of clinical history and examination alone, although investigations may be required where there is diagnostic doubt or in severe cases.
> - Management of mild gastro-oesophageal reflux involves advice to parents about overfeeding and instruction on positioning the child after feeds.
> - More severe cases may require treatment with feed thickeners, antacids, H_2-receptor antagonists and proton pump inhibitors, with specialist support.

ANSWER TO CASE 30
A 12-year-old boy presenting with weight loss and abdominal pain

Q1 What is the most likely diagnosis?

The correct answer is D. Inflammatory bowel disease.

The history provided followed by examination and investigations make inflammatory bowel disease (IBD) the most likely diagnosis. However, important diagnoses, such as appendicitis, should be excluded as there is a high risk of perforation and further complications.

A Gastroenteritis – Incorrect. This is an infective cause of abdominal pain and diarrhoea with an acute presentation. It is unlikely in this case, due to the chronicity of the symptoms presented.

B Appendicitis – Incorrect. This is an important differential to exclude, especially with right iliac fossa tenderness and an elevated CRP. However, vomiting would be more likely than loose stools, and the child with appendicitis is unlikely to present with weight loss, chronic abdominal pain, anaemia and low albumin.

C Mesenteric adenitis – Incorrect. Mesenteric adenitis has an acute presentation and often presents after an URTI.

D Inflammatory bowel disease – Correct. This is the most likely explanation for the child's symptoms, based on the chronic nature, systemic effects and biochemical results showing anaemia and inflammation.

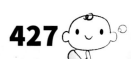

E Coeliac disease – Incorrect. This is an important differential diagnosis to exclude. The predominant symptoms in coeliac disease tend to be non-specific and are unlikely to involve tenderness in the right iliac fossa.

♀ Key Point

IBD tends to present in older children, with an insidious course and a mixture of gastrointestinal and systemic symptoms.

Q2 What one further investigation is most important to confirm the likely diagnosis?

The correct answer is B. Colonoscopy.

In IBD, definitive diagnosis relies on endoscopic and biopsy findings, which are obtained via colonoscopy or sigmoidoscopy. In Crohn's disease, biopsy reveals transmural inflammation and non-caseating granulomas. On endoscopy, there are skip lesions (discontinuous sites of pathology), the mucosa has a cobblestone appearance and there is fat wrapping of the intestine. In ulcerative colitis (UC), biopsy reveals mucosal and submucosal inflammation, with no granulomas, and distorted glands. On endoscopy, the disease is continuous, with crypt abscesses, and mucosal ulceration.

A Flexible sigmoidoscopy – Incorrect. Flexible sigmoidoscopy is useful in UC where the sigmoid colon and rectum are very inflamed and the risk of perforation is high. In the context of these clinical findings, ileocaecal involvement is likely; therefore, visualisation beyond the sigmoid colon is required.

B Colonoscopy – Correct. A colonoscopy allows the clinician to directly visualise the colon and take biopsies. As the tenderness is in the right iliac fossa, a colonoscopy is going to be the only method of directly visualising the ileocaecal valve.

C Antibody testing – Incorrect. Although some antibodies have been associated with IBD, the test sensitivity is low.

D Urea and electrolytes – Incorrect. Urea and electrolytes are useful if the patient is suspected to be fluid depleted or if fluids are to be given to the patient and the electrolyte balance needs to be known. In this case, the child is not dehydrated and fluids are unlikely to be prescribed.

E Faecal calprotectin – Incorrect. Although this is elevated in IBD, it is not diagnostic.

♀ Key Point

The best imaging should allow direct visualisation of the pathological parts of the bowel, while allowing biopsies to be taken for histological analysis.

ⓘ IMPORTANT LEARNING POINTS

- IBD is a lifelong condition that has a characteristic remitting-relapsing course.
- The main symptoms are abdominal pain, weight loss, failure to thrive and diarrhoea.
- Investigations should rule out important differential diagnoses and check for anaemia and malabsorption.
- Management of IBD involves patient education, inducing remission and maintaining remission.
- IBD is associated with long-term complications, such as colorectal cancer and osteoporosis.

ANSWER TO CASE 31
A pregnant lady with concerns about Down syndrome

Q1 In the UK, what are the components of the screening test that this pregnant woman is offered?

The correct answer is A. Nuchal translucency scan, β-hCG, PAPP-A.

Down syndrome is a genetic disorder caused by an autosomal chromosome abnormality leading to trisomy 21. It can result in complex medical conditions and learning difficulties. Antenatal screening is offered to all pregnant women in the UK. The antenatal screening for Down syndrome gives a woman a risk score which takes into account her age and can lead to further antenatal diagnostic testing.

A Nuchal translucency scan, β-hCG, PAPP-A – Correct. These three tests make up the combined screening test and should be offered to pregnant women between 11 and 13 weeks gestation. This is the most accurate test.

B β-hCG, uE3, AFP, Inhibin-A – Incorrect. These tests make up the quadruple test, which is offered if women present for screening after 13 weeks or if the combined test cannot be performed. The quadruple test is not as accurate as the combined test.

C Nuchal translucency scan, β-hCG – Incorrect. These are just two of the tests that make up the combined test and therefore would not be used for a full assessment of the risk of Down syndrome in pregnancy.

D Chorionic villus sampling – Incorrect. This is a diagnostic test, not a screening test. It can be used after the screening test if a high risk of Down syndrome is suspected. Complications include infection, miscarriage and heavy bleeding. The risk of miscarriage is about 1 in 100.

E Amniocentesis – Incorrect. This is the other diagnostic test that can be used after screening in pregnancies considered as high risk. Complications include infection and miscarriage. The risk of miscarriage in amniocentesis is also about 1 in 100.

♀ Key Point

Antenatal screening is available for Down syndrome. Screening calculates the probability of the foetus having Down syndrome. If the pregnancy is considered as high risk, the pregnant woman is offered antenatal diagnostic testing with chorionic villus sampling or amniocentesis. However, these procedures both have a risk of miscarriage.

Q2 In this case, what is her biggest risk factor for Down syndrome?

The correct answer is B. Older maternal age.

The most likely cause of Down syndrome is nondisjunction of chromosomes during meiosis, and the likelihood of this increases with maternal age. Other causes are an unbalanced Robertsonian translocation (involving chromosome 21) and mosaicism.

A Full term pregnancy – Incorrect. The length of the pregnancy has no impact on the development of Down syndrome, as Down syndrome is a genetic condition present from the moment of conception.
B Older maternal age – Correct. Oocytes in ovaries are arrested in the prophase stage of meiosis 1 for storage. When they mature and are ready for ovulation, the oocyte completes meiosis. As a woman ages, the chromosomes within the oocyte are less likely to split evenly into the gametes, forming some gametes with two of a particular chromosome and others with none. When fertilisation occurs, this can lead to 47 chromosomes in the fertilised egg rather than 46. If the trisomy affects chromosome 21, the resulting infant will have Down syndrome.
C Multiparity – Incorrect. The number of children does not increase the risk of Down syndrome.
D Previous child with autistic spectrum disorder – Incorrect. ASD leads to impairments in social interactions, communication and stereotyped behaviour. ASD is thought to be an acquired condition and is not linked to an increased risk of a subsequent child having Down syndrome or any other genetic syndrome. Nonetheless, this family may have difficulty coping with two children with learning difficulties.
E Previous smoking history – Incorrect. A previous smoking history is not associated with a higher risk of having a child with Down syndrome.

♀ Key Point

The risk of having a child with Down syndrome is increased in advanced maternal age, due to an increased rate of nondisjunction in meiosis. Note that paternal age also increases the risk.

Q3 What services should be involved in the care of patients with Down syndrome? Select all that apply.

The correct answers are A. Speech and Language Therapy, B. Physiotherapy, C. Paediatrician follow-up, D. Social services, and E. Dieticians.

Down syndrome requires a multidisciplinary care approach, predominantly managed in a community setting.

A Speech and Language Therapy – Correct. Speech and language therapy are important in managing difficulties in sucking or swallowing identified at birth through to managing communication difficulties in older age groups.
B Physiotherapy – Correct. Physiotherapy can help children with Down syndrome as development milestones for motor functions may be delayed and mobility can be restricted due to hypotonia and laxity in ligaments.
C Paediatrician follow-up – Correct. Children are often under the care of a community paediatrician who coordinates care and ensures that complications of Down syndrome are investigated and managed appropriately.
D Social services – Correct. Social care is important to ensure that families receive the support they need. Social services may also be useful for the child to help find supportive housing in adulthood.
E Dieticians – Correct. Children with Down syndrome are likely to become obese. Therefore, early input with dieticians can help children and their families reduce the likelihood of later obesity.

♀ Key Point

Down syndrome is associated with many complications and a multidisciplinary team approach is required to manage its medical, psychological and social effects.

ⓘ IMPORTANT LEARNING POINTS

- Down syndrome is the most common chromosomal abnormality with multiple physical characteristics and an increased prevalence of learning disabilities.
- Features include characteristic facies, with up-slanting palpebral fissures and epicanthic folds, an enlarged protruding tongue, hypotonia and singular palmar creases.
- Antenatal screening is offered to all pregnant women. The combined screening test is the most accurate and is offered to women who are 11 to 13 weeks pregnant. It involves an ultrasound scan and two blood tests.
- Infants can also be diagnosed at birth and chromosomal karyotyping should be carried out on all babies where there is high clinical suspicion of Down syndrome.
- Complications can present at birth, including congenital heart defects, gastrointestinal atresias and hypothyroidism, or they can present later in life, including type 1 diabetes and coeliac disease.
- Management involves coordinating care and ensuring that referrals to appropriate services are made as required, as well as screening and investigation for any complications of Down syndrome.

ANSWER TO CASE 32
A 9-year-old boy with acute onset testicular pain

Q1 What is the next step in the management of this child?

The correct answer is D. Refer to the surgical team (paediatric if available) to organise an urgent scrotal exploration, despite inadequate fasting.

An urgent surgical exploration, with rapid untwisting of the torsioned spermatic cord, is the only treatment that will save the testis. This procedure should therefore be performed as soon as possible. Any other investigations are of limited diagnostic value and will delay the start of this time-critical intervention.

A An USS of his scrotum to visualise testicular blood flow – Incorrect. An USS cannot rule out testicular torsion. Whilst specificity is close to 99%, the sensitivity is only 89%. Therefore the decision to treat should be based on the history and the examination, not the scan result.

B Commence IV antibiotics to treat possible epididymo-orchitis – Incorrect. The most likely diagnosis for this child is testicular torsion. Antibiotics are not administered pre-operatively, as torsion does not have an infectious component.

C Contact the anaesthetic team after the child has been appropriately fasted – Incorrect. As treatment of testicular torsion is time critical, the anaesthetic team needs to urgently assess this child and perform a rapid sequence induction to minimise the risk of aspiration.

D Refer to the surgical team (paediatric if available) to organise an urgent scrotal exploration, despite inadequate fasting – Correct. The only treatment for this condition is urgent surgical exploration with untwisting of the twisted blood vessels. This will allow reperfusion of the testis and might – if done within six hours of onset – save the viability of this testis.

E Prescribe analgesia, anti-emetics and scrotal support, and ask the family to come to the next available clinic appointment – Incorrect. None of these measures will treat the underlying condition. Adequate pain relief will be established once the testis is untwisted and the ischaemic pain dissipates. The same applies for vomiting, which occurs secondary to severe pain and vagal stimulation. If the testis has twisted, it will become non-viable within six hours.

⚲ Key Point

A child with acute onset testicular pain has acute torsion until proven otherwise.

Q2 Mark the following statements true or false.

A Testicular torsion is not related to trauma – False. Approximately 4-8% of all cases of testicular torsion are attributable to a preceding blunt trauma and a scrotal exploration should be performed without delay. The differential diagnosis is a testicular haematoma or testicular rupture.

B Doppler USS is 100% sensitive and 100% specific in the diagnosis of testicular torsion – False. Whilst the specificity of Doppler USS for testicular torsion is close to 99%, the sensitivity of the test is only 89%. This means that an USS is not always reliable to rule out testicular torsion. Decisions should be based on clinical assessment.

C At six hours post-torsion, approximately 85% of testes will survive – False. The salvage rate is close to 100% if the procedure is performed within six hours of onset of pain. This drops to less than 50% after six hours and to under 20% after 12 hours.

D Following operative detorsion of a twisted testis, the contralateral testis should undergo fixation – True. In theory, if the patient has abnormal testicular lie (congenital bell clapper deformity), this is present bilaterally. Therefore, the contralateral testis will be at high risk of torsion. It is necessary to fix the contralateral side once the diagnosis is established.

E If a paediatric orchidectomy is necessary, implantation of a suitable prosthesis should be carried out during the same operation – False. First, following orchidectomy for testicular torsion, the area is inflamed and swollen. This significantly increases the risk of infection. Second, a testicular prosthesis is a permanent fixture. It is important to wait until the child has reached puberty and his testis has reached its full adult size so the prosthesis is size matched.

⚲ Key Point

Once one testis has twisted, it is more likely for the contralateral side to twist as well. Standard practice is therefore to fix both sides once the diagnosis has been confirmed.

ⓘ IMPORTANT LEARNING POINTS

- In suspected testicular torsion, surgical referral should occur as quickly as possible, with a view to surgical exploration.
- The differential diagnosis for an acute painful scrotum includes:
  - Testicular torsion
  - Torsion of the hydatid of Morgagni
  - Epididymo-orchitis
  - Scrotal haematoma (if following trauma)
  - Testicular rupture (if following trauma)
  - Idiopathic scrotal oedema (if the scrotum is erythematous and oedematous, but relatively non-tender)

ANSWER TO CASE 33
A 2-month-old presenting with irritability and shortness of breath

Q1 Which of the following investigations is most useful in assessing the cause of the tachycardia?

The correct answer is A. ECG/cardiac monitoring.

All the tests suggested are potentially helpful, but the most important diagnostic test is an ECG. The patient is tachycardic and may have an infection, based on the history. However, the HR is much higher than expected, increasing the suspicion of an arrhythmia.

A   ECG/cardiac monitoring – Correct. This child has profound tachycardia in the absence of significant compromise. An ECG is a quick and effective method of determining the underlying cardiac rhythm.

B   Echocardiogram – Incorrect. It is often useful to obtain an echocardiogram to ensure there are no underlying structural causes for an arrhythmia, but it will not change the immediate management. In most units, an echocardiogram is not available immediately and the first priority should be stabilisation and treatment of the patient.

C   Arterial blood gas – Incorrect. An arterial blood gas would show an elevated lactate/low pH in significant cardiovascular compromise, but it will not give a diagnosis.

D   Chest X-ray – Incorrect. This is another useful investigation to check for signs of heart failure or other chest pathology, but again, it will not pick up an arrhythmia.

E   Blood glucose – Incorrect. Although it is important to routinely check a child's blood glucose in an emergency, this is neither the classic presentation of diabetic ketoacidosis nor of hypoglycaemia.

♀ Key Point

Always assess HR in the clinical context. If there isn't a clear secondary cause of tachycardia or the tachycardia is greater than expected, the likelihood of a primary cardiac cause is increased.

Q2 Which of the following rhythms is most likely with the above presentation?

The correct answer is D. Supraventricular tachycardia.

Supraventricular tachycardias are narrow complex tachycardias and the most commonly encountered tachyarrhythmia in children. They are most commonly caused by re-entry circuits within the heart which, in severe cases, may require cardiac ablation.

A   Ventricular tachycardia (VT) – Incorrect. This is a broad complex tachycardia originating in the ventricular myocardium. VT always requires immediate action. It is unlikely in this patient, as the baby is clinically relatively stable.

B   Ventricular fibrillation (VF) – Incorrect. This rhythm is characterised by utter disorganisation of ventricular waves on ECG and no ventricular contraction. VF is never seen in a stable patient, as the patient would rapidly become severely compromised.

C   Atrial fibrillation (AF) – Incorrect. AF is an irregular rhythm with an absence of discrete P waves. It is a specific type of supraventricular tachycardia caused by the atria oscillating and creating fibrilliform waveforms. Although this fits with the clinical presentation, atrial fibrillation is not common in the paediatric age group.

D   Supraventricular tachycardia (SVT) – Correct. SVT is a narrow complex re-entry tachycardia. It is characterised by lack of variability in HR (which would normally change with respiration and movement) and absent or abnormal P waves. Supraventricular tachycardia can present with non-specific symptoms and in patients who are otherwise relatively well. The key clue here is the degree of tachycardia, which is disproportionate to other parameters.

E   Sinus tachycardia – Incorrect. This is an increased HR with normal P wave morphology. This indicates an extra-cardiac cause for tachycardia and will be resolved when the cause is found and treated. Common causes include volume depletion and hypotension, sepsis, hyperthyroidism and anaemia. In this case, although sinus tachycardia is possible, the HR is much greater than would be expected.

♀ Key Point

Ventricular tachycardias are associated with severe compromise, and any patient in ventricular fibrillation will be in cardiac arrest.

Q3 What would be the initial treatment for the likely diagnosis?

The correct answer is E. Vagal manoeuvres.

Although the patient is currently unwell, he is stable; therefore, simple measures should be used initially. All the answers below (except eyeball pressure) are potentially part of the algorithm for managing an SVT, and it is important to be aware of them.

A   Synchronised DC cardioversion – Incorrect. This would be used later in the management if vagal manoeuvres and medical management were ineffective. It may be used secondarily to vagal manoeuvres if obtaining IV or IO access is delayed.

B   Amiodarone – Incorrect. This would be a second-line antiarrhythmic medicine and would be used following failure of vagal manoeuvres and no response to adenosine or DC cardioversion. It works by inhibiting adrenergic stimulation (alpha and beta blocking properties) and by decreasing AV conduction by prolonging the refractory period in myocardial tissue.

C Adenosine – Incorrect. This would generally be the first-line antiarrhythmic agent following vagal manoeuvres, but vagal manoeuvres should be attempted first. Adenosine works by slowing conduction through the AV node. Its onset of action is swift, and its duration is extremely short.

D Eyeball pressure – Incorrect. This is NEVER recommended in children, due to the high risk of sustaining ocular damage.

E Vagal manoeuvres – Correct. This patient is not cardiovascularly compromised at present, so vagal manoeuvres (e.g. a cold stimulus to the face) should be attempted prior to any medical therapy.

⚷ Key Point

In relatively well patients with SVTs, vagal manoeuvres should always be attempted before giving medications or attempting DC cardioversion.

ⓘ IMPORTANT LEARNING POINTS

- Sinus tachycardia is much more common than primary cardiac arrhythmias.
- SVTs are initially managed by vagal manoeuvres, but may require adenosine or DC cardioversion if severe or refractory to conservative treatment.
- After treatment and stabilisation, always repeat the ECG. There may an underlying, treatable cardiac abnormality (like Wolff-Parkinson-White syndrome) that could put the patient at long-term risk.

ANSWER TO CASE 34
A 7-year-old presenting with a murmur and fever

Q1 For each of the following clinical examination findings, choose one diagnosis which is the most likely from the list below:

A Systolic murmur heard over the right, second intercostal space, radiating to the carotids

The correct answer is v. Aortic stenosis.

This is the classical murmur of aortic stenosis, which accounts for approximately 6% of all congenital heart defects in children.

B Diastolic murmur with "opening snap" best heard at the apex, with no radiation.

The correct answer is vi. Mitral stenosis.

This is the classical murmur of mitral stenosis, a thickening or rolling of the mitral valve leaflets. Most cases of mitral stenosis are secondary to infection with rheumatic fever. In high income countries (such as the UK) with a very low prevalence of rheumatic fever, mitral stenosis may be congenital. Congenital mitral stenosis is associated with further congenital malformations of the heart.

C Systolic murmur best heard in the left second intercostal space, radiating to the centre of the back.

The correct answer is iii. Pulmonary stenosis.

This is the classical murmur for pulmonary stenosis, most often caused by thickened pulmonary valve leaflets.

D A continuous "machinery-like" murmur best heard over the left upper sternal edge.

The correct answer is ii. Patent ductus arteriosus.

This is the classical murmur heard in a child with a patent ductus arteriosus: a condition where the connection between the pulmonary artery and descending aorta, needed in utero, is still patent after birth.

E Soft systolic murmur heard over the left second intercostal space, varying in intensity on movement and deep breathing.

The correct answer is viii. Benign flow murmur.

Innocent murmurs are often heard in children when they are in a hyperdynamic state (e.g. febrile, with increased cardiac output).

⚷ Key Point

Innocent murmurs can be remembered by the seven S's: short, systolic, sweet (not harsh), swinging (variable in intensity), small (limited to a small area), single (no clicks or gallops), sensitive (changes with position).

Q2 You suspect infective endocarditis. What investigation(s) is/are essential to complete before treatment is commenced?

The correct answer is A. At least three separate sets of blood cultures.

A At least three separate sets of blood cultures – Correct. It is vital to take multiple blood cultures in patients suspected of suffering from infective endocarditis. A major criterion for diagnosis is a positive blood culture with typical bacteria (Viridans streptococci, *Streptococcus bovis*), HACEK group (*Haemophilus, Actinobacillus, Cardiobacterium hominis, Eikenella corrodens* and *Kingella*), *Staphylococcus aureus* or *enterococci* without primary focus. Antibiotic penetrance and efficacy can be difficult when treating infective endocarditis, so it is important to know the sensitivities of the organisms before starting treatment.

B Ophthalmology review to look for retinal emboli – Incorrect. Retinal emboli can be a feature of infective endocarditis, and any child in whom this diagnosis is suspected should have their fundi assessed, but this is not vital prior to commencing antibiotic therapy.

C ECG – Incorrect. Although important to assess for any conduction deficits in infective endocarditis, performing an ECG is not vital before treatment is started. It is usually done anyway, as it is a simple test.

D Echocardiogram – Incorrect. Although an echocardiogram aids the diagnosis of infective endocarditis, treatment may be commenced prior to obtaining this. The scan findings will not change immediately following treatment.

E Lung function testing – Incorrect. Lung function tests are not indicated in infective endocarditis.

Key Point

Diagnosis of infective endocarditis is reliant on blood culture results. As such, a minimum of three sets of blood cultures should be taken before starting antibiotic therapy.

Q3 Your team suspects a diagnosis of infective endocarditis. Which of the following is/are parts of the Modified Duke's criteria for diagnosing infective endocarditis and is/are essential to complete before treatment is commenced?

The correct answers are A. β haemolytic streptococci positive blood cultures, B. Temperature >38°C, and C. Predisposing cardiac condition.

Infective endocarditis is an infection of the heart valves and/ or endocardium, often associated with valvular vegetations and/or thrombus formation. It is notoriously difficult to diagnose and, although rare in children, should be excluded in a child with pyrexia of unknown origin. Clinicians use the modified Duke's criteria to guide diagnoses of infective endocarditis (p31). Although a recent dental procedure may be an event during which bacteria enter the blood stream, it is not a criteria for diagnosis. Splinter haemorrhages occur from micro-emboli originating from the cardiac vegetation. Although often present in infective endocarditis, they are rare in children, are non-specific and do not alone form a criterion for diagnosis.

(i) IMPORTANT LEARNING POINTS

- Innocent murmurs do not require further investigations and will usually disappear with time. Diastolic murmurs are never innocent murmurs.
- A flow murmur is a common innocent murmur. This is often secondary to infection, anaemia or dehydration, but the child should always be followed up to ensure the murmur has disappeared.
- Pathological murmurs always warrant further investigations with an echocardiogram.
- Infective endocarditis is a risk for all children, especially those with valvular heart lesions. If suspected, it is vital to send off at least three sets of blood cultures before starting antibiotics.

ANSWER TO CASE 35
A 4-month-old boy presenting with a possible UTI

Q1 Assuming no imaging studies have been performed, which of the following tests would be most useful to do first?

The correct answer is C. Renal USS.

The evaluation of UTIs in children requires:

1. *Accurate diagnosis often with limited, non-specific clinical history available, particularly in neonates.*
2. *Awareness that this may be the first presentation of congenital anomalies of the kidneys or urinary tract, such as dysplastic kidneys, vesico-ureteric reflux or posterior urethral valves that increase the risk of infection.*
3. *Careful consideration of potential complications of infection such as renal scarring.*

This patient has clear evidence of a UTI, as evidenced by two pure growths of E. coli in the urine, with an associated elevated urinary WCC. It is an atypical urinary tract infection, because although this organism is a common cause of UTIs, the patient has failed to respond to antibiotics after 48 hours. NICE guidelines (p306) would suggest that this scenario requires an acute USS, and both an MCUG and a DMSA scan should be strongly considered once the acute infection has resolved.

A MCUG – Incorrect. This contrast scan evaluates the presence of structural abnormalities (such as posterior urethral valves) and vesico-ureteric reflux. In an atypical UTI, it is important to consider vesico-ureteric reflux as the cause, as it may increase the risk of future infections. However, it should be performed after the acute infection has resolved, as it will not significantly alter acute management.

B DMSA – Incorrect. This radionuclide scan evaluates renal function. It can be used acutely to delineate pyelonephritis from cystitis, but acute changes can resolve as the infection is treated. The recommendations are to wait for three to six months following acute infection to evaluate potential renal scarring.

C Renal USS – Correct. USS will show anatomical abnormalities, such as hydroureteronephrosis (which may be due to posterior urethral valves in boys, for which an ablation procedure would be needed). Prophylactic antibiotics may also be initiated, depending on the abnormality identified.

D Abdominal X-ray – Incorrect. This is not indicated in further evaluation of a UTI, although it may potentially be useful in detecting radiolucent calculi if nephrolithiasis is suspected.

E CT-KUB – Incorrect. Although a CT-KUB would provide sophisticated imaging of the kidney and the renal tract, the radiation exposure limits its use to isolated cases of suspected renal trauma or renal calculi.

Key Point

UTIs in children less than 3-months-old or acutely unwell should be taken very seriously and they invariably need admission to hospital, intravenous antibiotics and further investigations. Male infants with posterior urethral valves can present with UTIs, although some cases are diagnosed in utero due to antenatal ultrasound scanning.

Q2 Which of the following would most strongly suggest an atypical UTI (rather than a typical UTI)?

The correct answer is D. Abdominal or bladder mass.

It is important to evaluate whether an infection is an atypical UTI, since this may mean more serious pathology and suggest a need for further evaluation.

A Failure to respond to 24 hours of antibiotics – Incorrect. A 48-hour trial of antibiotics would be needed before determining an atypical infection, as it can take up to two days to see a response to therapy.

B A pure growth of *E. coli* (10^5 organisms/mL) – Incorrect. *E. coli* is frequently seen in UTIs; therefore, isolating *E. coli* by itself does not merit further investigation.

C A mixed growth of organisms in two separate urine samples – Incorrect. A mixed growth indicates a likely contaminant; therefore, if a UTI is still suspected, another urine sample should be sent. Ensure that this is a clean catch sample to minimise the risk of contamination again and that the sample is taken directly to the microbiology laboratory without delay. This is a common problem with primary care or out-of-hours samples, as the delay between collection and analysis can lead to artefactual increases in organism counts.

D Abdominal or bladder mass – Correct. This indicates possible significant pathology. For example, the mass could be a multicystic dysplastic kidney, severe hydronephrosis or an unusual tumour.

E CRP of 64 mg/L – Incorrect. A high baseline CRP does not suggest an atypical infection. However, it is a useful marker of response to treatment on subsequent blood tests. Other concerns of an atypical UTI would be renal dysfunction, as this indicates either baseline renal pathology or acute kidney injury secondary to the UTI.

Key Point

Take the time to ensure that the best possible urine sample is collected. In older children, a mid-stream urine sample should be collected. In babies, a clean catch sample should be collected, or if that fails an "in-out catheter", or a suprapubic aspiration under ultrasound guidance can be used. Once the sample is collected, it should be sent to the laboratory as soon as possible to avoid inaccurate results.

Q3 Which of the following increases the likelihood of a urine sample being contaminated?

The correct answer is C. "Pad" sample being taken (compared to a clean catch sample).

Assessing whether a urine sample shows an infection or is a contaminant requires evaluation of the following:

a) *Mechanism by which the sample was obtained*
b) *Presence of WBC and epithelial cells in the urine*
c) *Quantity and name of the organism(s) that grow(s) on culture*
d) *Replication of result by a second urine sample taken concurrently*
e) *Time taken to get the sample to the laboratory.*

In general, a clean catch sample, with no epithelial cells, an elevated WCC, leukocytes/nitrites on a dipstick and a pure growth of one organism in multiple urine bottles will strongly suggest a UTI.

A No epithelial cells reported on microscopy (compared to epithelial cells being present) – Incorrect. Epithelial cells are contaminants that should not normally be present in significant amounts in the urine. Therefore, if epithelial cells are present, the sample is more likely to be contaminated.

B WCC 3+ being reported on microscopy (compared to white cells not being present) – Incorrect. An elevated WCC suggests an inflammatory response in the urine, which could potentially be caused by a UTI. It can also be a sign of glomerulonephritis.

C "Pad" sample being taken (compared to a clean catch sample) – Correct. Pad samples are liable to contamination from the perineal area and from the genitalia, although sterile pads which are removed as soon as micturition has occurred reduce the risk of contamination.

D Pure growth of a single organism (compared to mixed growth of several organisms) – Incorrect. This is suggestive of an infection with a single organism; therefore, this makes a contaminant less likely. Contamination from skin/faeces usually contain multiple organisms: this reflects the organisms normally present at that site.

E The same organism grown in two separate urine samples (compared to being grown in just one sample) – Incorrect. The same contaminant is unlikely to grow in two separate "contaminated" samples; therefore, this makes a contaminant less likely.

F The presence of both nitrites and leukocytes on a dipstick (compared to neither or just one) – Incorrect. Leukocytes and nitrites increase the likelihood of a UTI being present, particularly when both are positive.

Key Point

The urine dipstick itself is less reliable in babies than it is in adults. First, it is more difficult to get clean catch specimens, and other methods of obtaining urine are liable to contamination. Second, nitrites are less likely to be positive in children who are not yet continent of urine. This is because in order for bacteria to produce nitrites, urine has to be held in the bladder for at least 30 minutes. Therefore, initial microscopy results are very important to consider.

(i) IMPORTANT LEARNING POINTS

• UTIs are usually mild and respond well to short courses of oral antibiotics.

• The diagnosis can only be confirmed by urine cultures, although be wary of misleading results due to contamination. Clean catch specimens minimise the risk of false positives.

• For inpatients, it is important to follow up the results of any urine culture tests. It is very common for these results to be missed, leading to patients continuing on ineffective antibiotics, despite a test result demonstrating antibiotic resistance.

• In cases with severe, recurrent or atypical infections, be aware of possible complications and the need for further investigations.

ANSWER TO CASE 36
A 9-year-old boy presenting with primary nocturnal enuresis

Q1 Which of the following would you want to do in further assessing this child?

The correct answers are A. Full abdominal examination, B. Ask about John's fluid intake, C. Plot height and weight, D. Dipstick urine, and E. Take a social history and find out how John is getting on at school.

Nocturnal enuresis or bedwetting describes the involuntary wetting that can occur during sleep. The causes of bedwetting are not fully understood. They can include sleep arousal difficulties, polyuria and bladder dysfunction, and often bedwetting can run in families. Bedwetting has a negative impact on self-esteem; therefore, its treatment is very important for both the physical and mental wellbeing of the child.

A Full abdominal examination – Correct. This would be an important step in assessing the child for organic causes. Although the child may claim to have a normal bowel habit, palpable faeces may indicate constipation as the underlying cause of urinary incontinence.

B Ask about John's fluid intake – Correct. It would be important to do this, to check that John is not drinking excessively at night, or that he is not restricting his fluid intake in an attempt to stop the bedwetting. Fluid intake should be adequate and should vary depending on time of day, ambient temperature and amount of physical activity. Regular toileting should be encouraged and children should avoid caffeinated drinks.

C Plot height and weight – Correct. This is important to do during any consultation with a child. Growth is an important marker of general well-being. It can sometimes be the first indicator that something is wrong, and there may be an organic secondary cause.

D Dipstick urine – Correct. It is helpful to perform a urine dipstick to ensure there is no evidence of renal disease.

E Take a social history and find out how John is getting on at school – Correct. This is fundamental in this scenario. Bedwetting can be the first sign of bullying, problems at school or maltreatment.

Key Point

Primary nocturnal enuresis is common and usually does not have an organic cause, particularly in younger children. In contrast, secondary enuresis (where a previously continent child becomes incontinent) should always be thoroughly investigated.

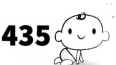

Q2 John's mother is very keen to work hard to get his problems under control. There are no problems at school and John's family is very supportive. Assuming that all the initial investigations are normal and John is clinically well, what would be the first line management for John?

The correct answer is E. Referral to an enuresis clinic for a bell pad alarm.

Treatment for bedwetting should focus on the fact that it is not the child's fault. Drinking habits should be reviewed. Bell pad alarms/reward systems are extremely effective, and desmopressin may be effective medical therapy in selected cases.

A   Desmopressin – Incorrect. In the case of John, whose mum seems keen to try other measures, desmopressin is not the first-line treatment. It can be used for social reasons (such as sleepovers), or in children where other treatment has failed, older children, or if the other treatment options are not suitable for the parents.

B   Referral for counselling – Incorrect. In children with underlying psychological disturbances, or in whom bedwetting is secondary to maltreatment, counselling and other forms of support may be necessary. The question clearly states, however, that this is not an issue for John.

C   Fluid restriction – Incorrect. Adequate fluid intake is important and fluid restriction, even in the evening, should be avoided. Regular toileting should be encouraged and children should avoid caffeinated drinks.

D   Trimethoprim to treat presumed UTI – Incorrect. There were no features to suggest infection in this scenario.

E   Referral to an enuresis clinic for a bell pad alarm – Correct. In families where this is acceptable, this would be the first line treatment, combined with reward systems. The key is that the child has to wake up to go to the toilet when the alarm goes off — parents should not be lifting their children. This would not be suitable for all families, but in those who are willing, there are excellent success rates. Sensors are placed in the bed and in the underwear of the child so that when the child starts to wet, the alarm goes off and wakes the child.

⚲ Key Point

For nocturnal enuresis, desmopressin may be required, but generally conservative measures such as bell pad alarms and reward systems are effective.

ⓘ IMPORTANT LEARNING POINTS

- Enuresis is common, particularly nocturnally, and in younger children.
- Although secondary enuresis may have a secondary cause, primary enuresis is something children usually grow out of.
- First-line treatment for nocturnal enuresis usually involves conservative measures, such as reviewing drinking habits, regular toileting and bedside alarms. This is extremely effective.

ANSWER TO CASE 37
A 3-year-old girl presenting with bloody diarrhoea and anuria

Q1 What would you do first in this scenario?

The correct answer is A. IV fluid resuscitation.

This child sounds very unwell and is in hypovolaemic shock secondary to gastroenteritis. The initial management of an acutely unwell patient is always the same: resuscitate using an airway, breathing and circulation approach. The question tells you that her airway is patent by proxy of the fact that she is responding to her mother. "B" has already been assessed and she is on oxygen. The next step of management is "C" – circulation.

A   IV fluid resuscitation – Correct. The question clearly states that she is peripherally shut down, tachycardic and anuric. A 20 mL/kg fluid bolus is needed to try to restore circulating volume. She should be monitored carefully for signs of fluid overload. In the presence of renal dysfunction, care must be taken in administering further fluid boluses.

B   IV antibiotics – Incorrect. The fluid bolus is the priority, but IV antibiotics should be considered in any shocked child with potential septicaemia. However, there is evidence of worsening prognosis by giving antibiotics in HUS, which is a potential diagnosis at this stage.

C   Oral fluid challenge – Incorrect. Although fluids are what this child needs, an oral fluid challenge would not act quickly enough; therefore, IV fluids should be given.

D   Paracetamol – Incorrect. Managing pain is less important than treating hypovolaemia.

E   Surgical opinion for her abdomen – Incorrect. This child has probable gastroenteritis and requires fluid resuscitation. There is nothing to suggest that there is any other intra-abdominal pathology requiring surgical intervention, but a detailed abdominal examination is needed. However, even if the abdominal examination revealed surgical concern (e.g. clinical suspicion of perforation), in the first instance, stabilisation with a fluid bolus should be commenced immediately.

⚕ Key Point

The management of any acutely unwell child, regardless of the possible underlying diagnosis, should start with resuscitation, using an ABC approach.

Q2 What is the most likely diagnosis?

The correct answer is E. Haemolytic Uraemic Syndrome.

This anuria is consistent with acute kidney injury. Of note, there are also low platelets and the history of a recent visit to a farm certainly raises the possibility of E. coli 0157 infection. This picture of severe gastroenteritis with bloody diarrhoea, acute renal failure and thrombocytopenia is classic of HUS.

A Glomerulonephritis – Incorrect. The history is not typical here and would be unlikely to present so acutely, with a shocked child in acute renal failure.

B Henoch-Schönlein Purpura – Incorrect. The child with HSP is typically very well with normal renal function. HSP is also associated with abdominal pain, arthralgia and a typical purpuric rash.

C Chronic kidney disease – Incorrect. Although we cannot definitely say that the renal failure is new, the presentation is acute and secondary to HUS. Of note, the urea is elevated in proportion to the creatinine, again suggesting a more acute picture. The low haemoglobin may be a result of the microangiopathic haemolytic anaemia seen in HUS.

D Gastroenteritis – Incorrect. Although, superficially, this child does have gastroenteritis, there are clues in the history that this is more complicated. Pure gastroenteritis would be unlikely to cause this degree of renal failure, and it does not cause thrombocytopaenia. This, combined with the possible *E. coli* 0157 exposure, makes HUS the most likely overriding diagnosis.

E Haemolytic Uraemic Syndrome – Correct. This is a rare condition that tends to occur in outbreaks due to exposure to *E. coli* 0157, often following exposure to infected farm animals.

⚕ Key Point

Patients with HUS usually present as severely unwell. Suspect this diagnosis particularly if there has been possible contact with *E. coli* 0157.

ⓘ IMPORTANT LEARNING POINTS

- HUS is defined by the triad of acute kidney injury, thrombocytopenia and microangiopathic haemolytic anaemia. It typically presents with bloody diarrhoea, abdominal pain and vomiting.

- It is a rare diagnosis, and gastroenteritis is a much more common cause of bloody diarrhoea. The important clues are on the blood test results (renal function, platelet count, haemoglobin), and the severity of the illness.

- Management is generally supportive, with fluid and electrolyte replacement. Referral to a specialist unit is required, as the child may require dialysis and intensive monitoring. In severe cases, seizure prophylaxis and blood products may be required.

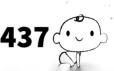

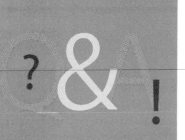

2.02
CLINICAL CASES: INTERMEDIATE
ALL AUTHORS

CONTENTS

CASE 1

A 5-year-old girl presenting with an acute neck swelling

A previously fit and well 5-year-old girl is reviewed in ED with a progressively enlarging, left-sided neck swelling. She reports having a sore throat and has a fever of 38°C, but observations are otherwise normal.

Questions

Q1 What clinical feature(s) below would be of concern and prompt further investigation?
  A Night sweats
  B Coryzal symptoms
  C Hepatosplenomegaly
  D Stridor
  E Weight loss

Q2 On examining the child, what finding(s) would suggest acute infection? Select all that apply.
  A Overlying erythema
  B Multiple, bilateral cervical lymph nodes.
  C Solitary, painless neck mass
  D Fluctuant mass
  E Fever

Q3 If a non-infective pathology is suspected, which three of the following should be organised as first-line investigations?
  A MRI scan of the neck
  B Ultrasound scan
  C Blood film
  D FBC
  E Excision biopsy

Q4 With regard to neck masses in children, mark the following statements true or false.
  A The most common histological feature on biopsy is reactive hyperplasia

  B Most palpable lymph nodes over 0.5 cm will require an excision biopsy
  C Branchial cysts most commonly present in the neonatal period
  D Supraclavicular swellings are common in children
  E Neck swellings are rarely associated with infectious mononucleosis

For answers see page 452

CASE 2

A 10-year-old boy with newly diagnosed diabetes

Jamie is a sporty and active 10-year-old. His mother noticed that recently his clothes have seemed too big for him, and he was always complaining of feeling tired. Jamie was very embarrassed to admit that he had wet the bed on two occasions this week. Observations are within normal limits.

On examination, Jamie is very thin, with signs of recent weight loss. Jamie's urine dipstick shows 4+ glucose, 2+ ketones, 1+ leucocytes and is negative for nitrites.

A new diagnosis of diabetes is suspected.

Questions

Q1 Which of the following best fits with a diagnosis of Type 1 diabetes in this child?
  A A high blood glucose, only if it is seen following a formal oral glucose tolerance test
  B A random blood glucose >11.1 mmol/L
  C The presence of polyuria and polydipsia
  D 4+ of glucose on urine dipstick
  E The presence of ketonuria

Q2 Regarding the aetiology of diabetes, mark the following statements true or false.
  A All diabetes in children is type 1
  B Type 1 diabetes mellitus is an autoimmune condition caused by damage to pancreatic alpha cells

439

C Pancreatic damage is mediated by T lymphocytes

D Type 1 diabetes can be associated with other autoimmune conditions such as Addison's disease, coeliac disease and hypothyroidism

E HLA-DR3 and HLA-DR4 are associated with an increased risk of developing diabetes

At hospital, it is confirmed that Jamie does have diabetes. He has a blood glucose level of 26 mmol/L. He is admitted to the paediatric ward to establish his insulin regime and to allow his mother to learn important principles for management of his condition. He is then discharged home on the same day and then regularly visited at home by the community nurses over the next few weeks.

Q3 Regarding insulin, mark the following statements true or false.

A Insulin is usually derived from the pancreas of pigs

B Injections must be confined to a certain location to ensure a consistent dose-response relationship

C Insulin is usually given as one injection per day

D Most children will require relatively small amounts of insulin in the months following diagnosis

E Insulin should be given to keep blood glucose within the normal range at all times

Q4 In addition to insulin administration, which of the following will also cause reductions in blood glucose? Select all that apply.

A Growth hormone secretion

B Glucagon

C Use of corticosteroid medication

D Consumption of alcoholic drinks

E Febrile illnesses

A few weeks after discharge, Jamie is awarded "man of the match" in his five-a-side team game, but his mother notices he appears withdrawn and quiet on the way home and he says he feels "funny". She checks his blood glucose and finds it is 2.8 mmol/L.

Q5 Which would be the next most appropriate action to manage Jamie's hypoglycaemia?

A IM glucagon

B Offer Jamie a sugary drink

C Withhold his insulin for the rest of the day

D Call an ambulance

E Give him a sandwich

It is now one year since Jamie's diagnosis, and he is making good progress, with no other emergency presentations to hospital. He is now giving some of his injections by himself

Time of day		Breakfast (08:00)		Lunch (13:00)		Dinner (18:00)		Bedtime (21:00)
		Pre	Post	Pre	Post	Pre	Post	
Mon.	Blood Glucose	11.7		4.1		3.8	7.2	5.8
	Insulin Dose (units)	4 (short acting)		5 (short acting)		6 (short acting)		10 (long acting)
Tues.	Blood Glucose	10.1		6.1				7.1
	Insulin Dose (units)	5 (short acting)		6 (short acting)		3 (short acting)		11 (long acting)
Wed.	Blood Glucose	12.9	6.1		6.0	11.9	9.0	
	Insulin Dose (units)	5 (short acting)		4 (short acting)		5 (short acting)		12 (long acting)

with his mother's supervision. He is seen in clinic by his consultant for his annual review.

Q6 What conclusion can you draw from the above glucose readings? (normal range 4-7 mmol/L)

A Jamie must be snacking overnight

B Jamie should skip breakfast

C Checking Jamie's blood glucose overnight for few nights will be helpful

D Jamie should cut out sugary food from his diet

For answers see page 453

CASE 3
A 14-year-old girl presenting with delayed puberty

A 14-year-old girl has primary amenorrhoea. On further questioning, the girl says she is tired and feels cold all the time. Her general development is normal and she attends mainstream school. She is an academically able child and is expected to do very well in her exams the following year. Observations are within normal limits. On examination, she is on the 50th centile for height, her BMI is 16.5 kg/m^2 (<10th centile), and is prepubertal (Tanner stage 1).

Questions

Q1 Which of the following findings are consistent with the likely underlying diagnosis? Select all that apply.

  A Lanugo hair

  B Hypertension

  C Bradycardia

  D Obsessional thoughts

  E Social withdrawal

Q2 Which of the following initial investigations would be helpful in this patient? Select all that apply.

  A LH and FSH concentrations

  B Thyroid function tests

  C MRI brain

  D Adrenal MRI

  E Chromosomal karyotyping

Q3 Which management option is best?

  A Watch and wait; follow up in 6 months

  B Start on antidepressants

  C Pubertal induction using oestrogen preparations

  D Start on GnRH agonist

  E Referral to child and adolescent mental health services

For answers see page 456

CASE 4
A 12-day-old baby presenting with poor feeding and vomiting

A 12-day-old boy presents with poor feeding and vomiting. There are no risk factors for neonatal sepsis. Parents are non-consanguineous, pregnancy was uneventful and antenatal scans were normal. The baby was born at term by spontaneous vaginal delivery with a birth weight of 3.4 kg. Family history is unremarkable.

On examination, the baby is lethargic and irritable, with dry mucous membranes. The RR is 61 breaths/min (tachypnoeic) with saturations of 93% in air, HR is 170 bpm (tachycardic) and the temperature is 37°C. His current weight is 3.0 kg. Clinical examination is unremarkable, with normal male genitalia and bilaterally descended testes. The scrotum appears hyperpigmented.

A full septic screen is performed and broad-spectrum antibiotics are started.

Initial capillary blood gas shows mild metabolic acidosis and lab results show Na 120 mmol/L, K 7.5 mmol/L, bicarbonate 16 mmol/L and glucose 2.3 mmol/L. Urea is 3mmol/L and creatinine is 40 μmol/L. A urine dipstick is negative for nitrites and leucocytes. His chest X-ray is normal. CSF microscopy and biochemistry are negative. WCC and CRP are normal, and blood cultures come back negative after 48 hours.

Questions

Q1 What is the most likely diagnosis?

  A Fulminant sepsis

  B Congenital adrenal hyperplasia (CAH)

  C Gastro-oesophageal reflux disease

  D Heart failure

Q2 Which of the following tests is most useful in establishing the diagnosis in this clinical scenario?

  A Karyotyping

  B Specific gene testing

  C 17-hydroxyprogesterone (17 OHP)

  D Pelvic ultrasound

Q3 Which of the following may be important aims in the treatment of this condition? Select all that apply.

  A Normalisation and maintenance of normal electrolytes

  B Glucocorticoid replacement

  C Mineralocorticoid replacement

  D Supporting normal growth and sexual maturation

For answers see page 457

CASE 5
A 5-year-old boy presenting with a headache

A five-year-old previously healthy boy presents with a four week history of intermittent headaches and vomiting that is worse in the morning. He has also become unsteady on his feet and often trips over things. He has not had a fever or diarrhoea and is otherwise well. Observations are within normal limits.

Questions

Q1 In this case, which clinical features suggest the presence of raised intracranial pressure? Select all that apply.

  A Early morning headaches

  B Unsteadiness

  C Persistent vomiting

  D Intermittent headaches

Q2 On examination, there is evidence of ataxia and past-pointing. Bilateral papilloedema is present on fundoscopy. What is the most likely underlying diagnosis?

  A Severe hypertension

  B Post-infectious acute cerebellar ataxia

  C Cerebral abscess

  D Brain tumour

  E Viral gastroenteritis

Q3 What would be your next investigation?

  A CT or MRI scan

  B Lumbar puncture

  C Blood culture

441

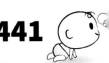

D Varicella serology

E EEG

Q4 The CT scan confirms an intracranial lesion. How would you manage this child in ED? Select all that apply.

A Corticosteroids

B Intravenous aciclovir

C Discharge with parental advice to return if symptoms are worsening

D Lumbar puncture to relieve the symptoms of raised ICP

E Referral to the nearest neurosurgical centre

For answers see page 458

CASE 6
A 13-month-old girl presents with severe pallor

A 13-month-old girl presents with severe pallor. She has been on cow's milk for the past six months and is a fussy eater with poor intake of solid food. HR is 165 bpm (tachycardic) but observations are otherwise normal. On examination, she was alert and active. She is not dysmorphic, appears well and has no bruises, lymphadenopathy or hepatosplenomegaly. Her urine dipstick is normal. Heart sounds are normal, and there was no peripheral oedema. Renal and liver function tests are normal. Full blood count shows haemoglobin of 61 g/L, with MCV 63 g/dL (microcytic). White cell count, platelets and LFTs, including bilirubin, are normal, and DAT is negative. Reticulocyte count is elevated.

Questions

Q1 What is the most likely underlying diagnosis?

A Acute lymphoblastic leukaemia

B Iron deficiency anaemia

C Aplastic anaemia

D Coeliac disease

E B12 deficiency

Q2 What would be your next investigations? Select all that apply.

A Bone marrow aspirate

B Iron studies

C Blood film

D Parvovirus screen

E Endoscopy

Q3 What would be your first-line management for the treatment of the above condition?

A Observation as an outpatient and advise

B Admit for blood transfusion

C Discharge, commence oral iron supplementation and observe

D Admit for IV iron supplementation

E Referral to gastroenterology for urgent endoscopy

Q4 What feature is not typical of this condition and should prompt rapid referral to a specialist team?

A Black tarry stools

B Poor diet

C Normal serum ferritin

D Severe pallor

E Exclusively breastfed

For answers see page 460

CASE 7
A 4-year-old presenting with thrombocytopenia

A 4-year-old previously healthy boy presents with bruising and a rash following a viral URTI one week ago. Observations are within normal limits. On examination, he appears well. He has a widespread petechial rash and several bruises on his arms, legs and trunk. He has no hepatosplenomegaly and no palpable lymphadenopathy. His BP, temperature and urine dipstick are all normal. Renal and liver function tests are normal. Full blood count shows haemoglobin of 120 g/L, a normal white cell count, and platelets 18 x 10^9/L. Clotting screen is normal.

Questions

Q1 What is the most likely underlying diagnosis?

A Acute lymphoblastic leukaemia

B Immune thrombocytopenic purpura

C Henoch-Schönlein purpura

D Systemic lupus erythematosus

E Meningococcal sepsis

Q2 What would be your next investigation?

A Bone marrow aspirate

B Blood film

C No further investigation

D Autoantibody screen

Q3 What would be your first-line management for the treatment of the above condition?

A Observation and advice

B Intravenous immunoglobulin

C Corticosteroids

D Splenectomy

E Platelet transfusion

Q4 What features are not typical of this condition? Select all that apply.

A White cell blasts on blood film

B Spontaneous resolution in 6-8 weeks

C History of a preceding febrile illness

D Platelet count 10 x 10^9/L

E Epistaxis

For answers see page 462

CASE 8
A 4-month-old boy presenting with severe respiratory distress

A 4-month-old boy presents to ED in severe respiratory distress. On examination, he is pale and cachectic. His weight falls below the 0.4th centile, despite a birth weight at the 50th centile. His RR is 60 breaths/min (tachypnoeic) with saturations of 92% in air. His HR is 175 bpm (tachycardic). Capillary refill time and BP are normal and his temperature is 37.3°C. Mum reports she believes his poor weight gain is the consequence of chronic diarrhoea.

Questions

Q1 What features in the history might make you suspect a primary immunodeficiency? Select all that apply.
- A Female sex
- B Faltering growth
- C Three upper respiratory tract infections per year
- D Family history of unexplained early death
- E Recurrent or resistant thrush

Q2 Which features on a chest X-ray would make you suspect a primary immunodeficiency? Select all that apply.
- A Pleural effusion
- B Bilateral pulmonary infiltrates
- C Absent thymus
- D Hyperinflation
- E Pneumothorax

Q3 Which three investigations would be most helpful in diagnosing a primary immunodeficiency?
- A Stool MC&S
- B Full blood count with differential white cell count
- C Immunoglobulins
- D Lymphocyte subsets
- E Blood cultures

Q4 Which of the following are key points in the management of a primary immunodeficiency? Select all that apply.
- A Antibiotic prophylaxis
- B Full immunisation
- C Splenectomy
- D Immunoglobulin infusions
- E Early use of blood products to support deficits

For answers see page 463

CASE 9
A 1-year-old boy presents with an itchy rash

A 1-year-old boy presents with vomiting and an erythematous crusting rash across the trunk and upper limbs. He is tachypnoeic at 55 breaths/min, tachycardic at 170 bpm, capillary refill time is 3 seconds, he is febrile at 38.8°C and lethargic. There is no wheeze. He has not passed urine today and has not been eating or drinking well. His skin turgor is markedly reduced.

He has a background of eczema and recurrent episodes of viral-induced wheeze. Urine dipstick and chest X-ray are both normal.

Questions

Q1 Which of the following are correct regarding eczema? Select all that apply.
- A Infantile eczema affects mainly the flexor surfaces and the nappy area
- B Most children with infantile eczema will have severe eczema throughout life
- C A family or personal history of allergic conditions is common
- D Heat, chemicals and stress can aggravate the condition
- E The mainstay of treatment is with topical emollients and corticosteroids

Q2 What features would support a diagnosis of secondary bacterial infection? Select all that apply.
- A Fever
- B Dry, erythematous plaques
- C Excoriated skin
- D Oedema and erythema of affected skin
- E Crops of fluid filled vesicles

Q3 Which of the following should be included in the initial management in this case of suspected infected eczema? Select all that apply.
- A A course of oral corticosteroids to control the exacerbation of eczema
- B Swabs of cutaneous lesions for microscopy and culture
- C Oral antibiotics (e.g. flucloxacillin) to cover common skin organisms such as *staphylococcus aureus*
- D Antihistamines to relieve pruritus
- E Antiviral therapy such as aciclovir

For answers see page 465

CASE 10
A 3-year-old boy presenting with possible appendicitis

Richard Peters is a 3-year-old boy who has been admitted with possible appendicitis to the Paediatric ward. He has been made NBM awaiting an ultrasound. The nurse in ED weighed him at 16 kg. His DOB is 03/06/2011, his hospital number is SM678112 and he has no allergies.

Question

The pharmacist has just approached you with a prescription chart (Chart 3a) which she says contains some errors.
Please re-prescribe this prescription chart, correcting any mistakes you find.

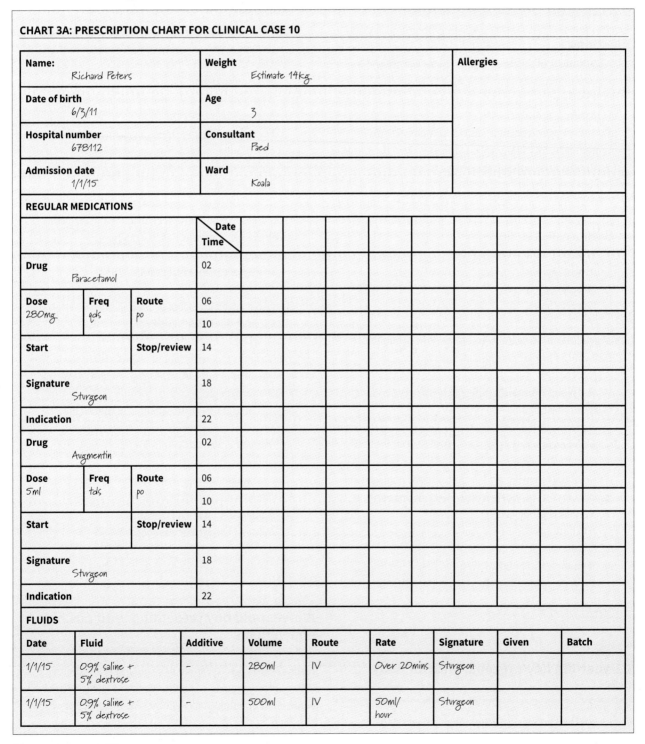

CHART 3A: PRESCRIPTION CHART FOR CLINICAL CASE 10

Name: Richard Peters	Weight Estimate 14kg	Allergies
Date of birth 6/3/11	Age 3	
Hospital number 678112	Consultant Paed	
Admission date 1/1/15	Ward Koala	

REGULAR MEDICATIONS

		Date / Time								
Drug Paracetamol		02								
Dose 280mg	**Freq** qds	**Route** po	06							
			10							
Start	**Stop/review**	14								
Signature Sturgeon		18								
Indication		22								
Drug Augmentin		02								
Dose 5ml	**Freq** tds	**Route** po	06							
			10							
Start	**Stop/review**	14								
Signature Sturgeon		18								
Indication		22								

FLUIDS

Date	Fluid	Additive	Volume	Route	Rate	Signature	Given	Batch
1/1/15	0.9% saline + 5% dextrose	–	280ml	IV	Over 20mins	Sturgeon		
1/1/15	0.9% saline + 5% dextrose	–	500ml	IV	50ml/ hour	Sturgeon		

For answers see page 466

CASE 11
A 6-hour-old girl presenting with bilious vomiting

A female infant was born at 36 weeks gestation, weighing 2.6kg. The mother never attended any antenatal appointments or scans. The baby had good Apgar scores and breastfed soon after birth. At 6 hours of age, the baby developed bilious vomiting. Observations are within normal limits.

Questions

Q1 Which of the following conditions could be in your list of differential diagnoses? Select all that apply.
- A Duodenal atresia
- B Malrotation
- C Meconium ileus
- D Oesophageal atresia
- E Jejunal atresia

Q2 Which of the following statements is correct? Select all that apply.
- A The colour of bile is green
- B An abdominal X-ray is the most important test to order
- C A contrast enema is the most appropriate test to order
- D The fact that the baby passed meconium after birth is a positive sign that a significant abnormality is unlikely
- E Abdominal distension and tenderness are worrying signs

The paediatric surgical registrar organises an urgent upper GI contrast, which confirms the diagnosis of malrotation with midgut volvulus.

Q3 Which of the following statements is correct? Select all that apply.
- A 6-12 hours should be spent resuscitating the patient; a laparotomy should be planned for the next day.
- B A unit of blood should be cross-matched and ready as soon as possible.
- C The parents should be counselled that prognosis is very good
- D The name of the procedure that is performed for malrotation is Ladd's procedure
- E The appendix should always be removed during surgery for malrotation.

For answers see page 468

CASE 12
A baby born at 32 weeks gestation

Mrs Smith is a 28-year-old lady who spontaneously went into labour at 32 weeks gestation. Her pregnancy had been uneventful, though she continues to smoke 20 cigarettes a day.

The baby's nasal flaring, grunting and intercostal recession are noted at birth. The RR is 75 breaths/min (tachypnoeic) with saturations of 92% in air, HR is 170 bpm (tachycardic) and the temperature is 37°C. The baby was empirically treated for sepsis, and started on CPAP respiratory support.

Questions

Q1 What is the definition of a premature delivery?
- A Baby born with a birth weight of less than 2.5kg
- B Baby born at less than 34 weeks gestation
- C Baby born at less than 32 weeks gestation
- D Baby born at less than 36 weeks gestation
- E Baby born at less than 37 weeks gestation

Q2 Which of the following are risk factors for premature delivery? Select all that apply.
- A Maternal smoking
- B Maternal alcohol abuse
- C Maternal infection/chorioamnionitis
- D Previous premature birth/miscarriage
- E Multiple pregnancy
- F Chronic maternal illness, e.g. diabetes/hypertension

Q3 Which of the following are common problems seen in preterm babies? Select all that apply.
- A Feeding difficulties/hypoglycaemia
- B Respiratory Distress Syndrome
- C Jaundice
- D Infection
- E Electrolyte disturbance
- F Hydrocephalus

Q4 The baby is discharged from the neonatal unit, and is seen in a follow-up clinic 12 weeks after being born. You are asked to plot the weight and height of the baby on a growth chart. What corrected age would you plot the baby at?
- A 12 weeks
- B 6 weeks
- C 4 weeks
- D 10 weeks
- E 11 weeks

For answers see page 469

CASE 13
An 11-month-old presenting with possible developmental delay

Maisy is an 11-month-old girl who has come to clinic for a follow-up appointment.

She was born at 28 weeks gestation via spontaneous vaginal delivery following a normal pregnancy with normal ultrasound scans. She required intubation for four days for RDS (respiratory distress syndrome), but was discharged home, feeding normally and with no respiratory support after eight weeks in hospital.

In her first follow-up appointment, she was making progress. She was 6-months-old (3 months corrected) and had good head control, some head rise when prone and had just started to smile.

You perform a developmental assessment on her in clinic today. You find:

> Gross motor: She can hold her head well, lift her chest with extended arms when prone, sit with a curved back when supported, and can roll front to back.

> Fine motor: She is reaching for objects. She can fix on and follow objects across 180 degrees. She can hold objects with a palmar grasp, but is not transferring between hands or bringing objects to the midline.

> Social/Self-care: She smiles, screams and laughs, but has not yet developed stranger awareness.

> Language: She is cooing but not babbling.

Questions

Q1 What best described Maisy's development status?
- A Isolated fine motor delay
- B Gross motor and speech delay
- C Isolated speech delay
- D Global developmental delay
- E Isolated gross motor delay

Q2 With regard to neurological development in ex-premature infants, mark the following statements true or false.
- A It is normal for a child to preferentially reach with their right hand for objects at this age
- B Children born prematurely do not have developmental delay unless they have had a neurological complication
- C Prematurity can be associated with poor concentration and hyperactive behaviour

Q3 What is the next best step in managing Maisy?
- A Send bloods for karyotyping
- B Refer for an MRI brain
- C Refer to Community Paediatrician and MDT assessment
- D Arrange a hearing test

Q4 With regard to normal development, mark the following statements true or false.
- A An average 8-month-old should sit unsupported
- B A 15-month-old not walking should be investigated
- C An average 2-year-old can draw a circle
- D An average 3-year-old can build a tower of nine bricks
- E Children should develop object permanence by 12-months-old

For answers see page 470

CASE 14
A 22-month-old presenting with delayed gross motor skills

Lily is a 22-month-old Afro-Caribbean girl who was referred to the paediatric clinic as she is still not walking. She is on the 2nd centile for weight and height but was born on the 25th centile. She is still being breastfed. Her parents are both clinically obese. She is making attempts to walk when holding onto furniture. The rest of her developmental assessment is normal, as is her neurological examination. Parents also have pointed out that her knees are wider apart than they should be. On examination, you confirm genus varum, a bowing appearance of the legs, and widening of her wrists. Vitamin D deficiency is suspected.

Questions

Q1 What further history would be most helpful to support the diagnosis of rickets?
- A Age at which parents started walking
- B Birth history
- C Dietary history

Q2 What investigations should be performed as part of her initial workup? Select all that apply.
- A Plotting height/length centile, and calculating mid-parental height
- B Full blood count
- C Checking thyroid function
- D Checking chromosomes
- E X-ray of the wrist

Q3 Which of the following are classically associated with rickets? Select all that apply.
- A Fractured ribs
- B Rachitic rosary
- C Pectus excavatum
- D Pectus carinatum
- E Intercostal recession

For answers see page 472

CASE 15
A 5-day-old baby with a genetic condition picked up on newborn screening

A baby born at 37 weeks gestation is tested in their first week of life using the routine Guthrie test. The baby's parents are given the results of the test, which shows a specific genetic condition has been identified. The doctor draws out the family tree to demonstrate the pattern of inheritance of the disorder and to explain to the parents how their child inherited the condition.

The pedigree diagram is shown below.

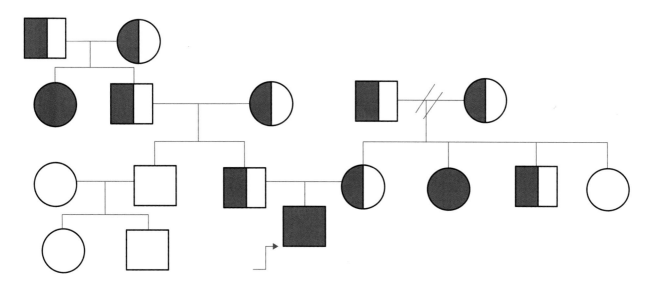

Questions

Q1 What type of inheritance is shown by the pedigree diagram?

  A Autosomal dominant

  B Autosomal recessive

  C X-linked dominant

  D X-linked recessive

Q2 With regards to the above inheritance pattern, mark the following statements true or false.

  A The condition affects both sexes equally

  B The condition can "skip" generations

  C The condition can only be passed from a mother to her children

  D If the child is affected, both parents must be carriers or affected themselves

  E This condition is more common where the parents are consanguineous.

Q3 Three years later, the mother has just given birth to a healthy daughter. However, she also had a miscarriage (cause unknown) whilst trying to conceive again. What symbols need to be added to the pedigree diagram?

  A An empty circle and a coloured triangle with a cross through it

  B A coloured circle and an empty square

  C A coloured square and a coloured triangle with a cross through it

  D An empty circle and an empty triangle with a cross through it

  E An empty circle and an empty diamond

For answers see page 473

CASE 16

A 9-year-old boy presenting with tight foreskin

A 9-year-old boy presents to ED with a four month history of progressive difficulty in passing urine. He states his penis is very sore, especially while passing urine. On examination, he has a red, inflamed foreskin that is scarred and fibrotic. Observations are within normal limits. A diagnosis of balanitis xerotica obliterans is made, and possible circumcision is discussed.

Questions

Q1 Mark the following statements true or false.

  A Circumcision can always be safely performed in the community

  B Balanitis xerotica obliterans is an indication for circumcision

  C Physiological phimosis is an indication for circumcision

  D Circumcision may be complicated by meatal stenosis

Q2 Please match the following conditions to their definitions or the appropriate management of the condition:

  A Priapism

  B Acute urinary retention

  C Paraphimosis

  D Phimosis

  E Post-circumcision haemorrhage

  i Can usually be reduced after the application of topical lignocaine and pressure

  ii A physiological condition of the prepuce that rarely requires surgery

  iii An erection lasting more than four hours that may or may not be painful

  iv Should stop after 10 minutes of continuous firm pressure

  v May require insertion of a suprapubic catheter

For answers see page 475

447

CASE 17
A 2-year-old presenting with bony deformities

A 2-year-old Afro-Caribbean girl presents with inability to walk properly. The child was born at 35 weeks gestation but did not suffer any perinatal complications. She was exclusively breastfed until she was 1-year-old and is a fussy eater. Observations are within normal limits. On physical examination, the child is irritable. Marked skeletal deformities are noted on both upper and lower limbs, including bowing of the legs, and the child is on the 25th centile for height.

Questions
Q1 What is the most likely diagnosis in this child?
  A Beriberi
  B Pellagra
  C Rickets
  D Scurvy
  E Kwashiorkor

Q2 What are the risk factors for the likely diagnosis? Select all that apply.
  A Fair skin
  B Coeliac disease
  C Breastfeeding with vitamin D supplementation
  D High altitude
  E Use of anticonvulsants

Q3 What are the clinical features of the likely diagnosis? Select all that apply.
  A Harrison's sulcus
  B Narrowing of the wrists
  C Enamel hypoplasia
  D Increased tendency of fractures
  E Bone pain

Q4 What biochemical changes are observed in the likely diagnosis? Select all that apply.
  A Decreased alkaline phosphatase level
  B Increased parathyroid hormone level
  C Increased plasma phosphate level
  D Decreased plasma calcium level

For answers see page 476

CASE 18
A 12-month-old presenting with faltering growth

A 12-month-old girl Sarah presents with poor weight gain. The child was eating foods appropriate for her age. She was introduced to solid food at eight months of age and had stopped being breastfed at ten months of age. The child was often irritable while eating. The mother reported that the child had been having frequent flatulence after feeding and loose bowel motions.

Sarah was born at term through normal vaginal delivery, weighing 3.3 kg, without any perinatal complications. There was no significant past medical history but there was a family history of coeliac disease. She had achieved her developmental milestones at appropriate ages. The mother described increasing sadness and having difficulty coping since the child was born. She denied any history of abuse or violence in the household.

Sarah's observations are within normal range. Weight is 6.8 kg (less than the 3rd percentile), height is 72 cm (15th percentile) and head circumference is 45 cm (50th percentile). She is alert and has good interaction with her mother. The abdomen is mildly distended and tender to palpate. She has some wasting of the buttocks. The rest of the physical examination is unremarkable. Laboratory investigations reveal mild anaemia.

Due to the family history, serology testing was performed and it was positive for antibodies against tissue transglutaminase, confirming coeliac disease.

Questions
Q1 Which of the following are commonly accepted definitions for faltering growth? Select all that apply.
  A Weight less than 65% of ideal weight for age
  B Weight less than 5th percentile for more than one occasion
  C Depressed length-for-head circumference
  D Weight gain of 120 g per week between three and six months of age
  E Deceleration of weight gain across two or more major percentile lines over time

Q2 Mark the following statements true or false.
  A Those in charge of management should assume there is either an organic cause or a non-organic cause of faltering growth, not both concurrently
  B Different standardised growth charts are needed for children from different racial and ethnic backgrounds
  C Inpatient care should be considered for children with faltering growth when there is severe psychosocial impairment at home
  D The fundamental mechanisms contributing to faltering growth are insufficient nutritional intake, inadequate absorption and decreased metabolic requirement
  E The deceleration in the growth velocity of head circumference independent of weight and length deceleration is suggestive of constitutional growth delay

Q3 Mark the following statements true or false.
  A Chronic diseases such as coeliac disease and cystic fibrosis impair the intestinal absorption of nutrients, thus resulting in faltering growth

B A single record of weight below ideal weight for age is sufficient to diagnose faltering growth

C The history provided by parents is always reliable for a child with suspicious features of child abuse or violence

D It is important to observe the interaction between the child and his/her parents, particularly during feeding

For answers see page 477

CASE 19
A 2-year-old presenting with a blue episode

A mother brings her 2-year-old girl to ED following episodes where she seemed to turn blue. The mother describes her as becoming breathless, turning a bluish colour and crouching down.

This has happened three times and each episode lasted for two minutes. Last time, it seemed to last longer and her mother became concerned and called an ambulance. On the ambulance crew's arrival, her daughter had completely recovered but she was brought to the hospital anyway. Observations are within normal limits.

She is new to the area, as the family are travellers. She tells you that before they moved, her daughter was under investigation for a condition called Tetralogy of Fallot (TOF). However, due to relocation, this was not followed up.

Questions
Q1 What are the structural features of TOF?

A Infundibular pulmonary stenosis, ventricular septal defect, atrial septal defect

B Right ventricular hypertrophy, atrial septal defect, aortic stenosis

C Right ventricular hypertrophy, ventricular septal defect, overriding aorta and infundibular pulmonary stenosis

D Overriding aorta, infundibular pulmonary stenosis, atrial septal defect

E Atrioventricular septal defect, coarctation of the aorta and mitral regurgitation.

Q2 What examination findings would you classically expect to see in a patient who is presenting for the first time with TOF (prior to receiving any treatment)?

A Harsh ejection systolic murmur, heard best at the left upper border of the sternum, radiating into the back

B Collapsing pulses and a wide pulse pressure

C No murmur audible

D Pansystolic murmur heard at the lower left sternal edge

E Low BP, bounding peripheral pulses and a constant machinery murmur.

As you are speaking to your senior, you can hear the child crying and becoming irritable. Suddenly, she stops shouting and you glance over to see her lying flat on the bed, struggling

to breathe and beginning to turn blue. A hypercyanotic spell is suspected.

Q3 What is your initial management?

A Place the child in the recovery position and insert an oropharyngeal airway before administering oxygen

B Gain IV access and administer a 10ml/kg fluid bolus immediately

C Administer a 150 microgram dose of IM adrenaline

D Lean the child over your knee and perform five back blows

E Place the child in a knees-to-chest position and administer oxygen

Q4 If this child had presented as a cyanosed newborn, what other conditions would be among your differential diagnosis?

A Transposition of the great arteries

B Total anomalous pulmonary venous drainage

C Ventricular septal defect

D Patent ductus arteriosus

E Truncus arteriosus

For answers see page 478

CASE 20
A 5-week-old girl presenting with respiratory distress and poor weight gain

You are asked to review a 5-week-old baby girl who has been referred in by her GP with respiratory difficulties and poor weight gain.

She is a breastfed infant and mum reports that recently she has been struggling with her feeds, becoming very breathless and sweaty during them. She has not been putting on weight well. She was born at term, with an uncomplicated antenatal period and a normal neonatal check. Her birth weight was 3.5 kg and she is now 3.6 kg.

The baby has a RR of 65 breaths/minute (tachypnoeic), with oxygen saturation of 95% on room air. Observations are otherwise normal.

The baby is alert, but irritable, with good tone and soft anterior fontanelle. She has moist mucosa and shows no signs of dehydration. She has warm peripheries and palpable, symmetrical femoral pulses. Her HR is regular, heart sounds have a gallop rhythm with a faint systolic murmur, best heard over the lower left sternal edge. There is mild recession, with no crackles or wheeze on auscultation. She has a soft abdomen, and a liver palpable 3 cm below the costal margin.

Questions
Q1 Which of the following conditions would be within your differential diagnosis? Select all that apply.

A Ventricular septal defect

B Total anomalous pulmonary venous drainage

449

C   Bronchiolitis

D   Cardiomyopathy

E   Atrial septal defect

Q2   When suspicious that a child is presenting in heart failure, what initial management is appropriate?

A   Intubate and ventilate the baby, preparing for transfer to a specialist cardiac unit

B   Intravenous fluid replacement

C   Urgent abdominal ultrasound

D   Close monitoring and trial of diuretic therapy

E   DC cardioversion

Q3   The baby has an echocardiogram which shows a ventricular septal defect. Her parents are concerned and want to know what the risk of a congenital heart defect would be if they had another child?

A   No increased risk

B   Slightly increased risk

C   Sibling will definitely have some form of congenital heart disease, but this may differ in severity and type

D   50% increased risk

E   Vastly increased risk, multiple and early scans offered and termination advised if defects detected.

For answers see page 480

CASE 21
A 4-year-old boy presenting with nephrotic syndrome

A 4-year-old boy presents with a three day history of facial swelling and generalised puffiness following a viral URTI last week. Observations, including a BP, are within normal limits. His urine dipstick shows 3+ proteinuria, and is negative for blood, leucocytes and nitrites. Baseline bloods show normal haemoglobin, white blood cell count, platelets, renal function and electrolyte tests. However, he has significant hypoalbuminaemia.

Questions

Q1   What is the most common cause of the underlying diagnosis?

A   Minimal change disease

B   Focal and segmental glomerulosclerosis

C   Membranous nephropathy

D   Post-infectious glomerulonephritis

E   IgA nephropathy

Q2   What would be the first-line management for the suspected underlying diagnosis?

A   High dose oral corticosteroids, antihypertensives

B   IV corticosteroids, IV antibiotics

C   High dose oral corticosteroids, penicillin prophylaxis, no added salt diet

D   Immunomodulatory agents

E   Antihistamines

Q3   In the treatment of the above condition, which of the following are complications of long-term treatment? Select all that apply.

A   Weight gain

B   Hyperactive behaviour

C   Abdominal striae

D   Adrenal suppression

E   Cataracts

Q4   If a renal biopsy was undertaken, what would be the most likely findings in the above child?

A   Podocyte foot process effacement

B   Scarring of parts of some of the nephrons

C   Thickened basement membrane but not hypercellular

D   Immune complex formation on the basement membrane

E   IgA deposition

For answers see page 481

CASE 22
An 11-year-old boy presenting with haematuria

An 11-year-old boy is taken to ED because his urine has changed colour (now rusty-coloured, like Coca-Cola), and he reported blood in it this morning. He has been more lethargic over the last week or so since developing an URTI. BP on presentation is 125/70 mmHg (hypertensive), but all other observations are within normal limits. The only abnormality found on examination is oedema of his face, feet and ankles. Blood tests show normal haemoglobin, white cell count, platelets, urea and electrolytes, albumin and liver function tests with CRP of 11 mg/L. Urine dipstick shows 3+ of protein, and 4+ of blood. Microscopy shows red cell casts, but no organisms.

Questions

Q1   What is the most likely diagnosis in this child?

A   IgA nephropathy

B   Nephrotic syndrome

C   Post-infectious glomerulonephritis

D   Urinary tract infection

E   Rapidly progressive glomerulonephritis

Q2   Which of the following tests would be best for confirming the suspected diagnosis?

A   Complement levels

B   Hepatitis serology

C   ASOT titres

D   Renal ultrasound

E Renal biopsy

F IgA levels

Q3 How would you manage this patient?

  A Discharge with diuretic therapy to offload the oedema

  B Refer for consideration of renal dialysis

  C Monitor haematuria, BP and renal function, with clinic follow-up.

  D Admit and monitor for 24 hours in hospital

For answers see page 483

CASE 23
A 5–year-old girl presenting with a purpuric rash

A 5-year-old girl attends ED with a two day history of painful knees and abdominal pain. On examination, she is haemodynamically stable, apyrexial and looks well. Observations are within normal limits. Abdominal examination is normal. She has diffuse areas of purpura on the extensor surfaces of her legs, which her mum says have been present since yesterday.

Questions

Q1 What is the most likely diagnosis?

  A Acute lymphoblastic leukaemia

  B Meningococcal septicaemia

  C Henoch-Schönlein Purpura

  D Immune thrombocytopenic purpura

  E Drug-related rash

Q2 Which three investigations would be useful in the further management of this child?

  A FBC

  B Renal USS

  C U&Es

  D Urine dipstick

  E Abdominal X-ray

Q3 Initial investigations are all normal. Given this, what is the best management of this child, assuming she is still haemodynamically stable?

  A Reassure and discharge

  B Admit for full septic screen and start IV antibiotics

  C Arrange urgent platelet transfusion

  D Speak to the local tertiary referral centre to arrange transfer

  E Advise, regular urine monitoring, and early follow-up

  F Oral corticosteroids and bring back to clinic in one week

For answers see page 485

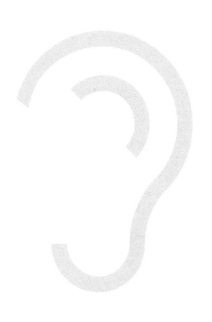

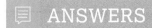

ANSWERS

ANSWER TO CASE 1
A 5-year-old girl presenting with an acute neck swelling

Q1 What clinical feature(s) below would be of concern and prompt further investigation?

The correct answers are A. Night sweats, C. Hepatosplenomegaly, D. Stridor and E. Weight loss.

Neck lumps are a common presenting symptom and may be encountered in primary care, as well as in the hospital setting.

A Night sweats – Correct. This may be a presenting feature of Hodgkin's Lymphoma or TB and warrants further investigation when encountered.

B Coryzal symptoms – Incorrect. URTIs are associated with a reactive cervical lymphadenopathy.

C Hepatosplenomegaly – Correct. Hepatosplenomegaly is associated with lymphoma or infectious mononucleosis.

D Stridor – Correct. This symptom requires urgent assessment in the ED if encountered in a child. Infected lymph nodes can result in deep neck space collections of pus that can, in rare cases, result in airway compromise. This can also occur with malignancy.

E Weight loss – Correct. This is an unusual feature in any child and may be suggestive of an underlying chronic inflammatory condition, such as TB or malignancy.

Key Point

"Red flag" features for a paediatric neck mass include: progressive increase in size, stridor, weight loss, night sweats and fever.

Q2 On examining the child, what finding(s) would suggest acute infection?

The correct answers are A. Overlying erythema, B. Multiple bilateral cervical lymph nodes measuring less than 1 cm, D. Fluctuant mass and E. Fever

A Overlying erythema – Correct. Acute inflammation is classically described as "calor, dolor, rubor, tumor" (heat, pain, redness and swelling). It is important to examine for overlying erythema and careful palpation will elicit the other features.

B Multiple, bilateral cervical lymph nodes – Correct. Bilateral cervical lymphadenopathy is very common, affecting approximately 50% of all children with an acute infection.

C Solitary, painless neck mass – Incorrect. A solitary, painless neck mass is not suggestive of acute infection but may be related to another underlying cause, such as malignancy.

D Fluctuant mass – Correct. Fluctuance in a neck swelling can often be a result of suppurative infection. Here liquefaction of the lymph node can result in abscess formation. This may be managed with broad spectrum intravenous antibiotics or incision and drainage. Superficial neck abscesses can progress to affect deep neck spaces, which can lead to airway compromise.

E Fever – Correct. Fever is a common systemic response to acute inflammation, and prolonged fever may be indicative of an abscess.

Key Point

Palpable bilateral cervical lymphadenopathy measuring less than 1 cm is common in children and does not warrant further investigation, particularly if there is an obvious infective cause.

Q3 If a non-infective pathology is suspected, which three of the following should be organised as first-line investigations?

The correct answers are B. Ultrasound, C. Blood film and D. FBC.

Initial investigation involves simple blood tests and non-invasive radiological testing. The most important differential to be concerned about is malignancy, although infection seems to be likely from the history.

A MRI scan of the neck – Incorrect. MRI is a highly specialist and expensive radiological investigation. This is not used as first-line when investigating cervical lymphadenopathy but has an indication in suspected lymphatic malformations.

B Ultrasound scan – Correct. Ultrasound is a widely available and simple radiological investigation that is well tolerated in children. As such, it is a first-line investigation that allows assessment of the location of pus and determination of the nodal distribution, shape, echogenicity, calcification, necrosis and vascular pattern to assist in diagnosis. This can often be combined with fine needle aspiration (FNA) if the child is able to tolerate the procedure (unless an atypical mycobacterium is a possibility).

C Blood film – Correct. A blood film is a useful adjunct test in evaluating a lymph node with suspicion of lymphoma. It allows the assessment of immature blast cells, which are a key feature of malignancy. A normal blood film does not exclude a diagnosis of lymphoma.

D FBC – Correct. An elevated white cell count and neutrophilia are associated with infection, and pancytopenia is associated with malignancy.

E Excision biopsy – Incorrect. Excision biopsy should be reserved for cases of diagnostic uncertainty when initial investigations have suspected but not confirmed a possible malignancy.

♀ Key Point

Investigation of a neck lump begins with a thorough history and precise examination. The most appropriate initial radiological investigation is an ultrasound scan. A normal ultrasound and blood tests do not exclude a malignancy, but they are useful for inclusion of other causes, e.g. infection. Further investigation may be required if the index of suspicion is high for malignancy.

Q4 With regard to neck masses in children, mark the following statements true or false.

Most lymphadenopathies are benign, even those cases that progress to lymph node biopsy. However, it is important to ensure that they are thoroughly evaluated, as even in a well child, lymphadenopathy could be an early sign of an underlying serious pathology, such as lymphoma.

A The most common histological feature on biopsy is reactive hyperplasia – True. Reactive hyperplasia is the most common biopsy finding in cases of lymphadenopathy in children. It is benign.

B Most palpable lymph nodes over 0.5 cm will require an excision biopsy – False. Palpable lymph nodes up to 2 cm in size are considered non-sinister in children in the absence of red flag symptoms. Excision biopsy may be warranted for a lymph node over 3 cm for a definitive pathological diagnosis.

C Branchial cysts most commonly present in the neonatal period – False. Lymphatic malformations are the most likely neck mass to present in the neonatal period, while branchial cysts are most often found in the teenage population.

D Supraclavicular swellings are common in children – False. Supraclavicular swelling is uncommon in children and should prompt further evaluation. It is associated with serious underlying pathology, such as lymphoma and TB. A chest X-ray may be helpful in identifying associated mediastinal lymphadenopathy and underlying respiratory disease.

E Neck swellings are rarely associated with infectious mononucleosis – False. Infectious mononucleosis is associated with diffuse bilateral cervical lymphadenopathy in children. A Monospot test should be requested if suspected. Advise patients to avoid contact sports if proven due to the risk of rupture of a potentially enlarged spleen.

♀ Key Point

Supraclavicular lymph nodes should always be examined in a paediatric neck examination, as they are much more likely to be associated with malignancy. Adequate exposure of the clavicles is recommended to ensure the area is not missed on palpation.

ⓘ IMPORTANT LEARNING POINTS

- "Red flag" features when assessing a paediatric neck mass include progressive increase in size, weight loss, night sweats, fever and stridor.
- Most cases of cervical lymphadenopathy are reactive, secondary to infection.
- An ultrasound scan is a widely available, simple radiological investigation that is well tolerated in children and is therefore the first line in lymph node evaluation. It is operator dependent and should be interpreted in the clinical context.

ANSWER TO CASE 2
A 10-year-old boy with newly diagnosed diabetes

Q1 Which of the following best fits with a diagnosis of Type 1 diabetes in this child?

The correct answer is B. A random blood glucose >11.1 mmol/L.

Type 1 diabetes is diagnosed by a random blood glucose, with a formal oral glucose tolerance test rarely being required. Children with Type 1 diabetes are also usually symptomatic at the time of diagnosis. Type 2 is becoming increasingly common amongst children, as the prevalence of obesity is rising.

A A high blood glucose only if it is seen following a formal oral glucose tolerance test – Incorrect. A formal glucose tolerance test is rarely required to make the diagnosis in children, but can be performed in borderline cases.

B A random blood glucose >11.1 mmol/L – Correct. According to WHO criteria, diagnosis can be made in a symptomatic child such as Jamie, with a random plasma blood glucose >11.1 mmol/L. This is not to indicate that any child with a blood glucose >11.1 mmol/L should be considered to have diabetes. Physiological stress, such as that encountered during an acute asthma attack, or gastroenteritis with release of endogenous corticosteroids, can induce transient hyperglycaemia, even in children who do not have diabetes.

C The presence of polyuria and polydipsia – Incorrect. Although excessive urination and thirst should lead to consideration of diabetes mellitus, this is not diagnostic

453

and other conditions such as habitual drinking and diabetes insipidus must also be considered.

D 4+ of glucose on urine dipstick – Incorrect. This indicates that the renal threshold of reabsorbing glucose has been exceeded; however, this is not a diagnostic criterion for diabetes.

E The presence of ketonuria – Incorrect. This also occurs during fasting states, not solely in diabetes.

Key Point

Diabetes in children and young people is usually diagnosed by means of a clinical history, and a random blood glucose. A formal OGTT is rarely required.

Q2 Regarding the aetiology of diabetes, mark the following statements true or false.

A All diabetes in children is type 1 – False. The majority of cases are type 1; however, type 2 diabetes is increasing in prevalence, particularly in obese and south Asian populations.

B Type 1 diabetes mellitus is an autoimmune condition caused by damage to pancreatic alpha cells – False. Type 1 diabetes is an autoimmune condition due to autoimmune damage to the insulin secreting beta cells of the pancreas. Alpha cells are responsible for secretion of glucagon, which raises blood glucose. The clinical syndrome of diabetes is only seen once over 80% of beta cells have been destroyed.

C Pancreatic damage is mediated by T lymphocytes – True. Beta cells in the pancreas are damaged by T lymphocytes.

D Type 1 diabetes can be associated with other autoimmune conditions such as Addison's disease, coeliac disease and hypothyroidism – True. Children are screened for these conditions following diagnosis.

E HLA-DR3 and HLA-DR4 are associated with an increased risk of developing diabetes – True. HLA-DR2 and DR5 appear to be protective. It has been determined that the HLA region on chromosome 6 is the predominant factor in determining genetic predisposition to developing type 1 diabetes.

Key Point

Type 1 diabetes is a condition resulting from immune mediated destruction of pancreatic beta cells. It is of multifactorial causation, with environmental factors inducing the clinical syndrome in those with a genetic susceptibility.

Q3 Regarding insulin, mark the following statements true or false.

A Insulin is usually derived from the pancreas of pigs – False. Insulin is usually synthetically produced. Most children are

on insulin analogues where the insulin molecule is slightly modified in order to achieve faster (rapid-acting analogues) or slower (long-acting analogues) action.

B Injections must be confined to a certain location to ensure a consistent dose-response relationship – False. Rotation of injection sites is an important practice. This avoids complications such as lipohypertrophy or lipodystrophy. Rates of absorption vary between sites, with quickest absorption being from the adipose tissue of the abdomen and slowest from the thighs.

C Insulin is usually given as one injection per day – False. A combination of insulin types will be required, with the usual regime consisting of a long acting insulin to suppress gluconeogenesis (e.g. Lantus) and shorter acting boluses (e.g. Novorapid) to cover meals. Most children will be on regimes requiring 3-4 separate daily injections.

D Most children will require relatively small amounts of insulin in the months following diagnosis – True. This is known as the "honeymoon period", as beta cell function has not yet been completely exhausted. Children usually require 1unit/kg/day of insulin in the long term; however, approximately 3-6 weeks following initiation of treatment, their blood glucose may be manageable on as little as 0.5units/kg/day.

E Insulin should be given to keep blood glucose within the normal range at all times – False. Overly tight control of blood glucose increases the risk of hypoglycaemia. Therefore, mild hyperglycaemia is tolerated acutely.

Key Point

Insulin requirements are determined by a combination of residual beta cell function, glucose consumption and energy expenditure.

Q4 In addition to insulin administration, which of the following will also cause reductions in blood glucose?

The correct answer is D. Consumption of alcoholic drinks.

Maintaining glucose levels requires careful attention not just to diet, but also health and lifestyle choices. Any new medications (e.g. corticosteroids) may have an effect on glucose levels or the effect of insulin, and this needs to be considered when adjusting doses.

A Growth hormone secretion – Incorrect. GH is a counter regulatory hormone, with actions opposing insulin, increasing blood glucose concentration. GH secretion increases during puberty, accounting for increased insulin requirements at this stage.

B Glucagon – Incorrect. Glucagon is secreted by the alpha cells of the pancreas. It causes glycogenolysis and gluconeogenesis, thus increasing glucose levels.

C Use of corticosteroid medication – Incorrect. Steroid ingestion increases blood glucose levels.

D Consumption of alcoholic drinks – Correct. It is important for young people who drink alcohol to be aware of this effect, as it can result in unpredicted hypoglycaemia.

E Febrile illnesses – Incorrect. Febrile illness is associated with hyperglycaemia, due to the actions of stress (counter-regulatory) hormones.

⚷ Key Point

Young people will transition into a more active role in the management of their condition as they become more mature and independent. It is important that they are educated on an ongoing basis about factors which affect their blood glucose to enable them to make well informed lifestyle choices.

Q5 Which would be the next most appropriate action to manage Jamie's hypoglycaemia?

The correct answer is B. Offer Jamie a sugary drink.

Hypoglycaemia can be a medical emergency, but in a well child, oral glucose is the first line management.

A IM glucagon – Incorrect. In an alert, conscious and co-operative child, this is not the recommended first step. Glucagon may be the next appropriate action if Jamie was unable or unwilling to take anything orally.

B Offer Jamie a sugary drink – Correct. This can be repeated after 10-15 minutes if there are ongoing concerns.

C Withhold his insulin for the rest of the day – Incorrect. This would be dangerous. Blood glucose levels should be closely monitored, with appropriate adjustment of insulin doses.

D Call an ambulance – Incorrect. This may be appropriate if, for example, there were concerns regarding Jamie's level of consciousness. Additionally if a child significantly overdoses on insulin, or if they ingest excess oral hypoglycaemic agents, urgent medical review would be required. A glucose infusion may be required.

E Give him a sandwich – Incorrect. Simple carbohydrates, such as juice, glucose gel or jam, are the priority as they immediately raise blood glucose. Complex carbohydrates, such as bread, should be given after this, to help maintain the blood glucose level.

⚷ Key Point

Most children with diabetes will suffer a hypoglycaemic episode at some point. Recognition of symptoms and sensible stepwise management protocols are essential principles that families will need to learn to manage their child's diabetes safely. First-line management in a well child is oral simple carbohydrates, like a sugary drink.

Q6 What conclusion can you draw from the above glucose readings?

The correct answer is C. Checking Jamie's blood glucose overnight for few nights will be helpful.

Maintaining a diary of blood glucose recordings can be an invaluable tool for troubleshooting, particularly in cases where glycaemic control appears to be suboptimal. Occasionally, a continuous glucose sensor can be inserted under the skin to measure interstitial glucose for few a days. The most common indications for this are: frequent/unpredictable hypoglycaemic episodes and hypoglycaemia unawareness.

A Jamie must be snacking overnight – Incorrect. Jamie has high blood glucose readings prior to eating in the morning, and this can be for a variety of reasons apart from food intake overnight. Counter-regulatory hormone release, e.g. cortisol, in the morning (Dawn phenomenon) can account for high morning blood glucose.

B Jamie should skip breakfast – Incorrect. If blood glucose is high, a correction dose should be offered, taking into account the additional carbohydrates consumed.

C Checking Jamie's blood glucose overnight for a few nights will be helpful – Correct. Jamie may need to adjust his night time insulin dose. Morning hyperglycaemia is usually associated with glucose release from the liver overnight. Growth hormone and sex steroid hormones during puberty can cause morning hyperglycaemia as well (dawn phenomenon). Hyperglycaemia may also be the result of nocturnal hypoglycaemia, and subsequent secretion of excess counter-regulatory hormones. This is called the Somogyi phenomenon.

D Jamie should cut out sugary food from his diet – Incorrect. In general, dietary guidelines are similar for children with diabetes as they are for the entire population. A healthy diet will consist of approximately 50% carbohydrates, 30-35% fat and 10-15% protein. A large proportion should consist of foods with a low glycaemic index: these foods release their glucose into the bloodstream at a slower rate than high glycaemic index foods. Carbohydrate counting (carb counting) is used to match the amount of insulin given at mealtimes to the amount of carbohydrate eaten.

⚷ Key Point

Even in well controlled diabetes, it is still important to check blood glucose levels. This ensures objective information is available for any changes in insulin therapy. Carbohydrate counting is used to match insulin dose to carbohydrate consumption.

ANSWER TO CASE 3
A 14-year-old girl presenting with delayed puberty

Q1 Which of the following findings are consistent with the likely underlying diagnosis?

The correct answers are A. Lanugo hair, C. Bradycardia, D. Obsessional thoughts and E. Social withdrawal.

Although nothing has been said about food avoidance or fear of gaining weight, this child is likely to have anorexia nervosa. Anorexia nervosa has both psychological manifestations, and physical manifestations as a result of inadequate oral intake. The low BMI and amenorrhoea strongly suggest the diagnosis. She is also tired and hypothermic, common findings in anorexia nervosa.

A Lanugo hair – Correct. Patients with anorexia nervosa are commonly found to have fine, downy lanugo hair on examination.

B Hypertension – Incorrect. Patients with anorexia nervosa are often hypotensive, not hypertensive.

C Bradycardia – Correct. Sinus bradycardia occurs in up to 95% of cases of anorexia nervosa.

D Obsessional thoughts – Correct. Obsessional thoughts are common in patients with anorexia nervosa and are not limited to food.

E Social withdrawal – Correct. Patients with anorexia nervosa may become withdrawn from their social circle or lose interest in activities they previously enjoyed.

⚲ Key Point

Common findings in patients with anorexia nervosa are prepubertal sexual characteristics, lanugo hair, low BMI and signs of systemic failure, such as hypotension, hypothermia and bradycardia.

Q2 Which of the following initial investigations would be helpful in this patient?

The correct answers are A. LH and FSH concentrations, B. Thyroid function tests and E. Chromosomal karyotyping.

Although, clinically, it may appear that this is a clear case of anorexia nervosa, investigations are required to assess other potentially treatable causes. This includes hypothyroidism, Turner's syndrome and hypogonadotrophic hypogonadism.

A LH and FSH concentrations – Correct. This will help to identify if the hypothalamo-pituitary-gonadal axis is intact and exclude primary gonadal failure. If LH and FSH are low, it implies the problem is hypothalamic/pituitary in origin (as seen in anorexia nervosa), whereas if they are high/normal, the problem is more likely to be primary gonadal failure.

B Thyroid function tests – Correct. Children with hypothyroidism may present with delayed puberty. They do not always present with typical weight gain.

C MRI brain – Incorrect. This is not a key initial investigation, although is very important in patients where there is a suspicion of a pituitary tumour.

D Adrenal MRI – Incorrect. An adrenal mass would present with precocious puberty, not delayed.

E Chromosomal karyotyping – Correct. Any girl with primary amenorrhoea should have her karyotype checked to rule out Turner's syndrome. Other rarer conditions, such as complete androgen insensitivity syndrome (i.e. a male genotype XY with a female phenotype because of androgen insensitivity) can present with primary amenorrhoea.

⚲ Key Point

- All girls with delayed puberty should have a karyotype done to exclude Turner's syndrome.
- Baseline LH and FSH measurements are useful first-line investigations to differentiate primary from secondary gonadal failure.

Q3 Which management option is best?

The correct answer is E. Referral to child and adolescent mental health services

The mainstay of treatment for anorexia nervosa is with child and adolescent mental health services. It is also important to treat anorexia nervosa from a medical perspective. There may be associated bradycardia or hypotension. Introducing feeding may be associated with refeeding syndrome, and so electrolytes need to be closely monitored. Severe cases will require admission to hospital for medical stabilisation and refeeding.

A Watch and wait; follow up in 6 months – Incorrect. Anorexia nervosa needs to be actively managed from the point of diagnosis.

B Start on antidepressants – Incorrect. Even if there was associated depression, talking therapies are first-line therapy, not medication.

C Pubertal induction using oestrogen preparations – Incorrect. In this case, inducing puberty using oestrogens does not solve the underlying diagnosis of anorexia nervosa. The patient has delayed puberty due to hypothalamic dysfunction secondary to anorexia.

D Start on GnRH agonist – Incorrect. This paradoxically suppresses gonadotrophin production, reducing FSH and LH levels. GnRH agonists are used in management of central precocious puberty.

E Referral to child and adolescent mental health services – Correct. Urgency of the referral in patients depends on evidence of systemic failure and rate of weight loss.

♀ Key Point

Patients with suspicion of anorexia nervosa should be referred to mental health services. The urgency of referral depends on the rate of weight loss and evidence of systemic failure.

ⓘ IMPORTANT LEARNING POINTS

- Delayed puberty may be the first presentation of anorexia nervosa.
- Delayed puberty is more likely to have a pathological cause in girls than in boys.
- All girls with delayed puberty need to undergo chromosomal analysis to exclude Turner's syndrome, even if they have no other features of the disease.
- Anorexia nervosa cases should promptly be referred to mental health services. If there is systemic failure, or very rapid weight loss, referral has a greater urgency, and inpatient admission may be warranted.

ANSWER TO CASE 4
A 12-day-old baby presenting with poor feeding and vomiting

Q1 What is the most likely diagnosis?

The correct answer is B. Congenital adrenal hyperplasia.

The differential for poor feeding and vomiting in a neonate includes infection, sepsis, congenital heart disease and bronchiolitis. However, the presence of hyponatraemia and hyperkalaemia should always prompt clinicians to rule out CAH.

A Fulminant sepsis – Incorrect. Sepsis is an important differential diagnosis because of lethargy and irritability. However, given i) no temperature, ii) negative cultures and iii) normal inflammatory markers, it is less likely than CAH. It is important to note that the absence of fever and negative blood cultures do not rule out sepsis. Therefore, even though it is not the top differential, this baby needs to be empirically treated for sepsis.

B Congenital adrenal hyperplasia – Correct. Hypoglycaemia, hyponatraemia, hyperkalaemia and dehydration in the neonatal period suggest CAH. Hyperpigmentation of scrotal skin is due to elevated ACTH concentration, which also fits with the diagnosis. This is the salt losing form of CAH.

C Gastro-oesophageal reflux disease – Incorrect. GOR may present with vomiting, particularly after feeds. However, it would not cause the electrolyte derangement noted in this case.

D Heart failure – Incorrect. Heart failure may present with poor feeding, but in this case there were normal antenatal scans, and a chest X-ray with no signs of heart failure. Additionally, the electrolyte derangement doesn't fit with heart failure.

♀ Key Point

The possibility of CAH should be considered in infants presenting with diarrhoea, vomiting and hypoglycaemia, especially when associated with hyponatraemia, hyperkalaemia, hypovolemia and metabolic acidosis.

Q2 Which of the following tests is most useful in establishing the diagnosis in this clinical scenario?

The correct answer is C. 17-hydroxyprogesterone.

It is important to collect the correct blood samples before starting corticosteroid replacement. It is often difficult in the dehydrated, shocked neonate to collect blood. 17-hydroxyprogesterone is one of the precursors accumulating in 21-hydroxylase deficiency, the commonest form of the disease. Other useful tests are ACTH (high), renin (high) and cortisol (inappropriately low). A urine steroid profile is also diagnostic. In countries with newborn CAH screening, 17-hydroxyprogesterone is measured in a blood spot.

A Karyotyping – Incorrect. Karyotyping may be required if there is doubt over gender, but it is not diagnostic.

B Specific gene testing – Incorrect. Gene testing is not routinely done in CAH. However, it is useful if the parents are planning for future pregnancy.

C 17-hydroxyprogesterone – Correct. 17OHP is a precursor in the adrenal biosynthetic pathway that is very high in 21-hydroxylase deficiency, the most common form of CAH.

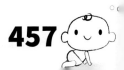

Q4 The CT scan confirms an intracranial lesion. How would you manage this child in ED?

The correct answer is E. Referral to the nearest neurosurgical centre.

This child has evidence of raised ICP which may be caused by a large tumour directly infiltrating the brain or by the tumour obstructing CSF flow.

A Corticosteroids – Incorrect. Corticosteroids will reduce oedema surrounding the tumour, thereby reducing ICP. This should only be given after discussion with neurosurgeons, since, if surgery is being done imminently, corticosteroids may increase risk of bleeding. In the presence of raised ICP, mannitol or hypertonic sodium chloride may also be used.

B Intravenous aciclovir – Incorrect. There is no indication for antiviral treatment, as the pathology is malignancy.

C Discharge with parental advice to return if symptoms are worsening – Incorrect. There are clearly symptoms and signs of raised intracranial pressure that require prompt recognition and management. If treatment is delayed, it could lead to cerebral herniation (coning), coma or death.

D Lumbar puncture to relieve the symptoms of raised ICP – Incorrect. Lumbar puncture is contraindicated in this instance, as a sudden reduction in pressure may precipitate cerebral herniation.

E Referral to the nearest paediatric neurosurgical centre – Correct. Urgent referral to the on-call paediatric neurosurgeon is required for management of raised ICP. If supportive measures and corticosteroids alone are not able to control ICP, emergency neurosurgical intervention may be required.

♀ Key Point

The most important initial management of a patient with a brain tumour is to safely control raised ICP. Emergency management of airway, breathing and circulation is required for children with reduced GCS, seizures or "Cushing's response", together with transfer to a specialist paediatric neurosurgical centre.

ⓘ IMPORTANT LEARNING POINTS

- Early symptoms of brain tumours in children can mimic those of common benign paediatric conditions.
- Symptoms and signs include headache, vomiting, visual symptoms and signs (including papilloedema, nystagmus and squint), motor symptoms and signs (including ataxia, weakness, swallowing difficulties and speech disturbance), behavioural change/drowsiness and seizures.

ANSWER TO CASE 6

A 13-month-old girl presents with severe pallor

Q1 What is the most likely underlying diagnosis?

The correct answer is B. Iron deficiency anaemia.

The key features here are the dietary history and the fact the child is found to be well, with no worrying features on examination.

A Acute lymphoblastic leukaemia – Incorrect. ALL is an important differential diagnosis for anaemic symptoms in children. Children with leukaemia will often present more unwell with additional features including pallor, tiredness, pain and lymphadenopathy. It is unusual, but possible, for children with ALL to present with an isolated anaemia. It is therefore essential for children presenting with abnormal FBC parameters to obtain an urgent blood film.

B Iron deficiency anaemia – Correct. Iron deficiency anaemia is the commonest cause of anaemia in an otherwise well child. There is often a history of excessive cow's milk intake in the older infant or inadequate dietary variety. Proteins in cow's milk disrupt iron absorption and whole milk proteins can cause an enteropathy, thus causing chronic blood loss.

C Aplastic anaemia – Incorrect. This is an important differential but very rare. It is usually associated with other abnormalities in the blood parameters.

D Coeliac disease – Incorrect. Coeliac disease may result in a microcytic anaemia but is also associated with weight loss, abdominal distension, irregular bowel habits and diarrhoea.

E B12 deficiency – Incorrect. B12 deficiency is associated with a macrocytic anaemia, not a microcytic anaemia.

♀ Key Point

Iron deficiency anaemia is the commonest cause of anaemia in children. The anaemia is not usually severe, but can be mild or moderate.

Q2 What would be your next investigations? Select all that apply.

The correct answers are B. Iron studies and C. Blood film.

A Bone marrow aspirate – Incorrect. A bone marrow aspiration would not be indicated in this child at this stage. If the anaemia fails to respond to a course of adequate iron therapy or there are other abnormalities in the blood count, then a bone marrow aspirate may be performed at a later stage.

B Iron studies – Correct. A low serum ferritin, low iron and elevated total iron binding capacity (TIBC) will help to confirm iron deficiency anaemia.

C Blood film – Correct. A blood film examination is essential to look at cellular morphology. The most important diagnosis to rule out is ALL, where a blood film may reveal lymphoblasts.

D Parvovirus screen – Incorrect. Parvovirus can cause aplastic anaemia, but it is not the most likely cause, particularly given that platelets and WBC counts are normal. It will also usually be associated with a low/normal reticulocyte count, as it affects the bone marrow.

E Endoscopy – Incorrect. Whilst an endoscopy may be required in adults presenting with severe iron deficiency anaemia, in children with a compatible history, dietary iron deficiency is most likely.

⚷ Key Point

Iron deficiency anaemia is confirmed by verifying a low serum ferritin, low iron, and an elevated TIBC. However, ferritin may be in the normal range if there is concurrent illness, as ferritin is elevated in acute inflammation.

Q3 What would be your first-line management for the treatment of the above condition?

The correct answer is C. Discharge, commence oral iron supplementation and observe.

Whilst local guidelines and policies may vary, the general principles are that a period of observation in hospital, along with adequate documentation of successful toleration of oral iron therapy, are important in children with this severe an anaemia.

A Observation as an outpatient and advise – Incorrect. Such a low Hb level necessitates treatment.

B Admit for blood transfusion – Incorrect. Normally, it is possible to avoid blood transfusion in the case of iron deficiency, regardless of how low the haemoglobin is. This child has anaemia but no heart failure and she is well compensated. If done, transfusion should be done cautiously.

C Discharge, commence oral iron supplementation and observe – Correct. The degree of anaemia necessitates oral iron supplementation, and improvement of diet.

D Admit for IV iron supplementation – Incorrect. IV iron is rarely used, as it has caused deaths by anaphylaxis. It would be reserved for cases where oral supplementation was not feasible or achieved.

E Referral to gastroenterology for urgent endoscopy – Incorrect. This child has a good consistent history for dietary iron deficiency, so endoscopy is not indicated.

⚷ Key Point

Children with severe iron deficiency anaemia do not necessarily need a blood transfusion, even if the haemoglobin is very low. In general, they should be started on oral iron supplementation and observed closely to ensure this is tolerated.

Q4 What feature is not typical of this condition and should prompt rapid referral to a specialist team?

The correct answer is A. Black tarry stools.

The presence of significant GI bleeding would be a very different entity and requires prompt endoscopic evaluation and gastroenterologist review.

A Black tarry stools – Correct. Black tarry stools suggest blood loss and could be suggestive of a Meckel's diverticulum. This should prompt urgent assessment by gastroenterologists. Iron supplements may cause black stools, but not tarry stools.

B Poor diet – Incorrect. Iron deficiency occurs in the context of an inadequately balanced diet. If the family report a well-balanced diet, other causes should be looked for.

C Normal serum ferritin – Incorrect. Serum ferritin is an acute phase reactant so it may be falsely elevated with intercurrent viral infections. A normal serum ferritin does not exclude iron deficiency, which is why measuring iron and TIBC is helpful.

D Severe pallor – Incorrect. The degree of pallor will be linked to the degree of the anaemia, not the underlying cause.

E Exclusively breastfed – Incorrect. After six months of age, exclusive breastfeeding can lead to iron deficiency. Cow's milk and human milk both have low iron contents but the bioavailability of iron from human milk is higher. Infants who are fed on formula milks are less likely to develop severe iron deficiency anaemia, as formula milk is supplemented with iron.

⚷ Key Point

Black tarry stools are suggestive of blood loss and further investigation needs to be carried out to rule out GI bleeding, e.g. from a Meckel's diverticulum.

ⓘ IMPORTANT LEARNING POINTS

- Iron deficiency anaemia is the most common cause of anaemia in childhood. The majority of cases are dietary in origin. It can result in severe anaemia.
- Exclusive breastfeeding after six-months-old or excessive cow's milk consumption in infants are risk factors for development of iron deficiency.
- Admission and supportive care during the initial stages of managing severe anaemia is important, even if supplementation is oral.

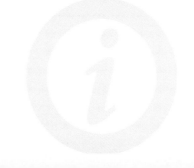

ANSWER TO CASE 7
A 4-year-old presenting with thrombocytopenia

Q1 What is the most likely underlying diagnosis?

The correct answer is B. Immune thrombocytopenic purpura.

Petechiae and bruising have a broad differential, with many sinister causes such as meningococcal sepsis, ALL and non-accidental injury.

A Acute lymphoblastic leukaemia – Incorrect. Children with leukaemia will often present as more unwell, with additional features including pallor, tiredness, pain and lymphadenopathy. It is unusual, but possible, for children with ALL to present with an isolated thrombocytopenia. It is therefore essential to obtain a blood film for any children presenting with thrombocytopenia.

B Immune thrombocytopenic purpura – Correct. ITP is characterised by rapid-onset bruising and petechiae in an otherwise well child. There is often a history of a recent viral infection or immunisations.

C Henoch-Schönlein purpura – Incorrect. HSP is a clinical diagnosis based on the identification of certain clinical features including an evolving palpable purpuric rash, joint pain and periarticular oedema. There may also be abdominal symptoms and renal involvement. It is a vasculitic disorder and may be precipitated by an URTI. Thrombocytopenia is not characteristic; conversely the platelet count may be elevated.

D Systemic lupus erythematosus – Incorrect. In older children and teenagers, thrombocytopenia is more often associated with autoimmune diseases and rheumatological conditions, such as SLE. Additional symptoms and signs include a characteristic facial "butterfly" rash, fatigue and arthralgia.

E Meningococcal sepsis – Incorrect. Early meningococcal infection can be difficult to recognise. Children presenting acutely unwell with a fever and non-blanching rash should be treated empirically with broad-spectrum intravenous antibiotics.

⚷ Key Point

ITP is the most common cause of thrombocytopenia in children. Diagnosis of ITP is made by exclusion of other more serious conditions, particularly ALL.

Q2 What would be your next investigation?

The correct answer is B. Blood film.

A blood film is key to ensuring leukaemia is not missed.

A Bone marrow aspirate – Incorrect. Bone marrow aspirate is not indicated in children diagnosed with classic ITP. It is an invasive test, often requiring general anaesthetic use. However, it may be considered after discussion with a paediatric haematologist when atypical features are present or if thrombocytopenia is unusually prolonged.

B Blood film – Correct. Blood film examination is essential to look at cellular morphology. The most important diagnosis not to miss is ALL where a blood film may reveal lymphoblasts.

C No further investigation – Incorrect. ALL needs to be ruled out.

D Autoantibody screen – Incorrect. Further investigations are only indicated in older children, or in patients with chronic ITP when autoimmune disorders and other rare conditions may be the cause of the thrombocytopenia.

⚷ Key Point

If atypical features of ITP are present, it is recommended that the patient is referred to a paediatric haematologist for a bone marrow aspirate.

Q3 What would be your first-line management for the treatment of the above condition?

The correct answer is A. Observation and advice.

The natural disease course for ITP is spontaneous resolution; therefore, in most cases, no specific treatment is needed.

A Observation and advice – Correct. The majority of children with ITP undergo spontaneous resolution within 6-8 weeks. Initial management should not depend on platelet count alone and is influenced by the presence of complications including significant haemorrhage. The parents should be advised to attend the ED if the child sustains a head injury.

B Intravenous immunoglobulin – Incorrect. Only in the case of severe symptoms and significant haemorrhage is intravenous immunoglobulin considered. This treatment has not been shown to influence the overall disease duration.

C Corticosteroids – Incorrect. Corticosteroids are only indicated in specific cases, e.g. significant haemorrhage. This treatment has not been shown to influence the overall disease outcome. Diagnosis of ITP must be certain before giving corticosteroids as this can have major adverse consequences should the patient turn out to have underlying leukaemia. Many specialists recommend BMA prior to starting corticosteroid treatment for this reason.

D Splenectomy – Incorrect. Splenectomy is very rarely required and only considered in cases of chronic ITP (>6 months duration) with impaired quality of life.

E Platelet transfusion – Incorrect. Due to the disease aetiology, transfused platelets will be quickly consumed. Therefore, transfusion should be reserved for patients with life-threatening haemorrhage.

⚲ Key Point

Initial management of ITP consists of observation, reassurance, parental education and support. The vast majority of cases resolve spontaneously, and significant haemorrhage is rare.

Q4 What features are not typical of this condition?

The correct answer is A. White cell blasts on blood film.

Atypical features may necessitate alternative treatment, or an alternative diagnosis. ALL is important to always rule out with a blood film.

A White cell blasts on blood film – Correct. The presence of white cell blasts on blood film is not a feature of ITP and is suggestive of leukaemia. This should prompt immediate referral to a paediatric haematologist for further management.

B Spontaneous resolution in 6-8 weeks – Incorrect. The natural course of uncomplicated ITP is for the disease to spontaneously resolve within 6-8 weeks.

C History of a preceding febrile illness – Incorrect. ITP is often associated with a recent URTI.

D Platelet count 10 x 10⁹/L – Incorrect. Platelet count can fall to extremely low levels with ITP. It is common for the platelet count to be <20 x 10⁹/L.

E Epistaxis – Incorrect. Epistaxis and mucosal bleeding can occur with thrombocytopenia. Severe complications, including intracranial haemorrhage, are rare.

⚲ Key Point

Leukaemia is the most common childhood cancer, and may in rare cases present as an isolated thrombocytopaenia.

ⓘ IMPORTANT LEARNING POINTS

- ITP is characterised by an isolated finding of low platelets, resulting in possible bleeding, bruising and petechiae formation.
- Most cases in children are mild and self-limiting, but if the platelet count drops dramatically, there is a risk of severe bleeding including intracranial haemorrhage.
- Management generally involves observation and advice, although rarely corticosteroids may be used first-line to increase the platelet count. In such cases, it is important to consider a bone marrow aspiration first to avoid masking a diagnosis of ALL.

ANSWER TO CASE 8
A 4-month-old boy presenting with severe respiratory distress

Q1 What features in the history might make you suspect a primary immunodeficiency?

The correct answers are B. Faltering growth, D. Family history of unexplained early death, and E. Recurrent or resistant thrush.

Although recurrent infections are the hallmark of a primary immunodeficiency, the average child with an intact immune system will have numerous GI and respiratory infections a year. This can make diagnosis tricky, but the clinician should be wary with children who develop serious infections or infections with normally benign organisms. A detailed family history is essential, as it may offer important clues to diagnosis and many of the primary immunodeficiencies display X-linked inheritance.

A Female sex – Incorrect. Seventy percent of primary immunodeficiencies occur in males, as X-linked inheritance is common to many syndromes.

B Faltering growth – Correct. Faltering growth is common; contributing factors include high energy expenditure due to hypermetabolism in infectious states, oral ulcers causing poor oral intake, and chronic diarrhoea.

C Three upper respiratory tract infections per year – Incorrect. The "normal" child has four to eight respiratory infections per year. Features of infection that should raise suspicion of a primary immunodeficiency include infection with opportunistic organisms (e.g. aspergillus), frequent courses of antibiotics with little effect, and unusual sites of infection, e.g. liver and skin abscesses.

D Family history of unexplained early death – Correct. There is a strong genetic component to many primary immunodeficiencies and a family history of early childhood death should be checked in any suspected cases.

E Recurrent or resistant thrush – Correct. Persistent candidiasis should alert the clinician to the possibility of a primary immunodeficiency, as this opportunistic fungal infection is common in immunodeficiency.

⚲ Key Point

Primary immunodeficiency should be suspected if there are concurrent infections at multiple sites, persistent infections resistant to antibiotics, atypical or unusual organisms causing infection, accompanying faltering growth or failure to thrive. Family history of unexplained early death should also raise suspicion.

 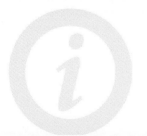

Q2 Which features on a chest X-ray would make you suspect a primary immunodeficiency?

The correct answers are B. Bilateral pulmonary infiltrates, and C. Absent thymus.

The presence of an infection on chest X-ray is not specific for an immunodeficiency. However, serial X-rays showing persistent infections may arouse suspicion. Features associated with infection with opportunistic organisms, such as Pneumocystis jirovecii *(bilateral pulmonary infiltrates), or the absence of lymphoid tissue strongly suggest an immunodeficiency.*

A Pleural effusion – Incorrect. Pleural effusion can be seen in pneumonia but is not specifically associated with primary immunodeficiency.
B Bilateral pulmonary infiltrates – Correct. This describes the classic chest X-ray appearance of infection with the opportunistic organism *Pneumocystis jirovecii*, a yeast-like fungus pathogenic in immune deficiency.
C Absent thymus – Correct. Hypoplasia of lymphoid tissue is a key feature of several primary immunodeficiencies, including SCID and Di George syndrome.
D Hyperinflation – Incorrect. This is commonly seen in asthma and has no strong link to immunodeficiency.
E Pneumothorax – Incorrect. This is associated with connective tissue disorders and has no strong link to primary immunodeficiency.

Key Point

Chest X-rays are not routinely ordered due to a suspicion of immunodeficiency, but they may bring up unexpected signs that increase the likelihood of one being present.

Q3 Which three investigations would be most helpful in diagnosing a primary immunodeficiency?

The correct answers are B. Full blood count with differential white cell count, C. Immunoglobulins, and D. Lymphocyte subsets.

Investigations that can demonstrate an infection, such as blood cultures and inflammatory markers, are not specific tests for immunodeficiency, although they are useful in clinical practice for patient management. Immunodeficiency can be investigated by exploring the number and function of key cells of the immune system.

A Stool MC&S – Incorrect. Stool cultures may identify the pathogen responsible for a particular episode of infection but cannot diagnose a primary immune deficiency, although infections with opportunistic organisms may arouse suspicion.

B Full blood count with differential white cell count – Correct. Persistent lymphopaenia or neutropaenia suggests immune deficiency, although a stand-alone measurement may represent an isolated infection in an individual with normal immune function.
C Immunoglobulins – Correct. Maternal IgG confers protection until six months of age, but following this, low levels of immunoglobulin can indicate humoral immune deficiencies. Poor production of antibodies in response to childhood vaccines such as pneumococcus, diphtheria and tetanus can also indicate a humoral immune deficiency.
D Lymphocyte subsets – Correct. The presence or absence of T or B lymphocytes or natural killer cells is key to the diagnosis of SCID and can be helpful in diagnosing other immunodeficiencies affecting cellular immunity. However, a normal level of lymphocytes does not exclude a cellular immunodeficiency as cells may be non-functional.
E Blood cultures – Incorrect. Blood cultures may identify the pathogen responsible for a particular episode of infection but cannot diagnose a primary immune deficiency, although infections with opportunistic organisms may arouse suspicion.

Key Point

Laboratory work up for a suspected immunodeficiency should include full blood count with differential white cell count, immunoglobulin levels (IgG, IgM and IgA), response to vaccines, HIV testing, complement levels, and lymphocyte subsets.

Q4 Which of the following are key points in the management of a primary immunodeficiency?

The correct answers are A. Antibiotic prophylaxis, and D. Immunoglobulin infusions.

Management centres on preventing infection and prompt, aggressive treatment of infection when it occurs. These children are particularly vulnerable to iatrogenic complications as treatments commonly used in immunocompetent children, such as live vaccines, may have devastating consequences in the immunodeficient child.

A Antibiotic prophylaxis – Correct. Antibiotic prophylaxis is crucial in primary immunodeficiency to prevent against infection, particularly with opportunistic organisms.
B Full immunisation – Incorrect. Immunisation with live attenuated vaccines such as BCG, rotavirus and poliovirus can cause overwhelming or fatal infections in the immunocompromised and should be avoided.
C Splenectomy – Incorrect. This is not a treatment for primary immunodeficiency but may be a cause of secondary immunodeficiency.

CLINICAL CASES: INTERMEDIATE

D Immunoglobulin infusions – Correct. Immunoglobulin infusions form part of the mainstay of treatment for many primary immunodeficiencies where defects in humoral immunity are present.

E Early use of blood products to support deficits – Incorrect. Blood products in patients with immunodeficiency should be used cautiously due to the possibility of graft-versus-host disease if blood products containing viable lymphocytes are used. Whenever necessary, irradiated, CMV-negative blood products should be used.

Key Point

Management of primary immunodeficiency requires prophylactic antibiotics for opportunistic infections, aggressive and early antibiotic treatment for infection, avoidance of live vaccines, and isolation precautions as deemed necessary.

ⓘ IMPORTANT LEARNING POINTS

- Immunodeficiencies are extremely rare, but delayed diagnosis has potentially catastrophic consequences for this vulnerable patient group. In the initial stage, it is more important to know when to suspect an immunodeficiency rather than how to clinically diagnose it.

- Immunodeficiency should be considered in i) all cases of infections with atypical or opportunistic organisms and ii) complicated infections with common organisms.

- Management is predominantly supportive. Other treatments that may be considered are: IV immunoglobulin, enzyme replacement, haematopoietic stem cell transplant and gene therapy.

ANSWER TO CASE 9
A 1-year-old boy presents with an itchy rash

Q1 Which of the following are correct regarding eczema?

The correct answers are C. A family or personal history of allergic conditions is common, D. Heat, chemicals and stress can aggravate the condition, and E. The mainstay of treatment is with topical emollients and corticosteroids.

Eczema is a chronic, inflammatory, itchy skin condition characterised by episodic exacerbations. It has a classic distribution pattern, but be wary of atypical presentations. Diagnosis is based on clinical features, family history and history of atopy.

A Infantile eczema affects mainly the flexor surfaces and the nappy area – Incorrect. Infantile eczema affects predominantly the face, scalp and extensor surfaces, typically sparing the nappy area. In older age groups, the flexor surfaces are more likely to be affected.

B Most children with infantile eczema will have severe eczema throughout life – Incorrect. Almost 40% of cases of infantile/childhood eczema will clear by adulthood.

C A family or personal history of allergic conditions is common – Correct. Eczema forms part of the atopic triad with asthma and allergic rhinitis.

D Heat, chemicals and stress can aggravate the condition – Correct. Exacerbating factors include heat, perspiration, stress and anxiety, rapid temperature changes, and exposure to chemicals or cigarette smoke.

E The mainstay of treatment is with topical emollients and corticosteroids – Correct. Emollients maintain hydration and should be applied liberally. Topical corticosteroids should be given to suppress inflammation as indicated.

Key Point

Differentiating eczema and psoriasis is important. Eczema is likely to be itchy, to run in families and to be associated with other allergic conditions, such as asthma and allergic rhinitis.

Q2 What features would support a diagnosis of secondary bacterial infection?

The correct answer is A. Fever.

Secondary infection of eczema is a common complication. In bacterial infections, there is classically honey coloured crusting (impetiginisation) of the skin around the site of the infected eczema. This always warrants urgent treatment.

A Fever – Correct. Fever is a sign of a systemic response to infection. If there are no other localising factors, the infection is likely to relate to the infected eczema.

B Dry, erythematous plaques – Incorrect. Dry plaques are seen in chronic eczema. Signs suggestive of bacterial infection include weeping, pustules and impetiginisation.

C Excoriated skin – Incorrect. Excoriated skin is commonly seen in eczema. This breech in the epidermal barrier may represent the mode of pathogen entry; however, it does not directly suggest a bacterial infection.

D Oedema and erythema of affected skin – Incorrect. Severe oedema and erythema indicate an acute exacerbation and may indicate a bacterial infection of the skin. However, mild oedema and redness secondary to inflammation is seen commonly in non-infected eczema

E Crops of fluid filled vesicles – Incorrect. Crops of fluid filled vesicles are suggestive of a viral infection with varicella zoster or herpes simplex and should be treated with antiviral agents. Such infections can be very severe, and there should be a low threshold for using intravenous therapy.

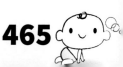

Q3 Which of the following should be included in the initial management in this case of suspected infected eczema?

The correct answer is D. Antihistamines to relieve pruritus.

This patient is septic, with the likely source being secondary bacterial infection of the eczema. Prompt treatment is required. This will involve fluid resuscitation and intravenous antibiotics. Topical corticosteroids should be introduced early to control the eczema itself. Symptomatic relief is also important, and so an antihistamine should be prescribed.

A A course of oral corticosteroids to control the exacerbation of eczema – Incorrect. Oral corticosteroids may be necessary to control severe exacerbations of eczema in the absence of severe infection. The priority here is to treat and prevent the rapid evolution of infection. Topical corticosteroids should be introduced early to control the eczema itself; failure to do that will put the child at risk of re-infection. Treatment with topical antiseptic creams and soap substitutes is also advised.

B Swabs of cutaneous lesions for microscopy and culture – Incorrect. Secondary bacterial infections in eczema are most frequently caused by organisms commonly present on the skin such as *Staphylococcus* and *Streptococcus* species; therefore, routine skin swabs are unnecessary and do not alter management. They may be useful in recurrent infections or infection refractory to treatment to isolate organisms and identify antibiotic sensitivities. All clinically septic children should have blood cultures taken preferably prior to commencing antibiotics.

C Oral antibiotics (e.g. flucloxacillin) to cover common skin organisms, such as *Staphylococcus aureus* – Incorrect. Prompt antibiotic therapy is needed as this child is clearly showing signs of sepsis. Although flucloxacillin would be an acceptable choice of antibiotic, the oral route is not appropriate here due to presentation with vomiting. It would also be sensible to add in benzylpenicillin to broaden the antibiotic cover against streptococcal infection as well.

D Antihistamines to relieve pruritus – Correct. Antihistamines can relieve itching and some may also have additional sedative properties which can ease discomfort

E Antiviral therapy such as aciclovir – Incorrect. If a bacterial infection is suspected, aciclovir has no role. However, it should be administered promptly in secondary viral infections.

♀ Key Point

All septic patients have a similar initial treatment pathway regardless of aetiology. It is important to give antibiotics and fluids early, take blood cultures and identify the source of infection. In the case of underlying eczema, appropriate strength topical corticosteroid therapy should be introduced early to control the exacerbation.

ⓘ IMPORTANT LEARNING POINTS

- Eczema is a chronic, inflammatory condition of the skin which has a relapsing and remitting clinical course.
- Disruption of the epidermal barrier of the skin and inflammation leads to erythematous patches which can be intensely pruritic, affecting the face, scalp and extensor surfaces in infants, but predominantly flexural areas in older children and adults.
- Secondary complications include superimposed bacterial and viral infections of the skin.
- Optimal management involves avoidance of exacerbating factors, restoration of hydration and the barrier function of the skin, and treatment with appropriate strength corticosteroids for the skin inflammation.
- Due to the chronic nature of eczema and the intensive treatment regimens required, patient education is critical.
- Like all skin conditions, eczema can have a considerable psychological burden on sufferers, the impact of which should be regularly assessed.

ANSWER TO CASE 10
A 3-year-old boy presenting with possible appendicitis

There are some relatively subtle errors on this chart.
- *The estimated weight needs to be updated to the actual weight. This will change all subsequent calculations.*
- *The allergies section is not completed, signed or dated.*
- *The hospital number is incomplete.*
- *No consultant is identified who will be responsible for Richard's care.*
- *Age does not state any units, eg. years or months*

The regular medication:
- Both paracetamol and augmentin have been prescribed orally for a patient who is nil by mouth and can be changed to IV. Even if it were correct, "PO" should not be used, "ORAL" should be used.
- Paracetamol has been prescribed at 20 mg/kg qds (although this has not been indicated). The maximum oral dose of paracetamol is 75 mg/kg/day, equivalent to 18mg/kg QDS. Hence this prescription would exceed the maximum dose. It must be re-written at 15 mg/kg/dose QDS IV (the maximum IV dose is 60 mg/kg/day).
- Timings have not been specified – this means the medications cannot be given.
- Start and stop dates must be supplied.
- The signature is illegible and no contact details are provided to correct the chart.
- Augmentin should be written as the generic name of "Co-Amoxiclav".
- Even if co-amoxiclav could be given orally, there is no indication of which formulation to use. This could be either

the 125/31 or 250/62 varieties. When written up as IV, the correct dose is 30 mg/kg.

The fluids:

> Normal saline (0.9% sodium chloride) is always used for a bolus.
> The amount of fluid in ml/kg should be quantified.

> New calculations required given the new weight of the patient.
> The maintenance fluids should specify that they are "full maintenance".
> The name should be printed, with contact details provided.

The full prescription is shown in *Chart 3b.*

CHART 3B: PRESCRIPTION CHART FOR CLINICAL CASE 10

Name: RICHARD PETERS	Weight 16kg	Known allergies
Date of birth 03/06/2011	Age 3 years	NO KNOWN DRUG ALLERGIES
Hospital number SM678112	Consultant DR ANDREWS	Signature: A.Jones Jones Blp 1234
Admission date 01/01/2015	Ward KOALA	Date: 1/1/15

REGULAR MEDICATIONS

		Date / Time	1/1	2/1	3/1	4/1	5/1	6/1	7/1	8/1	9/1
Drug PARACETAMOL 15mg/kg		00									
Dose 240mg	**Freq** QDS	**Route** IV	06									
			10									
Start 1/1/15	**Stop/review** 3/1/15	12									
Signature A.Jones JONES 1234		18									
Indication Abdominal pain		22									
Drug CO-AMOXICLAV (30mg/kg)		02									
Dose 480mg	**Freq** tds	**Route** IV	06									
			10									
Start 1/1/15	**Stop/review** 6/1/15	14									
Signature A.Jones JONES 1234		18									
Indication ? Appendicitis		22									

FLUIDS

Date	Fluid	Additive	Volume	Route	Rate	Signature	Given	Batch
1/1/15	0.9% SODIUM CHLORIDE (20ml/kg bolus)	–	320ml	IV	Over 20min	A.Jones JONES 1234		
1/1/15	0.9% SODIUM CHLORIDE +5% DEXTROSE (full maintenance fluids)	–	500ml	IV	54ml/ hour	A.Jones JONES 1234		

ANSWER TO CASE 11
A 6-hour-old girl presenting with bilious vomiting

Q1 Which of the following conditions could be in your list of differential diagnoses?

The correct answers are A. Duodenal atresia, B. Malrotation, C. Meconium ileus, and E. Jejunal atresia.

Bilious vomiting has a wide range of possible causes in the neonate. Any baby with any bilious vomiting should be investigated.

A Duodenal atresia – Correct. Babies with duodenal atresia may present with bilious or non-bilious vomiting. This depends on the atresia being pre or post ampullary (ampulla of Vater in the second part of the duodenum). Frequently, babies with the condition have a large visible mass in the left upper quadrant of the abdomen (very distended stomach). The diagnosis can be made antenatally with the history of polyhydramnios and a dilated distended abdomen on antenatal scans.

B Malrotation – Correct. Babies with malrotation are frequently otherwise well infants with no significant anomaly on antenatal scans. This is a true paediatric surgical emergency and can be life threatening if not treated immediately.

C Meconium ileus – Correct. This condition is frequently associated with cystic fibrosis. Occasionally, the parents have a family history of the condition. A contrast enema can be therapeutic in some instances, as it dissolves the inspissated meconium.

D Oesophageal atresia – Incorrect. Babies with TOF/OA present with frothing of mucus and saliva, and not with bilious vomiting.

E Jejunal atresia – Correct. Babies with this condition tend to have a moderately to severely distended abdomen on presentation (the more distal the atresia the more distended the abdomen). One always needs to remember that all these conditions may co-exist with malrotation.

♀ Key Point

Any obstruction that occurs after the ampulla of Vater (post ampullary, second part of duodenum) can lead to bilious vomiting.

Q2 Which of the following statements is correct?

The correct answers are A. The colour of bile is green, and E. Abdominal distension and tenderness are worrying signs.

A The colour of bile is green – Correct. This might be stating the obvious, but a recent study published in the

BMJ surveyed a huge number of parents and health care professionals. Worryingly, a "bilious vomit" was described as anything from white, yellow or green right through to dark brown. A "bilious vomit" is a dark green vomit that looks like classic "Fairy Liquid" washing-up detergent. This is always a worrying sign and should always be investigated.

B An abdominal X-ray is the most important test to order – Incorrect. Whilst an abdominal X-ray is useful for differentiating a proximal from a distal obstruction, ruling out perforation, diagnosing calcifications and checking the position of various tubes, the test is not diagnostic.

C A contrast enema is the most appropriate test to order – Incorrect. The most appropriate test to order is an upper gastrointestinal contrast study looking for malrotation. A contrast enema can be useful as a second line investigation after malrotation has been excluded.

D The fact that the baby passed meconium after birth is a positive sign that a significant abnormality is unlikely – Incorrect. A baby with malrotation can pass meconium after birth. As this is the most devastating of all differential diagnoses, passing meconium is not a positive sign. The passage of meconium also does not exclude a duodenal or small bowel atresia either.

E Abdominal distension and tenderness are worrying signs – Correct. Classically, the infant with malrotation and midgut volvulus presents with bilious vomiting only. The abdomen is scaphoid (sucked inwards) and non-tender. This is true for the early stage of the condition. Once the gut has twisted on its blood supply, venous engorgement, obstruction and gut ischaemia ensue. At this late stage, the abdomen can become distended and tender, and the baby can pass blood per rectum. It is a sign that damage to bowel has become irreversible and soon will be life-threatening.

♀ Key Point

Bilious vomit is dark green in colour. It is a paediatric surgical emergency until proven otherwise.

Q3 Which of the following statements is correct?

The correct answers are B. A unit of blood should be cross matched and ready as soon as possible, D. The name of the procedure that is performed for malrotation is Ladd's procedure, and E. The appendix should always be removed during surgery for malrotation.

A 6-12 hours should be spent resuscitating the patient; a laparotomy should be planned for the next day – Incorrect. Once the diagnosis of malrotation and midgut volvulus is confirmed, there should be absolutely no delay in taking this child for emergency laparotomy. Always remember that dead gut will lead to dead baby in under six hours!

B A unit of blood should be cross matched and ready as soon as possible – Correct. It is possible that this baby will require bowel resection and become haemodynamically unstable. An adult unit of blood should be ordered as soon as the diagnosis is suspected.

C The parents should be counselled that prognosis is very good – Incorrect. A midgut volvulus can have devastating consequences. Whilst some babies survive the condition with normal gut and absorptive capacity, other babies are not that lucky. On occasion, the entire small bowel (from the DJ flexure to the second third of the transverse colon) can be necrotic. This is not compatible with life. On other occasions, the baby has a short length of viable small bowel remaining. This is compatible with life but might require lifelong total parenteral nutrition, gut lengthening procedures or a small bowel and liver transplant. The morbidity and mortality associated with this condition is extremely high.

D The name of the procedure that is performed for malrotation is Ladd's procedure – Correct. This procedure involves division of peritoneal bands that hold the bowel in an abnormal rotation, broadening of the base of the mesentery, straightening the duodenum and removing the appendix. This procedure prevents reoccurrence of a midgut volvulus in 90% of cases.

E The appendix should always be removed during surgery for malrotation – Correct. When a Ladd's procedure is performed and the caecum and appendix are returned into the peritoneal cavity, their new position is the left upper quadrant. If the patient should develop acute appendicitis in the future, the clinical picture can be very confusing. The appendix is therefore removed during a Ladd's procedure.

Key Point

Surgical untwisting of the twisted gut should be performed urgently once midgut volvulus is diagnosed.

IMPORTANT LEARNING POINTS

- The classic clinical presentation of malrotation with midgut volvulus is bilious vomiting in 90% of patients. A minority will present with rectal bleeding or will be severely unwell with no vomiting.
- Aggressive speedy resuscitation is needed whilst the contrast study is organised.
- If the patient is too unwell for an upper GI contrast study, a laparotomy should be performed without delay. A patient is too unwell if they are haemodynamically unstable or have a distended peritonitic abdomen.

ANSWER TO CASE 12
A baby born at 32 weeks gestation

Q1 What is the definition of a premature delivery?

The correct answer is E. Baby born at less than 37 weeks gestation.

The definition of a preterm delivery is any baby born before 37 weeks gestation. The gold standard is to calculate the expected date of delivery from an antenatal dating scan, but it can also be calculated from the last menstrual period. Often, in resource poor settings, birth weight is used as a proxy marker for prematurity. This can be very inaccurate as the genetic differences across different populations mean there is a wide variation in expected "normal" term baby weights. Extreme prematurity is generally defined as any baby born before 28 weeks gestation.

Q2 Which of the following are risk factors for premature delivery?

The correct answers are A. Maternal smoking, B. Maternal alcohol abuse, C. Maternal infection/chorioamnionitis, D. Previous premature birth/miscarriage, E. Multiple pregnancy and F. Chronic maternal illness, e.g. diabetes/hypertension.

Prematurity is thought to be multifactorial in origin. All these factors are thought to contribute to its aetiology.

A Maternal smoking – Correct. Smoking during pregnancy has many negative effects on the foetus, including increasing the risk of prematurity. Smoking cessation support should be offered to all pregnant women. However, in the UK, approximately 10% of mothers will continue to smoke during pregnancy.

B Maternal alcohol abuse – Correct. Alcohol abuse has many complications for the foetus, including foetal alcohol syndrome and prematurity.

C Maternal infection/chorioamnionitis – Correct. Infection can be a trigger for preterm labour. Infections can be passed on to the baby during passage through the birth canal or before in the case of ascending infections.

D Previous premature birth/miscarriage – Correct. This is a strong risk factor for preterm labour. This can be due to genetic or environmental factors.

E Multiple pregnancy – Correct. There is a higher incidence of prematurity in twin pregnancies.

F Chronic maternal illness, e.g. diabetes/hypertension – Correct. Other chronic illnesses include epilepsy and severe heart disease. Antenatal care in these cases is led by an obstetrician.

Key Point

Premature onset of labour is a multifactorial process. It is a risk factor for infection and antibiotics should be considered in these babies.

Q3 Which of the following are common problems seen in preterm babies?

The correct answers are A. Feeding difficulties/Hypoglycaemia, B. Respiratory Distress Syndrome, C. Jaundice, D. Infection, and E. Electrolyte disturbance.

Preterm babies have more complications than term babies. This is due to the multisystemic effect of prematurity. The outcome in terms of morbidity and mortality improves as gestation increases.

A   Feeding difficulties/Hypoglycaemia – Correct. The suck reflex is poorly developed, and the gut is immature. Care must be taken to avoid the devastating complication of necrotising enterocolitis, which is more likely if enteral feeds are increased too quickly in premature babies. A poor sucking reflex in more premature babies means extra support may be needed. Due to the lack of glycogen storage and brown fat found in premature babies, they are less able to cope with even a short time without glucose from intravenous fluids or enteral feeds.

B   Respiratory Distress Syndrome – Correct. This is due to immature development of the lungs, and particularly surfactant deficiency. Antenatal steroids can boost the maturation of the type 2 alveolar cells in the foetal lungs that produce endogenous surfactant. Once the baby has been born, if the baby has significant respiratory distress, additional artificial surfactant can also be given. Premature babies may need extra respiratory support, including oxygen, CPAP or mechanical ventilation.

C   Jaundice – Correct. Higher packed cell volumes and liver immaturity are two reasons why premature babies are more at risk of developing jaundice.

D   Infection – Correct. Infection can trigger preterm labour. Premature babies also have weaker immune systems, can require long term indwelling venous catheters and endotracheal tubes and remain on the neonatal unit for months, all of which increase risk.

E   Electrolyte disturbance – Correct. Poor retention of electrolytes by the immature renal system leads to electrolyte disturbances that often need correction with additional supplements.

F   Hydrocephalus – Incorrect. Hydrocephalus can be seen after significant intraventricular haemorrhage, but it is not a direct risk of prematurity.

Key Point

A premature birth may affect any organ system in the baby's body. The management of the extremely preterm infant is complex and involves a multidisciplinary, patient-centred approach.

Q4 The baby is discharged from the neonatal unit, and is seen in a follow-up clinic twelve weeks after being born. You are asked to plot the weight and height of the baby on a growth chart. What corrected age would you plot the baby at?

The correct answer is C. 4 weeks.

Growth charts are used to ensure adequate growth and plan interventions in those with faltering growth or, more rarely, those whose growth velocity exceeds expectations. Babies born prematurely have their measurements and developmental milestone dates corrected for their gestation until the age of two years.

This is done as follows:
Baby's current age (weeks) - (40 weeks - baby's gestation at birth)
$=12-(40-32)$
$=4$ weeks

Therefore, for example, a baby born at 32 weeks gestation would not be expected to socially smile until 14 weeks of chronological age, which would be 6 weeks corrected.

> ### ⓘ IMPORTANT LEARNING POINTS
>
> - Prematurity is an important global cause of neonatal mortality and morbidity.
> - Premature babies are at increased risk of infection, particularly the extremely premature.
> - The effects of prematurity may be seen in any organ system of the baby.
> - It is important to correct for prematurity when assessing growth and development until the age of two.

ANSWER TO CASE 13
An 11-month-old presenting with possible developmental delay

Q1 What best described Maisy's development status?

The correct answer is D. Global developmental delay.

The two things that need to be done in this scenario are a) calculate Maisy's developmental age, and b) calculate her current developmental stage. Corrected gestational age is calculated by subtracting the number of weeks premature from their chronological age. In this example, Maisy is 11-months-old and was born 12 weeks early (full term = 40 weeks) with makes her corrected age about 8-months-old (11 minus 3).

With the description given the developmental level is:

Gross motor skills: 5-6 months
Fine motor skills: 3-4 months
Language skills: 3-4 months
Social skills: 5-6 months

This means that she is 2-5 months delayed across all areas, and has global developmental delay. Global developmental delay even after correction is a common finding with premature infants regardless of their neonatal course.

⚲ Key Point

It is paramount to calculate a corrected age before assessing development in premature infants. This is usually done until age 2.

Q2 With regard to neurological development in ex-premature infants, mark the following statements true or false.

A   It is normal for a child to preferentially reach with their right hand for objects at this age – False. Developing "handedness" before roughly a year, especially with a history of developmental delay, should be considered as a possible early sign of cerebral palsy.

B   Children born prematurely do not have developmental delay unless they have had a specific neurological complication – False. They are often delayed despite no significant neurological issues. This is thought to be related to formation of important neuronal connections and brain development happening ex utero instead of in utero.

C   Prematurity can be associated with poor concentration and hyperactive behaviour – True. This association is well recognised. There is a high prevalence of ADHD in ex-premature children.

⚲ Key Point

Premature infants are more likely to suffer complications in the neonatal period, as well as in childhood and later life.

Q3 What is the next best step in managing Maisy?

The correct answer is C. Refer for a Community Paediatric and MDT assessment.

Neonatal clinics will normally follow up a patient who has been on the Neonatal Unit until two years of age, even when referred to a Community Paediatrician. Other referrals to consider in the UK include Portage (an educational source for pre-school age children with complex needs who are likely to need significant educational support later on), and notification for a statement of special educational needs (SEN) which is now known as an Education, Health and Care Plan.

A   Send bloods for karyotyping – Incorrect. Although karyotyping may be considered at some point, it is not indicated at this stage as there is no strong suggestion she has a genetic disorder (with no dysmorphic features, and prematurity to explain her developmental delay). It would also not alter her current management. An array CGH is another test to consider — this is a blood test increasingly being used to identify possible genetic defects in those where there is no obvious cohesive syndrome but where a genetic abnormality is possible. It can detect many thousands of genetic defects by comparing test DNA with reference DNA and analysing the differences.

B   Refer for an MRI brain – Incorrect. Although an MRI may be relevant as part of her workup, it is not the most important next step, as she has no focal neurological deficit to imply a focal brain lesion/abnormality. If the brain is abnormal, it is likely to have been due to a static event perinatally and so detection, although important, will not alter outcome.

C   Refer to a Community Paediatrician and MDT assessment – Correct. Although all the management options are potentially valuable, referring to a Community Paediatrician and for an MDT assessment (physiotherapy, occupational therapy, and speech and language therapy) may improve her outcome. Each of these therapies may, in different ways, improve her strength and abilities at certain tasks, and guide parents in how to continue the support and exercises at home. The overall aim is to maximise the child's potential, helping her to become as independent as possible as an adult, and improve her quality of life.

D   Arrange for a hearing test – Incorrect. A hearing test should always be arranged when there is speech and language delay but in this context, with significant delay in all areas, hearing impairment is less likely to be the cause of the speech delay. This should be arranged as part of her management plan, but is not the most important next step.

⚲ Key Point

A multitude of different investigations need to be considered in global developmental delay, ranging from simple blood tests to MRI scans. However, in the majority of cases, the most useful management will be providing a package of care individualised to that patient, and this is usually coordinated and overseen by a Community Paediatrician.

 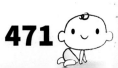

Q4 With regard to normal development, mark the following statements true or false.

Knowing when milestones are expected to be achieved is fundamental to assessing development. There is always a range in which these milestones can be achieved, and the range increases with age. A detailed summary of developmental milestones is given on p36.

A   An average 8-month-old should sit unsupported – True. Learning to sit is achieved in steps. It starts with a need for support and the baby having a curved back. Over a period of a few weeks to months, the baby can achieve sitting unsupported with a straight back and the ability to carry out many tasks simultaneously.

B   A 15-month-old not walking should be investigated – False. A 15-month-old not walking, although later than average, does not need investigating. Referral would be considered after 18 months. Often children that are bottom shuffling will walk later, as they can get around very efficiently without needing to walk.

C   An average 2-year-old can draw a circle – False. A 2 year-old is able to scribble back and forth and circularly but not draw a complete circle.

D   An average 3-year-old can build a tower of nine bricks – True. An average 3-year-old can build a tower of nine bricks after it is demonstrated to them. To remember this, it is roughly three times the age: an 18 month-old can build a tower of four bricks (1.5 x3 is 4 (ish)), a 2-year-old can build a tower of 6 and 3-year-old a tower of nine.

E   Children should develop object permanence by 12-months-old – True. Object permanence is a cognitive and visual milestone reached when there is awareness that an object can still exist despite having disappeared from view.

⚲ Key Point

Developmental assessment can be time-consuming, and full assessment can take up to an hour, which is not feasible in all paediatric assessments. However, it is important to be aware of key milestones and to make a crude assessment of developmental status in every professional encounter with a child.

ⓘ IMPORTANT LEARNING POINTS

- Always calculate the corrected gestational age of the child (up until 2-years-old) when doing a developmental assessment.
- Assess gross motor, fine motor, language and social skills in every developmental assessment.
- Global developmental delay requires long term, multidisciplinary team management. This should be initiated as soon as possible.

ANSWER TO CASE 14
A 22-month-old presenting with delayed gross motor skills

Q1 What further history would be most helpful to support the diagnosis of rickets?

The correct answer is C. Dietary history.

Vitamin D deficiency is an important, treatable cause of delayed walking. The history and ethnicity suggests a child with rickets. A clear indicator of rickets is the bowed legs. She is likely to be vitamin D deficient, leading to hypocalcaemia and rickets, along with other vitamin and mineral deficiencies such as iron. Given the parents' obesity, there is a suggestion of poor diet in the family.

A   Age at which parents started walking – Incorrect. Although this question may be asked, it is unlikely to be the most useful part of the history. There is some hereditary relationship with development but this is more seen in language development, and the story given suggests another cause is more likely.

B   Birth history – Incorrect. With no other developmental delay, and a normal neurological examination, a complication at birth is unlikely to be the cause of the delayed walking.

C   Dietary history – Correct. A dietary history, including whether or not she is still breastfed, would be important and help clarify the diagnosis. Note that some children can have vitamin D resistant rickets that is not related to diet.

⚲ Key Point

Vitamin D is mainly obtained from diet, especially in countries with limited sun exposure. It is important to think about when assessing developmental delay. It is now recommended that all children in the UK take vitamin D supplementation until 5-years-old.

Q2 What investigations should be performed as part of her initial workup?

The correct answers are A. Plotting height/length centile, and mid-parental height, B. Full blood count, and E. X-ray of the wrist.

Vitamin D levels and a bone profile will need to be checked in the work up for rickets. Although there may a strong clinical suspicion of Vitamin D deficiency, it is important to consider other diagnoses as well, as there may be more than one contributory factor to delayed walking.

A   Plotting height/length centile, and mid-parental height – Correct. This may give a clue as to a possible diagnosis. It is likely that both height and weight are affected in Vitamin D deficiency, with height potentially more affected due to bowing of the legs. In endocrine conditions like hypothyroidism, the child is often short and fat.

B Full blood count – Correct. A co-existent nutritional iron deficiency may exist, which may result in anaemia and associated faltering growth.

C Checking thyroid function – Incorrect. There is no clinical suspicion of thyroid dysfunction, and normally a child with hypothyroidism would be short and fat, rather than short and thin. This child is also likely to have had a thyroid function test at birth, as it is standard practice in the UK and elsewhere.

D Checking chromosomes – Incorrect. In the presence of short stature without other explanation, all girls should have their chromosomes checked to rule out Turner's syndrome. However, in this case, height was previously on the 25th centile, and treatment with Vitamin D may facilitate catch-up growth. Rickets should be excluded prior to genetic testing.

E X-ray of the wrist – Correct. In rickets, this will characteristically show metaphyseal splaying (opening out), cupping (cup shape to the bone) and fraying (appearing worn away), as well as generalised osteopenia.

Key Point

Don't develop a false sense of security from identifying a possible cause of developmental delay. Nutritional deficiencies, for example, commonly co-exist, so it is important to do a thorough assessment and work up.

Q3 Which of the following are classically associated with rickets?

The correct answers are B. Rachitic rosary, and C. Pectus excavatum.

Any child with a diet deficient in Vitamin D or calcium can develop rickets. It is particularly prominent in those with dark skin, premature babies, and in those taking medications which interfere with Vitamin D metabolism. It is important to recognise the disease, as it can usually be treated by simple dietary advice and supplemental vitamin D.

A Fractured ribs – Incorrect. This is not usually associated with rickets. However, if present, this may be a sign of NAI, particularly if there are posterior rib fractures. Severe vitamin D deficiency can increase one's risk of fractures in any location and vitamin D should be tested when there is doubt about the mechanism of injury.

B Rachitic rosary – Correct. This is the name given to the classical rib appearance in rickets. There is a nodular appearance at the costochondral junction due to lack of mineralisation and an overgrowth of the joint cartilage.

C Pectus excavatum – Correct. This is abnormal development of the rib cage, where the sternum is caved in, giving the appearance of a sunken chest wall. This may be associated with rickets, as well as Marfan's syndrome and scoliosis.

D Pectus carinatum – Incorrect. This is characterised by the protrusion of the chest over the sternum. It is not associated with rickets, but may be seen in chronic asthma.

E Intercostal recession – Incorrect. This is usually associated with acute respiratory distress, not rickets.

Key Point

Rickets is associated with the following signs:

- Delayed closure of the fontanelle
- Rachitic rosary
- Genu varus (bowing of legs) or genu valgum (knock knees)
- Harrison sulci
- Pectus excavatum
- Frontal bossing
- Kyphoscoliosis
- Increased fracture tendency
- Metaphyseal cartilage swelling at wrist, distal femur and distal tibia
- Delayed gross motor skills

(i) IMPORTANT LEARNING POINTS

- Always look for potential reversible causes when presented with a patient with developmental delay.
- There may be more than one concurrent pathology. For example vitamin D and iron deficiency anaemia may coexist.
- Vitamin D deficiency is a common and easily treatable disease. Guidelines in the UK now recommend that all children take vitamin D supplements until 5-years-old.
- Those with rickets should be followed up to ensure compliance with treatment, biochemical improvement and radiographic healing.

ANSWER TO CASE 15
A 5-day-old baby with a genetic condition picked up on newborn screening

Q1 What type of inheritance is shown by the pedigree diagram?

The correct answer is B. Autosomal recessive.

A Autosomal dominant – Incorrect. Autosomal dominant patterns usually affect every generation in a family and affect both genders equally. For a child to be affected, one of the parents must also be affected by the condition.

B Autosomal recessive – Correct. Autosomal recessive patterns occur when both parents are carriers of the recessive allele. Autosomal recessive patterns can "skip" generations and affect both genders equally.

473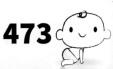

C X-linked dominant – Incorrect. X-linked dominant patterns usually affect every generation in the family and affect males and females equally. Fathers that are affected pass on the gene to their daughters, whereas mothers have a 50% chance of passing on the condition to any offspring.

D X-linked recessive – Incorrect. X-linked recessive patterns disproportionately affect male family members as they only have one X-chromosome, whereas female family members are likely to have a normal allele to compensate on the other X-chromosome.

⚲ Key Point

Pedigree diagrams can be used for explaining the inheritance pattern of a genetic condition, including the likelihood of it being passed on to future offspring.

Q2 *With regards to the above inheritance pattern, mark the following statements true or false.*

A The condition affects both sexes equally – True. Autosomal recessive conditions are due to an abnormality on one of the 22 autosomes that are present in every cell. As both males and females have the same 22 autosomes, the condition affects both males and females equally.

B The condition can "skip" generations – True. Autosomal recessive conditions are more common between siblings than between other family members of different generations. This is because both parents must be carriers of the defective allele.

C The condition can only be passed from a mother to her children – False. Autosomal recessive conditions can be passed along any line of inheritance, but they require both the mother and father to be carriers of the defective gene.

D If the child is affected, both parents must be carriers or affected themselves – True. Autosomal recessive conditions can only be passed on if both parents are carriers or if they are affected by the condition. This is because two affected gene copies are needed to produce the disease phenotype.

E This condition is more common where the parents are consanguineous – True. Autosomal recessive patterns are more common if the parents are consanguineous, as the chances of both parents being a carrier of the same gene defect is greater.

⚲ Key Point

Autosomal recessive patterns are a common pattern of genetic inheritance. The pattern can be seen by looking at the affected individual's pedigree diagram and looking for features like affecting both genders and missing out generations of the family.

Q3 *Three years later, the mother has just given birth to a healthy daughter. However, she also had a miscarriage (cause unknown) whilst trying to conceive again. What symbols need to be added to the pedigree diagram?*

The correct answer is D. An empty circle and an empty triangle with a cross through it.

A An empty circle and a coloured triangle with a cross through it – Incorrect. The empty circle is the correct symbol to identify an unaffected female; however, the coloured triangle with a cross through it implies the miscarriage was due to the identified genetic condition.

B A coloured circle and an empty square – Incorrect. The coloured circle means the daughter that they have had is affected, whereas we know she is healthy, and the empty square would suggest the miscarriage was a healthy boy who survived.

C A coloured square and a coloured triangle with a cross through it – Incorrect. The square is the symbol for a male family member, and we have been told that the child is female. A coloured-in symbol means the child will be affected and the daughter is healthy. The coloured triangle with a cross through it implies the miscarriage was due to the identified genetic condition, which we do not know.

D An empty circle and an empty triangle with a cross through it – Correct. The empty circle is the correct symbol for a healthy female, and the empty triangle with a cross through is the correct symbol for a foetus which miscarried due to an unknown cause. Please note that sometimes a small filled in circle is used to denote a miscarriage as well as a triangle with a cross through it.

E An empty circle and an empty diamond – Incorrect. The empty circle is the correct symbol for a healthy daughter, but the diamond is the symbol for a baby of unknown or indeterminate gender, not a foetus that miscarried.

⚲ Key Point

Pedigree diagrams should include miscarriages and terminations as well as live births.

ⓘ IMPORTANT LEARNING POINTS

- Patterns of inheritance can be seen by drawing out the pedigree diagram of a family and asking questions about the status of relatives from both the maternal and paternal families.
- An affected person has a coloured in symbol, whereas unaffected members have empty symbols.
- Miscarried or terminated pregnancies can be shown either as a small filled in circle or as a triangle with a cross through it for a miscarriage, with an extra horizontal line through the cross for a termination.
- Babies that are yet to be born should be noted with their estimated date of delivery and, if known, their gender.

ANSWER TO CASE 16
A 9-year-old boy presenting with tight foreskin

Q1 Mark the following statements true or false.

A Circumcision can always be safely performed in the community – False. Whilst many practitioners in the community have vast experience in performing circumcisions, this setting does not cater for the child that is concurrently unwell or that develops complications post procedure. Some cases (such as children with haemophilia or congenital heart disease) should be dealt with at hospital to reduce the risk of complications.

B Balanitis xerotica obliterans is an indication for circumcision – True. This is what the child in this case is likely to be suffering from. Clinical examination reveals a scarred fibrotic foreskin that does not "pout" with retraction. This is an absolute indication for circumcision as it prevents disease progression and is therapeutic.

C Physiological phimosis is an indication for circumcision – False. This condition will settle spontaneously by the time the child is 8 to 10-years-old. It has been noted that during peri-puberty (with the onset of erection/ejaculation), most foreskins become easily retractable. Less than 1% of boys are unable to fully retract their foreskin as teenagers. It is therefore important to assure children and their families that normal "tight" foreskins do not require circumcision. Instead, children should be encouraged to gently retract their foreskin on a regular basis (especially in the bath).

D Circumcision may be complicated by meatal stenosis – True. This complication can occur if the external urethral meatus is damaged during the procedure. It can also occur as a direct complication of having balanitis xerotica obliterans (BXO).

⚷ Key Point

BXO is the only definite indication for circumcision.

Q2 Please match the following conditions to their definitions or the appropriate management of the condition:

A Priapism
iii An erection lasting more than four hours that may or may not be painful.

This condition is common in boys with sickle cell anaemia during a sickle cell crisis. It can also occur following pelvic trauma.

B Acute urinary retention
v May require insertion of a suprapubic catheter.

Causes for acute urinary retention can be divided into two groups.

› Mechanical obstruction to flow of urine (e.g. bladder stones, trauma to the urethra).
› Abnormal innervation of bladder, leading to inability to empty the bladder adequately (e.g. cerebral palsy, spina bifida, spinal tumours).

C Paraphimosis
i Can usually be reduced after the application of topical lignocaine and pressure.

This condition results from forced retraction of the foreskin. The resulting constricting ring causes venous engorgement of the glans penis, followed by loss of arterial blood flow. If left untreated, the condition can lead to necrosis of the glans.

D Phimosis
ii A physiological condition of the prepuce that rarely requires surgery.

Phimosis is a narrowing of the opening of the foreskin, preventing full retraction of it. It can be treated with simple measures like gentle retraction of the foreskin and the application of topical steroids.

E Post-circumcision haemorrhage
iv Should stop after 10 minutes of continuous firm pressure.

Post-circumcision bleeding occurs in up to 10% of cases performed in the community. In resistant cases, an adrenaline soaked swab may be used for application of pressure. A minority of cases require hospital admission, a return trip to theatre or a transfusion. If bleeding does not stop after the regular measures are applied, underlying causes should be sought (e.g. undiagnosed haemophilia).

⚷ Key Point

Physiological phimosis is one of the commonest causes for presentation to primary care physicians and paediatric surgical clinics. The condition rarely requires surgical intervention.

ⓘ IMPORTANT LEARNING POINTS

- On examination of the foreskin, a healthy one will "pout" on retraction whereas an unhealthy one (BXO) will not.
- The only absolute medical indication for circumcision is BXO, although other reasons for circumcision may include recurrent infection, high grade vesicoureteric reflux and cultural factors.
- Pre-pubertal children should never have their foreskins forcefully retracted, as this might lead to scarring of the foreskin or a paraphimosis.

ANSWER TO CASE 17
A 2-year-old presenting with bony deformities

Q1 What is the most likely diagnosis in this child?

The correct answer is C. Rickets.

A Beriberi – Incorrect. This condition is caused by a deficiency in vitamin B1, also known as thiamine. It is traditionally classified into dry beriberi, mainly affecting the peripheral nervous system, and wet beriberi, which mainly affects the cardiovascular system.

B Pellagra – Incorrect. This condition is caused by a deficiency in vitamin B_3, also known as niacin. The symptoms are classically described as a triad of diarrhoea, dermatitis and dementia.

C Rickets – Correct. The history and clinical features of difficulty with gait, prematurity, prolonged exclusive breastfeeding, irritability, skeletal deformities and short stature are all consistent with the diagnosis of rickets.

D Scurvy – Incorrect. This condition is caused by vitamin C deficiency. Patients often present with malaise, lethargy, easy bruising, poor wound healing and gum and dental diseases.

E Kwashiorkor – Incorrect. Children with this condition, which is caused by severe insufficient dietary protein, frequently present with distended abdomen, diarrhoea, faltering growth, oedema, frequent infections and irritability.

♀ Key Point

Rickets is an important differential diagnosis in a child presenting with difficulty walking and skeletal deformities. In individuals with features of malnutrition, it is important to consider the coexistence of deficiencies in multiple nutrients.

Q2 What are the risk factors for the likely diagnosis?

The correct answers are B. Coeliac disease, and E. Use of anticonvulsants.

A Fair skin – Incorrect. The increased melanin in dark skin contains a natural sun protective factor and thus results in reduced cutaneous vitamin D synthesis compared to children with fair skin. However rickets can still occur in fair skinned individuals.

B Coeliac disease – Correct. Intestinal vitamin D absorption is reduced in conditions that impair fat absorption due to the fat-soluble nature of vitamin D. Therefore, rickets can occur in children with coeliac disease, inflammatory bowel disease and cystic fibrosis.

C Breastfeeding with vitamin D supplementation – Incorrect. Exclusive breastfeeding without vitamin D supplementation is associated with an increased risk of vitamin D deficiency due to the low level of this vitamin in breast milk. The insufficiency is further aggravated if the mother had low vitamin D levels during pregnancy or if the baby was born prematurely.

D High altitude – Incorrect. Vitamin D deficiency is associated with the winter season and high latitudes, not high altitudes. Beyond a latitude of 40 degrees and during winter, little or no ultraviolet-B radiation reaches the surface of the earth, making vitamin D deficiency relatively common at the end of winter.

E Use of anticonvulsants – Correct. Certain medications such as anticonvulsants and antiretrovirals increase the risks of vitamin D deficiency as these medications enhance the catabolism of 25-hydroxyvitamin D and 1,25-dihydroxyvitamin D.

♀ Key Points

The risk factors can be classified into four major categories: (1) decreased vitamin D synthesis secondary to lack of sun exposure, (2) decreased nutritional intake, (3) perinatal factors and (4) others. It is important to consider liver and kidney diseases, because vitamin D is converted into its active form through processes in these organs.

Q3 What are the clinical features of the likely diagnosis?

The correct answers are A. Harrison's sulcus, C. Enamel hypoplasia, D. Increased tendency of fractures, and E. Bone pain.

A Harrison's sulcus – Correct. Harrison's sulcus, also known as Harrison's groove, can be observed at the lower margins of the thorax in patients with rickets due to the muscular pull of the diaphragmatic attachments to the lower ribs.

B Narrowing of the wrists – Incorrect. The underlying impaired mineralisation and widening of the epiphyseal plate lead to widening of the wrists and knobby deformities on long bones and chest (known as rachitic rosary). The disorganisation of the growth plate produces characteristic cupping, splaying, formation of cortical spurs and stippling on X-ray.

C Enamel hypoplasia – Correct. Hypoplasia of the dental enamel is a very common finding in calcipaenic rickets. These children also suffer from delayed tooth eruption.

D Increased tendency of fractures – Correct. Fractures are relatively common in children with rickets due to impaired bone mineralisation.

E Bone pain – Correct. A physical examination often reveals tenderness in the bones.

Key Point

A child with vitamin D deficiency can present with hypocalcaemic manifestations, skeletal deformities, behavioural symptoms and delayed growth.

Q4 What biochemical changes are observed in the likely diagnosis?

The correct answers are B. Increased parathyroid hormone level, and D. Decreased plasma calcium level.

A Decreased alkaline phosphatase level – Incorrect. Alkaline phosphatase plays a role in the mineralisation of bone and growth plate cartilage. The serum level is usually markedly increased over the age-specific range in nutritional rickets.

B Increased parathyroid hormone level – Correct. Hypocalcaemia secondary to low vitamin D level stimulates the secretion of parathyroid hormone.

C Increased plasma phosphate level – Incorrect. Intestinal calcium and phosphorus absorption are both regulated by 1,25-dihydroxyvitamin D; thus, vitamin D deficiency results in decreased plasma calcium and phosphate level.

D Decreased plasma calcium level – Correct. See answer above.

♀ Key Point

Vitamin D deficiency can lead to secondary biochemical derangements in plasma calcium, phosphate, alkaline phosphatase and parathyroid hormone levels.

(i) IMPORTANT LEARNING POINTS

- Vitamin D is an essential fat-soluble nutrient that is mainly synthesised in the skin through exposure to sunlight. Reduced exposure to sunlight increases the risk of vitamin D deficiency.
- Exclusive breastfeeding, maternal vitamin D deficiency and prematurity are other important risk factors. Supplemental dietary sources and fortified products are important sources of vitamin D in children.
- Vitamin D deficiency can result in the derangement of plasma calcium, phosphate, alkaline phosphatase and parathyroid hormone.
- Children with vitamin D deficiency should be treated with replacement therapy and be followed up to ensure resolution.

ANSWER TO CASE 18
A 12-month-old presenting with faltering growth

Q1 Which of the following are commonly accepted definitions for faltering growth?

The correct answers are B. Weight less than 5th percentile for more than one occasion, and E. Deceleration of weight gain across two or more major percentile lines over time.

There is no clear consensus on the definition of faltering growth but the commonly accepted definitions are weight less than 5th percentile for more than one occasion, deceleration of weight trajectory across two or more major percentile lines over time and weight less than 80 percent of ideal weight for age.

A Weight less than 65% of ideal weight for age – Incorrect. An accepted definition for faltering growth is weight less than 80% of ideal weight for age, not 65%.

B Weight less than 5th percentile for more than one occasion – Correct. It is important to note that this persistence of weight in the range of less than 5th percentile should be recorded on at least two separate occasions.

C Depressed length-for-head circumference – Incorrect. An acceptable parameter for assessment is weight-for-length.

D Weight gain of 120 g per week between three and six months of age – Incorrect. This amount of weight gain is expected, but it is more important to assess the velocity of weight gain rather than the amount of weight gain.

E Deceleration of weight gain across two or more major percentile lines over time – Correct. This signifies significant departure from the expected trajectory of weight gain with age.

♀ Key Point

In order to assess a child with faltering growth, it is important to plot the weight, length and head circumference on a standardised growth chart and to observe the trend over a period of time rather than diagnosing the child in a single visit.

Q2 Mark the following statements true or false.

Regardless of whether the cause is organic or non-organic, the underlying mechanism of faltering growth is deficiency of nutrients available for growth. The management plan should recognise all the relevant risk factors and address them appropriately, including involving allied health services, to ensure that the child achieves catch-up growth. The majority of cases can be managed in an outpatient setting.

A Those in charge of management should assume there is either an organic cause or a non-organic cause of faltering growth, not both concurrently – False. The causes of failure to thrive are classically described as organic and non-organic but commonly there are multiple confounding factors in each case involving organic and non-organic components. In the clinical case above, the child tested positive for coeliac disease. This may be complicated by the mother's probable postpartum depression.

B Different standardised growth charts are needed for children from different racial and ethnic backgrounds – False. One set of growth charts are used for all racial and ethnic groups because studies revealed that environmental influences appear to contribute more to variations in growth than genetic factors do.

C Inpatient care should be considered for children with faltering growth when there is severe psychosocial impairment at home – True. Other groups that should be considered for inpatient care include those with failure of outpatient management and suspicion of child abuse or neglect.

D The fundamental mechanisms contributing to faltering growth are insufficient nutritional intake, inadequate absorption and decreased metabolic requirement – False. The former two are correct, but the latter should be increased metabolic requirement. This is most commonly caused by infection. During infection, deceleration in growth velocity can be observed, but it only results in faltering growth if the infections are recurrent, as growth normally catches up after the infection resolves. Other conditions that can increase metabolic requirements are congenital heart disease, chronic pulmonary disease and endocrine disorders such as diabetes mellitus and hyperthyroidism.

E The deceleration in the growth velocity of head circumference independent of weight and length deceleration is suggestive of constitutional growth delay – False. This is more typical of neurological disorders. Evaluation of proportionality between weight, length and head circumference can be helpful in determining the contributing factors.

⚲ Key Point

Faltering growth is often multifactorial in origin. Even in the presence of an organic cause such as coeliac disease, look for other factors that may be exacerbating faltering growth as well, such as poor nutrition.

Q3 Mark the following statements true or false.

A Chronic diseases such as coeliac disease and cystic fibrosis impair the intestinal absorption of nutrients, thus resulting in faltering growth – True. Examples of other medical conditions reducing absorption of nutrients from the gut are chronic liver disease and chronic diarrhoea.

B A single record of weight below ideal weight for age is sufficient to diagnose faltering growth – False. Although a weight of less than 80% of ideal weight for age is sometimes suggested as one of the definitions, a definite diagnosis should involve deceleration of growth velocity over time.

C The history provided by parents is always reliable for a child with suspicious features of child abuse or violence – False. If the parents are the offenders, they may provide history inconsistent with the injuries observed. In such cases, the child can be interviewed alone, if they can verbalise.

D It is important to observe the interaction between the child and his/her parents, particularly during feeding – True.

Important observations include the parents' response to the child's cues of hunger and satiety, swallowing difficulties or distractions during feeding, and the child's and the parents' behaviour while feeding.

⚲ Key Point

Complete history, examination and review of growth charts are essential for evaluating a child with faltering growth. Laboratory investigations are not always required in managing such cases but are often performed by the paediatrician and can be useful.

ⓘ IMPORTANT LEARNING POINTS

- The fundamental mechanism of faltering growth is deficiency in nutrition available for growth, secondary to insufficient intake, inadequate absorption, excessive metabolic requirement or psychosocial factors. All possible risk factors should be recognised and addressed.
- Detailed history, examination and evaluation of growth charts over time are essential in managing such patients.
- Nutritional guidance and behavioural management are often adequate, but allied health involvement and hospitalisation may be needed in some cases.

ANSWER TO CASE 19
A 2-year-old presenting with a blue episode

Q1 What are the structural features of TOF?

The correct answer is C. Right ventricular hypertrophy, ventricular septal defect, overriding aorta and infundibular pulmonary stenosis.

TOF is a condition made up of four cardiac abnormalities as described above, leading to potential cyanotic episodes. The other combinations of defects are not common, but they are possible. They have no common or eponymous terminology to describe them but could be classified as "complex congenital cardiac defects".

Q2 What examination findings would you classically expect to see in a patient who is presenting for the first time with TOF (prior to receiving any treatment)?

The correct answer is A. Harsh ejection systolic murmur, heard best at the left upper border of the sternum, radiating into the back.

A Harsh ejection systolic murmur, heard best at the left upper border of the sternum, radiating into the back – Correct. The murmur in TOF is generally not caused by the ventricular septal defect (VSD) but by the right ventricular outflow tract obstruction (pulmonary stenosis). It is therefore classically described as a harsh ejection systolic murmur, which can radiate to the back. The murmur diminishes as the obstruction worsens, which means less blood is passing out of the right ventricle into the pulmonary circulation.

B Collapsing pulses and a wide pulse pressure – Incorrect. These are classical descriptions of aortic regurgitation. This is rare in children but can be associated with a bicuspid aortic valve or with connective tissue disorders such as Marfan syndrome.

C No murmur audible – Incorrect. There will generally be a murmur present in TOF. The murmur diminishes as the obstruction worsens, and during hypercyanotic spells the murmur may not be audible.

D Pansystolic murmur heard at the lower left sternal edge – Incorrect. This is the classical murmur of a VSD. Although TOF does involve a VSD, this murmur is not the most likely one to be heard in TOF.

E Low BP, bounding peripheral pulses and a constant machinery murmur – Incorrect. This is the classical murmur of a patent ductus arteriosus (PDA). The ductus arteriosus connects the aorta and the main pulmonary artery, and is needed in foetal life to divert blood away from the pulmonary bed. After birth, this connection closes due to the fall in pulmonary vascular resistance, so that the pulmonary and systemic circulations can both function efficiently. In PDA, this communication remains. Indomethacin can be used to close the duct in premature infants, and occasionally prostaglandins will be required to maintain the patency of the duct. A PDA is temporarily required in "duct dependent" heart lesions, where the systemic circulation depends on receiving oxygenated blood through the open duct.

♀ Key Point

In a clinical setting, particularly outside of tertiary cardiac units, murmurs can be critical to diagnose congenital cardiac defects, as treatment may need to be commenced before an echocardiogram is available (for example, to keep a patent ductus arteriosus open). It is, however, important to remember that many cardiac defects have no accompanying murmur. In any compromised child, involve senior clinicians and evaluate the child based on all clinical findings, not just a murmur.

Q3 What is your initial management?

The correct answer is E. Place the child in a knees-to-chest position and administer oxygen.

This child is experiencing a hypercyanotic or "tet" spell. These occur during episodes of almost complete right ventricular outflow tract obstruction and are a medical emergency as they prevent adequate oxygenation of the body. This must be managed with a stepwise approach; each progressive step aims to increase blood flow to the pulmonary vasculature: optimal positioning to increase systemic vascular resistance is the first step (knees-to-chest position). If systemic vascular resistance is elevated, then blood will shunt to the pulmonary circulation. If this is ineffective, the next steps are administering IV morphine sulphate, giving a fluid bolus, and then considering IV beta blockers. If these three steps are ineffective, emergency cardiac surgery may be required. These spells tend to occur when an infant or young child is distressed or after strenuous exercise in older children. It is unusual to encounter children presenting with cyanotic episodes in high income countries like the UK as antenatal diagnosis and postnatal specialist management have become increasingly sophisticated.

A Place the child in the recovery position and insert an oropharyngeal airway before administering oxygen – Incorrect. If the child were unable to maintain their own airway then an oropharyngeal airway may be required. The goal of position in patients with a hypercyanotic spell is to increase systemic vascular resistance, as this will lead to shunting from the systemic to the pulmonary circulation. The recovery position doesn't achieve this.

B Gain IV access and administer a 10ml/kg fluid bolus immediately – Incorrect. Although administering a fluid bolus would increase the filling of the right ventricle and thus help to encourage blood flow into the pulmonary circulation, this is not the first step in the management of a hypercyanotic spell. Complete the management in a step wise progression as the simple steps can also be the most effective.

C Administer a 150 microgram dose of IM adrenaline – Incorrect. This would be an appropriate treatment for a child under six who was suffering from acute anaphylaxis. However, there is no evidence of anaphylaxis, and adrenaline would act as a pulmonary vasoconstrictor, reducing pulmonary blood flow even further.

D Lean the child over your knee and perform five back blows – Incorrect. This would be the correct action if the child was choking and conscious but unable to cough effectively. In this situation, it would most likely distress the child further and exacerbate her symptoms.

E Place the child in a knees-to-chest position and administer oxygen – Correct. This position increases systemic vascular resistance, thus leading to systemic to pulmonary shunting. Oxygen helps reduce pulmonary vascular resistance in the hypoxic patient.

♀ Key Point

Hypercyanotic spells should initially be managed conservatively, by optimising the child's position (knees-to-chest position) and administering oxygen.

Q4 If this child had presented as a cyanosed newborn, what other conditions would be among your differential diagnosis?

The correct answers are A. Transposition of the great arteries, B. Total anomalous pulmonary venous drainage and E. Truncus arteriosus.

Central cyanosis presents as bluish discolouration of the mucous membranes caused by a reduction in circulating oxygen. It generally corresponds with an oxygen saturation of approximately 85%.

A Transposition of the great arteries – Correct. Cyanosis occurs because deoxygenated blood is pumped out through the aorta, not the pulmonary artery.

B Total anomalous pulmonary venous drainage – Correct. In this situation, the pulmonary venous drainage is malpositioned, meaning the veins make connections with the systemic circulation. This results in deoxygenated blood entering the left side of the heart, causing cyanosis.

C Ventricular septal defect – Incorrect. In ventricular septal defects, there is additional blood flow from the left ventricle (oxygenated, high pressure) to the right ventricle (deoxygenated, low pressure). Therefore, cyanosis generally does not occur, unless the VSD is really large, i.e. in an AVSD.

D Patent ductus arteriosus – Incorrect. In this situation, there is additional blood flow from the aorta (oxygenated, high pressure) to the pulmonary artery (deoxygenated, low pressure). Therefore, cyanosis generally does not occur.

E Truncus arteriosus – Correct. This is characterised by a single arterial trunk emerging from both ventricles, causing mixing of oxygenated and deoxygenated blood, leading to cyanosis.

⚲ Key Point

The key difference between cyanotic and acyanotic heart disease is that cyanotic heart disease features mixing of deoxygenated blood into the systemic circulation.

ⓘ IMPORTANT LEARNING POINTS

- Congenital heart disease can be divided into cyanotic and acyanotic disease.
- The major cyanotic heart diseases to be aware of are Tetralogy of Fallot, transposition of the great arteries, hypoplastic left heart syndrome, truncus arteriosus and total anomalous pulmonary venous drainage.
- The major acyanotic heart diseases are: ventricular septal defect, atrial septal defect, atrioventricular septal defect, patent ductus arteriosus, and coarctation of the aorta.
- Tetralogy of Fallot comprises four defects: i) right ventricular hypertrophy, ii) ventricular septal defect, iii) overriding aorta, and iv) infundibular pulmonary stenosis.

ANSWER TO CASE 20
A 5-week-old girl presenting with respiratory distress and poor weight gain

Q1 Which of the following conditions would be within your differential diagnosis?

The correct answers are A. Ventricular septal defect, and D. Cardiomyopathy.

This child is presenting with features consistent with heart failure, but with no known cause. It can be caused by a congenital acyanotic cardiac defect, the most common of which is VSD. A VSD consists of an opening anywhere within the ventricular septum. VSDs account for approximately 30% of cases of congenital heart disease. Cyanotic heart disease also causes heart failure, but can be ruled out as the child is not cyanotic and has been relatively well since birth. Heart failure can also be caused by other conditions affecting the heart, like either primary cardiac disease (e.g. cardiomyopathy) or secondary to systemic phenomena (e.g. sepsis). The child will ultimately need an echocardiogram to discern the specific cause and severity of the heart failure.

A Ventricular septal defect – Correct. The majority of children affected by a VSD will be asymptomatic. Usually, these will be cases of small VSD. "Small" refers to a diameter narrower than that of the aortic valve. Children affected by a larger VSD may experience signs and symptoms of heart failure. The VSD creates a left-to-right shunt, reducing left ventricular output and creating back pressure in the right side of the heart.

B Total anomalous pulmonary venous drainage – Incorrect. This is a cyanotic heart disease, which would present much earlier, with significantly greater compromise.

C Bronchiolitis – Incorrect. This would be more likely to present with crackles and/or wheeze on auscultation with a hyperinflated chest and a wet cough.

D Cardiomyopathy – Correct. Cardiomyopathies are a group of conditions affecting the heart muscle itself causing failure of the pumping mechanism and thus symptoms of heart failure. This is an important differential diagnosis to consider when presented with a child in heart failure.

E Atrial septal defect – Incorrect. The vast majority of patients with these defects will be asymptomatic and upon clinical evaluation, will have a soft systolic murmur at the upper left sternal edge. Patients with a larger ASD may rarely present with heart failure.

Key Point

Before getting an echocardiogram, keep the differential for new onset heart failure wide, as there are usually several possible causes. Bear in mind that the larger the VSD, the more likely the patient is to go into heart failure. However, this means the murmur is less likely to be heard, since with a wider passage for blood to shunt through, turbulent blood flow is less likely. A chest X-ray can be useful, e.g. to look for cardiomegaly.

Q2 When suspicious that a child is presenting in heart failure, what initial management is appropriate?

The correct answer is D. Close monitoring and trial of diuretic therapy.

Heart failure is a clinical diagnosis, and the exact cause does not need to be established before treatment is commenced. Diuretic therapy to offload the heart may improve symptoms initially, but the definitive management for this child is likely to be surgical.

A Intubate and ventilate the baby, preparing for transfer to a specialist cardiac unit – Incorrect. Intubation and ventilation are not clinically needed. Tertiary cardiac input will be necessary, but even if the child has surgery, they need to be stabilised first.

B Intravenous fluid replacement – Incorrect. This treatment strategy is likely to worsen the baby's clinical condition, as intravenous fluids increase preload and exacerbate heart failure. If additional feeding is required, this should be given via nasogastric tube with fluid input monitored.

C Urgent abdominal ultrasound – Incorrect. The enlarged liver in this case is likely to be secondary to cardiac congestion and will reduce in size following appropriate diuretic therapy. An abdominal ultrasound is not required, unless there is doubt about the diagnosis.

D Close monitoring and trial of diuretic therapy – Correct. This baby has symptomatic heart failure and is struggling to cope with her current circulating volume. Low doses of diuretics are safe for neonates, and a loop diuretic like furosemide is generally very well tolerated.

E DC cardioversion – Incorrect. This child is alert and has a HR of 150 bpm. The child does not appear to be suffering from a compromising cardiac arrhythmia requiring cardioversion. An ECG may instead be a sensible step in the investigation and management of this child to look for underlying cardiac defects and to assess for any arrhythmia.

Key Point

Patients with heart failure generally require medical management before surgical intervention for any underlying lesion. Initial treatment is with diuretics.

Q3 The baby has an echocardiogram which shows a ventricular septal defect. Her parents are concerned and want to know what the risk of a congenital heart defect would be if they had another child?

The correct answer is B. Slightly increased risk.

If there is a strong family history of cardiac malformation, additional foetal echocardiography may be offered. Earlier scans may not be beneficial and medical professionals must always ensure they give unbiased and non-opinionated information to parents regarding termination. In reality, many variables and factors increase the risk of congenital heart disease.

Babies born at or below 37 weeks gestation have a significantly increased risk of congenital heart disease. Maternal diabetes, hypertension, thyroid disorders and alcohol use also increase risk. Certain medications, particularly antipsychotic medicines or anticonvulsive medicines, can increase risk.

(i) IMPORTANT LEARNING POINTS

- Children can present non-specifically with cardiac disease, so a high index of suspicion should be maintained. Liaison with a tertiary cardiac centre and an echocardiogram should be performed to exclude a cardiac cause.
- Volume of a murmur does not necessarily correlate with severity of condition, as it only reflects the degree of turbulence in blood flow. Therefore a patient may have a large VSD but a very quiet murmur, since there is minimal turbulence.
- The mainstay of management for heart failure is the use of diuretics and optimisation of nutrition. Surgical management can be considered but this is usually not done acutely, since it is better to improve the patient's overall health first to reduce any associated surgical risk.

ANSWER TO CASE 21
A 4-year-old boy presenting with nephrotic syndrome

Q1 What is the most common cause of the underlying diagnosis?

The correct answer is A. Minimal change disease.

Nephrotic syndrome is characterised by proteinuria, hypoalbuminaemia and oedema. He has proteinuria and hypoalbuminaemia with normal BP and renal function which fits with the clinical diagnosis.

A Minimal change disease – Correct. This would be the most likely finding in a child with a first presentation of nephrotic syndrome, with no atypical features.

B Focal and segmental glomerulosclerosis – Incorrect. This is a rarer cause of nephrotic syndrome; it carries a poorer prognosis and is less likely to be steroid-sensitive.

C Membranous nephropathy – Incorrect. This is more common in adults and again carries a worse prognosis, with immunomodulatory agents almost always required. As well as idiopathic aetiology, it is also associated with SLE, hepatitis and medications, including NSAIDs.

D Post-infectious glomerulonephritis – Incorrect. This usually presents 7-10 days following a streptococcal throat infection. There is a nephritic picture and the urine is usually dark. Corticosteroids are not generally indicated and antibiotic therapy is usually unhelpful by the time post-streptococcal glomerulonephritis develops. Supportive therapies may be required, but usually the prognosis is excellent.

E IgA nephropathy – Incorrect. This commonly presents with macroscopic haematuria but rarely can present with nephrotic syndrome. Treatment is usually supportive and aimed at managing any complications.

⚲ Key Point

Minimal change disease is the most common cause of nephrotic syndrome in children, accounting for around 80% of cases.

Q2 What would be the first-line management for the suspected underlying diagnosis?

The correct answer is C. High dose oral corticosteroids, penicillin prophylaxis, no added salt diet.

The treatment for a first episode of nephrotic syndrome is corticosteroids, penicillin prophylaxis (as pneumococcal peritonitis is a potential complication) and a no-added-salt diet. In the acute setting, if the child is hypovolaemic, an albumin infusion may be necessary. Fluid restriction should generally be avoided.

A High dose oral corticosteroids, antihypertensives – Incorrect. BP should be monitored but if normotensive there is no need for antihypertensives.

B IV corticosteroids, IV antibiotics – Incorrect. There is no evidence that intravenous corticosteroids are more effective than oral corticosteroids. Only prophylactic antibiotics are needed, as there is no evidence of a current infection.

C High dose oral corticosteroids, penicillin prophylaxis, no added salt diet – Correct. Children with nephrotic syndrome should be initially treated with four weeks of high dose oral corticosteroids with a reducing dose and may also be given antibiotics to protect against encapsulated infections. A no-added-salt diet can help with fluid balance.

D Immunomodulatory agents – Incorrect. If there are frequent relapses or there is no response to corticosteroids, immunosuppression may be required. Commonly used agents include levamisole, tacrolimus, cyclosporin, mycophenolate mofetil, cyclophosphamide and rituximab.

E Antihistamine – Incorrect. A common differential for an oedematous patient is allergy, but antihistamines are not indicated when the diagnosis is nephrotic syndrome. Remember to dipstick the urine of a child who presents with puffiness.

⚲ Key Point

Minimal change disease is considered steroid-sensitive; therefore, it usually responds to a course of corticosteroids.

Q3 In the treatment of the above condition, which of the following are complications of long-term treatment?

The correct answers are A. Weight gain, B. Hyperactive behaviour, C. Abdominal striae, D. Adrenal suppression, and E. Cataracts.

Oral corticosteroids are the first-line treatment for nephrotic syndrome, and are usually effective. However, steroid side effects are numerous.

A Weight gain – Correct. This is seen with corticosteroid treatment and is usually secondary to increased appetite.

B Hyperactive behaviour – Correct. This is a commonly reported side effect by parents.

C Abdominal striae – Correct. This can be seen following long-term usage.

D Adrenal suppression – Correct. This can be seen following long-term usage. Exogenous steroids lead to reduced ACTH (adrenocorticotropic hormone) production, and this leads to reduced endogenous corticosteroid production. With high dose corticosteroids, this is particularly problematic, as during acute infections, an adrenal crisis can be precipitated. This is because with a background of adrenal suppression, the body does not produce the increase in endogenous corticosteroids required to fight infection.

E Cataracts – Correct. Cataracts are associated with long-term corticosteroid usage.

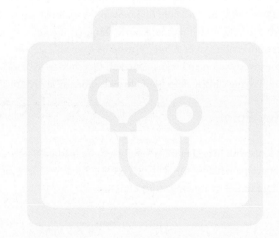

Key Point

Features of steroid toxicity include:

- Weight gain (increased appetite)
- Striae
- Acne
- Change in facial and body shape – "moon face" and "buffalo hump"
- Poor growth
- Behavioural changes
- Increased susceptibility to infections – especially varicella
- Adrenal suppression
- Hypertension –regular BP monitoring is needed (occasionally hypotension rather than hypertension can be seen secondary to adrenal suppression)
- Osteopenia
- Proximal myopathy
- Cataracts

Q4 If a renal biopsy was undertaken, what would be the most likely findings in the above child?

The correct answer is A. Podocyte foot process effacement.

Renal biopsy is usually only undertaken if there are atypical features or if there is no response to corticosteroid treatment. Minimal change disease is the most frequent renal biopsy finding in uncomplicated nephrotic syndrome – proteinuria results due to a breakdown of the glomerular basement membrane, meaning no barrier to albumin passage.

A Podocyte foot process effacement – Correct. This is the key feature of minimal change disease, which is seen on electron microscopy only. This would be the most likely finding in a child with a first presentation of nephrotic syndrome.
B Scarring of parts of some nephrons – Incorrect. This is associated with focal and segmental glomerulosclerosis.
C Thickened basement membrane but not hypercellular – Incorrect. This is associated with membranous nephropathy.
D Immune complex formation on the basement membrane – Incorrect. This is associated with post-streptococcal and membranoproliferative glomerulonephritis.
E IgA deposition – Incorrect. This is associated with IgA nephropathy.

Key Point

- Although minimal change disease has a typical electron microscopy appearance, it is not usually necessary to do a biopsy to confirm the diagnosis.

(i) IMPORTANT LEARNING POINTS

- There are multiple causes of oedema, including nephrotic syndrome as well as cardiac and hepatic failure. If oedema is localised, the most common cause is allergy or infection.
- The commonest cause of nephrotic syndrome is minimal change disease, and this is usually corticosteroid responsive. Prophylactic antibiotics should also be prescribed, as well as a no-added-salt diet.
- Patients with nephrotic syndrome are more vulnerable to infection, particularly pneumococcal disease, including pneumococcal peritonitis. Therefore, prophylactic antibiotics should be considered.

ANSWER TO CASE 22
An 11-year-old boy presenting with haematuria

Q1 What is the most likely diagnosis in this child?

The correct answer is C. Post-infectious glomerulonephritis.

This is the typical picture of post-infectious glomerulonephritis, which can be caused by group A Streptococcus. Typically it presents one to two weeks after streptococcal throat infection, or four to six weeks after a streptococcal skin infection, and causes the typical features of glomerulonephritis.

A IgA nephropathy – Incorrect. In children, the usual presentation is with macroscopic haematuria in a well child. Typically the signs and symptoms are the same as with post-streptococcal glomerulonephritis (change in urine colour, haematuria, oedema, lethargy), but it occurs along with an URTI rather than being one to two weeks following one. Complement levels are normal in IgA nephropathy but reduced with post-streptococcal glomerulonephritis. Interestingly, the serum IgA may be increased in IgA nephropathy.
B Nephrotic syndrome – Incorrect. This child has a normal serum albumin so this cannot be nephrotic syndrome, which typically does not present with haematuria.
C Post-infectious glomerulonephritis – Correct. This is the commonest glomerulonephritis seen in children in the UK. It is usually a result of a streptococcal infection elsewhere in the body causing nephritis. It commonly presents with oedema, hypertension, haematuria and general lethargy. The urine is typically described as Coca-Cola-coloured, or there may be macroscopic haematuria.
D Urinary tract infection – Incorrect. A UTI should be ruled out by a urine MC&S, but in this case, the initial dipstick is not suggestive of a UTI, and the symptoms are more suggestive of an alternative diagnosis. Typical presentation of a UTI would include fever, lethargy, poor feeding and offensive smelling urine.

483

E   Rapidly-progressive glomerulonephritis – Incorrect. The child is too well for this diagnosis and has normal renal function. A child with rapidly-progressive glomerulonephritis would be more likely to present with a severe nephritic picture and acute kidney injury.

⚷ Key Point

It is easy to get confused between nephrotic syndrome and nephritic syndrome. Remember that nephrotic syndrome requires hypoalbuminaemia as part of the diagnosis, and minimal change disease is uncommon in those over 10-years-old.

Q2 Which of the following tests would be best for confirming the suspected diagnosis?

The correct answer is C. ASOT titres

The key here is to pick the test which most likely suggests post-infectious glomerulonephritis. ASOT titres and anti-DNAse B are therefore correct, although a full screen for haematuria ought to be done, including FBC, clotting, U&Es, throat swab, ASOT titres, anti-DNAse B, renal ultrasound, with consideration of also checking complement levels, and auto-antibodies. Thyroid and lipid profile should also be checked, as well as albumin.

A   Complement levels – Incorrect. Typically there is reduced C3 and C4 in post-streptococcal glomerulonephritis, but complement levels can also be reduced in other types of glomerulonephritis, such as systemic lupus erythematosus, therefore making these measurements less specific.

B   Hepatitis serology – Incorrect. This would be important if the diagnosis was membranous nephropathy and may well be done in the initial diagnostic work-up, but in a child with a possible diagnosis of post-infectious glomerulonephritis, this will not help confirm or refute the diagnosis.

C   ASOT titres – Correct. This is the key investigation, since it demonstrates previous infection with Group A *Streptococcus*, although in an 11-year-old boy with previous infections, it is useful to repeat convalescence samples (after the infection) together with anti-DNAase B levels (which is another marker of previous exposure).

D   Renal ultrasound – Incorrect. Although the child may have a renal USS, this would not be diagnostic of post-infectious glomerulonephritis.

E   Renal biopsy – Incorrect. This would be reserved for children who did not follow the typical benign course of this illness, or who developed other features which put the diagnosis into question.

F   IgA levels – Incorrect. Although not diagnostic, these can be elevated in individuals with IgA nephropathy and it therefore may be a useful test. However, it does not help in confirming the suspected diagnosis in this case.

⚷ Key Point

A diagnosis of post-infectious glomerulonephritis requires recent streptococcal infection, which can be explored in the history and confirmed by ASOT testing and anti-DNAase B levels.

Q3 How would you manage this patient?

The correct answer is C. Monitor haematuria, BP and renal function, with clinic follow-up.

A   Discharge with diuretic therapy to offload the oedema – Incorrect. This is not the correct management for oedema, particularly in patients with mild oedema. It risks causing the patient to become intravascularly depleted and precipitates acute kidney injury.

B   Refer for consideration of renal dialysis – Incorrect. Renal function is normal.

C   Monitor haematuria, BP and renal function, with clinic follow-up – Correct. Management in this patient should be supportive, as the child is stable, with normal haematological, renal and electrolyte blood tests. The patient should receive careful follow up via the community nursing team to monitor the clinical situation (BP, urine dip, daily weights) and be seen in a clinic setting within the week.

D   Admit and monitor for 24 hours in hospital – Incorrect. There is no current concern that this patient will rapidly deteriorate. There is a clear history for PIGN; therefore, they can be sent home and followed up in the clinic. However, this would be the preferred option if the child was hypertensive.

⚷ Key Point

Well children with normal renal function and BP can be followed up in the clinic. They should be carefully monitored with the involvement of the community nursing team for BP, urine dip and weight. Fortunately, the prognosis is good for most children with spontaneous resolution expected.

ⓘ IMPORTANT LEARNING POINTS

- Macroscopic haematuria should always be taken seriously in a child. It can be caused by various pathologies, as well as by general haematological disorders.
- Post-infectious glomerulonephritis is the most common cause and requires evidence of streptococcal exposure. The prognosis is generally good, with supportive treatment usually only required.
- Patients with non-traumatic haematuria should be followed up closely.

ANSWER TO CASE 23
A 5–year-old girl presenting with a purpuric rash

Q1 What is the most likely diagnosis?

The correct answer is C. Henoch-Schönlein Purpura.

These are the differentials of a purpuric rash. Despite not knowing the platelet count for this question, the history and the description of the rash is very suggestive of Henoch-Schönlein purpura (HSP).

A   Acute lymphoblastic leukaemia – Incorrect. The child would typically be more unwell with a slightly longer history typically of tiredness and lethargy. The blood tests will show low platelets, plus abnormalities in haemoglobin and/or white cell count, and a blood film would be abnormal.

B   Meningococcal septicaemia – Incorrect. This would be a very acute presentation and if the child had a true purpuric rash of meningococcal sepsis, they would be moribund. The rash would typically affect the extremities first.

C   Henoch-Schönlein Purpura – Correct. This is an autoimmune IgA mediated vasculitis of childhood. It can affect many systems, typically causing abdominal pain (and rectal bleeding if severe), joint pains and a typical vasculitic rash. It can be preceded by a viral URTI but may occur without.

D   Immune thrombocytopenic purpura – Incorrect. This would fit with a relatively well child, but the other features in the history suggest HSP is a more likely diagnosis. A normal platelet count would exclude this diagnosis.

E   Drug-related rash – Incorrect. This is an unlikely diagnosis given the history and the description of the rash. There is no history of drug ingestion, and the rash is not urticarial in nature.

♀ Key Point

The characteristic feature of HSP is the rash. It is classically a raised purpuric rash on the buttocks and extensor limb surfaces.

Q2 Which three investigations would be useful in the further management of this child?

The correct answers are A. FBC, C. U&Es and D. Urine dipstick.

In general, the diagnosis of HSP is clinical and not based on any laboratory investigations. Some are important, though, to rule out other differentials and to ensure that there are no complications.

A   FBC – Correct. This is important to ensure that the platelets are normal given the purpuric rash.

B   Renal USS – Incorrect. This would be unnecessary in an uncomplicated case of HSP without renal involvement. There is nothing in the history suggesting that the kidneys are affected.

C   U&Es – Correct. Nephrotic syndrome is a rare complication of HSP and therefore baseline renal function is an important investigation.

D   Urine dipstick – Correct. Negative urine dipstick with normal BP and renal function excludes renal involvement (HSP nephritis) in the early stages. However, as this can occur later, continued monitoring for the first six weeks is important.

E   Abdominal X-ray – Incorrect. Abdominal pain is very common in children. HSP is associated with inflammatory changes in the coeliac plexus, but also more seriously, with intussusception. An abdominal X-ray is only helpful (in conjunction with an erect chest X-ray) if perforation is suspected. USS is the investigation of choice if intussusception is suspected.

♀ Key Point

Generally the most worrying concern with HSP is renal complications. It is therefore important to check renal function, BP and dipstick the urine.

Q3 Initial investigations are all normal. Given this, what is the best management of this child, assuming she is still haemodynamically stable?

The correct answer is E. Advise, regular urine monitoring, and early follow-up.

The blood picture in this child is essentially normal. Typical HSP is usually self-limiting and does not require any specific treatment. NSAIDs can be helpful for joint pain, but should be avoided if there is evidence of renal involvement. They offer symptomatic relief, but otherwise in typical cases, no other treatment is indicated. Early follow up is important to look for any renal involvement. Children may require admission if immobile due to pain or for pain control.

A   Reassure and discharge – Incorrect. Although the overall message to parents in an uncomplicated case of HSP is reassurance, follow up is necessary to check for resolution and to ensure there are no late renal complications.

B   Admit for full septic screen and start IV antibiotics – Incorrect. In a classic case of HSP, this is not necessary. If there is ever any doubt about the nature of a purpuric rash in an unwell child, the default is to treat for presumed meningococcal sepsis.

C   Arrange urgent platelet transfusion – Incorrect. Platelet count is normal. Even if idiopathic thrombocytopaenic purpura

485

was the diagnosis, platelet transfusions are rarely given as they are just consumed by the antibodies.

D   Speak to the local tertiary referral centre to arrange transfer – Incorrect. This would be one of the necessary steps in managing a new diagnosis of acute lymphoblastic leukaemia, or an atypical/complicated case of HSP.

E   Advise, regular urine monitoring, and early follow-up – Correct. A full explanation to parents is necessary as the rash can cause great anxiety. Follow up within a week is necessary, either in a day-care setting or with the primary care physician. Urine dipstick and BP should be checked, either by the parent or a community nurse. NSAIDs may be useful in symptomatic management of joint pain, provided the renal function is normal. If there is any evidence of renal involvement in the first six weeks, long term follow up is required.

F   Oral corticosteroids and bring back to clinic in one week – Incorrect. There is some evidence that oral corticosteroids can be used in HSP to reduce the duration of joint pain, but they are not standard management due to the potential side effects. In typical HSP, corticosteroids would not be recommended. Steroids may be helpful for severe abdominal involvement or if the rash becomes necrotic.

Key Point

The management of HSP is generally supportive, as it is usually a self-limiting disease.

IMPORTANT LEARNING POINTS

- HSP classically causes abdominal pain, arthralgia manifesting in difficulty weight-bearing, a characteristic purpuric rash and possible renal complications. One percent of patients progress to renal disease.
- Always be aware of meningococcal septicaemia in any patient with a purpuric rash. If they are unwell, then you should treat for meningococcal disease.
- Management of HSP is generally symptomatic with simple analgesia, although if there is more complex renal involvement other treatments may be considered.
- HSP is generally a benign condition with most patients fully recovering with no long term complications.

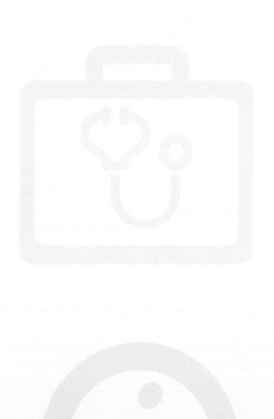

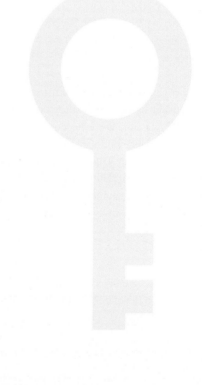

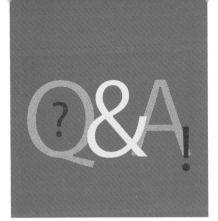
CONTENTS

CASE 1
A 2-year-old girl presenting with knee pain

Hayley is a 2-year-old girl who has been brought to ED by her parents. She banged her right knee on a table two weeks ago. It was sore at the time, but she has subsequently mobilised on it. She has been unable to weight-bear on her right leg for the last 48 hours and she has a swollen right knee. Her HR is 155 (tachycardic) and her temperature is 38.5°C, with observations otherwise within normal limits. She has been off her food for the last day and "hasn't been herself", according to her parents. Initial bloods show a white cell count of $13.1 \times 10^9/L$. On examination, her right knee is markedly swollen and is held in a flexed position (around 60°). She is reluctant to flex or extend the knee due to pain.

Questions

Q1 What should be the working diagnosis?
 A Fracture
 B Knee ligament injury
 C Septic arthritis
 D Transient synovitis
 E Osgood-Schlatter disease

Q2 What additional investigations might be helpful in establishing a diagnosis? Select all that apply.
 A X-ray right knee
 B CRP
 C ESR
 D Ultrasound right knee
 E X-ray right hip

Q3 What is the next best stage in management of this patient?
 A Immediately commence broad-spectrum antibiotics
 B Admit and observe the patient
 C Immediately commence broad-spectrum antibiotics and then aspirate the knee

D Refer to the orthopaedic team for knee aspiration/ washout and then commence broad-spectrum antibiotics

Q4 Given the patient's age, what are the most likely causes of septic arthritis? Select all that apply.

A *Staphylococcus aureus*

B *Neisseria gonorrhoea*

C Group B streptococci

D Gram negative bacilli

E *Haemophilus influenzae*

For answers see page 493

CASE 2
An 11-year-old boy presenting with a wrist injury

Peter is an 11-year-old boy who was playing football two days ago. He had a painful right wrist immediately after stopping a forceful shot at goal, and his father took him to a minor injuries unit the same day. HR is 130 bpm (tachycardic), but observations are otherwise within normal limits. He was sent home with analgesia, but has returned to the ED today with worsening pain, swelling and some pins and needles feeling in his index finger and thumb. An X-ray demonstrates an undisplaced extra-articular greenstick ulnar fracture.

Questions

Q1 What two pieces of information from the history are most important for the above scenario from the list below?

A Hand dominance

B Mechanism of injury

C Family history

D Time of last meal

E Weight

Q2 How would you assess the function of the anterior-interosseous nerve branch of the median nerve?

A Ask the child to spread their fingers, whilst the examiner tries to push them together

B Ask the patient to extend their wrist

C Ask the patient to make an "ok" sign with their index finger and thumb

D Test sensation over the anatomical snuff box area

E Test sensation over the regimental badge area

Q3 How would you manage this child?

A Closed reduction and percutaneous pinning

B Open reduction and internal fixation

C Futura splint for eight weeks

D Below elbow Plaster of Paris for 2-3 weeks

E Above elbow Plaster of Paris for 2-3 weeks

For answers see page 494

CASE 3
An 8-year-old boy presenting with groin and knee pain

Mark is an 8-year-old boy presenting with a two week history of right groin pain and knee pain exacerbated by exercise. His father suffered from similar problems during his childhood. Mark reports that he is bullied at school for being short. Prior to this, his gait had been normal. Developmental history is normal and he walked at 1-year-old.

Observations are within normal limits. On examination, he is reluctant to walk. With some encouragement, he demonstrates an antalgic gait, painful internal rotation and abduction of the hip and a leg length discrepancy.

Questions

Q1 What is the most likely differential diagnosis?

A Developmental dysplasia of the hip

B Slipped upper femoral epiphysis

C Perthes' disease

D Transient synovitis

E Septic arthritis

Q2 Which two of the following are risk factors for this condition?

A Breech presentation

B Obesity

C Low birth weight

D Female

E Short stature

Q3 Which of the following are the two most appropriate initial investigations?

A AP and lateral X-ray of the hip

B CT scan

C MRI scan

D FBC, CRP, ESR

E Ultrasound

Q4 How should this child be treated?

A Surgical containment of the femoral head

B Intravenous antibiotics

C Bed rest and traction

D Fixation of the epiphysis with threaded pins/ screws

E Conservative management with observation only

For answers see page 495

CASE 4
A 3-year-old boy presenting with short stature

Dylan is a 3-year-old boy with short stature. He was born by emergency caesarean section due to breech presentation and at six-hours-old, he became pale and floppy. His blood glucose was low and resolved with a feed. He had another hypoglycaemic episode at 12 hours of age and was then admitted to the neonatal unit, where he stayed for 24 hours with no further hypoglycaemia. Dylan's development has been normal and he has been otherwise healthy. Observations are within normal limits.

Family history has been unremarkable. Dad is 178 cm, and mum is 166 cm. Systemic examination is unremarkable, with no disproportion, dysmorphic features or body asymmetry.

Measurements from his growth charts are shown in *Figure 1*.

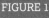
FIGURE 1

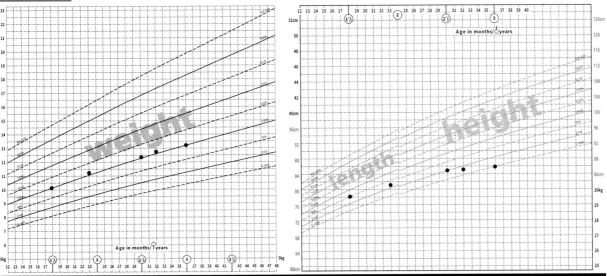

Height and weight plotted on standardised WHO charts.

Questions

Q1 Using the centile chart (*Figure 2a*) please calculate the centile of the mid-parental height.

    A 25th

    B 50th

    C 75th

    D 2nd

Q2 Which of the following suggest a pathological cause for short stature? Select all that apply.

    A Discrepancy between height and weight

    B Discrepancy in height centile and mid-parental centile

    C Poor height velocity

Q3 Which of the following is/are likely to yield useful information as to the cause of short stature? Select all that apply.

    A Birth weight

    B Neonatal hypoglycaemia

    C Neonatal jaundice

    D Floppy episodes during illness

Q4 Which investigation(s) should be requested for this patient? Select all that apply.

    A Thyroid function tests

    B Insulin-like growth factor 1 (IGF1)

    C Coeliac screen

    D IGFBP-3

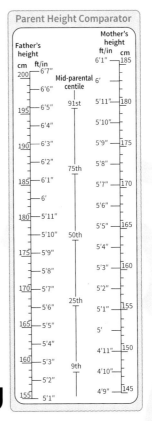

FIGURE 2A

Centile chart.

For answers see page 497

489

CASE 5
An 18-month-old girl presenting with an abdominal mass

An 18-month-old girl presents with a left sided abdominal mass. She is otherwise fit and well, with no significant past medical history. The mass was noticed incidentally by her mother whilst changing her. She has a normal bowel habit and has been passing urine normally. Heart rate, respiratory rate and temperature are within normal limits.

Q1 Which of the following might suggest that the abdominal mass may be a tumour? Select all that apply.
  A Severe pain
  B Rapid change in size of abdominal mass
  C Systemic symptoms such as fever, tiredness and weight loss
  D Presence of blood in the urine
  E Watery diarrhoea and sweating

On examination, she is well, although her abdomen appears asymmetrical. On palpation, you can feel a large, well-defined, left-sided mass. Her BP is 135/85 mmHg (above the 95th centile for her age and height) and her temperature is normal.

Q2 Which two of the following diagnoses are most likely?
  A Constipation
  B Neuroblastoma
  C Intussusception
  D Wilms' tumour
  E Splenomegaly

Q3 How would you further investigate this patient? Select all that apply.
  A Urinary homovanillic acid (HVA) and vanillylmandelic acid (VMA)
  B Laparoscopy
  C Abdominal ultrasound
  D Urine dipstick
  E Chest X-ray

For answers see page 499

CASE 6
A 28-day-old baby with projectile vomiting

A 28-day-old male infant presented to ED with a history of vomiting for one week. The baby was born at term with no significant antenatal history. His birth weight was 3.3 kg. He was formula fed since birth and tolerated all his feeds up until a week ago. The mother described the vomits as projectile, occurring approximately 20 minutes after each feed. She states that the vomits have always been milky white, never bilious or bloody. She also mentions that the baby has remained eager

to feed, but over the past few days his urine output and stool frequency have markedly decreased. He is currently on the 10th centile for height and weight.

On examination, the baby is thin and crying. The HR is 170 bpm (tachycardic), with observations otherwise within the normal limits. The baby is moderately dehydrated. Examination of the abdomen is normal. IV access is obtained and initial blood tests are taken.

Q1 Which of the following results is/are likely to be found? Select all that apply.
  A Hyponatraemia
  B Hyperkalaemia
  C Hypochloraemia
  D Metabolic acidosis
  E Acidic urine

Q2 What is/are the most appropriate next step/steps to confirm the diagnosis?
  A Ultrasound
  B Test feed
  C Contrast study
  D CT scan
  E Endoscopy

Q3 After the diagnosis of "pyloric stenosis with moderate dehydration" has been confirmed, which of the following should you do? Select all that apply.
  A Insert a nasogastric tube
  B Calculate and commence maintenance fluids
  C Insert a catheter
  D Allow the baby to formula feed
  E Place the baby on the emergency operating list

For answers see page 500

CASE 7
A 1-day-old boy with desaturations after feeds and drooling

A male baby is born via normal vaginal delivery at 37 weeks gestation. The baby had normal antenatal scans except for polyhydramnios. The baby was well at birth, but was subsequently noticed to be very "mucus-y". Mother tried to breastfeed the baby, but he desaturated every time. He responded well to some suction but started drooling excessively. His RR is 63 breaths/min (tachypnoeic), but other observations are within normal limits. The paediatric team is called to the postnatal ward.

Q1 Which steps/investigations would be useful in the acute management of this baby? Select all that apply.
  A Chest X-ray only
  B Chest and abdominal X-ray
  C Nasogastric tube

D HIDA scan

E Renal ultrasound scan

The diagnosis of oesophageal atresia is established. A Replogle tube is passed and placed on continuous suction. The baby is self-ventilating on room air. The paediatric surgical registrar now has time to fully examine the baby. The baby does not seem syndromic. She notices that the baby's abdomen has become progressively more distended over the past hour. She also notices that the baby has passed some meconium from his penis. On examination of the perineum, she finds that the baby has a skin dimple in the midline, but has no anus.

Q2 Regarding the management of this baby, mark the following statements true or false.

A If the baby desaturates again, bag and mask ventilation is first line of management

B A cross matched unit of blood should be ordered as soon as possible

C Surgery can be undertaken in a day or two, after the baby stabilises

D An echo should be performed post operatively

E Both conditions should be treated under the same anaesthetic

Q3 What other investigations are indicated in this baby? Select all that apply.

A Renal ultrasound scan

B CT of the abdomen and pelvis

C Ultrasound scan and X-ray of the back

D MCUG

E Genetic workup

For answers see page 501

CASE 8
A 4-year-old boy presenting with fever and a rash

A 4-year-old boy, Jacob, is brought into ED with a fever of 39.2°C. His mother reports a new rash on his abdomen and chest that did not disappear when she pressed a glass on it.

His respiratory rate is 50 breaths/min (tachyponeic), with subcostal recession. His saturations on room air are 92%. His HR is 174 bpm (tachycardic). BP is normal. He is peripherally cool, with a central capillary refill time of 4 seconds. Jacob is drowsy and difficult to wake, though he responds to pain. His blood sugar is 5.7 mmol/L. A non-blanching rash is present on his chest and abdomen. His estimated weight is 19 kg.

Jacob has been intubated and ventilated in ED. He has had two 20 mL/kg boluses of 0.9% sodium chloride and one dose of IV ceftriaxone. The retrieval team has been contacted, and arrangements have been made to transfer Jacob to PICU.

Initial settings are: PIP 18, PEEP 5, Rate 40, Oxygen 30%.

Questions

Q1 After being intubated and ventilated, Jacob's arterial blood gas shows a pH of 7.20, pO_2 of 10 kPa, pCO_2 of 8.2 kPa, and BE of -7. Which of the following adjustments will theoretically improve ventilation?

A Increase the oxygen concentration

B Reduce the respiratory rate

C Increase the peak inspiratory pressure

D Change the endotracheal tube to a laryngeal mask airway

E Increase the peak end expiratory pressure

Q2 Jacob's BP is stable, but his hands and feet are still cool to touch, with weak pulses. His capillary refill time remains three seconds. His HR is now 165 bpm. He has not produced urine despite being catheterised in ED. What should be done next?

A Prepare to commence haemofiltration

B Give another 20 mL/kg bolus of 0.9% sodium chloride

C Give 250 mL of colloid fluid

D Start inotropic support with milrinone

E Recheck his renal function

Q3 Jacob's mother is understandably distressed by his condition. She says he has not eaten all day, and she is worried about his nutrition. She asks if he can have some milk. What is the safest advice you can give in ED?

A Jacob can have some milk via a NG tube

B Jacob will have TPN started by NG tube

C Jacob will have TPN started via a central line in ED

D Jacob will not be fed at present, but will receive IV fluids

E A dietician will need to be consulted in ED before making a decision about feeding enterally

For answers see page 503

CASE 9
A 3-day-old baby presenting with weak femoral pulses

You are called to the postnatal ward to assess a 3-day-old male infant. During his routine postnatal check, the midwife tells you she found it very difficult to feel his femoral pulses. She also thinks she heard a murmur and would like you to assess him further.

The pregnancy had been low risk, with normal antenatal scans and serology. The baby was born in good condition via spontaneous vaginal delivery.

His initial observations show a respiratory rate of 55 breaths/min (normal), oxygen saturations of 75% in room air, a HR of 170 bpm (tachycardic), with a normal BP and temperature.

He has cool peripheries. Femoral pulses are faintly felt. The HR is regular, and there is a harsh systolic murmur loudest at the left upper sternal edge.

You immediately call for senior help and administer oxygen.

Questions

Q1 Which of the following investigations are essential in the assessment of this baby? Select all that apply.
   A Baseline bloods including CRP, blood cultures, and blood gas
   B Blood glucose
   C Four-limb BP
   D Echocardiogram
   E Electrocardiogram

Q2 Your team makes a diagnosis of coarctation of the aorta. Given this presentation, which two of the following options would you add to your management in addition to the general approach to an acutely unwell patient?
   A Prostaglandin infusion
   B DC cardioversion
   C Antibiotics in line with trust guidance on neonatal sepsis
   D Atropine
   E Indomethacin infusion

Q3 A medical student in the paediatric department asks for tips on feeling for pulses during the standard neonatal examination. Which of the following statements is correct?
   A Femoral pulses can be difficult to feel and if they are unsure, they should ask a senior to review the baby.

   B If the perfusion, colour and tone of the lower limbs is normal, palpation of the femoral pulses is not needed.
   C Weak and low volume femoral pulses are pathognomonic for coarctation of the aorta
   D It is best to feel for femoral pulses at the same time as assessing hip stability to save time.
   E When palpation of the pulses is impossible, often the pulse can be heard when the femoral area is auscultated with the bell of a stethoscope.

Q4 Four years later, you are a registrar in clinic and the same child comes to see you, having had corrective surgery. He is asymptomatic and thriving. What residual features would you expect to be present?
   A Absent femoral pulses
   B Brachio-femoral delay
   C Hypertension
   D Cyanosis
   E Rib notching on X-ray

For answers see page 504

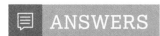 **ANSWERS**

ANSWER TO CASE 1
A 2-year-old girl presenting with knee pain

Q1 What should be the working diagnosis?

The correct answer is C. Septic arthritis.

Septic arthritis can have serious complications and is a key differential diagnosis in any febrile child presenting with acute joint pain.

A Fracture – Incorrect. Although there is a history of trauma, this occurred two weeks prior and the child did initially weight-bear on the leg.

B Knee ligament injury – Incorrect. Given the age of the child, mechanism of the initial injury and the fact that she has put weight on the knee since the injury, this is unlikely.

C Septic arthritis – Correct. The child has three of the five modified Kocher criteria (temperature >38.5°C, inability to weight-bear, white cell count >12 x 10⁹/L), which gives around a 90% chance of septic arthritis. The preceding trauma may be a red herring or may have caused a sterile haemarthrosis that has subsequently become infected.

D Transient synovitis – Incorrect. Differentiating septic arthritis from transient synovitis can be difficult. In the above case, there is no preceding illness and enough positive modified Kocher criteria are present to warrant concern regarding septic arthritis.

E Osgood-Schlatter disease – Incorrect. Osgood-Schlatter disease is caused by inflammation of the patella ligament at its insertion onto the tibial tuberosity at the knee. There is often a painful, palpable bump over the tibial tubercle. It predominantly affects sporty, male children between the ages of 9 to 16.

⚲ Key Point

Septic arthritis should be excluded in a child with preceding trauma as a haemarthrosis provides a rich medium in which organisms can grow.

Q2 What additional investigations might be helpful in establishing a diagnosis?

The correct answers are A. X-ray right knee, B. CRP, C. ESR and D. Ultrasound right knee.

Radiographs of the affected joint and baseline bloods including CRP are the first line investigations of choice in any acutely swollen joint.

A X-ray right knee – Correct. An AP and lateral X-ray of the affected joint is sensible to ensure no underlying fractures are missed. The lateral view may also demonstrate a lipohaemarthrosis.

B CRP – Correct. CRP is a useful marker of underlying inflammation.

C ESR – Correct. ESR is also an important inflammatory marker, and should be performed in addition to CRP.

D Ultrasound right knee – Correct. If there is diagnostic doubt, the ultrasound can confirm the presence of an effusion. Any synovial reaction identified is consistent with infection. Ultrasound can also be used to guide aspiration if needed. This would not be appropriate for pus in the knee as this requires a washout but may be useful in other rheumatological conditions. Ultrasound may also be useful to identify features of autoimmune disease associated with an effusion, such as synovial thickening although this depends on the skill of the ultrasonographer. An ultrasound should not delay knee washout where there is a high suspicion of septic arthritis.

E X-ray right hip – Incorrect. Given the history and clear knee pathology, an X-ray of the hip is unnecessary providing the child has no evidence of hip pain upon examination.

⚲ Key Point

Septic arthritis classically results in elevated inflammatory markers (CRP, ESR, white cell counts), pyrexia and an inability to weight-bear. The more factors present, the more likely the diagnosis.

Q3 What is the next best stage in management of this patient?

The correct answer is D. Refer to orthopaedic team for knee aspiration/washout and then commence broad-spectrum antibiotics.

Aspiration of the joint under sterile conditions is the definitive way to diagnose an infected joint. Antibiotics started prior to aspiration can eradicate organisms prior to culture making definitive diagnosis and targeting of antibiotic therapy difficult.

A Immediately commence broad-spectrum antibiotics – Incorrect. Although sepsis campaigns advocate the immediate commencement of intravenous antibiotics, in the case of joint infections early administration before aspiration can prevent accurate identification of a causative organism.

B Admit and observe the patient – Incorrect. The patient has a high probability of having a septic joint according to Kocher's modified criteria and, without treatment, is likely to deteriorate.

C Immediately commence broad-spectrum antibiotics and then aspirate the knee – Incorrect. Early antibiotic therapy can prevent accurate diagnosis of the causative organism.

D ~~Refer to the orthopaedic team for knee aspiration/~~ washout and then commence broad-spectrum antibiotics – Correct. Given the patient's age, an anaesthetic will be necessary. If there is frank pus aspirated under anaesthetic, a formal washout of the joint is needed. If there is no pus, as much fluid as possible should be aspirated and sent for urgent MC&S. Following aspiration, broad-spectrum antibiotics should be immediately commenced.

⚲ Key Point

Aspiration of a joint should be performed before commencing antibiotics as antibiotic therapy can eradicate organisms prior to culture.

Q4 Given the patient's age, what are the most likely causes of septic arthritis?

The correct answers are A. *Staphylococcus aureus* and E. *Haemophilus influenzae*.

Different organisms are more likely to affect each specific age group due to different exposures. Confirmation is via aspiration of joint fluid under sterile conditions and culture.

A *Staphylococcus aureus* – Correct. This is common in all age groups and is the most common organism to infect joints.
B *Neisseria gonorrhoea* – Incorrect. This primarily occurs in sexually active teenagers.
C Group B streptococci – Incorrect. This primarily occurs in neonates and children under one.
D Gram negative bacilli – Incorrect. This primarily occurs in neonates and children under one.
E *Haemophilus influenzae* – Correct. This is seen in 1 to 5-year-olds.

⚲ Key Point

Staphylococcus aureus is the most common causative organism in joint infections.

ⓘ IMPORTANT LEARNING POINTS

- Any child with a temperature and inability to weight-bear or with a swollen joint should be assessed for septic arthritis.
- A history of trauma does not exclude a subsequent septic arthritis.
- The child should undergo aspiration and joint washout prior to commencing antibiotics to allow identification of the infecting organism.

ANSWER TO CASE 2
An 11-year-old boy presenting with a wrist injury

Q1 What two pieces of information from the history are most important for the above scenario from the list below?

The correct answers are A. Hand dominance and B. Mechanism of injury.

A Hand dominance – Correct. Knowing the hand dominance of the child is important for practical reasons. The child and parent will need advice on casting and/or resting the injured side. This may require alterations to their school work, such as no sports or stopping writing for a short period.
B Mechanism of injury – Correct. In any child with a fracture, knowing the underlying mechanism of injury is vital for understanding both how to treat the fracture and to ensure there are no child protection issues.
C Family history – Incorrect. This is unrelated to fracture management, apart from in rare cases of pathological fractures where the underlying cause may have a genetic aetiology.
D Time of last meal – Incorrect. This is important in the context of urgent surgery, but doesn't apply in the above case.
E Weight – Incorrect. The weight of the child has no bearing on management.

⚲ Key Point

Understanding the link between mechanism of injury and likely pathology is vital to determining whether there are any child protection concerns.

Q2 How would you assess the function of the anterior-interosseous nerve branch of the median nerve?

The correct answer is C. Ask the patient to make an "ok" sign with their index finger and thumb.

Accurate examination and documentation of neurovascular status following a fracture are vital so that no nerve or arterial injuries are missed. The same should be documented following any reduction of the fracture.

A Ask the child to spread their fingers, whilst the examiner tries to push them together – Incorrect. This tests the motor function of the ulnar nerve.
B Ask the patient to extend their wrist – Incorrect. This tests motor function of the radial nerve.
C Ask the patient to make an "ok" sign with their index finger and thumb – Correct. The anterior interosseous branch of the median nerve innervates flexor pollicis longus, pronator quadratus and the radial half of flexor digitorum profundus.

D Test sensation over the anatomical snuff box area – Incorrect. This tests the sensory modality of the radial nerve.

E Test sensation over the regimental badge area – Incorrect. This tests the sensory modality of the axillary nerve.

Key Point

A full neurovascular examination should be conducted distal to any fracture. Nerves are rarely fully transected (neurotmesis) but instead are often compressed (neuropraxia) leading to a transient loss of function or paraesthesia which usually recovers in weeks to months.

Q3 How would you manage this child?

The correct answer is D. Below elbow Plaster of Paris for 2-3 weeks.

The anatomy and biomechanics of children's bones are unique, resulting in different fracture patterns, different healing mechanisms and different management compared to adults. Children's fractures have significantly lower rates of non-union. Adult fractures take four to six weeks to heal, whereas children's take approximately half this time.

A Closed reduction and percutaneous pinning – Incorrect. The injury is closed, extra-articular and is minimally displaced. In an 11-year-old child, this should heal quickly and is likely a stable injury. Operative intervention should be reserved for a) extra-articular injuries that are i) angulated or ii) associated with a deformity, and b) intra-articular injuries that are displaced.

B Open reduction and internal fixation – Incorrect. Operative intervention is not indicated.

C Futura splint for eight weeks – Incorrect. If the child is comfortable and the greenstick fracture is stable, a Futura splint for 2-3 weeks is an option, as it will immobilise the joint. However eight weeks is too long.

D Below elbow Plaster of Paris for 2-3 weeks – Correct. This is the appropriate management of a stable greenstick fracture, as the child is uncomfortable due to swelling and soft tissue injury. The fracture will heal over a 2-3 week period and a fiberglass below elbow cast allows the wrist to be protected if the child is likely to be active. Repeat X-ray at this time is unnecessary in stable undisplaced greenstick fractures and the child may return to have the plaster removed at the hospital or the parents may be given instructions to remove it themselves if they wish.

E Above elbow Plaster of Paris for 2-3 weeks – Incorrect. While the time period is correct, immobilising the elbow joint is unnecessary in a stable greenstick fracture and can lead to problems with stiffness upon removal of the cast.

Key Point

Undisplaced extra-articular fractures do not require operative intervention unless there is visible deformity or angulation, although this should be judged on a case-by-case basis.

(i) IMPORTANT LEARNING POINTS

- In any paediatric fracture, determining the mechanism of injury and understanding patterns of injury is vital to exclude any child protection issues.
- Neurovascular status should be carefully documented both pre and post any reduction. In the child with an upper limb injury, neurological status is best done by demonstrating movements, and then asking the child to copy them.
- Paediatric fractures heal quickly. Casts should be used to protect the fractured area from further trauma and to hold any unstable injury in a reduced position. Casts are associated with complications, such as joint stiffness; therefore, they need to be removed in a timely manner.

ANSWER TO CASE 3
An 8-year-old boy presenting with groin and knee pain

Q1 What is the most likely differential diagnosis?

The correct answer is C. Perthes' disease.

Perthes' disease is due to lack of blood flow to the growing femoral head and subsequent avascular necrosis. Hip, knee, groin pain and limp are common presentations in the 5 to 12-years-old age range.

A Developmental dysplasia of the hip – Incorrect. Congenital developmental dysplasia of the hip may be picked up before the child begins to walk by an observant parent. In later childhood, developmental dysplasia of the hip presents insidiously with an abnormal gait and excessive shoulder sway with minimal if any hip pain. Trendelenburg's sign is positive.

B Slipped upper femoral epiphysis – Incorrect. SUFE is the posterior-inferior displacement of the upper femoral epiphysis through the epiphyseal plate. It usually occurs in tall, overweight boys during the adolescent growth spurt.

C Perthes' disease – Correct. This child is displaying the signs and symptoms of Perthes' disease. Classically, it presents with insidious onset hip pain radiating down the thigh, associated with a limp. All hip movements are reduced and painful, especially internal rotation and abduction. Leg length discrepancy and muscle wasting may occur in severe disease.

D Transient synovitis – Incorrect. This presents more acutely, and is associated with minor trauma or viral infection. Pain is usually absent at rest and the limb is held in the position of greatest ease; usually flexed, abducted and slightly externally rotated. There will be no leg length discrepancy.

E Septic arthritis – Incorrect. Septic arthritis is a purulent infection of the joint space. It presents acutely, usually with fever, an exquisitely painful joint and an inability to weight bear.

♀ Key Point

Thorough history and examination, taking into account the child's age is paramount when a child presents with a limp. A diagnosis of transient synovitis should only be made after careful consideration of more sinister pathology.

Q2 Which two of the following are risk factors for this condition?

The correct answers are C. Low birth weight and E. short stature.

The exact cause of Perthes' disease is still unknown. A number of risk factors have been identified, such as low birth weight, short stature, family history, delayed skeletal age, and low socioeconomic status.

A Breech presentation – Incorrect. Breech presentation predisposes to developmental dysplasia of the hip, not Perthes' disease. Other risk factors for developmental dysplasia of the hip include family history, female sex, maternal oligohydramnios and first born child.

B Obesity – Incorrect. Associated with an increased risk of SUFE.

C Low birth weight – Correct. Risk factors for Perthes' disease also include a family history, low socioeconomic class and delayed skeletal age.

D Female – Incorrect. Perthes' is four times more common in boys.

E Short stature – Correct. Conversely, SUFE is more common in tall boys.

♀ Key Point

Childhood pathologies presenting with a limp are common and often share similar history and examination findings. Therefore, an awareness of the risk factors for these conditions can go a long way in narrowing down the differential diagnosis and preventing unnecessary investigations.

Q3 Which of the following are the two most appropriate initial investigations?

The correct answers are A. AP and lateral X-ray of the hip, and D. FBC, CRP, ESR.

Plain hip radiographs and baseline blood tests are standard initial investigations in the child presenting with new joint pain. Blood tests are primarily to exclude a septic cause or malignancy and radiographs may demonstrate features of Perthes' disease.

A AP and lateral X-ray of the hip – Correct. Plain radiographs are the most appropriate initial imaging study and the mainstay in the diagnosis of Perthes' disease. A limping child is a common presenting complaint with several differential diagnoses. Many of the causative conditions have characteristic X-ray appearances suggestive of a particular diagnosis. Radiological features of Perthes' disease include collapse of the femoral head, sclerosis and widening of the joint space. Later, the femoral head becomes fragmented and irregular.

B CT scan – Incorrect. Not typically used in the diagnosis of Perthes' disease.

C MRI scan – Incorrect. This would not be an initial investigation. However, MRI does have a role to play in the diagnosis of Perthes' disease if the history, physical examination and other imaging studies do not identify the source of the pathology. MRI is very sensitive at detecting early disease devoid of plain radiographic features.

D FBC, CRP, ESR – Correct. Elevated white cell count, CRP or ESR may suggest septic arthritis or osteomyelitis. If these tests are within their reference ranges, it strengthens the suspicion of Perthes' disease.

E Ultrasound – Incorrect. This investigation is of limited value in the diagnosis of Perthes' disease, but it may identify joint effusion, which would help in the broader evaluation of a limping child.

♀ Key Point

For any child with an atraumatic limp, have a low threshold for performing a hip X-ray and check baseline inflammatory markers. Septic arthritis is the most worrying differential, and although there is no perfect diagnostic test, normal inflammatory markers in an apyrexial patient makes it much less likely.

Q4 How should this child be treated?

The correct answer is A. Surgical containment of the femoral head.

The main aim of treatment is to keep the femoral head contained in the acetabulum, and maintain good hip movement. This is compromised in Perthes' disease by the changes in shape of the femoral head. In younger children, containment can usually be achieved conservatively, with observation, activity restriction, partial weight bearing, traction and physical therapy. In older children, conservative management is more likely to fail, and femoral and/or pelvic osteotomies (removing part of the bone) may be necessary.

A Surgical containment of the femoral head – Correct. Mild to moderate degree Perthes' disease is said to be present if there is less than 50% involvement of the femoral head with preservation of joint space. In younger children management is likely to be conservative with bed rest and traction. Severe disease occurs when there is more than 50% involvement of the femoral head and usually mandates surgical treatment.

B Intravenous antibiotics – Incorrect. Antibiotics are not used in the management of Perthes' disease. Instead, they are indicated in infective pathologies, such as septic arthritis and osteomyelitis.

C Bed rest and traction – Incorrect. Indicated in mild to moderate Perthes' disease in a child younger than 6-years-old.

D Fixation of the epiphysis with threaded pins/screws – Incorrect. This is the appropriate management of slipped upper femoral epiphysis with minor displacement of the femoral head.

E Conservative management with observation only – Incorrect. Conservative management may be appropriate for mild Perthes' disease. However, such conservative treatment includes bed rest, traction, analgesia and regular physiotherapy to increase muscle strength, not observation alone.

⚷ Key Point

A simple aide-memoire to remember the treatment of Perthes' disease is "half a dozen, half a head". So, if the patient is more than 6-years-old or has more than half the femoral head involved, surgical containment treatment should be considered.

ⓘ IMPORTANT LEARNING POINTS

- Any patient 4 to 8-years-old presenting with atraumatic hip or knee pain should be investigated for Perthes' disease.
- Remember that a child presenting with features suggestive of transient synovitis may in fact be an early presentation of Perthes' disease. Viral illnesses, such as upper respiratory tract infections, are very common in childhood: this may be a "red herring" in the history.
- Where diagnosis remains uncertain, MRI scans can be used, and early orthopaedic input should be sought.

ANSWER TO CASE 4
A 3-year-old boy presenting with short stature

Q1 Using the centile chart, please calculate the centile of the midparental height.

The correct answer is B. 50th centile.

Mid-parental height calculation is based on the calculation of the mean parental height correcting for sex as the mean sex difference is around 13 cm.

Therefore the following formulae are suggested:
➤ *Boys' sex-corrected height = (Father's height + mother's height + 13) / 2*
➤ *Girls' sex-corrected height = (Father's height + mother's height - 13) / 2*

Charts like that given simplify this process (*Figure 2b*). Note that this chart is for boys, and there is a separate chart for girls.

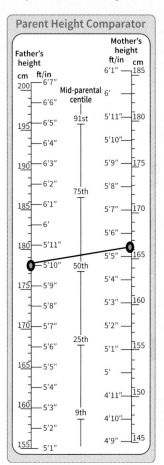

FIGURE 2B
Centile chart.

⚷ Key Point

Mid-parental height should always be corrected for the gender of the child.

Q2 Which of the following suggest a pathological cause for short stature?

The correct answers are A. Discrepancy between height and weight, B. Discrepancy in height centile and mid-parental centile, and C. Poor height velocity.

Accurate measurements and record keeping are paramount in the assessment of growth in children. Healthcare providers should always refer children to paediatricians when there is discrepancy between height and weight centiles, when height falls two centiles below or above the mid-parental height or when there is evidence of poor growth rate.

A Discrepancy between height and weight – Correct. When there is a discrepancy between height and weight, one needs to rule out endocrine causes of short stature, such as GH deficiency, thyroid disorders and Cushing's syndrome. Children with GH deficiency, Cushing's syndrome or hypothyroidism are usually short and fat. Children with no endocrine cause of obesity are tall and obese.

B Discrepancy in height centile and mid-parental centile – Correct. The greater the distance from the mid-parental height, the higher the possibility that height is abnormal. In cases where one parent is short, one needs to consider conditions inherited by autosomal dominant manner (e.g. skeletal dysplasia) that may have been undetected in the parent.

C Poor height velocity – Correct. Height velocity is calculated by the increase in height over a period of time (at least 6 months, best over one year). The denominator consists of the difference in decimal age.

Key Point

Endocrine problems often present with an obese child who is short for his family.

Q3 Which of the following is/are likely to yield useful information as to the cause of short stature?

The correct answers are A. Birth weight, B. Neonatal hypoglycaemia, C. Neonatal jaundice and D. Floppy episodes during illness.

Past medical history in the majority of children with short stature is unremarkable, but sometimes there are clues present, as described below.

A Birth weight – Correct. Children born SGA who fail to catch up can be offered GH treatment. Additionally, being born SGA might be part of a syndrome. On the other hand, in the context of tall stature, a large birth weight may be associated with an overgrowth syndrome, such as Beckwith-Wiedemann.

B Neonatal hypoglycaemia – Correct. GH deficiency can present in neonatal life with hypoglycaemia.

C Neonatal jaundice – Correct. Pituitary hormone deficiencies can be related to conjugated hyperbilirubinaemia (ACTH, GH) and unconjugated hyperbilirubinaemia (TSH).

D Floppy episodes during illness – Correct. Floppy episodes during illness might suggest episodes of hypoglycaemia.

Key Point

A detailed neonatal history may provide important clues for the identification of the aetiology of short stature.

Q4 Which investigation(s) should be requested for this patient?

The correct answers are A. Thyroid function tests, B. Insulin-like growth factor 1, and C. Coeliac screen.

Baseline tests are helpful to rule out conditions such as growth hormone deficiency, hypothyroidism, coeliac disease and Turner's in girls. Growth hormone is particularly of concern in this case, given that:

i   *The child is short with a disproportionately high weight.*
ii   *There is a history of neonatal hypoglycaemia.*
iii *Loss of height is occurring in the second to third year of life (a growth hormone driven phase).*

Other tests that are likely to be requested are a FBC, ESR, CRP, LFTs, bone profile, urea and electrolytes, and Vitamin D levels. This may identify chronic illness. If a pituitary lesion is suspected, then wider pituitary function tests should be checked, along with an MRI of the pituitary. A bone age X-ray is also helpful to see whether this is delayed or normal. In females, chromosome testing is required to rule out Turner's syndrome.

A Thyroid function tests – Correct. Hypothyroidism can present with short stature in children especially when longstanding.

B Insulin-like growth factor 1 – Correct. GH acts on its receptor on the liver to produce IGF-1. IGF-1 is a surrogate marker for GH action. It acts on the growth plates to promote linear growth.

C Coeliac screen – Correct. Coeliac disease may manifest with poor growth, thus tissue transglutaminase and anti-endomysial antibodies should be checked. Children with coeliac disease are usually underweight but this is not an absolute rule. Gastrointestinal manifestations may not always be present or reported therefore most clinicians include coeliac screening in the first line investigations for short stature.

D IGFBP-3 – Incorrect. GH circulates in a ternary complex with IGF1, IGFBP-3 and ALS (acid labile subunit). IGF1 is related to nutritional status, therefore in underweight children, IGFBP-3 might be helpful. However, it is not routinely checked.

Key Point

Thyroid function tests, IGF-1, coeliac screen, FBC, ESR, CRP, LFTs, bone profile, urea and electrolytes, and vitamin D levels are useful first-line investigations in the assessment of short stature. In girls, a karyotype should always be included to rule out Turner's syndrome.

> **ⓘ IMPORTANT LEARNING POINTS**
>
> - Accurate height and weight measurements should be obtained over multiple time points in all children with suspected weight or height abnormalities. The trend in both of these should be looked at from birth and compared to the mid-parental height.
> - There is more likely to be a pathological cause for short stature if i) growth velocity is poor, ii) height is significantly lower than mid-parental height centile, iii) if there is a discrepancy between height and weight centiles, and iv) if there are clues suggesting chronic illness in the history.
> - GH deficiency might present with transient hypoglycaemia in the neonatal period or infancy and then short stature later on (the second or third year of life).

ANSWER TO CASE 5
An 18-month-old girl presenting with an abdominal mass

Q1 Which of the following might suggest that the abdominal mass may be a tumour?

The correct answers are B. Rapid change in size of abdominal mass, C. Presence of systemic symptoms such as fever, tiredness and weight loss, D. Presence of blood in the urine, and E. Watery diarrhoea and sweating.

Doctors responsible for examining infants and children must be able to recognise the presence of an abdominal mass, as this may indicate underlying malignancy. Some tumours may only present with an abdominal mass (with no other symptoms). History and examination can help discriminate between potential malignant and benign pathology although all need investigation. The age of the child is also important as some tumours are more common in very young children (e.g. neuroblastoma and hepatoblastoma) and others are more common in older children (e.g. germ cell tumours).

A Severe pain – Incorrect. Painful masses are more suggestive of an abscess/abdominal collections, unless the mass has caused abdominal obstruction.

B Rapid change in size of abdominal mass – Correct. Again, a mass that is rapidly increasing in size is more suggestive of malignancy, although it may also represent an abdominal collection/abscess.

C Systemic symptoms such as fever, tiredness and weight loss – Correct. Although systemic symptoms are not always present, fever, tiredness and weight loss may suggest underlying malignancy.

D Presence of blood in the urine – Correct. Children with tumours affecting the renal tract (e.g. Wilms' tumour or rhabdomyosarcoma) may have microscopic or macroscopic haematuria. Microscopic haematuria is only diagnosed

after a urine dipstick test so a negative history is not always helpful.

E Watery diarrhoea and sweating – Correct. The presence of loose, watery stool may be caused by a neuroblastoma that secretes vasoactive intestinal peptide.

♀ Key Point

Abdominal malignancies are often associated with specific features:

- Haematuria – Wilms' tumour
- Hypertension – Wilms' tumour and neuroblastoma
- Urinary obstruction – rhabdomyosarcoma affecting the renal tract/bladder
- Watery stools and sweating – neuroblastoma

Q2 Which two of the following diagnoses are most likely?

The correct answers are B. Neuroblastoma and D. Wilms' tumour.

The presence of a well-defined mass and hypertension is strongly suggestive of cancer, most likely Wilms' tumour or neuroblastoma.

A Constipation – Incorrect. Constipation is common in children and can cause abdominal distension, pain and rarely a left-sided mass (which is sometimes "indentable"). However, there is no history of infrequent stools in this child.

B Neuroblastoma – Correct. Neuroblastoma commonly arises in the adrenal glands, abdomen or thorax. It can present with an isolated abdominal mass, or can be associated with pain, sweating, pallor, diarrhoea and hypertension.

C Intussusception – Incorrect. Intussusception is caused by the "telescoping" of one segment of small bowel into another. It causes acute paroxysms of pain often associated with vomiting. An abdominal mass may be present however the clinical presentation of this child is not consistent with intussusception.

D Wilms' tumour – Correct. Wilms' tumours commonly present with a painless palpable or visible mass in an otherwise well child. Other features include hypertension and haematuria.

E Splenomegaly – Incorrect. It should (but not always) be possible to distinguish between an enlarged spleen and renal mass by palpation. An enlarged spleen, unlike an enlarged kidney, is not ballotable and it is not possible to palpate above it. Splenomegaly, however, is not associated with hypertension.

♀ Key Point

Malignancies may present in a child that is otherwise asymptomatic.

 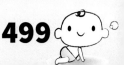

Q3 How would you further investigate this patient?

The correct answers are A. Urinary homovanillic acid (HVA) and vanillylmandelic acid (VMA), C. Abdominal ultrasound, D. Urine dipstick and E. Chest X-ray.

One of the most helpful initial investigations is an abdominal ultrasound scan. Ultrasound can reveal which organ the mass is arising from before being confirmed on more detailed imaging such as CT or MRI.

A Urinary homovanillic acid (HVA) and vanillylmandelic acid (VMA) - Correct. Urine levels of VMA and HVA (metabolites of catecholamines) are elevated in most cases of neuroblastoma.

B Laparoscopy – Incorrect. Laparoscopy is an invasive test which is not indicated, especially before imaging. Following diagnosis of an abdominal tumour on imaging and tumour markers, a biopsy may be planned, but this is not always the case.

C Abdominal ultrasound – Correct. This is the most useful initial investigation to determine the underlying cause. It will reveal which organ the mass originates from and provide diagnostic information before more detailed imaging can be arranged (CT or MRI). Ultrasounds are accessible, do not expose the child to radiation and do not require sedation.

D Urine dipstick – Correct. Some tumours affecting the renal tract may cause microscopic haematuria (including Wilms' tumour and rhabdomyosarcoma).

E Chest X-ray – Correct. A chest X-ray is required to look for the presence of lung metastases.

⚷ Key Point

Differentiating between organomegaly and abdominal tumours can be difficult based on examination findings alone. Investigations including ultrasound and tumour markers provide useful initial diagnostic information.

ⓘ IMPORTANT LEARNING POINTS

- Remember that otherwise well children with an asymptomatic abdominal mass may have a renal tumour.
- The location of the mass and presence of additional symptoms and signs can be useful for distinguishing between different tumour types. However, definitive diagnosis is always based on histology of the tissue.
- Diagnostic work-up includes imaging (ultrasound, CT/MRI), blood tests (FBC, U&E, LFT, clotting and tumour markers) and urine dipstick (for haematuria and urinary catecholamines).
- Suspected abdominal tumours in children should be referred to a paediatric oncology centre for specialist management.

ANSWER TO CASE 6
A 28-day-old baby with projectile vomiting

Q1 Which of the following results is/are likely to be found?

The correct answers are A. Hyponatraemia, C. Hypochloraemia, and E. Acidic urine.

The likely diagnosis in this case is pyloric stenosis. There is projectile, non-bilious vomiting, in a baby that is eager to feed. This classically presents with a hypochloraemic metabolic alkalosis. In this case, initial blood gas showed the following:

Na	133 mmol/L (133-146)
Cl	92 mmol/L (96-111)
K	3.3 mmol/L (3.5-5.5)
HCO$_3$	31.2 mmol/L (22-26)
pH	7.52 (7.35-7.45)

A Hyponatraemia – Correct. The characteristic biochemical change is a hypochloraemic metabolic alkalosis. This is mainly due to loss of gastric fluids (HCl contains hydrogen and chloride), along with smaller amounts of sodium and potassium. Typically, patients with pyloric stenosis are dehydrated with elevated serum pH and bicarbonate levels.

B Hyperkalaemia – Incorrect. There is loss of potassium from gastric fluids.

C Hypochloraemia – Correct. Due to loss of chloride from gastric fluids.

D Metabolic acidosis – Incorrect. A metabolic alkalosis is the typical finding; this is due to loss of the hydrogen ion in lost gastric secretions.

E Acidic urine – Correct. In pyloric stenosis, there is a paradoxical aciduria. Initially, the urine is alkaline to compensate for the metabolic alkalosis. As the condition progresses and dehydration worsens, the kidneys prioritise sodium conservation. As sodium is reabsorbed, potassium and hydrogen ions are excreted (due to the Na/K/H pumps in the kidney) resulting in "paradoxical" aciduria.

⚷ Key Point

The typical biochemical finding in babies with pyloric stenosis is a hypochloraemic metabolic alkalosis with paradoxical aciduria.

Q2 What is/are the most appropriate next step/steps to confirm the diagnosis?

The correct answer is B. Test feed.

If a palpable "olive" mass was found on examination, no further investigation would be needed. If the abdominal examination is normal, a test feed is the first-line investigation to confirm the diagnosis of pyloric stenosis, followed by an ultrasound if the diagnosis is still unclear. Many centres will do an ultrasound regardless, to confirm the diagnosis.

A Ultrasound scan – Incorrect. This is not the first line investigation. However, an ultrasound is often done in most centres to confirm the diagnosis. The following three criteria are needed to confirm pyloric stenosis on ultrasound: i) a pyloric muscle thickness >4 mm, ii) a pyloric muscle length >18 mm, and iii) failure of fluid passage beyond the pylorus despite vigorous gastric peristalsis.

B Test feed – Correct. A test feed should be performed prior to any other investigation. The baby's stomach should be empty. This can be achieved by inserting a nasogastric tube into the stomach and draining/aspirating the contents. The baby is then given a small feed of Dioralyte. At the same time, the examiner places their hand in the epigastrium, below the liver edge. The dextrose feed allows the baby's abdominal muscles to relax and the pylorus to contract. The pyloric tumour can be rolled under the fingers of the palpating hand. Occasionally, gastric peristalsis can be seen during the examination. If the pylorus is palpable, no further tests are needed. If, however, the test feed was not conclusive, an ultrasound scan is recommended. This is often performed by the paediatric surgeon rather than in the referral centre where an ultrasound is a more popular test due to lack of expertise in feeling the abdominal mass after a test feed.

C Contrast study – Incorrect. Contrast is usually reserved for cases where ultrasonography was inconclusive. The "string sign" is the diagnostic term given to the delayed passage of a small amount of contrast through a thin, long pyloric canal.

D CT scan – Incorrect. This test is not indicated for pyloric stenosis, as sufficient diagnostic information can be yielded from ultrasound/contrast studies.

E Endoscopy – Incorrect. This invasive procedure is not required for diagnosis.

Key Point

A positive test feed is sufficient to make the diagnosis of pyloric stenosis. This is usually carried out by the paediatric surgeon or an experienced paediatrician.

Q3 After the diagnosis of "pyloric stenosis with moderate dehydration" has been confirmed, which of the following should you do?

The correct answers are A. Insert a nasogastric tube and B. Calculate and commence maintenance fluids.

A Insert a nasogastric tube – Correct. A fine (6F or 8F) nasogastric tube should be inserted. Gastric contents should actively be aspirated in regular intervals, in the interim the tube should be allowed to freely drain into a bag.

This minimises the risk of aspiration and allows accurate replacement of gastric fluid losses.

B Calculate and commence maintenance fluids – Correct. Meticulous fluid management in babies with pyloric stenosis extremely important. There are three aspects to fluid management: a fluid bolus (as the baby is dehydrated), maintenance fluids (as being kept nil by mouth), and replacement fluids (to replace nasogastric losses).

C Insert a catheter – Incorrect. Insertion of a urinary catheter in infants can be traumatic and a source of infection and should be reserved for very sick babies. Therefore it is not routinely done.

D Allow the baby to formula feed – Incorrect. Babies with pyloric stenosis are very hungry, but it is very important to keep the infant fasting, along with a correctly placed nasogastric tube. Both actions insure an empty stomach and minimise the risk of aspiration.

E Place the baby on the emergency operating list – Incorrect. The standard treatment for pyloric stenosis is surgery, namely a pyloromyotomy. It is, however, very risky to subject a patient with a significant electrolyte/fluid imbalance to general anaesthetic. Therefore, surgery should only be undertaken once fluid and electrolyte imbalances have been resolved and the blood tests have normalised. This can take 48 hours or longer.

Key Point

Electrolyte imbalances in a baby can be dangerous. The first step in managing pyloric stenosis is active fluid resuscitation.

IMPORTANT LEARNING POINTS

- Pyloric stenosis is the commonest surgical cause of non-bilious vomiting in infants.
- It can be diagnosed clinically, or after a test feed. Otherwise, ultrasound is required.
- Pyloromyotomy is the definitive treatment for the condition, but the operation should only be performed once adequate fluid resuscitation has been achieved.

ANSWER TO CASE 7
A 1-day-old boy with desaturations after feeds and drooling

Q1 Which steps/investigations would be useful in the acute management of this baby? Select all that apply.

The correct answers are B. Chest and abdominal X-ray, and C. Nasogastric tube.

The nasogastric tube is inserted first. Typically, there is some resistance in passing it and caution must be taken not to perforate the oesophagus.

C Give 250 mL of colloid fluid – Incorrect. Fluid resuscitation should be with 0.9% sodium chloride, not with colloid, which is no longer recommended for use in children. Colloid may precipitate allergic reactions and is thus avoided.

D Start inotropic support with milrinone – Incorrect. Whilst inotropic support is likely to be needed on PICU, the emphasis in the immediate phase should be on aggressive fluid resuscitation. After a third bolus, dopamine may be considered as it can be given peripherally.

E Recheck his renal function – Incorrect. Sending a sample to the lab may give useful information, but will not influence the acute management.

⚷ Key Point

Recognising and promptly treating shock is of paramount importance. This starts with aggressive fluid resuscitation, and up to 60 mL/kg can be given in the first 30 minutes. Delays can result in children developing decompensated shock (with hypotension), which can be a pre-terminal event.

Q3 Jacob's mother is understandably distressed by his condition. She says he has not eaten all day, and she is worried about his nutrition. She asks if he can have some milk. What is the safest advice you can give in ED?

The correct answer is D. Jacob will not be fed at present, but will receive IV fluids.

In this situation, nutritional needs are secondary to acute resuscitation. The child may require imminent intubation, where an empty stomach is preferable. There may also be some gut ischaemia, as the child is in shock. Therefore, enteral feeding should be avoided.

A Jacob can have some milk via a NG tube – Incorrect. Jacob is clinically shocked, and is likely to have an element of gut ischaemia due to poor perfusion. Therefore, he should not be fed enterally for the acute phase, in order to avoid complications.

B Jacob will have TPN started by NG tube – Incorrect. TPN is administered via a central line.

C Jacob will have TPN started via a central line in ED – Incorrect. For TPN, Jacob would need to have a dedicated line with full aseptic precautions. It should therefore be started in a controlled fashion, with full aseptic precautions taken, rather than in the acute resuscitation phase. TPN is also potentially toxic, so a decision as to whether it is needed should be made once the likely disease course is noted.

D Jacob will not be fed at present, but will receive IV fluids – Correct. Jacob should not be fed enterally during the acute phase, in order to avoid complications. He will receive intravenous fluids (usually 0.9% sodium chloride with 5% dextrose) in order to maintain hydration and adequate blood glucose concentration.

E A dietician will need to be consulted in ED before making a decision about feeding enterally – Incorrect. This decision making skill should be within the doctor's skill set.

⚷ Key Point

Enteral feeding is preferred in the stable patient. In the shocked patient, however, it can result in adverse effects in the setting of gut tissue ischaemia due to poor perfusion.

ⓘ IMPORTANT LEARNING POINTS

- Resuscitation should follow an ABCDE approach.
- Resuscitation requires careful management of oxygenation and ventilation. These are manipulated slightly differently on the ventilator: oxygenation predominantly by changing mean airway pressure/FiO_2, and ventilation predominantly by changing peak inspiratory pressure and respiratory rate.
- In severe sepsis, it is important to aggressively fluid resuscitate early, with up to three fluid boluses required in the first 30 minutes. Dopamine can be started peripherally if needed.
- Acutely, nutritional needs come secondary to managing shock. Therefore patients should be made NBM in severe sepsis, with consideration of TPN if enteral feeding is delayed for a prolonged period.

ANSWER TO CASE 9
A 3-day-old baby presenting with weak femoral pulses

Q1 Which of the following investigations are essential in the assessment of this baby?

The correct answers are A. Baseline bloods including CRP, blood cultures, and blood gas, B. Blood glucose, C. Four-limb BP, D. Echocardiogram, and E. Electrocardiogram.

When presented with an unwell infant, consider common and serious differential diagnoses. In this case, the most likely differential diagnoses are sepsis or cardiac issues, although metabolic disorders can also present this way. Coarctation of the aorta is the most likely diagnosis. This is a narrowing in the descending aorta, which restricts the volume of oxygenated blood circulated to the body. This narrowing may cause back pressure through the heart and pulmonary circulation resulting in heart failure. These symptoms occasionally occur after 48 hours of life due to closure of the ductus arteriosus. Prior to the closure, the patent duct provided an additional route through which blood could escape, thus preventing the symptoms of heart failure. Other investigations must be undertaken as soon as possible. If a provisional diagnosis of "duct dependent cyanotic heart disease" is suspected, the management should be intubation, treatment with prostaglandin infusion and urgent transfer to a cardiac unit.

A Baseline bloods including CRP, blood cultures, and blood gas – Correct. The blood gas may show a metabolic acidosis due to hypoperfusion. Sepsis should be strongly suspected in any neonate that acutely deteriorates; therefore, broad spectrum antibiotics should be started.

B Blood glucose – Correct. Hypoglycaemia can exacerbate any existing problems and can in itself be fatal, if left untreated.

C Four-limb BP – Correct. Classically, when measuring four-limb BP (exactly as it sounds – measuring the BP in both arms and both legs) if an infant has coarctation, their upper limbs measure BP at least 20 mmHg greater than the lower limbs. This is again due to the increased pressure proximal to the narrowing of the aorta. Although a very valuable investigation if positive, this investigation is not a gold standard for diagnosis for coarctation of the aorta because of a high rate of false negatives.

D Echocardiogram – Correct. Though it is unlikely that an echocardiogram can be performed acutely in most peripheral hospitals, it will give a definitive diagnosis.

E Electrocardiogram – Correct. Cardiac monitoring and ECG may be useful investigations. They may show right ventricular hypertrophy. As the afterload increases in the systemic circulation, there is shunting across the foramen ovale from the left atrium to right atrium. This increases volume in the pulmonary circulation, and hence leads to right ventricular hypertrophy.

⚲ Key Point

Although a baby might be born with a coarctation, they often deteriorate around day three of life. This is due to a ductus arteriosus being patent before this, and allowing blood to shunt around the narrowing.

Q2 Your team makes a diagnosis of coarctation of the aorta. Given this presentation, which two of the following options would you add to your management in addition to the general approach to an acutely unwell patient?

The correct answers are A. Prostaglandin infusion, and C. Antibiotics in line with trust guidance on neonatal sepsis.

The acute deterioration implies a trigger that has worsened the underlying coarctation. This is most likely due to closure of the ductus arteriosus (given that it is on day three), but it may also be due to a possible infection. Therefore both these possibilities need to be covered.

A Prostaglandin infusion – Correct. This infant has presented on day three of life with symptoms suggestive of heart failure. This indicates that the duct closure has contributed to the symptoms. In order to alleviate these symptoms, it is reasonable to attempt to re-open the duct with a prostaglandin infusion. This treatment is not without risk, and a major common side effect is apnoea. Prostaglandin infusion should only be commenced at the request of a senior registrar or consultant and on discussion with a tertiary cardiology centre.

B DC cardioversion – Incorrect. There is no indication for DC cardioversion in this patient. He is conscious and has a regular HR.

C Antibiotics in line with trust guidance on neonatal sepsis – Correct. Neonatal sepsis can present in a myriad of different ways, and although we assume that this infant's heart failure is a result of his coarctation, it could also be sepsis. It is therefore prudent to take blood cultures and commence the baby on broad spectrum antibiotics as per local guidelines.

D Atropine – Incorrect. Atropine is a drug which speeds up conduction through the AV node within the heart thus increasing HR. It is not indicated in this scenario.

E Indomethacin infusion – Incorrect. Indomethacin is a cyclooxygenase inhibitor which is used to close a patent ductus arteriosus in premature infants. It does this by inhibiting prostaglandin synthesis.

⚲ Key Point

Do not forget that in any acutely unwell neonate, it is generally prudent to assume there may be an infection. Take blood cultures and commence intravenous antibiotics.

Q3 A medical student in the paediatric department asks for tips on feeling for pulses during the standard neonatal examination. Which of the following statements is correct?

The correct answer is A. Femoral pulses can be difficult to feel and if they are unsure, they should ask a senior to review the baby.

A Femoral pulses can be difficult to feel and if they are unsure, they should ask a senior to review the baby – Correct. Femoral pulse palpation in neonates is a simple screening test for coarctation of the aorta. It should be incorporated into every routine infant examination. It can, however, be very difficult to feel femoral pulses, especially in a crying baby. Sometimes, it can take a few moments to isolate where the femoral pulses are and palpate them adequately; even experienced clinicians often take a minute or so to ensure that this is done. Consider gently holding the baby's leg straight and exerting gentle pressure over the inguinal region with the index finger.

B If the perfusion, colour and tone of the lower limbs is normal, palpation of the femoral pulses is not needed – Incorrect.

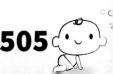

This is false as often babies will be able to perfuse their lower limbs despite a coarctation.

C Weak and low volume femoral pulses are pathognomonic for coarctation of the aorta – Incorrect. Although palpation of femoral pulses is a useful screening examination for coarctation, weak pulses do not always demonstrate a coarctation. An important differential is that of shock, as the definition of shock is poor perfusion, which would mean the pulse volume is low.

D It is best to feel for femoral pulses at the same time as assessing hip stability to save time – Incorrect. Try to concentrate on one aspect of the examination at a time to ensure that nothing is missed.

E When palpation of the pulses is impossible, often the pulse can be heard when the femoral area is auscultated with the bell of a stethoscope – Incorrect. The femoral pulses should not be audible. If the femoral artery can be auscultated, it would imply turbulent blood flow in that area, which could indicate other pathology.

⚷ Key Point

Coarctation of the aorta is a potentially fatal condition if not adequately managed. Newborn examinations are a vital time in which the diagnosis can be suspected, so always carefully check for femoral pulses.

Q4 *Four years later, you are a registrar in clinic and the same child comes to see you, having had corrective surgery. He is asymptomatic and thriving. What residual features would you expect to be present?*

The correct answer is C. Hypertension.

A Absent femoral pulses – Incorrect. Following repair of coarctation, there will no longer be a narrowing of the descending aorta and therefore no reason to find absent femoral pulses.

B Brachio-femoral delay – Incorrect. The brachio-femoral delay is caused by the position of the narrowing in the descending aorta (after the branches of the brachiocephalic, common carotid and subclavian arteries), resulting in higher pressure and volume of blood being delivered to the upper limbs. When the narrowing has gone, this issue will no longer exist.

C Hypertension – Correct. Several studies have investigated the presence of hypertension in children and young adults following successful repair of coarctation in infancy. The results show that hypertension remains despite adequate repair. It is hypothesised that this is due to reduced arterial reactivity, leading to a higher pressure of blood flow in order to gain vessel response.

D Cyanosis – Incorrect. Coarctation of the aorta is an acyanotic heart condition, and any signs of cyanosis should be thoroughly investigated as this would indicate significant hypoxia. This is not a recognised complication of coarctation repair.

E Rib notching on X-ray – Incorrect. Rib notching is an X-ray finding which becomes present in children 4 to 12-years-old with an untreated coarctation. It is caused by erosion of the posterior surface of the ribs by large collateral vessels which have developed to support the systemic circulation. In a neonate, these collaterals have not yet developed, and it takes time for these collaterals to alter the contours of the ribs. When a coarctation is treated early, large collateral vessels do not have the time to form.

⚷ Key Point

Patients with coarctation and other congenital heart disease may have lifelong complications, despite corrective treatment.

ⓘ IMPORTANT LEARNING POINTS

- It is important to assess femoral pulses on newborn examination, as this is an opportunity to diagnose coarctation of the aorta before it becomes symptomatic.
- Coarctation of the aorta typically presents on day three of life, but can occur anytime in the first two weeks of life, as the ductus arteriosus may close later. Prostaglandin infusions keep the duct open and can be lifesaving.
- Even in treated cases of coarctation, there may be long-term complications such as hypertension.

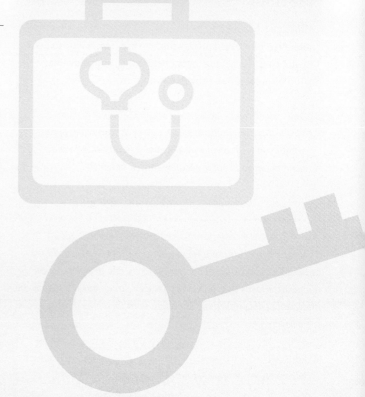

3.01
HISTORY TAKING

ZESHAN QURESHI, CHRISTOPHER HARRIS AND MICHAEL MALLEY

CONTENTS

INTRODUCTION

When approaching a potentially unwell child, it is important to remember that children are not just small adults. Bear in mind the following:

› The child's parents, relatives or carers may not have the whole story, especially if the child has been in someone else's care, so a collateral history may be necessary.

› The parents' "sixth sense" about their child's health should always be taken seriously. Equally, parents may underestimate the seriousness of their child's condition.

› Younger children may not be able to give any history, or the history given may be misleading.

› All children, but particularly younger infants, may have underlying congenital abnormalities that have remained undetected until presentation in extremis.

› Children can compensate physiologically for severe illness. As such, signs of deterioration may not be evident until late in the illness course.

› Children are dependent on adult carers for many things, particularly in early life. This can lead to opportunities for abuse, which can be easily missed if not specifically assessed.

› Decisions made during childhood with regards to health can impact on all areas of development.

› Pay special attention to putting the child at ease. The doctor should make a point of introducing themselves to the child individually, and perhaps let them lead introductions to the rest of the family. Toys are widely available in paediatric healthcare settings and they can be used effectively to relax younger children.

PREPARATION

Usually, there will be time to prepare before seeing a child. During this time, review any pre-existing information. This may include: ambulance triage notes, nursing triage notes, referral letters, previous clinic letters, hospital discharge letters and current hospital notes. Often, allergies or social concerns are automatically highlighted on hospital computer notes. There may also be a handover from a colleague: don't be afraid to ask them questions to clear uncertainty. Blood tests and imaging may have been requested, or recent investigation results may be available. This will give an initial impression of the key issues and the parent/patient agenda before going into the consultation.

Start by greeting the parents and child. Let them know who you are and why you are seeing them.

Throughout the consultation:

1 Be confident, using good eye contact and open body language.
2 Be empathetic, ensuring all those in the room are at ease.
3 Ensure that the parents and child understand what is happening in the consultation. Give them time to speak, and explore their feelings with regard to each pertinent issue.
4 Avoid medical jargon. Explain any unfamiliar words or concepts in simple terms.

PRESENTING COMPLAINT

History-taking should begin with open questions. It is worthwhile allowing the child or family member to explain the problem in their own words. Resist the temptation to intervene with questions too quickly. Once they have finished, both open and closed questions can be used to clarify information. What is the problem? How long has it been going on? Has the child been well between symptoms? How has this problem affected the child's development, schooling and home life?

Focus on the main symptoms. Mnemonics can be helpful to explore symptoms. Examples of those commonly used are shown in *Box 1*.

Think about relevant associated symptoms to the presenting complaint that may help "clinch" the diagnosis. It may be easier to think in terms of "boxes", or a group of questions which immediately elucidate particular presenting complaints. Examples are shown in *Table 1*.

Box 1: Helpful mnemonics for history taking

SOCRATES	ODPARA	P3MAFTOSA
Site.	Onset.	Presenting complaint.
Onset.	Duration.	Past medical history.
Character.	Progression of the main presenting	Personal history i.e. feeding/growth/
Radiation.	complaint.	development/birth history.
Associated features.	Aggravating factors.	Medicines.
Timing.	Relieving factors.	Allergies.
Exacerbating and alleviating factors.	Additional symptoms.	Family history.
Severity.		Travel history.
		Other factors.
		Social factors.
		Alleviating/relieving factors.

TABLE 1: Common symptoms to consider in history taking

Symptom	Key Points	Differential Diagnoses
Fever.	• Cough/coryza. • Difficulty breathing. • Vomiting/diarrhoea. • Urinary symptoms. • Rigors. • Rashes. • Joint pain/inflammation. • Signs of meningism, including infectious contacts. • Foreign travel.	• Upper respiratory tract infection (URTI). • Pneumonia/bronchiolitis. • Gastroenteritis. • Appendicitis. • Urinary tract infection (UTI). • Otitis media. • Septic arthritis/osteomyelitis. • Soft tissue infection, e.g. abscess, cellulitis. • Meningitis/encephalitis.
Vomiting.	• Timing (as related to feeds, or in early morning). • Substance vomited (bilious or bloody). • Diarrhoea. • Abdominal pain. • Obstructive symptoms. • Fever. • Urinary symptoms. • Signs of meningism. • Symptoms of diabetic ketoacidosis (DKA). • Foreign travel or infectious contacts. • Weight loss.	• Gastroenteritis. • Appendicitis. • Obstruction, e.g. volvulus, adhesions, malrotation, pyloric stenosis in neonates. • UTI. • Meningitis. • DKA. • Raised intracranial pressure (ICP).

Continued

TABLE 1: *Continued*

Symptom	Key Points	Differential Diagnoses
Wheeze.	• Onset and progress of wheeze. • Treatment at home. • Trigger. • Personal or family history of atopy. • Previous admissions and severity. • Effect on life (e.g. missing school).	• Asthma. • Bronchiolitis. • Viral induced wheeze. • Foreign body inhalation. • Anaphylaxis. • Gastro-oesophageal reflux. • Cardiac failure.
Faltering growth.	• Weight/height trajectory. Food in: • Diet content. • Diet volume. • Liquid intake. Food out: • Diarrhoea (including steatorrhoea). • Vomiting. • Reflux symptoms. Increased metabolic requirements: • Chronic illnesses. • Malignancy. Other factors: • Low socio-economic status or markers of neglect.	Broad range of differentials including: • Malabsorption. e.g. coeliac disease, inflammatory bowel disease (IBD), cystic fibrosis (CF), chronic liver disease, chronic diarrhoea/vomiting. • Perinatal factors. e.g. intrauterine growth restriction (IUGR), prematurity. • Endocrine. e.g. growth hormone deficiency, diabetes, thyroid disorders. • Genetic. e.g. Turner syndrome, achondroplasia, Russell-Silver syndrome. • Increased metabolic requirements. e.g. recurrent infections, cardiac disease. • Non-organic. e.g. neglect/child abuse, inappropriate diet.
Rash.	• Distribution. • First noticed when and where. • Itchy/non-itchy. • Blanching/non-blanching. • Type of lesion – macule/papule/vesicle/blister/ purpura. • Mucosal involvement. • Atopic history, allergic contacts. • Associated symptoms e.g. fever, joint pains, abdominal pain, bleeding symptoms.	Macular/papular rashes: • Viral rash (including measles/rubella). • Sandpaper rash = Streptococcal infection. • "Salmon pink" rash = Juvenile idiopathic arthritis (JIA). • Eczema. • Contact dermatitis. Vesicles: • Chickenpox/shingles. • HSV (think infection of underlying eczema: eczema herpeticum). Purpura: • Meningococcal sepsis. • Henoch-Schönlein purpura (HSP). • Idiopathic thrombocytopenic purpura (ITP). Wheal and flare: • Allergy. • Viral urticaria. Primary skin infection: • Cellulitis. • Hand-foot-and-mouth disease. • Impetigo. • Ringworm.
Seizure.	Think chronologically: • What happened before the seizure: aura, trauma, fever? • What happened during the seizure: absence, focal, generalised, tonic/clonic, tongue biting, incontinence? • Duration of seizure. • Medications given. • What happened after the seizure: post-ictal phase? • Previous seizures. • Red flag symptoms: weight loss, focal neurology, persistent reduced GCS post seizure, seizure >15 minutes duration, non-blanching rash or other signs of meningism, past history of trauma.	• Epileptiform seizure. • Febrile convulsion. • Non-epileptiform or pseudo-seizure. • Hypoglycaemia. • Electrolyte imbalance. • Infection. e.g. meningitis/encephalitis. • Malignancy. • Trauma/elevated intracranial pressure (ICP).
Limp.	• Pain. • Recent viral symptoms. • Fever. • Trauma. • Birth history (especially breech delivery). • Elevated BMI (particularly in teenagers).	Think in terms of age: All ages: • Septic arthritis. • Osteomyelitis. • Trauma or physical abuse. • Malignancies (e.g. leukaemia).

Continued

509

TABLE 1: *Continued*		
Symptom	**Key Points**	**Differential Diagnoses**
	• Any systemic symptoms e.g. diarrhoea, rashes, extra-articular manifestations of JIA. • Signs of malignancy, particularly haematological. Think: i) general sign, e.g. weight loss/malaise/growth delay; ii) red cell lineage, e.g. signs of anaemia; iii) white cell lineage, e.g. recurrent infections and iv) platelet lineage, e.g. bleeding/bruising). • Positive family history.	Under 5 years: • Developmental dysplasia of the hip. • Transient synovitis. • Haemophilia. 5–12 years: • Perthe's disease. • Transient synovitis. • IBD/rheumatological disease. >12 years: • Slipped upper femoral epiphysis. • Juvenile idiopathic arthritis. • Other rheumatological causes.
Blood in urine.	• Painful or painless. • Microscopic or macroscopic (frank). • Isolated or with proteinuria. • Infective symptoms e.g. fever, dysuria, frequency. • Abdominal pain. • Oedema/signs of nephrotic involvement. • Trauma. • Recent viral infections. • Other health concerns: HIV infection, hepatitis B infection, diabetes, haemoglobinopathy. • Menstrual cycle. • Signs of bleeding elsewhere. • Family history of renal disease.	Non-haematuria causes: • PV bleeding/menstruation. • Oxalate crystals in babies. • Myoglobinuria. Non-glomerular causes: • UTI. • Renal vein thrombosis. • Malignancy. • Renal stones. Glomerulonephritis: • Post-infectious glomerulonephritis. • IgA nephropathy. • HSP • Systemic lupus erythematosus (SLE).
Possible Non-Accidental Injury.	• Establish mechanism of injury and any complications. • Timing of injury and delay in presentation. • Witnesses of the injury. • Previous hospital visits. • Any other injuries. • Detailed social history including household members, carers. • Social worker involvement.	• Accidental injury (including pathological fractures, e.g. with osteogenesis imperfecta). • Non-accidental injury.

Be quantitative. As children often cannot report subjective things themselves, it is important to get objective evidence. In acute histories, ask how many times they have passed urine in the last 24 hours and establish their fluid intake, whether in bottles, cups or breastfeeds. Quantify the episodes of vomiting and diarrhoea in a similar manner.

PAST MEDICAL HISTORY

The past medical history not only gives important hints to the current diagnosis but also to the risk of future deterioration. For example, an infant who spent three months ventilated on the neonatal unit and is now presenting with wheeze is at high risk of rapid deterioration. Most children have no chronic illnesses, and those that do usually only have one condition to enquire about. Take a detailed history of each underlying disease. Key questions to ask in common chronic conditions are shown in *Table 2*. In general, for any chronic disease find out:

› Age at diagnosis.
› Current medication, and healthcare professionals involved in care.
› Hospital admissions associated with the disease, and treatment received.
› Specific treatment plans in place (e.g. children with

metabolic disorders usually have an algorithm in place for how they need to be managed in the event of deterioration).
› Progression of illness, i.e. stable/worsening/getting better.
› Impact of disease on the child's life.

Also ask about any operations. Other screening questions may include whether the child ever sees their primary care physician, and how often they have visited the emergency department (ED).

BIRTH HISTORY

At a minimum, ask the gestation of the pregnancy, any major complications in pregnancy or birth and whether the child was admitted to a neonatal unit. Note that birth history is less important in a clinically well child more than 2-years-old. Parents of neonates who had a prolonged stay in the neonatal unit are likely to keep a copy of their discharge letter. Note:

› Gestation at birth and any antenatal concerns (including anomalies on scans).
› Mode of delivery and indications.
› Need for resuscitation and initial APGAR scores (if known).
› Birth weight/centile, and whether this remained stable, deteriorated or improved.

TABLE 2: Examples of disease specific questions to ask	
Conditions	Key details
Asthma.	• Age at diagnosis, current management, recent investigations (including peak flow) and whether the disease is stable/worsening/improving. • Number and severity of hospital admissions (including use of intravenous therapy, and intensive care admissions). • Frequency of steroid treatment for acute exacerbations. • Frequency of salbutamol inhaler usage when well. • Triggers. e.g. household smoking. • Other impacts of the disease, e.g. poor exercise tolerance, weight loss.
Inflammatory bowel disease.	• Age at diagnosis and subtype of disease, including any endoscopy or imaging results. Recent investigations, current management and whether the disease is stable/worsening/improving. • Number and severity of acute exacerbations, including hospital admissions and treatment. • Other impacts of the disease, e.g. faltering growth.
Type 1 diabetes.	• Age at diagnosis and current management. • Quality of glycaemic control, including most recent HBA1c result. • Frequency of hypoglycaemic or hyperglycaemic episodes, including hospital admissions and diabetic ketoacidosis. • Other impacts of the disease, e.g. faltering growth.
Epilepsy.	• Age at diagnosis, current management and compliance. • Frequency/type of seizures, including hospital admissions and in-patient treatment. • Other impacts of the disease, e.g. side effects of medication.
Cerebral Palsy.	• Level of functionality, including any carers required and any assisted feeding. • Details of recent hospital admissions, and any long-term medications. • Ceiling of care, if in place.

➤ Any respiratory support required, including number of days with each treatment (e.g. intubated for five days).

➤ Significant diagnosis whilst an inpatient, e.g. group B streptococcus, necrotising enterocolitis.

➤ Fitness at discharge, including feeding or oxygen support.

➤ Medications given at discharge.

FEEDING HISTORY

Feeding history is most relevant to neonates. It is important to enquire whether they are breast fed or bottle fed, how often they feed and how much they consume. Other indicators of feeding quality are weight gain and number of wet nappies. In older children, going off food is relevant, but it is much more important to ensure they have adequate oral intake throughout illness (at least 50% of normal consumption).

DEVELOPMENTAL HISTORY

Simple screening questions may include: Do you have any concerns about your child's development? Has anyone else mentioned concerns? How does your child get on at school? How does he/she compare to his siblings? A child presenting with faltering growth requires a detailed assessment of all four developmental domains (gross motor, fine motor, vision/hearing and social/self-care). If presenting with a simple unrelated condition like a viral infection, a much briefer history is acceptable.

DRUG HISTORY AND IMMUNISATIONS

When taking a drug history, include doses and frequencies. Ask the parent if they have a list of their child's medications with them. Specifically inquire about allergies, including non-drug allergies and the nature of the allergic reaction. Check that the child is up-to-date with immunisations. Make note of over-the-counter medications and vitamin supplements. Compliance is also important, particularly with inhalers for asthma and insulin for diabetes, so ask if there are any issues with taking prescribed medications.

FAMILY HISTORY

Relevant questions include: *Do any illnesses run in the family? Is there any history of childhood death or recurrent miscarriage in the family?* It is also important to assess for consanguinity, and a polite way to ask this is: *Were the parents related before marriage?* Genetic conditions may present with sudden infant death or miscarriage that may go undiagnosed even at post mortem. This history should prompt further screening. Chronic illness in the family requiring medication can increase the possibility of accidental ingestion of medications by inquisitive young children or purposeful overdose by older children.

SOCIAL AND TRAVEL HISTORY

Social history provides insight into the child's normal day-to-day life. Relevant questions include: Who stays with the child? Who was looking after the child when they became unwell? Are any of those who live at the same address unwell? Are there any problems with damp or pests? Are there smokers in the household? Travel history is particularly relevant if the child is presenting with infective symptoms. The key question is: *Has the child travelled abroad recently?*

Do not feel awkward asking sensitively about a child's home situation. At a minimum, find out who lives with the child, and who else, if anyone, is involved in their care (e.g. au pairs, partners, grandparents). Ask about their progress in school. Ask about social services involvement. It can be useful to normalise this question and phrase this as: *This is a question we have to ask to everyone. Have you or Jamie ever had any help from social services or had a named social worker?* If the answer is yes, then explore the nature of these social concerns.

SYSTEMS REVIEW

Ask general questions about health, covering neurology (headaches, drowsiness, fits), cardiology (palpations, chest pain, dizzy episodes), gastrointestinal (vomiting, bowel movements, abdominal pain, weight loss), respiratory (wheeze, breathlessness, chest pain), skin (rashes), orthopaedics/rheumatology (joint/bone pain), genitourinary (pain on urination, increased urinary frequency, bed wetting), haematology (bruising, bleeding). This can be brief in a focused history.

CONCLUDING

Make sure the main ideas, concerns and expectations of the parent/child have been elicited: *Is there anything you think I've missed or anything you are particularly concerned about? Do you have any questions for me at the moment?*

To end, summarise the key points and give the parent/child an idea of what to expect now. This can be brief; for example: *So, just to summarise, Jamie has had three previous admissions with exacerbations of Crohn's disease and has presented today with diarrhoea and vomiting over the last 12 hours. You are worried he might have another exacerbation. I'll just examine Jamie and then we can discuss what is going on in more detail.*

PRESENTING YOUR FINDINGS

The history may be presented to a senior clinician for review, to a colleague at

handover, or to an examiner during an assessment. It is helpful to open with a summary of the history and then detail the important positive and negative findings of the history. After presenting the history, suggest your next steps, i.e. examination, investigations and initial therapy. For example:

Snapshot

"Alex is a 7-year-old boy, who presented with mum to ED this afternoon. He has a 24 hour history of difficulty in breathing, consistent with a mild-to-moderate exacerbation of asthma, requiring admission."

Current Presentation

"Alex has had a cough for two days and has developed progressive difficulty in breathing over the last 24 hours. He has a low grade temperature and a dry cough. He has been using two puffs of his salbutamol inhaler every four hours without improvement, but is still speaking in complete sentences."

Background about Asthma

"Alex is a known asthmatic, diagnosed at 3-years-old, and is on regular beclomethasone and PRN salbutamol. He has had three hospital admissions this year and four courses of oral steroids for acute exacerbations. Two years ago, he was admitted to the paediatric intensive care unit (PICU) for three days, receiving IV salbutamol, and being intubated. His known triggers are pet dander and URTI. He also has a history of eczema. His normal peak flow reading is around 300 L/min. He misses about two days of school per month due to his asthma."

Additional Background Information

"Alex was born at term without complication and there have been no concerns about his growth and development. He takes no other medications, has no allergies and his immunisations are up-to-date. Alex's mother has asthma and his father has hay fever. Alex lives in a flat with his parents and his 5-year-old brother. There are no

smokers in the house and the family have never had any involvement with social services."

Summary and Plan

"In summary, Alex is a 7-year-old boy presenting with a likely acute exacerbation of his asthma.

I would like to proceed to examine Alex, review his observation chart, perform a peak flow measurement and consider oral steroid/salbutamol therapy."

CLINICAL CASES

CASE 1
A 2-day-old baby presenting with jaundice

Doctor Briefing

You are asked to see Jamie, a 2-day-old baby on the postnatal ward who is jaundiced. Jamie is mum's first baby and she has had trouble establishing feeding. Please take a history from his mother, with a view to making a diagnosis.

Mother (actress) Briefing

Jamie is your first baby, and you delivered five days ago at Queen Hospital. The baby was born at 36 weeks, with a birth weight of 2300 g, by normal vaginal delivery, and cried at delivery. You had one temperature of 38.2°C during labour and one dose of antibiotics just before delivery. The pregnancy was fine from your perspective: all your scans and blood tests were normal. Your blood group is A+.

You have had difficulty establishing feeding and don't feel like Jamie has had a good feed yet, despite trying every two to three hours. In retrospect, you think the jaundice started yesterday on day 1 of life. You are in a stable relationship with your husband and are hoping to go home today.

You are concerned because you don't know what is causing the jaundice and because you are worried that you might have to bottle feed your baby if he doesn't take to the breast. If specifically asked, Jamie's dad has alpha-1-antitrypsin deficiency.

Assessment

For all scenarios:

› Introduction.

› Ask a mixture of open and closed questions.

› Ensure understanding throughout.

› Summarise your findings to the parents, and give them an opportunity to raise any other issues.

History of Presenting Complaint (Jaundice and Poor Feeding)

Question	Justification	Answer	Evolving thought process
When did you first notice the jaundice?	Jaundice on day 1 of life is more worrying and may relate to infection/haemolysis.	"Day 1."	A bit more worried, since early onset.
How are you feeding Jamie, how often, and how is that going? Is Jamie latching on to the breast? How long is each feed?	Dehydration worsens jaundice, and it is therefore important to optimise feeding.	"Breastfeeding 2–3 hourly, but not been latching on properly, and not lasting for more than a few minutes."	Poor feeding may be significantly contributing to this jaundice. Alternatively, the feeding may be poor as the child has an infection which has precipitated the jaundice.
Has the baby passed any wet and dirty nappies? If so, how many?	Wet nappies serve as marker of hydration status. Failure to pass meconium can indicate gastrointestinal obstruction.	"There has been one dirty nappy, and two mildly wet nappies."	
Has the baby been drowsy, had any funny movements or felt floppy?	May potentially be a result of dehydration, or if the jaundice levels are very high, may suggest the baby is at risk of kernicterus.	"No."	
How has Jamie's breathing been? Has he had any temperatures?	Jaundice may relate to an infection. Although remember there may be an infection without a temperature.	"Breathing is fine, and there have been no temperatures."	Sounds like the baby is systemically well.
Has Jamie had any other problems between delivery and now, other than the feeding and jaundice?	Screening for other problems that may be relevant.	"No."	

Obstetric and Birth History

Question	Justification	Answer	Evolving thought process
How was the pregnancy? Were there any problems on the scans? What is your blood group?	Antenatal diagnosis may be helpful. Maternal blood group will determine the risk of haemolytic blood disorders (O- is high risk).	"All scans were normal. Blood group is A+."	No additional concerns identified. There is a potential set up for ABO incompatibility, which may explain the jaundice. Will need to check the baby's blood group and check a direct antigen test (DAT).
How many weeks pregnant were you when Jamie was delivered? Was it a vaginal delivery, forceps or caesarean? Did he cry straight away or need help?	Premature babies are more vulnerable to jaundice. Forceps may result in cephalohaematoma that can give rise to jaundice. A baby requiring resuscitation may have an infection.	"Jamie was born at 36 weeks, by normal vaginal delivery, and cried straight away."	Prematurity may be contributing to the jaundice.
What was the birth weight?	Low birth weight infants are more likely to become jaundiced and to have difficultly feeding.	"2300g."	Low birth weight may be contributing to the jaundice.
Were any issues identified on the newborn baby check?	General screen for problems. The presence of jaundice is usually checked for on the baby check.	"No."	No additional concerns.
How long was it between the rupture of your membranes and delivery? Did you have any temperatures during labour? Were you given antibiotics during labour? Do you know if you've had a positive test for the bug Group B strep?	These are all risk factors for infection, which is particularly important in day 1 jaundice.	"Delivered within two hours of membrane rupture. One temperature of 38.2°C during labour, given one dose of antibiotics, just before delivery, and mum has never had a positive group B strep test."	Getting more concerned about possible infection, as we have day 1 jaundice, prematurity, and a temperature during labour (with inadequate antibiotics). As a result, this baby will need antibiotics.

Continued

Question	Justification	Answer	Evolving thought process
Do you have any other children? Any health problems with them now or in the past?	Group B strep infection in a previous child increases risk in subsequent births.	"First child."	Being a first time Mum may contribute to difficulty establishing feeding. Mum also likely to be particularly sensitive.
Do you (or dad) have any health problems that you are aware of?	Many causes of jaundice are hereditary, e.g. hereditary spherocytosis or alpha-1-antitrypsin deficiency.	"Dad has alpha-1-antitrypsin deficiency."	Alpha-1-antitrypsin deficiency is a cause of jaundice. It may be helpful to screen the child for this, particularly if the jaundice is prolonged or if mum is a carrier as well.

Drug History

Question	Justification	Answer	Evolving thought process
Is Jamie on any medication? Has he had Vitamin K? Does he have any allergies?	Unlikely to be on any medications, but useful to know as may have been started on antibiotics.	"No medications, no allergies, and has had one vitamin K injection."	No new concerns identified.

Social History

Question	Justification	Answer	Evolving thought process
Who is currently at home? Does Jamie have a social worker? Is dad around?	Find out if there are any social concerns or if wider support is needed.	"I live with Jamie's dad, and we are in a stable relationship. No social worker involved."	No social concerns at present.

Developmental history and immunisation history are not relevant in a baby at 2-days-old, as they are yet to meet the first milestone for either. It is appropriate to check the newborn examination record to see if any problems were identified.

Concluding

Question	Justification	Answer	Evolving thought process
Is there anything that I've missed, or anything that you are particularly concerned about? Do you have any questions for me at the moment?	May identify useful information that has been missed. Will also help framing communication with the mother.	"I'm really keen to breastfeed, but I am afraid it's failing. I am also worried that we don't know what has caused the jaundice."	Worth asking a breastfeeding midwife to give support. Need to take time to explain possible causes of jaundice to mum.

🔍 PRESENTING YOUR FINDINGS

Jamie is a 36 week 2300 g baby on day 2 of life, who has presented with jaundice beginning on day 1.

Jamie was born by normal vaginal delivery and required no resuscitation. Mum had one temperature during labour, with inadequate antibiotic cover. Antenatal scans are normal, and mum has blood type A+. This is mum's first baby and she is still establishing breastfeeding. Jamie has passed two mildly wet nappies today. Dad has alpha-1-antitrypsin deficiency. There are no social concerns.

My differential diagnosis is jaundice secondary to infection, or blood group incompatibility, exacerbated by prematurity and poor feeding.

I am going to cannulate Jamie, and then check serum bilirubin (SBR), full blood count (FBC), urea and electrolytes (U&Es), C-reactive protein (CRP) and blood cultures. I will start benzylpenicillin and gentamicin, and check the baby's blood group and DAT. I will make a decision about phototherapy when the SBR comes back, and if the CRP is high, I will consider a lumbar puncture. Blood sugars need to be monitored, and if breastfeeding cannot be established after further support, we will need start top-up feeds, either formula or expressed breast milk, at 90mL/kg/day.

CASE 2
A 6-week-old baby with a temperature

Doctor Briefing

You are asked to see Fred, a 6-week-old baby in the ED, who had a temperature at home of 39°C. He is otherwise well, but mum wants him checked just to be safe. Please take a history from his mother, with a view to making a diagnosis.

Mother (actress) Briefing

Jamie is your second baby, and you delivered six weeks ago at King's Hospital. The baby was born at 38 weeks, with a birth weight of 4 kg, by an elective C-section (due to breech presentation) and cried at delivery. You had one raised temperature of 39°C during labour and were given two doses of antibiotics. The pregnancy was fine from your perspective: all your scans and blood tests were normal.

Fred is feeding well, every three hours on the breast, for 15 minutes a time. He is putting on a good amount of weight, and is tracking the 50th centile on the growth chart.

You are in a stable relationship with your husband and are expecting to be sent home. Your other child is completely healthy and has never had any medical issues.

You are concerned because you don't know what is causing the temperature, and want reassurance that it's probably nothing. If specifically asked, you tested positive on a swab for group B streptococcus during the pregnancy.

Assessment

For all scenarios:

> Introduction.
> Ask a mixture of open and closed questions.
> Ensure understanding throughout.
> Summarise your findings to the parents, and give them an opportunity to raise any other issues.

History of Presenting Complaint (Temperature)

Question	Justification	Answer	Evolving thought process
When did you first notice the temperature? How high has it been, and for how long? Have you given anything to bring the temperature down?	Establishing the history of the temperatures gives clues as to the likelihood of there being an infection, and how many days it may have been present.	"He has only had one temperature this morning of 39°C. We didn't give anything for it."	Since the temperature is particularly high, it is more likely to be related to pathology. As it has only just manifested, a clinical focus may not be obvious yet.
How has Fred been in himself? Is he more sleepy or tired than usual? Has he had any floppy episodes, or funny movements?	Looking for general signs of being unwell that would be consistent with a clinically apparent infection	"He is completely well in himself."	Reassuring, although it is still concerning that he has an unexplained temperature.
How are you feeding Fred, how often, and how is that going? If breastfeeding, is Fred latching on to the breast? How long is each feed?	Septic babies are less likely to feed well.	"Breastfeeding is going well, Fred is latching on to the breast every 3 hours for 15 minutes."	Being reassured that this child is likely to be clinically well at present.
Has Fred passed any wet and dirty nappies? If so, how many?	Poor feeding can lead to dehydration, and a poor urine output is a marker of septic shock.	"There has been one dirty nappy and eight wet nappies in the last 24 hours, which is the same as normal."	
How has Fred's breathing been? Any cough, and if so is anything being coughed up? Any rashes or swellings anywhere? Any vomiting or diarrhoea? Any abnormal movements that could be fits?	Trying to localise the site of any possible infection.	"He has been completely well."	No specific focus of infection is identified.
Has Jamie had any other problems between delivery and now, other than this temperature?	Screening for other relevant problems.	"No."	Being reassured that Fred has generally been a well baby.

Obstetric and Birth History

Question	Justification	Answer	Evolving thought process
How was the pregnancy? Were there any problems on the scans?	Antenatal diagnosis may be helpful; for example, antenatally diagnosed pelviureteric junction (PUJ) obstruction increases the risk of urinary tract infections (UTIs).	"All scans were normal"	No additional concerns identified.

Continued

Question	Justification	Answer	Evolving thought process
How many weeks pregnant were you when Jamie was delivered? Was it a vaginal delivery, forceps or caesarean? Did he cry straight away or need help?	Premature babies are more vulnerable to infection. A baby requiring resuscitation may have had an occult infection.	"Jamie was born at 38 weeks, by elective C Section for breech, and cried straight away."	No additional concerns identified.
What was the birth weight?	Low birth weight infants are more likely to have infections.	"4kg."	No additional concerns identified.
Were any issues identified on the newborn baby check?	General screen for problems. The presence of jaundice is usually checked for on the baby check.	"No."	No additional concerns identified.
How long was it between the rupture of your membranes and delivery? Did you have any temperatures during labour? Were you given antibiotics during labour? Do you know if you've had a positive test for the bug Group B strep?	These are all risk factors for infection.	"Fred delivered within 4 hours of membranes rupturing. There was one temperature of 39°C during labour, but I was given two doses of antibiotics. I tested positive for Group B streptococcus during pregnancy."	Evidence for possible infection increasing, with maternal temperature and group B streptococcus. Adequate antibiotic cover was given. Vertically transmitted infections can potentially present late.

Past Medical/Surgical History

Question	Justification	Answer	Evolving thought process
Has Fred ever had any operations? Have you been to hospital with him since birth? Does he have any known medical conditions?	May all be linked to the temperature, e.g. recent surgery may mean a post-operative intra-abdominal collection.	"Fred has had no previous operations, no hospital attendances and no medical diagnoses."	No new concerns identified.

Drug History

Question	Justification	Answer	Evolving thought process
Is Fred on any medication? Does he have any allergies?	Unlikely to be on any medications, but useful to know as may have been started on antibiotics, and drug interactions should be considered. Drugs may also be a clue to underlying diseases. Allergies are unlikely in a six week old breast fed baby.	"No medications, no allergies."	No new concerns identified.

Developmental History

Question	Justification	Answer	Evolving thought process
Is Fred smiling? Can he fix his eyes on people/things he is interested in and follow them as they move?	At six weeks, a baby would generally be expected to fix and follow, and to social smile.	"He can do both."	No developmental concerns at present.

Family History

Question	Justification	Answer	Evolving thought process
Anyone currently ill in the family? Any recent travel? Any unusual foods eaten lately?	Infection can be highly contagious.	"Grandma and Granddad both currently have a cold."	Possible source of infection from grandparents.
Do you have any other children? Any health problems with them now or in the past? Do you (or dad) have any health problems that you are aware of?	Group B strep infection in a previous child makes it more likely this child will have it. There may be a history of Sudden Infant Death Syndrome (SIDS).	"No health problems with the other children or in the family."	No additional concerns identified.

Social History

Question	Justification	Answer	Evolving thought process
Who is currently at home? Does Fred have a social worker? Is dad around? Does anyone smoke at home?	Find out if there are any social concerns, or if wider support is needed. Smoking increases risk of infection in the child.	"My husband and I live together, and have been happily married for several years. We are both non-smokers, and there is no social worker."	No social concerns at present.

Immunisation history is not relevant in a six-week-old baby, as the first immunisations are at eight-weeks-old.

Concluding

Question	Justification	Answer	Evolving thought process
Is there anything that I've missed, or anything that you are particularly concerned about? Do you have any questions for me at the moment?	May identify useful information that has been missed. Will also help framing communication with the mother.	"I am really keen to go home."	Needs a careful and sensitive discussion about a management plan.

🔍 PRESENTING YOUR FINDINGS

Fred is term baby who presents at six weeks of age very well in himself, but with a one-off temperature at home of 39°C.

There is no difficulty in breathing, no seizures, no rashes, no vomiting and no diarrhoea. Fred is feeding well at the breast, with a normal number of wet nappies.

Jamie was born by an elective C-section for breech, required no resuscitation and went home with mum after a normal newborn baby check. Mum had one raised temperature during labour, and a background of Group B streptococcus, with two doses of antibiotics given during labour. Antenatal scans are normal. Fred is growing well, tracking the 50th centile. Grandma and granddad both currently have an upper respiratory tract infection (URTI), but there is no family history of note. This is mum's second child, and the other child is well. There are no social concerns.

I am concerned about possible infection, particularly considering the maternal background, although there is no clear focus for infection identified.

After doing a full examination, I will cannulate the baby, and check the FBC, U&Es, CRP and blood cultures. I will get a clean catch urine sample, and a chest X-ray if there are any signs of respiratory disease on examination. A nasopharyngeal aspirate will be helpful if the baby has signs of possible bronchiolitis. In view of the history of Group B streptococcus and fever, I would also perform a lumbar puncture. I will start broad spectrum antibiotics. Fred is currently feeding well, so I'd be happy for him to continue breastfeeding at present.

CASE 3
A 13-year-old boy presenting with a wheezy episode

Doctor Briefing
You are asked to see a boy, Steven, 13-years-old, in the ED who has started wheezing at home. Please take a history from his mother, with a view to making a diagnosis.

Mother (actress) Briefing
Steven is your only child, and you are worried about him because he is wheezing and has difficulty breathing. He is breathing fast and having to pause in the middle of sentences to catch his breath. His shortness of breath has come on gradually. He does not have a fever but he has had a bit of a cold for the last few days. He is off his food, but drinking about two-thirds of normal. Steven occasionally has had wheezy episodes in physical education lessons, but he usually gets better quickly.

Steven is otherwise well, is not on any medication and has never attended hospital before. He was born at 35 weeks by a normal vaginal delivery. He is up-to-date with his immunisations, developing normally, growing well and performing well academically.

You are a single mother, but are coping well. Steven stays with Dad every other weekend. You don't smoke. Dad and the paternal granddad both have eczema.

You are concerned because this is the worst you've ever seen Steven, and he can't talk to you properly. If specifically asked, you are also worried that his dad smokes and that this might contribute to the breathing problems.

Assessment
For all scenarios:
> Introduction.
> Ask a mixture of open and closed questions.
> Ensure understanding throughout.
> Summarise your findings to the parents, and give them an opportunity to raise any other issues.

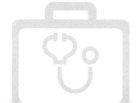

History of Presenting Complaint (Wheeze)

Question	Justification	Answer	Evolving thought process
When did the wheeze start? What was he doing at the time? Was it sudden/gradual? How has it progressed since it began?	Sudden onset wheeze could imply foreign body aspiration or anaphylaxis.	"The wheeze came on gradually whilst walking home, and is gradually getting worse and worse."	Unlikely to be foreign body aspiration, and less likely to be anaphylaxis, although both can present atypically.
How has his breathing been otherwise? Does he use more effort than normal to breathe? Has it affected his speech?	Children can be happy wheezers or in marked respiratory distress, and how their breathing affects them will influence treatment.	"Steven is breathing much faster than normal and struggling to keep up. He is unable to complete sentences."	There is significant respiratory distress, which will require urgent treatment.
Has he had a cough, and if so, is he coughing anything up? Any fevers? Has he had a runny nose, a sore throat or any ear pain or discharge?	A respiratory tract infection is a common cause of an asthma exacerbation, or viral-induced wheeze.	"No fever. He has had a cold for the last few days, with a cough and a snotty nose."	This appears like a viral infection has triggered a wheezy episode. It may or may not be asthma.
Any vomiting or diarrhoea? Any headache, neck stiffness, fits? Any pain, difficulty peeing, or change in the colour or smell of the urine? Any rashes or joint swelling?	Given the significant respiratory distress, it is worth enquiring about other possible sources of infection.	"None."	Likely to be an isolated respiratory issue.
Is he eating and drinking normally or less than normal? Is he peeing and pooing the same amount as usual?	Gives a measure of how unwell the child is, and any dehydration.	"He is completely off his food, but has had five cups of water today."	He is remaining sufficiently hydrated in this episode.
How was Steven before this episode? Has he ever wheezed before? Does he ever wheeze or cough while exercising, or at night? Has he ever had any tests for breathing issues before (X-ray, peak flow, lung function tests)?	Gives a measure of any underlying lung disease.	"He wheezes sometimes when playing sports. He has never had any tests looking at his lungs."	Makes underlying lung disease, i.e. asthma, more likely.

Past Medical/Surgical and Birth History

Question	Justification	Answer	Evolving thought process
Was Steven born on time or early? Were there any complications at birth?	Premature babies are more likely to develop asthma.	"He was born at 35 weeks, by a normal vaginal delivery, with no complications."	Prematurity might predispose to asthma.
Does Steven suffer from asthma, eczema or hay fever? Any other medical problems? Has he ever been admitted overnight to hospital or had to miss school with illness?	Atopic diseases are linked together. Previous admissions/medical disorders may explain current symptoms, e.g. heart disease or gastro-oesophageal reflux disease.	"He is otherwise completely well."	No other concerns.

Drug History

Question	Justification	Answer	Evolving thought process
Is Steven on any medication? Have you given him anything for this episode? Does he have any allergies?	Medications may be a clue to an underlying diagnosis. Even if he doesn't have any medications, parents may give a child another sibling's or a parent's medication, e.g. salbutamol inhaler.	"No medications, no allergies."	No new concerns identified.

Growth and Developmental History

Question	Justification	Answer	Evolving thought process
Are there any worries or concerns about Steven's development compared to his peers at school? Is he performing well in assessments?	There is no specific concern about his development in the initial history, but it is useful to get a broad idea of his current status.	"No concerns at all."	No new concerns identified.
Is Steven growing as expected for him?	Chronic disease can be associated with faltering growth.	"Yes, he is growing well (75th centile when plotted)."	Less likely to have a severe, chronic underlying disease.

Immunisation History

Question	Justification	Answer	Evolving thought process
Has Stephen had all of his immunisations?	Unimmunised children are at risk of childhood infections.	"Yes."	No new concerns identified.

Family History

Question	Justification	Answer	Evolving thought process
Is anyone currently ill in the family? Any recent travel?	Infection can be highly contagious, and may explain the presenting illness.	"None."	No new concerns identified.
Do you (or dad, or grandparents) have any health problems that you are aware of?	Atopic diseases run in families.	"Dad and granddad on the father's side have eczema."	There is a family history of atopic disease, making asthma more likely.

Social History

Question	Justification	Answer	Evolving thought process
Who is currently at home, and where does Steven stay? Does Steven have a social worker? Is dad around? Does anyone smoke at any place he stays?	Find out if there are any social concerns, or if wider support is needed. Smoking increases risk of infection in the child.	"I am separated from Steven's dad. Steven spends every other weekend with dad, who smokes. There is no social worker."	No social concerns at present, although dad's smoking may be contributing to this.

Concluding

Question	Justification	Answer	Evolving thought process
Is there anything that I've missed, or anything that you are particularly concerned about? Do you have any questions for me at the moment?	May identify useful information that has been missed. Will also help framing communication with the mother.	"Mum is concerned this may be related to Dad's smoking."	Needs a careful and sensitive discussion about smoking cessation for the father.

🔍 PRESENTING YOUR FINDINGS

Steven is an unwell 13-year-old boy that has presented with wheeze and difficulty in breathing, on a likely background of asthma.

The wheeze came on gradually whilst walking home and is associated with laboured breathing, leading to an inability to complete sentences. He has not taken any medications for his breathing. Over the last few days, he has had URTI symptoms. Oral fluid intake is around two-thirds of normal.

Steven was a premature baby (born at 35 weeks gestation), and although he has had a few mild wheezy episodes whilst exercising, he has had no major medical problems up until today. Dad and granddad have eczema. Growth and development appears normal, and immunisations are up-to-date. Steven splits time between mum and dad, who are divorced. Dad is a smoker.

The most likely diagnosis is a viral exacerbation of asthma, although other things to consider in a wheezy child are foreign body inhalation, anaphylaxis, heart failure and gastro-oesophageal reflux.

As this child appears very unwell, I would want to do a rapid, focused respiratory examination, and after that, begin treatment with oral corticosteroids and back-to-back nebulisers. I will cannulate Steven, get a venous blood gas, and baseline bloods including FBC, CRP and U&Es, knowing also that I might need the cannula for intravenous bronchodilator therapy afterwards. I will also arrange a chest X-ray, and if Steven is compliant, try to get a peak flow reading.

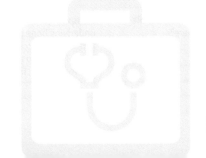

Question	Justification	Answer	Evolving thought process
Are you feeling unwell in any other way? For example, difficulty breathing, cough, headache, fits, drowsy episodes, pain elsewhere?	Abdominal pain may be part of a systemic pathology. Also may have referred pain in the abdomen e.g. from right lower lobe pneumonia.	"I feel fine otherwise."	Likely to be something abdominal causing the problem.

Past Medical/Surgical and Birth History

Question	Justification	Answer	Evolving thought process
Were you born on time, or early? Were there any complications around birth? Do you have any major medical problems? Any previous operations? Have you ever had to stay overnight in hospital, or had to miss school with illness?	Could explain the abdominal pain. Previous abdominal surgery often results in the appendix being taken out, even if it is not for an appendicectomy.	"I haven't been told about any problems with me as a baby. I have mild asthma, and take my asthma pump sometimes. I don't remember ever staying in hospital."	No other concerns identified.

Drug History

Question	Justification	Answer	Evolving thought process
Are you on any drugs for your health? Have you taken anything for this pain? Do you have any allergies?	Medications may hint at underlying diagnosis. It may also give clues as to possible overdoses in certain presentations. Analgesia so far can also give insight into level of pain.	"I take a blue inhaler for asthma when I feel wheezy— I don't know the name of it though. I don't have any allergies. I have not taken any drugs today."	Will need analgesia quickly, as has not had anything yet.

Growth and Developmental History

Question	Justification	Answer	Evolving thought process
What school do you attend? How is school going? Any problems with academic performance?	Unlikely to affect the differential diagnosis, but developmental problems could be identified at this stage and fed into appropriate support systems if needed.	"I am at St Bartholew's school, and things are going fine."	No new concerns identified.
Are you growing well in terms of your height and weight? Any recent weight loss?	Chronic disease may result in faltering growth and abdominal pain, e.g. inflammatory bowel disease.	"Yes, I am about average height and weight for my class. I haven't lost weight recently."	Less likely to have a severe, chronic underlying disease.

Immunisation History

Question	Justification	Answer	Evolving thought process
Have you had all of your immunisation jabs?	Unimmunised children are at risk of rarer infections.	"I don't know, but probably."	No new concerns identified.

Family History

Question	Justification	Answer	Evolving thought process
Do you (or parents or grandparents) have any health problems that you are aware of?	Certain gastrointestinal disorders, e.g. inflammatory bowel disease, have a familial tendency.	"None."	No new concern identified.

CASE 5: A 14-YEAR-OLD GIRL PRESENTING WITH ACUTE ABDOMINAL PAIN

Social History

Question	Justification	Answer	Evolving thought process
Where do you stay, and who do you live with? Do you have a partner at the moment? Can you tell me about them? Are mum or dad coming in today? Do you have a social worker?	Important to identify any possible social concerns, and will ideally need to contact parents about any interventions.	"I live with mum and dad, and am an only child. I'm dating a 17-year-old boy, and we love each other very much. I don't remember ever seeing a social worker. Mum is coming in later."	Is in a relationship with a significantly older partner. Has presented without parents, although mum is on her way. Maybe some child protection concerns, but need to find out more information.

Concluding

Question	Justification	Answer	Evolving thought process
Is there anything that I've missed, or anything that you are particularly concerned about? Do you have any questions for me at the moment?	May identify useful information that has been missed. Will also help framing communication with the mother.	"I'm very worried about being pregnant, and do not want mum or dad to know I am having sex or that I have a boyfriend. Please don't tell them."	Needs a careful and sensitive discussion about the next steps of management.

PRESENTING YOUR FINDINGS

Samantha is a 14-year-old girl who presents on her own to the ED with right iliac fossa pain and vomiting consistent with appendicitis.

The pain started two days ago, as a diffuse abdominal pain, but is now a sharp, severe pain localised to the right iliac fossa. It is made much worse on movement. She has also experienced three episodes of vomiting during this time. There is no diarrhoea, and she has recently opened her bowels. She is off her food and is hardly drinking, with a reduced urine output. Additionally, Samantha is currently sexually active with a 17-year-old partner, and her period is three days late. She reports no other symptoms of note.

Samantha has a background of mild asthma, treated with PRN salbutamol. She has no allergies, and all her immunisations are up-to-date. There are no concerns regarding her growth, nor regarding her development. She lives at home with mum and dad, and mum is coming in to see us.

At this point, the most likely diagnosis is acute appendicitis, but I would like to rule out ectopic pregnancy.

Initially, I would like to give adequate analgesia, and contact the general surgeons for review. I will do a detailed examination, particularly looking for signs of peritonism. I will insert a cannula, and take blood for FBC, clotting, U&Es, CRP and group and save. I would also like to dipstick the urine, and do a urine pregnancy test. Samantha may be Gillick Competent, but ideally I would like to speak to her parents and get the family on board with the management plan. There are also possible safeguarding issues that need to be addressed with regards to the older boyfriend, underage sex, and absent parents in ED (although we have been told mum is on her way).

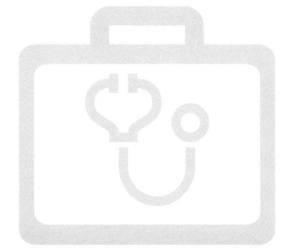

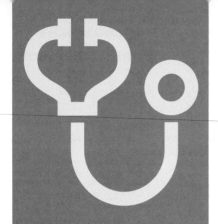

3.02
EXAMINATION
AMY MORAN AND ZESHAN QURESHI

CONTENTS

CONTENTS

INTRODUCTION

Paediatric examinations can be fun and are a chance to make your patient smile and laugh. They are a balance between systematic and opportunistic examination. Although some children can be unwilling or too upset to be examined, using play techniques can help win over any tantrum (*Figure 1-4*). For some children, this will be their first encounter with a doctor so keeping the interaction friendly helps to minimise fear. With older children, chat to them, find out their likes and dislikes and explain to them what you are going to do before you do it, at each stage. Wherever possible, remain at the same height as the child to reduce intimidation.

Practice is essential, particularly before a clinical exam. Use every opportunity

to examine lots of patients, including siblings of inpatients and young relatives. Practice will make it easier to combine clinical knowledge with examination findings to form a diagnosis – or at least it will draw some broad differentials.

The examination chapter is laid out in order of some of the key systems that feature in both acute, outpatient and exam settings. In nearly all circumstances all systems will need to at least briefly be assessed.

Certain rules apply to all examinations:

> Remember to wash hands before seeing a patient.

> Begin with an introduction to both the parent and the child.

> Explain what is going to be done before doing it.

> With younger children, take consent from parents. Tell the child what is going to be done. If the child is asked whether it is ok to examine their chest and they then say "no," it is then difficult to proceed. Instead say, "now I am going to listen to your chest."

> When examining for pain, look at the child's face to gauge their reaction rather than the part of the body being examined.

> When finished, thank the child.

MEDICAL DEVICES

Children will often have medical devices in situ. A good knowledge of it may identify relevant past medical history, as well as facilitate ongoing management (e.g. knowing where blood samples might be taken from).

Central Venous Access

> Portacath®. This is an implanted port that sits under the skin connected to a central venous catheter (*Figure 5*). The port is accessed with a specific needle (*Figure 6*). Medication can be given via the port and blood can be taken from it. It is seen most commonly in patients undergoing long-term intravenous treatments, such as chemotherapy, regular blood transfusions (e.g. sickle cell disease, thalassaemia) or regular intravenous antibiotics (e.g. cystic fibrosis). The

FIGURE 1

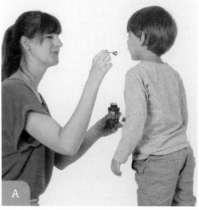

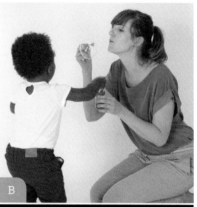

Asking a child to blow bubbles to help them relax (A) and for a younger child, blowing bubbles for them (B).

main complications are infection, port dislodging (the port can sometimes flip too), thrombosis or blockage of the catheter.

> Hickman line. This is a brand of tunnelled central venous catheters used for long-term treatment such as chemotherapy (*Figure 7*). Medication may be given via the line and blood can be taken from the line. If not used regularly, the lines should be flushed. As with any central venous device, blockage, dislodgement, thrombosis and infection can occur. The line can also split; it may sometimes be possible to repair small splits depending on their location. Note that a **Broviac line** is similar to a Hickman line, but the lumen is smaller, meaning it can be used in smaller children and infants.

> PICC (Peripherally Inserted Central Catheter) line. These may be inserted under local or general

527

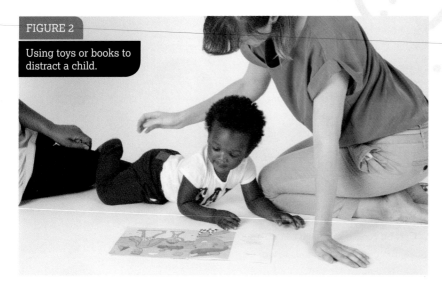

FIGURE 2

Using toys or books to distract a child.

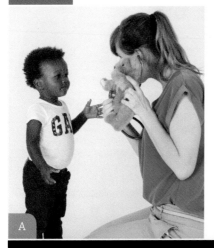
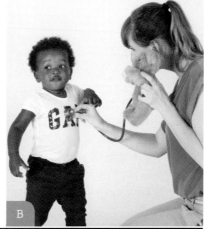

FIGURE 3

A   B

Here a teddy bear is used to turn auscultation into a game.

FIGURE 4

Thanking a child for persevering with an examination might keep them in a good mood!

anaesthetic, depending on the child's age (*Figure 8*). PICC lines tend to be in place for a few weeks, rather than months to years. They need to be flushed regularly to avoid blocking, and the complications are the same as for the other types of central venous devices. Note that Power PICC is a brand of PICC that allows contrast media to be injected for CT scans.

Respiratory Support

- CPAP (Continuous Positive Airway Pressure). This gives positive airway pressure to keep alveoli open and aid recruitment (*Figure 9*). It can be delivered via nasal prongs or a nasal mask. It can offer pressures of usually 4-8 cm H_2O in air or oxygen.

- Nasal cannula oxygen. This is a simple way to deliver oxygen to a baby (*Figure 10*). Increasingly, HFNC (High Flow Nasal Cannula Oxygen) is used as a means to generate pressure similar to CPAP. HFNC has the same indications as CPAP and is delivered via nasal cannula. A flow rate is set, usually in a range of 2 L/min to 8 L/min, again with oxygen or in air.

- Endotracheal tube. This is used in the severely unwell child/baby (*Figure 11*). It allows mechanical ventilation via a variety of techniques, such as high frequency oscillation and patient triggered ventilation.

- Tracheostomy. This is a type of surgical airway (*Figure 12*). There are a number of indications for its creation, such as vocal cord paralysis and tracheomalacia. A Swedish nose is a small cap attached to the tracheostomy to allow humidification.

Inhalers

- Inhaler. Inhalers deliver inhaled medication to airways. Different drug companies use different shapes.
  - Turbohalers. Bullet shaped, e.g. Pulmicort® and Bricanyl®: twisted by the patient to activate (*Figure 13*).
  - Metered dose inhalers. Traditional L-shaped inhalers. These are pressed during inhalation to

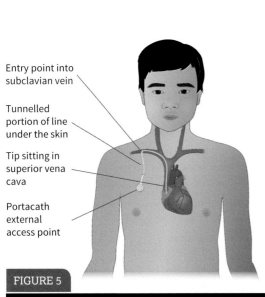

Entry point into
subclavian vein

Tunnelled
portion of line
under the skin

Tip sitting in
superior vena
cava

Portacath
external
access point

FIGURE 5

Portacath®. The port is visible by a small raised area, usually under an arm, the lateral chest wall or on the anterior chest wall.

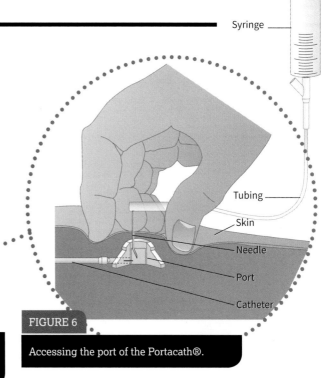

Syringe

Tubing

Skin

Needle

Port

Catheter

FIGURE 6

Accessing the port of the Portacath®.

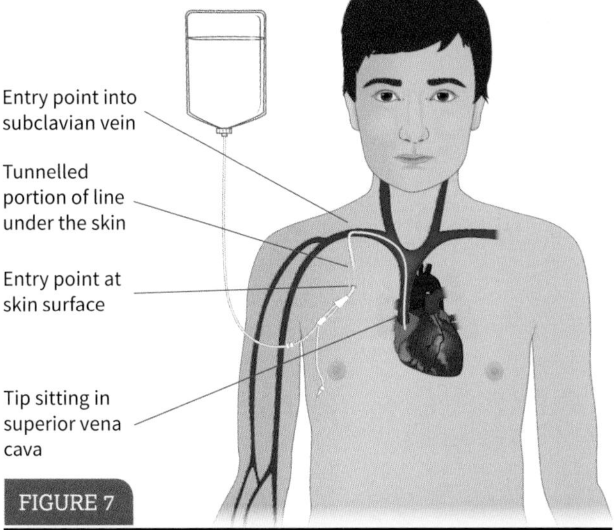

Entry point into
subclavian vein

Tunnelled
portion of line
under the skin

Entry point at
skin surface

Tip sitting in
superior vena
cava

FIGURE 7

Hickman line. It usually exits the lateral or anterior chest wall. There is a cuff beneath the skin to keep the catheter in place. Different numbers of lumens are available depending on the intended use of the line.

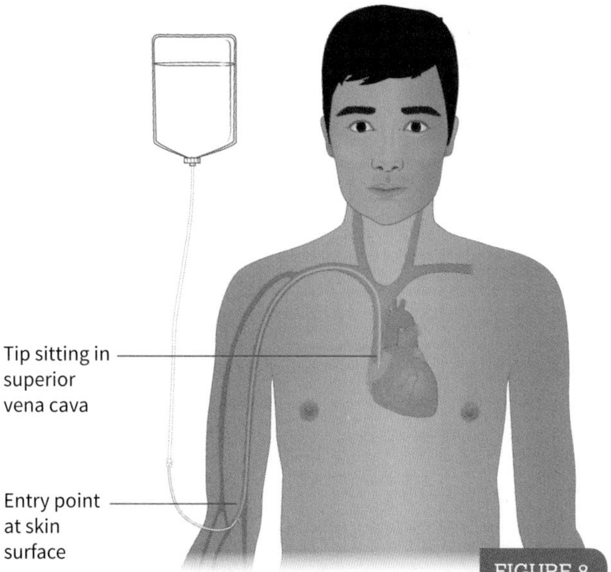

Tip sitting in
superior
vena cava

Entry point
at skin
surface

FIGURE 8

PICC line. This is usually inserted via the antecubital fossa, with the tip sitting in the SVC just outside the right atrium.

FIGURE 9

CPAP.

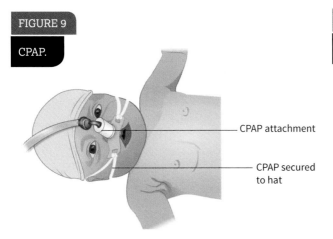

CPAP attachment

CPAP secured
to hat

FIGURE 10

Nasal cannulae.

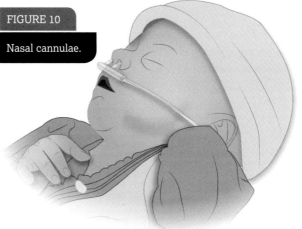

FIGURE 11

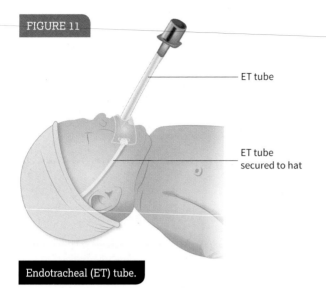

ET tube

ET tube
secured to hat

Endotracheal (ET) tube.

FIGURE 12

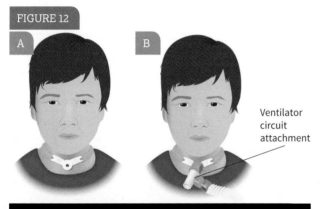

A

B

Ventilator
circuit
attachment

Tracheostomy. Not attached to ventilator (left), attached to ventilator (right).

deliver the drug, and should be used with a spacer (*Figure 14*).

> › Accuhalers. Round, circular inhalers e.g. Seretide™ or Flixotide™. They have a dose release lever on the side (*Figure 15*).

Different colours help to indicate type of drug:

> › Blue. Bronchodilator, e.g. salbutamol and terbutaline.
> › Brown. Corticosteroid, e.g. beclomethasone.
> › Purple. Combination, e.g. Seretide™ (salmeterol and fluticasone).
> › Green. Atrovent® i.e. ipratropium.
> › Orange. Flixotide™.
> › Red. Combination bronchodilator and corticosteroid, e.g. Symbicort® (formoterol and budesonide).

> Spacer. This is a plastic chamber that enhances inhaled drug delivery (*Figure 16*).
> Acapella®. This is a type of airway clearance used in cystic fibrosis as part of physiotherapy (*Figure 17*). It looks like a small spacer device. It has a mouthpiece that the child breathes into, generating positive end-expiratory pressure (PEEP) to open airways.
> Flutter®. This is similar to the above, but looks more like a large whistle (*Figure 18*).

Surgical Conduits

> Antegrade Continence Enema (ACE). This uses the appendix to create a passage from the colon that opens out onto the anterior abdominal wall as a small stoma. Catheters can be inserted through this to empty faeces from the colon. It is performed for example in spina bifida patients.
> Mitrofanoff. This uses the appendix to create a conduit from the bladder into a small stoma on the external abdominal wall for neuropathic bladders, such as in spina bifida. A catheter can then be passed directly through this new opening into the bladder to empty it.

FIGURES 13 and 14

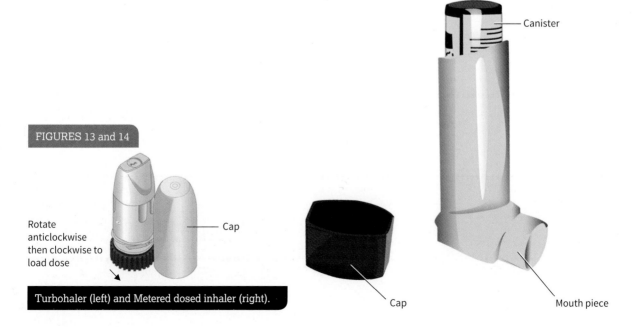

Rotate
anticlockwise
then clockwise to
load dose

Cap

Turbohaler (left) and Metered dosed inhaler (right).

Canister

Cap

Mouth piece

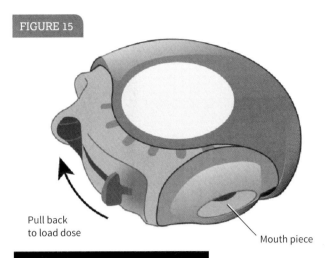

FIGURE 15

Pull back
to load dose

Mouth piece

Accuhaler.

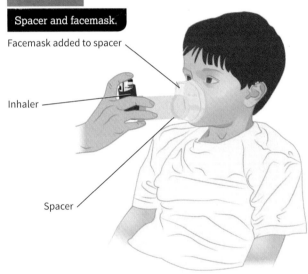

FIGURE 16

Spacer and facemask.

Facemask added to spacer

Inhaler

Spacer

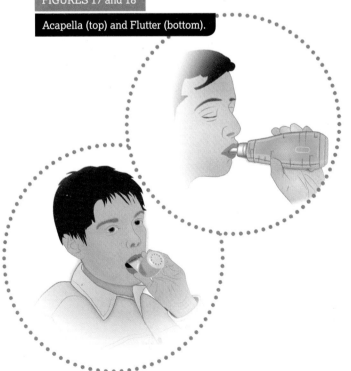

FIGURES 17 and 18

Acapella (top) and Flutter (bottom).

> Gastrostomy. This is a surgical opening into the stomach from the external abdominal wall (*Figure 19*). It is used for feeding or medication. It may also be referred to as PEG which refers to the operative method used – Percutaneous Endoscopic Gastrostomy.

> Jejunostomy. This is a surgical opening into the jejunum. It is used in patients for whom a gastrostomy is unsuitable or still results in significant gastro-oesophageal reflux symptoms. PEGs can be extended to create a PEG-J. Note: Distinguishing a jejunostomy from a gastrostomy is often difficult, but they may be labelled.

> Vesicostomy. This is a surgical opening into the bladder from the lower abdominal wall that allows drainage of urine from the bladder. It is performed in cases of neuropathic bladder or bladder outlet obstruction.

> Ileostomy/Colostomy. These bags collect faecal matter (*Figure 20*) out of a surgical opening. The higher up this is coming from in the GI tract, the more liquid the material is. Ileostomies are usually in the right lower quadrant, colostomies in the left lower quadrant. They may be associated with a refeeding fistula at a distal site, through which faecal matter is 'refed' into the distal bowel.

Neurosurgical

> Ventricular reservoirs. This is used to tap CSF for ventriculomegaly/progressive hydrocephalus (*Figure 21*).

> Ventriculoperitoneal Shunt (VP Shunt). This drains excess CSF from ventricles (*Figure 22*). The shunt may become blocked, infected or dislodged. Also look for a scar in the upper quadrant of the abdomen.

> External Ventricular Drain (EVD). This is unlikely to be encountered in an examination as it is used temporarily to drain excess CSF from ventricles (*Figure 23*). Antibiotics can be given through it, directly into the CSF. These are usually seen in PICU or NICU at neurosurgical centres on patients with obstructive hydrocephalus.

Mobility Aids and Orthoses

> Wheelchairs. These come in many variants (*Figure 24*). Self-propelled wheelchairs arc propelled by the users, meaning the user turns the wheels themselves. Powered wheelchairs are battery operated, and may be driven via a variety of controls including joystick, head control and breath-assisted devices. Additionally, a patient may need back, neck or head supports on the wheelchair.

> Walkers. These may have no wheels and need to be lifted to move (which offers the greatest stability) or may have two or four wheels, depending on level of mobility (*Figure 25*). Four-wheeled walkers may also have seats, allowing use for longer distances.

> Other mobility aids/contracture prevention. These may be in the form of special shoes, insoles or joint splints (*Figure 26*).

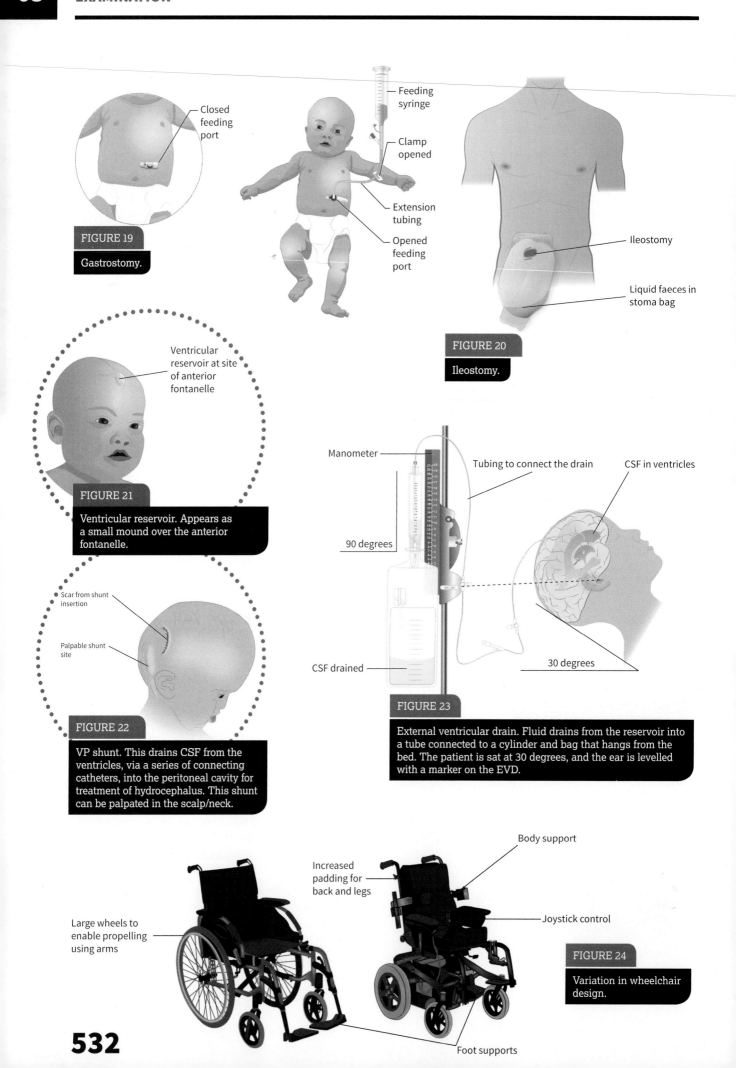

Closed feeding port

FIGURE 19

Gastrostomy.

Feeding syringe

Clamp opened

Extension tubing

Opened feeding port

Ileostomy

Liquid faeces in stoma bag

FIGURE 20

Ileostomy.

Ventricular reservoir at site of anterior fontanelle

FIGURE 21

Ventricular reservoir. Appears as a small mound over the anterior fontanelle.

Scar from shunt insertion

Palpable shunt site

FIGURE 22

VP shunt. This drains CSF from the ventricles, via a series of connecting catheters, into the peritoneal cavity for treatment of hydrocephalus. This shunt can be palpated in the scalp/neck.

Manometer

90 degrees

CSF drained

Tubing to connect the drain

CSF in ventricles

30 degrees

FIGURE 23

External ventricular drain. Fluid drains from the reservoir into a tube connected to a cylinder and bag that hangs from the bed. The patient is sat at 30 degrees, and the ear is levelled with a marker on the EVD.

Body support

Increased padding for back and legs

Joystick control

Large wheels to enable propelling using arms

FIGURE 24

Variation in wheelchair design.

Foot supports

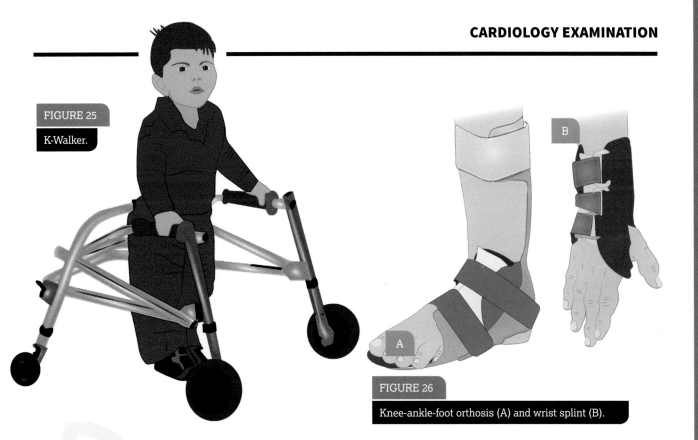

FIGURE 25

K-Walker.

FIGURE 26

Knee-ankle-foot orthosis (A) and wrist splint (B).

CARDIOLOGY EXAMINATION

All unwell children presenting to hospital will require a cardiovascular examination. Particular incidences where a more detailed assessment may be required include:

1 Child with possible pathological murmur of unknown cause. Often children (particularly newborns on their routine checks) are noted to have an incidental murmur. This needs to be assessed to identify its exact nature, and whether it is associated with signs of heart failure or any other indication of cardiovascular compromise.

2 Child presenting with an irregular heart rhythm or episodes of syncope or chest pain. This may be associated with underlying cardiac disease. Do they have valvular heart disease? Do they have heart failure (*Box 1*)?

3 Child who is acutely unwell. This may be a result of a critical cardiac lesion (e.g. coarctation of the aorta) or myocardial dysfunction secondary to sepsis or pericarditis for instance. Additionally, administration of intravenous fluids and boluses may cause circulatory overload tipping children into heart failure, so this needs to be continually reassessed for during resuscitation.

Common patients that are likely to appear in exams are shown in *Table 1*. Note that any child with a severe uncorrected cardiac defect is also likely to have faltering growth.

Starting the Examination

The examination begins by observing the child upon entering the examination room. On introduction to the child/parents, begin with a broad assessment:

1 Does the child look well or unwell? What colour are they? A corrected cyanotic heart lesion will not result in a completely pink child. Are they chatting with no shortness of breath? Are they sweating and uncomfortable?

2 Are there signs of chronic ill health? Do they look underweight? Are there any drains, central lines or long term feeding tubes in place?

3 Are there medications nearby? Is there a portable oxygen cylinder? Are they on a monitor?

4 Are there dysmorphic features? (*Table 2*)

Summary Checklist

Global assessment of child on approach.

Inspection. Hands, face, neck, chest, back, abdomen, legs.

Palpation. Apex beat, thrills and heaves, hepatomegaly.

Auscultation. Heart sounds, murmurs.

Bedside tests. Observation chart, plot height/weight, BP, ECG, urine dipstick.

Box 1: Clinical features of heart failure

- Shortness of breath/tachypnoea.
- Poor feeding.
- Sweating.
- Low oxygen saturations.
- Crackles/wheeze.
- Tachycardia.
- Third/fourth heart sounds.
- Apex may be displaced.
- Hepatomegaly.
- Peripheral oedema.

Inspection

In order to undertake a more focused inspection, the child needs to be exposed. In an older child, they may be wearing a vest and lifting this or moving it to one side when the necessary area is inspected is fine. It is not necessary for bras to be removed. Older children can be examined at a 45° angle, toddlers seated upright on a parent's lap, and a baby flat on the bed.

TABLE 1: Common patients that may appear in clinical examinations	
Diagnosis	**Possible clues**
Flow/Innocent murmur.	• Well child. • A soft ejection systolic murmur that does not radiate, may alter with respiration and position.
Ventricular septal defect.	• Well child. • A pansystolic murmur heard loudest at lower left sternal edge. • They may have a thrill at lower left sternal edge.
Pulmonary stenosis.	• Well child. • An ejection systolic murmur at upper left sternal edge, radiating to back. • They may have a thrill in the pulmonary region.
Atrial septal defect.	• Fixed splitting of the second heart sound. • An ejection systolic murmur at upper left sternal edge.
Aortic stenosis.	• An ejection systolic murmur at upper right sternal edge, radiating to the carotids. • They may have a thrill in the carotid region.
Patent ductus arteriosus.	• A continuous murmur throughout systole and diastole, loudest at the upper left sternal edge. • Bounding pulses palpable. • Wide pulse pressures.
Surgically corrected Tetralogy of Fallot.	• Possible cyanosis. • An ejection systolic murmur (residual pulmonary stenosis). • They may also have a diastolic murmur (pulmonary regurgitation) or a pansystolic murmur (residual VSD). • Midline sternotomy scar (from corrective surgery). • They may also have a lateral thoracotomy scar if a temporary shunt was placed before definitive surgery. • They may also appear malnourished/small for gestational age.
Surgically corrected transposition of the great arteries.	• An ejection systolic murmur (may have right ventricular outflow obstruction). • A midline sternotomy scar (from corrective surgery) and drain scars.
Surgically/ endovascularly corrected valve lesion.	• A midline sternotomy scar and drain scars OR groin scar. • They may have murmur from restenosis, a leaky valve, or a flow murmur across a new valve. There may also be a loud click if a metallic valve was inserted.

Hands

› Signs of general ill health. This will include wasting of the small muscles in the hands from chronic disease and scars from previous cannulation. Xanthoma is also important, due to the association of hypercholesterolaemia with both hypertension and Alagille syndrome.

› Capillary refill. (*Figure 27*). The examiner should push down for five seconds with their index finger on the pulp of the child's finger and count the number of seconds it takes for normal colour to return: it should take less than two seconds. Check centrally (over the sternum) as well.

› Clubbing. Clubbing will appear as a result of long standing cyanotic heart disease; therefore it does not appear in children under 6-months-old (*Figure 28*).

› Peripheral stigmata of infective endocarditis.

  › Splinter haemorrhages (nails) – also associated with SLE and trauma.

TABLE 2: Common syndromes associated with cardiac disease		
Syndrome	**Appearance**	**Associated cardiac lesions**
Turner syndrome.	• Webbed neck. • Wide-spaced nipples. • Shield-shaped chest. • Wide carrying angle of the arms.	• Coarctation of aorta. • Bicuspid aortic valve.
Williams syndrome.	• Small upturned nose. • Long philtrum. • Flat nasal bridge. • Wide mouth. • Small chin. • Small/widely spaced teeth. • May have stellate pattern to the iris.	• Peripheral pulmonary stenosis. • Aortic stenosis (supravalvular).
Trisomy 21.	• Single palmar crease. • Low set ears. • Flat nasal bridge. • Upslanting palpebral fissures.	• AVSD. • VSD.
Noonan syndrome.	• Low set/posteriorly rotated ears. • Widely spaced eyes (hypertelorism). • Down slanting palpebral fissures. • Webbed neck. • Ptosis.	• Pulmonary stenosis. • ASD.
Alagille syndrome.	• Broad, prominent forehead. • Deep sunken eyes. • Small pointy chin.	• Peripheral pulmonary stenosis. • Tetralogy of Fallot.
22q11.2 deletion.	• Long, narrow face. • Wideset/almond shaped eyes. • Cleft lip/palate. • Small/low set ears. • Small mouth.	• Tetralogy of Fallot. • VSD.

(AVSD = atrioventricular septal defect, VSD = ventricular septal defect, and ASD = atrial septal defect)

FIGURE 27

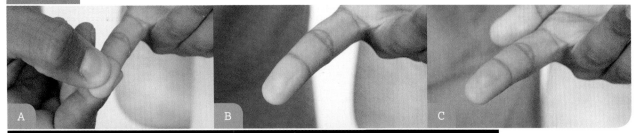

Capillary refill. Compressing the capillary bed (A), resultant pale finger (B), and colour returning (C).

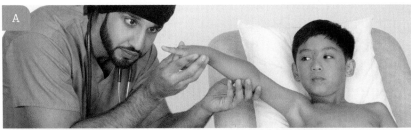

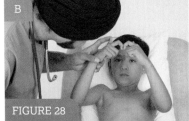
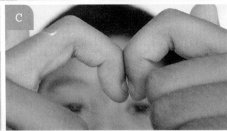

FIGURE 28

Testing for clubbing (in an unclubbed child) by two different methods.
A. Inspecting the outstretched fingers.
B/C. Asking the child to bend their index fingers, and bring the dorsal surfaces of the distal phalanx together. Demonstrate first. A diamond should be visible between the nail beds.

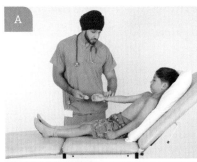

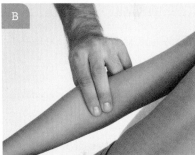

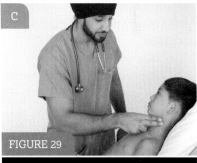

FIGURE 29

Palpating the pulses: Radial (A), brachial (B), and carotid (C).
Note that whilst measuring the pulse the respiratory rate can also be counted.

> › Janeway lesions (red, non-tender lesions on the palms).
> › Osler's nodes (painful lesions on the distal fingers).
> › Bony abnormalities. Absent thumbs or radius (Holt-Oram syndrome), absent radius (VACTERL syndrome).

Pulses and Blood Pressure

> › Radial pulse. Count the pulse rate for 30 seconds (*Figure 29*). Is it regular? Does it collapse on lifting the arm up (aortic regurgitation)? This pulse is difficult to feel in babies and therefore is usually not palpated in the examination. It is absent on the left side post a coarctation repair (if a subclavian flap is used).
> › Brachial pulse. Assess pulse volume. The brachial pulse is absent on one side when a coarctation repair has been made using the subclavian flap technique.
> › Blood pressure. The cuff width needs to be approximately two thirds the length of the upper arm, and when placed on it needs to encircle the upper arm completely (*Figure 30*). Normal ranges for heart rate and blood pressure are shown in *Table 3*.

TABLE 3: Normal values for HR and BP by age		
Age	Normal HR	Normal systolic BP
0 to 1-year-old	110-160 bpm	80-90 mmHg
1 to 2-years-old	100-150 bpm	70-95 mmHg
2 to 5-years-old	95-140 bpm	85-100 mmHg
5 to 12-years-old	80-120 bpm	90-110 mmHg
>12-years-old	60-100 bpm	90-120 mmHg

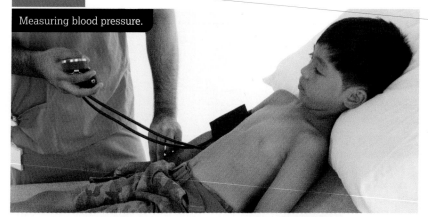

FIGURE 30

Measuring blood pressure.

FIGURE 33

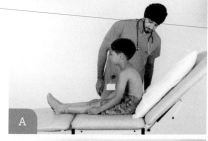

A

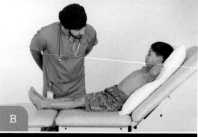

B

Inspecting the chest from the behind (A) and the front (B). Lift up each arm to inspect the axillae.

Face

- Dysmorphic features. Assess the face shape, the eyes, the ears, the mouth, the tongue, the lips and the chin (*Table 2*).
- Conjunctiva. Look for pallor (anaemia) (*Figure 31*).
- Xanthelasma. Yellow plaques around the eyelid. May be seen in familial hypercholesterolaemia.
- Polycythaemic appearance (very red). Associated with cyanotic congenital heart disease.
- Central cyanosis. Ask the child to stick out their tongue and look underneath it for blue discolouration. Also observe the colour of the gums and lips.
- Dental caries (decay). Indicates poor dental hygiene. This is a risk factor for infective endocarditis.

Neck

- Jugular venous pressure. This is only measured in older children (*Figure 32*).

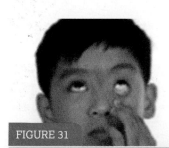

FIGURE 31

Assessing for anaemia. Ask the child to pull one of their lower lids down themselves and look up to the ceiling. To put the child more at ease, this can be demonstrated on the examiner or on the parent first.

Measure the height of the JVP from above the sternal angle.

- Carotid pulse. This is only measured in older children. Measure one side only. It is good for getting an appreciation of pulse volume and character (*Figure 29*).

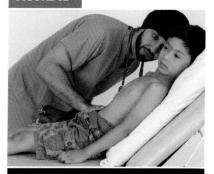

FIGURE 32

Measuring JVP. Position the child with their back at a 45° angle to the bed, with their head turned away from the side of the neck being inspected.

Chest

- Harrison's Sulcus. This is seen in conditions with increased pulmonary blood flow (and also chronic asthma). It appears as a groove along the lower chest where the diaphragm inserts onto ribs.
- Scars. Inspect the anterior chest, the axilla and the back. Look for drain scars, as well as surgical incision scars (*Figure 33-4*).
- Respiratory rate. Tachypnoea is associated with cardiac disease. Measure respiratory rate whilst measuring the pulse.

Back

- Oedema. Inspect for sacral oedema (*Figure 35*). It may be easier to do this when the patient is already sitting forward (e.g. after auscultating the base of the lungs).
- Basal lung crepitations. Auscultation of the lung bases can be done here to look for crepitation associated with left heart failure (*Figure 36*).

Abdomen

- Hepatomegaly. This is associated with right heart failure. It will be smooth rather than hard.

Groin

- Femoral pulse. An absent/reduced femoral pulse is associated with coarctation of the aorta. Whilst palpating the femoral pulse, palpate the brachial or radial pulse, looking for delay (*Figure 37*). Radio-femoral delay indicates coarctation of the aorta but can be harder to appreciate in children than in adults.
- Cardiac catheterisation scars. These will be small scars in the groin overlying the femoral arteries.

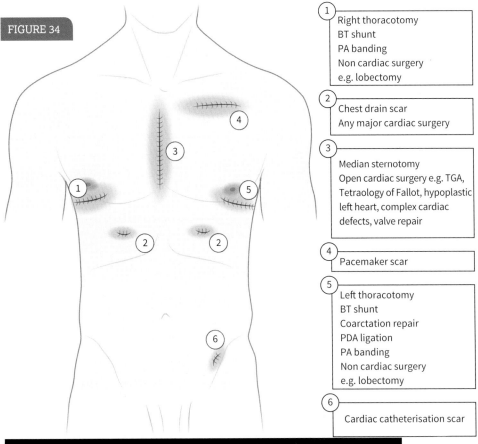

FIGURE 34

1. Right thoracotomy
   BT shunt
   PA banding
   Non cardiac surgery
   e.g. lobectomy

2. Chest drain scar
   Any major cardiac surgery

3. Median sternotomy
   Open cardiac surgery e.g. TGA,
   Tetraology of Fallot, hypoplastic
   left heart, complex cardiac
   defects, valve repair

4. Pacemaker scar

5. Left thoracotomy
   BT shunt
   Coarctation repair
   PDA ligation
   PA banding
   Non cardiac surgery
   e.g. lobectomy

6. Cardiac catheterisation scar

Surgical scars. TGA (transposition great arteries), BT (Blalock-Taussing), PDA (persistent ductus arteriosus), PA (pulmonary artery). Cardiac catheterisation procedures include valve surgery and PDA closure.

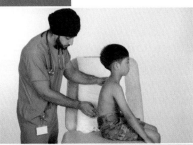

FIGURE 35

Inspecting for sacral oedema. Push down on a bony prominence such as the posterior superior iliac spines for five seconds and then release.

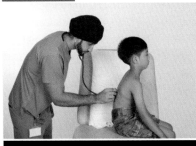

FIGURE 36

Auscultation for basal crepitations.

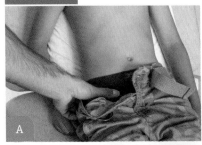
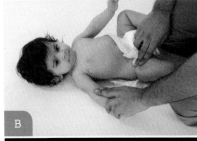

FIGURE 37

A

B

Palpating the femoral pulse. In older children, the femoral pulse should be palpable through the clothes and therefore modesty can be preserved (A). Palpating for brachio-femoral delay in a baby (B).

Legs

> Oedema. This may be present due to heart failure (*Figure 38*).

Palpation

> Apex beat (*Figure 39*). The apex beat should be in the midclavicular line, at the 4th-5th intercostal space. It may be in an abnormal position (e.g. displaced in cardiomegaly or on the right side in dextrocardia), or become more forceful (e.g. left ventricular hypertrophy).
> Ventricular heaves (*Figure 40*). These indicate ventricular hypertrophy.
> Thrills. These occur as a result of turbulent blood flow that can be felt as a vibration on the skin surface. Feel in the zones shown in *Figure 41*. Thrills suggest valvular or cardiac disease. Pulmonary stenosis may be associated with a thrill at the left sternal edge. A VSD may be associated with a thrill at the left lower sternal edge. Note that a thrill in aortic stenosis can often be felt in the suprasternal notch (*Figure 42*).

FIGURE 38

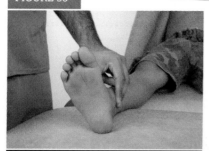

Assessing for pedal oedema. Palpate over the medial malleolus: push down for five seconds and then release.

FIGURE 40

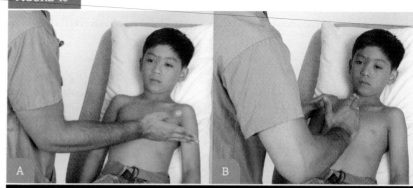

A   B

Feeling for: Left ventricular heaves. Horizontally place the ulnar side of the palm on the left side of the chest, at the level of the apex, feeling for impulses (A), and right ventricular heaves. Place the ulnar side of the palm vertically against the left sternal border (B).

FIGURE 39

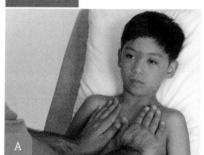

A

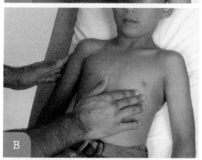

B

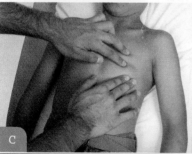

C

Feeling the apex beat: Feel both sides of the chest to identify which side the heart is on (A), localise the apex beat with one finger (B), and use the other hand to count the number of rib spaces from the sternal notch to the apex (C).

FIGURE 41

Sites to palpate for thrills.

- ● Suprasternal notch: aortic stenosis
- ● Subclavicular: patent ductus arteriosus
- ● Right upper sternal edge (2nd intercostal space): aortic lesions
- ● Left upper sternal edge (2nd intercostal space): pulmonary lesions
- ● Left lower sternal edge (5th intercostal space): tricuspid lesions/ VSDs
- ● Left midclavicular line (5th intercostal space): mitral lesions

FIGURE 42

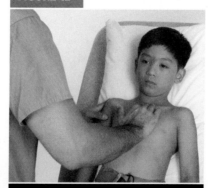

Feeling for a thrill of aortic stenosis with the tips of the fingers in the suprasternal notch.

Auscultation

In a baby that is sleeping, it may be prudent to auscultate first and then go back and carry out the rest of the examination. Smaller children may be anxious about a stethoscope, and various strategies can be employed to put them at ease (*Figure 43*). Listen in all of the same zones as were palpated for thrills (except the suprasternal notch) (*Figure 44*). Listen with the bell and the diaphragm in the mitral zone, and just the diaphragm elsewhere. Palpate a central pulse concurrently. Note that children are likely to find palpation of the carotid pulse uncomfortable for longer periods, so it may be preferable to palpate the brachial pulse.

FIGURE 43

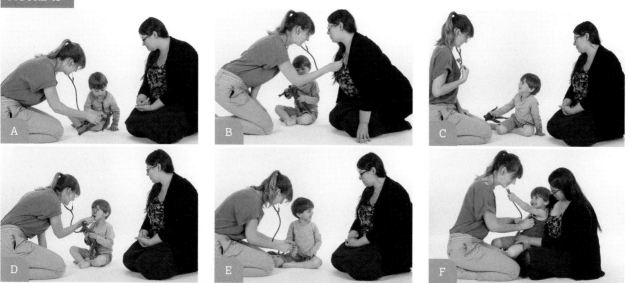

Examine a doll (A), examine the mother (B), and/or examine yourself (C) at the start if the child seems anxious. Then, before putting the stethoscope on the child's chest, put it in a more comfortable/comical place like their nose (D) or hand (E)! Even when doing the exam, let them be playful (F). There is a wide range of possibilities for entertaining/relaxing a child!

FIGURE 44

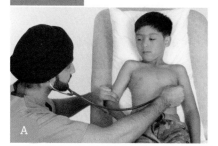
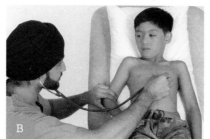
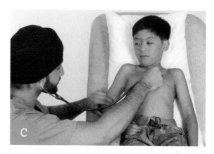

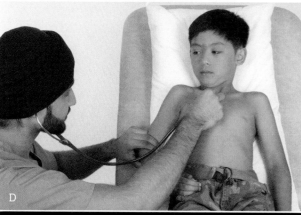

Auscultating for murmurs at: Mid clavicular line, 5th intercostal space (A), lower left sternal edge, 5th intercostal space (B), upper left sternal edge, 2nd intercostal space (C), and upper right sternal edge, 2nd intercostal space (D).

During auscultation, it is important to assess:

1 What heart sounds are present and whether they are normal or diminished. Fixed splitting of the second heart sound (no variation with respiration) is a feature of ASD and is best heard over ULSE. A loud second heart sound is associated with pulmonary hypertension or increased pulmonary blood flow, e.g. large VSD or PDA.

2 Presence of any additional heart sounds:
   a A third heart sound (S3) heard after the second heart sound can be normal but is also a possible sign of heart failure. It is best heard with the bell over the apex and will sound like "Kentucky," i.e. 1-2-3.
   b A fourth heart sound (S4) is rarely heard (it immediately precedes the first heart sound) but is pathological when present. It may indicate heart failure or pulmonary hypertension. This sounds like "Tennessee," in the order 4-1-2.
   c A gallop rhythm is heard in tachycardic patients with third and fourth heart sounds (sometimes just a loud third heart sound is heard as the third and fourth heart sounds have "fused" together).
   d Ejection clicks are associated with pulmonary and aortic stenoses due to the forceful opening of these valves.
   e A midsystolic click is associated with mitral valve prolapse. It occurs in the middle of systole, as the valve prolapses.
   f Opening snap. Heard after the second heart sound in mitral stenosis.

3 Whether any murmurs are present. Feel a central pulse simultaneously. If a murmur is present, assess:

a Loudness.

  i How loud is the murmur generally? This should be graded (*Table 4*).

  ii In which area of the chest is the murmur loudest?

  iii Check if the murmur gets louder with:

   1 Leaning forward (aortic lesions – *Figure 45*). Innocent murmurs may change with position (Still's murmur may be louder and venous hum quieter when the patient is supine).

   2 Inspiration (right sided lesions) /expiration (left sided lesions).

   3 Turning onto the left side (mitral lesions).

   4 Listening with the bell (mitral stenosis).

b Character. Harsh sounding murmurs are usually pathological.

c Timing. Systolic, diastolic, or continuous. Include length, i.e. ejection systolic vs. pansystolic.

d Radiation (*Figure 46*). Check if it radiates to the:

  i Back (pulmonary stenosis).

  ii Axilla (mitral regurgitation).

  iii Neck (aortic stenosis).

TABLE 4: Levine grading scale of cardiac murmurs

Grade	Thrill	Auscultation
1.	No.	Only faintly audible with a stethoscope.
2.	No.	Faint, but easily audible on auscultation.
3.	No.	Moderately loud and easily heard on auscultation.
4.	Yes.	Loud but not audible without a stethoscope.
5.	Yes.	Very loud but not audible without a stethoscope.
6.	Yes.	Audible without a stethoscope.

FIGURE 46

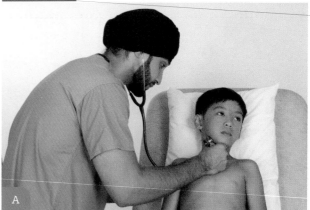
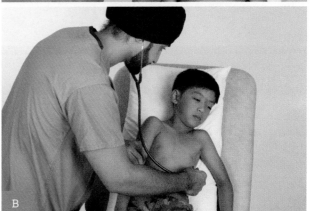
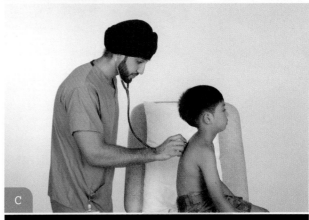

Auscultation for radiation to the: neck (A), axilla (B), and back (C).

FIGURE 45

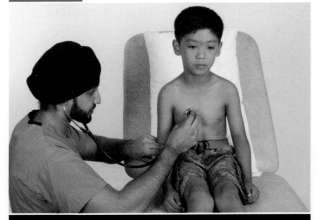

Leaning forwards to exaggerate aortic murmurs/ elicit positional variation for an innocent murmur.

Tables 5a-d below show some key cardiac lesions and their distinguishing features.

TABLE 5a: Pansystolic murmurs

Lesion	Site	Radiation	Additional features
VSD.	• LLSE.	• None.	• Squatting may make louder. • May have a thrill.
Mitral regurgitation.	• Apex.	• Axilla.	• Louder on expiration/rolling onto left.
Coarctation.	• ULSE/infrascapular.	• Back.	• Absent/reduced femoral pulses. • May also be a continuous murmur.

(LLSE = left lower sternal edge, ULSE = upper left sternal edge, VSD = Ventricular Septal Defect)

TABLE 5b: Ejection systolic murmurs

Lesion	Site	Radiation	Additional features
Pulmonary stenosis.	• ULSE.	• Back.	• Louder on (i) lying flat, and (ii) inspiration.
Aortic stenosis.	• URSE.	• Carotids.	• Louder on (i) sitting forward, and (ii) expiration.
ASD.	• ULSE.	• None.	• Fixed splitting of S2. • May be an associated diastolic tricuspid flow murmur if there is a large left-to-right shunt.
Pulmonary flow murmur.	• LLSE (usually).	• None.	• Soft, short, non-harsh, no thrill.

(LLSE = left lower sternal edge, ULSE = upper left sternal edge, URSE = upper right sternal edge, LLSE = left lower sternal edge, ASD = Atrial Septal Defect)

TABLE 5c: Diastolic murmurs

Lesion	Site	Radiation	Additional features
Mitral stenosis.	• Apex.	• Axilla.	• Mid diastolic. • Louder on (i) rolling onto the left, and (ii) expiration.
Aortic regurgitation.	• URSE.	• Also heard at LLSE.	• Early diastolic. • Louder on (i) sitting forward, and (ii) expiration. • Collapsing pulse.

(LLSE = left lower sternal edge, URSE = upper right sternal edge)

TABLE 5d: Continuous murmurs

Lesion	Site	Radiation	Additional features
PDA.	• Under left clavicle.	• Back.	• Bounding pulses.
BT shunt murmur (palliative procedure for TOF, pulmonary atresia, critical PS etc).	• URSE.	• Widespread.	• Will have right or left thoracotomy scar. • Child likely to be cyanosed.
Coarctation.	• ULSE/infrascapular.	• Back.	• Absent/reduced femoral pulses. • May also be pansystolic.

(URSE = upper right sternal edge, ULSE = upper left sternal edge, BT = Blalock–Taussig, TOF = Tetralogy of Fallot, PS = Pulmonary Stenosis)

Completing the Examination

> Do a general paediatric examination.

Bedside tests include:

> Review the observation chart.

> Plot the height and weight on an age and sex appropriate chart.

> ECG.

> Urine dipstick, looking for haematuria as evidence of endocarditis.

> Fundoscopy if endocarditis is suspected.

541

CASE SCENARIO

SCENARIO 1

Thomas is a six-year-old boy who has attended clinic today for review of his murmur. You have been asked to perform a cardiovascular examination on him and present your findings.

✔ EXAMINATION CHECKLIST

Domain	Findings	Evolving thought process
Global assessment of child.	• Well. • Some dysmorphic features. • Looks small.	• Unlikely to have an acute pathology. • May have an underlying syndrome, which may be associated with a cardiac disorder. • Needs to have height/weight plotted.
Inspection.	• Upslanting palpebral fissures. • Flat nasal bridge. • Not cyanosed. • No scars.	• Cardiac lesion not severe enough to require surgery or to cause cyanosis. • May have Trisomy 21, which is associated with VSD, ASD, and AVSDs.
Palpation.	• Normally placed apex. • No thrills or heave. • Normal pulses.	• No additional pathology identified.
Auscultation.	• Normal heart sounds. • No click. • 3/6 pansystolic murmur LLSE. • Does not radiate.	• Consistent with VSD.

DEVELOPMENTAL ASSESSMENT

This section will focus on performing a developmental assessment in a child under five years. A full assessment is usually only conducted by subspecialty paediatricians, so here broad assessments of each of the key domains will be touched upon. Within this, it should be possible to assess the developmental age of a child to within about six months. For each domain, given an approximate developmental age, establish what the child can do and importantly what they cannot do - although they may not display what they can do if they decide not to co-operate!

The developmental examination should answer:

1   Is this child's development appropriate for their age?
2   If there is delay, is it one domain or is it global?

TABLE 6: Patient conditions that may appear in clinical examinations

Condition	Possible clues
Cerebral Palsy – diplegia or hemiplegia.	• Isolated motor delay – gross and fine possibly.
Duchenne Muscular Dystrophy.	• Delayed motor milestones. • May also be speech delay.
Trisomy 21.	• Delayed motor milestones due to hypotonia. • May be hearing concerns. • Typical facial features.
Autism Spectrum Disorder.	• Delays in speech and social interaction.
Global developmental delay.	• Delay in more than two domains.
Normal child.	• No delay evident.

PRESENTING YOUR FINDINGS

Thomas is a 6-year-old boy seen in clinic for review today.

Thomas looks well and appears comfortable and acyanotic at rest. He has dysmorphic facies, with upslanting palpebral fissures and a wide flat nasal bridge.

Thomas has a normal pulse rhythm and volume with a rate of 92 beats per minute. He has no scars on his chest. His apex beat is non-displaced.

On auscultation of his chest, he has a 3/6 pansystolic murmur heard loudest at the lower left sternal edge that does not radiate. There is no evidence of cardiac failure.

These findings are consistent with a VSD in a child with Trisomy 21.

To complete my examination, I would like to plot Thomas' height and weight on an age and sex, trisomy 21 appropriate growth chart, measure his BP and perform an ECG. To confirm the diagnosis of a VSD, Thomas would need to be referred for an echocardiogram.

Summary Checklist
Global assessment of the child on the approach.

Gross motor skills. How the child moves overall.

Fine motor skills and vision. Interacting with objects, drawing, building blocks.

Language and hearing. Expressive and receptive language.

Social and self-care. Interactions with others.

Completing the examination. Testing other domains. If not done, a neurological examination may be appropriate.

Bedside tests. Plot height/weight, review observation chart.

3 If there is delay, is it significant or mild?

Common exam scenarios are shown in *Table 6*.

General Advice

When testing a child's development, here are some top tips:

▸ Have a logical schema in mind for assessing each of the domains. Leave gross motor skills to the end in the older child as this will involve getting them to run and jump and after this they may not be so willing to sit down and draw!

▸ Check that the child can speak/understand English, can see and can hear.

▸ If testing requires use of equipment, e.g. a pencil or bricks, observe what the child does with them first before asking for a specific task.

▸ Test what the child can do and test what the child cannot do to obtain the maximum developmental age.

▸ Get down to the same level as the child. An adult standing over a child is very intimidating.

▸ Involve the parent in the activity if the child is wary.

▸ Remove the equipment from one activity before moving onto the next so that there are not too many distractions for the child.

▸ If a child is unable to perform a task, then they are "unable to demonstrate to me today" rather than they cannot. It may be that they just did not want to perform on the day, so always base your summary on what you have seen today rather than dismissing the child completely.

Starting the Examination

Before examining the child, initial thoughts can be gathered. These will be specific to the child being examined, but may include:

1 Dysmorphic features. This may hint at a possible underlying cause for developmental delay.

2 Paraphernalia in the room. Mobility aids, e.g. wheelchairs imply motor delay. Medications around the bed may point to a possible diagnosis.

3 Interactions with parents, and general behaviour. Much of the developmental assessment may happen without formal assessment occurring. The child may be running and jumping around the room: instantly, the gross motor development is likely to be at least 3-years-old. They may be speaking in two word phrases to mum: speech development is at least 18-months-old.

4 Gross appearance of the child. From this initial observation, it should be possible to guess a rough age range for the child. It should be possible to tell roughly if a child is under 6-months-old, 6 to 12-months-old, 1 to 3-years-old or over 3-years-old, although of course with faltering growth, estimates may be misleading.

Gross Motor Skills

The tests below are roughly listed based on what is expected in younger children first. Start at what appears to be the most

appropriate stage. If the child looks under six-months-old, start at the beginning. If they demonstrated walking with a steady gait on entering the room, there is no need to test for developmental milestones achieved before this landmark.

1 Movements and position at rest. Are they moving all four limbs, and are they moving them equally? Can they roll over? (5 to 6-months-old).

2 Primitive reflexes (non-mobile child).

   a Moro. Sudden downward dropping of head (whilst supporting bottom) results in both arms being flexed/abducted (< 3-months-old).

   b Grasp. Examiner places finger in baby's hand, and the baby reacts by grasping it. (< 3-months-old).

   c Stepping. Holding the baby upright on a flat surface, the baby lifts one foot and then the other as if stepping/walking (< 4-months-old, and reappears at 12-months-old).

   d Asymmetrical tonic neck reflex. With the baby lying on their back: when their head moves to one side, the arm and leg on the side the head is turned towards extend, and the opposite arm and leg flex (< 6-months-old).

3 Place in ventral suspension. Is there any head lag?

   a Some head lag (6-weeks-old).

   b No head lag. Also able to lift head above midline (3-months-old).

4 Place them prone. Can they:

   a Lift head and/or raise chest resting on elbows? (3-months-old).

   b Raise chest with fully extended arms? (5 to 6-months-old).

5 Place the child in a sitting position. Can they:

   a Sit supported/unsupported with a curved back (5 to 6-months-old).

   b Sit unsupported with a straight back (8 to 9-months-old).

   c Crawl/bum shuffle (8 to 9-months-old).

6 Pull to a standing position. Can they:

   a Stay in a standing position? (10-months-old).

7 Moving on two legs. Can they:

   a Cruise. Walk while holding on to things (10-months-old).

   b Walk.

      i With an unsteady gait (12-months-old).

      ii With a steady gait (15-months-old).

   c Run (18-months-old).

   d Stoop down to pick things up (18-months-old).

   e Jump and kick a ball (2-years-old).

   f Ride a tricycle (3-years-old).

   g Hop (4-years-old).

   h Stand one foot for ten seconds (5-years-old).

8 Walking up and down stairs.

   a 2 feet per step (2-years-old).

   b 1 foot per step going up, 2 feet per step going down (3-years-old).

   c 1 foot per step going up, 1 foot per step going down (4-years-old).

9 Other.
- a Bounces and catches a ball (5-years-old).
- b May be able to ride a bike without stabilisers (5-years-old).

Fine Motor and Vision

Start by generally observing the child playing, and crudely assess what they can do. Assess them whilst on the same level as they are, and make sure that there are no distractions around (e.g. clear up building blocks when another test is being done). Give them a crayon and see what they draw. Then draw the different images (from a line to a triangle, depending on the child's age). Cover the image when drawing it so that the child cannot see how you have drawn it (*Figure 47*). This tests copying. If the child can see how you have drawn the image, this instead tests imitation, which happens earlier than copying. For each construction with the bricks, produce it for the child first, and then break the construction, and ask them to make it again (*Figure 48*). If they cannot do this, try asking them to imitate the construction, where they see how you have made it.

Fine motor landmarks are shown in *Table 7 and 8*.

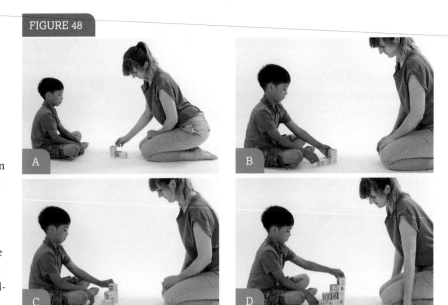

FIGURE 48

Demonstrating building a L-shaped train (A), child replicating a L-shaped train (B), child replicating 6 brick stairs (C), and child replicating ten brick stairs (D).

Additional skills tested include:

> Scissors.
>> Using both hands (2-years-old).
>> One handed (3-years-old).
>> Cuts a page in half. Cuts along a line progressing to cutting out shapes (4-years-old).
> Page turning.
>> Skimming pages (15 to 18-months-old).
>> Turning pages singly (2-years-old).
> Threading beads.
>> Can thread large beads (3-years-old).
>> Can thread small beads (4-years-old).

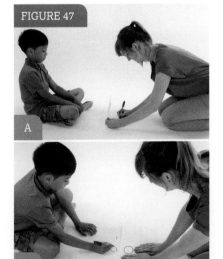

FIGURE 47

Drawing images in a manner that is hidden from the child (A), and exposing each image individually for the child to copy (B).

TABLE 7: Fine motor landmarks (Under 1)	
Age	**Action**
6 weeks.	• Holds hand in fist. • Grasps anything put in palm.
6 months.	• Palmar grasp. • Reaches out for objects. • Brings object to midline. • Hand to hand transfer (taking an object from one hand and putting it in the other). • Mouthing objects (putting them in their mouth).
9 months.	• Crude pincer grip.
10 months.	• Fine pincer grip.
12 months.	• Casts objects away. • Bangs objects together. • Object permanence (can be tested simply by dropping a toy and seeing if the child looks for a fallen object). • Points at things.

Vision

Test ability to fix and follow. Hold up an interesting (silent) object and see if the child follows it with their eyes. Children can follow to 90 degrees by six-weeks-old, and 180 degrees by three-months-old.

Speech, Language and Hearing

Ask/assess whether there are any concerns about hearing at the beginning and if English is the first language. Then speak to the child, getting them to speak back. Note landmarks described in *Table 9*. Useful props include picture books and small objects (e.g. bear, pencil and cup).

Social and Self-care

This comes from observing the child, playing games with them, and getting a thorough history from the parents (*Table 10*).

Completing the Examination

➤ Do a general paediatric examination.
➤ Perform a neurological examination.
➤ Examine the eyes and hearing.

Bedside tests include:
➤ Review the observation chart.
➤ Plot the height and weight on an age and sex appropriate chart.

TABLE 8: Fine motor landmarks (Over 1)

Age	Drawing		Building blocks	
15 months.	Marks paper (cylindrical grasp).		Tower of 2.	
18 months.	To and fro scribble.		Tower of 3.	
2 years.	Circular scribble.		Tower of 6.	
2.5 years.	Copies line.		–	–
3 years.	Copies circle (tripod grasp).		Tower of 9.	
			Train with chimney (L shaped).	
3.5 years.	Copies cross.		3 brick bridge.	
4 years.	Copies square.		6 cube stairs.	
5 years.	Copies triangle (and can draw person, house with chimney/windows/door).		10 cube stairs.	

TABLE 9: Speech and language milestones

Age	Understanding (receptive language)	Vocalising (Expressive language)	Age	Understanding (receptive language)	Vocalising (Expressive language)
Newborn.		• Crying.	2 years.	• Verbs and two part commands.	• 50 words and 2 word phrases.
6 weeks.	• Startles to noise.		2.5 years.	• Prepositions (e.g. put doll under table).	• 3-4 words together.
3-4 months.	• Turns to sound.	• Cooing.	3 years.	• Comparatives (e.g. which circle is the biggest?). • Adjectives (e.g. which one is red?). • Negatives (e.g. which is not a fork?).	• What/where questions. Can give full name and sex.
5-6 months.	• Turns to own name.	• Babbling.			
8-9 months.		• "Mama" "dada" said indiscriminately.			
10 months.	• Understands "no".				
12 months.	• A few simple nouns (e.g. "mum") and first name.	• A few individual words.	4 years.	• Follows three part/complex instructions (e.g. first give me the pencil, then grab the key and put it in the cup).	• Why/when/how questions. • Talks in narratives/ sequences. • 4-5 word sentences.
15 months.	• Follows simple commands. Points to body parts.				
18 months.	• Lots of simple nouns (e.g. leg). Knows 2-3 body parts.	• 10-20 words.	5 years.	• Enjoys jokes.	• Talks about past/ present/future.

TABLE 10: Social/self-care milestones	
Age	**Social**
6 weeks.	• Social smile i.e. child smiling back at you or when pleased.
8-9 months.	• Stranger anxiety (up until two years). • Plays peekaboo. • Holds/bites food.
12 months.	• Waves bye-bye. • Claps • Points. • Drinks from beaker.
18 months.	• Imitative play / domestic mimicry (copies parent's actions at home). • Symbolic play, e.g. brushes doll's hair, may feed/put doll to bed. • Removes socks / shoes.
2 years.	• Temper tantrums. • Plays alongside other children (parallel play). • Eats with spoon. • Starts toilet training. • Loses stranger anxiety.
3 years.	• Plays with other children. • Shares. • Eats with fork and spoon.
4 years.	• Dresses and undresses. • Concern/sympathy for others. • Understands turn-taking. • Eats with Knife and fork.
5 years.	• Very definite likes and dislikes. • Can amuse themselves for long periods of time. • Can care for pets. • Chooses best friends.

🔍 PRESENTING YOUR FINDINGS

Eva is a six-month-old corrected premature infant. She appears well, with no dysmorphic features.

On assessment of her gross motor skills, she demonstrated the ability to sit supported with a curved back. When held in ventral suspension, she demonstrated the ability to lift her head above the midline.

On assessment of her fine motor skills, Eva demonstrated the ability to bring both hands to the midline.

Socially, she demonstrated the ability to smile.

From my assessment of Eva, I would place her around the six month age based on her fine motor skills and between four and six months based on her gross motor skills.

I would like to assess the rest of Eva's development, plot her length, weight and head circumference on an appropriate centile chart and perform a neurological examination. If these were all normal, I would keep her development under review until the age of two years.

 ## CASE SCENARIOS

SCENARIO 2

Eva is an ex-premature infant, born at 28 weeks gestation, now nine-months-old (six-months-old corrected).

Observations during the developmental assessment are shown in *Figure 49*.

FIGURE 49

A. Placed in sitting position. B. Placed in ventral suspension. C. Observing hand movements. D. Observing social interactions.

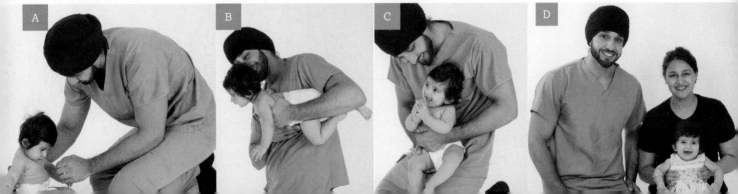

SCENARIO 3

James is an 18-month-old that has attended clinic today as a result of concerns about his development.

Observations during gross motor assessment are shown in *Figure 50*, and fine motor/vision assessment in *Figure 51*.

FIGURE 50

A. Moving along floor. B. Interacting with an object placed in front of him. C. Unsupported on both feet.

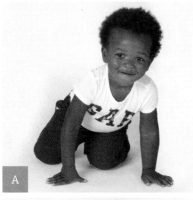
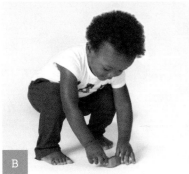
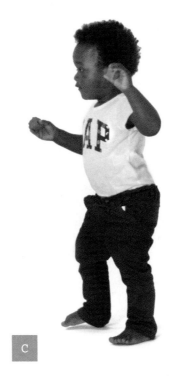

🔍 **PRESENTING YOUR FINDINGS**

James is an 18-month-old boy. He appears well, with no dysmorphic features.

On assessment of his gross motor skills, James demonstrated crawling and standing with a steady stance. He was able to stoop down to the floor to pick a toy up with good balance.

On assessment of his fine motor skills, James demonstrated to and fro scribbling but did not demonstrate circular scribbling. Although able to turn a thick-paged book, James skimmed multiple pages of a paper book at once.

From my assessment of James, I would place him around the 18 month age, based on his fine motor and gross motor skills.

I would like to assess the rest of James' development, plot his length, weight and head circumference on an appropriate centile chart and perform a neurological examination. If these were all normal, I would explore further what the specific development concerns were, and send off any appropriate investigations.

FIGURE 51

A. Using pen and paper. B. Using thick paged book. C. Using thin paged book.

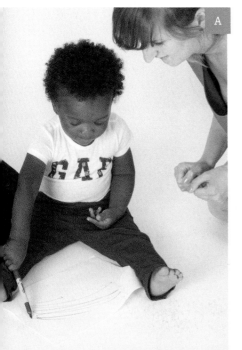
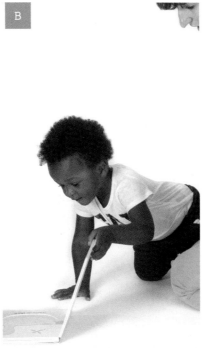
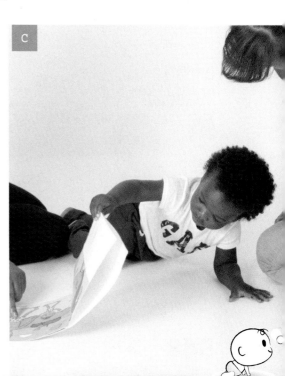

SCENARIO 4

Tristan has been brought to clinic today for a developmental review.

Gross motor assessment is shown in *Figure 52*. Fine motor/vision assessment is shown in *Figure 53-6*. Additionally, it is noted that he can copy a circle but not a cross. Speech and language assessment is shown in *Figure 57-9*. Social behaviour/self-care is shown in *Figure 60*. There was no stranger anxiety throughout the interaction.

FIGURE 56

Fine motor assessment. A. Turning pages of a book. B. Threading beads onto string. C. Cutting paper using scissors.

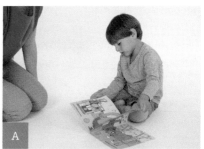

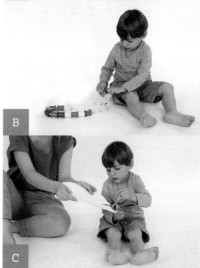

FIGURE 52

Gross motor assessment. A. Standing on one leg. B. Jumping. C. Kicking a ball.

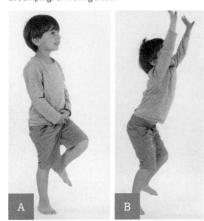

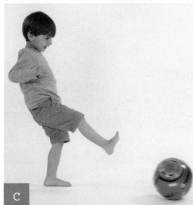

FIGURE 54

Fine motor assessment. A. Demonstrating a bridge, and driving a pen through it. B. Copying building a bridge a driving a pen through it.

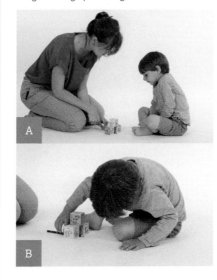

FIGURE 55

Fine motor assessment. A. Demonstrating six brick stairs. B. Attempting to copy six brick stairs.

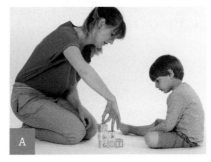

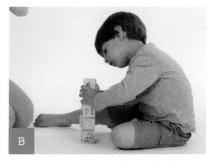

FIGURE 53

Fine motor assessment. A. Demonstrating a brick tower. B. Copying a tower of three. C. Copying a tower of six. D. Attempting to copy a tower of eight, but it becomes unstable.

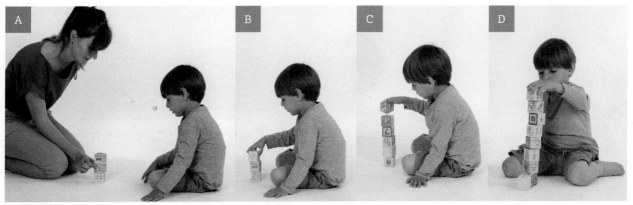

EXAMINATION

FIGURE 57

Tristan is asked questions surrounding a picture book.

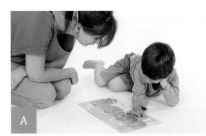

"Who is the biggest?"

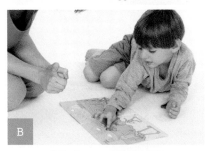

"Who is not on the beach?"

FIGURE 58

Tristan is asked to point to his head.

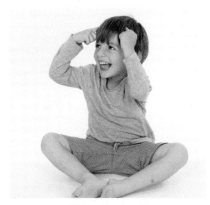

"Touch your head!"

FIGURE 59

Tristan is given instructions with a pen, cup and teddy bear in front of him.

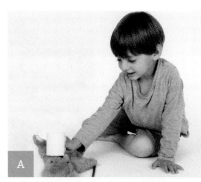

"Put the cup on the teddy!"

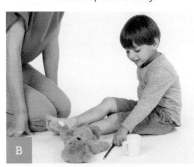

"Which one do you write with?"

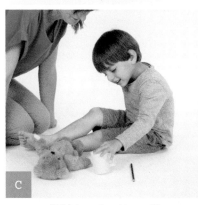

"Which one is not brown?"

FIGURE 60

A. Playing. B. Drinking.

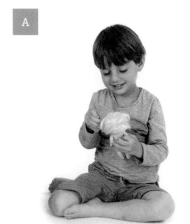

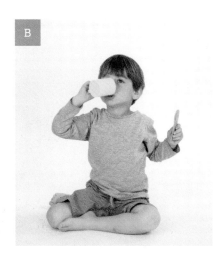

Q PRESENTING YOUR FINDINGS

I was asked to examine Tristan's development today. Tristan appeared well grown and there were no dysmorphic features.

Assessing Tristan's gross motor skills, he demonstrated standing on one leg, jumping and kicking a ball. This would put his gross motor skills at those of a 3-year-old.

Tristan demonstrated copying circles but not crosses. He demonstrated building a tower of six bricks and a three brick bridge. He did not demonstrate building a set of steps using six bricks, and on attempting to build an eight brick tower, the tower became unstable. Tristan turned book pages one at a time. He was able to thread large beads onto string and used scissors two-handed to cut. This would put his fine motor skills at those of a 3-year-old.

Tristan demonstrated knowledge and understanding of size comparatives, body parts, prepositions, object function and negatives. This would put his speech and language skills at those of a 3-year-old.

Finally, Tristan demonstrated symbolic play and was able to use a cup with one hand. There was no stranger anxiety throughout the interaction. I would like more information on social development, but it is likely to be in line with other parameters.

Overall, I would estimate Tristan's age to be 3-years-old. To complete my examination, I would like to plot his height, weight and head circumference on an appropriate centile chart and perform a neurological examination.

SCENARIO 5

Ritchie has been brought to clinic today due to parental concerns that his development is not as advanced as his peers.

Gross motor assessment is shown in *Figure 61*. Fine motor/vision assessment is shown in *Figure 62*. Additionally, it is noted that he can copy a triangle and build a ten brick staircase. Speech and language assessment is shown in *Figure 63-4*. Social and self-care are shown in *Figure 65*.

FIGURE 63

Receptive language. A brick, spoon and teddy bear are placed in front of the child.

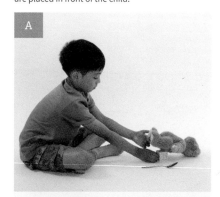

"Put the brick under the teddy!"

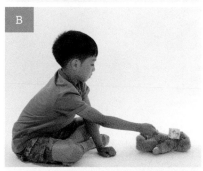

"Pick up the brick with the spoon and feed it to the teddy!"

FIGURE 61

Gross motor assessment.
A. Hopping. B. Ball catching.

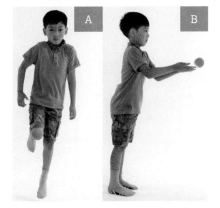

FIGURE 62

Fine motor assessment. Cutting technique.

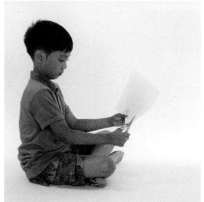

FIGURE 64

Using expressive language

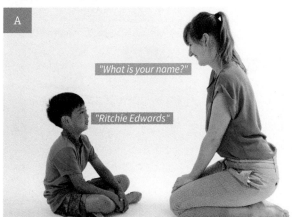

"What is your name?"

"Ritchie Edwards"

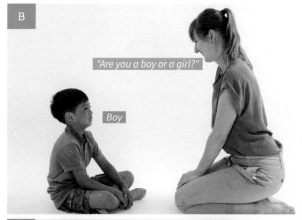

"Are you a boy or a girl?"

Boy

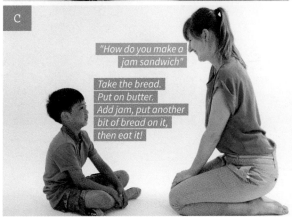

"How do you make a jam sandwich"

Take the bread. Put on butter. Add jam, put another bit of bread on it, then eat it!

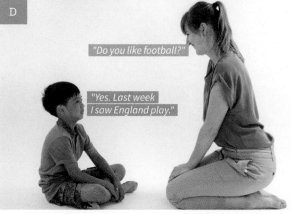

"Do you like football?"

"Yes. Last week I saw England play."

FIGURE 65

Social/self care assessment. A. Eating with a knife and fork. B. Doing up buttons.

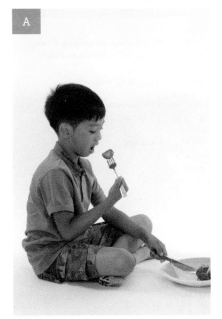

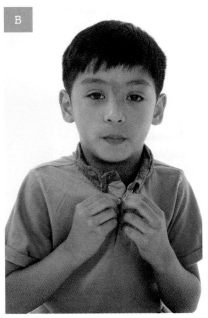

Q | PRESENTING YOUR FINDINGS

I assessed all four domains of Ritchie's development today. Ritchie appeared well grown and there were no obvious dysmorphic features. He has what appears to be a cafe-au-lait birthmark in centre of his forehead.

Assessing Ritchie's gross motor skills, he demonstrated hopping and catching a ball underarm. Mum tells me that he walks up and down stairs in an adult fashion. This would put his gross motor skills at those of a 5-year-old.

Assessing Ritchie's fine motor skills, he demonstrated building steps of 10 bricks. Ritchie demonstrated copying shapes including a triangle. He was able to cut in a straight-line using the scissors one-handed. This would put his fine motor skills at those of a 5-year-old.

Assessing Ritchie's speech, he was able to comprehend prepositions, and complex instructions, putting his receptive language at least at the level of a 4-year-old. His expressive language included knowing his name, and gender, as well as speaking in short sentences, with an appreciation for sequences of events. He was also able to talk about the past. His expressive language was at the level of a 5-year-old.

Ritchie demonstrated eating with a knife and fork and doing up buttons, which puts him at least at the level of a 4-year-old.

Based on my assessments today, Ritchie's development is in keeping with a child of 4.5 to 5 years of age.

To complete my examination, I would like to plot his head circumference, height and weight on a centile chart and perform a relevant neurological examination.

FIGURE 67

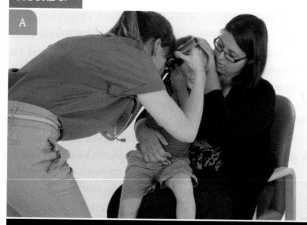

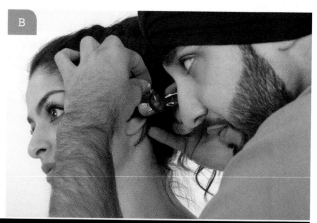

A. Positioning a young child for otoscopy. Younger children should be seated in their parent's lap, facing to one side. The parent should then place one arm around the child's body, and the other around the child's forehead. Ensure one finger from the hand holding the otoscope rests against the face to protect against sudden movements. The holding of the child both comforts them and prevents them from sudden movements. Pull the ear down and back to better visualise the eardrum. B. Positioning an older child for otoscopy. In older children, pull the ear up and back.

TABLE 12: Summary of otitis externa and otitis media

Otitis Externa	Otitis Media
• Ear pain.	• Ear pain.
• Hearing may be muffled.	• Fever.
• Ear may be itchy.	• May tug at ear.
• Red ear canal.	• Bulging tympanic membrane.
• Ear discharge.	• Effusion (purulent) behind tympanic membrane.
• Usually unilateral.	• Can be bilateral.

› Teeth and gums. A koplick spot is white spot found on buccal mucosa opposite the lower molars. It indicates measles. Oral thrush will result in a white coating/spots to the tongue and/or gums.

Completing the Examination

› Perform a general paediatric examination.

› Hepatosplenomegaly. In the context of an acute pharyngitis/tonsillitis is likely to indicate EBV infection.

› Rash. Examine the rest of the body for rash, including feet.

FIGURE 68

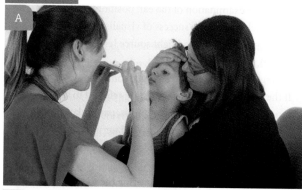

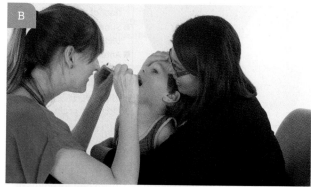

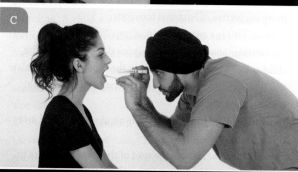

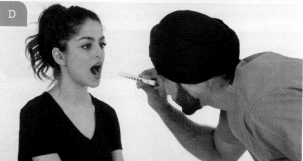

Throat examination. A/B. Younger child being positioned by parent, sat on their lap facing forward. The parent places one hand on the forehead and one arm around the child, enclosing both arms. C/D. Older child, with or without tongue depressor, depending on adequacy of view.

Bedside tests include:

> Review the observation chart.
> Plot the height and weight on an age and sex appropriate chart.
> Swab any discharge or tonsillar pus.
> Urine dip for proteinuria/haematuria as throat infections can cause a glomerulonephritis.

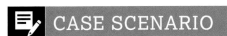
CASE SCENARIO

SCENARIO 6

Paul is a 2-year-old boy who has presented to ED with fever, coryza and reduced appetite. Please perform an ENT examination.

EXAMINATION CHECKLIST

Domain	Findings	Evolving thought process
Global assessment of child on approach.	• Alert. • Looks miserable. • Coryzal.	• May have an upper respiratory tract infection (URTI).
Inspection.	• Pulling at ear. • No discharge from ear. • Mouth closed. • No chest recessions.	• Ear pain, possible ear infection.
Palpation.	• Tachycardia. • Normal BP. • Small cervical lymph nodes. • Feels hot.	• Tachycardia secondary to pain/fever/possible sepsis.
Throat examination.	• Tonsils not enlarged or red. • No exudate.	• Tonsils not inflamed.
Ear examination.	• Right ear drum dull and bulging. • Ear canal red.	• Likely right otitis media.

PRESENTING YOUR FINDINGS

Paul is a 2-year-old boy whom I have seen in ED. He presented with a history of fever, coryza and a reduced appetite.

Paul appears to have an acute febrile illness and appears miserable with this. He is febrile and tachycardic, with a normal blood pressure. On examination, Paul is coryzal and is pulling at his right ear. He has some cervical lymphadenopathy.

Examining his right ear, the ear canal is erythematous and his tympanic membrane is red and bulging. His tonsils are normal.

These findings are consistent with an upper respiratory tract infection, specifically a right-sided otitis media. To complete my examination, I will examine for lymph nodes elsewhere, palpate for hepatosplenomegaly and examine for other possible sources of infection.

If his heart rate comes down after administration of analgesia/antipyretics, I would advise discharge, analgesia and antipyretics as needed and regular fluid intake. If it does not, he requires reassessment, as he may be septic or have an infection from another source.

EXAMINATION OF THE EYE

Eye examination is carried out in the following situations:

1 If there is a change in the quality or size of the visual field. In younger children, clues to this may be the child bumping into things or being more clumsy than usual.
2 If malalignment of the eyes is noted or there is double vision. This may be noticed by parents, or teachers.
3 If there are neurological signs/symptoms. This includes any other neurological features, such as headaches.

Common patients that are likely to appear in exams are shown in *Table 13*.

Starting the Examination

The examination begins by observing the child on entering the room. Begin with a broad assessment:

1 Does the child look well or unwell? Do they have any dysmorphic features (e.g. Trisomy 21 is associated with squints)? Any features of cerebellar disease (e.g. tremor)?
2 Does the child wear glasses? The use of glasses implies a partially correctable visual defect. If a refractive error is being corrected, the thickness of lenses is a good proxy marker for the severity of the defect.

TABLE 13: Common patients that may appear in clinical examinations	
Diagnosis	Possible clues
Squint (Strabismus).	• Most likely to be intermittent and related to refractive errors (child will have glasses).
Nystagmus.	• Can be congenital. • May be part of oculocutaneous albinism. • May be associated with cerebellar signs.
Cranial nerve palsy.	• III. Eye position is down and out, pupil may be dilated, and associated with ptosis. Can be congenital or secondary to tumour. • IV. Impaired depression of the eye from the abducted position. It can be congenital or acquired, e.g. due to head trauma. It often causes double vision and the head to be tilted. • VI. Impaired abduction (looking outwards) of affected eye. It can be congenital or acquired, e.g. trauma, raised intracranial pressure, or tumours.

Summary Checklist

Global assessment of child on approach.

Inspection. Glasses, eye position, pupil size/symmetry, eyelids, conjunctiva.

Visual acuity. Both eyes together and then each individually.

Visual fields. Test all four quadrants.

Eye movements. In eight directions.

Accommodation reflex. Look for convergence and constriction of pupils.

Pupillary reflexes. Direct and indirect.

Fundoscopy/slit lamp. Slit lamp via specialist.

Squint testing. Latent vs. manifest. Paralytic vs. non-paralytic.

Bedside tests. Review observations; plot height and weight.

Inspection

▸ Eye position. Look at where the pupils are in relation the rest of the eyes (*Figure 69*). In a squint, the pupils may be pointing in a different direction.

› Nystagmus will be demonstrated by rhythmic to and fro movements of the eye. It can be horizontal, vertical or circular in direction and is involuntary. Any nystagmus identified should prompt assessment of hearing and the cerebellum.

› Opsoclonus is brief, rapid movements of the eyes in all directions. It is described as "dancing eyes". Opsoclonus myoclonus syndrome is a condition of opsoclonus, myoclonus and ataxia that, in children, may be due to infection but importantly can be a paraneoplastic phenomenon of neuroblastoma.

▸ Pupil size/symmetry. The pupils should be equal in size, and neither dilated or constricted, although this will vary depending on the lighting.

▸ Ptosis. A droopy eyelid could be congenital or a sign of a facial nerve palsy.

▸ Conjunctiva. Conjunctivitis implies inflammation of the eye, which may relate to allergy or an infection. Conjunctivitis may be purulent, which implies an infective cause, or non-purulent. Non-purulent conjunctivitis is a feature of Kawasaki disease. It can be differentiated from uveitis,

which also causes a red eye, as the redness in conjunctivitis is usually greatest in the periphery of the eye. In uveitis, the redness increases approaching the limbus (the border between the sclera and the cornea) and is associated with pain and visual disturbances.

Special Tests

▸ Visual acuity. This should be measured for both eyes together, and then each eye individually. It should also be measured both with and without glasses if they are needed. Start at six metres, and if clear vision is not possible at this distance, progressively move in by one metre at a time. A Snellen chart is ideal, but for younger children picture charts might be used. In those with significant visual defects, detecting light and dark might be all that is possible.

▸ Visual fields. Initially test vision with both eyes open, and then test each eye individually. Test all four quadrants of vision. Confrontational testing should be used, whereby the examiner compares their visual fields to that of the patient as performed during cranial nerve examination (p587). Colour vision can be tested using a red pin, and similarly this can be used to map out the blind spot.

▸ Eye movements. (*Figure 132-5*).

▸ Rapid eye movements. Not routinely done, but may pick up nystagmus. (*Figure 70*)

▸ Accommodation. (*Figure 130*).

▸ Pupillary reflexes. (*Figure 131*).

▸ Fundoscopy/slit lamp examination. Fundoscopy is useful for assessing the red reflex (particularly in identifying congenital cataracts) (*Figure 71*). Look at the optic disc (particularly to identify papilloedema) (*Figure 72*). Slit lamp allows more detailed assessment by specialists.

Strabismus (malalignment of the eyes)

If strabismus (a squint) is noted, it is important to describe:

▸ Timing. Latent (intermittent, i.e. only appears when fixation is interrupted, e.g. covering the eye) or manifest (always

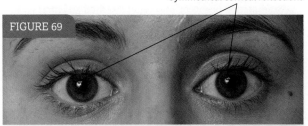

FIGURE 69

Symmetrical corneal reflections

Normal eyes. Note that the white light reflections (corneal reflections) are in identical positions in both eyes.

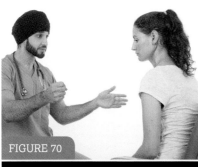

FIGURE 70

Rapid eye movements. Make a fist with one hand, and keep an open palm with the other hand. Position both hands about 1m apart, and alternatively state "fist" and "palm", asking the patient to look at each in response. This may elicit nystagmus. Do this with the hands separated in both the horizontal and vertical plane.

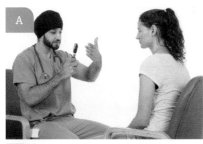

A

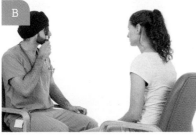

B

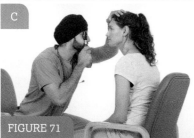

C

FIGURE 71

Fundoscopy. A. Use a hand to check the opthalmoscope is in focus. B. Start at a distance checking the red reflex. C. Move in closer (use the right eye to look at the patient's right eye). Stabilise the patient's head with the other hand.

visible when eyes both open). Phoria denotes a latent squint, trophia denotes a manifest squint.
> Direction. Upward vs downward vs convergent (going inward - eso) vs divergent (going outward -exo). This

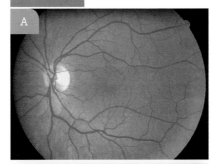

A

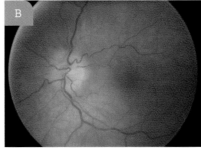

B

A. Normal optic disc. B. Papilloedema with blurred disc margins.

can be combined with trophia or phoria, e.g. an esotrophic squint is where the eye turns inwards.
> Eyes affected. Monocular (one eye) vs binocular (both eyes).
> Paralysis. Paralytic (nerve palsy/ muscle weakness) vs non-paralytic. Most squints are non-paralytic. An acquired paralytic squint is usually caused by a tumour or brain trauma.

The above can be identified by:
1 Inspection. A manifest squint will be obvious without any special tests.
2 Corneal reflections (*Figure 69*). These should be in identical positions on both eyes on top of the pupil. If not, they are malaligned.
3 Eye movements. Perform the H test to identify paralysis (p587).
4 Cover/uncover test. Ask the child to fix on an object approximately one metre away. Cover each eye in turn and observe for movement of the uncovered eye. Repeat twice to identify more subtle movement.
  a When there is a squint present already, if the normal eye is covered, the eye with a squint may (*Figure 73*):

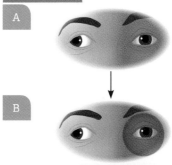

FIGURE 73A

A

B

Cover/uncover test. A. Divergent squint at rest. B. Squint does not disappear on covering the left eye. The squint is manifest and paralytic.

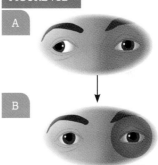

FIGURE 73B

A

B

Cover/uncover test. A. Divergent squint at rest. B. Squint disappears on covering the left eye. The squint is manifest and non-paralytic.

i Correct and fix on the object being focused on (non-paralytic squint). This is because the dominant eye is no longer receiving an image, and so the eye with the squint becomes dominant. On uncovering the normal eye, the manifest squint will reappear, and the dominant eye will take up fixation again.
ii Stay in the same position (paralytic). In this situation, e.g. cranial nerve II palsy, the eye cannot move because of a neuropathy.
Note that covering the eye with the squint should not make a difference to the normal eye, as the normal eye is already fixed on an object.
  b When there is no squint present at rest.

557

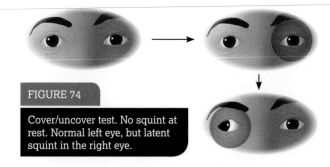

FIGURE 74

Cover/uncover test. No squint at rest. Normal left eye, but latent squint in the right eye.

i Covering a seemingly normal eye may reveal a latent squint. This is because fixation of that eye is interrupted. It can be identified by either looking through a semitransparent "cover" or by quickly removing the cover, and looking for correction of the eye.

CASE SCENARIOS

SCENARIO 7

Joy is a nine-year-old girl who has attended clinic today because of intermittent double vision. You have been asked to examine her eyes and present your findings.

✔ EXAMINATION CHECKLIST

Domain	Findings	Evolving thought process
Global assessment of child.	• Appears well. • No dysmorphic features. • Not using glasses.	• Unlikely to have an acute pathology. No obvious causes of double vision.
Inspection.	• Looks normal.	• Need to find out what positions result in double vision.
Visual acuity.	• Normal.	• Unlikely to relate to a refractive error.
Visual fields.	• Normal.	• Optic nerve likely normal.
Eye movements.	• Develops double vision on lateral gaze of right eye. • Unable to abduct right eye.	• Lateral rectus palsy on right.
Accommodation reflex.	• Normal.	• No optic/oculomotor nerve pathology identified.
Pupillary reflexes.	• Normal.	• No optic/oculomotor nerve pathology identified.
Fundoscopy/slit lamp.	• Normal.	• No additional pathology identified.
Squint testing.	• Squint only present when looking right, but always present. • Unaffected by cover/uncover test.	• Paralytic squint.

5 Alternate cover test. This tests for a latent squint (*Figure 74*). Again, have the child fix on an object ahead. Cover one eye and then move the cover to the other eye, observing for movement just as the eye is uncovered. Outward movement of the eye as it is uncovered means that when that eye was covered, the eye was turned inwards and vice versa.

Completing the Examination

➤ Do a general paediatric examination.

Bedside tests include:
➤ Review the observation chart.
➤ Plot the height and weight on an age and sex appropriate chart.

🔍 PRESENTING YOUR FINDINGS

Joy is a nine-year-old girl seen in clinic for review today.

Joy looks well and appears comfortable at rest. There are no obvious abnormalities with the eye at rest.

On examination of eye movements, Joy reports double vision, worst on lateral gaze and there is a paralytic squint of the left eye on looking laterally. Visual acuity, visual fields, pupillary reflexes, accommodation and fundoscopy are all normal.

This is consistent with a right sixth cranial nerve palsy. I would be concerned about a possible brain tumour and would like to complete a full neurological examination and request brain imaging (CT or MRI if available).

GASTROINTESTINAL EXAMINATION

This should be performed in all general paediatric examinations. Specifically consider:

1 A child reporting abdominal pain. Where is this child's pain most severe, how severe is it, and how might this help with diagnosis? Pain may be acute or chronic and palpation of the abdomen may localise it to an area, which will help narrow the differential, e.g. right iliac fossa pain in appendicitis. Consider whether the pain may be referred, e.g. lower lobe pneumonia causing abdominal pain.

2 Does this child have an acute abdomen? Assessment hinges on identifying signs of peritonism in the abdomen (*Box 2*). This is important to recognise as identification necessitates immediate treatment and surgical input. Such patients will not come up in medical school/post graduate assessments!

Common patients that are likely to appear in exams are shown in *Table 14*.

Summary Checklist

Global assessment of child on approach.

Inspection. Hands, wrists, face, neck/upper torso, abdomen, legs.

Palpation. Gross palpation, liver, spleen, kidney.

Percuss. Liver, spleen, kidneys, bladder, ascites.

Auscultate. Bowel sounds, bruits.

Completing the examination. Inspect anus, external genitalia, hernial orifices.

Bedside tests. Observation chart, inspect stool/urine, blood glucose, urine dipstick, plot height/weight.

Box 2: Signs of peritonism

- Severe tenderness.
- Guarding.
- Percussion tenderness.
- Abdominal rigidity.
- Fever.
- Abdominal distension.
- Tachycardia/hypotension.

TABLE 14: Common patients that may appear in clinical examinations

Disease	Possible clues
Sickle cell disease.	• Anaemia. • Jaundice. • Splenomegaly. • Afro-Caribbean ethnicity.
Thalassemia.	• Frontal bossing. • Anaemia. • Jaundice. • Hepatomegaly. • Splenomegaly. • Middle Eastern, Asian or Mediterranean origin.
Hereditary spherocytosis.	• Anaemia. • Jaundice. • Splenomegaly. • Caucasian origin.
Liver transplant.	• Abdominal scar in the upper zone. • Palpable liver, with regular, hard edge. • May have original liver retained (auxiliary transplant), with the new liver in an ectopic position.
Surgical patient.	• Abdominal scar, with location and type correlating with likely pathology.

Starting the Examination

The examination begins by observing the child upon entering the examination room. Whilst introducing yourself to the child/parents, begin with a broad assessment:

1   Does the child look well or unwell? Clues for this come from the child's colour (pallor), respiratory rate and activity. If they are able to jump/run around, they do not have a peritonitic abdomen, whereas if they are staying absolutely still for fear of pain or if they look lethargic, this is more worrying.

2   Are there any signs of chronic ill health? See if the child looks cachectic, whether they have any medication around the bed, and if they have any medical devices, long term lines or feeding tubes in place.

3   Has any initial treatment or monitoring been started? Is the child on oxygen or intravenous fluids? Are they on a monitor?

Inspection

The next phase is a more focused inspection. Ensure the child is exposed from the nipple to the knee. However, in older children, use a blanket to preserve their modesty. Babies should be fully undressed, taking care not to allow them to get cold.

Hands

› Signs of general ill health. This will include wasting of the small muscles in the hands from chronic disease and scars from previous cannulation.

› Clubbing. This is associated with chronic liver disease and malabsorption, e.g. inflammatory bowel disease.

› Pallor of palms. This indicates severe anaemia, e.g. in splenic sequestration in sickle cell disease.

› Palmar erythema. Redness of the palms due to increased vascularity is associated with excess oestrogen from chronic liver disease (rare in children).

› Leukonychia. White discolouration of the nails related to hypoalbuminaemia in chronic liver disease.

› Koilonychia. Spoon shaped nails, due to being thinned. Most commonly related to iron, B12 or folate deficiency.

Wrists

› Liver flap. (*Figure 75*) In hepatic encephalopathy, the hands will start to tremor.

› Pulse. Tachycardia, in any condition causing hypovolaemia, e.g. sepsis/GI bleeds, or pain e.g. appendicitis.

› Arteriovenous fistulae. This is used for renal dialysis.

Face

› Jaundice and pallor. Look for both in the conjunctiva (*Figure 76*). In an older child, ask them to pull their eyelid down themselves.

› Kayser-Fleischer rings. Rings seen around the iris as a result of copper deposition (Wilson's disease). Requires formal slit lamp assessment.

› Oral ulceration. This is associated with inflammatory bowel disease or poor nutrition (*Figure 77*).

› Breath. Hepatic fetor associated with liver disease, or "pear drop" breath associated with ketoacidosis.

FIGURE 75

Liver flap. Ask the child to cock their wrists back and hold them in that position for 30 seconds.

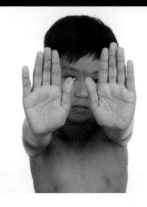

FIGURE 76

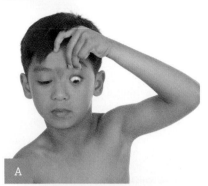

A. Exposing the sclera to look for jaundice. B. 10-year-old boy with jaundice.

FIGURE 77

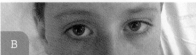

Inspect the mouth, looking mainly at dentition and for ulceration.

> Dentition. Poor dentition is associated with malnutrition.
> Glossitis. Inflammation of the tongue. This is associated with iron, B12 or folate deficiency.
> Angular stomatitis. Inflammation of the corner of the mouth. May relate to iron, thiamine, or B12 deficiencies.
> Freckling around the mouth. This is associated with Peutz-Jeghers syndrome, which can present with GI bleeding from polyps.
> Dysmorphic features. Facial features can give a clue as to possible pathology in a syndrome. For example, Alagille syndrome is associated with a broad forehead, sunken eyes, small chin and chronic liver disease.

Neck and Upper Trunk

> Lymph nodes. Palpate lymph nodes in the neck and supraclavicular fossa.
> Gynaecomastia. This may be from excess oestrogens in chronic liver disease. It is also a normal variant, particularly in pubertal boys.
> Spider naevi. This is a central red spot with extensions radiating out like a spider's web. It is due to dilated blood vessels, and occluding the central spot will result in seeing the emptied peripheral veins filling from the centre. Classically seen in the superior vena cava distribution.
> Central venous access devices. There may be a temporary central line, e.g. post liver transplant, or a long term tunneled line, e.g. those on long term TPN. If they have since been removed, scars might be seen.

Abdomen

Ensure that the child is lying flat with their arms by their sides. Ask them to point to the site of any pain. Inform the child that this will be examined last and

FIGURE 79

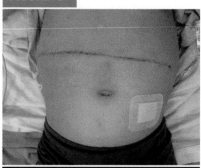

Transverse scar across the upper abdomen from a liver transplant.

FIGURE 78

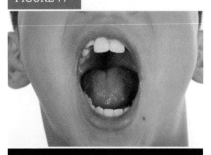

① **Kocher's incision**
Biliary/liver surgery e.g. Kasai procedure for biliary atresia. Extended transversely for liver transplant.

② **Midline laparotomy** Upper midline — upper GI surgery e.g. Nissen's fundoplication for GORD. Longer midline incisions are used for major abdominal surgery more generally.

③ **Transverse upper abdominal incision** Congenital diaphragmatic hernia repair. Splenic surgery.

④ **Pyloromyotomy scar** Pyloric stenosis surgery.

⑤ **Appendicectomy scar** Appendicitis surgery.

⑥ **Umbilical/sub-umbilical scar** Hernia repair, exomphalos repair. Gastroschisis repair has scar within/in place of the belly button.

⑦ **Point incision scar** Drains, ports, or biopsy sites.

⑧ **Inguinal scar** Hernia repair.

⑨ **Lateral thoracolumbar scar** Renal surgery e.g. nephrectomy.

⑩ **Hockey-Stick scar** Renal transplant.

Common abdominal scars in paediatrics.

if at any time it is too sore to continue, they should signal to stop.

> Distension. Distension may be secondary to flatus, fluid, fat, faeces, and do not forget foetuses in teenage girls.
> Dilated superficial veins. This is a sign of portal hypertension. They emanate from the umbilicus.
> Scars. Look anteriorly, posteriorly, in the flanks, and in the groin (*Figure 78-9*). These may be both operational incisions and from drains inserted at the same time.
> Drains. Surgical drains may still be in place post procedure, e.g. biliary drain post Kasai procedure for biliary atresia.
> Stoma bags. p531.
> Peritoneal dialysis catheter. This may be present in chronic renal disease. The catheter is inserted into the peritoneum, and left in situ.
> Antegrade colonic enema. p530.

Palpation

Abdominal palpation in children is tricky, since it is important to keep the child as relaxed as possible. It is very important to distract them with another conversation so they do not concentrate on the pain and guarding/rigidity can be palpated accurately. It can be help-ful to demonstrate the examination on a parent/teddy bear first. Another option is to turn the examination into a game, e.g. trying to feel/guess what they had for breakfast. Palpate as follows:

> Gross palpation. This is to assess for pain and for any masses (*Figure 80*). For neonates and small children, palpate four quadrants. In older children, palpate three upper, three middle, and three lower zones. Whilst palpating, look at the face for pain. For any masses, describe the size, site, tenderness and mobility. Consider also seeing if it transilluminates (e.g. hydrocele), or if there are overlying bruits (e.g. vascular legions). Possible causes of masses are shown in *Table 15*, and of pain in *Table 16*.
> Liver. (*Figure 81*). A normal liver can be felt up to two finger breadths below

TABLE 15: Causes of abdominal masses	
Upper abdomen	**Lower abdomen**
• Hepatomegaly. • Splenomegaly. • Liver transplant. • Renal mass/enlarged kidney. • Neuroblastoma. • Wilms' tumour.	• Impacted faeces. • Appendicular abscess. • Palpable bladder. • Renal transplant.

TABLE 16: Examples of how the site of abdominal pain may point to a diagnosis		
Disease	**Site of pain**	**Additional possible examination findings**
Constipation.	• Diffuse.	• Palpable faecal mass.
Acute appendicitis.	• Right iliac fossa.	• May have local or general peritonitis.
Gastroenteritis.	• Diffuse.	• Hyperactive bowel sounds. • May have fever.
Irritable bowel syndrome.	• Diffuse.	• No signs of peritonism. • Generally well.
Urinary tract infection.	• Suprapubic.	• Nitrites and leukocytes on urine dipstick. • Febrile.
Right lower lobe pneumonia.	• Right upper quadrant.	• Tachypnoea. • Decreased breath sounds. • Dull percussion note. • Crepitations in right lower zone of the lungs.

FIGURE 80

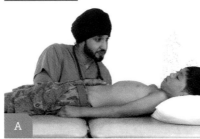
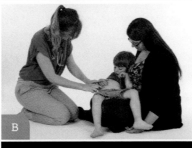

Abdominal palpation. A. Optimal position, at the same level as the child. Start away from the site of pain, and always do light palpation before deep palpation. Look at the child's face to observe for pain. B. Examination pragmatically done with the help of the mother.

FIGURE 81

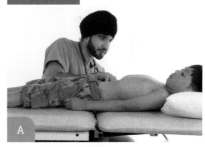
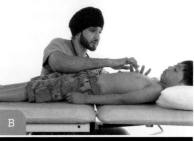

Assessing for hepatomegaly. A. As the patient inhales, slowly move the hand up the abdomen from the right iliac fossa towards the costal margin. If a liver edge is felt, describe whether it is smooth/rough and soft/hard. B. Percuss to confirm the position of liver, starting at the upper chest.

Box 3: Causes of hepatomegaly

- Inflammation.
  - Infectious hepatitis (virus, bacteria, fungi, parasites).
  - Autoimmune hepatitis.
  - Drug induced hepatitis.
- Malignancy.
  - Primary, e.g. hepatoma, hepatoblastoma.
  - Infiltrative, e.g. leukaemia/ lymphoma.
- Vascular congestion.
  - Right heart failure.
  - Constrictive pericarditis.
  - Budd Chiari syndrome.
- Biliary obstruction.
  - Biliary atresia.
  - Choledochal cysts.
  - Tumours.
  - Cystic fibrosis.
- Storage disorders.
  - Gaucher disease (lysosomal storage disease).
  - Glycogen storage disease.
  - Wilson's disease.
  - Hemochromatosis.
  - Alpha 1 antitrypsin deficiency.

FIGURE 82

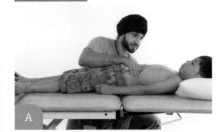
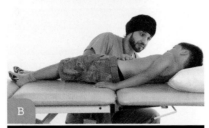

Assessing for splenomegaly. A. Start at the right iliac fossa, using the same technique as for the liver, but this time moving left and upward towards the left upper quadrant. B. If the spleen cannot be felt, ask the patient to rotate onto their right and repeat, as this may make the spleen palpable. Percuss to confirm.

Box 4: Causes of splenomegaly

- Portal hypertension, e.g. secondary to chronic liver disease, or congestive heart failure.
- Malignancy, e.g. leukaemia, lymphoma.
- Infection, e.g. malaria, tuberculosis, EBV.
- Connective tissue disease, e.g. SLE.
- Haematological e.g. sickle cell, thalassaemia, haemolytic anaemia.
- Storage disease, e.g. Gaucher disease.

FIGURE 83

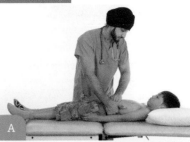
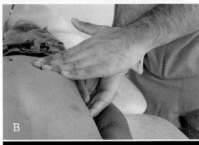

Balloting the kidneys. Push up with the fingers of the hand that are on the back to move the kidney upwards so that it can be felt by the hand on the anterior abdomen.

Box 5: Causes of an enlarged kidney

- Hydronephrosis.
- Wilms' tumour.
- Polycystic kidney disease.
- Renal cyst.
- Renal vein thrombosis.
- Tuberous sclerosis.

TABLE 17: Differentiating the kidney and spleen

Spleen	Kidney
• Notch present. • Moves diagonally towards the right iliac fossa on inspiration. • Cannot get above it. • Dull to percuss. • Not ballotable.	• No notch present. • Moves down on inspiration. • Can get above it. • Resonant to percuss. • Can be bimanually ballotable.

the right costal margin. Causes of hepatomegaly are shown in **Box 3**.

▸ Spleen. Assess for splenomegaly. (**Figure 82**). Normal can be 1-2cm below costal margin. Causes of splenomegaly are shown in **Box 4**. If splenomegaly is found, look for lymphadenopathy elsewhere.

▸ Kidneys. Ballot the kidneys between your hands in each of the flanks (**Figure 83**). Causes of an enlarged kidney are shown in **Box 5**. Differentiating the kidney and spleen can be difficult, and key differences are shown in **Table 17**.

▸ Bladder. Palpate for an enlarged bladder in the suprapubic region.

Note also that in a complete abdominal examination, the heart should be palpated. If dextrocardia is present, the child may have situs inversus.

Percussion

▸ Liver and spleen. Percuss the liver and the spleen. This will help assess the upper margin and confirm the lower margin.

▸ Ascites. If there is suspected ascites, assess for either shifting dullness (**Figure 84**) or a fluid thrill (**Figure 85**).

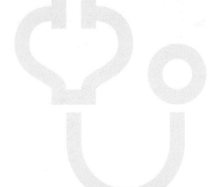

EXAMINATION

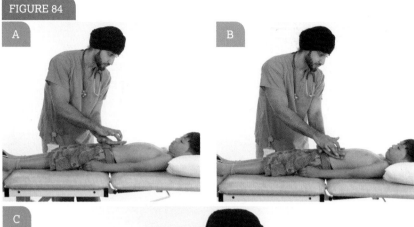

FIGURE 84

A

B

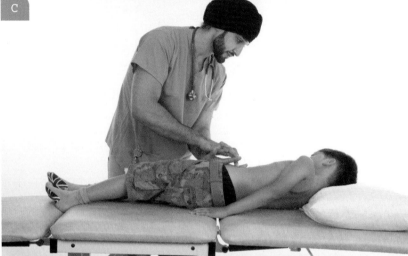

C

Assess for shifting dullness as follows: A. Percuss from the centre of the abdomen outwards, until a dull percussion note is found (representing fluid). B. Pinpoint the location where the note becomes dull. C. At this point, the examiner should keep their hand in the percussed position, whilst rolling the patient towards them. Wait 30 seconds, and then re-percuss. If the note is resonant, this implies that the fluid has shifted under gravity. Confirm this by rolling the patient back into their original position and re-percussing. The percussion note should become dull again.

FIGURE 85

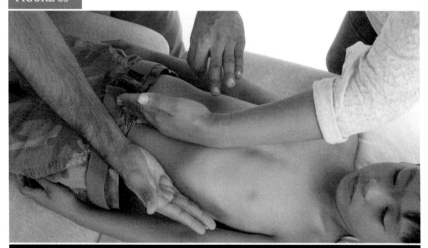

Assessing for a fluid thrill. Ask a parent to place a hand over the centre of the abdomen (to prevent conduction through the skin). Firmly flick the abdomen on one flank and feel for a 'thrill' on the other side.

> Bladder. The bladder is dull to percuss, and if enlarged, can be measured by percussion up from the suprapubic region.

Auscultation

Listen around 2 cm above the umbilicus:
> Bowel sounds. These may be normal, tinkling e.g. bowel obstruction, or absent e.g. peritonitis.
> Renal bruit. Present in renal artery stenosis.

Completing the Examination

Depending on the presenting symptoms, as well as performing a general paediatric examination, it is important to also inspect:
> The anus. Looking for fistula/skin tags (associated with Crohn's disease).
> The external genitalia and hernia orifices. Abdominal pain could be referred pain, e.g. from testicular torsion.
> Rashes. e.g. purpura (HSP), pyoderma gangrenosum and erythema nodosum (IBD).
> Pitting oedema. This may be from hypoalbuminaemia, e.g. chronic liver disease.

Bedside tests include:
> Review the observation chart.
> Plot the height and weight on an age and sex appropriate chart.
> Stool sample.
> Urine dipstick.
> Blood glucose.

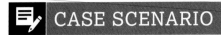 CASE SCENARIO

SCENARIO 8

Claude is a 4-year-old boy, who attends the renal outpatient clinic for routine review. You are asked to perform an abdominal/renal examination on him, and present your findings to the consultant.

✔ EXAMINATION CHECKLIST

Domain	Findings	Evolving thought process
Global assessment of child on approach.	• Alert, active, and looks well.	• Unlikely to have an acute pathology.
Inspection.	• Previous central venous access scar. • Gastrostomy in situ. • Small scar to the right of his umbilicus. • Midline laparotomy scar.	• Has had major abdominal surgery in the past, which is likely to be the time when central venous access was acquired. Gastrostomy implies that there are current/past feeding difficulties. • Scar to the right of the umbilicus may relate to a previous surgical drain.
Palpation.	• Egg-shaped mass over midline. • Laparotomy scar.	• Likely transplanted kidney. Given this information, the scar to the right of the umbilicus may have been a site of peritoneal dialysis.
Percussion.	• No organomegaly. • No ascites.	• No additional pathology identified.
Auscultation.	• Normal.	• No additional pathology identified.
Completing the examination.	• Normal.	• No additional pathology identified.
Bedside tests.	• Awaiting.	• Although looks well, possible faltering growth suggested by previous chronic disease (necessitating renal transplant), and gastrostomy being in situ. • May have blood/protein in urine with any renal pathology.

MUSCULOSKELETAL EXAMINATION

A partial musculoskeletal or locomotor examination is undertaken in every paediatric assessment: gait is more often than not observed, as is an assessment of muscle bulk and gross movements. Consider the following more specific circumstances:

1. In a child presenting with joint pain, stiffness, or loss of function (e.g. difficulty with handwriting). Is this an isolated joint pathology/injury or part of a wider problem?
2. Screening for associated musculoskeletal involvement in a child with a predisposing condition. For example, psoriasis, IBD.
3. Assessment of hypermobility.

Signs and symptoms of joint disease are shown in *Box 6*. Common patients that are likely to appear in exams are shown in *Table 18*.

Box 6: Clinical features of joint disease

- Pain.
- Swelling.
- Stiffness.
- Erythema.
- Locking.
- Instability.
- Loss of ability/function.

🔍 PRESENTING YOUR FINDINGS

Claude is a 4-year-old who was seen in the renal clinic for review.

He looks well. He has evidence of previous central venous access. He has a gastrostomy in situ, a small scar to the right of his umbilicus and a midline laparotomy scar. The abdomen is soft and non-tender throughout, with no clinically detectable organomegaly. There is a firm, non-tender, egg-sized mass underlying the laparotomy scar. There was no associated bruit. He has no other stigmata of disease.

These findings are consistent with a renal transplant. The scar to the right of his umbilicus is probably from previous peritoneal dialysis. It is not clear why he has a gastrostomy, but it could be for gastrointestinal or neurological pathology.

To complete my examination, I would like to review the observation chart, dipstick the urine and formally plot Claude on a growth chart.

Summary Checklist
Global assessment of the child on approach.

pGALS screening. Gait, arms, legs, spine.

Hypermobility screening. Beighton score.

Inspection. Hands, skin, eyes, spine, individual joints.

Palpation. Each individual joint.

Movement. Passive then active movement of joint in question.

Function. For important activities e.g. doing up buttons.

Completing the examination. Auscultate heart (if hyperflexibility), palpate abdomen (if malignancy/inflammatory arthritis suspected).

Bedside tests. Review observations; plot height and weight.

TABLE 18: Common patients that may appear in clinical examinations	
Diagnosis	**Possible clues**
Juvenile idiopathic arthritis (JIA). (*Table 19*).	• Often symmetrical. • Joints swollen, tender, movement restricted. • May be eye signs e.g. uveitis. • May be hepatosplenomegaly if systemic onset JIA.
IBD related arthritis.	• Often knees, ankles, wrists. • Associated signs of IBD e.g. oral ulcers, erythema nodosum, abdominal scars, colostomy at present or previously. • May appear malnourished.
Enthesitis related arthritis.	• Boys. • Large joint involvement including hip and sacroiliac joint. • Spine involved. • Dactylitis and uveitis may be seen.
Psoriatic arthritis.	• May be asymmetrical, often involves hands. • Psoriasis rash. • Psoriatic nail changes. • Dactylitis.
Marfan/ Ehlers-Danlos syndrome.	• Hypermobility. • Scars, bruising, elastic skin. • May have a heart murmur of aortic regurgitation or mitral valve prolapse.
Osteogenesis imperfecta.	• Blue sclera. • Bony limb deformities. • May have an affected parent. • Short stature and/or teeth affected (discolouration/damage).

Begin with the pGALS screening examination (paediatric Gait, Arms, Legs, Spine) to identify any difficulties in the school-aged child. This should be performed in:

› An unwell child with pyrexia.
› A child with a limp.
› A child with regression of motor milestones/clumsiness.
› A child with chronic disease with musculoskeletal presentations (e.g. inflammatory bowel disease, but also inflammatory arthropathies).

pGALS

Screening Questions

1 Do you have any pain or difficulty moving your arms, legs, back or neck? This is associated broadly with a musculoskeletal problem.
2 Can you get dressed without any help? This is associated with difficulty in fine and gross motor skills.
3 Can you walk up and down stairs without any problems? This is associated with weakness in abductor muscles.

The child will need to be exposed, ideally in shorts and girls in shorts and a vest top. Inspect the child standing upright from the front, back and sides (*Figure 86*).

› Skin rashes. e.g. psoriasis.
› Asymmetry. Difference in muscle bulk and leg length.
› Posture.

Starting the Examination

The examination begins by observing the child upon entering the examination room. During introductions to the child/parents, make a broad assessment:

1 Does the child look well or unwell? Are they in obvious pain? Do they have a major injury?
2 Are there signs of chronic ill health, do they look underweight? There may be an underlying inflammatory disorder contributing to the problem.
3 Are there limb supports around? e.g. walker, splints, wheelchair. The illness may already be diagnosed and partially managed.
4 Are there any dysmorphic features? e.g. Marfan's syndrome.

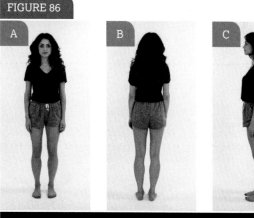

FIGURE 86

Inspection from: A. Front. B. Back. C. Side.

TABLE 19: Differentiating features of JIA			
Juvenile Idiopathic Arthritis			
Systemic Onset (Still's disease)	**Oligoarticular**	**Polyarticular RF positive**	**Polyarticular RF negative**
• Often symptoms from <5 yrs. • Systemic symptoms before joint involvement, e.g. weight loss, lymphadenopathy, HSP, anaemia. • No uveitis. • Fever for six weeks. • Rash – salmon pink, non-pruritic. • Polyarticular. • RF and ANA negative.	• Symptoms from early childhood 2yrs-5yrs. • Female predominance. • Large joints affected. • Swollen joints, may not be painful. • Erythema not as much a feature. • Uveitis. • ANA positive.	• Female predominance. • Begins in late childhood. • Symmetrical. • Hands and feet often involved. • No uveitis. • Often severe with joint destruction. • RF and ANA positive. • May be HLA DR4 positive.	• Female predominance. • Involves more than 4 joints. • Symmetrical. • Sacral joints not involved. • TMJ can be involved. • Can be ANA positive but RF negative.

> ‣ Scoliosis. Look from the side and from the back. The only clue may be an asymmetry in shoulder height or skin creases.
> ‣ Knees. They may be knock-kneed (valgus) or bow-legged (varus).

Gait

For each movement, walk with the child to ensure that they are not going to fall over (*Table 20*). Observe for any pain in the movements.

TABLE 20: GALS: Gait	
Instruction	**Illustration**
The child should walk away from the examiner, turn and then come back. Look for difficulty in turning. A hypermobile child may pronate and roll their feet in as they walk.	
Walk on heels.	
Walk on tiptoes. Observe the foot arches. A hypermobile child may be flat-footed.	

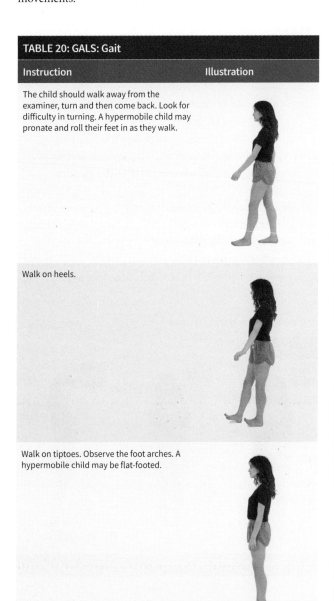

Arms

Have the child facing the examiner. For each movement, get the child to copy actions (*Table 21*).

TABLE 21: GALS: Arms	
Instruction	**Illustration**
Ask the child to stretch out their arms, palm up. Briefly inspect the hands, including nails, and arms. Look for muscle bulk, muscle wasting, rashes, nail changes, joint swelling and deformity.	
Ask them to turn their hands over as far as possible and make a fist. This tests supination at the wrist and elbow joints and flexion of the fingers.	
Ask the child to pinch their thumb and each finger in turn together to test their co-ordination and dexterity.	
Ask the child to turn the hand back over and squeeze the MCP joints, looking to see if there is any pain.	
Ask the child to make a prayer position, with their hands palm to palm and their elbows held up. This tests elbow flexion, finger extension, and wrist extension. Excessive movement may indicate hypermobility.	
Ask the child to put the backs of their hands together, keeping the elbows up. This tests wrist flexion.	

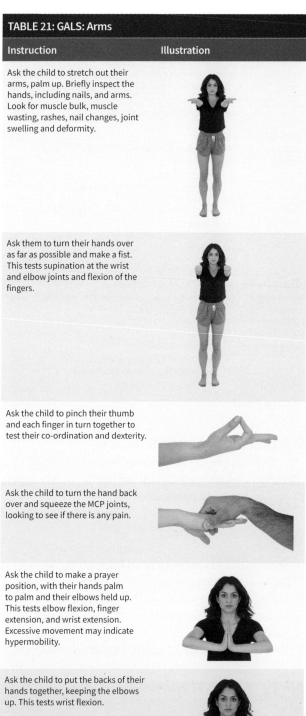

Continued

TABLE 21: *Continued*

Instruction	Illustration
Ask the child to raise their arms straight up to the ceiling to test extension of the shoulders and elbows.	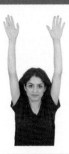
Ask the child to look up to the ceiling. This tests neck extension.	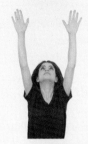
Ask the child to put their hands behind the head to test elbow flexion, shoulder abduction and shoulder external rotation.	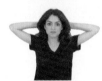
Ask the child to try and touch their shoulder with their ear, one side at a time, to test lateral flexion of the neck.	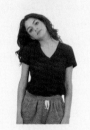
Ask the child to open their mouth as wide as they can and insert three fingers. Look for any asymmetry in mouth opening. This movement looks for temporomandibular joint disease.	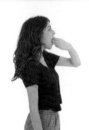

TABLE 22: GALS: Legs

Instruction	Illustration
Feel the warmth of each knee, comparing one side to the other.	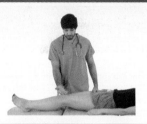
Check for knee effusion by: a Milk any fluid from the lower thigh and press each patella in turn (patella tap).	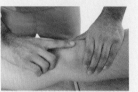
b Perform the sweep test. This can be used to identify smaller effusions. Stroke firmly along the medial side of the knee (shown), distal to proximal, and then quickly repeat on the lateral side, proximal to distal. If the fluid bulges on the medial side, the test is positive.	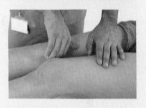
Ask the child to bend their leg, bringing their heel to their bottom.	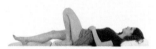
Ask the child to straighten their leg to ensure it can be extended. Compare movement of each side.	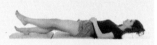
Flex the hip fully.	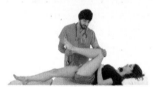
Check external rotation of the hip (moving leg in across body) with the hip flexed at 90 degrees.	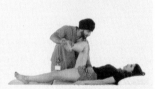
Check internal rotation of the hip (move the leg outwards across the body) with the hip flexed at 90 degrees.	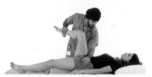
Place the child's leg back down on the examination couch and assess full extension of the knee.	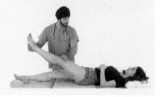

Legs

Have the child lie flat on the bed. Roll up the shorts to expose more of the leg. Ask again about any pain in the leg before performing each movement. Briefly look from hip to soles for muscle wasting, differences in leg length, foreign bodies in the soles of the feet. The technique is described in *Table 22*.

Spine

A brief assessment of the spine should be made (*Table 23*).

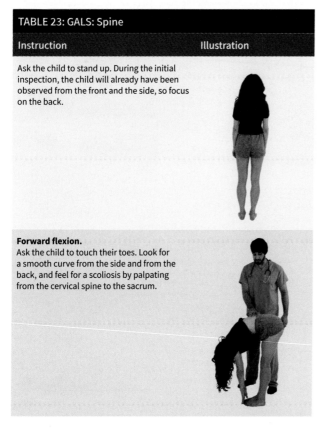

TABLE 23: GALS: Spine

Instruction	Illustration
Ask the child to stand up. During the initial inspection, the child will already have been observed from the front and the side, so focus on the back.	
Forward flexion. Ask the child to touch their toes. Look for a smooth curve from the side and from the back, and feel for a scoliosis by palpating from the cervical spine to the sacrum.	

Specific joints will now be examined in more detail. Remember to compare sides and if pathology is identified, examine the joint above and below.

Inspection

Hands

›   Clubbing. This may be due to inflammatory bowel disease.
›   Splinter haemorrhages. These are vertical lines of bleeding beneath the nail. Occurs in rheumatoid arthritis and psoriasis.
›   Nail bed telangiectasia. This is seen on the finger, adjacent to the cuticle, and is a feature of dermatomyositis, SLE and scleroderma.
›   Psoriatic nail changes.
 ›   Nail pitting. Small pits in the nail.
 ›   Onycholysis. Separation of the nail from the nail bed with resulting white discolouration of the nail.
 ›   Dactylitis. Sausage shaped swelling of the entire finger.
›   Koilonychia. This is due to iron deficiency, where the nails are 'spoon-shaped'.
›   Arachnodactyly. This describes long, slender fingers and toes seen in Marfan Syndrome.
›   Finger length. Pseudohypoparathyroidism is characterised by short 4th and 5th fingers.

Face

›   Blue sclera. This is seen in osteogenesis imperfecta.
›   Uveitis. This is seen in JIA and IBD.

›   Heliotrope rash. This is seen in dermatomyositis. It is a purple discolouration and swelling of the upper eyelids.
›   Oral ulcers. These are associated with IBD.
›   Malar rash. This describes an erythematous rash over the cheeks and nose seen in SLE.
›   Dentinogenesis imperfecta. This describes yellow/grey transparent teeth seen in some children with OA type 1.

Additional Skin Features

The skin often reveals disease specific signs:
›   Corticosteroid use.
 ›   Striae.
 ›   Abdominal obesity.
 ›   Moon face.
 ›   Interscapula fat pad.
›   Psoriasis.
 ›   A scaly pink rash is seen on extensor surfaces.
›   Dermatomyositis.
 ›   Gottron papules. Purple coloured areas are seen on bony prominences.
 ›   Scaly red or purple patches are seen on sun exposed areas.
 ›   Calcinosis. This is seen as hard white or yellow nodules, particularly on the fingers or joints.
 ›   Raynaud's phenomenon.
›   Systemic Lupus Erythematosus (SLE).
 ›   Discoid lupus. Disc-shaped, plaque-like lesions are seen in sun-exposed areas.
›   Juvenile idiopathic arthritis (*Table 19*).
 ›   Salmon-pink rash. This is usually on the limbs and torso, in small patches.
›   Ehlers-Danlos syndrome.
 ›   Bruising and scarring of skin is seen.
 ›   Hyperelastic skin.

Joint in Question

›   Erythema. This may be due to acute inflammation or infection.
›   Swelling. This signifies an acutely inflamed joint.
›   Scarring. This may be seen from tendon release surgery, e.g. in cerebral palsy.
›   Muscle wasting. This is commonly due to disuse or chronic inflammatory arthritis.
›   Joint deformities.
 ›   Joint subluxation/ulnar deviation may be seen in inflammatory arthropathies.
 ›   Claw hand deformity. Hyperextension of the MCP joint and lack of extension of the PIP and DIP joints in the little and ring finger due to interossei muscle weakness. This can be due to a brachial plexus injury sustained at birth or an ulnar nerve palsy.
›   Leg length. *Figure 87*. Causes of leg length changes are shown in *Table 24*.
›   Flat feet. Over six years of age, this may indicate hypermobility or lax ligaments. Below this age, flat feet are often a normal variant.

FIGURE 87

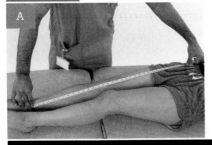
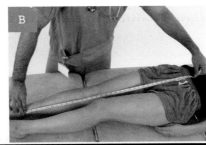

Leg length measurement: A. Measure from the anterior superior iliac spine to the medial malleolus to measure true leg length. B. Apparent leg length is taken from the umbilicus to the medial malleolus.

TABLE 24: Causes of leg length changes			
Legs short (compared to torso)	Legs long (compared to torso)	Unilateral shortened leg	Unilateral lengthed leg
• Skeletal dysplasia. • Rickets.	• Scoliosis.	• Fracture (particularly through a growth plate). • SUFE.	• Chronic inflammatory arthritis, e.g. juvenile idiopathic arthritis. • Hemihypertrophy.

Range of movement is formally measured with a goniometer. Start with active movements, and then if there is a limitation, or for movements that might be difficult, assist the patient in moving (passive movement).

Observe for:

› Pain. Watch the child's face.
› Limitation of movement. This is both for active and passive movement.
› Hypermobility. This is where the joint can be moved passively beyond the expected range of movement.
› Crepitus. Feel for crepitus in any painful joint (*Figure 88*). This implies an arthritic process.
› Muscle tone. Assess muscle tone during passive movement.

Palpation

› Temperature. An inflamed or infected joint may be hot. Feel for this using the back of the hand.
› Swelling. Look for any obvious swelling, particularly at the elbow and knee. Palpate for a joint effusion, particularly at the knee.
› Joint tenderness. Palpate the bony landmarks. Watch the child's face at this point to observe for their reaction.

Movement

Ask the child to perform the movements described in *Table 25* after being demonstrated by the examiner. Compare the range of movement on one side with the other.

FIGURE 88

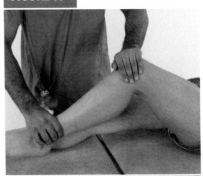

Feeling for crepitus in the knee.

TABLE 25: Assessing movement in main joints			
Body part	Movement	Instruction	Illustration
Shoulder.	Flexion/abduction (180 degrees).	"Reach your hands up to the ceiling".	
	External rotation (70 degrees).	"Scratch your back".	

Continued

TABLE 25: *Continued*			
Body part	**Movement**	**Instruction**	**Illustration**
	Internal rotation (80 degrees).	"Put your hand behind your back, with the palm against the back".	
	Adduction (45 degrees).	"Hug yourself".	
Elbow.	Flexion (150 degrees).	"Touch your shoulders".	
	Extension (5 degrees).	"Straighten your arms".	
Wrist.	Extension (80 degrees).	"Bend your elbows, and put your hands together like you are praying".	
	Flexion (90 degrees).	From the above position, "now do the same with your hands pointing downwards".	
Fingers.	Flexion (should be able to flex into a fist).	"Make a fist".	
	Extension (90 degrees).	"Bend your fingers back as far as you can".	

Continued

TABLE 25: *Continued*

Body part	Movement	Instruction	Illustration
	Abduction (30 degrees).	"Spread your fingers".	
Hip.	Flexion (120 degrees).	With the patient on their back, "lift up your leg".	
	Extension (30 degrees).	With the patient on their front "lift up your leg".	
	Abduction (50 degrees).	Move the leg out away from the body whilst keeping the pelvis stable.	
	Adduction (30 degrees).	Move the leg across to the other side of the body whilst keeping the pelvis stable.	
	External rotation (60 degrees).	Move the leg in, across the body, with the hip flexed at 90 degrees.	
	Internal rotation (30° - 60°: decreases with age).	Move the leg outwards, across the body, with the hip flexed at 90 degrees.	
Knee.	Flexion (140 degrees).	"Bring your foot to touch your bottom".	
	Extension (up to 5 degrees of hyperextension).	"Straighten your leg".	
Ankle.	Plantar flexion (50 degrees).	"Point your foot towards the floor".	
	Dorsiflexion (20 degrees).	"Pull your foot towards your head".	

If a joint can move further passively than when the child actively moves the joint themselves, ask them what stops the movement. If it is weakness, then neurological causes should be considered. If it is stiffness or pain, then think of nerve/muscle/joint pathology.

Causes of hip pain and restricted movement in children are shown in *Table 26*.

Function

When examining the musculoskeletal system, it is important to test function as this will impact on day-to-day activities.

➤ Arms.
  › Use of cutlery or cup.
  › Drawing/writing with pencil.
  › Grip.
  › Buttons.

➤ Spine.
  › Picking an object up off of the floor.
  › Putting on shoes and socks.
➤ Lower limbs.
  › Gait.
  › Getting out of a chair.
  › Standing.
  › Stairs.

Hypermobility

This is assessed using the Beighton score from 0-9. Hypermobility ranges from mild to severe. It can cause symptoms of:

➤ Clumsiness.
➤ Difficulty with grip and poor handwriting.
➤ Delayed walking and joint pain, particularly in the knees and ankles.

The Beighton score is assessed with the movements shown in *Figure 89*. Scoring more than four suggests hypermobility, but it should be considered in conjunction with a history of symptoms.

Completing the Examination

Depending on the findings:

➤ Examine the joint above and below.
➤ Measure the leg length.
➤ Auscultate the heart if Ehlers-Danlos or Marfan syndrome are suspected for mitral valve prolapse and aortic regurgitation.
➤ Palpate the abdomen for hepatosplenomegaly if not already done so, particularly if JIA or malignancy suspected.
➤ Perform a general paediatric examination.

Bedside tests include:

➤ Review the observation chart.
➤ Plot the height and weight on an age and sex appropriate chart.

TABLE 26: Differentials of paediatric hip pain	
Condition	**Possible clues**
Slipped Upper Femoral Epiphysis (SUFE). • Unstable: unable to weight bear. • Stable: able to weight bear.	• Adolescents, often boys that are overweight. • Groin, thigh or knee pain. • There is an antalgic gait with the foot turned out. • The affected limb may be shortened. • On flexion, the affected leg externally rotates. • Reduced internal rotation.
Perthes disease.	• Boys aged 4 to 8-years-old reporting knee pain but also groin and thigh pain. • Trendelenburg gait in late disease. • Reduced internal rotation and abduction.
Transient synovitis.	• Limping toddler. • Recent URTI. • Reduced internal rotation, pain/spasm on rolling leg.
Developmental Hip Dysplasia (if not detected early).	• The left hip is affected more than the right hip. • Girls are affected more than boys. • It is associated with breech birth. • The child may walk with the leg externally rotated or on tiptoes of the affected leg. • A waddling gait is seen in bilateral dislocation. • There is a discrepancy in leg length. • There is reduced abduction of the leg.
Septic arthritis.	• Systemically unwell child of any age, febrile. • Antalgic gait or non-weight bearing. • Tender, swollen, hot joint. • Elevated inflammatory markers.

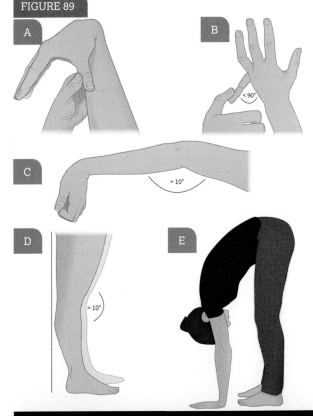

FIGURE 89

The Beighton Score. A. Touching thumb to forearm. Score 1 for each side. B. Extending the little finger more than 90° at the MCP joint. Again score 1 for each side. C. Straightening the arm and extending the elbow more than 10° beyond neutral. Score 1 for each side. D. Straightening the leg and extending the knee more than 10° beyond neutral. Score 1 for each side. E. Touching the palms to the floor. Ensure that the feet are flat and that the legs are straight. Score 1 for this.

CASE SCENARIO

SCENARIO 9

Leann is an 11-year-old girl who has presented to clinic today with a longstanding history of knee and hand pain. Please examine her and present your likely diagnosis.

✔ EXAMINATION CHECKLIST

Domain	Findings	Evolving thought process
Global assessment of the child.	• Appears well grown. • Comfortable at rest.	• No evidence of an acute pathology.
pGALS screening.	• Normal gait, legs and spine. • Some swelling of the fingers and reduced grip.	• Appears to have hand pathology, need to examine this in more detail.
Inspection.	• Nail pits. • Dactylitis of right 4th finger, swollen DIP joints of left hand. • Psoriatic plaques over arms. • No uveitis.	• Psoriatic hand changes evident.
Palpation.	• Swollen, tender DIP joints, 2nd and 3rd fingers on left hand. • Swollen right 4th finger.	• Inflammation of DIP joints on 2nd and 3rd fingers on left and of whole 4th finger on right.
Movement.	• Reduced flexion of fingers.	• Inflammation is causing limitations of movement.
Function.	• Difficulty with buttons and pencil grip.	• May be affecting school and getting dressed/undressed.

EXAMINATION OF A NECK MASS

Neck masses have a wide range of possible causes and may be discovered incidentally. Common patients that may appear in exams are shown in *Table 27*.

Summary Checklist

Global assessment of child.

Inspection. Neck and mouth.

Palpation. Lymph nodes, and any neck mass.

Special tests. Sticking tongue out and swallowing.

Auscultation. Mass for bruit.

Completing the examination. General lymphadenopathy, hepatosplenomegaly.

Bedside tests. Review observations, plot height and weight.

Q PRESENTING YOUR FINDINGS

Leann is an 11-year-old girl I saw in clinic this morning.

Leann looks well grown for her age and appears comfortable at rest. On pGALS screening, I identified pathology in Leann's hands, and therefore proceeded to examine the hands in more detail.

On examination of her hand, Leann has evidence of psoriatic changes with nail pits bilaterally and dactylitis of the fourth finger on her right hand. She also has psoriasis plaques on both of her elbows. On palpation, the distal interphalangeal joints of the 2nd and 3rd fingers on the left hand are tender and swollen. Leann has reduced flexion of her fingers and a weak grip, which causes difficulties with undoing buttons and holding a pencil.

My findings are consistent with psoriatic arthritis. To complete my examination, I would like to examine Leann's other joints for evidence of further joint involvement and plot her height and weight.

TABLE 27: Common patients that may appear in clinical examinations

Disease	Possible clues
Thyroglossal cyst.	• In midline. • Moves upward on sticking out tongue.
Sternocleidomastoid tumour.	• Occurs in infants. • Just above clavicle. • Torticollis towards opposite side of the lesion.
Lymphadenopathy. • Reactive. • Infective. • Lymphadenitis.	• Often small. • May be painful with other signs of infection elsewhere. • Painful, swollen, overlying skin red.
Lymphoma.	• Painless enlargement of lymph node. • Associated fever, night sweats, weight loss, skin rashes. • Look for other enlarged nodes and hepatosplenomegaly.
Branchial cyst.	• Side of neck. • Can develop abscess, may be discharging. • Can swell during times of URTI and then recede.
Haemangioma.	• Red or bluish in colour. • Can ulcerate.
Autoimmune thyroiditis.	• Goitre. • Short. • May be clinically euthyroid or hypothyroid. • Often a girl.
Graves' disease.	• Goitre. • Signs of hyperthyroidism, although may be euthyroid. • Proptosis. • Lid lag.

Starting the Examination

The examination begins by observing the child upon entering the examination room. On introduction to the child/parents, begin with a broad assessment:

1 Does the child look well or unwell? Many children with a neck lump will be otherwise asymptomatic, but bear in mind the child may have a severe infection.
2 Are there any signs of systemic disease? Look particularly for any suggestion of thyroid disease.

Inspection

As for all examinations, begin inspection on entering the room by making a broad assessment if the child appears unwell and if there is any monitoring attached or treatment already in progress. Then focus on the neck and mouth:

Neck

› Scars. This may be from previous thyroid surgery/lymph node excision.
› Neck masses. Identify the location and size.

Mouth

› Tooth decay/gum disease. This can be a cause of infection resulting in a neck lump.

Palpation

› Lymphadenopathy. Palpate from behind the anterior cervical, posterior cervical and submandibular chains (*Figure 66/90*). If lymph nodes are present, are they small and reactive? Define their size. Lympahdenopathy indicates that there may be an infective process, particularly if they are painful. Painless lymphadenopathy may indicate lymphoma.

For any mass identified in the neck, comment on:

› Size.
› Shape.

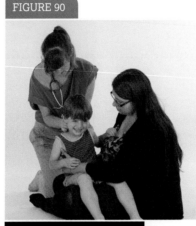

FIGURE 90

Palpating lymph nodes.

› Surface.
› Skin.
› Consistency. e.g. firm, soft.
› Tenderness.
› Temperature.
› Mobility.
› Transillumination. Cystic masses transilluminate.
› Pulsatility. Indicates a vascular lesion.
› Relation to surrounding structures. e.g. trachea.
› Movement. This includes with sticking out the tongue (thyroglossal cyst) and with swallowing (thyroid mass).

Auscultation

› Thyroid bruit. This may be heard in Graves' disease.

Completing the Examination

› Examine for lymphadenopathy in axillae and groin and hepatosplenomegaly.
› If a thyroid lump is suspected, assess the patient's thyroid status.
› Perform a general paediatric examination.

Bedside tests include:
› Review the observation chart.
› Plot the height and weight on an age and sex appropriate chart.

✎ CASE SCENARIO

SCENARIO 10

Andrew is a two-year-old boy who has attended clinic today with a neck swelling. You are asked to examine the mass and present your findings.

✔ EXAMINATION CHECKLIST		
Domain	**Findings**	**Evolving thought process**
Global assessment.	• Appears well grown. • No dysmorphic features.	• No pathology identified.
Inspection.	• Mass right side of neck, along border of sternocleidomastoid muscle, 2cm x 1cm, central punctum that appears to be discharging yellowish fluid.	• Not in midline, therefore unlikely to be a thyroglossal cyst or thyroid mass. Appears to be discharging/ possibly infected.
Palpation.	• Smooth, fluctuant mass, slightly tender, no associated lymphadenopathy.	• Could be a branchial cyst.
Special tests.	• Position not altered by swallowing. • Child would not co-operate with sticking tongue out.	• No additional pathology identified.
Auscultation.	• No bruit heard.	• No additional pathology identified.

EXAMINATION

Q PRESENTING YOUR FINDINGS

Andrew is a two-year-old boy who has presented to the clinic today with a neck mass.

Andrew appears well and is comfortable at rest. He has a 2 cm x 1 cm swelling on the right side of his neck along the lower anteromedial border of the sternocleidomastoid muscle. The mass has a central punctum, which is discharging yellow fluid. The mass is smooth, fluctuant and slightly tender to palpate. The position does not change upon swallowing and there is no audible bruit.

The mass is consistent with a right sided branchial cyst that may be associated with a sinus tract, in view of the discharge.

To complete my examination, I would like to plot Andrew's height and weight on a growth chart. To investigate the mass, I would like to refer Andrew for an ultrasound and surgical review.

NEUROLOGICAL EXAMINATION

A neurological assessment of one form or another is merited in most paediatric presentations, both acute and in outpatients. Situations when you might be expected to perform a complete neurological examination include:

1 The child presenting with seizures or syncopal episodes. Do they have an underlying neurological disorder? Is there a space occupying lesion?
2 The child presenting with bladder/bowel disturbance, e.g. chronic constipation, enuresis.
3 Headaches. This may be a presentation of a space occupying lesion.
4 An obvious neurological deficit, e.g. foot drop, balance disturbance.
5 Developmental delay.

A key distinction in examining the limbs is whether an upper or lower motor neurone lesion is present (*Table 28*). This

---

Summary Checklist
Global assessment of child on approach.

Inspection. Upper limbs, face, torso, back, legs.

Upper limbs. Power, tone, reflexes, sensation, coordination, function.

Lower limbs. Power, tone, reflexes, sensation, coordination, function.

Gait. Walking, tip toeing, running, walking on heels.

Cranial nerves. I–XII.

Cerebellar examination.

Bedside tests. Review observations, plot height, weight and head circumference.

---

section will also outline a focused assessment of a child in a wheelchair, and a schematic for examination of a child's head.

Common patients that are likely to appear in exams are shown in *Table 29*.

TABLE 28: Distinguishing between upper and lower motor neurone lesions

Domain	Upper Motor Neurone Lesion	Lower Motor Neurone Lesion
Inspection.	• Pronator drift.	• Fasciculation (small muscle twitches, involuntary) and muscle wasting.
Tone.	• Increased (may be reduced initially).	• Decreased.
Power.	• Reduced.	• Reduced.
Reflexes.	• Brisk/normal.	• Reduced/absent.
Clonus.	• Yes.	• No.
Plantar reflex.	• Up going.	• Down going.

TABLE 29: Common patients that may appear in clinical examinations

Disease	Possible clues
Duchenne Muscular Dystrophy.	• Male. • Waddling gait or walking on tiptoes. • Lumbar lordosis. • Hypertrophied calves. • Gower's sign. • Absent knee jerk but ankle jerk remains present. • May be speech delay.
Hemiplegic cerebral palsy.	• Arm held flexed on walking, more pronounced on running. • One side of body affected. • Increased tone. • Brisk reflexes.
Diplegic cerebral palsy.	• Scissoring gait. • Increased tone, more in legs than arms. • Brisk reflexes in legs.
Spina bifida.	• May be in a wheelchair or need a frame to walk. • Scar over the lower spine. • May have scoliosis. • Muscle wasting in legs. • Reduced tone and power in lower limbs. • Absent reflexes. • Presence of a shunt.
Post-viral cerebellitis.	• Well child. • Wide gait. • Romberg positive. • Incoordination. • Normal reflexes.
Hereditary Sensory and Motor Neuropathy.	• High stepping gait and foot deformities. • Distal muscle wasting 'inverted champagne bottle' legs. • Weakness more in legs than arms. • Absent reflexes. • Reduced proprioception.

Starting the Examination

For all the neurological examinations that follow, the examination starts on entering the room by inspecting the child in their surroundings and making a broad assessment.

1 Are they in a wheelchair? If so, how is it controlled and what supports are needed? A child requiring trunk, neck and head support infers a more severe phenotype. If not, have they walked into the room, and what is their gait like?

2 Is the child comfortable or in pain? Contractures can be very painful, and loss of function can result in the development of pressure sores.

3 Is the child cachectic or well grown? Chronic disease is associated with faltering growth.

4 Are there any devices, such as feeding tubes? The child may have poor swallowing.

5 Is there any obvious scoliosis? An "S" shaped curvature of the spine. In lordosis, the lower spine curves inward and the abdomen may be pushed forward. Kyphosis is the abnormal curvature of the upper spine giving a "hunched over" impression to the posture.

6 Are there any neurocutaneous markers? This includes café au lait spots, ash leaf macules, shagreen patches, neurofibromatosis, and port-wine stains.

7 Are there any obvious scars? e.g. spina bifida surgery.

8 Are there any dysmorphic features?

Ask about the child's normal function: can they walk unaided? If not, what do they require for support?

Examination of Upper Limbs
Inspection

Next is a more focused inspection concentrating on the arm but also looking at the patient as a whole. Both arms need to be exposed to compare left to right. Look at the natural movements as well as the resting posture. Look for:

› Scars. These may be due to contracture release surgery.

› Neurocutaneous lesions. Neurofibromatosis is associated with café au lait macules. Cutaneous neurofibromas and axillary freckling develop from adolescence onwards. Look at the nails for subungual fibromas seen in tuberous sclerosis (p233).

› Muscle wasting. This implies lack of use or a peripheral neuropathy.

› Contractures. This is particularly associated with cerebral palsy.

› Casts, splints or orthoses. These may be used in cerebral palsy to improve function.

› Movements. Lack of movement of one arm may indicate hemiplegia.

› Relative proportion of arms, trunk and legs. In achondroplasia, the limbs are relatively short compared to the trunk. Achondroplasia is also associated with decreased upper arm length (compared to lower arm), and decreased thigh length (compared to lower leg).

In children under one:

› Is there a hand preference? Hand preference under 18 months of age should prompt assessment for hemiplegia.

› How is coordination? Look how they are playing and reaching for objects (*Figure 91*).

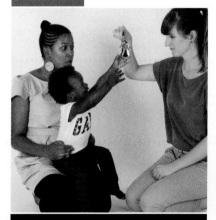

FIGURE 91

Good coordination, good truncal tone, antigravity movement (power at least 3/5), and using both arms equally so no obvious weakness/arm preference.

Tone

Check that it will not hurt the child to move their arm. Let them know they should ask you to stop if it hurts.

Hold the patient's hand in a handshake position, and use the other hand to support the elbow taking the weight of the arm.

Test tone (*Figure 92*):

› Flexing the elbow.

› Supinating the wrist.

› With wrist circumduction.

Tone may be increased (e.g. spastic cerebral palsy or acquired brain injury), normal, or decreased (e.g. ataxic cerebral palsy or myopathy).

Power

Compare left to right, looking for reduced power (*Box 7*). Aim to test all of the spinal nerve routes and the peripheral nerves (radial, ulnar and median nerves). If the child is non-compliant, get them to do any task involving movement of the arms, and observe.

Examination in older children is illustrated in *Figure 93-7*.

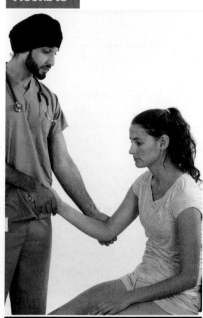

FIGURE 92

Testing for tone.

EXAMINATION

Box 7: Grading of Power

0. Paralysis, no contraction.

1. Flicker of contraction.

2. Can move with gravity excluded.

3. Can move against gravity but not against resistance.

4. Can move against some resistance but weaker.

5. Normal power.

FIGURE 95

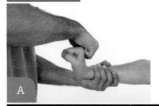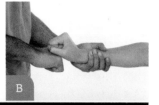

Wrist flexion and extension (C6-7), and radial nerve (wrist extension). Get the child to make a fist. The examiner should make a fist, then push down on the child's fist (extension- A) and then up against it (flexion- B). During these movements, the child should try to resist movement.

FIGURE 93

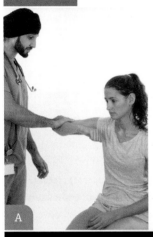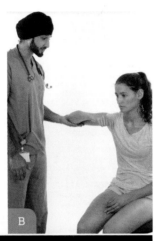

Shoulder abduction (C5) and adduction (C6-8). Ask the child to hold their arms out at 90° to body, elbows bent, like 'chicken wings'. Ask them to push their arms up (abduction-A) and then pull their elbows into their body (adduction- B) against resistance.

FIGURE 96

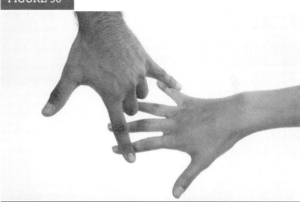

Finger abduction (T1/ulnar nerve). Ask the child to spread their fingers. The examiner should try to push them back together, whilst asking the child to resist.

FIGURE 94

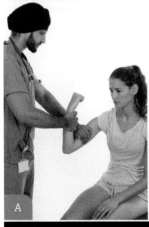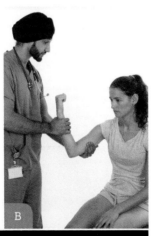

Elbow flexion (C5-6) and extension (C7-8). Ask the child to bend their arms up in front of their body. Hold their wrists and ask the child to pull the examiner towards them (flexion-A) and then push them away (extension- B).

FIGURE 97

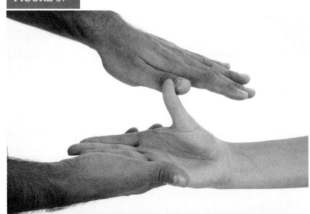

Thumb abduction (T1/median nerve). Ask the child to place the hand on a surface with the palm facing the ceiling. Ask them to then point their thumb directly to the ceiling, and then whilst pushing it down, ask the child to resist.

Additional features may be noted if there is a suspected peripheral nerve injury (*Figure 98-100*).

FIGURE 98

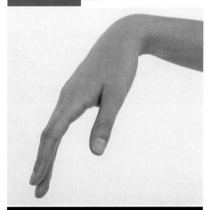

Radial nerve palsy. Wrist drop.

FIGURE 99

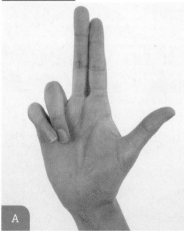

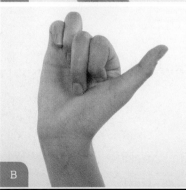

Ulnar nerve palsy "claw hand." At rest (A) and when trying to make fist (B). Note that both pictures show full extension of the 4th and 5th MCPs. These joints are not able to flex due to loss of function of the medial two lumbricals.

FIGURE 100

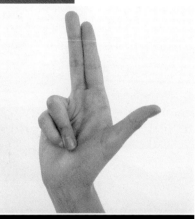

Median nerve palsy "Hand of Benedict". This only occurs on trying to make a fist. There is full flexion of the 4th and 5th MCP joints. However, the index and middle finger cannot flex at the PIP, DIP or MCP joints due to loss of function of the lateral two lumbricals.

In children under one:

> Pull infant from lying to sitting using their arms. One hand should support the head, the other hold the arms.

> Grasp. Assess this by asking the child to grab something, e.g. a finger.

> Place the child on their front; can they lift themselves up? Do they support their head when doing this? Do they lift themselves up onto their forearms or onto their hands?

Reflexes

The child must be relaxed to elicit reflexes. Arm reflexes are shown in *Figure 101-4*. First explain the test, and demonstrate it, showing that the tendon hammer is not painful. If it is difficult to elicit the reflex, ask the child to clench their teeth, screw up their eyes or count backwards from 100.

In patients under one-year-old, the above can all be attempted, as well as assessing for the presence of primitive reflexes (*Table 30*):

> In an age appropriate infant, asymmetry may indicate a problem with that limb, e.g. an asymmetrical Moro reflex could be due to a brachial plexus injury sustained at birth (Erb's palsy). The affected arm will not move.

FIGURE 101

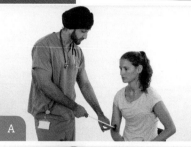

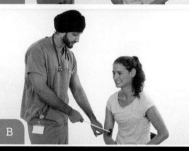

Biceps reflex (C5-6). With the arm bent and relaxed (e.g. across the lap), place a finger or thumb on the biceps tendon and strike it with the tendon hammer. Observe for contraction of the biceps muscle and/or elbow flexion. This is shown with (B) and without (A) reinforcement by clenching the teeth.

FIGURE 102

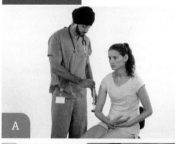

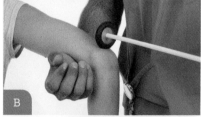

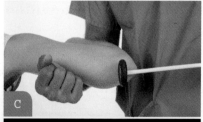

Triceps reflex (C6-7). Several techniques to elict this are shown, as it is often difficult. Observe for contraction of the triceps muscle, and/or elbow extension. A. With the child's arm bent, supporting the distal arm. B. Letting the arm dangle at the elbow. C. Supporting the forearm and the upper arm.

FIGURE 103

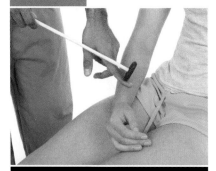

Supinator reflex (C5-6) Rest the child's arm on their lap. Strike the arm directly above the wrist on the radial side, proximal to the styloid process. Observe for contraction of the brachioradialis, flexion of the elbow, supination of the forearm, and/or flexion of the fingers.

TABLE 30: Examples of primitive reflexes		
Reflex	What is it?	Abnormal after..
Moro.	• Sudden movement of baby's head downwards results in limb extension then flexion.	• 3 months.
Asymmetrical tonic neck reflex.	• With the baby lying on their back, and the head to one side, two things happen. • The arm and leg, on the side the head is turned towards, extend. The opposite arm and leg flex.	• 6 months.
Grasp.	• Place a finger in the palm of the baby's hand. • They will grasp it, increasing their grip if you try to pull away.	• 3 months.
Stepping.	• Hold the baby upright, with their feet touching a firm surface. They will imitate walking.	• 4 months. • This reappears at about one year of age.

FIGURE 104

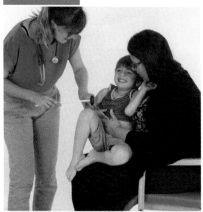

Getting help from a mother, and working with a younger child to elicit the biceps reflex.

▸ Presence of primitive reflexes beyond a certain age is abnormal and could indicate developmental delay.

Pronator Drift

Pronator drift tests for upper motor neurone lesions (*Figure 105*). This is because upper motor neurone lesions cause a relatively greater weakness in supination compared to prona-tion. Cerebellar lesions can also cause this sign.

Co-ordination

See cerebellar exam for more detail (p591):
▸ Past pointing (dysmetria) and intention tremor (*Figure 106*).
▸ Dysdiadochokinesis (*Figure 107*).

FIGURE 105

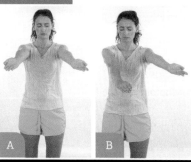

Pronator drift. A. Ask the child to put both their arms out, palm up (supinated), as if they were holding a pizza. Ask them to close their eyes and count to 10, keeping their arms in place. B. In a positive test, the affected arm will pronate and fall.

FIGURE 106

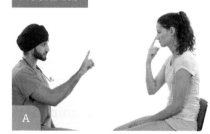

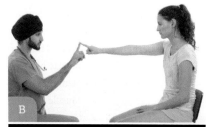

Finger-nose testing. Ask the child to touch the tip of their nose with their finger (A), and then to touch the examiner's finger (B). The examiner's finger should be held at full arm's length from them and moved around as the exercise is repeated.

FIGURE 107

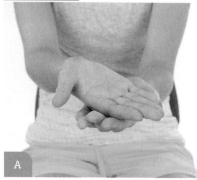

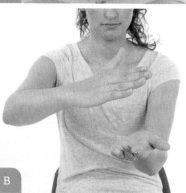

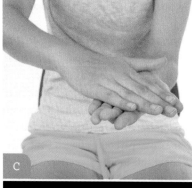

Ask the child to place one hand, palm up, with the other hand on top of it (A). Then ask them to rapidly lift it up (B) and down (C) from the palm, alternating between pronation and supination.

Power

Compare left to right, looking for reduced power (*Box 7*). Aim to test all the spinal nerve routes, as well as the peripheral nerves (*Table 31*), although they are more difficult to isolate than with the upper limbs. If the child is non-compliant, get them to do any task involving movement of the legs, and observe. Tests are shown in *Figure 113-6*. The examiner should oppose each movement accordingly.

FIGURE 113

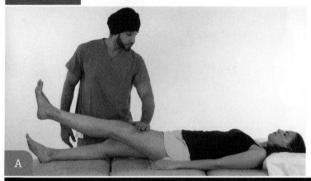
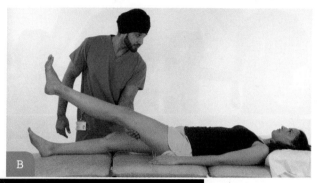

A. With the child lying flat on the bed, they should be asked to lift their leg straight up, whilst the examiner resists it (hip flexion L1-3). B. Then, from this position, they should be asked to push their leg back onto the bed, with the examiner's hand now underneath the thigh, trying to resist movement (hip extension L4-S1).

FIGURE 114

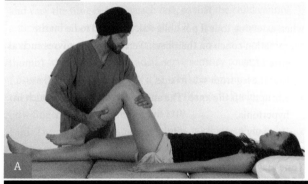
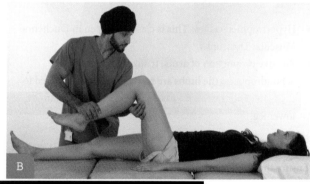

Ask the child to bend their leg. A. Ask them to pull their heel into the bottom (knee flexion L5-S1). B. Ask them to then kick out as if kicking a football (knee extension L3-4).

FIGURE 115

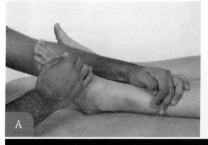
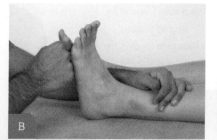

A. Ask the child to point their foot towards their head (left ankle dorsiflexion L4-5) against resistance. B. Then ask them to point it towards the floor (plantar flexion S1-2), against resistance.

FIGURE 116

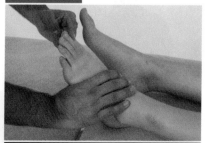

Ask the child to extend the big toe against resistance (extension of big toe (L5)).

In children under one:
> Pull to stand; can they support their weight?

Reflexes
These are described in *Figure 117-21*. As for arms, the child must be relaxed. If difficult, reinforce the reflex by asking the child to grip their fingers together and try to pull them apart (*Figure 122*).

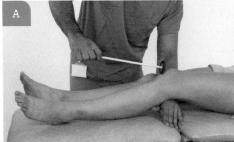
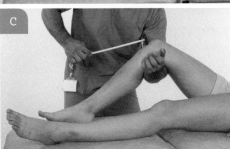
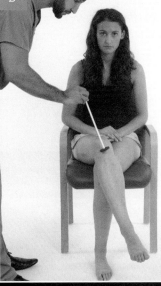

Knee jerk (L3-4). The leg will kick out if the reflex is present, or alternatively contractions may be just visible in the quadriceps muscle. In a toddler, where the tendon is more difficult to isolate, place a finger in the area and strike this instead. Several techniques shown: A. Roll one arm over the one leg and under the other. B. With the legs crossed over sat in a chair. C. Lift up one leg at the knee, taking its entire weight.

FIGURE 118

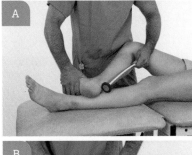
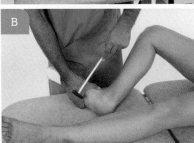
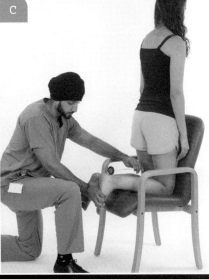

Ankle jerk (S1). Hold the foot with one hand, slightly dorsiflexed. Observe for downward movement of the foot and contraction of the gastocnemuis muscle. Several positions are shown: A. The knee is bent and the hip externally rotated. B. As above, but the sole of the foot is struck rather than the tendon directly. C. Kneeling on chair.

FIGURE 119

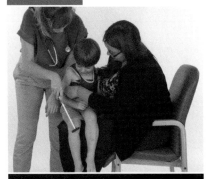

Getting help from a mother, and working with a younger child to elicit knee reflex.

FIGURE 120

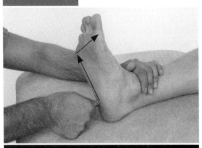

Plantar reflex. Warn the child that this may tickle. Run a finger nail from the heel, up the outside of the sole of the foot to the little toe, and then across from the base of the little toe to the base of the big toe. Observe for flexion of the toes. Extension of the big toe is consistent with an upper motor neurone lesion. It is normal in children less than 1-year-old.

FIGURE 121

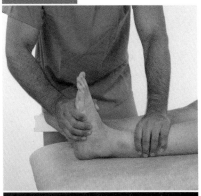

Ankle clonus. Rapidly dorsiflex the foot (upwards). On stopping, there may be involuntary upwards beats of the foot, which is called clonus. Although a few beats of clonus may be normal, particularly in children under one-year-old, sustained clonus suggests an upper motor neurone lesion.

583

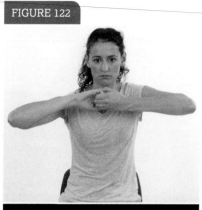

FIGURE 122

Reinforcement.

In under 1:
> Primitive reflexes as described in *Table 30*.

Sensation

Light Touch, Pain, and Temperature (Spinothalamic Tract)
> Light touch, pain and temperature are all tested as described in the arms section. Dermatomes for the legs are shown in *Figure 123*.

Proprioception and Vibration Testing (Dorsal Column)
> Proprioception. Hold the big toe either side of the interphalangeal joint, and perform this test as shown with the arms. If proprioception is not intact at the interphalangeal joint, test it at the carpometarsal joint, then the ankle, and then the knee.

> Vibration sensing. Vibrate a tuning fork and place it on the big toe, and perform this test as shown for the arm. If they cannot identify this, repeat on the malleolus, and then the tibial shaft, the tibial tuberosity, and finally the anterior iliac crest.

Sensation tests are summarised in *Figure 124*.

Peripheral nerves are less commonly damaged in the lower limbs than the upper limbs. However things to look out for are shown in *Table 31*.

Co-ordination
> Heel-shin test. *Figure 125*.

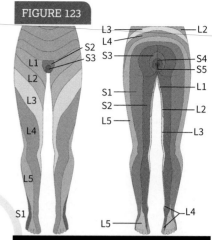

FIGURE 123

Dermatomes of the leg.

TABLE 31: Peripheral nerves of the lower limb		
Nerve	Motor loss	Sensory loss
Obturator nerve (L2-4).	• Hip adduction.	• Medial thigh.
Femoral nerve (L2-4).	• Hip flexion. • Knee extension.	• Anteromedial thigh. • Medial lower leg, to medial malleolus.
Common peroneal nerve (L4-S3).	• Foot dorsiflexion loss gives characteristic foot drop. • Foot eversion loss gives inverted posture.	• Anterolateral lower leg. • Dorsum of foot/toes.
Sciatic nerve (L4-S3).	• Paralysis of all muscles below knee- gives foot drop from weight of foot (via tibial and common fibular branches).	• Posterolateral/anterolateral lower leg. Plantar surface of foot (tibial branch). • Lateral lower leg, and dorsal foot (common fibular branch).

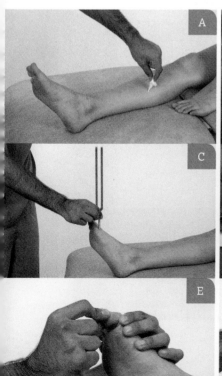

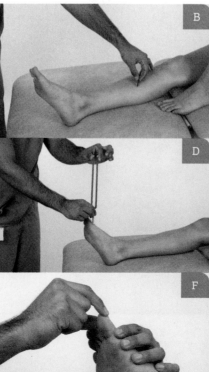

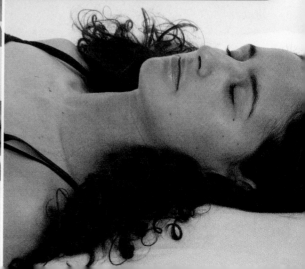

FIGURE 124

Sensation testing, whilst the patient's eyes are shut. A. Light touch with cotton wool. B. Pain with a neurotip. C. Vibration sense with a tuning fork, vibrating. D. Vibration sense with a tuning fork, stopping the vibration. E. Proprioception in the "down" position. F. Proprioception in the "up" position.

FIGURE 125

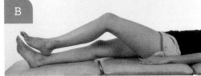

A

B

C

Demonstrate this first. With the child lying down, lift their heel up and onto their other leg, just below the knee (A), run it down the shin (B) and then bring it back to the start (C) and repeat.

FIGURE 126

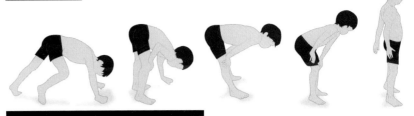

Gower's sign.

FIGURE 127

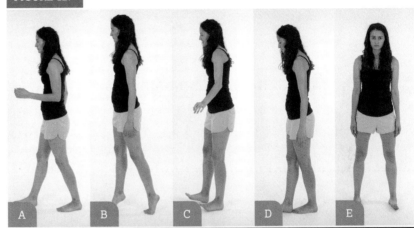

A   B   C   D   E

Going from left to right: A. Walk unaided. Assess movement of legs, arms, and trunk. Then ask the child to walk quickly and then run. This will make a subtle hemiplegia more pronounced, with flexion of the arm on the affected side more obvious. **B. Walk on tiptoes.** Again this will make a hemiplegia more pronounced, as well as testing plantar flexion and muscle strength. **C. Walk on heels.** This will exaggerate any difficulty in dorsiflexion. **D. Heel-toe walk.** Ask the child to walk as if on a tight rope, with the one foot in front of the other. Show them first and stay with them as they perform it, in case they fall. A child with ataxia will find this exercise much more difficult. **E. Walk on the outside of their feet (Fogg test).** This will make a hemiplegic gait more pronounced.

Gower's Sign

Ask the child to lie on the floor on their back. Then ask them to stand up without using their hands, if possible. If the child turns first onto their front and then rises from the floor by crawling up their legs, this is Gower's sign. It indicates proximal muscle weakness such as in Duchenne Muscular Dystrophy (*Figure 126*).

In children under one:

➤ Observe age appropriate activities e.g. bringing feet to mouth and crawling.

➤ Ensure the movements are smooth and equal on both sides.

Finally assess function of the legs. This is usually done by observing walking/running.

Examination of Gait

It is crucial that this is done knowing what the child is capable of. Ensure the child is supported so that if they fall, they may be caught. The child should be asked to move in the manners demonstrated in *Figure 127*. Different types of gait are shown in *Table 32*.

If there is an ataxic gait, use Romberg's test to help differentiate between cerebellar and sensory ataxia (*Figure 128*).

TABLE 32: Different types of gait

Types of Gait	Signs	Cause
Foot drop "high stepping" neuropathic gait.	• The leg on the side affected has to be lifted high to avoid the foot dragging along the floor.	• Common peroneal nerve palsy. • L5 radiculopathy. • Peripheral mono/poly neuropathy.
Waddling gait.	• The pelvis drops on the contralateral side to the leg being lifted (Trendelenburg sign). • The abdomen is pushed forward due to lumbar lordosis.	• Congenital hip dislocation. • Proximal myopathy, e.g. Duchenne muscular dystrophy.
Dyskinetic gait.	• Irregular, jerky, involuntary movements.	• Cerebral palsy. • Basal ganglia lesion.
Stomping gait.	• The feet are slammed onto the floor, and sometimes lifted high up to achieve this. • This is made worse in the dark (since visual compensation cannot be applied).	• Loss of proprioception, e.g. B12/folate deficiency.
Ataxic gait.	• Unsteady. • Broad based. • Difficulty heel-toe walking.	• Cerebellar cause, e.g. post viral cerebellitis.

Continued

TABLE 32: *Continued*		
Types of Gait	**Signs**	**Cause**
Spastic hemiplegia.	• The arm is held flexed, adducted, and is internally rotated, with the hand held in a fist. • The leg is in extension, stiff, and in plantar flexion. • The leg is dragged in circumduction (in a semi-circle).	• Cerebral palsy. • Acquired brain lesions, e.g. stroke.
Spastic diplegia.	• Tightness of adductors causes the knees to come together/legs to cross at midline, giving a "scissoring gait". • Dragging of both legs. • Narrow base. • Circumduction on both sides.	

FIGURE 128

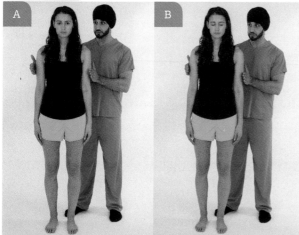

Romberg's test. A. The patient stands, feet together, eyes open, and hands by their side. B. The patient closes their eyes, and is observed for one minute whilst the examiner looks for loss of balance and swaying.

In cerebellar ataxia, vision cannot compensate for the ataxia, but in sensory ataxia it can. Therefore, with cerebellar ataxia, there will be difficulty with standing even with eyes open, but in a sensory ataxia, the loss of balance will not become evident until the eyes are closed.

The test is positive if the child can stand normally with their eyes open, but loses balance on closing their eyes.

Grading Motor Ability

The General Motor Function Classification System (GMFCS) is a grading system from 1-5 used to classify motor ability in children with four limb motor disorders (the majority of which are cerebral palsy) (*Table 33*). It distinguishes the need for different assist devices and is therefore a comment on quality of movement. It can also have some prognostic use as older children are unlikely to change their GMFCS.

Cranial Nerve Examination

Inspection

A lot can be achieved in the cranial nerve assessment from general observation:

> Dysmorphic facies. Rare syndromes such as Goldernhar syndrome are associated with both dysmorphic features (incomplete development of the ear, nose, soft palate, lip and mandible), and cranial nerve palsies (e.g. VII and VIII).
> Eyes. Look for presence of glasses, and any obvious squint.
> Look for possible signs of cranial nerve abnormalities.
>> Ptosis (III).
>> Eye/pupil position (III, IV, VI).
>> Pupil symmetry (II, III).
>> Facial symmetry (VII).
>> Speech (V, VII, IX, X, XII).
>> Sternocleidomastoid/trapezius bulk (XI).

The cranial nerves can either be tested in order, or by flow of movement down the face, e.g. after CN VII, test CN XII sticking their tongue out, then move down to test CN XI by turning their head.

CN I (Olfactory Nerve)

> Generally assessed from history rather than formal examination.
> Ask about smell, and test if necessary, e.g. with coffee, although ideally standardised smelling salts should be used.

TABLE 33: General Motor Function Classification System	
GMFCS grade	**Description of function**
I.	No restriction in walking but may have difficulties with coordination or balance.
II.	No devices needed when walking, may need a rail for stairs and find outdoor terrain more tricky, running difficult.
III.	Needs a mobility device such as crutches, may be able to use a manual wheelchair.
IV.	Uses wheelchair most of the time, wheelchair is controlled by the user.
V.	Severely limited mobility, including of head and neck, even when supporting aids are used, e.g. wheelchair bound with head support.

(Adapted from Palisano et al. (1997) Dev Med Child Neurol 39:214-23 CanChild: www.canchild.ca).

CN II (Optic Nerve)

Acuity

- Check that the child can actually see with both eyes first.
- If the child is wearing glasses, test vision with the glasses on.
- Use a Snellen chart if available; otherwise ask them to read something in the room, e.g. a book or a sign on the wall.

Visual Fields

The technique for this is shown in *Figure 129*.

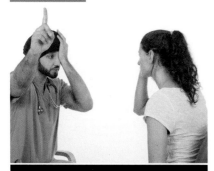

FIGURE 129

Visual fields testing.

- The examiner should sit opposite the child 50 cm-1 m away, and ask the child to cover one of their eyes using the palm of their hand. At the same time, the examiner covers their opposite eye (i.e. the examiner covers their right eye if the child is covering their left eye).
- Whilst the child looks at the examiner's nose, the examiner moves a wiggling finger inwards from outside of their visual field from the upper right corner, lower right corner, upper left corner and lower left corner: this tests all four quadrants. It is crucial that the examiner's finger starts outside of their visual field: this is confrontational testing, so if the finger is outside of the examiner's visual field (which is assumed to be normal) it should be outside of the child's visual field as well.
- Ask the child to "yes" when they can see the finger. The examiner should swap hands when moving from

medial to lateral visual fields (i.e. use the right hand to wiggle for the left lateral visual field, and the left hand to wiggle for the left medial visual field) so that the arm does not cross the field of vision.

Fundoscopy

- Red reflex. This is lost in the presence of cataracts, or white if there is a retinoblastoma (*Figure 71*).
- Optic disc. A pink disc with clear margins should be seen. Blurred margins are seen in papilloedema, which is associated with raised intracranial pressure (*Figure 72*).

Reflexes

- Test for accommodation (*Figure 130*) and pupillary reflexes (*Figure 131*).
- These both rely on the optic nerve for sensory input, and the oculomotor nerve for the motor limb.

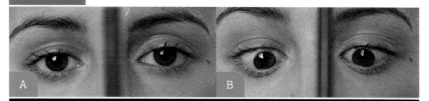

FIGURE 130

Accommodation tested using a pencil. A. Hold a finger or an object (e.g. pencil) in front of the child's face. Ask them to look off into the distance, and then suddenly focus on the pencil. B. The pupils should constrict and converge.

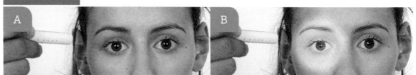

FIGURE 131

Pupillary reflexes. Shine a pen torch in each eye (A) and observe the effect (B). Look for constriction of the pupil (direct reflex) and then constriction of the opposite pupil (indirect reflex). Shine the pen torch in each eye twice, once for the direct reflex, once for the indirect reflex.

CN III (Oculomotor Nerve), CN IV (Trochlear Nerve) and CN VI (Abducens Nerve)

- This can be remembered as the "H test".
  - Sit in front of the child, resting one hand on their head or chin. The examiner should place their finger 50cm from the child's face, asking them to keep their head still and follow the finger with their eyes only (*Figure 132-3*).
  - The examiner should move their finger slowly in the shape of an "H", forming a horizontal line across the visual field and two vertical lines at the periphery (*Figure 134*). This will demonstrate the full spectrum of extraocular eye movements (*Figure 135*). For completeness, it is useful to ask the child to look directly up and directly down as well.
- Look for the position of the pupil and any nystagmus. Ask the patient if they have any pain or any double vision at any point. Note:
  - The position of the pupil.
  - Is there a delay in or incomplete movement indicating a palsy?
  - Is there any double vision? At extremes of vision this is normal.
  - Are the eye movements painful?
  - Is there any nystagmus?

FIGURE 132

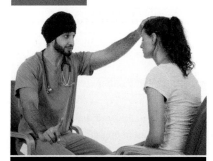

Eye movement assessment.

FIGURE 135

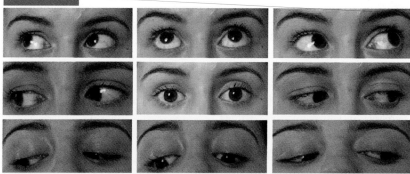

Assessing eye movements looking in eight directions.

FIGURE 133

A

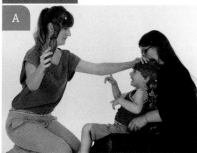

B

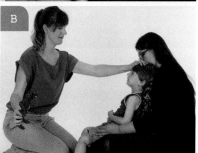

Adapting to a younger child. Using toys and mum to help elicit clinical signs.

FIGURE 136

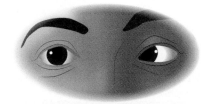

Example of a right sided 6th nerve palsy (patient asked to look right).

FIGURE 137

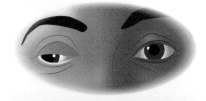

Example of a right 3rd nerve palsy: lid lag, pupil down and out. Older children will complain of diplopia. In a complete 3rd nerve palsy, the pupil will be dilated and not react to light. It can be congenital or acquired due to infection, trauma, space occupying lesion or hypertension.

FIGURE 138

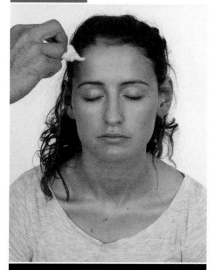

Sensation to the V_1 division of trigeminal nerve.
1. With the child's eyes closed, gently touch their face with cotton wool in each division of the trigeminal nerve.
2. Ask them to say "yes" when they can feel it.

FIGURE 134

Inferior oblique — Superior rectus

Up

Medial rectus ← *G a z e* → Lateral rectus

Down

Superior oblique — Inferior rectus

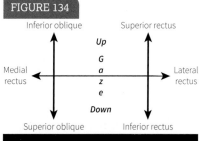

Eye movements.

Examples of third and sixth nerve palsy are shown in *Figure 136* and *137*.

CN V (Trigeminal Nerve)

➤ Sensory division. Test each of the trigeminal nerve divisions: ophthalmic, maxillary and mandibular, i.e. forehead, cheeks, jaw.

Test left and right but do not go in an obvious order. Then ask if it felt the same on both sides (*Figure 138*).
➤ Motor division. Ask the child to clench their jaw. Palpate the side of the face (masseter muscle) and the temples (temporalis muscle), looking for loss of muscle bulk/strength (*Figure 139*).
➤ Jaw jerk reflex. This is not routinely tested but should be offered (*Figure 140*).

➤ Corneal reflex. Involuntary blinking of the eyes when the cornea is stimulated. The efferent limb (i.e. the blinking) occurs as a result of facial nerve activity. This is not routinely tested (*Figure 141*).

CN VII (Facial Nerve)

➤ Test each individual branch, as shown in *Figure 142*. A lower motor neurone lesion, e.g. Bell's palsy, will affect all of the face. An upper motor neurone lesion, e.g. cerebral palsy, will affect the lower face only; i.e. the forehead is spared.

FIGURE 139

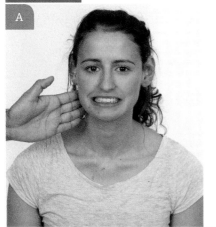

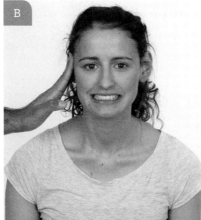

Clenching teeth and testing: A. Masseter (left). B. Temporalis (right).

FIGURE 143

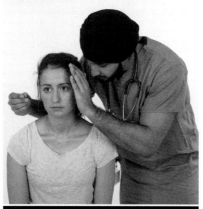

Testing hearing. Cover the patient's eyes with one hand (so they cannot lip read), and occlude the ear not being tested (by pushing on the tragus, and rubbing the fingers together over that ear to create white noise). Whisper a number in the ear being tested. Get increasingly louder until the child can hear the number.

FIGURE 140

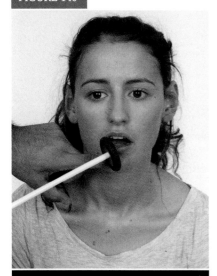

Jaw jerk. With the mouth slightly open, tap the space between the chin and the lower lip with a tendon hammer. This should result in masseter contraction.

FIGURE 141

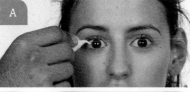

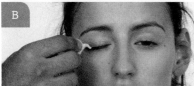

Corneal reflex. Touch the cornea with cotton wool (A) and look for blinking (B).

> Test the taste supply to the anterior 2/3 of the tongue. It can be tested using salt/sugar on the lateral side of the tongue, with the mouth rinsed in between. This is not routinely tested.
> Examine the ears for vesicles if there is a facial palsy. This is associated with Ramsey-Hunt syndrome, which is Herpes Zoster reactivation in the facial nerve.

CN VIII (Vestibulocochlear Nerve)
> Test hearing. Basic props may be used for crude testing of hearing in younger children (*Figure 143-4*).

> Rinne's and Weber's tests. These can be performed in older children. This differentiates between conductive and sensorineural deafness and requires a 512 Hz tuning fork. Activate the tuning fork first by tapping it on a hard surface/knee. Subsequent steps are shown in *Figure 145*.
> Assess balance. This is not routinely tested.

FIGURE 142

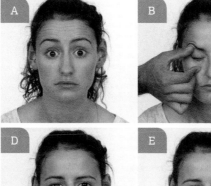
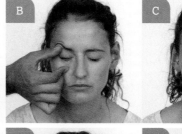
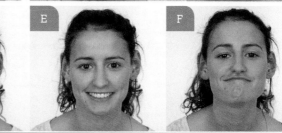

Facial nerve testing. From left to right, ask the child to: A. Raise their eyebrows (temporal branch). B. Close their eyes tightly, and then as the examiner, try and open them (zygomatic branch). C. Blow their cheeks out (buccal branch). D. Whistle (mandibular branch). E. Bare their teeth (mandibular branch). F. Stick forward their chin as if shaving (cervical branch).

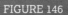
FIGURE 144

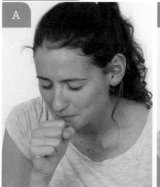
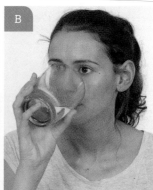

Crude hearing test. A. Use keys to make a sound, making sure the child cannot see them initially. B. Positive test if the child turns to the sound.

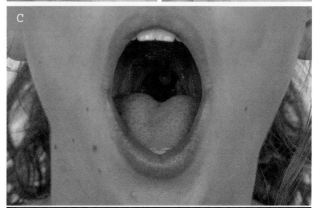
FIGURE 146

Asking the patient to: A. Cough. B. Swallow water. C. Say "ahh" to look in the mouth.

CN IX (Glossopharyngeal Nerve) and CN X (Vagus Nerve)

> Gag reflex. Gently check for sensation in the posterior pharyngeal wall on both sides. Then stick the tongue depressor into the back of the throat to elicit a gag reflex. Not usually tested.

> Swallowing water. IX is the sensory limb, X is the motor limb (*Figure 146*).

> Cough. Not a very sensitive test, as multiple factors affect cough, e.g. respiratory muscle strength, but tests vagal nerve function as well (*Figure 146*).

> Opening the mouth and saying "aaahh". Look for uvula deviation, and symmetrical rising of the soft palate (both

FIGURE 145

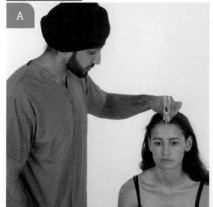
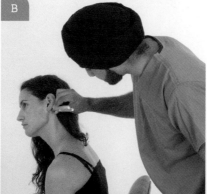
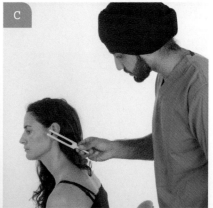

A. Weber's test. Tap the tuning fork, and place the base at the centre of the forehead. Ask the patient if they hear it loudest in the middle (normal), to the left, or the right. In a conductive deafness, Weber's test is louder in the affected ear, but in sensorineural deafness, it is loudest in the unaffected ear. B/C. Rinne's test. Tap the tuning fork, and place it on the bony mastoid process behind the ear (B), and then over the ear (C). In normal hearing and sensorineural deafness, conduction over the ear (air conduction) is better, whereas bony conduction is better in conductive deafness.

testing vagus nerve function). Deviation to the right suggests paralysis on the left (*Figure 146*).

CN XI (Accessory Nerve)
▸ Shrugging and turning head against resistance. This is tested as shown in *Figure 147*.

CN XII (Hypoglossal Nerve)
▸ Tongue inspection. Look for tongue wasting and fasciculation while the mouth is open and the tongue is still in the mouth (relaxed). Ask the child to stick out their tongue. Look for any deviation (*Figure 148*).
▸ Tongue movement. Get the child to move their tongue from side-to-side, and look for any weakness. Ask them to push the tongue into their cheeks (*Figure 149*).

FIGURE 148

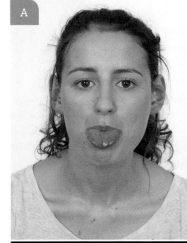
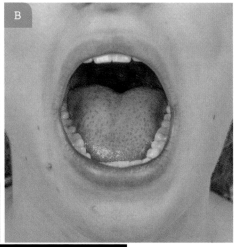

Inspection of the tongue sticking out and in the mouth.

FIGURE 147

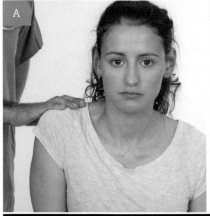
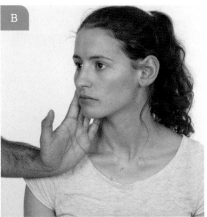

A. Ask the child to shrug their shoulders against resistance. This will show any weakness in the trapezius muscle. B. Ask the child to turn their head against your hand. This will show any weakness in the sternocleidomastoid muscle.

FIGURE 149

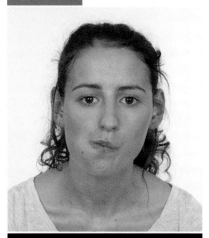

Tongue pushed into the cheek to assess power.

Cerebellar Examination
Cerebellar examination would be required in the child who appears to have "lost their balance". The commonest reason for this is a post-viral cerebellitis, often post-varicella infection, but it is important to look for signs of other causes such as inherited ataxias or a space occupying lesion. A helpful mnemonic for cerebellar signs is "DANISH Pastry":

D - dysdiadochokinesia
A - ataxia
N - nystagmus
I - intention tremor
S - slurred/staccato speech
H - hypotonia
P - past-pointing

General Inspection
▸ Walking aids. These may suggest gait abnormalities.
▸ Posture and baseline movements. There may be truncal ataxia and tremor.
▸ Look for clues suggesting an underlying aetiology.
  › Chronic liver disease, e.g. spider naevi, palmar erythema.
  › Alcohol intoxication.
  › Ataxic telangiectasia. Look for telangiectasia, particularly on the face/eyes.

Eye Signs
▸ Extraocular muscle movements. Use H testing (*Figure 132-5*). Get the child to hold their gaze in the lateral and vertical positions to try and illicit nystagmus.

- Rapid eye movements. Not routinely done, but may pick up nystagmus (*Figure 70*).

Speech

- Dysarthria. Slurring of speech can be identified by saying phrases such as "baby hippopotamus" or "British constitution." Staccato speech will be apparent, meaning each sound/note is sharply detached from the others.

Upper Limb Examination

- Tone. Hypotonia is associated with a cerebellar lesion.
- Power. Normally not significantly affected, but poor coordination can impair this.
- Reflexes. There may be diminished reflexes in Friedreich's ataxia.
- Intention Tremor. Ask the child to pick up an object. A tremor may become obvious on "intention" or "movement".
- Pronator drift. (*Figure 105*).
- Cerebellar rebound. (*Figure 150*).
- Past pointing (dysmetria) and intention tremor. (*Figure 106*).
- Dysdiadochokinesis. (*Figure 107*).

Lower Limb Examination

- Tone. Hypotonia is associated with a cerebellar lesion.
- Power. Power is not normally significantly affected.
- Reflexes. There may be diminished reflexes in Friedreich's ataxia, along with an upgoing plantar reflex.
- Heel-shin test. (*Figure 125*).

Gait

- Ataxic gait. An ataxic gait with a broad base, and difficulty balancing, particularly on heel-toe walking is seen.
- Romberg's test. Romberg's test is positive in sensory ataxia, but it is negative in cerebellar ataxia (*Figure 128*).

Examination of the Head

Head examination is not routinely done in older children, but is more relevant to babies/toddlers and those that have undergone surgical procedures.

Inspection

- Head size. (*Figure 151*).
- Head shape. (*Figure 152*).
- Dysmorphic features.

FIGURE 150

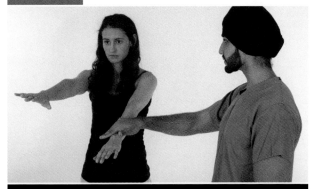

Cerebellar Rebound. With the patient's hands held out in front of them, press one arm down and then let go. Ask the child to try and put the arm back in the original position. In cerebellar rebound, this is very difficult, and the arm "overshoots" on correction.

FIGURE 151

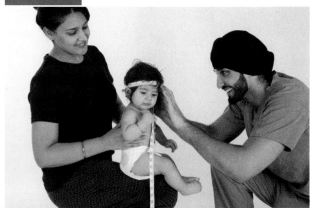

Measuring head circumference. Measure with a tape measure, going around the occiput, and above the eyebrows.

Normal

Plagiocephaly

Brachycephaly

Dolichocephaly

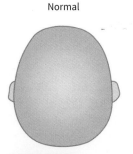

FIGURE 152

Head shapes.

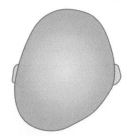

Plagiocephaly. An asymmetric and oblique deformity of the head.

Brachycephaly. Short wide head, with flattened occiput, i.e. a relatively short anteroposterior diameter.

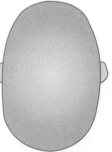

Dolichocephaly. Disproportionately long anteroposterior diameter.

Palpation

- Palpate the sutures and the fontanelles (*Figure 153*). Fusion of the sutures (craniosynostosis) may occur prematurely. It is usually isolated, but it may occur as part of a syndrome, e.g. Apert syndrome or Crouzon syndrome.
- Fontanelles can be:
  › Sunken. This is most commonly due to dehydration.
  › Bulging. This is associated with raised intracranial pressure, e.g. meningitis, hydrocephalus or crying.
  › Delayed closure. e.g. congenital hypothyroidism, trisomy 21, rickets.
  › Premature closure. This is associated with craniosynostosis and microcephaly. The posterior fontanelle usually closes before the child is two-months-old. The anterior fontanelle between 4 and 26-months-old.
- Palpate for any surgical procedures.
  › Ventriculoperitoneal (VP) shunt. This is usually a U shaped incision, 3 cm posterior/superior to the pinna of the ear, but it may vary depending on age. The catheter is palpable going to the abdomen/thorax. Look for an associated scar in the abdomen/thorax as well. The abdominal site is usually a vertical incision at the right subcostal margin.

FIGURE 153

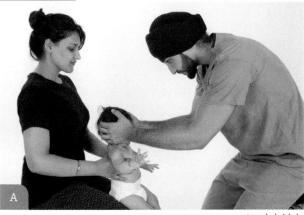

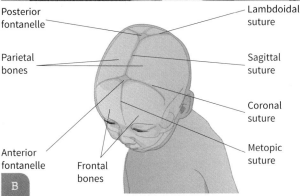

A. Palpating the skull sutures and fontanelles in an infant. Keep the head well supported while palpating and employ the parent's assistance if needed. B. The underlying anatomical landmarks.

The Child in the Wheelchair

A child may need to be examined whilst in a wheelchair. Most information can be deduced without putting the child onto an examination couch. The other neurological examinations or slightly adapted versions of them can be performed on the child who is wheelchair bound.

Inspection
Wheelchair

- Type of wheelchair (*Figure 24*).
  › Manual self-propelled. This needs good strength and co-ordination in upper body for operation.
  › Electric power wheelchairs. There are two broad types:
    ◻ Controlled via a hand device, e.g. joystick. This requires relatively good strength in hands, and reasonable hand-eye co-ordination.
    ◻ Controlled by a headswitch, chin joystick or breath assisted controls. This indicates a severe motor deficit, as the child cannot use their hands to control the joystick.
- Wedges or braces used to support, and if so, where? Truncal, neck and head supports indicate hypotonia; e.g. a child with cerebral palsy may be hypertonic in their arms and legs but have truncal hypotonia requiring a brace. Duchenne Muscular Dystrophy patients may require spinal support.

Face and Head

- Head size. e.g. a child with macrocephaly may have hydrocephalus, particularly if a shunt is present.
- Shunts. VP shunt in hydrocephalus.
- Dysmorphic facies.
- Obvious nystagmus or squint.

Arms

- Tremor.
- Abnormal posturing.
- Dystonic movements. e.g. chorea, athetosis.

Abdomen

- Scars. These can be seen from VP shunt placement.
- Gastrostomy or jejunostomy. These may either be in situ or scars may be visible from removal.
- Urinary catheter in place. This is common in spina bifida.

Palpation
Head

- Head circumference.
- Shunts. Palpate for any shunts or reservoirs.

Arms/Legs

- Tone and power can be grossly assessed by holding the child's hands/feets.
- Reflexes can also be assessed in the wheelchair.

Completing the Examination

> Perform a general paediatric examination.
> If the child is in a wheelchair, ideally perform a full neurological examination of the patient's arms and legs with the patient out of the wheelchair and on the bed.

Bedside tests include:

> Review the observation chart.
> Plot the height and weight on an age and sex appropriate chart.

CASE SCENARIOS

SCENARIO 11

Joe is a 7-year-old boy who has come to the outpatient clinic for review. He was born prematurely and has been regularly seen in the clinic. Please examine his lower limbs.

EXAMINATION CHECKLIST

Domain	Findings	Evolving thought process
Global assessment of child on approach.	• Alert, looks well, no supports.	• Not acutely unwell.
Inspection.	• Walks with legs turned inwards, more on tiptoes. • Scar over Achilles. • Loss of muscle bulk in the legs.	• Appears to have a diplegic gait. • May have had tendon release surgery. • Pathology likely to be chronic.
Tone.	• Increased.	• Likely upper motor neurone lesion, but with good function.
Power.	• 4/5 throughout.	
Reflexes.	• Brisk, with upgoing plantars.	
Pronator drift.	• Positive.	
Coordination.	• Good.	
Function.	• Good.	
Sensation.	• Normal to light touch, and joint position sense.	• Isolated motor pathology.

SCENARIO 12

Phoebe is an 8-year-old girl who presents to ED with drooping of the right side of her face. Please examine her cranial nerves.

EXAMINATION CHECKLIST

Domain	Findings	Evolving thought process
Global assessment of child.	• Appears well, not in pain, well grown for age.	• Lesion not impacting on general health.
Inspection.	• Drooping of right side of face. No dysmorphic features. • Normal gait on entering room.	• Possible facial nerve palsy.
Individual cranial nerves.	• Cannot close right eye tightly. • When smiles, right side does not lift. • Rest normal.	• Appears to have a unilateral facial palsy affecting all of that side of the face.

PRESENTING YOUR FINDINGS

Joe is a 7-year-old boy who I examined in clinic today.

He appears well and comfortable at rest. He has no obvious dysmorphic facies and no mobility aids. Joe has a diplegic gait. He has scars over his Achilles, consistent with tendon release surgery. Joe has signs of an upper motor neurone lesion affecting both his lower limbs, with increased tone, brisk reflexes and upgoing plantar reflex. Power is 4/5 throughout. His arms do not appear affected but I would need to formally examine them.

These findings are consistent with a spastic diplegia, which may be a result of cerebral palsy or an acquired brain injury.

To complete my examination, I would like to review the observation chart, perform a musculoskeletal and vascular examination of the lower limbs, examine the arms and examine cranial nerves. I would also like to plot his height and weight on a growth chart.

Phoebe is an 8-year-old year old girl who has presented to ED today with drooping of the right side of her face. Phoebe appears well grown for her age and grossly does not appear to have any other neurological signs. Her facial movements are asymmetrical, with lack of movement on the right side of her face. The rest of her cranial nerves are intact.

I believe that Phoebe has a right-sided facial nerve palsy caused by a lower motor neurone lesion. The most common cause for this would be a Bell's Palsy.

To complete my examination, I would like to perform fundoscopy, perform a cardiovascular exam, including blood pressure, examine the spine, and perform a formal neurological examination of her arms, legs, and gait.

RESPIRATORY EXAMINATION

The lungs are not the only organs in the thorax and other systems can produce respiratory signs, e.g. wheeze and crackles due to fluid overload secondary to cardiac failure. Do not look for solely a respiratory diagnosis when asked to perform a respiratory examination.

Particular incidences when a more detailed assessment might be required include:

1 Does the child in respiratory failure need immediate intervention? See *Box 8* for signs of respiratory distress. Be aware of signs of a tension pneumothorax, as this only requires clinical diagnosis before treatment is initiated.

2 Are there signs of chronic underlying respiratory disease or other chronic medical diseases that may impact the respiratory system? For example, a child with four limb cerebral palsy and scoliosis is likely to have reduced reserve for coping with a chest insult such as a lower respiratory tract infection.

Box 8: Signs of respiratory distress

- Head bobbing in infants.
- Nasal flaring.
- Grunting. This is a result of a child breathing through a closed glottis in order to increase their end expiratory pressures.
- Too breathless to speak.
- Stridor. This is a high pitched sound, indicating airway obstruction. It may be inspiratory, expiratory or biphasic.
- Tracheal tug.
- Intercostal recessions.
- Subcostal recessions.

3 Does this child with wheeze/respiratory distress require further treatment, or are they improving? This is one of the commonest assessments required in paediatrics, and often involves determination of whether bronchodilator therapy needs to be escalated, or whether it can be reduced.

Common acute presentations are shown in *Table 34*. Common cases for exams are shown in *Table 35*.

TABLE 34: Common acute respiratory presentations

Disease	Possible clues
Bronchiolitis.	• Usually under 6-months-old, but up to 1- to 2-years-old. • Increased work of breathing +/- oxygen requirement. • Crackles and wheeze on auscultation. • Reduced feeding.
Viral induced wheeze.	• Preschool-age children. • Associated coryzal symptoms. • Wheeze responding to salbutamol. • May be family/personal history of atopy.
Exacerbation of asthma.	• School-aged children. • Increased work of breathing, wheeze +/- oxygen requirement. • Breathless on speaking in severe exacerbation.
Lower Respiratory Tract Infection.	• Fever. • Increased work of breathing. • Crackles mainly, but there may also be wheeze.
Anaphylaxis.	• Trigger may be known. • May be airway compromise. • Wheeze. • May be associated rash and facial swelling.

TABLE 35: Common patients that may appear in clinical examinations

Disease	Possible clues
Cystic fibrosis.	• May be underweight. • Central line/gastrostomy visible. • Pancreatic enzymes around the bed. • Nasal polyps. • Clubbing.
Asthma.	• Harrison's sulcus. • Hyperexpanded chest. • May be no signs to see at all!
Bronchiectasis. • Congenital, e.g. CF, PCD • Acquired, Post infective, Obstruction e.g. foreign body, Connective tissue disease	• Wet cough. • Productive sputum. • Crackles. • Wheeze. • Faltering growth. • Clubbing.
Chronic lung disease (due to prematurity).	• Younger child. • Venepuncture scars on hand. • Chest drain scars. • Home oxygen. • Other signs of prematurity, e.g. head shape, developmental delay.
Kartagener syndrome.	• Bronchiectasis (as above). • Dextrocardia. • Situs inversus. • Nasal polyps. • Sinusitis. • Rhinorrhea.

Summary Checklist

Global assessment of child on approach.

Inspection. Hands, face, chest, abdomen.

Palpation. Lymph nodes, apex, chest expansion.

Percuss. Lungs, front and back.

Auscultate. Chest sounds throughout the lung fields.

Completing the examination. ENT assessment.

Bedside tests. Observation chart, peak flow, inhaler technique, plot weight/head circumference, inspect sputum sample.

Starting the Examination

The examination begins by observing the child. Begin with a broad assessment:

1 Does the child look unwell? Is the child playing happily or too breathless to even speak? Is there a cough or stridor? Any colour change to the skin? Is there an altered respiratory rate?

2 Are there any signs of chronic ill health? Determine if the child looks cachectic, whether they have any medication around the bed, and if they have any medical devices, long-term lines or feeding tubes in place. Is the child attached to a portable oxygen device? Is there a sputum pot?

3 Has treatment already been started? Are they attached to oxygen? Is a nebuliser currently being administered?

Inspection

Hands

› Clubbing. For causes and grading, see *Box 9* and *10*. In an older child, ask them to hold their thumbs together, nail-to-nail, and look through the diamond shaped space that is formed to assess loss of this normal curvature (*Figure 154*).

› Peripheral cyanosis.

Box 9: Causes of clubbing

Respiratory.
• Bronchiectasis (inc CF).
• Empyema/lung abscess.
• Pulmonary TB.
• Fibrosing alveolitis.

Cardiac.
• Cyanotic congenital heart disease.
• Bacterial endocarditis.
• Atrial myxoma.

GI.
• IBD.
• Biliary cirrhosis.

Other.
• Malignancy.

Box 10: Grading of clubbing

Stage 1. Fluctuant bogginess of nail bed.

Stage 2. Nail fold angle lost.

Stage 3. Nail bed has an increased curve.

Stage 4. Distal phalanx of finger enlarged.

FIGURE 154

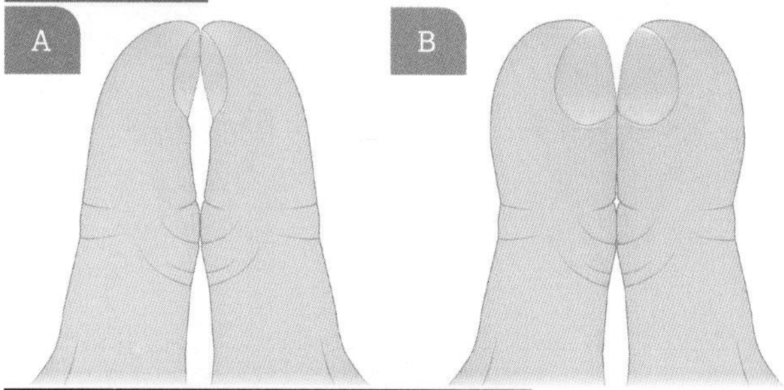

A   B

Clubbing. A. Normal. B. Clubbed.

› Radial pulse. Check this in an older child. Feel for 30 seconds and count the pulse rate. Tachycardia can be caused by sepsis, respiratory distress, or secondary to salbutamol use.

Face

› Dysmorphic features.

› Central cyanosis. This is best seen by asking the patient to open their mouth and lift their tongue. Cyanosis is seen in advanced cystic fibrosis, bronchiectasis or cyanotic congenital heart disease.

› Nasal polyps. Look in the nose. Bilateral polyps are often seen in patients with cystic fibrosis.

› Ask the child to cough and to huff. This will give an indication of whether there is a prolonged expiratory phase, or if there are significant lung secretions, e.g. cystic fibrosis.

› Hearing aids. Children may have associated hearing impairment with primary ciliary dyskinesia.

Neck

› Cervical lymphadenopathy. Palpate the anterior and posterior chains. Lymphadenopathy may indicate an acute illness or chronic inflammation.

› Tracheal position. (*Figure 155*).

Abdomen

› Gastrostomy. This may be present or there may be a scar from previous gastrostomy. It is used in children with cystic fibrosis with faltering growth to increase calorie intake and aid growth.

› Palpate liver. Is there hepatomegaly or has the liver been pushed down by hyperexpansion? Usually this would be performed at the end of the examination after the chest has been auscultated.

FIGURE 155

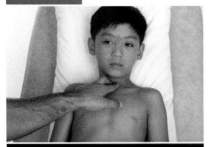

Tracheal palpation. Demonstrate the examination technique first. Place one finger either side in the sternal notch to see if the sternum is in the midline. Do not press too hard as it can be uncomfortable.

Chest

Start with anterior chest examination first.

- Respiratory rate. Count it over 30 seconds.
- Chest wall shape.
  - Pectus excavatum. Sternum pushed in, hollowed chest.
  - Pectus carinatum. Sternum pushed out, "pigeon chest".
- Obvious hyperinflation. This could be due to bronchiectasis, chronic asthma, cystic fibrosis, or chronic lung disease.
- Harrison's sulci. This refers to grooves along the lower border of the chest. It is seen in chronic airway disease and poorly controlled asthma.
- Scoliosis. This is particularly exaggerated in children with cerebral palsy, but it may not be obvious until the child is seen from behind.
- Central venous access device. This may be present in children with cystic fibrosis or bronchiectasis, who require prolonged courses of intravenous antibiotic treatment for exacerbations.
- Chest wall recessions. This indicates increased work of breathing.
- Scars. These may be from cardiac or lung surgery (*Figure 156*). Remember to lift up each arm and look in the axilla, as lateral thoracotomy scars may be hidden.

Palpation

- Chest expansion. Assess from the side. In asthma, the anteroposterior diameter may be increased (indicating obstructive airway disease)

FIGURE 156

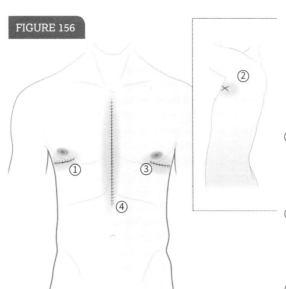

① **Right thoracotomy**
Right sided, may be axillary only. Could indicate a modified Blalock-Taussig shunt, a lobectomy performed due to congenital pulmonary airway malformation or repair of a tracheo-oesophageal fistula

② **Chest drain scar**
May be in multiple sites in axillary triangle. Usually small scars similar to venepuncture scars

③ **Left thoracotomy**
Blalock-Taussig shunt, lobectomy, coarctation repair, PDA ligation, pulmonary artery banding

④ **Median sternotomy**
Bypass surgery e.g. correction of major cardiac defects

Common chest wall scars in children.

FIGURE 157

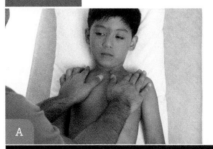
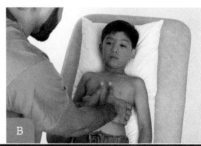

Both AP expansion and lateral expansion can be tested. A. AP expansion. Place the palms of the hands on the chest. Note how much the hands are raised when the child breathes in and out. B. Lateral expansion. Place the palms of both hands on the anterolateral chest wall either side of the midline with thumbs apart and pointing towards the head. Note how far apart the thumbs move as the child breathes in and out.

(*Figure 157*). In school-aged children, chest expansion is usually 3-5 cm.

- Feel for apex beat of heart. Altered position of apex beat may indicate mediastinal shift or dextrocardia.

Percussion

Percussion is not so useful in infants, but in older children it is performed. Percuss over the clavicles, in the upper, middle and lower zones on each side of the chest (both front and back), and in both axillae (*Figure 158*). Listen for the differences in the two sides. The note may be:

- Dull. This may be the case in consolidation or effusions (stony dull).
- Hyperresonant. This occurs with pneumothoraces.

FIGURE 158

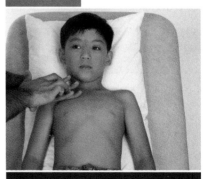

Place the middle finger of left hand over the site to percuss. With the middle finger of the right hand, tap 2-3 times onto the other finger. The wrist must be kept loose.

Auscultation

Work down from top to bottom comparing right to left. Auscultate in six zones on the anterior chest (upper left, upper right, middle right, middle left, bottom left, bottom right), both axillae, and repeat on the back (*Figure 159*). Abnormal sounds may include:

> Crackles. This indicates consolidation, collapse, bronchiectasis, pulmonary oedema or fibrosis.

> Wheeze. This is an expiratory sound due to airway narrowing, commonly due to bronchiolitis, viral-induced wheeze or asthma. If focal, consider an inhaled foreign body, particularly in preschool aged children.

> Reduced or absent air entry. This may be due to consolidation, effusion or poor lung expansion.

> Pleural rub. This is caused by inflamed pleura rubbing together. It is a creaking sound that can be heard in expiration and inspiration. Causes include pneumonia and pulmonary emboli.

Tactile vocal fremitus may be tested for at this stage, if relevant (suspected consolidation/collapse) (*Figure 160*).

Completing the Examination

> Repeat the above inspection through to auscultation, for posterior chest. This is less disruptive than palpating the front of the chest and then the back of the chest, and then listening to the front of the chest, listening to the back of the chest, etc.

> Examine the ENT system.

Bedside tests include:

> Review the observation chart.
> Plot the height and weight on an age and sex appropriate chart.
> Perform a peak flow.
> Collect sputum sample for culture.

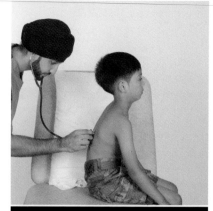
FIGURE 159

Auscultating the chest.

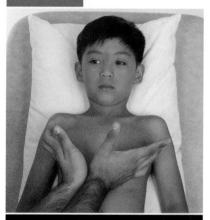
FIGURE 160

Place the medial, ulna border of the hand on the chest wall, palm side up. Feel for how the sound is transmitted to your hand. In older children, you can get them to say "ninety-nine". It will be increased in consolidation.

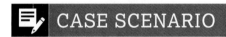
CASE SCENARIO

SCENARIO 13

Millie is a 14-year-old girl who has attended clinic today for review. Please perform a respiratory examination.

✔ EXAMINATION CHECKLIST		
Domain	Findings	Evolving thought process
Global assessment of child on approach.	• Alert, active, and looks well. • Looks underweight.	• Unlikely to have an acute pathology. • May have a chronic underlying disease.
Inspection.	• Small cervical lymph nodes, non-tender. • Little subcutaneous fat. • Normal RR. • Pancreatic enzymes by bed. • Empty sputum pot by bed.	• May be malnourished. In keeping with a chronic underlying systemic disease, could this child have cystic fibrosis?
Palpation.	• Normally placed apex. • Hyperinflated.	• Respiratory pathology identified, no evidence of Kartagener's syndrome.
Percuss.	• Normal.	• No additional pathology identified.
Auscultate.	• Few scattered crackles.	• May have a chest infection.

PRESENTING YOUR FINDINGS

Millie is a 14-year-old girl seen in the paediatric outpatients.

Millie appears underweight with little subcutaneous fat. However, I would like to plot her height and weight on a centile chart to confirm this. She appears comfortable at rest, has a normal respiratory rate and is not cyanosed. She has some small cervical lymph nodes palpable and a normally placed apex. Millie's chest is hyperexpanded, with a few scattered crackles heard on auscultation. I note that she has an empty sputum pot and pancreatic enzymes by her bedside.

These findings are consistent with a diagnosis of cystic fibrosis, particularly supported by the pancreatic enzyme supplements. She does not appear to have an exacerbation at present and there is no evidence of bronchiectasis.

To complete my examination, I would like to review the observation chart, plot Millie's height and weight on a growth chart as aforementioned, obtain a sample of sputum for microscopy, culture and sensitivity, and perform a peak flow test.

THYROID EXAMINATION

Thyroid examination may be performed in children with a suspected thyroid neck lump, or with clinical features of thyroid disease (*Table 36*). Common patients likely to appear in exams are show in *Table 37*.

TABLE 36: Clinical features of thyroid disease	
Hyperthyroidism	**Hypothyroidism**
• Weight loss. • Sweating. • Heat intolerance. • Increased appetite. • Diarrhoea. • Anxiety. • Tachycardia. • Hypertension. • Hand tremor. • Exophthalmos. • Lid lag.	• Weight gain. • Cold intolerance. • Constipation. • Bradycardia. • Slow relaxing reflexes. • Short stature. • Delayed puberty.

TABLE 37: Common exam patients	
Disease	**Possible clues**
Autoimmune (Hashimoto's) thyroiditis.	• Goitre. • Short. • Patient may be clinically euthyroid or hypothyroid. • Often female.
Graves' Disease.	• Goitre. • Signs of hyperthyroidism, although may be clinically euthyroid. • Proptosis. • Lid lag.
Thyroglossal cyst.	• Mass in midline. • Mass rises when tongue is stuck out.

Starting the Examination

The examination begins on entering the room. Whilst introducing yourself, make a broad assessment:

1   Does the child look well or unwell? Hyperthyroidism can be associated with cardiac arrhythmias.

2   Are they restless and sweaty? Do they have any tremors? These are all associated with hyperthyroidism.

Summary Checklist
Global assessment of child.
Inspection. Hands, face, eyes, teeth.
Palpation. Goitre.
Percussion. Sternum.
Auscultation. Goitre for bruit.
Completing the examination. BP, reflexes, proximal myopathy.
Bedside tests. Review observations, plot height and weight.

3   Are they an appropriate size for their height? Hypothyroidism is associated with being short and fat.

4   Are they appropriately dressed for the room temperature or wearing lots of layers? Temperature intolerance is reflected in clothing.

Endocrine examinations are often easier to carry out going from one body part to the next, and so this is how the thyroid examination will be presented.

Inspection and Palpation

Hands

➤ Pulse rate and rhythm. The patient who is hyperthyroid can be tachycardic, or in atrial fibrillation. Bradycardia is associated with hypothyroidism.

➤ Palmar erythema. This is seen in hyperthyroidism.

➤ Sweaty palms. This is seen in hyperthyroidism. Feel this.

➤ Blood pressure. In hyperthyroidism, there may be a high systolic pressure and wide pulse pressure.

➤ Thyroid acropachy. This is subperiosteal new bone formation of the digits which manifests as clubbing. It is associated with Graves' disease.

➤ Vitiligo. Look for other signs of autoimmune diseases such as vitiligo.

➤ Tremor. There may be a fine tremor if the patient is hyperthyroid (*Figure 161*).

FIGURE 161

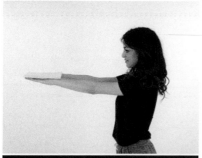

Ask the patient to hold out both their hands, arms outstretched. Look for a tremor. Putting a piece of paper over the hands will help make this more obvious.

Face

› Signs of thyroid eye disease. Look for these both from the front, the side and stand behind the child and look over and down (*Figure 162*):

  › Exophthalmos. This describes bulging of the eyeballs out of the orbit. Assess from the side, and by looking over the top of the patient from behind.

  › Ophthalmoplegia. This indicates pathology of cranial nerves III, IV and VI.

  › Lid lag. (*Figure 163*).

  › Lid retraction. If the eyelids are retracted, the sclera will be visible above the iris.

  › Oedema of the eyelid and conjunctivae. Conjunctival oedema is known as chemosis.

Neck

› To fully inspect the neck, look from the front, back and from both sides. Exposure of the chest is required to assess the sternal notch.

FIGURE 162

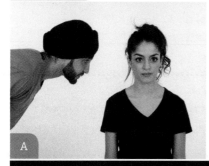
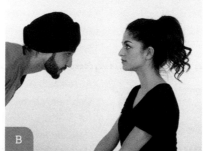
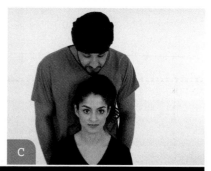

Inspect the eyes from: A. Side. B. Front. C. Above.

FIGURE 163

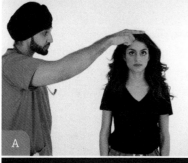
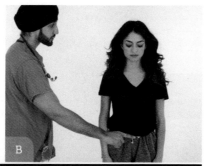

Lid lag. Ask the child to follow the examiner's finger (positioned horizontally) as it is moved rapidly from an up (A) to a down (B) position. The eyelid will lag behind the movement of the eye and so when the child looks down, the sclera will be more visible.

FIGURE 164

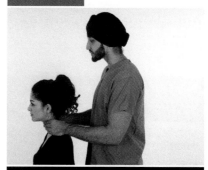

Palpating for a goitre.

FIGURE 165

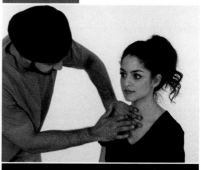

Percussing for retrosternal extension.

› Lymphadenopathy. Feel the anterior and posterior cervical chains for lymphadenopathy.

› Masses. Describe any masses as shown on p574. Palpate any goitre whilst standing behind the child (*Figure 164*), but warn them beforehand. Particularly assess for:

  › Size. Assessing this requires percussion down onto the chest to identify any retrosternal extension (*Figure 165*).

  › Shape/Surface/Consistency. There may be nodules.

  › Tenderness. This is suggestive of infection.

  › Transillumination. This is suggestive of a cyst.

  › Bruits. Bruits are associated with hyperthyroidism (*Figure 166*).

FIGURE 166

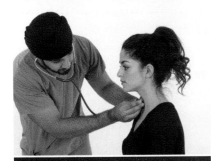

Auscultating for bruits.

FIGURE 167

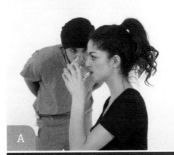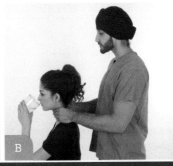

Ask the child to take a sip of water, hold it in their mouth and then ask them to swallow. Does the goitre move on swallowing? Inspect (A) and palpate (B) when doing this.

▷ Scars. A scar would indicate previous thyroid surgery.
▷ Swallow test. Thyroid goitres will move up with swallowing (*Figure 167*).
▷ Sticking out tongue. Ask the patient to stick out their tongue (*Figure 168*). A thyroid mass will remain in its position on tongue protrusion, whereas a thyroglossal cyst will move up.

Completing the Examination

▷ Reflexes. These may be slow-relaxing in hypothyroidism. Test one, e.g. knee jerk (*Figure 169*).
▷ Pretibial myxoedema. This is seen in Graves' disease. Bilateral, firm, non-pitting, asymmetrical plaques/nodules.
▷ Proximal muscle weakness. This is associated with hypothyroidism (*Figure 170*).
▷ Perform a general paediatric examination.

Bedside tests include:
▷ Review the observation chart.
▷ Plot the height and weight on an age and sex appropriate chart.

FIGURE 168

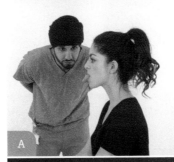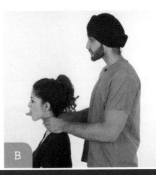

Assessing for thyroglossal cyst. Observe from the side (A), and palpate (B) to see if the mass rises on tongue protrusion.

FIGURE 169

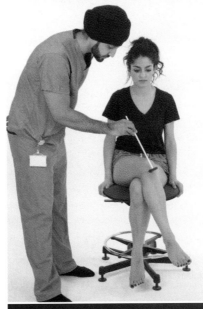

Assessing reflexes.

FIGURE 170

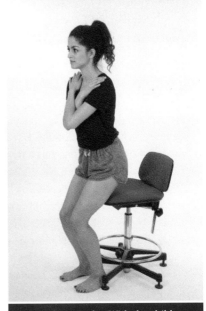

Proximal myopathy. With the child seated in a chair, ask them to stand up without using their arms (e.g. ask them to cross their arms whilst doing it).

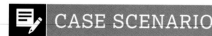

CASE SCENARIO

SCENARIO 14

Judy is a 14-year-old girl who has come to outpatient clinic with a neck mass. Please examine her neck and proceed as necessary.

✔ EXAMINATION CHECKLIST

Domain	Findings	Evolving thought process
Global assessment of child on approach.	• Appears well, obvious neck mass in midline. • Appears overweight.	• Not acutely unwell. Could the mass be a goitre?
Hands.	• Normal pulse rate. No peripheral stigmata of thyroid disease.	• May not be a thyroid mass, or could be thyroid disease well controlled.
Face.	• No lymphadenopathy. • Normal eye examination.	
Neck.	• Solid 2 cm x 2 cm mass, non-tender, diffusely enlarged, smooth, no bruits, not fluctuant, and not extending into the chest. • Mass moves up on swallowing, does not move on sticking out tongue.	• Likely thyroid mass. • Only sign suggesting it is hypothyroidism is that she appears overweight.

🔍 PRESENTING YOUR FINDINGS

Judy is a 14-year-old girl who has presented to clinic today with a neck mass.

Judy appears well but overweight. She has a neck mass in the midline that elevates on swallowing, but not on tongue protrusion. The mass is 2cm x 2cm, smooth, non-tender and not fluctuant. There is no retrosternal extension or thyroid bruit. There are no thyroid eye signs, or other signs of illness.

To complete my examination, I would like to plot Judy's height and weight on an age and sex appropriate growth chart.

My impression is that Judy has a thyroid goitre. I believe her to be hypothyroid in view of her short stature but would like to take a history to assess her thyroid status. The commonest cause of hypothyroidism with a goitre is autoimmune thyroiditis. To confirm this diagnosis, I would need to measure her T4 and TSH levels.

REFERENCES AND FURTHER READING

General

1   Bedwani SJ, Anderson CJR, Beattie RM. MRCPCH Clinical: short cases, history taking and communication skills. Third edition. Cheshire: PasTest; 2011.

2   Thomson A, Wallace H, Stephenson T. Short cases for the MRCPCH. Edinburgh: Churchill Livingstone; 2005.

3   Barakat N, Buchdahl R. Get Through. MRCPCH Part 2: 125 questions on clinical photographs. Florida: CRC Press; 2005.

4   Stanford School of Medicine. Newborn photo gallery. newborns.stanford.edu/PhotoGallery/

5   MRCPCH2009. Dysmorphic atlas. www.mrcpch2009.com/educational-materials/dysmorphic-atlas-1

6   Harris W. Examination Paediatrics. 4th Ed. New South Wales: Churchill Livingston; 2011.

7   Stephenson T, Wallace H, Thomson A. Clinical Paediatrics for Postgraduate Examinations. 3rd edition. Edinburgh: Churchill Livingstone; 2003.

Development

1   Sharma A, Cockerill H. From birth to five years: practical developmental examination. Fourth edition. Abingdon: Routledge; 2014.

Cardiology

1   Samuels M, Wieteska S. Advanced Paediatric Life Support. The Practical Approach. Fifth edition. Chichester: Wiley-Blackwell; 2005.

Musculoskeletal

1   Arthritis Research Council. pGALs. http://www
.arthritisresearchuk.org/health-professionals-and-students
/video-resources/pgals.aspx.

2   Wheeless' Textbook of Orthopaedics. www.wheelessonline
.com/ortho.

3   Houghton KM.Review for the generalist:evaluation of pae-
diatic hip pain. Pediatr Rheumatlo Online J. 2009;7:10.

4   Soucie JM et al. Range of motion measurements: reference and a database for comparison studies. Haemophilia.
2011;17:500-7.

5   Bandy W and Reese N. Joint Range of Motion and Muscle
Length Testing. Second edition. Missouri: Saunders
Elsevier;2013.

Neurology

1   Palisano R, Rosenbaum P, Walter S, Russell D, Wood E,
Galuppi B. Development and reliability of a system to clas-
sify gross motor function in a child with cerebral palsy. Dev
Med Child Neurol. 1997;39:214-23.

2   Cunningham ML, Heike CL. Evaluation of the infant with
an abnormal skull shape. Curr Opin Pediatr. 2007;19:645-51.

3.03

COMMUNICATION

ANNA CHADWICK AND MICHAEL MALLEY

CONTENTS

INTRODUCTION

Throughout medical training, the importance of communication skills is continually emphasised. Paediatrics has the additional challenges of communicating with children across all age groups, with parents and carers, and especially with children who cannot verbalise. *Table 1* shows the key differences between paediatric and adult communication. Teenagers can be treated more like adults. This chapter is designed to illustrate common components of effective communication in the paediatric setting.

TABLE 1: Communication with children and adults	
Children	**Adults**
Often indirect, through a parent/carer.	Usually directly from patients.
Children may not know why they are in hospital.	Adults usually self-present to medical care.
Child-focused language is required to explain complex ideas. It may be difficult to convince a child of the importance of something, and distraction/restraint techniques are often necessary.	More likely to understand medical terminology, and appreciate the need for procedures such as examination or blood taking.
Establishing rapport often involves being fun, playful and friendly towards the child.	Establishing rapport may involve a more serious, conservative approach.

THEORIES OF COMMUNICATION

It is important to recognise the limitations of applying communication models in practice. Patients are unlikely to interact well with a doctor who recites information or comes across as formulaic, so intuition and adaptation are key to communicating well. However, the foundations of good communication can be recognised within models and theory. Two models are described below.

Five Components of Communication

This theory helps frame the purpose and manner of the communication scenario (*Example 1*).

Ideas, Concerns, Expectations (ICE)

This theory helps identify any initial thoughts the patient might have, allowing communication to be tailored to this (*Example 2*). In paediatrics, this tool must incorporate the concerns of both the parents and the child.

KEY COMPONENTS OF COMMUNICATION

Communication with any patient, carer or staff member can benefit from addressing the following factors.

Preparation and Location

Choose an appropriate setting. Ideally, for a sensitive conversation, choose a quiet side-room, free from interruptions. Remove potential distractions, such as a pager, and read the medical notes and any test results prior to the discussion if possible. Similarly, think about the seating arrangements. Creating a comfortable setting that implies equality amongst the participants is likely to encourage effective communication. Get down to the child's level, rather than standing over them. Decide who should be present. Some discussions are best held with both parents present, while others may not be appropriate in front of the child. It is good practice to have an allied health professional present when breaking bad news, and it is always useful to establish beforehand what the patient or carers already know.

EXAMPLE 1

An illustrated example of the 'five components of communication' model.

		Element	Explaining the need for oral antibiotics for a 5-year-old with an ear infection in the Emergency Department (ED)
1		**Whom** – By whom is the communication initiated?	Here, the paediatric doctor will initiate the discussion.
2		**What** – What content is to be communicated?	The content to be explained is the need for antibiotics and how the prescription should be administered.
3		**How** – How is the content delivered?	The content is communicated verbally with written prompts (i.e. prescription on the bottle of antibiotics), and non-verbal skills are used throughout.
4		**Who** – Who is receiving the content?	The parent and child are the recipients of the content.
5		**What effect** – What is the outcome of the communication?	The hoped for outcome is that the parent will understand why antibiotics are needed and will feel reassured and confident in giving them.

EXAMPLE 2

An illustrated example of the 'Ideas, Concerns and Expectations' model. Explaining the diagnosis of type 1 diabetes to a 12-year-old girl and her mother.

Type 1 diabetes: new diagnosis	Possible questions to ask	Child	Parent
Ideas	What do you think might be going on?	May not know about diabetes. May not appreciate they are unwell.	May know this is diabetes already. May be more concerned about weight loss or other features.
Concerns	Is there anything in particular you are concerned about?	May be worried about injections or changing diet.	May be concerned her daughter won't know how to manage hypoglycaemia episodes. May have a relative with diabetes, and be worried about diabetic complications.
Expectations	What do you think might be the best plan of action?	She may want to be the one in charge of managing her diabetes. She may need more time to come to terms with the diagnosis.	She may expect tertiary specialist care. She may expect a cure. She may expect regular contact from diabetic specialists.

Creating Rapport

A simple introduction with a handshake and a smile or kneeling down to chat to a toddler before taking a history can create a comfortable rapport. In some settings, establishing a rapport may take longer — for example, when breaking bad news to a patient or carer you have not met before. Making an effort to put the patient and their carers at ease will improve the dialogue and working relationship.

Acknowledging Agenda

When entering into a new scenario, recognise the agendas of each of the people involved, as this may affect the outcome of the situation. For example, a parent who brings their child with a cough and fever to ED may be expecting a prescription for antibiotics: this is their agenda. However, the clerking doctor will be assessing the child's health and making a tailored decision about the appropriateness of antibiotics. Without recognising the parent's agenda, the doctor may miss an opportunity to discuss the lack of a role of antibiotics in a viral infection. If the parent feels their agenda has not been acknowledged, they may feel their expectations have not been met and may lose confidence in the doctor's clinical judgement.

The agenda underlying each interaction may not be obvious, but quick assumptions of culture or values impact the overall interaction with patients, carers and colleagues. Using non-judgmental and open questioning, providing clear information and offering the chance to ask questions should eliminate the risk of missing any key concerns.

Verbal Skills

Avoid beginning with closed questions and limit the use of jargon. If jargon is unavoidable, explain any such terms. When covering sensitive or confrontational topics, have an appropriate tone of voice. Recognise the effect of language barriers on good communication and use an impartial interpreter if needed. Although occasionally unavoidable in an emergency, using a bilingual paediatric patient to communicate to their non-English speaking parent can risk incorrect translation.

Non-Verbal Skills

Eye contact encourages trust and the appropriate use of body contact can be empathic. Don't be afraid of silence. Pauses in a conversation may feel uncomfortable, but are useful for processing information, particularly in the context of breaking bad news, and they may lead readily to the next stage of the conversation.

Paediatricians often need the ability to interpret the non-verbal skills of their patients, whether limited by age or cognitive ability. The appreciation of basic posture and behaviours (e.g. grimacing, back arching) may give essential information that cannot otherwise be communicated by the patient. The use of expert skills, such as occupational therapy (i.e. sign language, picture cards) and play therapy, can optimise communication in the absence of verbal skills.

Active Listening

Active listening not only involves critically analysing what is being said, but also letting the speaker know that they are being heard, both through encouraging words and behaviours. Similarly, it is important to ensure that any information or advice offered is registered. A useful tool is to ask the recipient to summarise in their own words the information imparted. This strategy can also be used when taking a clinical history or handover to a colleague.

COMMUNICATING WITH CHILDREN OF DIFFERENT AGES

Baby

In newborns, variations in the tone of a cry can indicate different needs. A high-pitched cry may signify pain or distress.

Parents/carers are often able to recognise cries due to hunger or tiredness. A happy baby may coo and babble or offer a smile. When communicating with a baby, use exaggerated non-verbal skills to reassure and comfort, like big smiley faces, gentle soothing noises and good eye contact. Use the parents to help console the infant, or consider examining during a feed if the baby is crying.

Pre-verbal Child

Toddlers may have stranger anxiety or be miserable if unwell. A direct introduction to the patient is important, crouching down to their level. Use a toy for distraction. Place a stethoscope on the parent's chest/the child's arm before formal auscultation. This helps introduce the instrument as being playful and non-painful. Cheerful smiles and a relaxed disposition can calm young children, but separation anxiety is common at this age, so allow parents to comfort the child as they wish. Avoid disturbing the child if they are nervous or agitated. Play therapists can be invaluable in communicating with children in these younger age groups.

Verbal Child

Ask a few questions; for example, enquire about their age or the names of any dolls they may have with them. Older children are more likely to follow instructions, so talk to them rather than their parents during examination. Try to continue the dialogue, using age-appropriate language (such as "sore" rather than "painful"), and ask the child to point to or describe any symptoms they have. The child may be able to describe symptoms or localise pain.

Adolescent/Young Person

This age range provides a variable challenge, as some teenagers will be open to communication and others less so. Talk directly to the patient. Work out whether the parents need to be present for the whole consultation. Offer to see the young person on their own. Some questions may be difficult to answer in front of parents, such as those involving sexual activity, drug and alcohol use, feelings of low mood and suicide attempts. If appropriate, find common ground to help develop a rapport, but maintain professionalism and appreciate the young person's boundaries.

Parents

The key here is to maintain an "adult" conversation whilst also simultaneously adapting to the child. Use empathic language to acknowledge concerns, and give clear, concise information where appropriate. Ensure understanding by asking the parent/carer to feed back the main points of the conversation.

COMMUNICATION CHALLENGES

Communication can be challenging when a child has developmental delay, autistic spectrum disorder (or other disorders of communication) or mental health problems. Using

the techniques for pre-verbal children is insufficient, as the child's understanding may be greater than suggested by their behaviour. Allow more time to assess the likely cognitive age of the patient. Ask the parents how they normally communicate with their child, or if there is anything the child particularly dislikes. Some children with autism, for example, do not like to be touched on certain parts of their body. The use of sign language, such as Makaton or picture cards, can be helpful. A play therapist may assist when performing essential tasks, such as examination or venepuncture. Always maintain eye contact where appropriate and try to involve the child in the consultation as much as possible. Do not be afraid to give them a break and return later, when discussion may be less distressing and information quicker to obtain.

CLINICAL CASES

CASE 1
A newborn baby presenting with ambiguous genitalia

Candidate Briefing

You are a junior doctor on the labour ward and you are paged to review a baby immediately after delivery. On arrival, you find the baby is clinically stable and is wrapped in a towel and being warmed on the resuscitaire. The midwife asks to speak to you outside the labour room and tells you that she thinks the baby's genitalia are abnormal. She explains that the first-time parents are expecting a baby girl and are unaware of the abnormality so far.

You return to the room to examine the infant, and find a well baby with ambiguous genitalia. The midwife asks you to explain the findings to the mother, as the father has popped outside to tell family members about the new arrival.

Patient/Actress Briefing

You are Sarah Thompson, a first-time mother who has just had a normal delivery at 39 weeks. The pregnancy was generally fine, although you were taking some medication for depression in the first few months before you realised you were pregnant. All scans and blood tests have been normal and the anomaly scan revealed you were having a baby girl. You have never smoked and stopped drinking when you found out you were pregnant. You work as a teaching assistant and live with your partner, the baby's father.

Your partner is supportive and although the baby was unplanned, you are both excited about becoming parents.

You are yet to hold your child as the midwife has said she would like the doctor to take a quick look, although she hasn't explained why. Initially, you are worried your baby is unwell following the birth, and you are anxious to hold her.

You don't understand how there can be any question over the gender, especially as you were told you were having a girl by the sonographer at your 20 week scan.

Questions to ask:

▸ How can the gender be ambiguous?

▸ What tests will be needed? Will the baby need surgery?

▸ Was there anything I did that could have caused this?

▸ Why was I told I was having a girl?

▸ Should I raise the baby as a boy or a girl for now?

Only if specifically asked, tell the doctor that you'd ideally like to wait for your baby's father to come back before having the conversation, but that he's told you that he's held up and you must speak alone for now.

✔	EXAMINER CHECKLIST	
Domain	**Comments**	
Introduction	• Introduces self by name and role. • Checks identity of the mother/infant. • Explains need to discuss an important finding and asks if the mother would like anyone else present.	
Explaining Findings	• Establishes what the mother has been told already. • Clearly explains that the infant's genitalia are ambiguous. • Explains that the anomaly scan is not a definitive method of predicting infant gender. Apologises for the upset this may have caused. • Explains that this means the gender of the infant cannot yet be confirmed. • Explains the need for senior review. • Explains that this may be the result of a genetic abnormality or a medical condition, i.e. congenital adrenal hyperplasia. • Reassures that this is not the parents' fault. • Explains the need for further investigations, such as genetic testing. • Acknowledges the need for possible medical or surgical intervention at a later date.	
Verbal Skills	• Speaks clearly and concisely when giving information. • Uses compassionate, caring language throughout. • Does not use medical jargon. • Uses silences appropriately. • Allows time for questions.	
Non-Verbal Skills	• Maintains good eye contact throughout. • Promotes active listening and responds to the actor's cues.	
Summary	• Summarises what has been said. • Ensures understanding of the main issues. • Clarifies the next step. • Offers further support and a follow-up meeting.	

CASE 2
A 3-day-old baby with a new diagnosis of Down Syndrome

Candidate Briefing

You are a junior doctor in the neonatal outpatient clinic. Mrs Jones is waiting to talk to you about her 1-day-old baby, Jamie. Jamie was floppy at birth and has mild dysmorphic features. Karyotyping has confirmed a diagnosis of Down syndrome (Trisomy 21). Mrs Jones does not know the diagnosis. Please inform Mrs Jones that the karyotype is positive and answer any questions she may have.

Patient/Actress Briefing

You are Mrs Jones. You are 32-years-old and gave birth to your first baby, Jamie, four weeks ago. The pregnancy was smooth and unremarkable. You gave birth at 38 weeks via a normal vaginal delivery. You were told you had a low risk of Down Syndrome, and antenatal scanning revealed no abnormalities.

You first thought something was wrong when Jamie struggled to breastfeed on day one and appeared floppy. The doctor mentioned that Jamie might have some "special facial features", but you do not really see them. You are currently breastfeeding but requiring bottle top-ups.

You live with Jamie's father and have a good support network. You work as a park attendant. You do not drink or smoke. You have no involvement with social services.

You were informed at the time of Jamie's birth that he might have Down Syndrome. You don't know much about it and think children with Down syndrome "look different" and need "lots of support".

Questions to ask:

▸ What is Down Syndrome?

▸ How do children get it?

▸ Why did this happen?

▸ Is it my fault? Is there anything I could have done differently?

▸ Why did the antenatal scans not pick this up?

▸ If I have any more children, will they also have Down Syndrome?

▸ What support is available to help me?

If specifically asked, you are worried that Jamie will never live a "normal life" and that he might "die young".

✔	EXAMINER CHECKLIST	
Domain	**Comments**	
Introduction	• Introduces self by name and role. • Checks identity of the mother/infant. • Explains the need to discuss the results of genetic tests and asks if the mother would like anyone else present.	
Discussing the Situation	• Explains that the test for Down syndrome is positive. • Explains Down syndrome is a chromosomal/genetic abnormality. Avoids jargon. • Mentions at least two complications of Down's syndrome when asked (e.g. learning difficulties, cardiac, bowel or neurological issues, leukaemia). • Explains the high likelihood of developmental delay (in over 90% of patients). • Explains Down syndrome is a life-long condition with no cure. • Reassures that many children with Down syndrome live a fulfilling life and can live to middle age. • Mentions medical support that is available: multidisciplinary team [MDT; e.g. occupational therapist (OT), physical therapist (PT), dietitian]. • Mentions non-medical support that is available (e.g. support groups, Down Syndrome Association, special schools). • Explains that testing in pregnancy gives a probability, but is not a guarantee.	

(Continued)

✔ EXAMINER CHECKLIST

Domain	Comments
	• Explains the relationship between maternal age and risk of Down Syndrome. • Reassures that it is not mother's fault. • Explains that the chance of having a second child with Down syndrome is slightly increased.
Verbal Skills	• Speaks clearly and concisely when giving information. • Uses compassionate, caring language throughout. • Does not use medical jargon. • Uses silences appropriately. • Allows time for questions.
Non-Verbal Skills	• Maintains good eye contact throughout. • Promotes active listening and responds to the actor's cues.
Summary	• Summarises what has been said. • Ensures understanding of the main issues. • Clarifies the next steps. • Offers further support and a follow-up meeting.

CASE 3
A woman at 29 weeks gestation requiring counselling for pre-term delivery

Candidate Briefing

You are the junior doctor and have been asked to see Mrs Patel on the labour ward. Mrs Patel is 29 weeks pregnant and has severe pre-eclampsia, but currently the baby is a good size for gestational age. The obstetric team members are worried she may need an emergency caesarean section if her blood pressure cannot be controlled. The midwife asks you to counsel her on what to expect from a preterm delivery and answer any questions she has.

Patient/Actress Briefing

You are Shushma Patel, a 31-year-old accountant. You are 29 weeks pregnant and this is your second pregnancy: two years ago, you had a miscarriage at 10 weeks. You have been told you are having a baby boy. Your husband frequently works abroad and is currently away due to work, and you haven't yet told anyone else that you are in labour.

You have never smoked and don't drink alcohol. This is a planned pregnancy and you have followed all advice from your midwifery team. You have received two doses of steroids to help develop the baby's lungs. You are very concerned about the risks to your baby of being born so early and are distressed that your husband won't be here to support you.

Questions to ask:
➤ Why is the baby coming early?
➤ Will the baby be able to breathe on his own?
➤ Will the baby be brain damaged?
➤ Will I be able to stay with my baby after he is born?

If prompted for further questions, you should ask if there are any studies on preterm delivery outcomes. Only if specifically asked should you explain the situation with your husband.

✔ EXAMINER CHECKLIST

Domain	Comments
Introduction	• Introduces self by name and role. • Checks identity of the patient. • Explains the need to discuss a potential preterm delivery and asks if the patient would like anyone else present.
Discussing the Situation	• Establishes what the patient has been told already and confirms the gestation of the pregnancy. • Explains that a senior paediatrician will attend the delivery and that the baby will be taken to a resuscitaire for stabilisation prior to transfer to the neonatal unit. • Explains the need to keep the baby warm using an incubator. • Explains that the baby is likely to require breathing support in the form of either continuous positive airway pressure (CPAP) or intubation. Acknowledges the importance of steroids in foetal lung development. • Explains that the baby will need to have blood tests and a cannula and will require feeding support. • Explains that further treatment will depend on the condition of the baby at birth. • Explains that the mother will be able to visit freely and will be close by on the postnatal ward. • Enquires about family situation, and explores possible ways to support the mother. • Explains the risks associated with preterm delivery but reassures that the chances of survival at this gestation are good. • If asked, offers to discuss the results of studies on outcomes of preterm deliveries.
Verbal Skills	• Speaks clearly and concisely when giving information. • Uses compassionate, caring language throughout. • Does not use medical jargon. • Uses silences appropriately. • Allows time for questions.
Non-Verbal Skills	• Maintains good eye contact throughout. • Promotes active listening and responds to the actor's cues.
Summary	• Summarises what has been said. • Ensures understanding of the main issues. • Clarifies the next step. • Offers further support and a follow-up meeting.

CASE 4
A 4-year-old boy inadvertently given the wrong dose of paracetamol

Candidate Briefing

You are the general paediatric junior doctor on call. You are asked to see a 4-year-old boy on the ward who has recently been brought up from ED, having been admitted with a first episode of viral-induced wheeze. In the ED, he was given twice the recommended dose of paracetamol for his age and the nurse on the ward has just noticed the mistake on the drug chart. She asks you to explain the mistake to the parents and answer any questions they may have.

Patient/Actress Briefing

You are Mr Lemarde, father to Theo, a 4-year-old boy admitted with his first wheezy episode. You are extremely concerned about him as he has had trouble breathing for the last two days. Theo was initially seen by a primary care physician, who sent you home with a salbutamol inhaler. You have brought him

609

in overnight as his breathing became more laboured and he developed a fever. So far, Theo has been given some paracetamol and salbutamol nebulisers before being transferred to the ward.

Theo is your only child and is usually fit and well. He has no other medical problems and is rarely unwell. He has no allergies.

When informed about the drug error, you are initially angry and confused about how this has happened. You are concerned about the effects an overdose may have on Theo and want to make a formal complaint.

Questions to ask:

> Why was the large dose prescribed and given?
> Why are there no procedures in place to prevent this kind of error?
> Who is accountable for the mistake?
> What effect might the overdose have on Theo? Does he need any tests or treatment?

Only if specifically mentioned, you should ask how to make a formal complaint.

✔ EXAMINER CHECKLIST	
Domain	Comments
Introduction	• Introduces self by name and role. • Checks the identity of the patient and his father. • Explains the need to discuss a drug error that has occurred involving Theo. • Asks if Mr Lemarde would like anyone else present.
Discussing the Situation	• Establishes what Mr Lemarde has been told so far. • Explains that a drug error has occurred, where Theo was given twice the recommended dose of paracetamol whilst in ED. • Apologises unreservedly for the error and acknowledges the shared responsibility amongst the medical team. • Explains that these errors are uncommon due to protocols in place for checking prescriptions but that these have failed on this occasion. • Establishes whether Theo is more unwell after the paracetamol overdose. • Explains that the amount of paracetamol given is unlikely to have a health impact on Theo, and that the total amount of paracetamol given per kg of body weight will be calculated to decide if any further tests are needed. • Explains that the drug error will be discussed with the members of staff involved, the nurse in charge and the admitting consultant, and will be reported internally via the incident reporting system. • Explains that an adverse clinical incident form will be filled in so that it will be looked into. • Offers advice on making a formal complaint, such as the contact details for the patient advice and liaison service (PALS).
Verbal Skills	• Speaks clearly and concisely when giving information. • Apologises clearly. Uses compassionate, caring language throughout. • Does not use medical jargon. • Uses silences appropriately. • Allows time for questions.

(Continued)

✔ EXAMINER CHECKLIST	
Domain	Comments
Non-Verbal Skills	• Maintains good eye contact throughout. • Promotes active listening and responds to the actor's cues.
Summary	• Summarises what has been said. • Ensures understanding of the main issues. • Clarifies the next steps. • Offers further support and a follow-up meeting.

CASE 5
A 15-year-old girl non-compliant with her diabetes medication

Candidate Briefing

You are a junior doctor in the diabetic outpatient clinic. Dawn Firth is a 15-year-old girl with type 1 diabetes who has come in for her annual review. Her mother is waiting for her outside the clinic room. Dawn has had diabetes since she was 8-years-old and is on a basal bolus regime.

Recently, there have been concerns that Dawn is not taking her insulin appropriately. In the past six months, she has had two admissions to hospital for diabetic ketoacidosis. Today, her glycated haemoglobin (HbA1c) is 75 mmol/mol; her other blood results are normal and her urine dipstick is clear. Her previous HbA1c was 53 mmol/mol.

You are asked to see Dawn and talk to her about her diabetes control. Please discuss the concerns and provide advice on how to optimise her current treatment in light of her results.

Patient/Actress Briefing

You are Dawn Firth, a 15-year-old with type 1 diabetes. You were diagnosed at 8-years-old after a two week history of weight loss, increasing thirst and passing more urine than usual. You are attending the clinic for your annual review with your mother who is waiting outside. You have had some blood and urine tests, with results pending.

Your current treatment plan is a basal bolus regime: you take your background insulin at night, but you have been concerned about your weight after hearing some nasty comments made by other girls at school. Having read on the internet that reducing your insulin causes weight loss, you have been omitting some insulin doses around mealtimes and running your blood sugars around 10–12 mmol most days, and sometimes higher. You have been admitted to hospital twice recently, feeling unwell and having high blood sugar levels. You have been advised to increase your insulin doses. Initially, you are reluctant to admit that you haven't followed this advice and instead feel that you would rather have high blood sugar levels than gain weight.

Areas for discussion:

> Initially be reluctant to discuss your diabetic control.
> If asked directly, explain that you have been omitting insulin doses in order to control your weight.

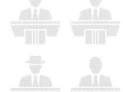

- Ask why having a low HbA1c is important.
- Explain how upset you are about your weight and that you feel that because you have diabetes you cannot act like a normal teenager.

Only if specifically asked about the weight loss, mention being upset by the comments made by other girls at school.

✔ **EXAMINER CHECKLIST**

Domain	Comments
Introduction	• Introduces self by name and role. • Checks identity of the patient. • Explains the need to discuss the diabetes, and asks if the patient would like her mother present.
Discussing the Situation	• Establishes what the patient has been told already and explains the blood and urine results. • Explains that HbA1c is a marker of long-term blood sugar control, and that the latest result is high and has increased since the previous annual review. • Asks whether the patient has any ideas about why this has happened. • Explores the reasons for the patient running high blood sugars and her understanding about the impact this has on her health. • Explains that chronically high blood sugars are likely to cause irreversible damage, such as problems with eyesight, kidney disease, nerve damage, and heart problems. • Explains that acutely high blood sugars can be dangerous and may require admission to a high dependency unit/intensive care unit (HDU/ITU) for treatment. • Acknowledges that the patient may also experience low sugar symptoms if control is poor. • Explores the psychological impact of having a chronic disease and appreciates the impact of having diabetes on daily life. • Offers to refer the patient to a dietician for more advice on healthy weight control and signposts to a clinical nurse specialist/support groups for young people with diabetes.
Verbal Skills	• Speaks clearly and concisely when giving information. • Uses compassionate, caring language throughout. • Does not use medical jargon. • Uses silences appropriately. • Allows time for questions.
Non-Verbal Skills	• Maintains good eye contact throughout. • Promotes active listening and responds to the actor's cues.
Summary	• Summarises what has been said. • Ensures understanding of the main issues. • Clarifies the next step. • Offers further support and a follow-up meeting.

CASE 6
A 6-month-old boy who has not been vaccinated due to parental choice

Candidate Briefing

You are the junior doctor in ED. Mrs Stevens has brought her 6-month-old son Bobby to hospital after he developed a fever at home. You diagnose him with a viral upper respiratory tract infection (URTI) and plan to send him home. During clerking,

you establish that Bobby has not had any vaccinations. Before discharging Bobby, please discuss this with his mother and answer any questions she may have.

Patient/Actress Briefing

You are Mrs Stevens, a 29-year-old office manager, and have brought your son Bobby to hospital because he developed a runny nose and high fever over the last couple of days. You have been seen by the paediatric team and are expecting to be discharged home today.

You have not given Bobby any routine vaccines as you don't believe that they work and think that they may cause him harm. Your niece had meningitis at 1-year-old, despite receiving the meningitis vaccine as part of the routine schedule, and you are adamant that this proves they are ineffective. You also have many friends whose children have suffered with fever and diarrhoea following the vaccines and have decided that, overall, it is better not to vaccinate Bobby.

Bobby was born at term and is usually well. You have already had discussions with your primary care physician regarding vaccinations but believe it is ultimately your right to refuse them because you do not believe they are suitable for your son.

Areas for discussion:
- Initially be reluctant to discuss the reasons for refusing vaccines as you have already talked this through with your primary care physician.
- Explain that you believe vaccines to be ineffective, giving the example of your niece contracting meningitis.
- Explain that you are also concerned that they may have side effects such as fever.
- Ask why it matters as you believe conditions like whooping cough are treatable, and he is too old for it anyway.
- Ask what the common side effects of vaccinations are.

Only if asked about your concerns should you state that you are worried about the vaccines being very painful.

✔ **EXAMINER CHECKLIST**

Domain	Comments
Introduction	• Introduces self by name and role. • Checks identity of the patient/parents. • Requests permission to discuss the mother's refusal to vaccinate, and asks if she would like anyone else present.
Discussing the Situation	• Establishes what the mother understands regarding immunisation schedule. • Explores the reasons for her refusal to vaccinate her son. • Accepts the mother's concerns as valid and offers to explain the nature of the immunisation schedule to ensure she is making an informed decision. • Explains that many of the diseases infants are vaccinated against have become dormant since the introduction of routine vaccination and as such public health has improved.

(Continued)

✔ EXAMINER CHECKLIST

Domain	Comments
	• Explains that vaccines protect against diseases that can be fatal, e.g. whooping cough, and that these diseases have re-emerged due to the reduced uptake of vaccinations. • Explains that the current meningitis vaccine does not protect against all strains of meningitis, so although the rates of bacterial meningitis have reduced dramatically, it is still possible to develop the disease, although new vaccines are being implemented. • Explains that although the vaccines frequently cause children to develop a mild fever and be unsettled, this is temporary and should not be a reason to avoid vaccination. • Acknowledges the mother's right to refuse the vaccine schedule but emphasises the clinical importance to protect both her son and other children around him.
Verbal Skills	• Clear and concise when giving information. • Uses compassionate, caring language throughout. • Does not use medical jargon. • Uses silences appropriately. • Allows time for questions.
Non-Verbal Skills	• Maintains good eye contact throughout. • Promotes active listening and responds to the actor's cues.
Summary	• Summarises what has been said. • Ensures understanding of the main issues. • Clarifies the next step. • Offers further support and a follow-up meeting.

REFERENCES AND FURTHER READING

1 Tate P, Tate L. The Doctor's Communication Handbook. Seventh Edition. London: Radcliffe Publishing Ltd.; 2014

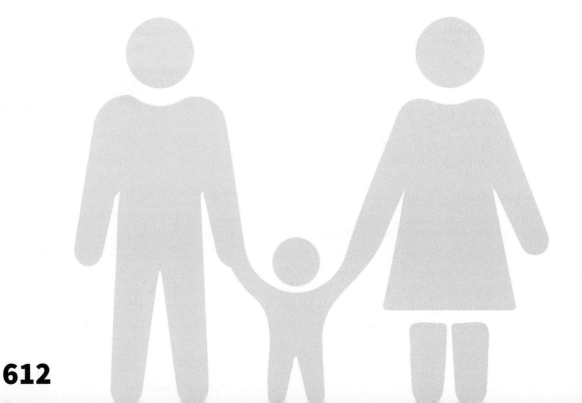

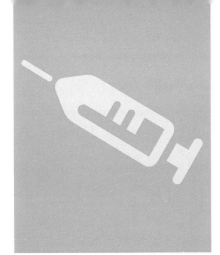

3.04
PRACTICAL SKILLS

**MICHAEL MALLEY, ZESHAN QURESHI,
ANITA DEMETRIOU AND MARIE MONAGHAN**

CONTENTS

INTRODUCTION

The key to success is preparation and practice. The best way to accomplish this is to discuss the procedure with a senior colleague and observe the skill in order to understand the process, before performing it under supervision. In addition to knowing the steps, it is important to know the indication for a procedure and its impact on management. This chapter contains a brief "how to" guide for each of the key competencies expected of junior doctors and paediatric trainees.

Important themes common to all procedures include:

- Explanation. Explain in lay terms what is going to be done, and why, to the child and parents. Invite questions.
- Consent. Gain informed consent and ensure the patient and parents are aware of any serious or common side effects. Consent may be written or verbal depending on the procedure.
- Pain relief. This may involve the use of oral/intranasal/intravenous/topical anaesthesia, cold spray, or oral sucrose.
- Distraction. Nearly all procedures are better tolerated with the use of appropriate distraction beforehand. Involve the play specialist team where possible. If unavailable, utilise smartphone apps/videos/toys as appropriate.
- Aseptic technique. Observe aseptic or sterile conditions as appropriate.
- Keep calm. Ensure adequate preparation, with appropriate support to hand. Being calm increases the likelihood of success. Know what to do in the event of any unexpected events.
- Post-procedure. After each procedure, clear the equipment, follow-up results and act on results as necessary.

A flow chart for performing procedures is shown in *Figure 1*.

VASCULAR ACCESS

Capillary Blood Gas ("heel prick")

Arterial blood gases are rarely performed in paediatrics unless from a secure arterial line in a high dependency setting. As a result, capillary gases fulfil an important role in the assessment of the ill child. Capillary blood gases are one of the most readily available objective barometers of a child's health. They are quick and easy to obtain, with almost immediate results.

Indications

- Acutely unwell patient, e.g. respiratory compromise, severe sepsis.
- Checking glucose, bilirubin, haemoglobin or electrolytes.
- Post intubation or for assessing the efficacy of ventilation.

Assessment

Early identification of the need for an invasive procedure. Involve play specialist. Early application of local anaesthetic when needed. Depending on age, check child has an understanding of what needs to be done.

Preparation

If parents wish to be actively involved, begin to get child into any appropriate holding position. Check that all equipment and team-members are ready. Ensure the child is actively distracted.

Teamwork

Distractor (play specialist or holder) should be the lead voice for communicating/coordinating between medical staff and child, reducing unfamiliarity for the child. Check that the team is ready: holder, distractor, person doing the task and parents (if opting to be present). Minimise the number of people in the room.

Implementation

Where possible, use a procedure room. If appropriate, ask the child if they would like a warning, e.g. "quick scratch coming" for cannulation.

Post Procedure

Thank the child and praise their efforts, e.g. with cheering, a high five, a sticker or a bravery certificate. Explain to the child why any bandage is on and ask parents to supervise it. Explain the ongoing plan again clearly, e.g. time to wait until blood results or admission details. Check if there are any questions. Perform any safety checks afterwards (e.g. flush cannula to ensure patency, request X-ray for position of ET tube)

FIGURE 1

Flowchart for performing an invasive procedure.

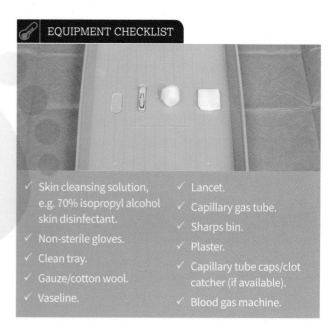

EQUIPMENT CHECKLIST

- ✓ Skin cleansing solution, e.g. 70% isopropyl alcohol skin disinfectant.
- ✓ Non-sterile gloves.
- ✓ Clean tray.
- ✓ Gauze/cotton wool.
- ✓ Vaseline.
- ✓ Lancet.
- ✓ Capillary gas tube.
- ✓ Sharps bin.
- ✓ Plaster.
- ✓ Capillary tube caps/clot catcher (if available).
- ✓ Blood gas machine.

STEP-BY-STEP GUIDE

1 Introduce oneself to the patient/family and explain the purpose of the procedure.

2 Wash hands and put on gloves.

3 Identify the best place to perform the test:
   › In a neonate, this will be a heel prick. This means selecting a spot around the periphery of the inferior aspect of the heel. Steer clear of the centre of the heel, where there are fewer capillaries and more nerve fibres (*Figure 2*).

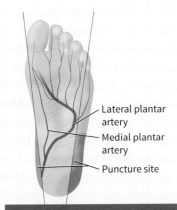

Lateral plantar artery
Medial plantar artery
Puncture site

Figure 2. Puncture sites for a heel prick. Avoid the centre of the heel.

   › In a child over six months, it may be easier to use the lateral aspect of the thumb, fingers or toes.

4 Gently rub the site and/or gently push down at the intended site a few times to improve capillary blood flow. Check for any previous site of capillary blood sampling that will still bleed without requiring another piercing of the skin.

5 Place a paper towel under the intended puncture site to catch any spillages.

6 Clean the area and allow it to dry (*Figure 3*).

7 Apply a thin layer of Vaseline over the area to be punctured (note this is optional and not used in some neonatal units). This will ensure that the blood stays in a bleb around the needle prick site rather than smearing elsewhere, making it easier to collect.

8 Take a mildly firm hold of the heel or digit and stretch the skin. Use the lancet to pierce the desired area (*Figure 4*).

9 Gently squeeze the area rhythmically, starting distally from the site of puncture and allowing reperfusion between squeezes. This should produce a steady bleb of blood from the site.

10 Hold the capillary tube horizontal or a little elevated. Holding it at a downhill angle may mean air bubbles are sucked in as the blood is collected quicker than it is produced. Holding it level or "uphill" from the patient will prevent this (*Figure 5*).

11 Gently move the end of the capillary tube to the bleb of blood and fill it to the end. Aim to only collect blood if it is free flowing so that clots are less likely to enter the capillary tube. If air bubbles enter, empty the capillary tube up until the point of the air bubble on gauze and refill the tube.

12 Once filled sufficiently, put the gas tube on a tray. Wipe the puncture site with some cotton wool or gauze to remove any remaining blood and any Vaseline (*Figure 6*).

13 Apply a plaster if needed (*Figure 7*). Note that this will not stick if Vaseline is still present.

14 If available, put a cap on both ends of the capillary tube as this will prevent spillage on transfer to the gas machine.

15 Thank the parents/patient and take the sample to the blood gas machine.

16 Remove the caps from the gas tube and put a clot catcher on the end to be inserted into the gas machine (if required).

17 Place lancet and capillary tube in a sharps bin.

18 Once the gas result has been obtained, immediately record it and make a plan based on the findings.

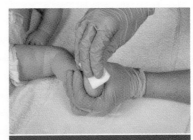

Figure 3. Paper towel placed under foot and skin surface cleaned.

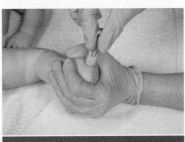

Figure 4. Tightened skin punctured with lancet.

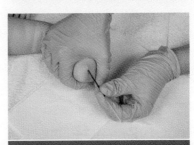

Figure 5. Collect blood in the capillary tube. Note the capillary tube is held horizontally, not down-slanting.

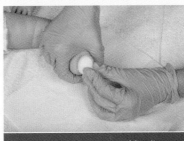

Figure 6. Compress to stop bleeding with cotton wool.

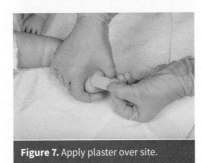

Figure 7. Apply plaster over site.

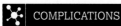

Note that this technique can also be used for sending blood samples for biochemistry and haematology testing. It is neither suitable for blood cultures as the blood sample is contaminated by the skin, nor for clotting studies as clotting factors are activated following skin contact. Blood bottles can be adapted by having a "scooper" on top. This makes it easier to collect the blood as it emerges.

COMPLICATIONS

This is generally a safe procedure, but complications may include:
- Infection.
- Pain, particularly with prolonged squeezing of the heel.
- Erroneous results from prolonged squeezing of a poorly perfused periphery (classically, erroneous hyperkalaemia or high lactate).
- Soft tissue injury.
- Rarely, bone infection/injury (from puncturing the calcaneus, particularly if central heel punctured).

TOP TIPS

- Vaseline is very helpful at preventing blood spillage and making it easier to "catch" in the capillary tube. However, some hospitals may not use Vaseline because of a possible risk of infection. If Vaseline is used, ideally each baby should have their own tube to minimise this risk.
- A common mistake is to hold the foot of a neonate tightly immediately after pricking it. After the initial prick, allow the child to kick their foot a little as this will promote blood flow and greatly settle the patient.
- Remember that blood is subject to the laws of gravity. Positioning the foot as low as possible may aid collection.

Venous Blood Sampling

Venepuncture is performed by several different techniques in paediatrics. In older children, the technique is exactly the same as for adults. In neonates and younger children, because the veins are much smaller, using adult techniques may cause the veins to collapse. Both methods are described below. Unlike with adults, venepuncture is usually very traumatic for a child. Therefore, in some circumstances, it is worth cannulating the child at the same time, as long as this doesn't compromise taking the blood sample. Taking the blood via a cannula can be more difficult in some children.

Indications

Indications for venepuncture are wide-ranging, and include:
- Performing a wide range of bloods tests as an investigation process for many conditions.
- Checking electrolytes in a child on intravenous fluid therapy.
- Measurement of drug levels, e.g. gentamicin.
- Taking a cross-match sample for blood transfusion.

Older Child

EQUIPMENT CHECKLIST

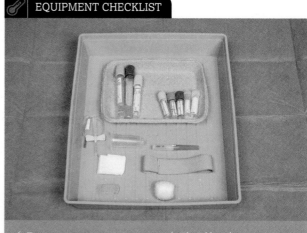

- ✓ Tray.
- ✓ Non-sterile gloves.
- ✓ Disposable tourniquet.
- ✓ Skin cleansing solution.
- ✓ Venepuncture needle/ Vacutainer or butterfly needle.
- ✓ Blood bottles.
- ✓ Cotton wool.
- ✓ Plaster.
- ✓ Sharps bin.
- ✓ Topical anaesthesia (e.g., cold spray, or Ametop cream).

🦶 STEP-BY-STEP GUIDE

1 Apply anaesthetic cream (if being used) 30-40 minutes before the procedure (*Figure 8*).

2 Wash hands and assemble equipment:
   i. Attach vacutainer to venepuncture needle/butterfly needle (depending on technique) (*Figure 9*).
   ii. Place blood bottles in draw order.
   iii. Cut a piece of tape to size.

3 Put on gloves.

4 Place the child in a comfortable position. This may involve putting a pillow under their arm. In younger children, positioning requires careful thought. The key is to immobilise the child, prevent them from watching the procedure and to facilitate distraction by having them look in another direction (*Figure 10*).

5 Place the tourniquet 7-10 cm proximal to the proposed insertion point (*Figure 11*).

6 Select the vein. This can be done by inspection and palpation. The antecubital fossa may be the best site to use, ideally in the non-dominant arm. However, in smaller children, it may be easier to hold their arm extended and access the veins on the dorsum of the hand. This is an easier position for keeping a child restrained.

7 Clean the site using the skin cleansing solution and then leave it to adequately dry.

8 If cold spray is being used, apply this now, in and around the intended puncture site (*Figure 12*).

9 Puncture the vein, making an effort not to re-palpate the site around the vein which has just been cleaned.

10 Draw blood by placing the blood tubes in the vacutainer (*Figure 13*). Invert the bottles. A similar technique is used with butterfly needles (*Figure 14*).

11 Remove the tourniquet (*Figure 15*).

12 Remove the needle and immediately dispose of any sharps.

13 Apply pressure to the puncture site with cotton wool until bleeding stops. Then secure it with tape.

14 Label bottles at the bedside.

15 Inform the child/parents to let staff know if they have any concerns, particularly with regard to pain or ongoing bleeding. Let them know that the dressing can be removed after a few hours.

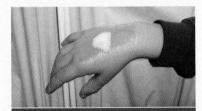
Figure 8. Ametop cream applied to skin over the site of a vein.

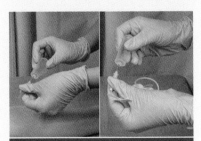
Figure 9. Assembling vacutainer (left), and butterfly needle (right).

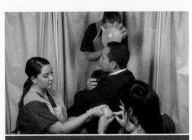
Figure 10. Ask a parent or a nurse to help with positioning. Sit the child in their lap, being cuddled, and facing away from the arm. Feed the arm under the holder's armpit so that the arm is isolated. In a particularly active child, a third person might be required to hold the arm still. Be creative with distraction techniques!

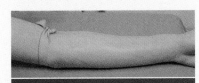
Figure 11. Apply the tourniquet.

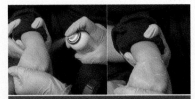
Figure 12. Applying cold spray (left), and awaiting crystal formation (right) before inserting the needle.

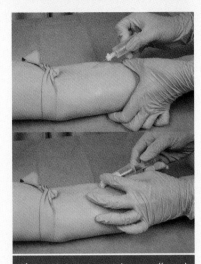
Figure 13. Insert vacutainer needle and then bottle.

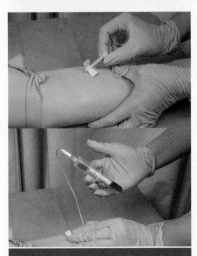
Figure 14. Inserting butterfly needle and then attaching the bottle.

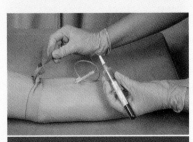
Figure 15. Remove the tourniquet as soon as last bottle of blood collected.

Note that this technique can be modified by using a butterfly needle attached to a syringe or by using a needle and syringe to draw blood.

EQUIPMENT CHECKLIST

- ✓ Tray.
- ✓ Non-sterile gloves.
- ✓ Skin cleansing solution.
- ✓ 23 gauge needle.
- ✓ Blood bottles.
- ✓ Cotton wool.
- ✓ Plaster.
- ✓ Sharps bin.
- ✓ Sucrose (if available).

COMPLICATIONS

- Infection.
- Pain.
- Soft tissue injury, e.g. skin extravasation.
- Venous thrombosis.
- Anaemia (if large recurrent blood samples are taken).

TOP TIPS

- In an older child who has had multiple blood tests before, it can be helpful to ask them if there are any sites that are particularly good for blood sampling.
- In a sick baby, it may be better to obtain blood samples from heel pricks. This saves the veins for cannulation and central lines. If venous blood sampling is needed, it is better to use smaller peripheral veins rather than larger central veins, as larger veins should ideally be saved for cannulation/central lines.
- Ensure that a suitable number of helpers are present before starting. Holding the child's hand and placing lids on the blood bottles can be difficult to do without adequate assistance.

Technique in a Neonate/Infant

STEP-BY-STEP GUIDE

1. Introduce oneself to the parents and explain the purpose of the procedure.
2. Wash hands and put on gloves.
3. Select the vein. This can be done by inspection and by palpation. The back of the hand is usually the best site for neonates, as larger veins are often reserved for central lines. Placing some cotton wool in the palm and gently squeezing the hand gives a tourniquet-like effect and will make the veins more prominent.
4. Clean the site using the skin cleansing solution and then leave it to dry (*Figure 16*).
5. Administer sucrose to the baby as analgesia if available (*Figure 17*). This could be done by asking the mother to put some on her finger or by putting it on the end of a dummy. Another option is getting the mum to breastfeed during the procedure. Note that some parents don't like this, because of the association of blood taking with breast feeding.
6. Puncture the vein with the needle. Once in the vein, blood will drip out of the other end of the needle.
7. Collect blood by placing the blood tubes underneath the needle, so that the blood drips into the tubes (*Figure 18*). For obtaining blood cultures, a separate needle and syringe should be used to aspirate blood from the back of the needle, and then afterwards put it into a blood culture bottle (follow local blood culture taking protocol). To improve blood flow, the hand may need to be squeezed and released intermittently.
8. Remove the needle, and immediately dispose of all sharps.
9. Apply pressure to the puncture site with cotton wool until bleeding stops (*Figure 19*), and then apply a plaster if needed (*Figure 20*).
10. Label bottles at the bedside.
11. Inform the parents to let staff know if they have any concerns, particularly with regard to pain or ongoing bleeding. Let them know that the dressing can be removed after a few hours.

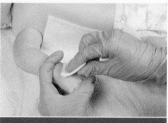

Figure 16. Clean site.

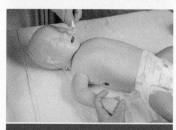

Figure 17. Drip sucrose into the mouth.

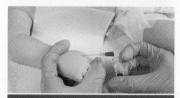

Figure 18. Allow blood to gently drip into the bottle.

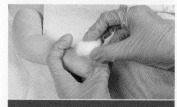

Figure 19. Apply pressure to stop any bleeding.

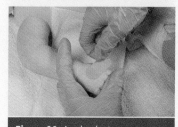

Figure 20. Apply plaster.

Arterial Line Sampling

Arterial line sampling is commonly required in NICU/PICU, and represents a common task which junior doctors may be expected to do.

Indications

- Arterial blood gas.
- Routine blood tests in patients with an arterial line in place.

EQUIPMENT CHECKLIST

- ✓ Port cleansing solution, e.g. 2% chlorhexidine.
- ✓ Non-sterile gloves.
- ✓ Gauze.
- ✓ Tray.
- ✓ 3 x syringes.
- ✓ 0.9% sodium chloride ampoule.
- ✓ Draw up needle.
- ✓ Sharps bin.

COMPLICATIONS

- Infection.
- Haemorrhage.
- Thromboembolism.
- Hypovolaemia.
- Arterial spasm.

TOP TIPS

- Calculate exactly how much blood is required in advance, and then draw up this exact amount from the arterial line. This ensures no blood is wasted, which is particularly important in small preterm babies with relatively small circulating volumes. Smaller babies will often have a chart documenting the volume of all blood taken off the arterial line, so be very careful.

- Sometimes, after arterial line sampling, the distal extremity can appear pale/white. Take this seriously and monitor very closely over the next five minutes. Consider asking for senior support or removing the arterial line if the colour has not returned to normal after this time.

STEP-BY-STEP GUIDE

1. Wash hands and put on gloves. Open packaging of syringes. Draw up sodium chloride flush in to one of the syringes using the draw up needle, and then dispose of the needle in the sharps bin.

2. Rotate the three-way tap so that it is open to the sampling port and the patient. The blood pressure reading should disappear from the monitor at this point (*Figure 21*).

3. Place sterile gauze under the three-way tap of the arterial line.

4. Clean the sampling port with the port cleansing solution.

5. Draw off 2-3 mL of blood from the arterial line into one of the syringes (*Figure 22*). Draw it off slowly, 0.5 mL at a time. In older children, this blood can be discarded, but in neonates it is replaced. If replacing it, inspect the syringe, ensuring that any air bubbles are expelled. Put the blood-filled syringe into its original packaging, ensuring it remains as sterile as possible- this blood will be returned to the patient.

6. Draw off the required sample volume in the second syringe. Do this slowly, and keep an eye on the colour of the distal extremities. If they change colour, it may be that blood is being drawn off too quickly and is being "stolen" from the distal blood supply.

7. Replace the first blood sample back into the arterial line, 0.5 mL at a time (*Figure 23*).

8. Flush the arterial line with the 0.9% sodium chloride, ensuring that no blood is left in the line (*Figure 24*).

9. Clean the port again with the port cleansing solution.

10. Switch the position of the three-way tap so that the sampling port is closed off again (*Figure 25*).

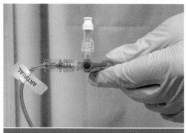

Figure 21. Turn three-way tap so that it is open to the sampling port.

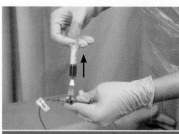

Figure 22. Draw off blood for replacement, and then, in a separate syringe, draw the blood for sampling.

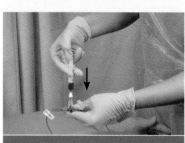

Figure 23. Return the initial replacement blood.

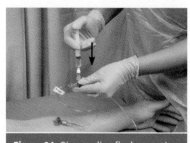

Figure 24. Give a saline flush, ensuring the line is clear of blood.

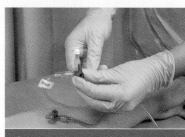

Figure 25. Close tap off to port.

Intravenous Cannulation

Although cannulation is done for the same indications in both children and adults, it can be much more difficult in children. This is because, particularly with younger children, co-operation can be an issue. It is important to ensure before the procedure takes place that the child is adequately distracted, a strategy is in place for analgesia and the proposed cannulation site is immobilised.

Indications

› Intravenous fluids (maintenance, replacement or bolus).
› Intravenous medications.

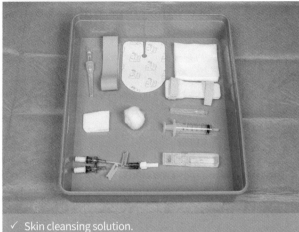

EQUIPMENT CHECKLIST

✓ Skin cleansing solution.
✓ Draw up needle.
✓ Syringe.
✓ 0.9% saline ampoule.
✓ Sterile adhesive dressing.
✓ Cannula.
✓ Disposable tourniquet.
✓ Cotton wool.
✓ Non-sterile gloves.
✓ Tray.
✓ Sharps bin.
✓ Splint and splint bandage (depending on age).
✓ Intravenous extension set (+ bung/connector).
✓ Gauze.

STEP-BY-STEP GUIDE

Preparing the Equipment

1 Wash hands and put on non-sterile gloves.
2 Attach the draw up needle to the syringe.
3 Remove the top from the 0.9% sodium chloride and draw it up into the syringe (*Figure 26*).
4 Expel any air from the syringe by tapping it or advancing the plunger.
5 Discard the needle in the sharps bin and flush through the intravenous extension set (*Figure 27*).
6 Leave the flush connected to the intravenous extension set and place it in the equipment tray alongside the other cannulation equipment.

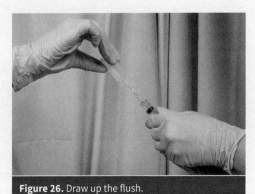

Figure 26. Draw up the flush.

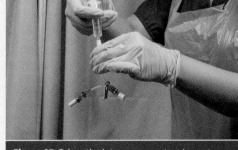

Figure 27. Prime the intravenous extension set.

STEP-BY-STEP GUIDE

Inserting the Cannula

1. Remove the cannula from its packaging and open the packet of sterile gauze.
2. Place the tourniquet approximately 7-10 cm proximal to the site of insertion.
3. Select an appropriate vein.
4. Clean the proposed site using skin cleansing solution and then leave it to dry.
5. Tether the chosen vein beneath the insertion site and insert the cannula at approximately 15° using an aseptic technique (*Figure 28*).
6. Advance the cannula until flashback is obtained.
7. Once flashback has been seen, advance the cannula slightly further (1-2 mm). This ensures the cannula tubing is within the vein before advancing it forwards, over and off the needle.
8. Hold the needle still and advance the cannula over it, all the way into the vein. No part of the cannula tubing must be seen at the point of entry.
9. Occlude the vein proximal to the cannula insertion site with firm pressure and then gently remove the needle (this will reduce blood loss when the needle is removed from the tubing) (*Figure 29*).
10. Dispose of the needle straight into the sharps bin.
11. Take off any blood samples needed from the end of the cannula (*Figure 30*).
12. Release the tourniquet.
13. If the child is very mobile or vigorous, it may help to secure the cannula in place at this stage with one piece of tape as a temporary measure. It can be formally secured once its position is confirmed.
14. Attach the intravenous extension set to the end of the cannula (*Figure 31*). Slowly flush the cannula through the extension set, 1 mL at a time, checking to see that the fluid is not going into subcutaneous tissue, and that there is minimal resistance to pushing the fluid through the cannula (*Figure 32*).
15. As the last millilitre goes through, clamp the extension set.
16. Dispose of the syringe in the sharps bin.
17. Wipe away any blood that may have leaked around the cannula with sterile gauze.
18. Apply tape and sterile adhesive dressing (*Figure 33*). Use tape and cotton wool to further secure the cannula even more if needed.
19. Apply a splint to the cannula and thoroughly bandage it so that it is inaccessible to the child.
20. Remove gloves and wash hands.

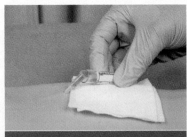

Figure 30. Collect blood sample.

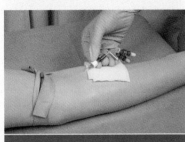

Figure 31. Attach IV extension set.

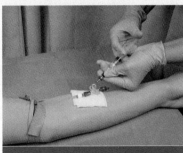

Figure 32. Flush cannula.

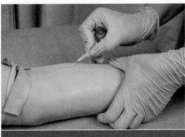

Figure 28. Insert cannula.

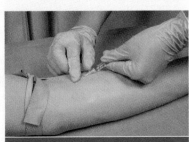

Figure 29. Occlude vein while removing needle.

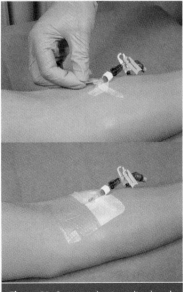

Figure 33. Secure using tape (top) and sterile adhesive dressing (bottom).

COMPLICATIONS

- Infection.
- Pain.
- Soft tissue injury, e.g. skin extravasation.
- Venous thrombosis.

 TOP TIPS

- Children will often attempt to pull cannulas out. Do not leave until the cannula is definitely stuck down and covered.
- Adhesive dressings may not stick to sweaty skin if the child is hot and vigorous. Using a barrier preparation such as Cavelon can overcome this. Apply the barrier preparation to the skin before sticking the adhesive dressing on top.
- One of the most common reasons for failing to insert a cannula is choosing the wrong vein. Spend time assessing the best veins on each limb. Remember also to select a vein which can be easily immobilised – choosing veins overlying joints (e.g. wrist or antecubital fossae) may prove difficult due to the child's movements.
- If struggling to find a vein, revert to anatomical sites common to almost all children. Consider the long saphenous vein anterior to the medial malleolus or "houseman's vein" on the lateral border of the wrist. In neonates, remember that scalp veins may yield extra unutilised possibilities.
- In a non-emergency situation, after two unsuccessful attempts at peripheral cannulation, ask a more experienced colleague to attempt cannulation.
- In emergency situations, after three unsuccessful attempts at peripheral cannulation, attempt intraosseous access instead.

Umbilical Venous and Arterial Catheterisation

Umbilical venous catheterisation (UVC) is a relatively common procedure in neonates and is usually relatively straightforward with practice. UVCs can be inserted in the first week of life, although the earlier the better, due to the declining patency of the umbilical cord. Umbilical arterial catheterisation (UAC), if needed, is usually done at the same time as inserting the UVC. This is often more difficult, as the artery is more muscular, with a smaller lumen.

Indications
UVC

> For administration of TPN in small babies.
> For giving high glucose concentrations to hypoglycaemic babies.
> For administration of certain drugs that may be poorly tolerated peripherally, e.g. dopamine.
> For performing exchange and partial exchange transfusions.

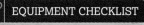 EQUIPMENT CHECKLIST

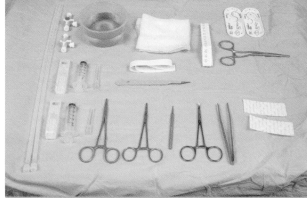

Ensure sterility:

✓ Sterile gown.
✓ Sterile towel.
✓ Sterile gloves.

Preparing to insert the UVC and UAC:

✓ Tape measure.
✓ 2 x appropriately sized umbilical catheters.
✓ 2 x three-way taps.
✓ 2 x 5 mL syringe.
✓ 2 x 0.9% sodium chloride ampoule.
✓ Draw up needle.
✓ Skin cleansing solution, e.g. 0.05% chlorhexidine gluconate aqueous solution (appropriate strength to avoid chemical burns).

✓ Umbilical tape.
✓ Scalpel.
✓ Sterile drapes.*

Inserting the UVC and UAC:

✓ Fine non-toothed forceps.*
✓ Blunt end dilator.*
✓ 2 x artery forceps.*
✓ Sterile gauze.*

Securing the catheter:

✓ 2 x sutures.
✓ 2 x Steri-Strips.
✓ Scissors.*
✓ Suture holder.*

*May all be included in a blunt dissection pack

- For immediate access in an emergency, when peripheral cannulation is difficult.

UAC

- Frequent arterial blood gas measurement/blood sampling.
- Continuous blood pressure reading.
- Exchange transfusion.

Exomphalos is a contraindication, but otherwise there are very few absolute contraindications.

The process for inserting a UVC and a UAC at the same time is described below.

Preparation

1   Lay the baby supine, and estimate the length of the two catheters (*Figure 34*).
2   Wash hands, dry them with a sterile towel, and put on a sterile gown.
3   Prepare the UVC and the UAC.
    i   Attach the three-way tap to the catheter.
    ii Draw up the sodium chloride in the 5 mL syringe using the draw up needle (*Figure 35*), and prime all the ports of the catheter, making sure it flushes all the way through (*Figure 36*). Immediately dispose of the draw up needle in the sharps bin.

iii Leave the catheter in the sterile packaging, ensuring that the distal end is not open to the atmosphere.

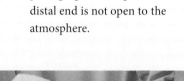

Figure 35. Drawing up the flush.

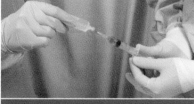

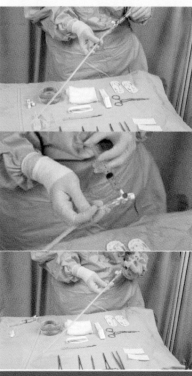

Figure 36. Priming the arterial line (red) and the venous line (blue) with saline. Note both ports of both catheters need to be flushed through.

4   Clean the umbilical cord area with the skin cleansing solution.
5   Place the sterile drapes around the umbilicus, leaving the feet/ head exposed. Clean again (*Figure 37*).
6   Tie the umbilical tape around the base of the umbilicus (*Figure 38*). This helps keep the cord upright, and also minimises any blood loss. Be careful not to make it too tight, as this may make passing the catheter harder.

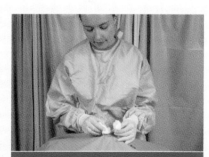

Figure 37. Create a sterile field and, while holding the cord with sterile gauze, clean around it.

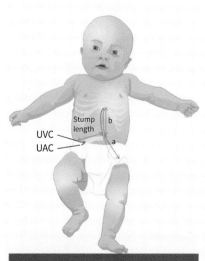

Figure 34. Cord lengths:
UVC: stump length + b.
UAC: stump length + 2a + b:
a= distance from umbilicus to mid-inguinal point.
b= distance from umbilicus to xiphoid.

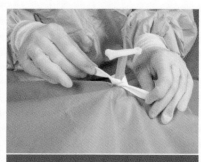

Figure 38. Tying the cord at the base.

Inserting the Umbilical Lines

1   Cut the umbilical cord with the scalpel in one clean motion. Try to make the cut surface as even as possible (*Figure 39*). It is important that the cord is not too long or too short. The longer the cord, the more difficult it is to insert the catheter. If the cord is too short, then there will not be space for a second attempt (i.e. cutting the cord again). Approximately 2-3 cm from the umbilicus is ideal.

2   Identify the vessels (*Figure 40*). The umbilical vein is the single, thin walled, peripheral, larger vessel. There are two arteries, which are muscular with a narrower lumen. Massage the cord from the base to the top to remove any debris in the vessels. Use gauze to stop any bleeding.

3   Pick the more favourable umbilical artery to attempt cannulation in first. Arterial forceps can be used to hold the cord upright. Any umbilical artery is likely to require prolonged, deep dilatation before proceeding, so do not rush. To dilate, use (*Figure 41*):

   i.   Fine non-toothed forceps or arterial forceps. To dilate the opening very superficially.
   ii. Blunt ended dilators. To dilate the vessel more distally.

4   Advance the first catheter into the umbilical artery up until the premeasured level. Non-toothed forceps can help give greater control (*Figure 42*). Check that blood aspirates into the syringe (*Figure 43*). Problems may arise:

   i.   By having the umbilical tape too tight. In this case, loosen the tape, and then re-advance.
   ii. By the umbilical cord being too mobile. In this case, hold it in place with one or two artery forceps (held by the non-dominant hand).

   iii. By creating a false passage, with the catheter going through the vessel wall, and into the stump. In this scenario, it is helpful to recut the cord more proximally and try again.
   iv. At 1-2 cm. Where the umbilical artery turns downwards. Use gentle pressure, and also try turning the umbilical stump towards the baby's head, to straighten the vessel.
   v.   At 4-5 cm. May be due to spasm/ kinking at the iliac vessels. Overcome with gentle pressure.

5   Inspect the baby's legs/toes: if they are blue or white, the catheter may be obstructing blood flow, and therefore needs to be removed.

6   Ensure haemostasis has been achieved. A second umbilical tape may be needed in some cases.

7   Secure the catheter (see "Securing the Catheter").

8   Grasp the umbilical cord with the curved artery forceps to hold it upright and straight again. Re-inspect the umbilical vein. It may be that a catheter can be inserted into

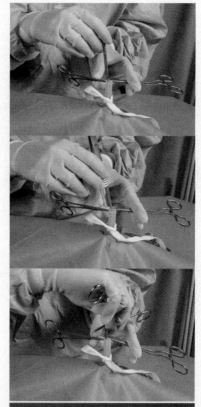

Figure 41. Hold the cord up using artery forceps if needed. Dilation of the vessels can be achieved with a blunt ended dilator (top), fine non-toothed forceps (middle), or arterial forceps (bottom).

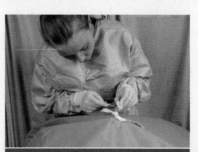

Figure 39. Cut the cord as close to the clamp as possible, approx 2-3 cm from the skin.

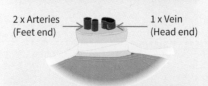

2 x Arteries (Feet end) ← → 1 x Vein (Head end)

Figure 40. Identify the vessels: two narrow muscular arteries (feet end) and one thinner walled vein (head end).

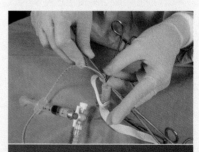

Figure 42. Advancing the UAC. Note that the syringe is still attached.

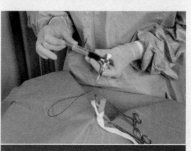

Figure 43. After reaching measured length, aspirate blood.

Continued

STEP-BY-STEP GUIDE

the vein with no manipulation of the vessel: it is usually much easier than for the artery. Prepare the umbilical vein for catheterisation if needed, as done with the artery.

9   Advance the second catheter into the umbilical vein, up until the premeasured level, ensuring blood aspirates (*Figure 44*). Problems may arise:

i.   Meeting a kink in the umbilical vein. This may occur

1-2 cm beyond the abdominal wall. Gentle traction should overcome this.

ii.   Getting coiled up/wedged in the portal system. Pull back part of the way and re-advance.

10   Secure the catheter (see "Securing the catheter"), ensuring that the sutures remain entirely separate. As with the UVC, check after insertion that the babies legs/toes haven't changed colour (if so the catheter

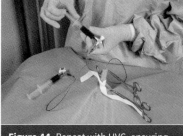

Figure 44. Repeat with UVC, ensuring blood aspirates.

will need to be removed). Ensure haemostasis has been achieved.

 STEP-BY-STEP GUIDE

Securing the Catheter

1   Using the suture holder, pass the suture through the stump of the cord, avoiding the vessels. Tie a secure knot to firmly fix the suture to the stump (*Figure 45*).

2   Loop the suture around the catheter, and then tie another knot, ensuring there is minimal slack in the suture (*Figure 46*). Repeat this again, two or three times, at 0.5 cm increments, giving a total of three or four knots (*Figure 47*).

3   Gently pull on the catheter to ensure that it is secure, and then cut the suture with the scalpel, leaving

tails of approximately 1 cm on either end (*Figure 48*).

4   Use steristrips to tape the knots against the cord, ensuring that

the sutures are taught whilst stuck down (*Figure 49*).

5   Gently pull on the catheter again to check that it is secure.

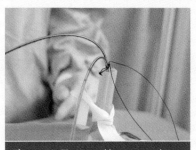

Figure 46. Tie second knot around base of catheter to secure it.

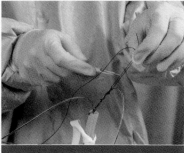

Figure 48. Cut the loose thread.

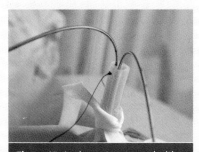

Figure 45. Anchor suture to cord with first knot.

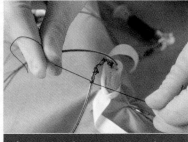

Figure 47. Tie knots approximately every 0.5cm.

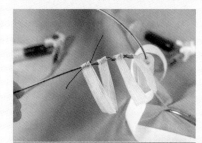

Figure 49. Use Steri-Strips to fix the knots to the catheter.

Finishing off

1. To keep the lines patent, an infusion of fluid should be set up to run at a slow rate, e.g. 0.5-1 mL/hr of 0.9% sodium chloride.

2. Perform an X-ray to check the position of the two catheters. The UVC goes straight up, whereas the UAC dips down first towards the pelvis, before going up. The UVC should be around T9-T10, and the UAC should be between T6 and T10. A low UAC can be between L3-5, but never leave at L1 as this is the level of the renal arteries (*Figure 50*).

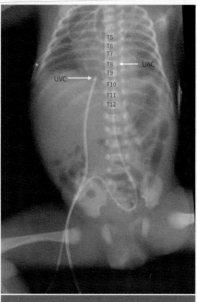

Figure 50. X-ray showing position of umbilical lines. UVC at T10, and UAC at T8 (Reproduced with kind permission from Radiopedia).

- Infection.
- Haemorrhage.
- Vessel perforation.
- Air/catheter tip embolism.
- Portal vein thrombosis.
- Cardiac/hepatic haematoma.
- Cardiac arrhythmia/perforation/tamponade (if catheter is advanced into the heart).

- Advancing the catheter gently but firmly from the tip will help prevent the creation of a false passage.
- Be very gentle when dilating the vessels: this will also reduce the risk of false passage.
- Most clinicians prefer putting the UAC in first. The UAC is technically more difficult, and the cord may need to be cut multiple times to successfully gain access, which is a lot easier if the UVC is not already in situ.

Emergency Umbilical Venous Catheterisation

Insertion of an umbilical venous catheter is a key life-saving skill that may be required during the resuscitation of a neonate. In the emergency setting, this is not a sterile procedure, but once the baby has been transferred to the neonatal unit, this can then be replaced in a sterile manner with a new catheter and secured properly.

Indications

▸ For fast, central access to administer drugs and fluids (e.g. adrenaline, bicarbonate, sodium chloride, blood), as peripheral cannulation in this scenario can be challenging.

- ✓ Umbilical catheter.
- ✓ 10 mL syringe of 0.9% sodium chloride.
- ✓ Umbilical tape.
- ✓ Scalpel.
- ✓ Fine non-toothed forceps.
- ✓ Gauze.
- ✓ Tape.

1. Flush the catheter with sodium chloride.

2. Tie the umbilical tape loosely around the base of the umbilicus.

3. Hold the umbilical cord straight up by holding the cord clamp (which will already have been placed by the midwife/obstetrician). Using the scalpel, make a single cut across the cord proximal to the clamp.

4. If there is significant blood oozing from the stump, tighten the umbilical tie. Use a piece of gauze to dab at any oozing, and identify the umbilical vein.

5. Dilate the umbilical vein superficially if needed. Insert the catheter 4-5 cm past the umbilical ring and ensure blood can be aspirated before it is used. Make a note of how far the catheter has been advanced and tape it to the abdomen. This can now be used to administer emergency drugs, fluids or blood.

6. If ongoing umbilical access is required, then a definitive umbilical catheter should be inserted in a sterile manner and sutured into place. If not required, the umbilical venous catheter can be gently withdrawn, with the umbilical cord-tie still in situ.

- Do not wait for X-ray confirmation before using this line. It is an emergency and position is confirmed by aspirating blood back.

Intraosseous Needle Insertion

Intraosseous needle insertion is the quickest way to give rapid fluid resuscitation in a peripherally shut down child. It also functions as central access, allowing inotropes to be administered in emergency situations. It is usually done in an emergency situation, and this is the process that will be described below. In a conscious child, use of local anaesthetic should be considered before the procedure.

EQUIPMENT CHECKLIST

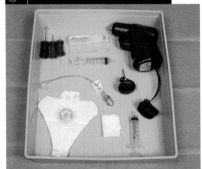

- ✓ Manual intraosseous (IO) needle or battery operated IO drill.
- ✓ IO needle (15 mm needle (pink) for patients under 40 kg, or 25 mm needle (blue) for more than 40 kg).
- ✓ Non-sterile gloves.
- ✓ Skin cleansing solution.
- ✓ Adhesive dressing (for securing IO needle).
- ✓ 5 mL syringe.
- ✓ Specimen bottle.
- ✓ Sharps bin.
- ✓ Equipment tray.
- ✓ Intravenous extension set:
  - ◊ Intravenous extension set.
  - ◊ Three-way tap.
  - ◊ 0.9% sodium chloride ampoule.
  - ◊ Draw up needle.
  - ◊ 5 mL syringe.

STEP-BY-STEP GUIDE

1. Wash hands. Put on non-sterile gloves.
2. Remove the top from the 0.9% sodium chloride and draw it up into the syringe.
3. Expel any air from the syringe by tapping it/advancing the plunger.
4. Discard the needle in the sharps bin and flush through the intravenous extension set (*Figure 51*).
5. Leave the flush connected to the intravenous extension set, and place it in the equipment tray.
6. Chose the site of access. Usually the anteromedial tibia is the first choice and presents a stable, flat surface (*Figure 52*). The anterolateral femur is the next most commonly selected site. Avoid areas of infected skin/wounds. Other contraindications include:
   - Fracture in targeted bone or proximal to site of insertion.
   - Excessive tissue or absence of adequate anatomical landmarks.
   - Previous, significant orthopaedic procedure at site (e.g. prosthetic limb/joint).
   - IO access in targeted bone within past 48 hours.
7. Clean with skin cleansing solution.
8. Immobilise the relevant limb, ensuring that the hand immobilising the limb is not placed under the limb in the process.
9. Insert the IO needle at 90° to the surface of the skin. There should be a loss of resistance (a "give") on entering the cortex of the bone. This may be done manually (*Figure 57*) or with a drill (*Figure 53*). If successful, the needle should be firmly attached.
10. After ensuring the needle is stable, remove the trocar from the needle: immediately dispose into the sharps bin.
11. Attach a syringe, and aspirate bone marrow if possible

(*Figure 54*). Samples cannot be put through a blood gas analyser and should be sent to the laboratory marked as bone marrow aspirate. Tests that may be performed include:
- › Red blood cell count.
- › Chloride.
- › Haemoglobin and haematocrit.
- › Total protein.

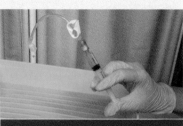
Figure 51. Prime the intravenous extension set.

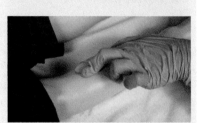
Figure 52. Palpate the anatomical landmark.

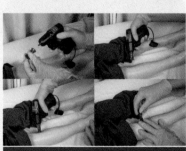
Figure 53. Insertion of intraosseous needle using the easy IO drill.

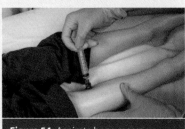
Figure 54. Aspirate bone marrow (attempt).

Continued

627

> Glucose.
> Albumin.
> Urea.
> Lactate.
> Creatinine.

12 Fix the IO needle with the adhesive dressing (*Figure 55*).

13 Attach the pre-primed intravenous extension set, and flush through with sodium chloride, checking there is no extravasation (*Figure 56*).

14 Administer medication/fluids as needed. Infusion of fluids is often painful for patients responsive to pain; therefore, following the IO needle insertion, IO anaesthetic (2% preservative-free lignocaine) may be considered for use.

15 Continue at least hourly observations of the access site for possible complications.

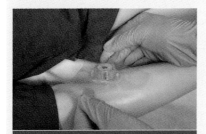

Figure 55. Secure with dressing.

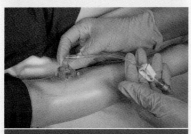

Figure 56. Attach intravenous extension set.

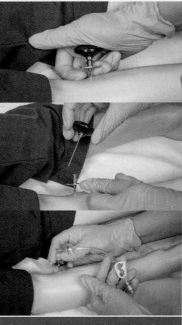

Figure 57. Same procedure using the manual intraosseous needle. Inserting the needle by twisting and pushing downwards (top), removing the trocar (middle) and attaching the intravenous extension set (bottom).

- Extravasation of fluid/medication, which can lead to compartment syndrome.
- Infection.
- Pain.
- Skin necrosis.
- Fractures.

- If a child is coming to ED following cardiac arrest or is significantly compromised, have everything set up to establish intraosseous access, as it is highly likely that it will be needed.

- There is nothing to prevent multiple IO needles being put in the same child at various sites; indeed multiple ports of access will frequently be required in an emergency.

- Intraosseous samples should never be run in a blood gas machine (the machine will break). If sending to the lab, the sample must be very clearly labelled so the laboratory staff can process it appropriately (if they think they are looking at a blood film, they are likely to report a leukaemic picture with the large number of blasts present!).

AIRWAY PROCEDURES

Bag-Valve-Mask Ventilation

Bag-Valve-Mask (BVM) Ventilation is a life-saving method of administering non-invasive positive pressure to inflate the lungs. The BVM's greatest attribute is that it is portable and does not require a gas supply to function.

Indications

> Respiratory arrest.
> Hypoventilating patient, i.e. a patient who is breathing either too slowly or too shallowly to be effective.

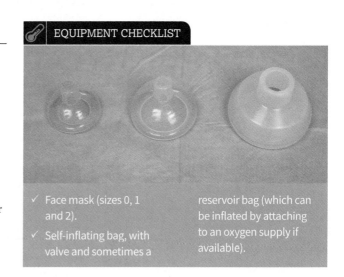

✓ Face mask (sizes 0, 1 and 2).
✓ Self-inflating bag, with valve and sometimes a reservoir bag (which can be inflated by attaching to an oxygen supply if available).

STEP-BY-STEP GUIDE

1 Pick the correct size mask (*Figure 58*). A tight seal is crucial. The mask should cover the nose and mouth, without pressing on the eyes (which may promote a vagal response or cause local trauma) or overhanging at the chin.

2 Pick the correct size bag. There are generally three sizes of self-inflating bag; infant, child and adult. In larger adolescents, use the adult size.

3 Two possible techniques can be used:

a One person technique (*Figure 59*):

Figure 58. Sizing the mask: too small (top), correct size (middle), too big (bottom).

i Place the face mask over the nose and mouth, creating a good seal and being careful not to press over the eyes.

ii With the left hand, create a C-shape with the thumb and forefinger. Place this on top of the mask, pressing it downwards onto the face.

iii The third, fourth and fifth fingers should be used to support the mandible. Be careful not to compress the soft tissues of the upper airway when performing this manoeuvre, by ensuring that fingers are placed on the bones of the jaw only (*Figure 59*). Some people are able to simultaneously perform a jaw-thrust; this needs practice.

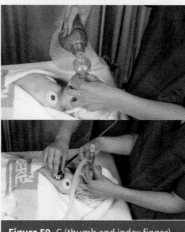

Figure 59. C (thumb and index finger) and E (little, ring and middle finger) grips, while ventilating a baby using a bag-valve-mask (top), and using a T-piece (bottom).

iv Compress the bag with the right hand. Watch for chest wall rise and listen for leak around the edge of the mask. The bag may only need to be compressed by a third or half of its volume for each breath. Adjust positioning as required.

b Two-person technique: this makes it easier to adequately create a seal, and to utilise the jaw thrust (*Figure 60*):

i Using both hands, press the mask down onto the face with the thumbs (+/- index fingers).

ii The other fingers can then perform a jaw-thrust on both sides.

iii The second person can then compress the bag.

4 Consider the need for a definitive airway or other forms of ventilatory support (invasive or non-invasive). If the patient is spontaneously breathing, they may require high flow oxygen, or alternatively in the acute newborn situation, they may recover very quickly and self-ventilate in air.

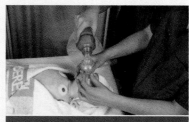

Figure 60. Two person technique.

COMPLICATIONS

• Pneumothorax.

• Aspiration (from stomach inflation).

TOP TIPS

• It can be helpful to place an oropharyngeal airway (Guedel airway) first, as this will draw the tongue forwards and prevent it from obstructing the airway. This will only work if the patient is sufficiently unconscious to not have a gag reflex.

• Bag-valve-mask ventilation can be a tiring process, so ask a colleague to take over when necessary.

• Make sure that when holding the mask over the patient's face, the bag is actually being compressed; otherwise no air/oxygen will be delivered to the patient, effectively suffocating them (the valve is closed at rest).

Nasopharyngeal Airway Insertion

Airway adjuncts are used in children with reduced consciousness and those that are difficult to ventilate. They are simple, effective ways to open the airway. Below, nasopharyngeal (NP), oropharyngeal (OP) and laryngeal mask airways are described.

A NP airway comprises a flange, body and bevelled opening (*Figure 61*).

1 Correctly size the NP airway (*Figure 62*). The size is indicated by the number printed on the side of the airway. Make sure the flange is large enough to anchor the NP airway in the nose. To be correctly sized, the bevelled opening should fit comfortably into the nostril, and the length should approximate the distance from the tragus of the ear (or angle of the jaw) to the nostril. The other way of sizing the tube is choosing a diameter that is approximately the same size as the diameter of the patient's little finger.

2 Put lubricant on the bevelled end of the NP airway (*Figure 63*).

3 Introduce the NP airway (bevel end first) into one of the nostrils and advance it along the floor of the nasal passage (*Figure 64*).

4 Continue until only the flange remains at the opening of the nasal passage.

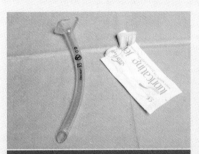

Figure 61. An NP airway, and lubricant.

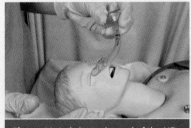

Figure 63. Lubricate the end of the NP airway.

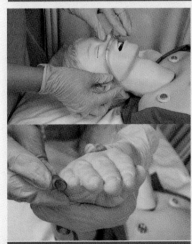

Figure 62. Sizing an NP airway from the nostril to the angle of the jaw (above) and comparing to size of little finger (below).

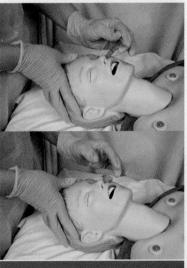

Figure 64. Inserting the NP airway.

Oropharyngeal Airway Insertion

An OP airway comprises a curved tube with a bit block and a flange (*Figure 65*).

 STEP-BY-STEP GUIDE

1. Correctly size the OP airway (*Figure 66*). They are colour coded according to size. To be correctly sized, the OP airway should measure from the angle of the jaw to the middle of the incisors.
2. Insert the OP airway, holding it by the flange, into the mouth (*Figure 67*). Initially, advance it upside down to avoid pushing back the tongue. Once in, rotate by 180 degrees. In neonates/small children, insert it with a laryngoscope/tongue depressor pushing down the tongue, with the OP airway in the direction it will sit, i.e. pointing downwards.

This also provides the opportunity to examine the oropharynx for foreign material.

3. Advance it into the mouth until the bit block rests between the teeth.

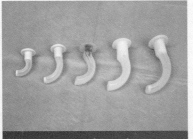

Figure 65. Range of sizes of OP airways.

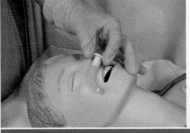

Figure 66. Sizing a guedel. Left: too short. Right: still a little short of the angle of the jaw, but much better fit.

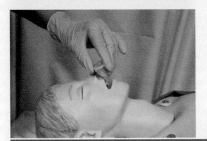

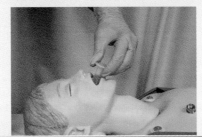

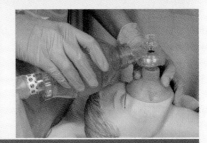

Figure 67. Inserting the OP airway: in an older child, insert it upside down (left) and then twist round 180 degrees to put in final resting position (middle). Once in, ventilate as normal (right).

Laryngeal Mask Airway

A laryngeal mask airway (LMA) is an example of an advanced airway (*Figure 68*). It is a supraglottic airway device. These airway devices offer increased airway protection compared to NP/OP airways, as they sit above the larynx.

 STEP-BY-STEP GUIDE

1. Deflate and lubricate the cuff (*Figure 69*).
2. Insert the LMA, holding it like a pen, until resistance is felt at the back of the pharynx (*Figure 70*).
3. Inflate the cuff using room air (via a syringe) (*Figure 71*).
4. Ventilate with the LMA in place, assessing for breath sounds and chest movement to ensure the LMA is in a good position (*Figure 72*).

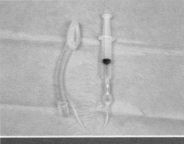

Figure 68. LMA (inflated) attached to syringe.

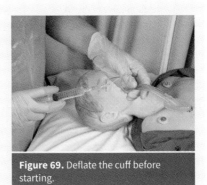

Figure 69. Deflate the cuff before starting.

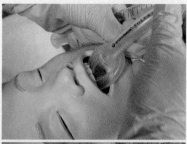

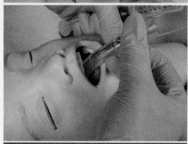

Figure 70. Insert the LMA like a pen.

Another example of a supraglottic airway device is the iGel. It is inserted held like a pen, until resistance is felt at the back of the pharynx. An iGel has the advantage of allowing an NG tube to be passed through it.

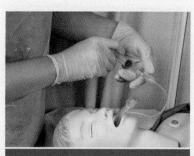

Figure 71. Inflate the cuff.

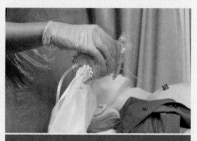

Figure 72. Ventilate.

Neonatal Intubation

Neonatal intubation of term and pre-term neonates is a key skill for any paediatric trainee. It can be performed with or without premedication. Premedication is preferred to make the procedure easier, and to reduce the cortisol response in the neonate. Common pre-medications include morphine, atropine and suxamethonium. Sometimes, in an emergency, there is no time to retrieve, prepare and give drugs in advance.

Indications

▸ Failure of oxygenation.
▸ Failure of ventilation (CO_2 clearance).
▸ To facilitate the administration of surfactant.
▸ Specific conditions requiring immediate intubation at birth, such as congenital diaphragmatic hernia.
▸ To secure the airway during resuscitation (if not able to move the chest despite airway manoeuvres or if the resuscitation is prolonged).

EQUIPMENT CHECKLIST

✓ Correctly fitting facemask.
✓ T-piece (attached to pressure limited gas flow device, e.g. neopuff), or self-inflating bag.
✓ Endotracheal (ET) tube (ideally three sizes, to cover a possibly larger and smaller baby than expected).
✓ Introducer (stylet).
✓ Appropriately sized straight blade (00, 0, 1) attached to a working laryngoscope.
✓ Suction circuit and suction catheter.
✓ Stethoscope.
✓ Oxygen saturation monitor.
✓ Scissors.

Method for securing tube (one example is shown below, but many exist):
✓ Hat with strings either side.
✓ Soft plastic flange, with a hard plastic clip.
✓ Forceps (to close the clip).

For premedication:
✓ IV access.

✓ Premedication drugs: note that these vary between units, but one combination commonly used is:

  a. Atropine (to treat any vagal response to intubation).
  b. Suxamethonium (muscle relaxant).
  c. Fentanyl or morphine (analgesia).

An assistant is essential to:
✓ Keep an eye on any monitoring.
✓ Pass the suction catheter.
✓ Pass the ET tube.
✓ Administer cricoid pressure if needed.
✓ Confirm placement of the tube with a stethoscope.

Capnometer (end-tidal CO_2) may help confirm the position of the ET tube. However, it may be misleading, particularly if there is reduced cardiac output or failure of adaptation of the neonatal circulation.

STEP-BY-STEP GUIDE

Preparation

1 Put the introducer in the ET tube, ensuring that the introducer is not protruding from the end of the tube (where it may cause tissue damage). Wrap the introducer around the hard plastic connector of the ET tube to ensure it is secure (*Figure 73*).

2 Ensure all equipment is working, including laryngoscope, light source, air/O$_2$, and suction circuit.

3 Check that the cannula is working. Draw up all premedication in advance.

4 If there is an NG tube in place,

5 aspirate the stomach contents. Position the neonate on a flat surface, head in the midline, with the neck slightly extended.

6 In a non-emergency intubation, optimise ventilation by using intermittent positive pressure ventilation (e.g. with a bag-valve-mask) and aim to fully saturate the baby before beginning.

7 Suction any visible secretions from the mouth.

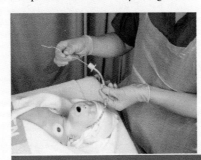
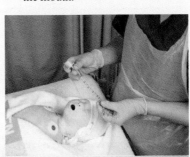

Figure 73. Putting introducer into ET tube.

STEP-BY-STEP GUIDE

Inserting the ET tube

1 Place the laryngoscope into the oropharynx. Initially place it low, putting it over the oesophagus. Gently pulling out anteriorly should reveal the vocal cords in the superior part of the view (*Figure 74*). An assistant pushing on the cricoid may be needed to bring the cords into view.

2 Suction any blood/secretions that may be present around the vocal cords.

3 Ask for the ET tube, and advance it through the cords. There is a black mark on the ET tube, which should just go through the cords (*Figure 75*).

4 Hold the tube firmly against the hard palate so that it does not move while removing the introducer (*Figure 76*).

5 Look for chest wall movement, and ask an assistant to listen for equal air entry. If there is more marked air entry on one side, gently withdraw

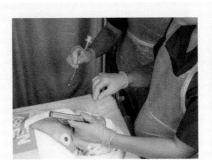
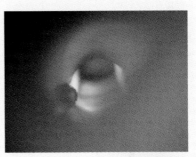

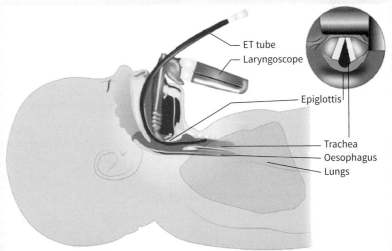

Figure 74. Visualising the vocal cords (with ET tube ready) (top left). Note the white vertical cords on either side of the airway (top right). Aim straight between these with the ET tube, with the tube finishing below the cords (bottom).

633

STEP-BY-STEP GUIDE

the tube by half a centimetre at a time until the air entry is equal. If the saturations improve, this is a good indication of correct position. Be careful not to extubate the baby.

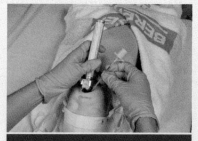

Figure 75. Inserting the tube.

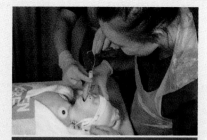

Figure 76. Holding the tube against the hard palate whilst the introducer is removed.

STEP-BY-STEP GUIDE

Securing the ET Tube

Described below is one common method of securing an ET tube. Different units use different techniques, including specially designed adhesive tapes and, in older children, the Melbourne strapping technique using Elastoplast.

1 Keep a secure hold on the tube whilst an assistant passes the soft plastic flange over the ET tube. Use the forceps to clamp the clip on the flange tight around the ET tube (*Figure 77*).

2 Attach a capnometer (if available) to the ET tube to check that CO_2 is being expelled (*Figure 78*).

3 Attach the ET tube to a ventilator circuit (or to a bag and mask).

4 Cut the tube to a reasonable length to reduce dead space (and resistance of the tube).

5 Tie the strings of the hat to the flange, securing the ET tube to the head (*Figure 79*). The tube is now secure and it no longer has to be held against the hard palate.

6 Auscultate again to check the tube is still in the correct position (*Figure 80*).

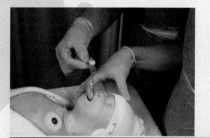
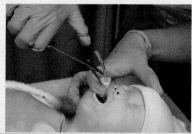

Figure 77. Placing flange over the tube, and tightening it in place.

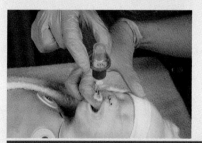
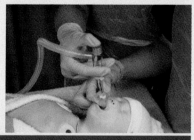

Figure 78. Attaching CO_2 monitor, and then the T-piece to connect to the ventilator. Note that the tube is firmly pushed against the hard palate as it is still not secure.

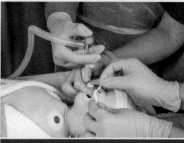
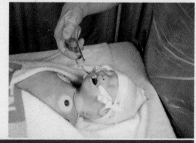

Figure 79. Tying the ET tube to the cap, and then releasing grip on the hard palate once secure.

STEP-BY-STEP GUIDE

7 Arrange a chest X-ray to assess the position of the tube. The tip of the ET tube should be 1 cm above the carina. If the carina cannot be visualised, then a position of T2-3 is adequate (*Figure 81*).

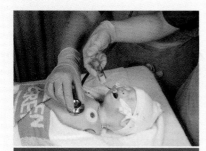

Figure 80. Final position confirmation by auscultation.

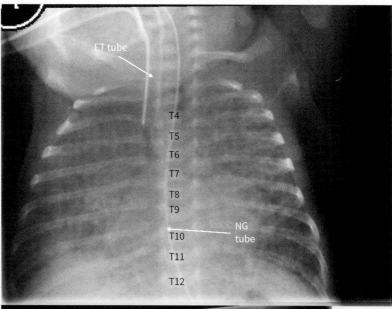

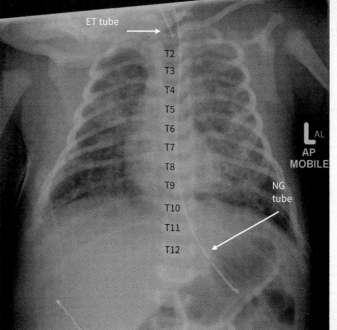

Figure 81. X-ray confirming ET Tube position.
TOP: Low position at T4 (although may be acceptable as head flexed during X-ray).
BOTTOM: High position at T1.

COMPLICATIONS

- Laryngospasm.
- Pneumothorax.
- Oesophageal intubation.
- Haemorrhage.
- Hypotension (from vagal stimulation).
- Lung collapse (from ET tube being too far advanced).
- ET tube obstruction (e.g. from blood/secretions).
- Oedema of the cords.
- Cord paralysis.
- Lung damage from barotrauma.

TOP TIPS

- Don't rush the procedure. Take time trying to visualise the cords before taking the ET tube. Have an assistant on hand to watch the monitor and keep a close eye on the saturations.
- Take no more than 30 seconds for each intubation attempt before withdrawing and re-oxygenating.
- The person holding the tube against the palate should have no other job. Otherwise, the tube is at risk of slipping in either direction.
- If possible, pass an NG tube first, as this will make the position of the oesophagus clear and can be used as a guide (as well as deflating the stomach).

- It may be tempting to try to advance the tube without having a good view of the cords. Do not do this, and instead ask a more experienced colleague to attempt the procedure. It will risk laryngospasm, local airway trauma and potentially a prolonged period of hypoxia.
- Consider "plan B" regarding any difficult airway. Can a smaller tube be used? Does a different size laryngoscope blade need to be used? Identify who can be called for help (PICU, anaesthetics, paediatric registrar covering another area of the hospital). Have an appropriately sized bag-valve-mask ready.

Surfactant Administration

Surfactant is administered via an ET tube in neonates. It significantly improves outlook in respiratory distress syndrome by increasing the compliance of premature lungs. Usually it is done in babies that are already intubated, but some centres will intubate purely to give surfactant and then extubate. Other indications are shown below.

Indications

› Respiratory distress syndrome.
› Meconium aspiration.
› Pulmonary haemorrhage.

EQUIPMENT CHECKLIST

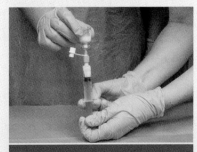

✓ Surfactant vial.
✓ Surfactant administration kit (surfactant tube, syringe, vial adaptor).
✓ Sterile gloves.
✓ Sterile scissors.
✓ Bag-valve-mask/T-piece for ventilation.

 STEP-BY-STEP GUIDE

Preparation

1 Confirm ET tube position, place the baby supine, and check that the bag-valve-mask or T-piece is working correctly.
2 Suction through the ET tube if needed to clear any secretions.
3 Calculate and prescribe the appropriate surfactant dose.
4 Check the length of the ET tube, and note this down.

 STEP-BY-STEP GUIDE

Drawing up the Surfactant

1 Place all equipment in the sterile area.
2 Wash hands and put on sterile gloves.
3 Cut the surfactant tube to the required length for the ET tube. It should be long enough to reach the bottom of the ET tube. The surfactant tube can be folded in half to enable measurement from markings already on it.
4 Attach the vial adapter to the surfactant vial, and ask an assistant to turn this upside down. Draw up the required surfactant volume into the syringe (*Figure 82*).

5 Attach the syringe to the tube (*Figure 83*).
6 Check again that the baby is optimally ventilated, with a good heart rate and good oxygen saturations.

Figure 82. Drawing up surfactant with assistant.

STEP-BY-STEP GUIDE

7   Ask the assistant to disconnect the ventilator from the baby, and quickly feed the surfactant tube down the ET tube.

8   Rapidly put the surfactant tube down the ET tube, and administer the surfactant (*Figure 84*). As soon as it is administered, ask the assistant to give intermittent positive pressure ventilation to the baby.

9   Once the baby is stable, reattach them to the ventilator.

Ensure a blood gas is repeated within an hour of giving any surfactant, as the ventilator requirement can rapidly change as the surfactant takes effect. The ET tube should also not be suctioned for at least an hour post surfactant administration, unless there is a clinical concern of obstruction.

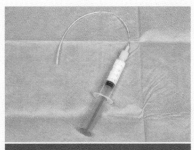

Figure 83. Surfactant ready to administer.

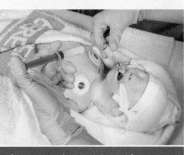

Figure 84. Administering surfactant.

TOP TIPS

- If giving a large volume of surfactant, divide it into two doses, and give intermittent positive pressure ventilation in between.

ASTHMA

Asthma Inhalers

The different varieties of inhalers can be confusing. A good practical summary can be found on most asthma association websites. Most inhalers in hospital will be the traditional metered dose inhalers, so their use will be described here. They should be used in conjunction with a spacer to optimise delivery, in all age groups.

Indication

Treatment of reversible obstructive airways disease (predominantly asthma, viral-induced wheeze and bronchiolitis).

EQUIPMENT CHECKLIST

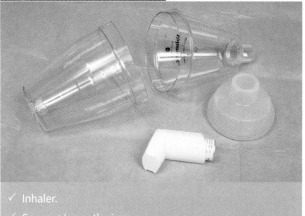

✓ Inhaler.
✓ Spacer +/- mouth piece.
✓ Assistant to help hold younger less cooperative children.

👣 STEP-BY-STEP GUIDE

1 Shake the inhaler well and place into the end of the spacer (*Figure 85*).
2 The next steps depend on the age of the child:

> In an older child, ask them to exhale completely and to then put their mouth firmly over the mouthpiece with a tight seal. Press the canister to release a dose into the spacer and then ask the patient to take one slow breath in and hold for ten seconds (or as long as comfortable) (*Figure 86*).

> In a younger child, a face mask may be required (*Figure 87*). This should be placed over the child's mouth and nose. Expel one puff into the chamber and count five breaths before releasing a second puff.

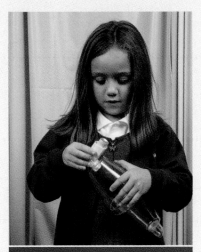

Figure 85. Assembling the spacer.

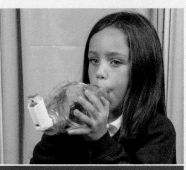

Figure 86. Taking one slow breath in after the canister has been pressed.

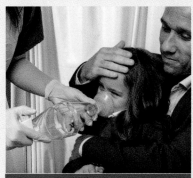

Figure 87. Using a facemask to administer inhaler.

👣 STEP-BY-STEP GUIDE

Complications

Steroid inhalers:
> Oral candidiasis. Advise the child to wash their mouth with water after use.
> Poor growth with prolonged use. However this risk is very small compared to oral doses.

Beta agonists:
> Tachycardia.
> Tremors.
> Headaches.

🚩 TOP TIPS

• Try to make the process fun, if at all possible. Use active distractions. The child may be comfortable watching a TV or smart phone videos. Make the spacer into a toy, offer stickers to make it more accessible, and let children play with it first to familiarise themselves with it.

• Do not get disconcerted if the child screams violently, as very few small children tolerate inhalers/spacers well. It can help to reassure the parents that this reaction is normal, and that when children cry they take deeper breaths and may actually open up their lungs to the medication as a by-product!

• If children are very difficult to engage, holding them in the same manner as one would for an ENT examination can be helpful: ask the parent to give them a big hug with one hand across both their arms and another on their forehead.

• Remember that when spacers are cleaned they should be left to drip-dry to avoid the build-up of static which can prevent medication reaching the patient.

Peak Flow Measurement

Peak flow can be a useful though crude measurement of respiratory function. It can be particularly useful in obstructive airway disease where the rate of exhalation is impaired by narrowed airways. Peak flow is about the maximum rate of flow generated, not the capacity of the lungs. The lower the peak flow reading, the greater degree of obstruction predominantly in the large airways (e.g. bronchoconstriction), which prevents effective exhalation. The test is very effort-dependent as forcing the maximal exhalation requires the use of numerous accessory skeletal muscles. Children have to be old enough to understand how to use the peak flow meter (at least 5-years-old).

Indication

> Acute asthma exacerbation.
> Asthma control monitoring in clinic.

EQUIPMENT CHECKLIST

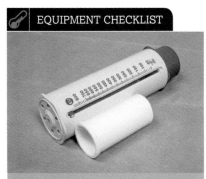

✓ Peak flow meter.
✓ Mouth piece.
✓ Height of the patient.
✓ Expected peak flow chart/peak flow calculator.
✓ Patient peak flow diary (if available).

TOP TIPS

- The score is all about the velocity of expiration rather than the capacity, so emphasise that the child needs to blow out as hard and fast as possible.
- Be familiar with the British Thoracic Society asthma management guidelines which use peak flow percentages as one factor in delineating the severity of an asthma exacerbation.

STEP-BY-STEP GUIDE

1. Assemble the peak flow meter, and mouth piece (*Figure 88*).
2. Explain the task. Often the technique will be likened to "blowing out the candles on your birthday cake" and it may help to pretend to be "blown away" by how hard the child can blow. Make it into a competition to see if they can beat their score with each attempt, and at every stage be encouraging and fun.
3. Ask them to stand up tall and blow as hard as they can into the mouthpiece, keeping their fingers clear of the measuring marks and movable parts (*Figure 89*).
4. Congratulate them on their performance but tell them you think they can do better. Try the same process three times and take the best score.
5. Plot the score on the chart of expected peak flow values for height (*Table 1*) or against the child's personalised previous scores.

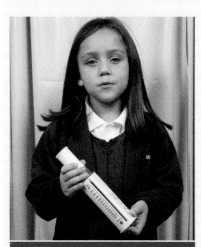

Figure 88. Assembling the peak flow meter and mouthpiece.

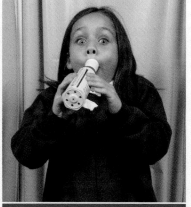

Figure 89. Blowing long and hard into the mouth piece.

TABLE 1: Interpreting peak flow values by height (adapted from www.peakflow.com, for use with EU/EN13826 peak flow meters).	
Height (m)	Predicted PEFR (L/min)
0.85	87
0.90	95
0.95	104
1.00	115
1.05	127
1.10	141
1.15	157
1.20	174
1.25	192
1.30	212
1.35	233
1.40	254
1.45	276
1.50	299
1.55	323
1.60	346
1.65	370
1.70	393

ADDITIONAL PROCEDURES

Lumbar Puncture

Lumbar punctures (LP) are most commonly done in patients with suspected meningitis. The technique in children is similar to that in adults, and is actually often easier since the intervertebral spaces are relatively larger. The technique in a neonate is described below. Older children are positioned in a similar manner to adult patients, and cold spray or lignocaine infiltration can be utilised as analgesia if desired.

Indication

› A clinical suspicion of meningitis/ encephalitis in the absence of contraindications.

› Tertiary neurological or metabolic investigations.

CONTRAINDICATIONS

- Suspicion of raised intracranial pressure and/or space occupying lesions (e.g. reduced consciousness level, focal seizures/neurology, papilloedema, Cushing's triad).
- Deranged clotting factors.
- A clinically decompensating or unstable patient.

EQUIPMENT CHECKLIST

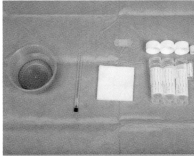

✓ Sterile drapes.
✓ Sterile gauze.
✓ Sterile gloves.
✓ Non-sterile apron.
✓ Skin cleansing solution, e.g. chloroprep.
✓ Lumbar puncture needle.
✓ Minimum of three universal collection pots (sterile white containers).
✓ Glucose bottle (the same blood bottle used to test blood glucose in the lab).
✓ Plaster.

Ensure an experienced colleague is present to hold the child effectively.

STEP-BY-STEP GUIDE

1 Check the patient's blood glucose level. This is required to accurately interpret the CSF glucose.

2 Wash hands, put on sterile gloves and apron.

3 Ensure you have consent for the procedure.

4 Position the patient effectively by ensuring:
  i The head is to the left side (if the doctor is right handed).
  ii The child is as close to the edge of the bed as possible.
  iii The child's back is parallel with the edge of the bed and at a right angle to the mattress (i.e. not tilted towards or away from the doctor).

5 Clean the area around L3-L4 in a circumferential manner. Also clean the area around the uppermost iliac crest.

6 Identify the iliac crest. Draw an imaginary line between the iliac crests: this will act as the anatomical marker. Identify a vertebral space one above or one below this imaginary line: this will be the site for the lumbar puncture (*Figure 90*).

7 Insert the spinal needle in the centre of the disc space, angled slightly proximally to slip between the vertebral bodies. Insert this parallel with the flat surface of the bed. It may be helpful to keep a finger on the iliac crest while doing this, for stability and as an anatomical landmark. It can be helpful to aim towards the umbilicus (*Figure 91*).

8 A slight "give" may be felt on progression through the spinal ligaments. At this stage, remove

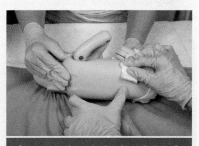

Figure 90. Clean the back, and identify a space above or below the line of the iliac crest.

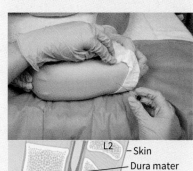

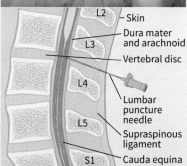

L2 — Skin
— Dura mater and arachnoid
L3 — Vertebral disc
L4 — Lumbar puncture needle
L5 — Supraspinous ligament
S1 — Cauda equina

Figure 91. Inserting the needle whilst curving the spine (top) with anatomical landmarks shown (bottom).

👣 STEP-BY-STEP GUIDE

the stylet of the needle and look for CSF in the same way you might look for flashback from a cannula (*Figure 92*). If no CSF is present, replace the stylet and reposition the needle. Continue to check for flashback each time.

9 When CSF is found, catch approximately eight drops in each of the three universal containers and approximately six drops in the glucose container (*Figure 93*).

10 Replace the stylet before removing the entire needle (*Figure 94*) and compressing the site with gauze (*Figure 95*). Place a plaster over the

puncture site as required (*Figure 96*). Note that use of a transparent quick drying film spray (e.g. Opsite) is an alternative.

11 Thank the patient and/or parents.

12 Carefully label the samples, send them to the lab and chase the results.

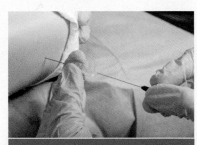
Figure 94. Reinsert the stylet.

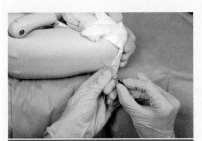
Figure 92. Remove the stylet while holding the lumbar puncture needle firmly.

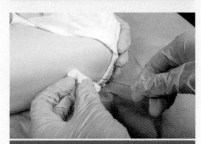
Figure 95. Remove the needle and quickly compress with gauze.

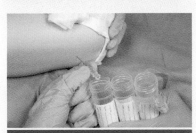
Figure 93. Drip CSF into bottles held by assistant.

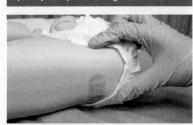
Figure 96. Place a plaster over the entry site.

⚛ COMPLICATIONS

- Bleeding.
- Infection.
- Swelling/bruising.
- Headaches.
- Unsuccessful procedure (dry tap/bloody tap).

🚩 TOP TIPS

- The LP can look like a traumatic procedure and observers can put the person performing it under undue pressure. Advising the parents to wait outside is beneficial for all parties.

- Correct positioning is key. Do not insert the needle until happy that the child is lying parallel with the bed and at a right angle to the mattress. Do not be afraid to ask the person holding the child to reposition as required.

- Adjust the bed to the most convenient height for the person doing the LP.

- The patient may flinch as the needle touches the skin. Be confident with this first movement, as being tentative may cause the patient more discomfort and make the procedure more difficult.

- When counselling the parents in advance, it is helpful to advise them that the procedure may not be successful. It is not uncommon to obtain a bloody tap or a dry tap, despite appropriate technique.

- If the CSF is flowing very slowly, rotating the needle gently so the bevel faces the child's head can sometimes yield a more effective flow.

- If a bloody tap is obtained, it can be helpful to wait a few seconds to see if the blood clears slightly. Some taps start off looking like whole blood but clear slightly to leave blood stained CSF.

Non-Invasive Blood Pressure Measurement

Blood pressure measurement can be challenging in a child who is upset, particularly since this may artificially increase the blood pressure. Distracting and calming the child is key.

Indication

Blood pressure should be checked as part of the routine observations in any patient seeking hospital care. It is particularly important in:

> Sepsis.
> Shock.
> Suspicion of raised intracranial pressure.
> Suspicion of renal impairment.
> Suspicion of congenital cardiac disease (four limb blood pressures).

EQUIPMENT CHECKLIST

✓ Sphygmomanometer "sphyg".
✓ Appropriate size of blood pressure cuff (inner surface of cuff should encompass 90-100% of the arm).
✓ Stethoscope.

TOP TIPS

• Attempt to settle the patient as much as possible. If attempting the procedure on a small baby, it may help if they are fed either during or just before the procedure and kept warm throughout.
• Ensure the right size cuff is used, as a slightly missized cuff can yield significantly erroneous results.

STEP-BY-STEP GUIDE

1 Place the cuff around the bicep muscle if measuring on the upper limb (preferred) or around the calf on the lower limb (*Figure 97*).

2 Place the stethoscope over a distal pulse. If in the arm, this will be the brachial pulse, and in the leg, the posterior tibial or dorsalis pedis pulse.

3 Ensure that the valve on the sphyg is closed. Inflate the cuff until the pulse is no longer heard (*Figure 98*). Inflate a further 20 mmHg beyond this.

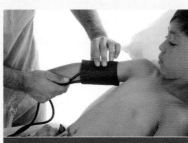

Figure 97. Place BP cuff in appropriate position.

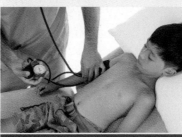

Figure 98. Inflate cuff until pulse is no longer heard through the stethoscope.

4 Gently open the valve of the sphyg and allow the cuff to deflate in a consistent and controlled manner. Continue to auscultate the distal pulse.

5 Mark the point at which turbulent blood flow (Korotkoff sounds) can be heard. This represents the return of the arterial flow and is the systolic blood pressure.

6 Continue deflating the cuff slowly. The sounds may become slightly more blowing in nature before returning to a harsh tapping.

7 The sounds will become abruptly muffled and subsequently disappear altogether. Classically (especially in adults), this disappearance is recorded as the diastolic pressure. However in children under 13-years-old, these sounds may not disappear altogether until the cuff is completely removed. In this case, the diastolic pressure should be recorded at the point the sounds became significantly muffled.

8 Estimate the mean blood pressure from these values:

Mean Blood Pressure (MAP)
= Diastolic Blood Pressure
$+ \frac{1}{3}$ (Systolic Blood Pressure - Diastolic Blood Pressure)

9 Record the reading in the medical notes/observation chart.

Nasogastric Tube Insertion

Nasogastric tubes are commonly used, particularly in neonates, where the more premature babies invariably require a period of NG feeding. Insertion is more challenging in children due to compliance difficulties. Placement into the lungs is a possibility, but feeding through this should be a never event.

Indication

> Gastric drainage/relief of bowel obstruction.
> Feeding.
> Prevention of vomiting.

EQUIPMENT CHECKLIST

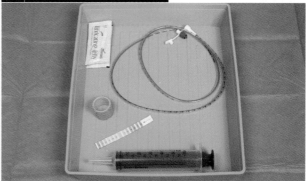

✓ Non-sterile gloves.
✓ Disposable apron.
✓ Lubricant gel.
✓ NG tube.
✓ 60 mL syringe and pH strip.
✓ Sticky tape.
✓ Drainage system.
✓ Cup of water (in older children).

STEP-BY-STEP GUIDE

1   Ideally have the child sitting up.
2   Wash hands, and put on gloves and an apron.
3   Estimate the length of the tube by measuring from the tip of the child's nose to the xiphisternum, passing the tragus of the ear (*Figure 99*).
4   Lubricate the end of the NG tube (*Figure 100*).
5   Slide the tube along the floor of the nasal cavity, initially aiming towards the occiput. There is usually slight resistance as the tube passes into the oesophagus (*Figure 101*).
6   In an older child, ask them to repeatedly swallow or offer them sips of water. This aids advancement of the NG tube.
7   Advance the tube to the pre-determined distance.
8   Attempt to aspirate gastric fluid into the syringe (*Figure 102*) and test it on a pH strip (*Figure 103*).
9   Securely tape the NG tube to the nose (*Figure 104*).
10 Attach the tube to a drainage system or spigot, as directed.

Checking the position of the NG tube can be done by several methods. First, the pH of the NG aspirate can be checked. If the pH is <5.5, then the NG tube is likely to be aspirating stomach fluid.

The most definitive way to check is with an X-ray (e.g. if stomach fluid cannot be aspirated or has a pH>5.5): a correctly positioned NG tube should be seen passing below the diaphragm (*Figure 105*). Feeding through an incorrectly placed NG tube is entirely avoidable through appropriate checks as above.

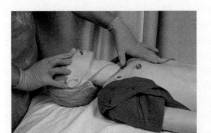

Figure 99. Measuring the NG tube.

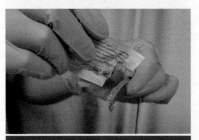

Figure 100. Lubricating the tip of the NG tube.

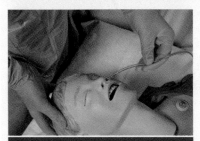

Figure 101. Advancing the NG tube.

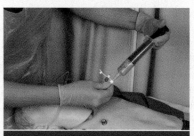

Figure 102. Aspirating the contents.

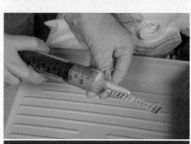

Figure 103. Checking the pH.

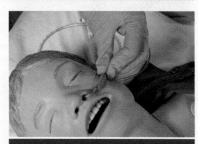

Figure 104. Securing the tube.

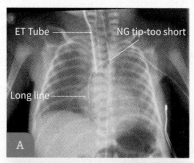

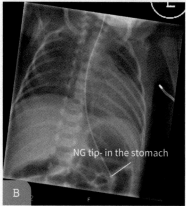

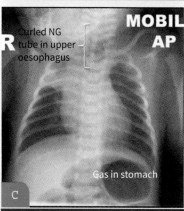

Figure 105. A. Short NG tube. B. NG tube in correct position. C. NG tube coiled in oesophagus due to oesophageal atresia.

- Use plenty of lubricant as this will minimise upset to the child. Local anaesthetic spray can be applied to the back of the throat pre-procedure: this reduces pain as well, but if this is done the child should not be asked to swallow water as the anaesthetic can give an unsafe swallow.

Urinalysis

Urinalysis is usually performed in paediatrics in the context of suspected infection. It is a simple test that often leads to a diagnosis, informing ongoing management.

Indication

- Suspected UTI.
- Haematuria.
- Abdominal injury (to check for renal damage).
- Suspected nephrotic syndrome.
- Urinary electrolytes.
- Urinary ketones.
- Toxicology.
- Pregnancy test.

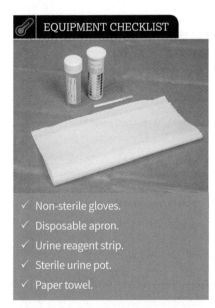

EQUIPMENT CHECKLIST

- ✓ Non-sterile gloves.
- ✓ Disposable apron.
- ✓ Urine reagent strip.
- ✓ Sterile urine pot.
- ✓ Paper towel.

👣 STEP-BY-STEP GUIDE

Obtaining a Urine Sample

A mid-stream urine sample is the gold standard. It is suitable for older, compliant children, and is obtained as follows:

1 Give the patient a sterile urine pot.
2 Ask them to clean their external genitalia with water and tissue.
3 Ask them to collect the urine sample next time they go to the toilet. The first part of the urine stream should not be collected, but then, without stopping the flow of urine, the subsequent urine should be caught in the bottle, filling it to the line.
4 The cap should then immediately be placed on the urine pot.

Clean catch urine samples are performed in babies or small children who are unable to give a mid-stream urine sample. The child is stripped down so that the urethra is exposed, and the genitalia are cleaned. The parent sits close to their child with a urine pot and catches the urine as soon as the child urinates. Sterile samples can also be performed by inserting a catheter, or by suprapubic aspiration.

Obtaining a "bag" sample is another option. A urine bag is placed over the genitalia so as to catch the urine as soon as the baby/child urinates. This is not suitable for suspected UTIs as the risk of skin/faecal contamination is high. However it may be suitable for other tests, such as urinary protein/electrolytes. Another similar method involves putting cotton wool in the front of the nappy, and then squeezing collected urine out of it.

👣 STEP-BY-STEP GUIDE

Performing a Urinalysis

1 Wash hands. Put on gloves and apron.
2 Inspect the urine sample. Note the appearance – does it look cloudy, dark yellow, red or have any sediment?
3 Remove the cap of the urine pot. Note the odour.
4 Check the expiry date of the dipstick on the container and remove one dipstick.
5 Place the dipstick in the urine for 2-3 seconds ensuring all of the reagents on the dipstick are immersed in the urine (*Figure 106*).
6 Remove the dipstick.
7 Place the dipstick horizontally onto a flat surface to ensure that the chemicals do not mix. Leave it to dry for the specified time (found on the reagent strip container) (*Figure 107*).

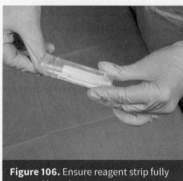

Figure 106. Ensure reagent strip fully covered by urine.

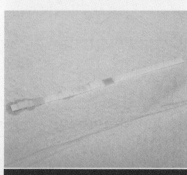

Figure 107. Dab on paper towel to dry stick.

8   Look at each reagent on the dipstick in turn. With each reagent, look at the corresponding colour on the tub (the tub will have a colour code on its side so that you can interpret the results) and identify if the value is normal or high (*Figure 108*).

9   Remove gloves and wash hands.

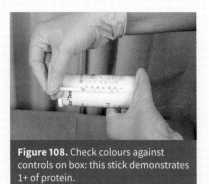
Figure 108. Check colours against controls on box: this stick demonstrates 1+ of protein.

•   Don't expect the same volume of urine in a baby as you would an adult. More is always better, but a few drops are sufficient to perform urinalysis.

BABY CARE

Changing a Nappy

This may be required of a doctor when performing a newborn examination, particularly if the mum is unwell or in severe pain.

✓ Clean nappy.

✓ Cotton wool/water or baby wipes.

Removing the Dirty Nappy

1   Wash hands.

2   Lay the baby on a towel or changing mat (*Figure 109*).

3   Unfasten the tabs on the dirty nappy, and fold them over to prevent them sticking to the baby (*Figure 110*).

4   Pull down the front half of the nappy. Whilst doing this, the front half of the nappy can be used to wipe off the bulk of any faeces from the bottom. It may be worthwhile putting a cloth/gauze over the genitals at this stage to prevent being urinated on (*Figure 111*).

5   Put the front half of the nappy on top of the bottom half of the nappy (clean side up). Do this by lifting the baby up, and folding the nappy underneath them (*Figure 112*).

6   Clean the baby's front. This can be done using cotton wool and water, or baby wipes. It is important in girls particularly to wipe from front to back: this reduces the likelihood of stool contaminating the urinary tract.

7   Clean the baby's bottom. Lifting the legs and/or rolling the baby onto one side should facilitate this. Ensure that the skin creases and thighs are cleaned as well (*Figure 113*).

8   Leave the skin to air dry, and remove the dirty nappy.

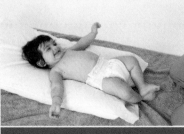
Figure 109. Position baby on towel/changing mat.

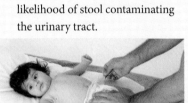
Figure 110. Unfasten tabs, folding them over.

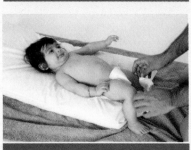
Figure 111. Pulling down the front of the nappy, and covering genitalia with gauze.

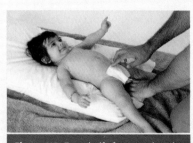
Figure 112. Front half of nappy placed on bottom half.

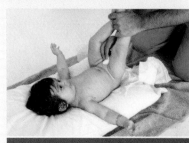
Figure 113. Cleaning the bottom.

STEP-BY-STEP GUIDE

Putting on the Clean Nappy

› Place the back half of the nappy under the baby, with the tabs on either side (*Figure 114*).

› Pull the front half up across the abdomen. Ensure that the part of the nappy around the legs is spread comfortably. Avoid covering the umbilical stump in newborns. In boys, it is helpful to point their penis down to stop them urinating out of the top of the nappy (*Figure 115*).

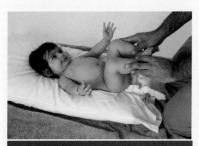

Figure 114. Back half of nappy placed under baby.

› Fasten the nappy on both sides, ensuring the tabs aren't sticking to the baby's skin (*Figure 116*).

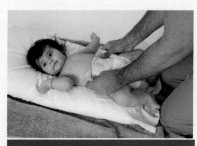

Figure 115. Front half pulled up across abdomen.

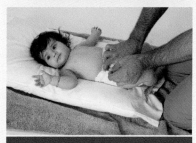

Figure 116. Nappy fastened on both sides.

Dressing and Undressing a Baby

When examining a baby, often the responsibility falls upon the doctor to undress them and dress them back up again afterwards.

General advice includes:

› Ask the parents if they are able to help/can undress/dress the baby themselves.

› Put the baby on a comfortable, safe, flat surface.

› Handle the baby gently, working slowly through the process. Avoid overextending the arms/legs, or putting the baby into uncomfortable positions.

› Ensure appropriate layers of clothing. As a general rule, babies should wear one more layer than an adult would, as they lose heat faster.

STEP-BY-STEP GUIDE

Dressing a Baby

Being gentle and slow is a must. If any outfit requires buttoning up at the back, turn the baby onto their front first. A technique for putting a babygrow on is shown below, but the technique varies depending on the particular clothing.

1 Unbutton the outfit (*Figure 117*).

2 Collapse down the sleeve of one arm of the babygrow to the point where the arm opens up for the hand. Gently grasp the baby's hand, and string it through the arm of the babygrow (*Figure 118*).

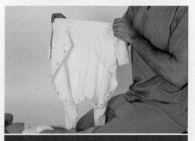

Figure 117. Unbutton and open up clothing.

3 Put on the second sleeve: collapse down the arm, and whilst grabbing the baby's hand, pull it through the sleeve in the same way as previously done (*Figure 119*).

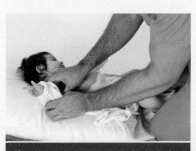

Figure 118. String one arm through the babygrow.

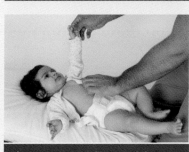

Figure 119. Put on the second sleeve.

4 Put each leg into the babygrow individually (*Figure 120*).

5 Button up the middle of the babygrow (*Figure 121*).

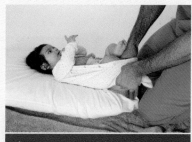

Figure 120. Put each leg individually into the openings for the lower limbs.

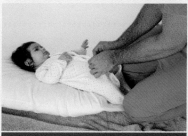

Figure 121. Button up the middle.

Preparing Baby Milk Formula

Formula milk may have to be provided by healthcare staff in hospital if the parents are unavailable. It may also be needed to be given if the mum is not producing any breast milk and the baby is dehydrated. Note that a full bottle is eight ounces.

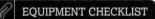

EQUIPMENT CHECKLIST

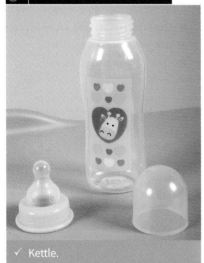

✓ Kettle.
✓ Steriliser.
✓ Baby bottle, teat, and cap.

STEP-BY-STEP GUIDE

Undressing a Baby

Start by undoing any buttons. Be gentle, slow and controlled throughout. For a top or some babygrows, it may be easiest to start by removing the sleeves, and then pulling the whole thing over the baby's head. Ensure that the head and body are supported with one hand when removing clothes with the other.

STEP-BY-STEP GUIDE

Step-by-Step Guide

1 Fill a kettle with fresh cold tap water, and bring to the boil.
2 Leave the water to cool for 15-30 minutes (ensuring the temperature of the water is above 70^{0}C).
3 Wash hands.
4 Take out the baby's bottle, teat and cap from a steriliser.
5 Stand the baby bottle on the cleaned work surface.
6 Follow the manufacturer's instructions for the formula using the specified amount of formula powder and hot water (hot water first).
7 Put the teat onto the bottle, holding the edge.
8 Screw the teat onto the bottle (*Figure 122*).
9 Place the cap over the teat.
10 Shake the bottle firmly until the powder has dissolved.
11 Allow the formula to cool quickly by running the bottle under a cold tap.
12 Test the temperature of the formula using the inside of your wrist. The formula should be at body temperature so should feel tepid to the touch, not hot.

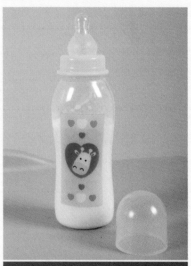

Figure 122. Milk ready to give.

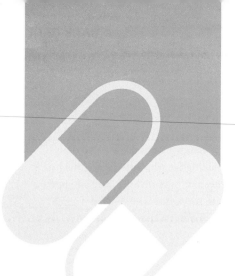

3.05
PRESCRIBING

MICHAEL MALLEY AND MARIE MONAGHAN

CONTENTS

THE IMPORTANCE OF GOOD PRESCRIBING

Good prescribing is essential for safe, effective clinical practice. It remains, however, a common source of potentially harmful errors. This chapter will focus on the art of paediatric prescribing and discuss common pitfalls. Almost all errors may be avoided by being meticulous and thoughtful. Prescriptions will be checked by pharmacy and nursing staff before being administered, but the ultimate responsibility remains with the prescriber.

Remember:

> Do not become complacent. It is easy to feel that prescribing common medications is a mundane chore which does not require full attention. Try to remember that every prescription is a complex process. There is no shame in looking up drug doses and no honour in prescribing medications solely from memory.

> Never prescribe an unfamiliar medication. Do not prescribe a drug at the behest of a nurse or senior colleague, as ultimately the prescriber takes responsibility for it. Look up the drug, and know its indications and side effects before prescribing. If still unsure, seek advice from a senior doctor or pharmacist.

> Always check the allergy status of the patient before prescribing. This should always be filled out on the drug chart, and this simple step can prevent potentially fatal consequences.

> Be aware of local and national protocols and know where you can access the dose, regimen, side effects and contraindications of each drug you prescribe. In the UK, the British National Formulary for Children (BNFc) is the universal reference point, whilst individual hospitals will have their own specific guidelines.

DIFFERENCES BETWEEN ADULTS AND CHILDREN

A number of subtle yet important differences exist between adult and paediatric prescribing. These are outlined below.

Drug Metabolism

Pharmacokinetics of medicines differs considerably in children and adults. For example:

> The kidneys do not achieve their peak glomerular filtration rate until the child is around 6-months-old, after which it gradually deteriorates into old age. Hence, renal excretion of medications may be impaired in the first few weeks of life. However, after 6–months-old, renal excretion is generally more efficient in children than adults. Safe and effective dosages will change accordingly.

> The rate of maturation of the cytochrome P450 (CYP450) enzymes in an infant affects medication metabolised by the liver. The expression of certain CYP450 enzymes may be absent or excessive in early childhood, requiring a different dosing strategy. A classic example is carbamazepine, where the expression of CYP3A4 is enhanced in children, leading to faster clearance compared to an adult.

> Infants have a relatively greater extracellular fluid compartment compared to intracellular fluid. This may affect the dosing and frequency of medication required to maintain adequate plasma levels.

Licensing

Many medications are not officially licensed for children, but are widely used based on smaller studies, clinical experience and historical practices. This is due to few research studies conducted in children, meaning that data must be extrapolated from older patients. However, if used frequently, such doses are usually supported by local protocols or national guidelines.

Dosage

Children are smaller than adults and are constantly growing. Hence, doses are almost always worked out in terms of weight or surface area, e.g. milligrams per kilogram (mg/kg) or, rarely, milligrams per metre-squared (mg/m^2). Update prescriptions at regular intervals as the child's weight changes. Doses can become inadequate quickly as the patient grows. It is perfectly reasonable to round doses of chronic medicines up slightly to allow room for the patient to grow. Body composition changes with age. Therefore, a child of the same weight but of a different age may receive a different dose of the same drug. IV aciclovir is a classic example of this.

The volume of the drug administered may remain the same despite differences in the dose, due to different liquid formulation strengths. For example, children aged 1-6 years receive 5 mL of the 125/31 suspension of co-amoxiclav (125mg amoxicillin plus 31mg of clavulanic acid), whilst children aged 6-12 years receive 5 mL of the 250/62 suspension (double the dose in the same volume). To ensure clarity, always write the strength of the medication on the prescription (i.e. 250/62) instead of merely "5mL Co-amoxiclav TDS". Alternatively, express the dosage in terms of mg, which is unambiguous.

Some medications may have a maximum dosage. For example, the dose of prednisolone in asthma is 1-2mg/kg. However, the maximum daily dosage is 40mg. Therefore, for a child weighing 25kg, the dose they receive will be 40mg, not the calculated 50mg.

Formulation

In younger children, liquid formulations are often more acceptable than tablets or capsules. An oral syringe should be used for accurate measurement and controlled administration of liquid medicines. The converse may be true for less palatable medications like flucloxacillin, where the tablet form may be better tolerated. Try to take steps to optimise the patient's compliance where possible.

What to Avoid in Children

Some medications should not be used in children. For example:

> Aspirin is linked to Reye's syndrome in children, causing potentially fatal liver failure (although it may still be prescribed for specific conditions, like Kawasaki disease).

> Tetracyclines are avoided in those under 12 because they discolour developing teeth.

> Ceftriaxone is often avoided in infants under 1–months-old, particularly those with jaundice, due to the risk of biliary stasis.

> Nitrofurantoin is contraindicated in infants less than 3-months-old due to the risk of haemolytic anaemia.

GENERAL PRESCRIBING

Involving the Patient and the Team

> Discuss the prescription with the patient and/or family. Not involving the patient can lead to non-adherence. Young children will generally not be able to consent to treatment; therefore, the parent/guardian should be asked to consent on their behalf. This involves a sensitive and honest discussion of the benefits and risks of each medication.

> Give the patient/family a chance to ask questions before prescribing.

> Inform the appropriate nurse what medication has been prescribed and check that they understand the prescription.

Renal or Hepatic Impairment

Be aware of patient co-morbidities, such as renal and hepatic impairment. Many renally-excreted drugs will have altered administration schedules, even in moderate renal impairment. Gentamicin is the classic example. Seek advice on dose adjustments from a pharmacist if no information is available.

Approaching the Prescription Chart

Always ensure the prescription chart contains the following information:

> Patient name.
> Patient hospital number.
> Patient date of birth.
> Allergy status.
> Address of the medical centre (for outpatient prescriptions).

The risk of error is reduced by:

> Writing in black ballpoint pen.
> Writing legibly in capital letters.

649

EXAMPLE 1

Prescribing antibiotics for a neonate

Drug. BENZYLPENICILLIN (50mg/kg)			Date Time	1/3	2/3	3/3	4/3	5/3	6/3	7/3	8/3	9/3
			02									
Dose. 150mg	Freq. BD	Route. IV	(06)									
			10									
Start. 1/3/15		Stop/review. 3/3/15	14									
Signature A.Jones		JONES 2134	(18)									
Indication. Suspected sepsis: review with blood culture results.			22									
Drug. GENTAMICIN (5mg/kg)			Date Time									
			02									
Dose. 15mg	Freq. OD	Route. IV	(06)			◯						
			10			Pre dose level						
Start. 1/3/15		Stop/review. 3/3/15	14									
Signature A.Jones		JONES 2134	18									
Indication. Suspected sepsis: review with blood culture results.			22									

> Signing each entry, and printing the prescriber's name.
> Giving a clear contact number (in case clarification is needed).
> Clearly writing the timing of medication.

Review the prescription once complete. This is particularly important for electronic prescribing, where automatic rules may change the original intention, e.g. a once-daily drug, where the first dose needs to be given immediately, has defaulted to 6 a.m. the next day. *Example 1* shows a typical prescription.

Logistical Considerations

> Cross out any administration boxes on the days where a prescribed drug should be omitted. For example, amphotericin B, when used as antifungal prophylaxis, is only given three days a week. Be particularly careful with once weekly drugs like methotrexate, which can be fatal if administered daily in error.
> Cross out any boxes where the drug has already been given. This is particularly important if a child has been given their first dose in ED and has been transferred to the ward.
> Indicate when drug levels will need to be measured and what actions need to be taken. For example, gentamicin is a potent antibiotic with potentially serious side effects (mainly nephrotoxicity and ototoxicity). Gentamicin trough levels need to be tested, checked regularly and acted upon if high. If concerned about renal toxicity, instruct to "trough and hold"; otherwise, a dose may be administered if the intent is not clear. To avoid gentamicin-related errors, most hospitals have a special gentamicin chart.
> If the standard prescription does not seem clear, do not be afraid to write free-text, provided this will aid the safe administration of the drug. For example, prescribing infusions can often be complex and their exact indications vague. Writing in long hand "Please use X mg of dopamine diluted in X mL of 0.9% NaCl. Start at 5 micrograms/kg/minute and titrate to keep a systolic blood pressure above 90mmHg" will increase the likelihood of the desired effect being achieved. Clear instructions also give a clear handover of prescribing intent to inform staff on subsequent shifts.

Avoid Shorthand

> Write out any units in full, other than "mL", "mg" and "g". For example "micrograms" and "nanograms": avoid symbols like µg, mcg or ng which may be mistaken for "mg". This also applies to the word "units" – fatal doses of insulin have been prescribed when the abbreviation "u" is mistaken for "0" or "iu" is mistaken for "1u" or "10".

> When documenting allergies, include a description of the reaction, e.g. a rash or confirmed anaphylaxis, and ensure this is likely to be a genuine allergic reaction. A parent may have falsely attributed a vomit after taking penicillin as an allergy. Differentiating this from true anaphylactic reactions will mean that the child has access to penicillin-based antibiotics should they become unwell.

Controlled Drugs

When prescribing controlled drugs, specify the drug name, strength, formulation and dose. Write out the total quantity to supply in words as well as figures (e.g. morphine sulphate 10mg tablets, 10 mg 4-6 hourly PRN. Please dispense a total of 14 (fourteen) tablets). Alternatively, specify the total quantity in milligrams, e.g. 140mg (one hundred and forty milligrams).

This rule does not apply to hospital prescriptions. However, this is a legal requirement in places like the UK for all discharge and outpatient prescriptions.

Oxygen

Oxygen is technically a drug and needs to be prescribed in the same manner as any other medication (*Example 2*). There is frequently a special section for this on the drug chart. It will ask you to specify:

> The mode of delivery (e.g. nasal cannula, facemask).

> The range of flow (e.g. from 1-5 litres/minute).

> The target saturations (usually above 92 or 94%).

When to prescribe oxygen causes confusion for students starting in paediatric units after completing adult respiratory blocks.

When treating the acutely unwell child, it is almost always appropriate to give high flow oxygen and titrate down as required. It is more dangerous not to give oxygen to a child who needs it than to give oxygen to a child who does not require it. There are very few scenarios where giving supplementary oxygen to a child will cause harm. Exceptionally few children rely on their "hypoxic drive" to breathe in the same way as adults with chronic type II respiratory failure. This is very rarely a consideration in general paediatrics. Problems may arise with:

> Inappropriately liberal oxygen delivery to very preterm infants (particularly under 32 weeks gestation). This may contribute to retinopathy of prematurity (neovascularisation of the developing retina, causing visual problems and treated with laser therapy).

> Inappropriately liberal oxygen given to children with duct-dependent heart disease. "Duct dependent" means that these patients rely on a patent ductus arteriosus (connecting the pulmonary artery and aorta to bypass the lungs in foetal life) to sustain oxygenation and perfusion to the tissues. The trigger for the duct to close is rising oxygen tension; hence, high-flow oxygen can theoretically cause this lifeline to obliterate. Given the mixing of oxygenated and deoxygenated blood in cyanotic congenital heart disease, aiming for saturations of 75-85% in these patients is appropriate.

Infusions

To prescribe an infusion, the following information is needed:

1   Drug name.

2   Diluent fluid name and volume (e.g. 0.9% sodium chloride or 5% dextrose).

EXAMPLE 2

Oxygen prescription

Drug. OXYGEN.			Date Time	1/1	2/1	3/1	4/1	5/1	6/1	7/1	8/1	9/1
			02									
Flow rate. 1-5 Litres/min.	**Target. Sats:** >92%.	**Route.** Nasal Cannula.	06									
			10									
Start. 1/1/15.		**Stop/review.** 2/1/15.	14									
Signature A.Jones		**JONES** 2134	18									
Indication. Pneumonia.			22									

3   Route of administration.

4   Rate of infusion and likely the acceptable range of a variable infusion (e.g. 5-20 micrograms/kg/min).

5   Patient's weight and age.

From this, the infusion can be calculated as per *Example 3*.

EXAMPLE 3

Prescription of a salbutamol loading dose and maintenance infusion in a severely asthmatic 5-year-old boy. Weight =20 kg.

Date	Drug	Dose	Route	Signature	Given	Batch
1/1/15	SALBUTAMOL (200 micrograms/mL)	250 micrograms (1.25mL)	IV	A. Jones JONES 1234		

Date	Fluid	Additives	Volume	Route	Rate	Signature	Given	Batch
1/1/15	0.9% SODIUM CHLORIDE	SALBUTAMOL 10mg	50mL	IV	6mL–30mL/hr (60–300 micrograms/kg/hr)	A. Jones JONES 1234		

Loading dose:

15 micrograms/kg (maximum dose 250 micrograms)
= 15 micrograms/kg x 20 kg
= **250 micrograms** (300 micrograms, rounded down to the maximum dose).

Using a standard solution of 200 micrograms/mL, this is equivalent to 250 micrograms ÷ 200 micrograms/mL = 1.25 mL. It is subsequently prescribed on the once-only section of the prescription chart.

Maintenance dose:

Lower limit= 60 micrograms/kg/hr (1 microgram per kg per minute)
Upper limit= 300 micrograms/kg/hr (5 micrograms per kg per minute)

For this case, 10mg of salbutamol is diluted in 50mL of 0.9% sodium chloride, at a concentration of **200 micrograms/mL** to generate a standard solution. This solution is then used to deliver the required dose.
   Infusions are prescribed at a rate of millilitres per hour (or minute); therefore, the maintenance dose has to be converted to millilitres.

In this case:
Lower limit = 60 micrograms/kg/hr ÷ 200 micrograms/mL = 0.3mL/kg/hr, i.e. 0.3mL of salbutamol contains 60 micrograms of salbutamol.
Upper limit = 300 micrograms/kg/hr ÷ 200 micrograms/mL = 1.5mL/kg/hr

These figures are then multiplied by the weight to get the tailored dose for the child:
Lower limit = 0.3 mL/kg/hr x 20 kg = 6mL/hr
Upper limit = 1.5 mL/kg/hr x 20 kg = 30mL/hr

It is subsequently prescribed on a fluid chart.

FLUID PRESCRIBING

Fluids are prescribed very differently in paediatrics than in adults. However, the formula is very simple once you know it. Fluids are almost always prescribed in 500mL bags. Prescription has three essential components:

1   The fluid constituents and bag size e.g. NaCl 0.9% + dextrose 5% + KCl 10mmol (500mL).

2   The rate at which to administer it, in mL/hr to achieve the desired 24-hourly fluid requirement.

3   The signature of the prescriber.

There should also be a record of:

1   Body weight, including weight change over previous 24 hours.

2   Fluid input (oral, nasogastric, intravenous) and output (urine, vomiting, drains, stomas, diarrhoea, insensible losses-particularly with fever/dehydration/hyperventilation) over previous 24 hours.

3   Assessment of fluid status (dehydrated, oedematous, euvolaemic).

4   Relevant blood results [full blood count (FBC), urea & electrolytes (U&Es), chloride, glucose, and urinary electrolytes, if measured].

Note that fluid and electrolyte calculations are almost always based on weight. However, if accurate calculation of insensible losses is critical (e.g. with acute or chronic kidney disease, with cancer, or with weight above the 91st centile), consider using body surface area for the calculations instead (insensible losses (300–400 mL/m^2/24 hours) plus urine output). Surface area is calculated based on height and weight, and can be looked up on a reference chart.

Neonatal Fluid Management

Neonatal fluid requirements can be defined as enough fluid to keep the baby euvolaemic (i.e. replacing measured and insensible losses). As a rule of thumb, use the fluid requirements in *Table 1*. These figures come from research with babies born at term, but are often used for babies of all gestations. These volumes also apply when giving nasogastric feeds. Factor in the clinical state of the baby, which includes urine output, weight gain and plasma sodium level.

The fluid usually prescribed to neonates is 10% dextrose, which addresses glucose requirements as well as fluid requirements. After the first one to two days, it is important to provide electrolyte support as well. This involves the addition of

TABLE 1: Fluid requirements in a neonate	
Day of life	**Maintenance fluid requirements**
1.	50-60mL/kg/day.
2.	70-80mL/kg/day.
3.	80-100mL/kg/day.
4.	100-120mL/kg/day.
5.	120-150mL/kg/day.

sodium (3mmol/kg/day) and potassium (2mmol/kg/day). Some neonatal units will also add calcium (1mmol/kg/day).

Calculation of electrolyte doses can be tricky at first, as the correct amount has to be added to the 500mL 10% dextrose bag in order to get the daily requirement. The key is to first work out the daily requirement of electrolytes (total mmols/day), and the daily requirement of fluids (mL/day). Then use the ratio between the total daily requirement of fluids and 500mL to work out how much goes into each bag. If the daily requirement of fluid is 250mL, ensure that the 500mL bag has the requirement for two days of electrolytes in it (*Example 4*). *Table 2* summarises the number of mmol of electrolytes to be

---

EXAMPLE 4

Fluid requirement calculation: A 4-day-old baby, weighing 3.5kg, with normal electrolytes and requiring maintenance fluids.

Date	Fluid	Additives	Volume	Route	Rate	Signature	Given	Batch
1/1/15	10% DEXTROSE (120mL/kg/day)	12.5mmol NaCl (3mmol/kg/day) 8.3mmol KCl (2mmol/kg/day)	500mL	IV	17.5mL/hr	A. Jones JONES 1234.		

Fluid = 120mL/kg/day = 120 x 3.5 = 420mL/day = 17.5mL/hr
Sodium = 3mmol/kg/day = 3 x 3.5 = 10.5mmol/day
Potassium = 2mmol/kg/day = 2 x 3.5 = 7mmol/day

The correct amount of potassium and sodium needs to be added to the 500mL dextrose bag. If 420mL of fluid is given in 24 hours, then every 420 mL of fluid needs to contain 10.5mmol sodium and 7mmol potassium. Therefore:

Sodium per 500mL bag = 10.5 x 500/420 = 12.5mmol
Potassium per 500mL bag = 7 x 500/420 = 8.3mmol

TABLE 2: Number of mmol of electrolytes to add to a 500mL bag of dextrose for different daily fluid and electrolyte requirements						
		Fluid requirement				
		40 mL/kg/day	60 mL/kg/day	90 mL/kg/day	120 mL/kg/day	150 mL/kg/day
Electrolyte requirement.	1 mmol/kg/day.	12.5 mmol	8.3 mmol	5.6 mmol	4.2 mmol	3.3 mmol
	2 mmol/kg/day.	25.0 mmol	16.7 mmol	11.1 mmol	8.3 mmol	6.7 mmol
	3 mmol/kg/day.	37.5 mmol	25.0 mmol	16.7 mmol	12.5 mmol	10.0 mmol
	4 mmol/kg/day.	50.0 mmol	33.3 mmol	22.2 mmol	16.7 mmol	13.3 mmol

653

added to a 500mL bag of 10% dextrose for different maintenance fluids infusion rates. Note that this is the same, regardless of the weight of the baby, as it is based on the ratio of fluid to electrolyte requirements, which is independent of weight. This is a useful reference on any neonatal job.

The above guidance is the generally employed practice across most neonatal units for most babies; however, local guidelines may be slightly different and should always be checked. Always consider every baby's individual fluid considerations before prescribing fluids and check with a senior colleague if in doubt.

Be aware also that some babies, particularly on surgical units, may be given total parenteral nutrition (TPN) for some time, instead of routine fluids. This is a specialist fluid regime and each patient will generally have an individualised regime calculated carefully between senior doctors and the pharmacy team, and ordered from a central supply accordingly.

Paediatric Fluid Management

After the neonatal period, children normally receive a mixture of sodium and dextrose – the typical combination is a premade bag of "0.9% Sodium Chloride + 5% Dextrose". Hypotonic fluids are avoided, as they have the potential to cause sudden fluid shifts into cells from the plasma, as well as risking hyponatremia. Glucose is required as children are more vulnerable than adults to hypoglycaemia. Potassium is usually added, adjusted according to serum levels – normally as a starting point 10 mmol potassium chloride is added to each 500 mL bag. *Table 3* shows how maintenance fluids over 24 hours are calculated in this age group. This means that for the first 10 kg of ANY child's weight, they will require 100 mL/kg. For the second 10 kg, they require 50 mL/kg and they will need 20 mL/kg for every kg after this.

Examples 5 and 6 demonstrate how this is done in practice. A shortcut is knowing that children require 1500 mL for the first 20 kg of weight inclusive plus "20 x the remaining weight".

TABLE 3: Fluid requirements in children. Be aware that over a 24 hour period, females rarely need more than two litres, and males rarely need more than 2.5 litres, so adjust fluid prescriptions accordingly.

Weight	Fluid requirement
0-10 kg	100 mL/kg
10-20 kg	50 mL/kg
Above 20 kg	20 mL/kg

Note that in cases of respiratory distress (e.g. lower respiratory tract infection), often only two-thirds of the normal fluid intake are given due to a theoretical possibility of the syndrome of inappropriate antidiuretic hormone secretion (SiADH) and fluid overload.

Fluid Boluses

For children, the typical fluid bolus is 20 mL/kg of 0.9% sodium chloride. Typically, boluses are given over less than ten minutes, although recent World Health Organisation (WHO) guidelines have suggested that it may be advisable to give boluses over a longer duration, due to the potential risk of fluid overload, particularly in developing world settings. Smaller boluses of 10 mL/kg are used in special groups e.g. neonates, those with cardiac disease, diabetic ketoacidosis and trauma. Be extremely cautious with fluid boluses in situations where rapid shifts of fluid can have disastrous consequences (e.g. cerebral oedema in diabetic ketoacidosis or pulmonary oedema in heart failure/myocarditis). Always reassess the child's fluid requirements after administration of a bolus. Generally, if a child has required three boluses (i.e. 60 mL/kg), call for anaesthetic support in case the child deteriorates into pulmonary oedema. The patient may still require more fluid if significantly shocked, but may also require invasive respiratory support.

Dextrose boluses in the hypoglycaemic child are usually given at 2 mL/kg of 10% dextrose. The glucose level should then be rechecked and the dose can be repeated, or a dextrose

---

EXAMPLE 5

Fluid requirement calculation: maintenance fluid in a 13kg child.

Date	Fluid	Additive	Volume	Route	Rate	Signature	Given	Batch
1/1/15	0.9% SODIUM CHLORIDE + 5% DEXTROSE + 10mmol KCl	–	500mL	IV	48mL/hr	A. Jones JONES 1234		

First 10 kg = 100 mL/kg/day = 100 x 10 = 1000 mL
Next 3 kg = 50 mL/kg/day = 50 x 3 = 150 mL
Total = 1150 mL in 24 hours
= 48 mL per hour

EXAMPLE 6

Fluid requirement calculation: maintenance fluid in a 26kg child.

Date	Fluid	Additive	Volume	Route	Rate	Signature	Given	Batch
1/1/15	0.9% SODIUM CHLORIDE + 5% DEXTROSE + 10mmol KCl	–	500mL	IV	67.5mL/hr	A. Jones JONES 1234		

First 10 kg = 100 mL/kg/day = 100 x 10 = 1000 mL.
Second 10 kg = 50 mL/kg/day = 50 x 10 = 500mL.
Next 6kg = 20 mL/kg/day = 20 x 6 = 120 mL.
Total = 1620 mL in 24 hours.
= 67.5 mL per hour.

---

infusion started. Remember that, in persistently hypoglycaemic children, a full hypoglycaemia screen should be sent whilst they are actually hypoglycaemic. This is because hypoglycaemia may be a result of a transient change, e.g. in insulin levels.

Replacement and Redistribution Fluids

Often, patients with surgical drains in place will require replacement fluids for ongoing losses. For example, nasogastric (NG) losses in a child with pyloric stenosis may be replaced mL for mL with 0.9% sodium chloride and 10% KCl. Gastric fluid is rich in chloride and potassium; hence, both must be replaced. Some replacement fluids will discount "normal losses"; for example, the decision might be made that stoma losses will be replaced only above 20mL/kg/day in a neonate. Additional fluid may also need to be prescribed on top of maintenance for redistribution of fluids, e.g. tissue oedema in sepsis.

Sodium Balance

Hyponatremia is common, particularly with hypotonic fluids. If it is asymptomatic, change any hypotonic fluid to isotonic fluid. Restrict IV maintenance fluids to 50-80% of normal if the child is hypervolaemic or at risk of hypervolaemia (e.g. SiADH). Acute symptomatic hyponatraemia (headache, nausea/vomiting, confusion/disorientation, irritability, lethargy, reduced consciousness, convulsions, coma, apnoea) requires immediate expert input, but may be treated with 2mL/kg boluses of 2.7% sodium chloride (given over 10-15 minutes), which can be repeated up to three times if the child is still symptomatic and the sodium is still low. When the child becomes asymptomatic, it is important to ensure that the sodium does not go up by more than 12mmol/L per day, as over-rapid correction can precipitate cerebral demyelination and brain damage.

Hypernatraemia is a less common complication of fluid therapy. Management depends on the fluid status. In hypernatraemic dehydration, the fluid deficit should be replaced (with 0.9% sodium chloride) over 48 hours. If the patient is not dehydrated, then consider going from hypertonic fluid (e.g. 0.9% sodium chloride/5% dextrose) to hypotonic fluid (e.g. 0.45% sodium chloride/5% dextrose). Urinary sodium/osmolality can help assess dehydration if it is unclear: urinary sodium is low and osmolality is high in hypovolaemia. It is important to ensure that the sodium does not go down by more than 12mmol/L per day: over-rapid correction can precipitate cerebral oedema.

Blood Products

Blood products are prescribed much less frequently for children than for adults. Cytomegalovirus (CMV) negative blood should be considered in those who may become compromised by CMV infection (which is normally harmless), e.g. neonates or the immunocompromised. Irradiated blood cells (where white blood cells are irradiated) may be required in those with a high risk of transfusion-related graft-versus-host disease (GvHD), e.g. neonates requiring exchange transfusion or the immunocompromised.

Blood products are summarised in *Table 4*, and *Example 7* shows an example prescription.

TABLE 4: Blood products and indications

Blood product	Indication	Prescription	Additional considerations
Red blood cells.	• Acute blood loss. • Transfusion dependent children, e.g. those with thalassaemia major. • Post chemotherapy. • Paediatric intensive care patients.	• Unlike with adults, red cells are prescribed in mL, not in units. • Packed red cell volume (mL) = desired rise in haemoglobin (g/dL) x 4 x weight (kg). • The maximum infusion rate is normally 5 mL/kg/hr, up to a maximum of 150 mL/hour.	• There is a potential risk for fluid overload, so furosemide should be considered halfway through the transfusion.
Fresh frozen plasma.	• Patients with coagulopathy (e.g. from chronic liver disease). • Before an invasive procedure. • If there is active bleeding.	• 10-15 mL/kg. • Given at a rate of 10-20 mL/kg/hr.	• Rarely, cryoprecipitate may be needed, for example, if there is active bleeding associated with a low fibrinogen and a raised D-dimer. • This might happen in disseminated intravascular coagulopathy (DIC).
Platelets.	• Low platelets have a variety of causes, including sepsis, iatrogenic (e.g. chemotherapy), and malignancy.	• Platelets are prescribed not in "pools" like in adults, but in mL. • Platelet volume= 15mL/kg over two to three hours.	• In idiopathic thrombocytopenic purpura (ITP), platelets are generally not prescribed, as they are likely to be destroyed by the disease process.

EXAMPLE 7

A 6-year-old sickle cell patient has a haemoglobin of 6 g/dL. Her normal haemoglobin is 8 g/dL. She requires a transfusion. Note that a different formula is used specifically for sickle cell transfusions (as below). Increasing the haematocrit excessively increases the risk of hyperviscosity, fluid overload and vaso-occlusive events.

The maximum rate of transfusion in sickle cell is 250mL/hr, and this is not exceeded. However since blood is normally given over a minimum of two hours, the above prescription would be prescribed as 60mL/hr not 100mL/hr.

Date	Fluid	Additive	Volume	Route	Rate	Signature	Given	Batch
1/1/15	PACKED RED CELLS	–	120ml	IV	60mL/hr	*A. Jones* JONES 1234		

$$\text{Packed red cell volume (mL)} = \text{Desired rise in haemoglobin (g/dL)} \times 3 \times \text{weight (kg)}$$
$$= (8-6) \times 3 \times 20$$
$$= 2 \times 3 \times 20$$
$$= 120mL$$

$$\text{Maximum Rate (mL/h)} = \text{Weight (kg)} \times 5$$
$$= 20 \times 5$$
$$= 100 \text{ mL/hr}$$

Table 5 gives a summary of common prescribing errors.

This chapter contains many 'dos and don'ts', but the take home message is that prescribing is one of the most important jobs performed by a clinician. A thoughtful and conscientious approach coupled with a willingness to ask for help will ensure safe, considerate and effective prescribing.

TABLE 5: Classic prescribing errors

Drug/situation	Type of Error
Wrong weight.	• Do not always assume the documented weight is accurate. • If a patient is unable to be weighed on admission, a weight may be estimated. • Have a marker or "normal" weight of children of different ages and question if it seems abnormally high or low.
Calculation errors.	• Check and double check calculations, particularly if complex. • Factor of 10 errors are common but can have catastrophic effects if administered.

continued

TABLE 5: *Continued*

Drug/situation	Type of Error
Misinterpreting dosing information.	• Be careful to read the whole monograph. For example, is the dose 100 mg/kg three to four times a day or 100 mg/kg/day in three to four divided doses? • Another common mistake is that formularies may break down different doses for different indications, e.g. amoxicillin IV dosing for listerial meningitis is listed after the IV section for "susceptible infections." The latter is sub-therapeutic for listeria but is commonly prescribed as it is the first dose listed.
Prescribing drugs in "mL".	• Wherever possible, medicines should be prescribed in mg or the most appropriate dose units. • Liquid medicines may come in a range of licensed and unlicensed forms and strengths. A common example is furosemide liquid which is available in 5 mg/mL, 20 mg/mL, 40 mg/mL and 50 mg/mL formulations. Writing 5 mL may mean 5-50 mg, depending on the strength of liquid available. • Some medication may be prescribed in mL, e.g. lactulose, co-amoxiclav. However the compound strength must be specified.

Penicillins.	• When prescribing "Tazocin" or "Augmentin" to penicillin-allergic patients.
	  • Tazocin = Piperacillin (a penicillin) + Tazobactam.
	  • Augmentin = Amoxicillin + Clavulanic acid.

Methotrexate.	• This is a very toxic drug used in inflammatory or neoplastic conditions. • It is a once WEEKLY drug. The classic mistake is to prescribe it daily.
Ibuprofen.	• Avoid prescribing this in asthma due to risk of bronchospasm.
Primary and secondary care interface.	• Information flow between primary and secondary care is a common source of omissions and errors. Ensure the drug history on admission is as complete as possible, and that any additional necessary information is acquired as soon as possible. • Ask about inhalers, topical preparations, vitamin supplements and vaccinations. • For discharge prescriptions, complete all medications, including previous regular medication. Specify liquid strengths if possible. Ensure that the discharge letter includes information about any medication stopped or changed during the admission.
G6PD.	• Numerous drugs may precipitate glucose-6-phosphate dehydrogenase deficiency (G6PD) crises. • Classic examples are ciprofloxacin, nitrofurantoin and the sulphonamides.
Drug-drug interactions.	• Remember the inducers and inhibitors of CYP450 enzymes. A common scenario is the prescription of clarithromycin, an enzyme inhibitor, which will increase the plasma concentration of anti-epileptics like carbamazepine and valproate.
Copying a previous incorrect prescription.	• Always recalculate prescriptions when re-prescribing. There may be a change in weight, or there may have been an error in the previous prescription.

REFERENCES AND FURTHER READING

1 Paediatric Formulary Committee. *BNF for Children* 2015. London: BMJ Group, Pharmaceutical Press and RCPCH Publications; 2015.

2 NICE guideline NG29: Intravenous fluid prescription in children and young people in hospital. 2015. https://www.nice.org.uk/guidance/ng29.

3 Maitland K et al. Mortality after fluid bolus in African children with severe infection. New EnglJ Med.2011; 364:2483-95

4 WHO. Paediatric emergency triage, assessment and treatment. 2016. http://apps.who.int/iris/bitstream/10665/204463/1/9789241510219_eng.pdf.

5 TOXBASE. www.toxbase.org.

6 The Cochrane Collaboration. www.cochrane.org.

7 Food and Drug Administration (FDA). www.fda.gov.

8 NHS Evidence. www.evidence.nhs.uk.

9 Joint United Kingdom Blood Transfusion and Tissue Transplantation Services Professional Advisory Committee (JPAC). 2015. Effective Transfusions in Paediatric Practice. http://www.transfusionguidelines.org.uk/transfusion-handbook/10-effective-transfusion-in-paediatric-practice/10-3-transfusion-of-infants-and-children.

4.01
UNDERGRADUATE AND POSTGRADUATE ASSESSMENTS IN PAEDIATRICS

MICHAEL MALLEY AND MARIE MONAGHAN

EXPECTATIONS OF A MEDICAL STUDENT

Although most medical students will not become paediatricians, doctors encounter children in most specialties, such as primary care, ENT and other surgical specialties, and emergency medicine, amongst others.

For undergraduates, senior clinicians want the student to approach the rotation in "good faith." This means feeling that the student has tried their best, made the most of their time on the ward and shown a measurable improvement in performance. This is not demonstrated in a one-off assessment, but continually throughout the attachment. In terms of competence, it is important the student is confident that they:

> Are aware of the basic management and recognition of common paediatric problems.

> Appreciate the differences between the management of children compared to adults, including communication challenges.

> Understand the differences in adult and paediatric basic life support.

> Are aware of child protection issues and start to understand their management.

> Have completed the requisite range of assessments (which may require organisation on the part of the student).

Before a supervisor meeting at the end of the placement, it is important to think about the main learning points from the rotation, as well as what has gone well, and not so well. Demonstrate evidence of engagement with the children, and the paediatric team. Be aware that supervisors will usually take advice from other paediatric staff to make a holistic assessment of each student.

For postgraduates, educational supervisors have a long list of criteria to "tick off". Become familiar with this list. Other factors to consider include evidence of quality improvement projects (e.g. audits), managerial experience (e.g. rota co-ordination), teaching experience, exam success and reflective practice. This should all be apparent in the trainee's learning portfolio. More generally, remember assessments are increasingly recognised as learning opportunities. Prepare

CONTENTS

for them thoroughly and ask for extensive and personalised feedback on how to improve afterwards.

WORK BASED ASSESSMENTS

Work-based assessments are changing at the time of writing, with new assessments added frequently. The basis of undergraduate and postgraduate assessment, however, remains CBDs (case-based discussions), CEXs (clinical evaluation exercises) and DOPS (directly observed procedural skills). The key is to empower the trainee to complete assessments that aid development and reflection. To ensure the best feedback, aim to have any assessment form filled out contemporaneously. This sounds simple but a surprising number of assessments occur opportunistically, but never get formally documented.

Selecting an Assessor

In practice, the quality of assessments varies greatly. Some supervisors will expect too little and others may expect too much. Do not choose someone because they are an "easy target". Instead, choose a familiar doctor, who is aware of the assessment process, will be fair, and will give detailed, honest feedback. It might be tempting to opt for a better grade over an honest appraisal, but in reality, constructive feedback is more beneficial in the long-term.

Case-Based Discussions

Case based discussions (CBDs) are an opportunity to discuss a case at length, from initial presentation to examination to management. CBDs encourage discussion of the approach to each part of the patient journey, with the aim of improving the student's knowledge and thought process along the way. When done properly, they can be time-consuming, so arrange to meet with a willing consultant or supervisor at a mutually convenient time. Ensure patient notes and investigation results are accessible. Present a pre-prepared overview of the case.

Mini Clinical Evaluation Exercises

Mini clinical evaluation exercises (Mini-CEXs) are designed to give juniors the opportunity to be observed in a clinical setting, e.g. communication, history taking or examination. Be opportunistic and take advantage of situations where natural observation occurs, e.g. on a ward round/in clinic. If appropriate, ask for an opportunity to repeat the assessment later to demonstrate improvements in practice.

Directly Observed Procedural Skills

Directly observed procedural skills (DOPS) are more common at the postgraduate level. They involve observation performing a clinical procedure, from blood taking to more advanced procedures, like chest drain insertion. Again, prepare in advance and make sure you get dedicated time to debrief after the procedure is complete.

OBJECTIVE STRUCTURED CLINICAL EXAMINATIONS (OSCEs)

History Taking

General Approach

History taking stations are common. Check what is expected in advance. These stations should be straightforward. There is a clear rubric to follow, and plenty of opportunities to practice in advance.

There are three "S's" in SucceSS:

> Structure. Replicate the same format for every history station.
> Smoothness. Practise fluently moving from one section of the history to the next.
> Sensitivity. Remember that the parent is potentially anxious/scared. Elicit their main concerns and give them a chance to speak – don't just ask closed questions.

Before entering the station, decide whether to take a focused history of a particular condition or a more general history. Use the information in the briefing to inform an initial differential diagnosis. Write down any key questions that spring to mind.

Elicit all the main concerns of the patient/carer (this may be an actor for the OSCE). One way to ensure nothing is missed is to ask, *Is there anything I've missed or anything else you are concerned about? Do you have any questions for me now?* To end, summarise the key points and state what will happen next. *So to summarise, Jamie has had three previous admissions with asthma and has come in today with wheeze and difficulty breathing over the last 12 hours. You are worried he might have pneumonia. I'll examine Jamie and then we can discuss what is going on in more detail.*

Presenting Findings

The presentation is key and this short soliloquy can dramatically alter the final grade. One suggestion is to stand with hands behind the back. Speak slowly and deliberately. Look at the examiner and speak with confidence. Open with a simple introduction. For example: *I met Mrs. Brown today, who presented with her son Alex. Alex presents with a history of …* followed by the headline symptoms. Then state the important positive and negative findings of the history. It is not a recollection of every word, but of information gathered. Ensure that the summary is no longer than one minute. After relaying the history, suggest the next steps. This will usually involve a full examination of the relevant systems and an investigation strategy. Think of any other information which may be helpful, for example the red book/growth chart, previous discharge summaries or medication lists, and request them as well. If there is still additional time, finish with a one sentence summary.

An example presentation is shown in *Box 1*, alongside a mark scheme in *Table 1*.

Box 1: Presenting a history

I met Mrs. Brown today, who brought her 7-year-old son Alex to ED with a 24 hour history of difficulty breathing and wheeze.

Alex is known to have asthma. He has had a cough for two days and has developed progressive difficulty in breathing and wheeze over the last 24 hours. He has a low grade temperature and a dry cough. He has been using two puffs of his salbutamol inhaler every four hours without improvement.

Alex has had many previous admissions to hospital, the most serious of which required IV salbutamol two years ago. His last admission was two months ago. His known asthma triggers are pets and upper respiratory tract infections, and he also has a history of eczema. His normal peak flow reading is around 300 mL/min. He misses about two days of school per month due to his asthma.

Alex was born at term without complication and there have been no concerns about his development.

Alex takes two puffs of a beclomethasone inhaler twice per day and uses his salbutamol inhaler when required. He takes no other medications. He has no known drug allergies and his immunisations are up-to-date.

Alex's mother has a history of asthma and his father has hay fever.

He lives in a flat with his parents and his 5-year-old brother. There are no smokers in the house and the family have never had any involvement with social services.

In summary, Alex is a 7-year-old boy who presents with a likely acute exacerbation of his asthma.

I would like to proceed to examine Alex, view his observations chart, perform a peak flow measurement and initiate bronchodilator therapy.

TABLE 1: History taking mark scheme

Domain	Mark				
Conduct of the consultation. To include: • Introduction, clarifies role. • Rapport. • Empathy and respect.	*(Clear Pass)*	Pass	Bare fail	Clear fail	Unacceptable
History taking. To include: • Clear history of presenting complaint. • Appropriate style. • Fluent and comprehensive history. • Explores and responds to concerns/feelings. • Summarises and checks understanding.	*(Clear Pass)*	Pass	Bare fail	Clear fail	Unacceptable
Differential diagnosis and initial management. To include: • Appropriate range of differentials appropriate for age. • Accuracy of information/ clinical knowledge.	Clear Pass	*(Pass)*	Bare fail	Clear fail	Unacceptable
FINAL GRADE.	*(Clear Pass)*	Pass	Bare fail	Clear fail	Unacceptable

Examination

Examination stations cause anxiety amongst undergraduate and postgraduate candidates alike. What if the child isn't co-operative or cries? What if signs are missed? Candidates often think they will be heinously penalised for forgetting pallor or lymphadenopathy or missing grade one clubbing. They aren't! Remember that the overall conduct of the examination counts more than the sum of its individual minutiae. Be professional, sensitive, structured and observant. The examiner will be asking the question: *Is this person appropriate for the next level?* Students should act like a junior doctor; junior doctors should act like a middle-grade doctor.

Before the Examination

Practise. A lot. Become familiar with the important components of each examination, and practice under supervision with real patients. This will ensure technique is committed to muscle memory, making it easier to concentrate on picking up relevant clinical signs.

The first and last minute of each station are crucial. Therefore, practise the introduction and take time to put the patient at ease. Then practise presenting the examination findings in one minute. Practise presenting both real and imaginary patients. Practise to the mirror, to friends, and to colleagues.

Patients suitable for examinations nearly always have chronic conditions and are clinically stable. Contemplate what signs they may have and make a list of the common underlying diagnoses (*Table 2*). Ask senior students what they encountered in their exams. It may be helpful to create maps of common differential diagnoses to consolidate key findings. *Figure 1* is an example for abdominal examination.

Starting the Station

Do simple tasks well. Remember: the first minute is critical. Hands should be washed before touching the patient. Give a cheery introduction to the child and parent, acknowledging everyone in the room. For older children, it is appropriate to introduce yourself to the child first. Ensure the patient is adequately positioned and appropriately exposed from the start. This will reduce awkwardness later and make important signs more apparent. This also helps build initial rapport with the patient.

Observing the Patient

Make a show of this – and excuse it by saying: *Right before I look at you, I'm just going to have a good look around. Don't worry—I'm not ignoring you!* Look for obvious clues, like wheelchairs/walking aids/medication/modified shoes and scars. Look carefully at the armpits and the back. Learn the meaning of surgical scars carefully; know at least two underlying causes per scar.

Examining the Patient

Examining children requires a balance between systematic and opportunistic examination. In clinical practice, opportunistic examination is often the way forward, but in time-pressured exams, be as structured as possible, working from peripheral signs to central examination. However, when examining an uncooperative child, do the components requiring

TABLE 2: Common examination findings in paediatric exams

System	Key Conditions	Key Signs	Key Knowledge
Cardiology.	• Congenital heart disease (especially coarctation, tetralogy, transposition). • Valvular abnormalities. • Septal defects. • Marfan syndrome. • Down syndrome (with ventricular or atrioventricular septal defect; VSD/AVSD).	• Cyanosis (not common in exams). • Clubbing. • Scars (sternotomy/ thoracotomy/ central lines). • Heart murmurs. • Signs of failure (e.g. hepatomegaly; not common in exams).	• Types of murmurs and their positions. • Grades of murmurs. • Operation scars. • Broad overview of common congenital defects. • Management of common cardiac defects (conservative/medical/surgical).
Respiratory.	• Cystic fibrosis (CF). • Bronchiectasis. • Asthma. • Chronic lung disease.	• Clubbing. • Hyperinflation (chronic obstructive disease, e.g. asthma). • Lung sounds. • Extrapulmonary signs, e.g. clubbing • Finger prick marks for diabetes in CF. • Medication (e.g. inhalers). • Failure to thrive. • Portacaths.	• Causes of clubbing. • Extrapulmonary signs of chronic respiratory diseases. • Management of asthma and cystic fibrosis.
Abdominal.	• Haemoglobinopathies. • Polycystic kidneys. • Ex-premature babies post necrotising enterocolitis (NEC) surgery. • Crohn's/Ulcerative colitis. • Nephrotic syndrome. • Post kidney transplant. • Antegrade colonic enema (ACE) stoma.	• Clubbing. • Organomegaly. • Abdominal scars. • Transplanted kidney. • Oedema. • Stomas.	• Differentials of hepatomegaly, splenomegaly and hepatosplenomegaly. • How to differentiate a spleen and a kidney on examination. • Management of haemoglobinopathies, inflammatory bowel disease, nephrotic syndrome.
Neurological.	• Muscular dystrophies. • Cerebral palsy (hemiplegia, diplegia, quadriplegia, ataxia). • Seventh cranial nerve palsy. • Neurofibromatosis. • Stroke. • Brain tumour.	• Increased/decreased tone. • Weakness. • Cerebellar signs. • Past pointing. • Brisk or absent reflexes. • Abnormal sensation. • Abnormal gait. • Gower's sign. • Congenital neurocutaneous markers (e.g. café-au-lait spots, freckling, Shagreen patches). • Wheelchairs/walking aids. • Modified shoes/footwear.	• Differentiate upper vs. lower motor neurone lesions. • Causes of upper vs. lower motor neurone lesions. • Dermatomal and myotomal innervations. • Reflex origins. • Management of cerebral palsy, and role of multidisciplinary team in any neurodisability.
Common multi-system conditions.	• Down Syndrome. • Turner Syndrome. • Neurofibromatosis. • Tuberous Sclerosis Complex. • Achondroplasia.	• Many signs depending on the condition.	• Learn the main associated signs for each condition so that they can be recognised if they appear in combination.

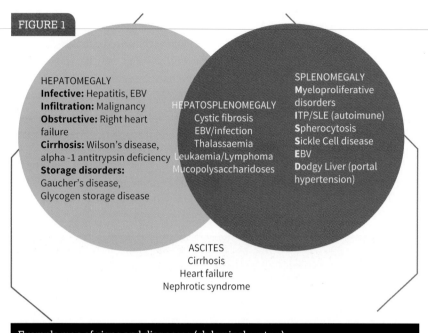

FIGURE 1

HEPATOMEGALY
Infective: Hepatitis, EBV
Infiltration: Malignancy
Obstructive: Right heart failure
Cirrhosis: Wilson's disease, alpha -1 antitrypsin deficiency
Storage disorders: Gaucher's disease, Glycogen storage disease

HEPATOSPLENOMEGALY
Cystic fibrosis
EBV/infection
Thalassaemia
Leukaemia/Lymphoma
Mucopolysaccharidoses

SPLENOMEGALY
Myeloproliferative disorders
ITP/SLE (autoimune)
Spherocytosis
Sickle Cell disease
EBV
Dodgy Liver (portal hypertension)

ASCITES
Cirrhosis
Heart failure
Nephrotic syndrome

Example map of signs and diagnoses (abdominal system).

quiet (e.g. listening for chest sounds) in the most convenient order. Explain to the examiner: *As Katie is currently settled, I would like to start centrally and examine peripherally afterwards.* Equally, leave anything potentially painful or distressing to the end of the examination (e.g. ENT assessment or palpation of a tender abdomen). Always get down to the level of the patient when examining, particularly when performing exams which may cause discomfort, such as palpating the abdomen.

Most importantly, be kind, be gentle, be considerate and treat the child as exactly that — a child and not an exam prop. Talk to the child, comment on their clothes, interact a little and the child is more likely to be at ease!

Concluding

Tell the child and the parent when the examination has finished and offer to help them re-dress. State the next steps in the assessment. For example: *To finish my abdominal examination I would like to check the external genitalia, the hernia orifices and take a urine dip. I'd also like to take a full history, perform a full multi-system examination and get a set of observations.*

Presenting Findings

Present the case to the examiner. A general opening could go along the lines of: *I examined Katie who is 3-years-old and appears well-grown, although I would like to confirm this on an appropriate growth chart.* Emphasise positive and important negative findings. Try to build a picture of related findings rather than saying them in isolation. For example: *Katie has a pansystolic murmur. There are, however, no signs of hepatomegaly, oedema or basal crepitations to suggest heart failure.* After presenting findings, offer a differential diagnosis, by stating: *These findings may be consistent with….* Then, offer a simple management plan. Start with investigations that can be done immediately (examination, observations, bedside tests), then state more complicated management (bloods, imaging, specialist referrals).

Finish with a one line summary: *To summarise, Katie is a 3-year-old girl who may have a ventricular septal defect (VSD), with no evidence of heart failure.*

An example presentation is shown in *Box 2*, alongside a mark scheme in *Table 3*.

Communication

Communication skills are vital in clinical practice. Thus, communication

has become more important in clinical examinations at both undergraduate and postgraduate level. Each scenario will vary, but some general advice is applicable to most settings.

Possible Scenarios

› **Patients.** Likely to be a teenager in paediatric exams (as a younger patient is less likely to be able to replicate the scenarios) or an actor playing a carer. Consider:
  › Explaining medical diagnoses, e.g. epilepsy, diabetes.
  › Consent issues, e.g. contraception/ Gillick competence.
  › Psychological issues, e.g. suicidal ideation.
› **Parents.** The most common scenario. Consider:
  › Breaking bad news, particularly chronic conditions, e.g. trisomy 21, cystic fibrosis, diabetes.
  › Information giving, e.g. first fit/ febrile convulsion, management of chronic conditions (e.g. asthma, eczema), breastfeeding in a HIV-positive mother.
  › Complaints, e.g. parent unhappy with service.
  › Ethical dilemmas, e.g. confidentiality and a child.
  › Safeguarding concerns, e.g. non accidental injury, Gillick competence.
  › Drug errors, e.g. double dose of gentamicin.
› **Nurses.** An increasingly popular station in undergraduate examinations. As a junior doctor, your relationship with nurses will determine your success and happiness! Consider:
  › Handover of a patient being admitted to the ward.
  › Discussion of a difficult case, e.g. withdrawal of care.
› **Medical students/junior colleagues.** Teaching skills are increasingly sought-after and examined. Be confident delivering concise teaching on core topics. A classic example is explaining the audit cycle.

Box 2: Presenting examination findings

I examined Adeolu today, a 4-year-old-boy, Afro-Caribbean in origin, who presented with his father.

He appears well grown for his age, although I would like to plot this on the appropriate growth chart. He is comfortable and pain-free at rest.

On peripheral examination, he has a resting heart rate of 92 bpm with mild pallor of the conjunctivae and jaundice.

On examination of his abdomen, he has a three centimetre non-tender hepatomegaly and a palpable spleen, with no other organomegaly or lymphadenopathy. I note a scar under his right clavicle which may represent a previous central line insertion.

To finish my examination, I would like to examine his hernial orifices and external genitalia. I'd like to ensure there was no bony tenderness anywhere, or any signs of respiratory compromise.

These findings would be consistent with a haemoglobinopathy – most likely sickle cell disease. I would also like to exclude any infectious or lymphoproliferative processes.

TABLE 3: Examination mark scheme

Domain	Mark				
Conduct of the examination. To include • Rapport, putting child at ease. • Appropriately professional. • Empathy and respect. • Appropriate communication.	_Clear Pass_ (circled)	Pass	Bare fail	Clear fail	Unacceptable
Clinical Examination. To include: • Appropriate technique. • Identifies appropriate signs. • Appropriate confidence. • Able to demonstrate signs.	_Clear Pass_ (circled)	Pass	Bare fail	Clear fail	Unacceptable
Discussion. To include: • Differential diagnosis. • Appropriate investigations. • Management considerations.	Clear Pass	_Pass_ (circled)	Bare fail	Clear fail	Unacceptable
FINAL GRADE.	_Clear Pass_ (circled)	Pass	Bare fail	Clear fail	Unacceptable

General Approach

Before starting, check which role the candidate is taking (e.g. medical student, junior doctor, senior doctor) and learn the patient's name. Write this down if needed. Wash hands, give an introduction and check the identity of the patient. Perhaps say at the outset that: *I've left my beeper with a colleague so we shouldn't be interrupted.* During the consultation, remember:

› **Be human!** If someone has just had a baby, say *congratulations* at the beginning! Empathise with the patient's story.

› **Check what the patient knows first.** It's easy just to say: *Before we get started, can you tell me where you're up to so far?* Use this to plan the station.

› **Set your agenda.** *I'm here to discuss the test results today, if that's okay. Feel free to jump in and ask any questions along the way* or *Would it be helpful if I explained a bit about this condition and address any concerns you might have?* This allows for the formation of a mutually agreed plan.

› **Don't give a monologue.** Actively interact. Stop at intervals and check that the patient is following the conversation. It is easy to ask: *Am I making sense so far? Do you have any questions at this point?* Remember: this is a two-way conversation and not a viva.

› **Prepare for common complex stations.** Many candidates don't know where to start with complex conditions like trisomy 21 or cystic fibrosis. Write down four sentences about each chronic, complex topic phrased in a way that is absolutely clear. Then ask: *Would it be helpful if I told you a little bit about X condition?* and deliver the information, modifying it slightly based on the expectations/age of the patient. For example, four sentences on Trisomy 21 might look something like: *Trisomy 21 is commonly called Down syndrome. This is caused when babies inherit a bit of extra genetic material from their parents. This is no one's fault and can't be predicted. This has many effects ranging from mild learning difficulties to more significant effects on the heart and internal organs. It's a common genetic condition and there is a huge amount of support available including medical teams, special schools and parental groups. Someone will be with you every step of the way. With this support, many children live happy, fulfilled lives well into their fifties and sixties.*

Finishing Off

Have a plan for the warning bell. Think about common things that are missed, or things that are best left to the end:

› **Ideas/concerns/expectations.** Ask *Do you have any other concerns that you'd like to mention?* This may uncover an important point that has been completely missed.

› **Summarise the key points of the consultation into two sentences.** This is an important component of a high-scoring station.

‣ Offer leaflets, mention parent support groups, make a plan for follow up.
For example: *I know this has been a lot to take in, so why don't we meet up again tomorrow to discuss this further?* Provide contact details. Make a positive plan to move forward – for example after discussing a difficult case with a medical student, suggest they spend time in a specialist clinic to learn more.

A possible mark scheme is shown in *Table 4*.

Practical Skills
Obtain clinical experience in the relevant skills before the assessment. Step-by-step guides to common procedures are shown on p613. Other practical skills that may be assessed are listed below.

Plotting a Growth Chart
Growth charts are simple but must be learned prior to the exam. Be aware that there are a number of different growth charts. These are primarily age-related, including neonatal, 0 to 4-years-old, and 2 to 18-years-old. However, there are also condition-specific charts, including Down syndrome and achondroplasia. Be prepared to plot serial growth measurements on these charts and be prepared to talk about differentials for faltering growth (p247).

Prescribing
Prescribing is increasingly being recognised as a neglected skill in medical education. Know how to calculate fluid requirements. Know how to use common reference sources (e.g. BNF) to calculate appropriate drug dosages (these do not need to be memorised). This station is not just about the drug prescription itself, but also the rest of the drug chart e.g. patient details, such as allergies, hospital number, address, name and date of birth. More detailed prescribing guidance is shown on p648.

DR ABCDE (acute assessment and resuscitation of the unwell child)
In an acute scenario, remember to be systematic. Assess airway, breathing, circulation, disability and exposure. This is done in the same way for every case, so practice and be confident. Ensure each letter of the alphabet is addressed before moving to the next. Treat each problem as soon as it is identified, and reassess from the beginning after each intervention. A common structure within each letter is to *"look, feel, listen, measure, treat"*. Practise this structure for the airway, breathing and circulation components.

Key points to consider include:
‣ Ask for the observations at the very beginning. The main benefits of this are two-fold. It offers a crude idea of what system is affected, depending on which observations are most deranged. It also provides an opportunity to call for help early in response to abnormal observations.
‣ If appropriate, give oxygen during the assessment of "Airway".
‣ Remember the scenario puts the candidate in the position of team leader. Others in the scenario will be role-playing so use them wisely.
‣ Remember the parents in the scenario. They may help calm the child down, but they also need to be updated with progress throughout.
‣ Reassess thoroughly after every treatment.
‣ Never forget to check the glucose, as this is a common yet reversible cause of acute deterioration.

A detailed guide on the assessment of the acutely unwell child is shown on p7.

TABLE 4: Communication mark scheme					
Domain	**Mark**				
Conduct of the consultation. To include: • Introduction, clarifies role. • Agrees aims and objectives. • Rapport. • Empathy and respect.	⟨Clear Pass⟩	Pass	Bare fail	Clear fail	Unacceptable
Explanation and information. To include: • Clear explanation, no jargon. • Assesses patient's prior knowledge. • Appropriate style. • Explores and responds to concerns/feelings. • Summarises and checks understanding.	Clear Pass	⟨Pass⟩	Bare fail	Clear fail	Unacceptable
Accurate information giving. To include: • Appropriate selection of information, including level/age-appropriateness, etc. • Accuracy of information/clinical knowledge.	⟨Clear Pass⟩	Pass	Bare fail	Clear fail	Unacceptable
FINAL GRADE	⟨Clear Pass⟩	Pass	Bare fail	Clear fail	Unacceptable

4.02
A GUIDE TO BEING A JUNIOR DOCTOR IN PAEDIATRICS

MARIE MONAGHAN AND MICHAEL MALLEY

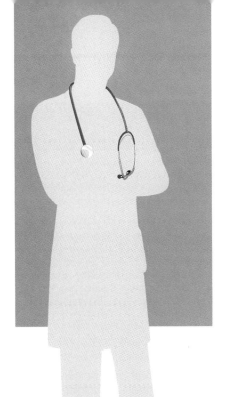

CONTENTS

GENERAL PREPARATION

Paediatrics is a fulfilling and stimulating career, offering the potential to bring joy to children and their families. A unique specialty with its own diverse range of conditions, paediatrics requires a flexible approach, an appreciation for the breadth of medicine, and a dextrous hand for the wide range of procedures involved. As much as it demands, it rewards. Paediatricians laugh, play games and most certainly become familiar with the most popular Disney films and children's TV shows!

Although exciting for those already familiar with paediatrics, not surprisingly, those starting out can find this field incredibly daunting after an education focused on adult-centred medicine (*Table 1*).

Before starting a general paediatric or neonatal job, practitioners may benefit from attending a paediatric life support course. These are usually incorporated into paediatric induction training. Being confident in resuscitation will lead to increased confidence when facing the most demanding situations. This training can also lend a structured approach to the care of any child and provide advice on the most effective way to communicate and interact in resuscitation scenarios. Induction training will also offer a good opportunity to explore the specific working environment of the paediatric department.

Table 2 shows the key areas in Paediatric units, and *Table 3* shows those areas that aid in coordinating patient care. Multidisciplinary teamwork is extremely important in paediatrics, meaning that effective communication is paramount for ensuring all parties are up to date with developments in a child's care. Being open with colleagues about previous levels of experience will help them tailor teaching, day-to-day task allocation and senior support.

The main chapters of the book give detailed information on key conditions encountered in paediatrics and key skills required for assessing and treating children. What follows is additional practical information to help with adaptation to life on paediatric wards.

TABLE 1: Examples of similarities and differences between adult and paediatric medicine

Similarities	Differences
Certain conditions that affect adults also affect children; for example, infection, asthma, diabetes and fractures (although the management of these are often specific to children).	In paediatrics, many conditions, such as diabetes or asthma, are diagnosed for the very first time in a patient's life, rather than forming part of their past medical history. Many rare conditions can also occur, like those with a genetic, developmental or metabolic origin, which are diagnosed in the paediatric population but are not associated with survival to adulthood.
Resuscitation training is a requirement in both adult and paediatric medicine.	Children, unlike adults, rarely undergo resuscitation due to a primarily cardiac cause. Most severe illnesses stem from respiratory or systemic causes, like asthma or sepsis. These contrasting causative factors mean that resuscitation is focussed on supporting the airway and breathing in the sick child. In terms of resuscitation outcomes, children are regarded as being better able to compensate for illness, respond to resuscitative efforts and recover after significant physiological insults. Similarly, ward admissions are often brief for children (one to two days) following response to appropriate medical intervention. The increasing use of ambulatory care, where patients are cared for on a ward–attender basis or are given medical care in the home, can potentially avoid the need for inpatient admission.
A structured examination approach and comprehensive history-taking are required in adult and paediatric medicine.	In paediatrics, history-taking has a broader social emphasis, and it includes paediatric-specific topics such as birth history, developmental history, immunisation status and safeguarding concerns. The source of the history is generally caregivers rather than the child, but a history may also be taken directly from the child, depending on their age and level of development. In paediatric examinations, while a thorough examination is required, the course of the examination is often opportunistic and adaptive – for convenience and to maintain the ease of the child. An example of this might be the examination of a child's gait as they walk into an examination room, unaware of observation, or the auscultation of an infant's heart sounds as they lie asleep.
	The majority of paediatric inpatient admissions are to a non-specialist, general paediatric ward, where care is managed by an admitting general paediatric consultant with an accompanying medical team, plus any necessary specialist input required.
	Planned simple procedures in paediatrics, when invasive, require preparation (for example, topical analgesia) and often the assistance of nursing staff and play specialists. Junior doctors in paediatrics are not expected to be accomplished in intravenous cannulation and are not expected to perform these procedures independently at the outset. Procedural skills are developed with senior support. Paediatrics also has a wider range of advanced procedures, such as endotracheal intubation, chest drain insertion, cranial ultrasounds, and central line insertion (umbilical or long line access).

TABLE 2: Locations in paediatric hospital care

Location	Function
Playroom.	Full of many toys and games, with activities organised by play therapists. Often a place where children are hiding when they can't be found!
Teenage room.	May contain age-appropriate activities for teenagers, such as books and computer games.
Treatment room.	Procedures are done here: this helps the bed space remain a safe, comfortable environment for the child and means that a distressed child can be managed in privacy.
School room.	Dedicated teachers provide ongoing education for inpatients.
Parents' room/ accommodation.	A room is often provided for parents to stay in. This may be within the ward, or it might be in a separate nearby building. A room with basic facilities for sitting and relaxing may also be available.
Hospital at home.	Children may remain under hospital care, but be visited by "hospital at home" nurses for ongoing treatment, such as intravenous antibiotics. These patients are discussed at a daily virtual hospital ward round.
Sensory room.	Contains interesting lights and colours, and soft floor padding. Provides a relaxing space; particularly great for younger children and those with learning difficulties.
Short stay unit.	For children being admitted for 24- 48 hours, although some allow for slightly longer durations of stay.
Day care unit.	Usually for patients not requiring an overnight stay or attending for a short period; for example, attending for allergy testing, for antibiotics, or for a sleep study or day surgery. Often primarily nurse-led.
Milk room.	For preparation and storage of milk, both formula and breast.

Continued

TABLE 2: *Continued*

Location	Function
Labour ward/Obstetric theatre.	Where pregnant women go to deliver.
Postnatal ward.	Where mother and babies go after delivery.
Cubicle.	For infectious/immunocompromised patients to isolate them from other patients.
Paediatric Emergency Department.	Often there is a separate dedicated area of the Emergency Department (ED) just for paediatrics.
Resuscitation area.	The ED will have a dedicated paediatric resuscitation (resus) bay, as well as resus areas on the postnatal and paediatric wards. Incubator spaces in the NICU contain most resuscitation equipment, but a separate resus area is available where the more stable babies can be brought if they deteriorate.

TABLE 3: People available to help deliver care. Units vary in which personnel are actually available and their roles.

	Colleague	Role
Paediatric ward.	Child protection (safeguarding) nurse/doctor.	There is an allocated child protection nurse and doctor in every paediatric unit.
	Children's community nurse.	Works alongside families to provide nursing support and monitor the effectiveness of any care package. May be important in discharge planning.
	Clinical support worker.	Works alongside allied health professionals (e.g. physiotherapists) to prepare for and deliver therapy.
	Dietician.	Gives advice on feeding and nutrition.
	Health visitor.	Their role primarily involves visiting families in their homes, and they routinely visit all new parents. Concerns about vulnerable children identified in the hospital may be followed up by a health visitor.
	Healthcare assistant/ Auxiliary nurse.	Works under the supervision of a nurse/midwife to help deliver care, including things like taking observations and washing/dressing patients.
	Occupational therapist.	Helps provide practical solutions for any child with a physical or psychiatric impairment. This may involve providing equipment or home adaptation.
	Orthoptist.	Helps manage eye movement problems, e.g. squints, alongside ophthalmologists.
	Paediatric nurse practitioner/Site manager.	Responsible for coordinating care through all paediatric wards and the ED. Helps facilitate discharges and achieve conflict resolution.
	Parent.	A parent usually resides most of the time with a sick child in hospital. The parent will often help to deliver care and may provide a vital observation indicating that the child has deteriorated.
	Police.	May be involved in child protection cases. Present in the ED for out-of-hospital cardiac arrests.
	Pharmacist/Pharmacy technician.	Can provide advice on specific dosing and formulation of drugs. Can also liaise with families and primary care physicians on exact regular medications. Vital source of help for doing difficult prescriptions, and they will check all prescriptions regardless. Pharmacists need to be alerted early about any discharges so they can prepare medications.
	Physician's assistant.	Trained to support doctors in the medical management of children. Roles vary depending on experience.
	Physiotherapist.	Helps patients with balance and mobility problems. Chest physiotherapy is particularly helpful in cystic fibrosis.
	Play specialist.	Experts in child-appropriate play. Vital support in distraction for practical procedures.
	Psychologist.	Clinical psychologists will assist in management of mental health problems, behavioural problems and patients with difficulty adjusting to a new diagnosis/illness. Educational psychologists (usually working in the community) address psychological issues to enhance a child's learning ability.

Continued

TABLE 3: *Continued*

	Colleague	Role
	Specialist nurse.	Nurses have wide ranges of potential specialities, including common diseases such as diabetes, cystic fibrosis and asthma, as well as more esoteric areas like small bowel transplants. Specialist nurses may review patients on the ward and see them in follow-up clinics independently.
	Social worker.	Provides support to vulnerable children/families. For any child protection concerns, it is worth checking to see if they are known to social services already. Social workers are crucial in coordinating child protection investigations.
	Speech and language therapist (SALT or SLT).	Helps those with speech and language problems, wider communication difficulty and feeding problems.
	Staff nurse.	Doctors work more closely with the nursing staff than any others. The staff nurses deliver overall care for the patient, including administering medication, performing observations/investigations and highlighting the deteriorating patient.
	Nurse-in-charge.	The nurse-in-charge actively manages the activity on the ward. Regular updates are helpful for the nurse-in-charge regarding management of the ward patients, particularly discharges.
	Ward sister.	Supervises the work of the nursing/health care assistant team. As experienced paediatric nurses, they are a great source of advice if you are stuck!
	Ward clerk.	Able to retrieve notes, book appointments, answer phone calls, and welcome patients/families to the ward.
Labour ward and post-natal ward.	Midwife.	Leads delivery of low risk pregnancies and supports resuscitation of sick newborns. Trained in newborn life support (NLS). Able to provide advice on many aspects of neonatology, particularly normal variations in newborns and feeding issues.
	Obstetrician.	Will make decisions on any urgent deliveries. May request counselling for a mother before a preterm delivery, and may hold discussions about bed status in the NICU before a delivery is planned or pregnant women with high risk deliveries are admitted to the ward.
	Anaesthetist.	Present in theatre for Caesarean sections. May often help in neonatal resuscitations, but aren't necessarily qualified in NLS.
	Breastfeeding advisor.	Able to provide specific guidance to mothers with difficulty establishing feeding.
	Nursery nurse.	Often available on the postnatal ward and will help deliver basic care to newborn babies.

GENERAL PAEDIATRIC WARDS

Completing Ward Rounds

Ward rounds take place daily on a paediatric ward and are led by the consultant or the registrar. The average length of stay for children is two days, and about 50% of patients stay less than 24 hours. The role of the junior doctor on the ward round is to:

> Ensure blood test/investigation results are available.
> Ensure patient details are written on every sheet of the written patient notes.
> Document information gathered (history, examination, observations, blood results, parental/patient thoughts).
> Document action plans.
> Document who was responsible for decisions.
> Ask questions if anything appears to have been missed/is unclear.

A typical ward round entry is shown in *Box 1*.

Parents, carers and nurses should be present on ward rounds wherever possible to help effectively communicate the care of the paediatric patient. Multidisciplinary ward rounds also take place, and ensure coordinated care from the multiple professionals involved in any child's care.

Reviewing a Patient

Junior doctors in paediatrics are neither intended nor expected to manage acutely unwell children independently. However, they are often the first members of the medical team to initially assess a patient. If asked to review an unfamiliar patient, ask for a brief SBAR (Situation, Background, Assessment and Response) format handover (*Box 2*), as this aids the prioritisation and management of the review. Abnormal observations will often have independently generated a medical review based on the recommendations of the now widely used Paediatric Early Warning Score systems in use on nurses' observation charts.

One common reason for review is to consider "stretching" a wheezy patient on salbutamol therapy. This is carried out to determine whether a patient is improving or deteriorating on current therapy. In cases where the patient's breathing is improving, the aim is to reduce the frequency of the medication (e.g. moving from two-hourly to three-hourly salbutamol).

Box 1: Typical ward round entry. Note patients details usually provided with a pre-printed sticker. There is also often a separate parent communication sheet to document discussions.

29.6.15	WR Fred Smith (Consultant)	Sarah King
10.54 a.m.		P54030493
		29.3.15

3 month old boy, admitted 28.6.15

Diagnosis: D3 RSV+ve Bronchiolits

            Ex prem (32 weeks)

Investigations: CRP<2

Management so far: Started on 20cc of nasal cannula oxygen, NBM, 2/3 maintenance IV fluids.

Current Observations: HR 160, RR 60, Temp 37.5, BP 90/60 Saturations 95%.

Looks much improved compared to last night: more active, and respiratory distress settling. Nasal cannula oxygen has been weaned from 30cc to 20cc. No temperatures, no apnoeas. Mum senses improvement in condition. No nursing concerns noted.

O/E Pink. Active. Normal heart sounds. Bilateral wheeze/crackles, but good air entry throughout. Abdomen soft and non tender. Good femorals. Good tone.

Plan

1. Wean oxygen down to 10cc, and if saturations remain above 95%, aim off oxygen later today.
2. Start on 50% (of maintenance) hourly NG feeds (maternal expressed breast milk) and 50% IV fluids
3. Review in evening, re. stopping fluids.
4. Update the parents when they come inthis morning

Sarah Johnson

Sarah Johnson

ST1 Paediatrics. Bleep 343

Box 2: SBAR handover

Situation, Background, Assessment and Recommendation (SBAR)

SBAR is a way to effectively communicate patient care to colleagues and is highly recommended as a tool for escalation of patient care and for enhancing the quality of handovers between teams.

An example of an SBAR handover used to escalate patient care:

"Hello, is that Dr. Smith? It's Dr. Right, the junior doctor. I'd like to tell you about a patient I'm concerned about.

The **situation** is that I am here with a 6-year-old girl called Sally Jones in the Paediatric Emergency Department and she is demonstrating marked respiratory distress.

The **background** is that she has a history of asthma and is not on regular medication but has a history of once being admitted to a HDU and receiving intravenous medication for her asthma.

My **assessment** is that her observations are concerning, with tachypnoea of 60 breaths per minute and oxygen saturations in air of 90%. I have examined her and she has signs of accessory muscle use and wheeze suggestive of a severe acute asthma exacerbation.

My **recommendation** is that she requires treatment for severe asthma. I have started her on back-to-back therapy with salbutamol nebulisers driven by oxygen, but I require your senior medical input and I would like you to come urgently, please."

At this review, assess whether the patient's work of breathing has improved sufficiently that they can safely be "stretched" one further hour. This assessment requires a focussed respiratory examination, an observation chart review, a check with the nursing staff and parents, and an understanding of the treatment delivered so far. This process continues until the patient has been "stretched" to a four-hourly regimen of salbutamol inhaler via a spacer device: a frequency which can be managed safely at home. While improvement in a patient's work of breathing is generally expected, deterioration can also occur, requiring escalation of care and increased frequency of medication.

If concerns remain, escalate care using an SBAR style handover. This same SBAR format can be used for evening/morning handovers and can be used by all members of staff.

Discussing a Patient with Another Hospital or Subspecialty

This task will occasionally be delegated to a junior doctor familiar with the details of a patient's presentation and inpatient management.

Before calling another hospital for advice, clarify the question needing to be asked and collate relevant information to allow a clear discussion of the patient. This may include:

> - Observation charts.
> - Drug chart.
> - Blood results.
> - Imaging reports.
> - Medical notes.
> - Contact details of the patient (telephone number/address).
> - GP details.
> - The consultant responsible for the patient at the referring hospital and the other hospital (if already known).

To contact the tertiary hospital, check if any listed contact numbers are already in the patient's notes. If not, use the hospital switchboard operator or search the internet. If unsuccessful on the first attempt, consider alternatives: Are there any other relevant professionals at that hospital who can be reached, such as other members within the team being called? A junior doctor, a secretary or a nurse in charge on the relevant ward may provide useful advice. At the end of the discussion, document the details of the conversation, ideally with relevant contact names and numbers for future reference.

Referring a patient for an inpatient review requires similar preparation. Always take the name and contact details of the specialist spoken to, as well as a realistic estimate of when they will be able to come. If a time-critical review is required (e.g. for suspected testicular torsion), ensure that the urgency is conveyed clearly and ask for an estimate of the wait, in order to act on any delays and escalate care should these occur.

Discharging a Patient and Arranging a Follow-up Review

Where possible, discharge letters should be prepared in advance of a child being medically fit, so as not to delay their discharge. The discharge letter is key in the communication of a child's health to all relevant parties. It needs to include information for primary care physicians and parents, as well as any medical person who may encounter the patient. The discharge letter should contain an overview of:

> - The status of the child at discharge, which is back to their baseline level of health in the vast majority of cases.
> - Ongoing management in the community, e.g. length of discharge medication, weaning regime for salbutamol inhalers.
> - Any follow-up needed within primary care services, including whether any medications need to be commenced or continued.
> - Any follow-up appointments.
> - Any outstanding investigations and the dates of such investigations.
> - What has been communicated to the parents.
> - Contact details of the hospital/medical team in charge of the child's care.

Often discharge letters are electronic and follow a set template.

Updating Parents and Caregivers about Progress

All doctors should strive to keep patients and caregivers actively involved in the medical management of a sick child. However, this may be inappropriate in the context of an emergency resuscitation of an acutely unwell young child. In such a situation, the best strategy may be for a healthcare professional to remain with the parents to provide support and assurance that the medical team are providing the best possible care. The actual presence or absence of parents during an active resuscitation will be at the discretion of the clinician leading the resuscitation.

NEONATAL UNITS

Neonatology is a sub-specialty of paediatrics, but it is a key rotation in the earlier stages of training for most paediatricians. In a large tertiary hospital, the unit will comprise three levels of intensity, ranging from the high intensity of the Intensive Therapy Unit (ITU) where the majority of patients are ventilated or clinically unstable, through to a High Dependency Unit (HDU) and then on to a lower dependency unit named the Special Care Baby Unit (SCBU). As attendance on the labour ward for deliveries is a daily occurrence, scrub clothing is expected.

The following sections will give advice on various aspects of work on the Neonatal Intensive Care Unit and Postnatal Wards. Aim to do an NLS course before starting on neonates.

Morning Neonatal Unit Handover and Night Summaries

Handover of the NICU patient is structured and systematic. Every handover of a patient starts with their name, age, corrected gestational age and original gestational age with birth weight and then their current condition, presented system-by-system, as shown in *Table 4*.

Attending Deliveries and Neonatal Crash Calls

The presence of a paediatrician is not expected at every delivery, but one will be called upon for certain situations such as:

> Emergency Caesarean sections.

> Instrumental deliveries (forceps or ventouse/"Kiwi").

TABLE 4: Example neonatal unit handover. Note that there is often a specific proforma for this		
Name, gestational age, age, corrected gestational age		**Mark Jacobs** 25+5→ d14 →27+5 corrected.
Current problems.		1. Prematurity. 2. Establishing feeds. 3. Suspected sepsis. 4. Bilateral Grade III. Intraventricular haemorrhage. 5. Respiratory distress syndrome. 6. Jaundice. 7. Small PDA.
Status overnight.		Has had a stable night.
Background.		Born by SVD, after SROM for 24 hours. Adequate antenatal steroids given. Magnesium sulphate given. Intubated at delivery and given one dose of surfactant before being extubated on day three to CPAP. Required ionotropic support for 24 hours. Has had one episode of culture-negative sepsis at birth, treated with three days of benzylpenicillin and gentamicin.
Respiratory.	• Support required: none, continuous positive airway pressure (CPAP), bilevel positive airway pressure (BiPAP), intubated and mechanically ventilated. • Oxygen requirement. • Blood gases.	Currently on CPAP, at a pressure of 6, in air. Respiratory rate is between 40 and 60, with no increased work of breathing. The last gas 6 hours ago was satisfactory. CXR yesterday showed ongoing RDS.
Cardiovascular.	• Heart rate/blood pressure. • Inotropic support. • Echocardiograms. • Electrocardiograms.	Heart rate is between 140-160 bpm. Mean arterial pressure is 30mmHg. No inotropes since day one. Echocardiogram on day three showed a 2mm PDA.
Fluids/feeding.	• Type and volume (mL/kg/d), e.g. total parenteral nutrition (TPN), intravenous dextrose, nasogastric feeding, bottle feeding, breast feeding. • Rate of increasing any feeds. • Vomiting, NG tube aspirates, diarrhoea. • Urine output, fluid balance, and weight changes. • Fluid boluses (including type and volume).	On 150mL/kg/day of TPN. NBM in view of active sepsis concerns. Urine output is 3mL/kg/hr over the last 12 hours, fluid balance in +15mL over the last 12 hours, and weight is unchanged from yesterday.
Sepsis.	If there are current septic concerns: • Number of days of treatment, drugs being used, and reason for starting treatment. • Cultures sent, and results back so far. • Any skin colonisation. • Changes in temperature. • Changes in C-reactive protein (CRP).	D3 of Vancomycin and Cefotaxime, started after recurrent episodes of bradycardia/desaturations, associated with a CRP rise to 30. Old long line tip growing Coagulase negative Staphylococcus from 5 days ago, sensitive to Vancomycin. Blood cultures negative so far. CRP overnight 65. Temperature stable.
Access.	Note the presence of lines (and if relevant tip position on X-ray): • Peripheral venous cannula. • Long line. • Umbilical venous catheter. • Umbilical arterial catheter. • Peripheral arterial line.	2 peripheral venous cannulae, plus a long line in the right antecubital fossa— the tip is at T2 on X-ray.

Continued

TABLE 4: *Continued*		
Blood results.	• Highlight any abnormal results not already mentioned. • Electrolyte results will be important for TPN prescriptions. • Haemoglobin, platelets and coagulation will determine transfusions. • CRP is useful for suspected sepsis, if not already mentioned.	Haemoglobin is 140, platelets are 100 and INR is 1.2. Na is 142, K is 5.0, Ca is 2.4, PO₄ is 1.6, Mg is 1.3.
Jaundice.	• Maternal and baby blood group. • Direct antigen test (DAT) result. • Latest serum bilirubin (SBR) and rate of rise if increasing. • Current treatment.	Last SBR was stable, but still 20 above the treatment line, and so single phototherapy continues. Mum and baby are both O-ve. DAT is –ve.
Neurological.	• Abnormal neurological activity, e.g. seizures, changes in tone, abnormal posturing. • Neurological investigations, e.g. cranial ultrasound scan (USS), magnetic resonance imaging (MRI), cerebral function analysing monitor (CFAM), electroencephalogram (EEG).	Bilateral grade III IVH seen on cranial USS 5 days ago.
Medications.	• List all medications, including route, dose, drug levels and any changes.	D3 Vancomycin and Cefotaxime Caffeine.
Social.	• Any child protection issues? Any restrictions on visiting?	No current social concerns.
Parental communication.	• When were the parents last updated? • Is there any new information they need to be told about?	The parents were fully updated yesterday and are happy with the ongoing plan.
Plan for the day.	• Suggested course of action.	1. Minimum 7 day course of antibiotics. 2. Repeat cranial ultrasound. 3. Blood gas once a shift. 4. Bloods overnight. 5. Chase cultures. 6. Review feeding/consider restarting trophic feeds if sepsis resolved.

> Shoulder dystocia.
> Meconium.
> Foetal distress, as demonstrated either on CTG (cardiotocograph) or on FBS (foetal blood sample) monitoring.

Induction should cover use of the Resuscitaire equipment. The equipment in theatres can be different to that on a labour ward, so become familiar with both before attending deliveries independently. A midwife is usually available to assist. For extremely sick neonates, bring the relevant resuscitation equipment from the neonatal unit. This should all be readily available in a resuscitation equipment bag and should include equipment for:
> Intubation.
> Umbilical venous access.
> Oxygen saturation monitoring.
> Temperature monitoring.

POSTNATAL WARDS

Postnatal wards provide a useful opportunity to get to know "the well baby"; as such, the most important task for the junior doctor is carrying out newborn baby checks.

Performing Baby Checks

To perform a baby check, the following are necessary:
> An ophthalmoscope with a good working light (if the light is dim, no red reflex can be elicited).
> A tape measure for head circumference check.
> A list of babies requiring a "baby check", highlighting the ones to be discharged that day so they can be prioritised.

The process of performing a baby check is described on p187. Important positive findings in a newborn examination may include:
> Absent red reflex.
> Absent femoral pulses.
> Unstable hips during the Barlow and Ortolani examinations.
> Heart murmur.
> Absent anus.

A healthcare assistant can be assigned to help bring the appropriate patients, parents and related documentation for mother and child to the examination room. Ideally, the babies should arrive complete with mother's antenatal notes, baby's medical notes, baby's personalised health record (previously referred to as "the red book"). The baby should be undressed to the nappy and covered with blankets for efficient examination. A translator should be booked if mother/parents do not speak English or have hearing difficulties.

The paediatrician now also has an opportunity to identify concerns that were potentially missed; for example, risk factors for sepsis, abnormal antenatal scans (e.g. hydronephrosis) and whether feeding is well established. Other important screening questions relate to family history (e.g. developmental dysplasia of the hip, congenital heart disease, sensorineural deafness, haematological conditions, and any other childhood/inheritable disease).

Reviewing Babies on the Postnatal Ward

Many additional duties are expected of the postnatal doctor; the following are some of the more common ones.

› Jaundice. Management of jaundice is discussed on p198. All doctors, midwives and healthcare assistants have the responsibility to assess each baby for jaundice every time they are reviewed. Any new onset of jaundice needs a formal measurement of bilirubin. Early jaundice should prompt consideration of haemolysis, including ABO incompatibility.

› Babies with deranged observations/acutely unwell. This may include abnormal temperature, tachypnoea or tachycardia. Perform a full set of observations (including oxygen saturations), and review the patient using an ABC approach. Review the medical notes, particularly risk factors for sepsis. A capillary blood gas may be helpful to check the partial pressure of carbon dioxide, pH, lactate and base excess.

› Suspected sepsis. All babies should be assessed for risk factors for sepsis. These include:
  › Prematurity.
  › Prolonged rupture of membranes (over 18 hours).
  › Maternal history of Group B Streptococcus carriage on a high vaginal swab.
  › History of pyrexia in the mother during her labour.
  › Maternal UTI.

Even in a well baby, the presence of risk factors for sepsis may prompt empirical treatment for infection (p200).

› Hypoglycaemia. Babies at high risk of hypoglycaemia will have blood glucose routinely monitored by their responsible midwife, and if low, may require a feeding plan and/or admission to the neonatal unit for intravenous dextrose and closer monitoring (p209). Babies at high risk include infants of diabetic mothers, premature babies, low birth weight babies and maternal labetalol use.

› Vomiting. Vomiting typically occurs in a well baby. However, sinister causes include oesophageal atresia, necrotising enterocolitis and malrotation with volvulus (p354). Check the observations, maternal antenatal notes, particularly the foetal anomaly scan and the baby's medical notes. Examine the baby, including a careful examination of the abdomen, looking for distension, tenderness, and the presence of an anus. Check the colour of the vomit, as a green/bilious colour should prompt discussion with a NICU registrar for exclusion of surgical causes.

› Delayed passage of meconium. A neonate who has not passed meconium within the first 48 hours of life may have an underlying cause, e.g. Hirshprung's disease or a CF-related meconium plug. Antenatal scans should be reviewed, and the baby should be examined for abdominal distension and the presence of a normal anus.

› Hepatitis B/HIV treatment. Check maternal status, and treat the baby appropriately (p201).

› A baby with abnormal antenatal scans. Often an antenatal plan will be made for action by the postnatal paediatric doctor; for example, with hydronephrosis, an antenatal plan may include prophylactic antibiotics, repeat ultrasound of the kidneys, ureters and bladder, and review by the paediatric urologists or local paediatric team.

› Safeguarding concerns. Several neonates may be born into complicated social situations; for example, domestic violence, homelessness, substance misuse or previous children with social services input. These concerns are usually identified before delivery, allowing establishment of a safeguarding plan in advance. The ongoing care of the neonate will require long-term joint input from the medical team, the safeguarding team and social services. A court order may be required prior to discharge.

› Neonate at risk of withdrawal. Infants born to mothers taking certain drugs/medications (e.g. morphine/heroin) are at risk of withdrawal after birth. A urine sample should be sent from the baby to check for toxicology as soon as possible after birth for future reference by social services. Signs of withdrawal include:
  › Inability to feed/poor weight gain.
  › Poor sleep.
  › High pitched cries.
  › Vomiting.
  › Objective measures of heart rate, respiratory rate, temperature and blood glucose.

Signs of withdrawal can be reduced by minimal handling, regular feedings and minimal lighting/noise disturbances. In severe cases, morphine treatment and admission to the neonatal unit may be required to relieve symptoms.

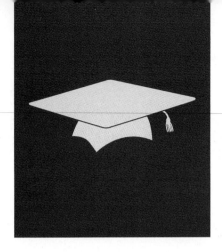

4.03

CAREERS IN PAEDIATRICS

MARIE MONAGHAN AND MICHAEL MALLEY

CONTENTS

EXPOSURE TO PAEDIATRICS

Paediatric clinical experience at medical school can be rather limited. As a result, those interested in paediatrics might have difficulty in attaining the desired amount of exposure to the specialty. Approach an educational supervisor or a paediatric consultant about getting more experience in the paediatric ED or general paediatric ward. Often, these environments seem like chaotic places but be proactive and offer to clerk in patients for the paediatric team. This can contribute to history taking and can be a useful way to gain feedback.

Current junior doctors can arrange a "taster week". This is a dedicated week of study leave arranged through an educational supervisor to give exposure to a speciality of interest. Talk to paediatricians, exploring what they love and hate about their career (*Table 1*). When on a placement, try to develop practical and communication skills. What may at first seem impossible, such as cannulating a 4-year-old, can become a highlight of the job. Note also that specialties like ED, primary care, ENT and many others come with exposure to paediatric patients.

Volunteer. Most cities have charities aimed at supporting young people. How about using a free afternoon to mentor a pupil? Volunteering will not only improve interaction skills with children, but will also generate meaningful experiences to draw on to support a paediatric speciality application. Incorporate paediatrics into a medical elective: this will provide an alternative perspective on paediatric practice and will be a useful experience to draw upon.

Aside from hands-on experience, getting involved in any research or audits taking place in the paediatric department is also a good idea. These can form the basis for departmental or regional presentations and could even be submitted to paediatric regional or national conferences. While in medical school, students should see if there is a paediatric society to join and become active members. If there isn't, they could perhaps establish one, with the aims of hosting paediatric teaching events at their university.

CAREER OPTIONS WITHIN PAEDIATRICS

There are two types of clinical paediatric jobs: general paediatricians and sub-specialists (*Table 2*).

TABLE 1: Pros and cons of doing paediatrics

Pros	Cons
Working with children adds an exciting dimension to practising medicine, with dynamism and humour considered great assets.	While helping children to get well can be elevating, it can be emotionally challenging when children have incurable or chronic severe illness or where children have been victims of non-accidental injury.
Paediatrics offers a wide variety of medicine with many sub-specialties for a satisfying intellectual aspect.	The training time to reach the consultant level is long and involves much out-of-hours work.
There are committed, enthusiastic and friendly nursing and auxiliary medical staff.	The work may not be as familiar as adult medicine initially.
Children, unlike many older adults, can recover completely from serious illnesses, which can add to a sense of job satisfaction.	Procedures can be practically difficult and emotionally challenging; for example, intravenous cannulation on chronically ill children with poor venous access or in particularly needle-phobic children.
Paediatric teams tend to be friendly and approachable.	No patient-doctor dialogue is possible in neonates.
Regular interaction with the broader multidisciplinary team (including physiotherapists, dieticians, nurse specialists, health visitors and primary care physicians) supports a holistic approach to patient management.	Interaction with patients' relatives (namely parents/carers) is more common and in depth. Stress can occasionally arise from situations where parent/carer views differ from the views of the paediatric team.

TABLE 2: Advantages of being a general paediatrician and of being a sub-speciality paediatrician

General Paediatrician	Sub-Specialty Paediatrician
General paediatricians are responsible for a wide variety of patients, from managing neonates on the hospital's Neonatal Unit to patients with varied illnesses on the paediatric ward.	Sub-specialty paediatricians are responsible for a wide variety of patients limited to the sub-speciality of interest. This means that they see the full spectrum of presentations and rarer complications for a condition within their field.

Sub-specialty paediatricians are often considered as national experts in their chosen sub-speciality of paediatrics. This can potentially give more influence in research or policy development in that topic. |
| Having a broad range of responsibilities helps to maintain clinical skills and knowledge as well as providing a satisfying variety to everyday work. | A wide range of sub-specialty jobs is available, which can vary depending on clinical interest and time commitments (*Table 3*). |

General Paediatricians

General paediatricians are exactly that; they cover all areas of paediatrics from primary care referrals, to patients admitted to the general ward, to the neonates seen in the local hospital's Neonatal Intensive Care Unit (NICU). This means they have an extensive knowledge base that encompasses all areas of paediatrics and are able to practice a diverse range of skills. They utilise their sub-specialty colleagues in tertiary units to guide more complex care and are often coordinators of care for children with complex, multi-system and/or social needs. In local hospitals, they often have special interests, e.g. respiratory, epilepsy, diabetes and safeguarding, which they practice with the oversight of tertiary hospital services in clinic settings and on the ward.

Sub-Specialty Paediatricians

As with adult medicine, paediatrics has many sub-specialties specific to it which cover some of the more complex and rarer diseases. As such, sub-specialty paediatricians often operate out of tertiary hospital centres with links to clinics in local hospitals, working alongside general paediatricians with special interests. *Table 3* summarises the range of possible potential sub-specialties.

TABLE 3: Sub-speciality jobs in paediatrics

Sub-Specialty	Description
Neonatal medicine.	The majority of neonatal admissions can be managed at the local hospital level in Special Care Baby Units (SCBUs) or Level 2 Neonatal Intensive Care Units (NICUs). Neonates at increased risk (e.g. due to extreme prematurity, antenatally-diagnosed congenital malformations or those born in very poor condition due to perinatal hypoxia) must have care delivered in Level 3 (tertiary) NICUs that have appropriate levels of experience.
Allergy.	Allergists manage patients with severe allergic reactions as part of a multi-disciplinary team.
Audiovestibular medicine.	Paediatric audiology deals with hearing and balance problems.
Cardiology.	Paediatric cardiology involves the management of children with complex heart problems. Increasingly, it involves performing interventional procedures. Training is through paediatric or adult (cardiological) sub-specialty training.
Clinical genetics.	Paediatric clinical genetics involves the diagnosis and management of genetic problems.

Continued

TABLE 3: Sub-speciality jobs in paediatrics.	
Sub-Specialty	**Description**
Community child health	Community paediatrics is a specialty that provides care for medically stable children with complex, long-term disability. Conditions vary from cerebral palsy to learning disability to mental health conditions such as autistic spectrum disorder (ASD) or attention-deficit hyperactivity disorder (ADHD). Children being investigated for safeguarding concerns may also receive care under the lead of the Community Child Health teams, and there are roles related to public health and audiology.
Child mental health.	Child mental health paediatricians utilise their medical knowledge to best support the mental health needs of paediatric patients. They work closely with psychiatrists but have distinct training pathways and responsibilities.
Clinical pharmacology and therapeutics.	Pharmacology is a small specialty dedicated to the pharmacological aspects of paediatric medications, with opportunities for research and development.
Diabetes and endocrinology.	Paediatric endocrinology includes the multi-disciplinary management of diabetic patients, as well as the diagnosis and management of conditions involving the hypothalamic-pituitary axis.
Emergency medicine.	Emergency medicine involves aspects of managing the acutely unwell child but also interfaces with primary care and secondary care. This specialty can also be reached at the consultant level by a sub-specialty branch of adult emergency medicine.
Gastroenterology and nutrition.	Gastroenterology involves the care of patients with disorders such as inflammatory bowel disease and coeliac disease. Nutrition covers patients with complex requirements, e.g. short bowel syndrome-related total parenteral nutrition (TPN) dependence.
Haematology.	Haematology involves managing blood disorders such as anaemia, platelet disorders and clotting disorders. It also involves the treatment of blood cancers such as leukaemia. Training in the UK is via adult sub-speciality training.
Hepatology.	Hepatologists manage conditions such as autoimmune hepatitis, biliary atresia and cirrhosis.
Infectious diseases.	Infectious disease specialists are experts in the diagnosis and treatment of infections.
Immunology.	Immunology is a field that covers a wide range of conditions, from inherited to acquired immune defects.
Inherited metabolic medicine.	Metabolic medicine is a relatively new but growing field that deals with children with inborn errors of metabolism. Conditions can present as acutely unwell children in the neonatal period or may present with failure to thrive or other disability in older children. Increasingly, these disorders are being picked up during newborn screening.
Nephrology.	Nephrology in the paediatric group can relate to inherited disorders such as autosomal recessive polycystic kidney disease, through to glomerulonephritis and complex nephrotic syndrome management. Dialysis and transplant management are also important areas in this field.
Neurodisability.	Neurodisability relates to the multidisciplinary management of children with chronic disabilities such as those arising from cerebral palsy or spina bifida.
Neurology.	Neurology relates to the medical management of children with a wide range of conditions including epilepsy, myasthenia gravis, Guillain-Barré syndrome and inherited defects.
Oncology.	Oncology deals with childhood cancers. This can involve the management of blood cancers (e.g. leukaemia) and solid tumours (e.g. neuroblastoma).
Paediatric intensive care medicine.	The care provided in paediatric intensive care medicine is highly specialised and involves the essential multi-system support needed for severely unwell children; for example, those post cardiac surgery or those suffering life-threatening sepsis, asthma or diabetic ketoacidosis.
Palliative medicine.	Children may have serious illness stemming from a range of acquired or inherited conditions, such as neuromuscular disorders or malignancy. Patients and their families benefit from symptom management, respite care and hospice services. In addition to these well recognised sources of support, the palliative care team provides assistance in coping with uncertainty and helps patients and their families start to prepare for a range of eventualities associated with terminal illness.
Paediatric surgery.	Paediatric surgery is distinct from paediatric training, typically necessitating a surgical training pathway. However, paediatric surgeons work closely alongside paediatricians in covering a broad and interesting range of conditions that span the neonatal period through to adolescence.
Respiratory medicine.	Respiratory medicine involves the care of children with inherited conditions such as cystic fibrosis and primary ciliary dyskinesia, as well as acquired conditions such as bronchiectasis, tuberculosis and severe asthma.
Paediatric radiology.	Paediatric radiology involves all radiological modalities investigating childhood illness. This specialty is typically reached through radiological training with a sub-specialty in paediatrics.
Rheumatology.	Rheumatology involves the management of musculoskeletal disorders ranging from inherited defects of collagen in Ehlers-Danlos Syndrome to multi-system illness, such as systemic lupus erythematosus or juvenile idiopathic arthritis.

TABLE 4: Utilising paediatric skills outside of clinical medicine.	
Area	**Description**
Academic work.	This can involve experimental research in expanding areas (such as the management of neonates with hypoxic ischaemic encephalopathy) and, as such, may involve dedicated study as part of a Master's or PhD degree.
Charity work.	Charity work can range from local educational programmes through to work abroad, e.g. establishing neonatal units, providing vaccination programmes and general paediatrics work.
Consultancy and management.	Consultancy may include the internal structure and functioning of a paediatric department or advising international hospitals on the logistical design of new services.
Politics / Advisory role.	Advocacy is essential; for example, trainee representation within paediatric schools ensures trainees' needs are addressed. This is also the case nationally; for example, in the design of healthcare policies.
Education.	Medical education can be practiced via the paediatric college (e.g. in question-writing for post-graduate examinations) or via university medical schools through the supervision of undergraduate and post-graduate students. Education may also be provided privately by a paediatrician; for example, by the design of a taught revision course or through the writing of medical textbooks.

Broader Paediatric Careers

As with all fields of medicine, skills acquired in paediatrics are transferrable to other areas of work (*Table 4*).

APPLYING TO PAEDIATRICS

Preparing for a career in paediatrics can begin in medical school or as a doctor prior to committing to specialty training. A rotation in paediatrics as a junior doctor is not mandatory for applying to paediatrics in the UK. However, specialty applications can seek evidence relating to prior paediatric clinical experience and, more broadly, commitment to the speciality. This can take the form of courses, clinical audits, management skills, academic achievements, publications, presentations, teaching skills and a supporting personal statement.

Specialty training length is variable internationally. In the UK, the training is eight years long and is "run through" all the way up to Consultant level. Areas to consider for an application are described below.

Professional Examinations

In the UK, post-graduate examinations in paediatrics are called the Membership of the Royal College of Paediatrics and Child Health (MRCPCH) exams. They consist of three written examinations and one clinical exam. The three written papers are called the "Foundation of Practice", "Theory and Science", and "Applied Knowledge in Practice". They are expensive and require dedicated revision. These are compulsory examinations for any paediatrician, and passing them shows ability and commitment to the specialty. It is possible to sit these initial examinations prior to starting paediatric training; however, this is not mandatory.

Paediatric Courses

Resuscitation skills are mandatory for all paediatricians, regardless of grade. Courses include Advanced Paediatric Life Support (APLS), Neonatal Life Support (NLS) and the European Paediatric Life Support Course (EPLS). Other educational non-resuscitation courses include those relating to paediatric sub-specialties or supporting the development of the skill set required for a paediatrician. It is financially prudent to apply for these courses when eligible for an educational study budget.

Teaching Skills

Demonstrating skills as a teacher shows an appreciation for education and an interest in developing skills as an effective communicator. There are various ways to become involved in teaching, such as peer-led teaching groups for mock examinations or by running evening lectures with guest speakers. Sessions can be designed and run independently, or jointly designed and run with the local university or hospital teaching societies. Contact local paediatric teaching leads to identify opportunities.

Clinical Governance

Clinical governance is important for maintaining high standards in healthcare. Partaking in clinical governance can take the form of guideline development or updating, as well as auditing current practice to improve services. Importantly, audits (comparison of current practice to a set standard) are deemed most beneficial when shortcomings are explored, changes implemented and a *re-audit* is performed to check that standards have improved. This allows completion of the *audit cycle*. As a first step in performing an audit, it is advisable to find an appropriate supervisor and propose an area of current practice which can be measured and compared to a local or national guideline.

Research

Research can be, but does not have to be, conducted as part of a dedicated research programme. Research can be incorporated into medical degrees by way of an intercalated degree with laboratory-based projects. There are also non-laboratory–based forms of research, such as translational research, clinical trials, observational studies and epidemiological studies. The best way to get involved in research may be to ask supportive lecturers, educational supervisors or consultants if any suitable projects are available for student involvement. Simple publications can come from a case report or a literature review.

Posters, Publications and Presentations

A poster can be presented at a local, regional, national or international conference. It does not have to be research; it can also be an audit or a quality improvement project. Tertiary centres are good places to present regional audits. The information from these types of audits may have wider relevance to national meetings or international conferences. Equally, this information may be relevant for publication in a peer-reviewed journal. Literature reviews or case reports are also publishable in peer-reviewed journals.

REFERENCES AND FURTHER READING

1 The Royal College of Paediatrics and Child Health. Available from: www.rcpch.ac.uk.

2 International Paediatric Association. Available from: http://www.ipa-world.org.

3 American Academy of Paediatrics. Available from: www2.aap.org/international.

4 Royal Australasian College of Physicians – Paediatrics and Child Health Division. Available from: www.racp.edu.au/about/racps-structure/paediatrics-child-health-division.

Index

Page numbers followed by *f* indicate figures.